Comprehensive
Clinical Endocrinology

Multimedia CD-ROM
Single User License Agreement

1. NOTICE. WE ARE WILLING TO LICENSE THE MULTI-MEDIA PROGRAM PRODUCT TITLED **Comprehensive Clinical Endocrinology, 3ʳᵈ edn** ("MULTIMEDIA PROGRAM") TO YOU ONLY ON THE CONDITION THAT YOU ACCEPT ALL OF THE TERMS CONTAINED IN THIS LICENSE AGREEMENT. PLEASE READ THIS LICENSE AGREEMENT CAREFULLY BEFORE OPENING THE SEALED DISK PACKAGE. BY OPENING THAT PACKAGE YOU AGREE TO BE BOUND BY THE TERMS OF THIS AGREEMENT. IF YOU DO NOT AGREE TO THESE TERMS WE ARE UNWILLING TO LICENSE THE MULTIMEDIA PROGRAME TO YOU, AND YOU SHOULD NOT OPEN THE DISK PACKAGE. IN SUCH CASE, PROMPTLY RETURN THE UNOPENED DISK PACKAGE AND ALL OTHER MATERIAL IN THIS PACKAGE, ALONG WITH PROOF OF PAYMENT, TO THE ATHORISED DEALER FROM WHOM YOU OBTAINED IT FOR A FULL REFUND OF THE PRICE YOU PAID.

2. **Ownership and License**. This is a license agreement and NOT an agreement for sale. It permits you to use one copy of the MULTIMEDIA PROGRAM on a single computer. The MULTIMEDIA PROGRAM and its contents are owned by us or our licensors, and are protected by U.S. and international copyright laws. Your rights to use the MULTIMEDIA PROGRAM are specified in this Agreement, and we retain all rights not expressly granted to you in this Agreement.

   - You may use one copy of the MULTIMEDIA PROGRAM on a single computer
   - After you have installed the MULTIMEDIA PROGRAM on your computer, you may use the MULTIMEDIA PROGRAM on a different computer only if you first delete the files installed by the installation program from the first computer.
   - You may not copy any portion of the MULTIMEDIA PROGRAM to your computer hard disk or any other media other than print-ing out or downloading non- substantial portions of the text and images in the MULITMEDIA PROGRAM for your own internal informational use.
   - Your may not copy any of the documentation or other printed materials accompanying the MULTIMEDIA PROGRAM.

   Neither concurrent use on two or more computers nor use in a local area network or other network is permitted without separate authorisation and the payment of additional license fees.

3. **Transfer and Other Restrictions**. You may not rent, lend, or lease this MULTIMEDIA PROGRAM. Save as permitted by law, you may not and you may not permit others to (a) disassemble, decompile, or otherwise derive source code from the software included in the MULTIMEDIA PROGRAM (the "Software"), (b) reverse engineer the Software, (c) modify or prepare derivative works of the MULTI-MEDIA PROGRAM (d) use the Software in an on-line system, or (e) use the MULITMEDIA PROGRAM in any manner that infringes on the intellectual property or other rights of another party.

   However, you may transfer this license to use the MULTIMEDIA ROGRAM to another party on a permanent basis by transferring this copy of the License Agreement, the MULTIMEDIA PROGRAM, and all documentation. Such transfer of possession terminates your license from us. Such other party shall be licensed under the terms of this Agreement upon its acceptance of this Agreement by its initial use of the MULTIMEDIA PROGRAM. If you transfer the MULTIMEDIA PROGRAM, you must remove the installation files from your hard disk and you may not retain any copies of those files for your own use.

4. **Limited Warranty and Limitation of Liability**. For a period of sixty (60) days from the date your acquired the MULTIMEDIA PRO-GRAM from us or our authorised dealer, we warrant that the media containing the MULTIMEDIA PROGRAM will be free from defects that prevent you from installing the MULTIMEDIA PRO-GRAM on your computer. If the disk fails to conform to this warranty you may as your sole and exclusive remedy, obtain a replacement free of charge if you return the defective disk to us with a dated proof of purchase. Otherwise the MULTIMEDIA PROGRAM is licensed to you on an "AS IS" basis without any warranty of any nature.

   WE DO NOT WARRANT THAT THE MULTIMEDIA PRO-GRAM WILL MEET YOUR REQUIREMENTS OR THAT ITS OPERATION WILL BE UNINTERRUPTED OR ERROR-FREE. THE EXPRESS TERMS OF THIS AGREEMENT ARE IN LIEU OF ALL WARRANTIES, CONDITIONS, UNDERTAKINGS, TERMS AND OBLIGATIONS IMPLIED BY STATUTE, COMMON LAW, TRADE USAGE, COURSE OF DEALING OR OTHERWISE ALL OF WHICH ARE HEREBY EXCLUDED TO THE FULLEST EXTENT PERMITTED BY LAW, INCLUDING THE IMPLIED WARRANTIES OF SATISFACTORY QUALITY AND FITNESS FOR A PARTICULAR PURPOSE.

   WE SHALL NOT BE LIABLE FOR ANY DAMAGE OR LOSS OF ANY KIND (EXCEPT PERSONAL INJURY OR DEATH RESULTING FROM OUR NEGLIGENCE) ARISING OUT OF OR RESULTING FROM YOUR POSSESSION OR USE OF THE MULTIMEDIA PROGRAM (INCLUDING DATA LOSS OR CORRUPTION), REGARDLESS OF WHETHER SUCH LIABIL-ITY IS BASED IN TORT, CONTRACT OR OTHERWISE AND INCLUDING, BUT NOT LIMITED TO, ACUTAL, SPECIAL, INDIRECT, INCIDENTAL OR CONSEQUENTIAL DAMAGES. IF THE FOREGOING LIMITATION IS HELD TO BE UNEN-FORCEABLE OUR MAXIMUM LIABILITY TO YOU SHALL NOT EXCEED THE AMOUNT OF THE LICENSE FEE PAID BY YOU FOR THE MULTIMEDIA PROGRAM. THE REMEDIES AVAILABLE TO YOU AGAINST US AND THE LICENSORS OF MATERIALS INCLUDED IN THE MULTIMEDIA PROGRAM ARE EXCLUSIVE.

5. **Termination.** This license and your right to use this MULTIMEDIA PROGRAM automatically terminate if you fail to comply with any provisions of this Agreement, destroy the copy of the MULTIMEDIA PROGRAM in your possession, or voluntarily return the MULTI-MEDIA PROGRAM to us. Upon termination you will destroy all copies of the MULTIMEDIA PROGRAM and documentation.

6. **Miscellaneous Provisions.** This Agreement will be governed and construed in accordance with English law and you hereby submit to the non-exclusive jurisdiction of the English Courts. This is the entire agreement between us relating to the MULTMEDIA PROGRAM, and supersedes any prior purchase order, communi-cations, advertising or representations concerning the contents of this package, No change or modification of this Agreement will be valid unless it is in writing and is signed by us.

Comprehensive
Clinical
Endocrinology

Third Edition

G Michael Besser MD, DSc, MD (Turin, honaris causa), FRCP, FMedSci
Professor of Medicine Emeritus
St Bartholomew's and the Royal London School of Medicine and Dentistry
Queen Mary College
University of London; and,
Honorary Consultant Physician
St Bartholomew's Hospital
London
UK

Michael O Thorner MB, BS, DSc, FRCP, FACP
Henry B Mulholland Professor of Internal Medicine
Chair, Department of Internal Medicine
University of Virginia Health System
Charlottesville, VA
USA

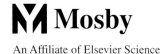
Mosby
An Affiliate of Elsevier Science

MOSBY
An affiliate of Elsevier Science Limited

First Edition 1984
Second Edition 1994
Third Edition 2002
Reprinted 2002

ISBN 0 7234 3185 X

British Library Cataloguing in Publication Data
A catalogue record for this book is available from the British Library

Library of Congress Cataloging in Publication Data
A catalog record for this book is available from the Library of Congress

Note
Medical knowledge is constantly changing. As new information
becomes available, changes in treatment, procedures, equipment
and the use of drugs become necessary. The editors, contributors,
and the publishers have taken care to ensure that the information
given in this text is accurate and up to date. However, readers
are strongly advised to confirm that the information, especially
with regard to drug usage, complies with the latest legislation and
standards of practice.

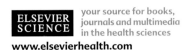
your source for books,
journals and multimedia
in the health sciences
www.elsevierhealth.com

Printed in Spain

Commissioning Editor	Deborah Russell and Cathy Carroll
Project Development Manager	Paul Fam
Project Manager	Hilary Hewitt
Illustrations Manager	Mick Ruddy
Illustrators	Robin Dean and Jenni Miller
Design Manager	Jayne Jones
Page Layout	Alan Palfreyman

The
publisher's
policy is to use
**paper manufactured
from sustainable forests**

Contents

Contributors

Melissa Aylstock AA
Founder and Executive Director
Klinefelter Syndrome and Associates
Roseville, CA
USA

Eugene J Barrett MD, PhD
Professor of Medicine
Department of Internal Medicine
University of Virginia
Charlottesville, VA
USA

Peter H Baylis BSc, MD, FRCP, FMedSci
Dean of Medicine
Professor of Experimental Medicine
Consultant Endocrinologist
The Medical School
University of Newcastle
Newcastle upon Tyne
UK

G Michael Besser MD, DSc, MD (Turin, honaris causa), FRCP, FMedSci
Professor of Medicine Emeritus
St Bartholomew's and the Royal London
   School of Medicine and Dentistry
Queen Mary College
University of London; and,
Honorary Consultant Physician
St Bartholomew's Hospital
London
UK

Joanne C Blair MB, ChB, MRCP
Research Fellow Paediatric Endocrinology
Department of Endocrinology
St Bartholomew's Hospital
London
UK

Stephen R Bloom MD, DSc, FRCP, FRCPath
Professor of Medicine
Department of Metabolic Medicine
The Hammersmith Hospital
Imperial College School of Medicine
London
UK

Keith E Britton MSc, MD, FRCR, FRCP
Professor of Nuclear Medicine
Department of Nuclear Medicine
St Bartholomew's Hospital
London
UK

Mary Brim
The Cushing's Support and Research
   Foundation
Boston, MA
USA

Julian Britton
Trustee
Thyroid Eye Disease Association
Winchelsea Beach
East Sussex
UK

Charles GD Brook MA, MD, FRCP, FRCPH
Emeritus Professor of Paediatric
   Endocrinology, University College London
The Middlesex Hospital
London
UK

John D Brunzell MD
Professor of Medicine
University of Washington
General Clinical Research Center
Seattle, WA
USA

Karen Campbell
The Cushing's Support and Research
   Foundation
Boston, MA
USA

Cathy Carbone
The Cushing's Support and Research
   Foundation
Boston, MA
USA

Lisa A Cerilli MD
Assistant Professor of Pathology
Department of Pathology
University of Virginia Health Sciences
   System
Charlottesville, VA
USA

Alan Chait MD
Edwin L Bierman Professor of Medicine
University of Washington
Division of Metabolism Endocrinology
   and Nutrition
Seattle, WA
USA

Adrian JL Clark DSc, FRCP, FMedSci.
Professor of Medicine
Department of Endocrinology
St Bartholomew's Hospital
London
UK

Peter E Clayton BSc, MB, ChB, MD, FRCP, FRCPCH
Professor of Child Health and Paediatric
   Endocrinology
Endocrine Science Research Group
University of Manchester
Manchester
UK

Janet E Dacie MB BS, FRCP, FRCR
Emeritus Consultant Radiologist
Department of Diagnostic Imaging
St Bartholomew's Hospital
London
UK

Terry F Davies MD, FRCP
Professor of Medicine
Director, Division of Endocrinology,
   Diabetes, and Bone Diseases
Mount Sinai School of Medicine
New York, NY
USA

Ann D Dunn PhD
Research Associate Professor of Medicine
University of Virginia Health System
Charlottesville, VA
USA

John T Dunn MD
Professor of Medicine
University of Virginia Health System
Charlottesville, VA
USA

John A Eaddy MD
Emeritus Professor of Family Medicine
Department of Family Medicine
University of Tennessee Graduate School
   of Medicine
Knoxville, TN
USA

Jane Edwards
The Cushing's Support and Research
Foundation
Boston, MA
USA

Raymond Edwards BSc, PhD
Consultant Biochemist
St Bartholomew's Hospital
London
UK

Eric A Espiner MD FRACP, FRS(NZ)
Emeritus Professor
Department of Medicine
Christchurch School of Medicine and
    Health Sciences
Christchurch
New Zealand

James A Fagin MD
Head Professor of Medicine
Division of Endocrinology and Metabolism
Vonta Center for Molecular Sciences
University of Cincinnati College of
    Medicine
Cincinnati, OH
USA

Simon J Fisher MD PhD
Endocrine Fellow
Beth Israel Deaconess Medical Center
Joslin Diabetes Center
Boston, MA
USA

**Stephen Franks MD, FRCP, Hon MD
    (Uppsala), FRCOG (ad eundem),
    F Med Sci**
Professor of Reproductive Endocrinology
Department of Reproductive Science and
    Medicine
Imperial College of Science, Technology
    and Medicine
Institute of Reproductive and
    Developmental Biology
Hammersmith Hospital
London
UK

Tam Fry
Honorary Chairman
Child Growth Foundation
London
UK

Robert F Gagel MD, Head (ad interim)
Division of Internal Medicine
Professor of Medicine
Department of Endocrine and Hormonal
    Disorders
MD Anderson Cancer Center
Houston, TX
USA

Mohammad A Ghatei PhD
Reader in Regulatory Peptides
Department of Metabolic Medicine
The Hammersmith Hospital
Imperial College School of Medicine
London
UK

James Gibney MB, MRCPI
Clinical Research Fellow in Endocrinology
Garvan Institute of Medical Research
St Vincent's Hospital
Sydney, NSW
Australia

Carole Gilling-Smith MRCOG, PhD
Consultant Gynaecologist
Director of the Assisted Conception Unit
Chelsea and Westminster Hospital
London
UK

James E Griffin MD
Professor of Internal Medicine
The University of Texas Southwestern
    Medical Center
Dallas, TX
USA

**Ashley B Grossman BA, BSc, MD, FRCP,
    FMedSci**
Professor of Neuroendocrinology
    Department of Endocrinology
St Bartholomew's Hospital
London
UK

Sherri A Groveman JD, LLM
San Diego, CA
USA

Lora Hammer
Assistant Director for Membership
The Thyroid Foundation of America, Inc.
Boston, MA
USA

Jennifer A Harvey MD
Associate Professor of Radiology
Department of Radiology
University of Virginia
Charlottesville, VA
USA

Victor M Haughton MD
Professor of Radiology
University of Wisconsin
Department of Radiology
University of Wisconsin Hospitals
    and Clinics
Madison, WI
USA

Ken KY Ho MD, FRACP
Professor of Medicine Chairman
Department of Endocrinology
St Vincent's Hospital
Sydney; and,
Garvan Institute of Medical Research
St Vincent's Hospital
Sydney, NSW
Australia

Yancey R Holmes MD
Clinical Fellow
Division of Endocrinology and Metabolism
Vonta Center for Molecular Sciences
University of Cincinnati College of
    Medicine
Cincinnati, OH
USA

**Vivian HT James DSc, FRCPath,
    HonMRCP**
Emeritus Professor of Chemical Pathology
University of London
London
UK

John A Jane Jr MD
Professor of Neurosurgery
Chair, Department of Neurological Surgery
University of Virginia
Charlottesville, VA
USA

C Ronald Kahn MD
President and Director
Joslin Diabetes Center
Boston, MA
USA

Gregory Kaltsas MD, MRCP
Consultant Endocrinology - Diabetologist
George Genimatas Hospital
Athens
Greece

Deana Kenward
Co-ordinator
Addison's Disease Self-Help Group UK
Guildford
UK

Grace Kim MD
Associate in Medicine
Mount Sinai School of Medicine
New York, NY
USA

Susan E Kirk MD
Assistant Professor in Internal Medicine
    and Obstetrics/Gynecology
Division of Endocrinology and Metabolism
University of Virginia Health System
Charlottesville, VA
USA

Robert Knutzen MBA
Chairman and CEO
Pituitary Network Association
Thousand Oaks, CA
USA

Peter G Kopelman MD, FRCP
Professor of Clinical Medicine
Deputy Warden
Barts and The London
Queen Mary's School of Medicine
    & Dentistry
University of London
London
UK

Edward R Laws Jr MD, FACS
Professor of Neurosurgery
Department of Neurosurgery
University of Virginia
Charlottesville, VA
USA

D Lynn Loriaux MD, PhD
Chairman, Department of Medicine
Oregon Health Sciences University
Portland, OR
USA

John C Marshall MD, PhD
Professor of Medical Science
Director Arthur and Margaret Ebbert
    Center for Research in Reproduction
University of Virginia Health System
Charlottesville, VA
USA

Marcia McDuffie MD
Associate Professor of Microbiology and
    Internal Medicine
University of Virginia Health System
School of Medicine
Microbiology and Internal Medicine
Charlottlesville, VA
USA

Shlomo Melmed MD
Professor of Medicine Senior Vice
    President
Academic Affairs Professor and Director
Cedars-Sinai Research Institute
UCLA School of Medicine
Los Angeles, CA
USA

Ram K Menon MD
Associate Professor of Pediatrics
Division of Endocrinology
Metabolism and Diabetes Mellitus
Children's Hospital of Pittsburgh
Pittsburgh, PA
USA

John P Monson MD, FRCP
Professor of Clinical Endocrinology
Department of Endocrinology
St Bartholomew's Hospital
London
UK

Gregory R Mundy MD
SBC Chair in Cancer Research
Director, Institute for Drug Development
San Antonio, TX
USA

Jerry L Nadler MD
Professor of Medicine
Chief Division of Endocrinology and
    Metabolism
Division of Endocrinology and Metabolism
University of Virginia Health System
Charlottesville, VA
USA

**Stephen O'Rahilly MD, FRCPI, FRCP,
    FMedSci**
Professor of Metabolic Medicine
University of Cambridge
Department of Medicine & Clinical
    Biochemistry
Addenbroke's Hospital
Cambridge
UK

Louise Pace
President and Founder
The Cushing's Support and Research
    Foundation
Boston, MA
USA

Todd Peebles MD
Assistant Professor of Radiology
Fletcher Allen Health Care
Medical Center, Hospital of Vermont
Burlington, VT
USA

Julian Pearce BSocSci, RN, MN, FRCNA
CAH Support Group of Australia Inc
    (CAHSGA)
Highton
Australia

**P Nicholas Plowman MA, MD, FRCP,
    FRCR**
Senior Consultant Clinical Oncologist to
    St Bartholomew's Hospital and the
    Hospital for Sick Children
London Hospital for Sick Children
London
UK

Toni R Prezant PhD
Assistant Professor of Medicine
Cedars-Sinai Medical Center and
    UCLA School of Medicine
Division of Endocrinology
Los Angeles, CA
USA

Miriam T Rademaker BSc, PhD
Senior Research Fellow
Christchurch Cardioendocrine Research
    Group
Department of Medicine
Christchurch School of Medicine & Health
    Sciences
Christchurch
New Zealand

Gerald M Reaven MD
Professor of Medicine
Stanford University School of Medicine
Stanford, CA
USA

Seymour Reichlin MD, PhD
Professor of Medicine, Emeritus
Tufts University
Vail, AZ
USA

Rodney H Reznek MBchB, FRCP, FRCR
Professor of Diagnostic Imaging
Academic Department of Radiology
St Bartholomew's Hospital
London
UK

Richard J Santen MD
Professor of Medicine
University of Virginia Health Sciences
  System
Charlottesville, VA
USA

**Martin O Savage MA, MD, FRCP,
  FRCPCH**
Professor of Paediatric Endocrinology
Department of Endocrinology
St Bartholomew's Hospital
London
UK

Mark A Sperling MD
Professor of Pediatrics
University of Pittsburgh
Division of Endocrinology, Metabolism and
  Diabetes Mellitus
Children's Hospital of Pittsburgh
Pittsburgh, PA
USA

Andrew F Stewart MD
Professor and Chief of Endocrinology
University of Pittsburgh School of
  Medicine
Pittsburgh, PA
USA

Paul M Stewart MD, FRCP, FMedSci
Professor of Medicine
Division of Medical Sciences
University of Birmingham
Queen Elizabeth Hospital
Birmingham
UK

Shahrad Taheri BSc, MSc, MB BS, MRCP
Wellcome Trust Research Fellow
Department of Metabolic Medicine
The Hammersmith Hospital
Imperial College School of Medicine
London
UK

**Rajesh V Thakker MD, FRCP, FRCPath,
  FMedSci**
May Professor of Medicine
The Oxford University Institute of
  Musculoskeletal Sciences
Botnar Research Centre
Nuffield Department of Clinical Medicine
Nuffield Orthopaedic Centre
Oxford
UK

Kamal Thapar MD, PhD, FRCS (C)
Attending Neurosurgeon
University Health Network
Toronto Western Hospital;
Staff Scientist
Arthur and Sonia Labatt Brain Tumor
  Research Center
Hospital for Sick Children; and
Assistant Professor
Division of Neurosurgery
University of Toronto
Toronto, ON
Canada

**Michael O Thorner MB, BS, DSc, FRCP,
  FACP**
Henry B. Mulholland Professor of Internal
  Medicine
Chair, Department of Internal Medicine
University of Virginia Health System
Charlottesville, VA
USA

Peter J. Trainer MD, FRCP
Consultant
Christie Hospital
Manchester
UK

Ehud Ur MB, FRCP
Associate Professor of Medicine
Division of Endocrinology
Queen Elizabeth II Health Sciences Centre
Dalhousie University
Halifax, NS
Canada

**Klaus von Werder, MD, FRCPProf,
  Dr. med, FRCP**
Professor of Medicine
Schlossparkklinik Teaching Hospital of the
  Charite
Humboldl University
Berlin
Germany

John AH Wass MA, MD, FRCP
Professor of Endocrinology
Consultant Physician
University of Oxford
Radcliffe Infirmary
Oxford
UK

Anthony P Weetman MD, DSc, FRCP
Professor of Medicine
Clinical Sciences Centre
University of Sheffield
Sheffield
UK

Jean D Wilson MD
Clinical Professor of Internal Medicine
The University of Texas Southwestern
Medical Center
Dallas, TX
USA

Foreword

I was initially attracted to the field of endocrinology because it so beautifully integrates physiology, biochemistry, and cell signaling with patient care. Clinical manifestations can usually be explained by understanding the physiologic role hormones – whether deficient or excessive. The fact that many endocrine disorders are amenable to cure or effective treatment also makes the practice of endocrinology especially satisfying.

Armed with a conceptual framework for understanding hormone secretion, hormone action, and principles of feedback control systems, the practitioner can elicit key elements of a patient's history and embark on a logical diagnostic approach. Despite these conceptual advantages in endocrinology, most glands are inaccessible to physical examination, with the exception of the thyroid and testes. Consequently, more than some specialties in medicine, endocrinology requires an astute observer who is trained to detect subtle physical signs that distinguish true endocrine disease from problems that masquerade as such. For example, deciding which obese patients should be screened for Cushing's syndrome is aided by knowledge that a patient with cortisol excess will usually manifest specific findings, such as central fat redistribution, striae, and proximal muscle weakness, in addition to features seen commonly in the general population. Similarly, endocrinologists have learned to recognize subtle clinical features suggestive of Graves' disease or acromegaly. Increasingly, the challenge is to identify endocrine disorders at their earliest stages rather than the when the clinical manifestations are flagrant. Terms like subclinical hypothyroidism, impaired glucose tolerance, and incidental adrenal or pituitary adenoma have crept into our vocabulary and have changed our approach to patients. Laboratory testing remains the primary diagnostic tool in endocrinology and it takes on added importance as we attempt to diagnose increasingly subtle forms of disease. We rely on increasingly sensitive hormone measurements to interrogate hormonal dynamics and we use various imaging studies to evaluate glandular anatomy. Guidelines for screening patients for osteoporosis, hyperlipidemias, diabetes, and hypothyroidism reflect the need to use objective laboratory tests to detect patients at risk for these and other disorders.

The rapid changes in medicine mandate that physicians continuously update their knowledge base and clinical skills. Fundamentally, we acquire new medical information in three main ways: 1) supervised patient care (apprenticeship); 2) lectures; and, 3) textbooks and journal articles. As society transitions to a new media age, our learning is increasingly visual. Lectures have evolved from slides with typed lists and the occasional photograph to animated PowerPoint presentations, or even web-based streaming videos. Textbooks have generally changed more slowly. However, *Comprehensive Clinical Endocrinology* has made impressive use of visual tools to aid the learning process. Though a cliché, the phrase "a picture is worth a thousand words" remains all too true. Through patient photographs, colorful schematic illustrations of physiology and cell biology, and with practical summaries of diagnostic and treatment approaches, the 3rd Edition of *Comprehensive Clinical Endocrinology*, takes full advantage of the many attributes of endocrinology to breathe life into the printed page. The book also highlights the latest advances in genetics and molecular biology and incorporates these into disease pathophysiology and patient management.

The Editors, G. Michael Besser and Michael O. Thorner, teach based on extensive personal experience, combined with insights gleaned from their involvement in cutting edge clinical and basic research. Their classic studies demonstrating how dopamine agonists, such a bromocriptine, suppress prolactin secretion and decrease tumor size, represent a paradigm for linking basic science with clinical medicine. Three decades after this important observation, endocrinology has many similar examples of translational research. This book emphasizes how new insights into physiology can enhance patient care. The Editors are joined by an international group of experts who are subspecialists in various endocrine diseases. Despite the number of authors, the quality of the information and illustrations is uniformly excellent.

There are many unique elements in the design of *Comprehensive Clinical Endocrinology*. There is a clear focus is on the clinical presentation of patients. The writing style is clear and direct. The multicolor figures are designed in a consistent manner and are remarkably informative. Several very strong chapters in this book have few counterparts in other texts. For example, the discussion of the "Endocrinology of the Placenta, Fetus, and Pregnancy," sets the stage for many developmental endocrine disorders, as well as acquired problems seen in infants of diabetic mothers and in neonatal thyrotoxicosis. The three chapters on "Imaging" are particularly comprehensive and are a welcome contribution to the field, as we increasingly use radiologic procedures in endocrinology. We can anticipate even more examples of MRI in the next edition. Perhaps most innovative is the series of "Patient Perspectives". These poignant testimonials recount the experiences of patients with androgen insensitivity syndrome, Graves' disease, diabetes, growth hormone deficiency, and several other endocrine disorders. These compelling essays provide invaluable information about physician–patient relationships, highlight the social and psychological impact of endocrine disease, and relate a few clinical pearls from those with life-long experience with these disorders. The message in these articles is at least as important as classic discussions of pathophysiology, diagnosis, and medical management. Useful websites and addresses for disease-oriented patient groups and professional organizations are also listed.

Comprehensive Clinical Endocrinology is current, authoritative, and practical. The format of the book, with its many illustrations and succinct well-organized text, helps the student digest topics that can be daunting when first encountered. For more experienced readers, there is much new information here and the fresh presentation makes it enjoyable to revisit familiar topics. A CD-ROM supplied with the book provides the illustrations that can be exported for use in PowerPoint. I plan to keep this colorful and interesting book close at hand as a tool for teaching and for up to date information on clinical management. Selected figures and the patient perspectives will also be valuable for communication with patients.

J Larry Jameson, MD, PhD
Irving S Cutter Professor and Chairman
Department of Medicine
Feinberg School of Medicine
Northwestern University
Chicago, Illinois

Preface

This third edition of *Comprehensive Clinical Endocrinology* is an expanded and logical extension of the earlier two editions. It is presented with a CD-ROM containing the illustrations that we trust will prove a valuable contribution, particularly as an aid to teaching. We have made several major changes to the content and format and have included a section of four chapters on diabetes mellitus.

Of major impact is the new section 'Patient Perspectives'. We believe this the first medical textbook to have such a section and that it will set a precedent for future textbooks. It is an acknowledgement that patients are more knowledgeable about their diseases and, properly, are more involved in determining their care. We earnestly believe that we as doctors have a great deal to learn from the patients about their perspective of their diseases, their experiences and interactions with the health care system, and the impact of their condition on them and their families. We are convinced that it is important to teach this aspect of clinical care as well as the more traditional aspects of endocrine, and other, disease processes.

The dramatic advances of recent years in the understanding of the normal physiology of human endocrinology and, as a consequence, of its pathological processes and their management, have continued unabated. This has largely been as a result of improvements in analytical techniques and the specificity and sensitivity of hormone assays and of the dramatic new knowledge acquired from application of the powerful molecular biological weapons. These innovations have allowed separation and accurate measurement of the relevant endocrine factors in blood, CSF and tissues, new immunocytochemical procedures for cellular localization of hormones and identification of the structure and functions of genes, gene products, receptors and their ligands and their disturbances in disease. Neuroendocrinology has become a clinical science with elaborations of profound new concepts of the relationships between mind and body, and the mechanisms governing the body's homeostasis and its alterations in disease. These developments were behind the design of the first edition of this textbook originally planned with the late

Andrew Cudworth, who tragically died so young. The principles have been continued and developed in both the second and this new more comprehensive and expanded third edition.

As before, the text is highly illustrated using new techniques developed by the Publishers. The work was initially conceived as a slide atlas and the principal messages of the book that have been developed from it are conveyed in the diagrams and pictures, and explained and expanded by the text. It has now evolved into a CD-ROM of the illustrations for creating slides for teaching and presentations. Normal physiology is the starting point of each section so that the pathological and clinical features of the disorders, their investigation and management can be based on this fundamental knowledge. Special attention has been given to the radiology and neuroradiology of endocrine diseases and the interrelationships between the behavioral and emotional features of the disorders and the chemical changes that have induced them. Wherever possible, the molecular basis of events considered is described. Diabetes mellitus and its closely related topics including disorders of lipids have now been included in this comprehensive third edition.

We acknowledge the dedication and invaluable help of Patrick Purcell in the compiling of the chapters. The staff of Elsevier Science has been long-suffering during the production of this textbook and accompanying CD-ROM, and we wish to extend our gratitude to them for their expert attention and help, especially to Paul Fam and Deborah Russell in the formulation of the concept and planning of this edition, Hilary Hewitt in production, Mick Ruddy in design and illustration and Cathy Carroll in editorial.

We wish to thank Professor Larry Jameson for writing the foreword, which encapsulates the essential elements of this text. Our greatest debt is to the multiple authors who have contributed so generously to make this volume so easy to read, up to date and beautifully illustrated.

G. Michael Besser
Michael O. Thorner

Endocrine Normal Ranges

The ranges given here are guidelines only, because laboratories use different reagents and therefore may obtain somewhat different values in the same situations. Each laboratory must derive its own normal ranges. Conversion factor (cf) is shown.

ADRENAL STEROIDS

	Traditional Units	cf	SI Units
Aldosterone			
Normal diet			
upright (4 h)	12–30ng/dL	27.7	330–830pmol/L
supine (30 min)	5–14.5ng/dL		135–400pmol/L
Cortisol			
09.00 h	7–25µg/dL	27.6	200–700nmol/L
18.00 h	3.5–10µg/dL		100–300nmol/L
24.00 h (asleep)	<1.8µg/dL		<50nmol/L
low/dose dexamethasone suppression test (2mg/day for 48 h)	<5µg/dL		<140nmol/L
after insulin-induced hypoglycemia (blood glucose <2.2mmol/L or <40ng/dL)	>21µg/dL		>580nmol/L
11-deoxycortisol	0.9–1.6µg/dL	28.8	24–46nmol/L
Dehydroepiandrosterone (DHEA)			
09.00	2–9µg/L	3.4	7–31nmol/L
DHEA-sulphate			
women	1100–4400ng/mL	0.0027	3–12µmol/L
men	750–3700ng/mL		2–10µmol/L
pre-pubertal	<185ng/mL		<0.5µmol/L
Androstenedione			
adults	0.9–2.3µg/L	3.49	3–8nmol/L
prepubertal children	<0.3µg/L		<1nmol/L
17-hydroxyprogesterone			
males	0.3–3µg/L	3.3	1–10nmol/L
females:			
follicular	0.3–3µg/L		1–10nmol/L
luteal	3–6µg/L		10–20nmol/L
Neonatal (i.e. from 32 weeks gestation to 2 weeks post-partum)	<24µg/L		<80nmol/L
Estradiol			
prepuberty	<6pg/mL	3.6	<20pmol/L
women:			
postmenopausal	<30pg/mL		<100pmol/L
follicular phase	55–110pg/mL		200–400pmol/L
mid-cycle	110–330pg/mL		400–1200pmol/L
luteal	110–274pg/mL		400–1000pmol/L
men	<50pg/mL		<180pmol/L
Progesterone			
women:			<57pmol/L
follicular phase	<3ng/mL	3.2	<10nmol/L
luteal	>10ng/mL		>30nmol/L
men	<2ng/mL		<6nmol/L
Testosterone			
prepubertal children	<0.2ng/mL	3.46	<0.8nmol/L
women	0.14–0.87ng/mL		0.5–3nmol/L (median 18nmol/L)
men	2.5–10ng/mL		9–35nmol/L (median 1.5nmol/L)
Dihydrotestosterone (DHT)			
women	0.087–0.27ng/mL	3.44	0.3–9.3nmol/L
men	0.29–0.76ng/mL		1–2.6nmol/L

PANCREATIC AND GUT HORMONES

	Traditional Units	cf	SI Units
Gastrin	<120pg/mL	0.45	<55pmol/L
Insulin			
overnight fasting	<16µU/mL	7.18	<114µmol/L
after hypoglycemia (blood glucose < 2.2 mmol/L or < 40ng/dL)	<3µU/mL		<21µmol/L
Carcinoembryonic antigen (CEA)	<5ng/mL	1	<5µg/L
Vasoactive Intestinal Polypeptide (VIP)	<72pg/mL	0.42	<30pmol/L
Pancreatic Polypeptide (PP)	<1260pg/mL	0.24	<300pmol/L
Glucagon	<175pg/mL	0.28	<50pmolmol/L

ANTERIOR PITUITARY HORMONES

	Traditional Units	cf	SI Units
Adrenocorticotrophic Hormone (ACTH) (plasma)			
09.00	<80pg/mL	0.22	<18pmol/L
Follicle Stimulating Hormone (FSH)			
women:			
follicular phase	2.5–10mU/mL	1	2.5–10U/L
midcycle	6–25mU/mL		25–70U/L
luteal phase	0.3–2.1mU/mL		>0.32–2.1U/L
postmenopausal	>30mU/mL		>30U/L
men	1–7mU/mL		1–7U/L
prepubertal children	<5mU/mL		<5U/L
Growth Hormone (GH)			
basal, fasting and between pulses	<0.3ng/mL	3	<1mU/L
after hypoglycemia	>7ng/mL		>30mU/L
Luteinising Hormone (LH)			
women:			
follicular phase	2.5–10mU/mL	1	2.5–10U/L
midcycle	25–70mU/mL		25–70U/L
luteal phase	<1–13mU/mL		<1–13U/L
postmenopausal	>30mU/mL		>30U/L
men	1–10mU/mL		1–10U/L
prepubertal children	<5mU/mL		<5U/L
Prolactin (PRL)	<18ng/mL	20	<360mU/L
Thyroid Stimulating Hormone (TSH)	0.4–5µU/mL	1	0.4–5mU/L

THYROID HORMONES

	Traditional Units	cf	SI Units
Thyroglobulin	<1.2ng/mL		N/A
Thyroxine T$_4$			
free	0.8–1.8ng/mL	12.9	10–22pmol/L
total	5–12µg/mL		58–174nmol/L
Triiodothyronine T$_3$			
free	3.5–6.5pg/mL	1.54	5–10pmol/L
total	70–220ng/mL	0.015	1.07–3.18nmol/L

CATECHOLAMINES (plasma, lithium heparin)

(lying and with venous catheter in place for 30 min prior to collection of sample)

	Traditional Units	cf	SI Units
Adrenaline (epinephrine)	0.01–0.25ng/mL	5.46	0.03–1.31nmol/L
Noradrenaline (norepinephrine)	0.08–0.75ng/mL	5.99	0.47–4.14nmol/L

Age related insulin-like growth factor-I (IGF-I)

	Traditional Units	cf	SI Units
0–3yrs	7–100ng/mL	7.5	0.9–13.3nmol/L
4–6yrs	14–175ng/mL		1.9–23.3nmol/L
7–9yrs	42–210ng/mL		5.6–28.0nmol/L
10–12yrs	50–280ng/mL		6.7–37.3nmol/L
13–15yrs	70–420ng/mL		9.3–56.0nmol/L
16–18yrs	70–420ng/mL		9.3–56.0nmol/L
20–40yrs	56–280ng/mL		7.5–37.3nmol/L
40–60yrs	42–175ng/mL		5.6–23.3nmol/L
over 60 yrs	25–175ng/mL		3.3–23.3nmol/L
Parathyroid Hormone (PTH)	9–54ng/L	10	0.9–5.4pmol/L
Alpha-Fetoprotein (AFP)	<10mg/dL	1	<10U/L
Beta Human Chorionic Gonadotrophin (β-hCG)	<50mU/mL	1	<50U/L
Calcitonin (plasma lithium heparin)	<80pg/L	1	<80ng/L

URINARY VALUES

	Traditional Units	cf	SI Units
Aldosterone	5–19µg/24h	2.8	14–53nmol/24h
Calcium	<300mg/24h	0.025	<7.5mmol/24h
Cortisol	20–100µg/24h	2.76	55–250nmol/24h
5-Hydroxyindoleacetic Acid (5-HIAA)	<9mg/24h	5.24	<75µmol/24h
Metanephrins	<12mg/24h	5.46	<63µmol/24h
Vanillyl Mandelic Acid (VMA)	1–7mg/24h	5	5–35µmol/24h
Adrenaline (epinephrine)	26µg/24h	5.46	<144nmol/24h
Noradrenaline (norepinephrine)	97µg/24h	5.46	<570nmol/24h
Dopamine	<585µg/24h	5.27	<3100nmol/24h

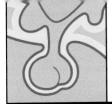

Section 1 Hypothalamus and Pituitary

Chapter 1

Neuroendocrine Control of Pituitary Function

Seymour Reichlin

INTRODUCTION

Secretion of each of the known anterior pituitary hormones is controlled by one or more releasing or inhibitory factors, which arise in the hypothalamus. These hypothalamic factors, termed 'hypophysiotropic hormones', interact at the level of the pituitary cell with the feedback effects of target gland hormones. All of the hormones are peptides with the exception of dopamine, a catecholamine. Hypophysiotropic hormones influence both the release of preformed pituitary hormones and the rate of synthesis of new hormones. They also regulate pituitary cell growth and pituitary cell receptors. Thyrotropin-releasing hormone (TRH) was the first of the hypophysiotropic hormones to be chemically characterized (1969) and, between that time and 1982, peptides regulating secretion of gonadotropins, corticotropin and somatotropin (growth hormone) were isolated and their structures elucidated. These discoveries validated the hypothesis proposed by Harris over five decades ago, that chemical substances carried from the hypothalamus to the anterior pituitary by way of the hypophysial–portal vessels are the means by which the brain controls pituitary function. These substances, and their analogs, can be used to stimulate or inhibit pituitary hormone secretion selectively for diagnostic and therapeutic purposes.

Pituitary regulatory substances of the hypothalamus are synthesized within specialized neurons by a process known as neurosecretion. The general concept of neurosecretion is the basis of our understanding of the way in which neural information is transduced into chemical messages. The idea of neurosecretion was first proposed by Scharrer and colleagues in the late 1920s. They recognized that certain nerve cells in the brain of insects and fish, and in the neurohypophysial system of mammals, resembled gland cells. Scharrer suggested that some nerve cells were capable of acting like glands of internal secretion and so introduced the term neurosecretion to describe this phenomenon.

In general, all neurons are neurosecretory in that they release a synthesized product from their terminals (**Fig. 1.1**). Within the brain and spinal cord the neuronal product is released into the confines of the synaptic cleft while the neurosecretory neurons of the hypothalamic hypophysiotropic neurons release their product into the blood that supplies the anterior pituitary gland. A third group of neurosecretory neurons, those of the neurohypophysis, secrete their products, vasopressin (VP) and oxytocin (OT), into the general circulation. Neurosecretions that enter the blood are also called *neurohormones*. Conventional neurotransmitter and neuromodulatory neurons synapse with the neurohypophysial and hypophysiotropic neurons and regulate them by secretion of neurotransmitters and neuropeptides.

ANATOMY OF THE HYPOTHALAMO-PITUITARY UNIT

Owing to its complex embryologic origin, the pituitary gland has four component regions (anterior lobe, intermediate lobe, neural lobe, pars tuberalis), which differ in relative size and function among various species. The anterior lobe is a purely glandular structure derived from the anterior wall of Rathke's pouch (an evagination of primitive oral ectoderm) to take up an intimate anatomic relationship with the floor of the hypothalamus at the site of appearance of the anlage of the neural lobe. The intermediate lobe, which in humans is virtually absent, is derived from the posterior wall of Rathke's pouch, its few constituent cells being dispersed in the anterior lobe. The neural lobe of the pituitary gland (also known as the posterior pituitary or neurohypophysis) consists mainly of dilated and enlarged endings of nerve cells whose cell bodies are in well-defined nuclei of the hypothalamus (**Fig. 1.2**). These nerve terminals are enmeshed in a highly vascular matrix of supportive cells termed pituicytes, which resemble glial cells of the brain. The principal secretions of the neurohypophysis are oxytocin (OT, uterus-contracting hormone/milk let-down hormone) and vasopressin (VP, antidiuretic hormone); both are synthesized as part of prohormones that include distinctive prohormone sequences originally termed neurophysins. The neurophysin–oxytocin and neurophysin–vasopressin prohormones are transported from the cell body peripherally in the form of packaged granules, to be stored in the nerve endings of the posterior pituitary. From their storage site, they are released in response to appropriate physiologic signals. Secretion of both hormones is mediated by neural reflexes and by the hormonal milieu: VP release is determined by blood osmolality, effective blood volume, nauseating agents and stress; OT is released in response to suckling and during labor. VP secretion is regulated as part of a negative feedback loop by glucocorticoids, while oxytocin secretion is stimulated by estrogens.

The anterior pituitary (also known as the adenohypophysis or pars distalis) is also controlled by the brain but, unlike the neural lobe, does not have a direct nerve supply. Rather, as noted above, neural information from the brain is transduced in the form of chemical messages by specialized hypothalamic cells and then released into the blood supply of the pituitary. Transfer of neuroregulators from hypothalamic neurons to the pituitary blood supply takes place in an anatomically specialized region of the ventral hypothalamus known as the median eminence or tuberoinfundibular region (**Fig. 1.2**). Neurons that project to this region are called *tuberoinfundibular neurons*. These terminate in

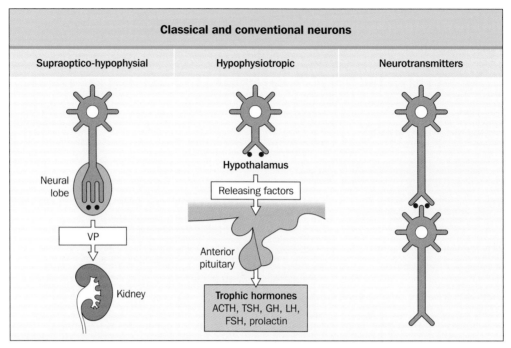

Figure 1.1 Classical and conventional neurons. Neurosecretory peptidergic neurons involved in pituitary regulation and conventional neurotransmitter synapses. (Left panel) The classic neurohypophysial system. Nerves project from cells of origin in the supraopticohypophysial and paraventriculohypophysial nuclei and end in the neural lobe. Oxytocin and vasopressin (VP, antidiuretic hormone) are synthesized on the endoplasmic reticulum as part of a large prohormone (which includes the specific oxytocin- and VP-related neurophysins) and are then packaged into granules, stored in nerve endings and subsequently released into the peripheral blood. Since they affect tissues at a remote site, they are classified as neurohormones. (Center panel) The hypophysiotropic neurons that arise in the hypothalamus and terminate in the median eminence in contiguity to the specialized capillary blood vessels of the hypophysial–portal circulation. Their secretions are also considered to be neurohormones, since they are secreted into blood and act remotely. (Right panel) Conventional neurons may secrete the same substances as those that are released into the blood by the classic neurosecretory neurons. The main difference, however, is that their products are secreted into a synaptic cleft. At receptors on neurons, neuropeptides can act as classical neurotransmitters or as neuromodulators. A neuromodulator is a substance that modifies neuronal responses to neurotransmitters. ACTH, adrenocorticotropin-releasing hormone; FSH, follicle-stimulating hormone; GH, growth hormone; LH, luteinizing hormone; TSH, thyroid-stimulating hormone. (Modified from Reichlin S. Introduction. In: Reichlin S, Baldessarini RJ, Martin JR, eds. The hypothalmus. New York: Raven Press; 1977.)

proximity to capillary walls within the median eminence that drain into a few larger veins, which in turn supply the sinusoids of the pituitary. By analogy with the venous supply of the liver, this vascular system is referred to as the hypophysial–portal system.

The anatomic distribution of the tuberoinfundibular neuron system has been elucidated by retrograde tracing of markers injected in the median eminence (**Fig. 1.3**) and by immuno-histochemical staining of neurons containing hypophysiotropic peptides (**Fig. 1.4**). By using mRNA probes that code for the hypothalamic factors, *in situ* hybridization methods can demonstrate the anatomic distribution of the hypothalamic hormones and determine the factors that regulate specific mRNA synthesis (**Figs 1.5 & 1.6**).

Tuberoinfundibular neurons are influenced by nerve fibers from many parts of the brain, e.g. those that integrate homeostasis, stress responses, mating, and reproduction. In addition, the tuberoinfundibular neurons are regulated by

feedback effects of classical target gland hormones (thyroid, adrenal cortex, gonads), by pituitary hormones themselves such as prolactin, by a growth-hormone-dependent factor arising from the liver (insulin-like growth factor I [IGF-1]), from fat cells (leptin), and from cells of the immune system (interleukin-1 [IL-1], interleukin-6 [IL-6], tumor necrosis factor-α).

The gross anatomic relations of the hypothalamus and pituitary, and abnormalities in disease, can be visualized by CT (computerized tomography) scanning and by nuclear magnetic resonance imaging (MRI; **Fig. 1.7**) (see also Chapter 39).

Each of the known anterior pituitary hormones is regulated by one or more hypothalamic hormones and in some instances a single hypothalamic hormone (sometimes referred to as 'releasing factor' or hypophysiotropic hormone) can influence more than one pituitary hormone. The main pituitary hormones and their regulating hypothalamic hormones are listed in **Figure 1.8**.

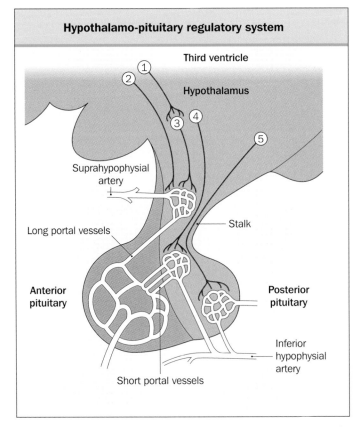

Hypothalamo-pituitary regulatory system

Figure 1.2 Hypothalamo-pituitary regulatory system. The products of the posterior pituitary are synthesized in the supraoptic and paraventricular nuclei (5). After packaging, they are transported as granules, by axoplasmic flow, to the nerve terminals in the posterior pituitary, where they are released directly into the circulation to act as classical neurohormones on distant target sites. The mechanism of control of anterior pituitary hormone secretion is entirely different. The anterior pituitary hormone-releasing or release-inhibiting hormones of the hypothalamus are synthesized within the nuclei of the hypothalamus (1–4) and transported to the median eminence, from where they travel to the anterior pituitary via the dense capillary network and the long portal veins. These hypothalamic factors occupy specific receptors on pituitary cells and lead either to the release or inhibition of the pituitary hormones. (Modified from Gay VL. The hypothalamus: physiology and clinical use of releasing factors. Fertil Steril. 1972;23:50–63. Courtesy of the American Fertility Society, Baltimore.)

STRUCTURE OF THE HYPOPHYSIOTROPIC HORMONES OF THE HYPOTHALAMUS

Isolation and chemical identification of hypothalamic factors with anterior pituitary-regulating properties has focused on extracts of hypothalamic tissues. Initially, they were known as 'releasing factors' after the first description in 1955 of corticotropin-releasing factor (CRF). The term 'releasing factor' was introduced by Saffran and Schally to describe a substance extracted from the neural lobe that stimulated the release of adrenocorticotropic hormone (ACTH) from pituitary fragments maintained in organ culture. In 1981, the chemical nature of this substance was elucidated by Vale and colleagues. By convention, most workers use the term releasing hormone to designate releasing factors whose chemical structures have been identified.

The amino-acid sequence of five well-established and one putative peptide hypophysiotropic hormones are shown in **Figure 1.9**. The sixth factor, Ghrelin is probably the so-called growth hormone secretagogue (GHS) and may be present in at least two different forms. It is uncertain whether it is produced in the hypothalamus in addition to the stomach. It appears also to increase appetite in addition to stimulating growth hormone (GH) secretion. Its physiologic role, in 2001, is yet to be determined. Not shown in the figure are the prolactin-releasing hormones (PRH). Vasoactive intestinal peptide (VIP) is the best established PRH, but there are several other putative PRHs, including two amidated peptides, one of 20 and the other of 32 amino acids in length, whose physiologic significance remains to be proved. Dopamine (**Fig. 1.10**) can also be classified as a hypophysiotropic pituitary hormone since it is present in hypophysial–portal vessel blood in sufficient concentrations to duplicate all its known inhibitory effects on the secretion of prolactin. At this time, government regulators in one or more countries have approved the clinical use of oxytocin, vasopressin, TRH, gonadotropin-releasing hormone (GnRH), corticotropin-releasing hormone (CRH), and growth-hormone-releasing hormone (GHRH), and analogs of vasopressin, GnRH, and somatostatin.

Many other active peptides and neurotransmitters can be isolated from the hypothalamus (**Fig. 1.11**) and have now shown to be also co-secreted with the known hypophysiotropic hormones or are found in neurons that project into the hypothalamus from other parts of the brain. Indeed, the hypothalamus contains a wider variety, and a higher concentration, of neuropeptides and neurotransmitters than any other part of the brain.

Most of the hypophysiotropic peptides that were first isolated from the hypothalamus have now also been shown to be formed within pituitary cells, where they form intrinsic paracrine (cell-to-cell) and autocrine (cell-to-self) regulatory systems. They are also found outside the hypothalamus, where they may act as mediators of affective state and biologic rhythms or as regulators of visceral function, activity, body temperature, and eating and drinking behavior.

In addition to dopamine, which inhibits prolactin secretion, at least one other hypothalamic factor, somatostatin, exerts physiologically significant inhibitory actions on growth hormone and thyroid-stimulating hormone/thyrotropin (TSH). These inhibitory factors interact with the respective releasing factor to exert dual control of secretion of prolactin, growth hormone, and TSH). The action of each of the hypophysiotropic hormones is not limited strictly to a single pituitary hormone: for example, TRH (the physiologic releaser of TSH) is a potent releaser of prolactin and, in some circumstances, releases adrenocorticotropic hormone (ACTH) and GH; gonadotropin-releasing hormone (GnRH) releases both luteinizing hormone (LH) and follicle-stimulating hormone (FSH); and somatostatin inhibits secretion of GH, TSH, and a wide variety of other nonpituitary hormones. The principal inhibitor of prolactin secretion is dopamine, but this potent bioamine, acting directly on the pituitary, also inhibits TSH and gonadotropin secretion. Additionally, under some circumstances, it inhibits GH secretion.

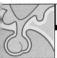

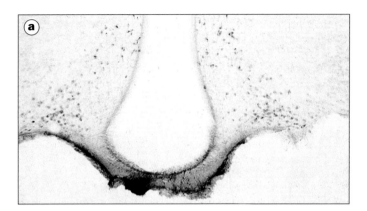

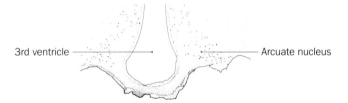

3rd ventricle — Arcuate nucleus

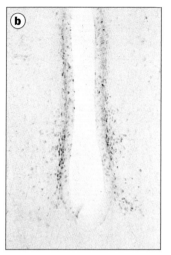

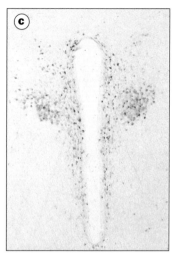

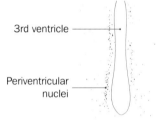

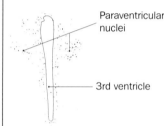

3rd ventricle —

Periventricular nuclei —

Paraventricular nuclei

3rd ventricle

Figure 1.3 Anatomy of the tuberoinfundibular system in the rat, demonstrated by retrograde transport of a tracer compound. A tracer compound, wheat germ agglutinin (which is taken up by nerve endings), was injected into the median eminence of a rat. Several hours later, the animal was killed and the brain sectioned and stained immunohistochemically with an antibody to wheat germ agglutinin. The tracer was found in cell bodies located in three main areas: (a) the arcuate nucleus; (b) the periventricular nucleus, which comprises a rich plexus that is several cells deep immediately under the ependymal layer of the third ventricle; and (c) the paraventricular nuclei. Many of the arcuate cells are dopaminergic and most periventricular cells are somatostatinergic. The paraventricular nucleus is complex and includes cells that secrete vasopressin, oxytocin, thyrotropin-releasing hormone, somatostatin, neurotensin, corticotropin-releasing hormone, vasoactive intestinal peptide, and many other hormones. In addition to projecting to the median eminence (for control of anterior pituitary secretion), the paraventricular nucleus projects to other regions of the neuroaxis where other visceral regulating functions are carried out. (Courtesy of Dr R Lechan.)

CHEMISTRY AND FUNCTION OF THE INDIVIDUAL HYPOTHALAMIC HORMONES

Thyrotropin-releasing hormone

The chemical structure of TRH was elucidated by groups of investigators led by Andrew Schally and Roger Guillemin. Their work, which was the culmination of more than a decade of effort to identify the nature of the thyrotropin-releasing activity of crude hypothalamic extracts, made neuroendocrinology credible to the general scientific and clinical community and was ultimately recognized by the award of a Nobel Prize. The discovery of TRH had a much greater significance than merely the demonstration of a factor regulating a particular pituitary hormone. The discovery validated neuroendocrinology as a field of research, validated the hypophysial–portal theory of anterior pituitary control, stimulated the search for other hypothalamic regulators, and revealed the potential value of releasing hormones as diagnostic and therapeutic agents.

Thyrotropin-releasing hormone, a tripeptide amide – (pyro) Glu-His-Pro-NH$_2$ – is a relatively simple substance. Although some substituted forms are potent, an intact amide and the cyclized glutamic acid terminal are essential for activity. TRH is chemically stable but it is rapidly degraded in plasma by circulating enzymes. Following injection of TRH in humans or rats, blood TSH levels rise rapidly and dramatically, a change being detected within 3min; peak values are normally attained between 10 and 20min after injection in normal subjects (**Fig. 1.12**) and sometimes later in subjects with hypothalamic or pituitary disease. The hormone is very potent: as little as 15µg yields a detectable response and maximal effects are achieved with a dose of 400µg. The standard clinical dose administered as an intravenous bolus injection is 200–500µg. Transient mild nausea, a sense of urinary urgency, and moderate (rarely marked) increases in blood pressure occur as side effects of injection. The surge of TSH release induced by TRH injection leads to a detectable rise in plasma triiodothyronine (T$_3$) and also an increase in thyroxine (T$_4$) release, although the latter is usually not large enough to be reflected in a significant increase in circulating levels of T$_4$

A striking feature of the TRH-induced TSH response is that its effects are blocked by prior treatment with thyroid hormone. Indeed, the interaction of the negative feedback effects of thyroid hormone on the pituitary with the stimulating effects of TRH is a major element in the feedback control of TSH secretion (**Fig. 1.13**).

In addition to stimulating TSH release, TRH is also a potent prolactin-regulating factor (PRF; **Fig. 1.14**). The time course of response of blood prolactin levels to TRH and the dose–response characteristics and suppressibility (by thyroid hormone pretreatment) of TRH all parallel changes in TSH secretion.

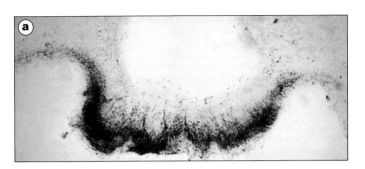

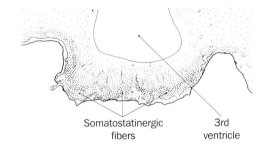

Somatostatinergic
fibers

3rd
ventricle

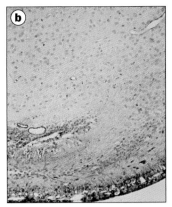

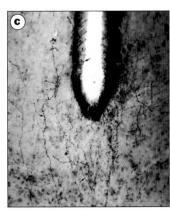

Median
eminence

3rd
ventricle

Somatostatinergic
fibers

GnRH
neurons

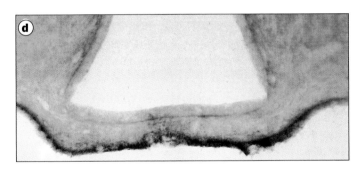

3rd
ventricle

TRH-containing
nerve endings

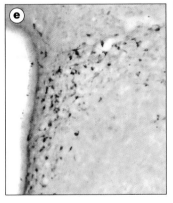

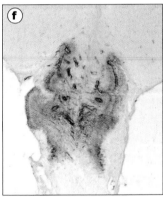

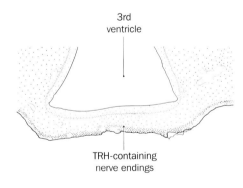

TRH in
paraventricular
neurons

GHRH
neurons

Median
eminence

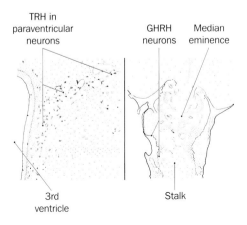

3rd
ventricle

Stalk

Figure 1.4 Hypophysiotropic neurons in the hypothalamus, demonstrated by immunohistochemical techniques using the Sternberger peroxidase antiperoxidase complex (PAP) method.
(a) The immunohistochemical appearance of somatostatinergic fibers in a frontal section of the hypothalamus of the rat at the level of the median eminence. (b) The sagittal section of the hypothalamus of the rat, showing somatostatinergic fibers. (c) Gonadotropin-releasing hormone peptidergic pathways in a horizontal section of the rat hypothalamus. (d) Thyrotropin-releasing-hormone (TRH)-containing nerve endings in the median eminence of the rat (frontal section). (e) TRH-containing neurons in the paraventricular nucleus of the rat (frontal section). (f) Anatomic localization of growth hormone releasing hormone in the stalk and median eminence of the Rhesus monkey. (Courtesy of Drs R Lechan, L Alpert, and J King.)

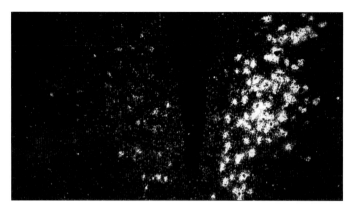

Figure 1.5 *In situ* hybridization of thyrotropin-releasing hormone mRNA in the paraventricular nucleus of a hypothyroid rat. The paraventricular nucleus on the left has been injected with a minute pellet of triiodothyronine (T$_3$), whereas an inert substance was injected into the right nucleus. The striking suppression of the hybridization signal indicates that T$_3$ acted locally to suppress synthesis of mRNA and is thus indicative of a hypothalamic locus for the suppression of the hypothalamic–pituitary–thyroid axis. (With permission from Dyess EM, et al. Triiodothyronine exerts direct cell-specific regulation of thyrotropin-releasing hormone gene expression in the hypothalamic paraventricular nucleus. Endocrinology. 1988;123:2291–7.)

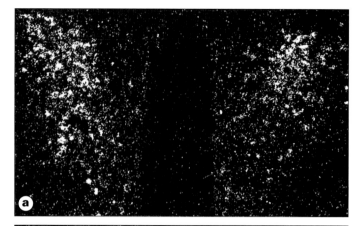

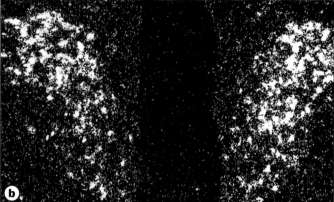

Figure 1.6 *In situ* hybridization of corticotropin releasing hormone (CRH) mRNA in the paraventricular nucleus of a rat. (a) *In situ* hybridization of CRH mRNA in the paraventricular nucleus of a normal rat. (b) Hybridization of CRH mRNA in a rat following the intracerebroventricular administration of recombinant human interleukin-1β (100ng, followed by an infusion of 20ng/h for 12 hours). When compared with (a), there is readily detectable activation of CRH neuronal activity. (Courtesy of Dr R Lechan.)

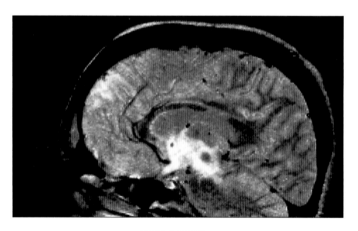

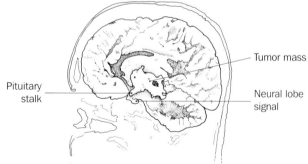

Figure 1.7 Magnetic resonance imaging scan of the brain and pituitary of a patient with eosinophilic granulomas of Langerhans' cell histiocytosis that have densely infiltrated the hypothalamus and thalamus. The patient was deficient in all anterior pituitary functions and had diabetes insipidus, but the lesion did not directly involve the pituitary region.

Nevertheless, there is reason to believe that TRH is not an important regulator of prolactin secretion under normal circumstances; for example, the prolactin secretory response to breastfeeding (in women and experimental animals) is unaccompanied by changes in plasma TSH levels, suggesting that this neurogenic reflex does not involve TRH. The prolactin-release-stimulating effects of TRH, however, may be responsible for the occasional occurrence of hyperprolactinemia (with or without galactorrhea) in patients with hypothyroidism. This finding can be attributed to increased sensitivity of prolactin-secreting cells to TRH in the hypothyroid state, and to an increase in TRH secretion.

In normal individuals, TRH has no influence on pituitary hormone secretion other than on TSH and on prolactin secretion. It can, however, stimulate release of ACTH in patients with Cushing's syndrome; and GH in acromegalics (**Fig. 1.14**).

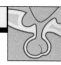

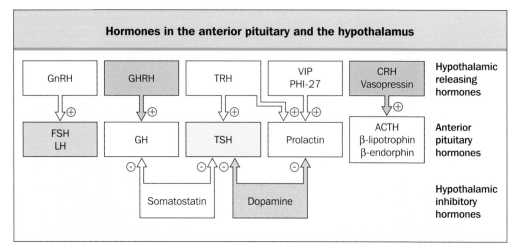

Figure 1.8 Hormones in the anterior pituitary and the hypothalamus. Summary of the hormones produced in the anterior pituitary and the hypothalamic hormones that regulate their secretion. ACTH, adrenocorticotropin-releasing hormone; CRH, corticotropin-releasing hormone; FSH, follicle-stimulating hormone; GH, growth hormone; GHRH, growth-hormone-releasing hormone; GHS, growth hormone secretagogue; GnRH, gonadotropin-releasing hormone; LH, luteinizing hormone; VIP, PHI-27, TRH, thyrotropin-releasing hormone; TSH, thyroid-stimulating hormone; VIP, vasoactive intestinal peptide.

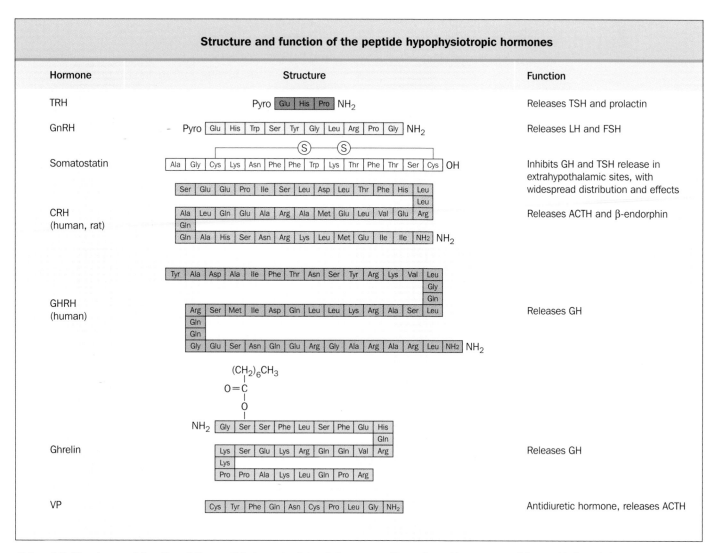

Figure 1.9 Structure and function of the peptide hypophysiotropic hormones. The amino-acid sequences of the peptide hypothalamic hypophysiotropic hormones are illustrated. ACTH, adrenocorticotropin-releasing hormone; CRH, corticotropin-releasing hormone; FSH, follicle-stimulating hormone; GH, growth hormone; GHRH, growth-hormone-releasing hormone; GHS, growth hormone secretagogue; GnRH, gonadotropin-releasing hormone; LH, luteinizing hormone; TRH, thyrotropin-releasing hormone; TSH, thyroid-stimulating hormone; VP, vasopressin.

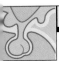

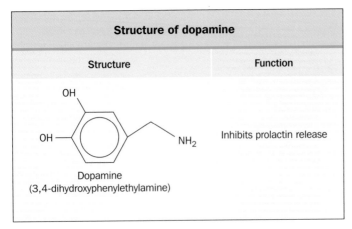

Figure 1.10 Structure of dopamine. Dopamine, the principal prolactin-inhibiting factor, is a biogenic catecholamine secreted by a distinct group of cells in the ventral hypothalamus. It serves as an important neurotransmitter in other regulatory pathways of the brain that are not related to the pituitary.

The 'paradoxical' GH response is a useful indicator of acromegaly (occurring in 70% of patients) and of the state of remission after therapy. TRH also releases GH in some patients with depression.

After a brief period of enthusiasm for its use in treatment of depression, amyotropic lateral sclerosis ('Lou Gehrig's disease'), and shock, it is now clear that TRH has no established therapeutic use. It is of limited value in endocrine diagnostic testing. Its greatest diagnostic value is in the differential diagnosis of thyrotoxicosis in borderline cases of mild thyroid overactivity. Since thyroid hormones inhibit TSH response to TRH, TRH effects are blunted or blocked in the presence of even mild degrees of hyperthyroidism. In current practice, the TRH test, which had been widely used in the evaluation of difficult diagnostic problems in the past, has been largely supplanted by the ultrasensitive TSH immunoassays, which allow measurement of basal or unstimulated TSH values in the full range of normal and below.

It might have been anticipated that TRH would be useful as a diagnostic agent to differentiate between pituitary and hypothalamic causes of TSH deficiency. Indeed, many patients with

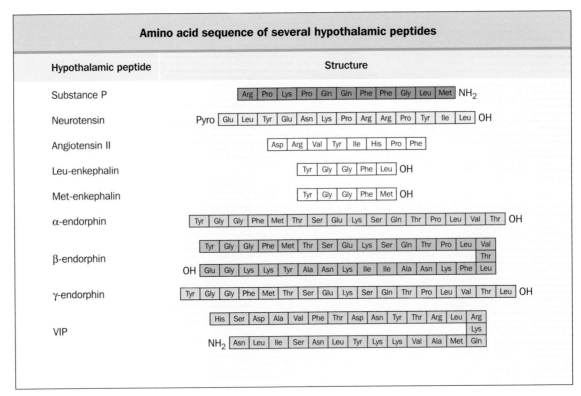

Figure 1.11 Amino acid sequence of several hypothalamic peptides. Many physiologically potent peptides have been isolated from the hypothalamus and are found to be localized in neurosecretory vesicles in hypothalamic neurons. They are also found in the brain outside the hypothalamus in many different projection systems where they perform functions unrelated to pituitary regulation. Changes in visceral function, appetite, and emotional state can be induced by these substances. Most of the peptides shown here are also secreted by pituitary cells themselves, where they form an intrinsic 'paracrine' (cell-to-cell) communicating system. The endogenous opioid peptides are a large group of substances that act like morphine by binding to various classes of opioid receptors. Included in this category are the enkephalins and the endorphins. All the peptides listed (and many others not shown) influence pituitary activity, but their function in normal regulation is not fully understood. Acting on the hypothalamus, substance P stimulates the release of growth hormone (GH) and luteinizing hormone (LH); neurotensin stimulates the release of GH; angiotensin II stimulates the release of adrenocorticotropic hormone (ACTH) and vasopressin; and the endogenous opioids stimulate the secretion of ACTH, prolactin, and GH, and inhibit LH. Vasoactive intestinal peptide (VIP) is an important prolactin-regulating factor responsible (at least in the rat) for response to stress and in part to suckling.

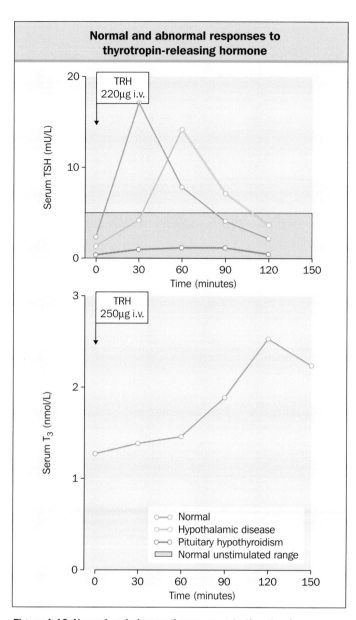

Figure 1.12 Normal and abnormal responses to thyrotropin-releasing hormone. (Top panel) The delayed thyroid-stimulating hormone (TSH) response to thyrotropin-releasing hormone (TRH) in a patient with hypothalamic disease. Peak plasma TSH values are reached at approximately 60min following exogenous TRH, compared to the normal, where the peak occurs at 20–30min. In pituitary hypothyroidism, TSH reserve may be severely reduced and there may be only a slight, or no response, to exogenous TRH. (Bottom panel) The normal rise in circulating plasma triiodothyronine (T_3) following an injection of TRH. The T_3 response lags behind the TSH response, reflecting the fact that T_3 rises secondary to stimulation of the thyroid gland by the released TSH.

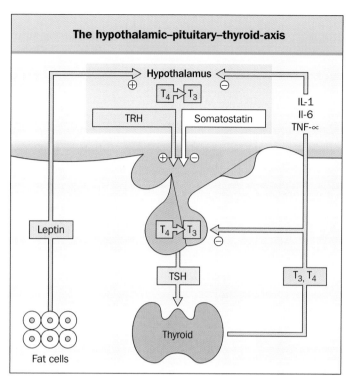

Figure 1.13 The hypothalamic–pituitary–thyroid axis. The thyroid gland is stimulated by thyroid-stimulating hormone (TSH) secreted by the anterior pituitary. Secretion of TSH is stimulated in turn by hypothalamic thyrotropin-releasing hormone (TRH) and is inhibited by the hypothalamic factor somatostatin. TSH secretion is also inhibited by the principal secretions of the thyroid (thyroxine, T_4 and triiodothyronine, T_3, thus forming a negative feedback loop. In addition to exerting direct inhibitory actions at the pituitary level, the thyroid hormones inhibit the secretion of TRH and stimulate the secretion of somatostatin, thus adding a hypothalamic level of negative feedback control of TSH secretion. The regulatory system is made even more complex by the intrahypothalamic and intrapituitary conversion of T_4 to the more-potent T_3, a process that is regulated by thyroid hormones and by the hypothalamic factors. TRH synthesis and secretion is also stimulated by leptin, a peptide secreted by peripheral fat depots and inhibited by proinflammatory cytokines interleukin-1 (IL-1), interleukin-6 (IL-6), and tumor necrosis factor-α (TNF-α). (Modified from Reichlin S. Neuroendocrinology. In: Wilson JD, Foster DW, eds. Williams textbook of endocrinology, 7th edn. Philadelphia, PA:WB Saunders; 1985.)

disease of the hypothalamus that has caused TRH deficiency show responses to injected TRH, while others with pituitary disease fail to respond to TRH (see **Fig. 1.12**). There are, however, a sufficient number of cases not showing the classic or predicted response to prevent clear-cut differential diagnosis. In such cases, accurate radiologic studies and other endocrine evaluations are required for diagnosis.

When TRH was chemically sequenced and synthesized, it became possible to use specific and sensitive methods to study its tissue distribution. One of the most surprising findings to arise from this work was that TRH was distributed widely outside the classic thyrotropic area of the hypothalamus. TRH has been found in: virtually all parts of the brain, including the cerebral cortex; the spinal cord; nerve endings abutting upon the ventral motor horn cells and upon the intermediolateral column of the spinal cord; the neurohypophysis; and the pineal gland. TRH has also been found in pancreatic islet cells and in various parts of the gastrointestinal tract. Although present in low concentrations in these areas, the aggregate in extrahypothalamic tissue far exceeds the total amount in the hypothalamus.

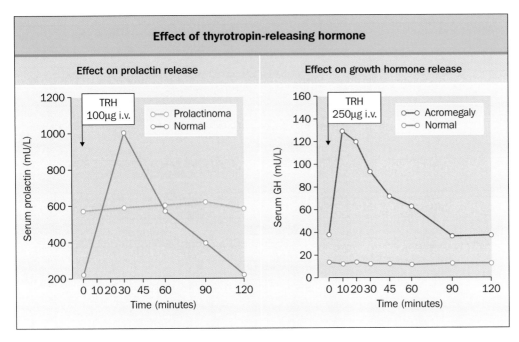

Figure 1.14 Effect of thyrotropin-releasing hormone. The effects of thyrotropin-releasing hormone (TRH) on release of prolactin and growth hormone (GH) are illustrated in normal subjects and in patients with pituitary tumors. (Left panel) TRH stimulates the release of prolactin in a normal subject while having no effect in a patient with prolactinoma (the usual response in such patients). (Right panel) TRH has no effect on plasma GH levels in a normal individual while it stimulates GH release in a patient with acromegaly.

The extensive extrahypothalamic distribution of TRH, its localization in nerve endings, and the presence of TRH receptors in brain tissue suggest that this peptide acts as a neurotransmitter or neuromodulator outside the hypothalamus. In particular, its distribution in the spinal cord at nerve endings of the intermediolateral column, which contain the cells of origin of the sympathetic nervous system, may explain the elevation of blood pressure that follows injections of TRH and may be relevant to clinical benefits claimed in treatment of shock and depression.

Gonadotropin-releasing hormone

It had been known from the work of McCann (1960) and of Campbell and co-workers (1964) that extracts of hypothalamic tissue contain a biologically active substance capable of stimulating the release of gonadotropic hormones from the pituitary. This material was isolated from the hypothalami of stockyard animals, and the structure was finally elucidated by Schally's group in 1971. Like TRH, the amino terminal of GnRH is a substituted amide. A terminal amide group is characteristic of a number of other small peptide hormones, including vasopressin, oxytocin, calcitonin, gastrin, and glucagon; in all these hormones (including TRH and GnRH), the amide group is needed for full hormonal activity. Most reproductive neuroendocrinologists now believe that the GnRH decapeptide is the only hypothalamic gonadotropin regulator and that observed dissociations of secretion of LH and FSH are due to the interacting effects of prior hormone status, steroid pretreatment, and patterns of GnRH administration.

Abnormalities in the embryogenesis of GnRH neurons account for gonadotropin failure in the human disorder Kallmann's syndrome (congenital hypogonadotropic hypogonadism). Uniquely among other hypophysiotropic neurons, those secreting GnRH arise in early development in the olfactory placode in the nasal cavity and take up their final position in the preoptic hypothalamus. Kallmann's syndrome is attributable to a mutation(s) in one of the proteins that guide the growing neuron as it tracks over this long distance.

Following intravenous injection, GnRH triggers a prompt, dose-related increase of LH and FSH in humans (**Fig. 1.15**) and in all vertebrate species in which it has been tested. After a single bolus injection, FSH release is usually delayed compared with LH secretion, the values peaking 10–30min after injection. The response of LH and FSH to GnRH is markedly influenced by the prior GnRH secretory state, by the gonadal steroid milieu, by the state of gonadal activity, by the time course of GnRH injection (i.e. single dose, multiple pulse, or constant infusion), and by the patient's genetic sex. Through secondary effects of pituitary activation, and under appropriately defined conditions, GnRH can induce spermatogenesis and testosterone production in men with hypothalamic hypogonadotropic hypogonadism, and ovulation in women with hypothalamic amenorrhea.

GnRH has been extensively tested as a diagnostic agent in differentiating between the causes of hypogonadism. It has proven to be a relatively poor diagnostic agent in differentiating hypothalamic from pituitary causes of hypogonadism. Although patients with complete pituitary failure fail to release gonadotropins after a single injection of GnRH, this can also be true for some patients with long-standing hypothalamic dysfunction even in the absence of intrinsic pituitary disease. Furthermore, in patients with clinically important hypogonadism due to pituitary disease, GnRH may induce a gonadotropin response within the normal range. Long-standing hypothalamic dysfunction can lead to poor or absent pituitary responsiveness. For these reasons, therefore, a single bolus injection of GnRH is a poor differential diagnostic agent. As a practical matter in clinical differential diagnosis, imaging studies are usually preferred to establish the site of disordered hypothalamic-pituitary dysfunction.

On the other hand, GnRH and its analogs have important clinical applications in the treatment of infertility, precocious puberty and prostate cancer. Intermittent injections of GnRH, which mimic the intermittent release of GnRH by the normal hypothalamus, will stimulate gonadotropin secretion and lead to normal pituitary–testicular and pituitary–ovarian function in

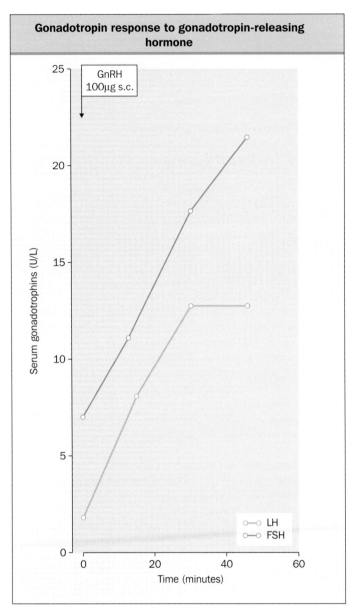

Figure 1.15 Gonadotropin response to gonadotropin-releasing hormone. The response is shown in a woman with galactorrhea–amenorrhea due to prolactinoma. This patient responded to an injection of gonadotropin-releasing hormone (GnRH) with a brisk release of follicle-stimulating hormone (FSH) and luteinizing hormone (LH).

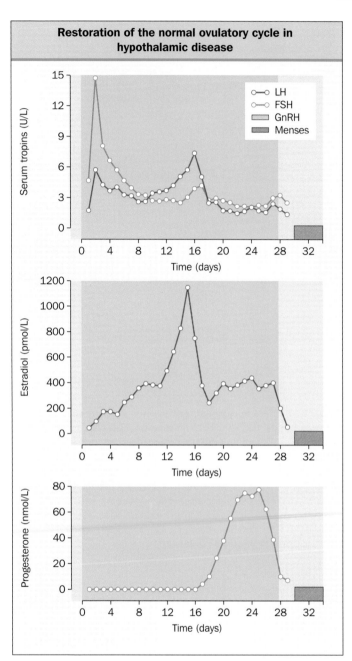

Figure 1.16 Restoration of the normal ovulatory cycle in hypothalamic disease. A normal ovulatory cycle was restored in a woman with hypothalamic disease, using intermittent gonadotropin-releasing hormone (GnRH) injections. Intermittent doses of GnRH were administered at 90min intervals by a pump. These findings indicate that mimicking of the normal pulsating release of GnRH can restore normal cyclical function. FSH, follicle-stimulating hormone; LH, luteinizing hormone. (Modified with permission from Crowley WF Jr, MacArthur JW. Stimulation of the normal menstrual cycle in Kallman's syndrome by pulsatile administration of luteinizing hormone-releasing hormone (LHRH). J Clin Endocrinol Metab. 1980;51:173–5.)

individuals with hypothalamic failure (**Fig. 1.16**). This application is clinically the most important of the hypothalamic hormones thus far and is widely used in suitable patients with hypogonadotropic hypogonadism by means of a portable programmed pump.

In contrast, administration of GnRH at a constant rate leads to reduced gonadotropin secretion (**Fig. 1.17**). This phenomenon, attributed to downregulation of GnRH receptors, has been exploited for the treatment of idiopathic precocious puberty and to inhibit pituitary–gonad function in men with prostate cancer. In patients with precocious puberty disorder, the use of a 'super agonist' of GnRH reversibly inhibits gonadal function to

prepubertal levels and is the treatment of choice. In men with carcinoma of the prostate, super agonists of GnRH can inhibit testosterone secretion without surgical castration or the feminizing effects of estrogens.

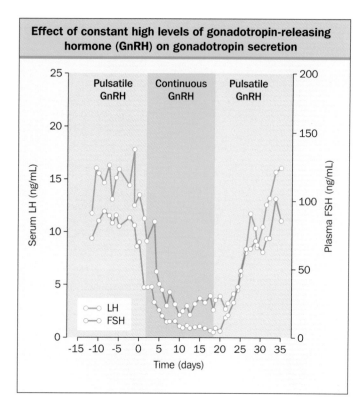

Effect of constant high levels of gonadotropin-releasing hormone (GnRH) on gonadotropin secretion

Figure 1.17 Effect of constant high levels of gonadotropin-releasing hormone (GnRH) on gonadotropin secretion. Data from a monkey show that continuous infusions of GnRH suppress luteinizing hormone (LH) and follicle-stimulating hormone (FSH) release while pulsatile injections restore it. Similar suppressive actions can be exerted by long-acting 'super agonist' doses of GnRH. (Modified with permission from Belchetz PE, Plant TM, Nakai Y, et al. Hypophysial responses to continuous and intermittent delivery of hypothalamic gonadotrophin-releasing hormone. Science. 1978;202:631–3. Courtesy of the American Association for the Advancement of Science, Washington, DC.)

The stimulating actions of GnRH interact with the effects of the gonadal steroids and with peptide secretions of the gonads – termed inhibins (see Chapter 11). These substances also exert actions on the synthesis and secretion of GnRH in the hypothalamus. Under particular circumstances, estrogens sensitize the pituitary to the stimulating effects of GnRH (the mechanism underlying the midcycle ovulatory surge) but can also inhibit GnRH responsiveness. Important negative feedback effects on the gonadotrope cells are exerted by the inhibins which selectively inhibit FSH secretion but not LH secretion.

Unlike TRH and somatostatin, almost all of the GnRH in the brain of mammals is restricted to the hypothalamus and related neural structures. Small amounts are found in the circumventricular organs of the brain, including the pineal gland. GnRH has also been found in milk, suggesting that the breast, a dermally derived structure, may have embryologic origins analogous to the primitive neuroectoderm, the source of neuroendocrine cells. The most important central-nervous-system effect of GnRH may be that involved in the regulation of mating behavior. Direct injection of GnRH into the hypothalamus has been reported to enhance female sexual responsivity, even in animals without a

pituitary (which are therefore incapable of responding with gonadotropin–ovarian hormone activation). Studies of the effect of GnRH on sex drive in humans have been unconvincing. In such studies it is essential to differentiate between a direct effect of GnRH at the level of the hypothalamus with indirect effects on sex steroid secretion mediated by the pituitary–gonad axis.

Growth-hormone-releasing hormone

Efforts to identify the chemical nature of GH-releasing hormone (GHRH) from hypothalamic extracts were unsuccessful for a long time. A clinical insight by Thorner and his colleagues led to the diagnosis of acromegaly due to ectopic secretion of GHRH from a pancreatic islet tumor from which it was isolated in 1982. Two different molecules have been identified by Vale and by Guillemin and their respective collaborators in GHRH-secreting pancreatic adenomas, one consisting of 44 amino acids and the other of 40 amino acids. Identical hormones have been isolated from the hypothalamus.

Administration of GHRH stimulates a brisk release of GH after intravenous injection (**Fig. 1.18**). GHRH has been used to treat GH deficiency in hypopituitary patients with short stature. It can stimulate GH secretion in many patients with GH deficiency caused by proven hypothalamic disease, or in the syndrome of idiopathic GH deficiency. The most common form of acquired GH deficiency is due to hypothalamic disease or rupture of the pituitary stalk. Most cases of 'idiopathic' GH deficiency are of hypothalamic origin. In theory, such cases could be treated with GHRH as well as with GH.

Growth hormone secretagogue (Ghrelin)

During studies of synthetic analogs of the metenkephalins in the 1970s, Bowers and colleagues found some that were potent stimulators of GH release with physiologic effects quite dissimilar to the classical GHRH. The activity of growth-hormone-releasing peptides suggested that there would be specific GH secretagogue receptors in the pituitary. Identification of these receptors made it possible to identify a novel class of endogenous growth hormone secretagogues, which were designated Ghrelin by their discoverers, Kojima and colleagues. Unlike GHRH, GHS peptides are not active in patients with GHRH deficiency due to hypothalamic disease, and, in contrast to GHRH, GHS responses *in vivo* are relatively greater than they are *in vitro*. GHS potentiates the effects of GHRH. Because GHS receptors (GHS-R) are present in the hypothalamus as well as in the pituitary, it is likely that GHS acts at both levels. GHS-R is clearly a part of the feedback control of the GH regulatory system, as shown by inhibition of its expression in the pituitary when blood levels of GH are elevated. Since Ghrelin is secreted by the stomach and other gastrointestinal tissues, it is likely to be a part of a gut–hypothalamic–pituitary regulatory system.

Somatostatin

During the course of efforts to isolate GHRH from hypothalamic extracts, Krulich and McCann discovered a fraction that inhibited GH release from pituitary incubates *in vitro*. They named the factor 'growth hormone release inhibitory factor' and postulated that GH secretion was regulated by a dual control system, one stimulatory and the other inhibitory. Relatively little

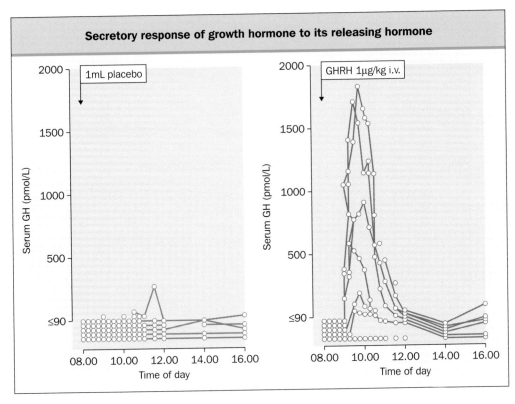

Figure 1.18 Secretory response of growth hormone to its releasing hormone. Human pancreatic growth-hormone-releasing hormone (GHRH) was injected into six normal men and was shown to stimulate the release of growth hormone (GH). (Modified from Thorner MO, Rivier J, Spiess J, et al. Human pancreatic growth hormone releasing factor selectively stimulates growth-hormone secretion in man. Lancet. 1983;1:24–28.)

attention was paid to this concept when first described since it was thought by most workers to be a nonspecific effect. Several years later, however, Brazeau and collaborators, while working in Guillemin's laboratory on the attempted isolation of GH-releasing factor, again observed the inhibitory factor. With the background in methodology gained from earlier studies of TRH and GnRH, they were able, in a relatively short time, to isolate and identify a potent peptide from hypothalamic extracts that inhibited GH release. The material, to which the name 'somatostatin' was applied, is a peptide containing 14 amino acids that lacks the amide and pyroglutamic acid termini characteristic of GnRH and TRH but contains a disulfide bridge similar to that of vasopressin and oxytocin. Other molecular forms of somatostatin have been isolated, including a peptide of 28 amino acids (the last 14 amino acids are identical to those in somatostatin-14) and a still larger form, the prohormone, with a molecular weight of approximately 15 000.

Somatostatin has been shown to be an important physiologic regulator of GH release (**Fig. 1.19**). It also inhibits the secretion of TSH and that of virtually all of the glands of the pancreas and gastrointestinal tract, including glucagon, insulin, gastric acid, and intestinal enzymes (**Table 1.1**). Furthermore, it inhibits salt/water transport across the intestine. Somatostatin is present in almost every tissue, in nerve terminals, and/or in specialized glandular cells on which it acts. It is widely distributed in tissues, where it acts in some situations as a paracrine secretion (i.e. control of one cell by secretion of an adjacent cell) and in others as a neuro-endocrine secretion (e.g. in the tuberohypophysial neurons of the hypothalamus).

Of the hypophysiotropic hormones isolated so far, somato-statin has the most extensive extrahypothalamic distribution in the central nervous system and in extraneural structures, especially in

the gastrointestinal tract. Since there is a relatively large amount of somatostatin in the brain, much effort has been made to determine its role in neural function, although no clear-cut generalizations have as yet emerged.

Several highly potent somatostatin analogs have been designed that are highly resistant to proteolytic digestion and exert selective effects on one or more of the five known somatostatin receptors. The best studied of these analogs, octreotide, has an established use in the suppression of hormone secretion in acromegaly, carcinoid tumors, and hypersecretory tumors of the gastrointestinal tract (such as VIPomas and glucagonomas). Radiolabeled preparations of somatostatin analogs are selectively bound to tissues and organs that possess somatostatin receptors and have been used to image metastases from neuroendocrine tumors (**Fig. 1.20**). Somatostatin receptors are also expressed in several types of immunocompetent cell, where they modulate immune function; radiolabeled octreotide has been used to outline and stage several forms of lymphoma, including Hodgkin's disease.

Corticotropin-releasing hormone

Although CRH (initially referred to as corticotropin-releasing factor) was the first of the hypophysiotropic factors to be recognized and to be given the generic name 'releasing factor' (by Saffran and Schally in 1955), its chemical nature was only determined in 1981 by Vale and collaborators.

Patients injected with CRH respond with increased ACTH and plasma corticosteroid levels (**Fig. 1.21**). In addition, the peptides β-lipotropin and endorphin are stimulated; these are synthesized in the corticotrophs, together with ACTH, as part of the precursor molecule pro-opiomelanocortin (POMC).

The availability of synthetic CRH has made it possible to answer several classical questions about hypothalamic–pituitary–adrenal

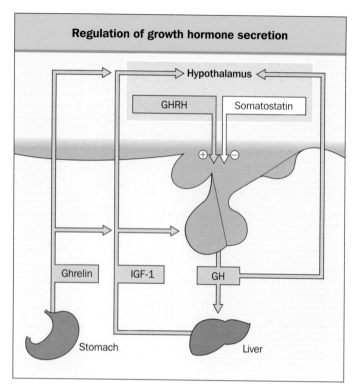

Regulation of growth hormone secretion

Hypothalamus

GHRH   Somatostatin

⊕   ⊖

Ghrelin   IGF-1   GH

Stomach   Liver

Figure 1.19 Regulation of growth hormone secretion. The secretion of growth hormone (GH) is stimulated by growth-hormone-releasing hormone (GHRH) and inhibited by somatostatin both secreted from the hypothalamus. Ghrelin is produced by the stomach and is then transported to the hypothalamus, where it probably serves as a releasing factor, and to the pituitary, where it acts as a paracrine GH stimulator. The hypothalamic hormones are secreted by distinct populations of tuberoinfundibular neurons. At the level of the pituitary, the stimulating effect of GHRH is modulated by insulin-like growth factor-I (IGF-I), a peptide formed in the liver and in many other tissues that are under the influence of GH; thus, IGF-I becomes part of the negative-feedback loop control of GH secretion. The release of somatostatin by the hypothalamus is stimulated by both GH and IGF-I, thus comprising the hypothalamic component of the negative feedback loop for GH regulation. Ghrelin secreted by stomach cells releases GH by direct action on the pituitary and indirectly by stimulating the release of GHRH.

Biological actions of somatostatin		
Acts on	**Inhibits secretion of**	**Other actions**
Pituitary	Growth hormone	
	Thyroid-stimulating hormone	
Gastrointestinal tract	Gastrin	
	Secretin	
	Gastric inhibitory peptide	
	Motilin	Inhibition of gall bladder emptying, gastric emptying, intestinal absorption, and gastrointestinal blood flow
	Vasoactive intestinal peptide	
	Gastric acid	
	Pancreatic bicarbonate	
	Pancreatic enzymes	
Pancreas	Insulin	
	Glucagon	

Table 1.1 Biologic actions of somatostatin. Some of the biologic actions of somatostatin outside the central nervous system are listed.

specific methods. Its distribution indicates that CRH can be regarded (as is the case of TRH and somatostatin) as a gut–brain peptide. Unlike other hypophysiotropic factors, CRH is bound in neurons and in blood (during pregnancy) to a specific binding protein. The highly potent effects of CRH in inducing psychologic changes in experimental animals and the evidence that CRH levels may be increased in patients with depression suggest that this peptide may be a factor in depression.

Prolactin-regulating factors

In keeping with the observation that the hypothalamus exerts tonic inhibitory effects on prolactin secretion is the finding that crude hypothalamic extracts inhibit prolactin release. This bioactivity was termed prolactin-inhibiting factor (PIF) by Meites (1966). PIF has been identified in portal vessel blood (1971), thus satisfying one of the critical requirements for proof of physiologic significance of a hypophysiotropic hormone. Although a number of substances that can inhibit prolactin release have been isolated from the hypothalamus, most workers believe that dopamine is the principal factor.

Evidence that acute prolactin release, as occurs in stress or in response to sucking, is due to a PRF is convincing. Several potent PRFs have been isolated, including VIP and TRH. A distinct PRF is found present in intermediate lobe/posterior pituitary extracts but its nature has not been identified. In addition two peptides, one 20 and the other 31 amino acids in length, have been isolated from intestine by using an orphan GH-receptor-like molecule as a screening procedure. The relative importance of these various prolactin releasers has not been clarified. It is likely that chronic 'tone' of prolactin secretion is determined by dopamine and that, in acute release situations, hypothalamic dopamine is suppressed and one or more of the PRFs is released.

control. The effects of CRH on the pituitary are inhibited by cortisol, thus confirming a direct pituitary feedback effect (**Fig. 1.22**). Vasopressin, which had previously been shown to have CRH-like activity, has now been shown to potentiate CRH action and in some settings may be even more important than CRH as a stimulator of ACTH release. An important element in the negative feedback control of ACTH secretion by cortisol is the striking inhibitory effect of this steroid on the synthesis and secretion of CRH and vasopressin. Among the most potent stimulators of CRH secretion is acute inflammation, shown to be mediated by the inflammatory cytokines IL-1, IL-6, and tumor necrosis factor-α. The cytokine–CRH–pituitary feedback response serves to modulate the pituitary–adrenal response to inflammatory stimuli such as bacterial endotoxin.

Extrahypothalamic distribution of CRH, long suspected from the results of bioassay studies, has now been confirmed by more

Visualization of a metastatic neuroendocrine tumor of the pancreas

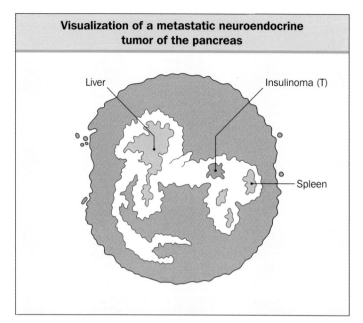

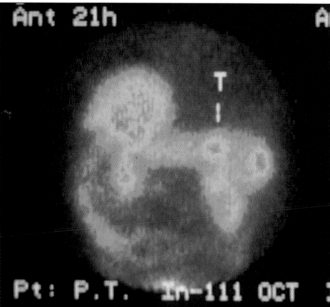

Figure 1.20 Visualization of a metastatic neuroendocrine tumor of the pancreas. An insulinoma (T) is shown, utilizing an indium-111-radiolabeled octreotide preparation that binds selectively to the somatostatin receptor.

Adrenocorticotropic hormone and its releasing hormone

Figure 1.21 Adrenocorticotropic hormone and its releasing hormone. Six normal men were injected with 100µg of corticotropin-releasing hormone (CRH). The initial rise in mean plasma adrenocorticotropic hormone (ACTH) was followed by an increase in mean serum cortisol. Control values after saline injections are also shown. (Modified from Grossman A, Kruseman ACN, Perry L, et al. New hypothalamic hormone, corticotropin-releasing factor, specifically stimulates the release of adrenocorticotrophic hormone and cortisol in man. Lancet. 1982;1:921–2.)

NEUROTRANSMITTER REGULATION OF HYPOTHALAMIC HORMONES

The hypophysiotropic neurons themselves are regulated by hormonal, neuropeptide, and neurotransmitter influences, the last arising from well-defined bioaminergic pathways that originate in the hypothalamus and elsewhere in the brain (**Fig. 1.23**). As noted above, dopamine is both a neurotransmitter and a hypophysiotropic hormone and arises in the hypothalamus from a group of tuberohypophysial neurons. As a hypophysiotropic hormone it is secreted by a selective group of tuberohypophysial neurons that differ from other dopaminergic neurons in the brain in that they have receptors for prolactin and form part of the feedback control of pituitary prolactin secretion. It is secreted into the portal vessel blood and inhibits prolactin secretion. Other biogenic amines, such as norepinephrine, epinephrine, serotonin, and histamine, influence other pituitary secretions by their effects on hypophysiotropic neurons. Central adrenergic pathways are important, not only for regulation of pituitary function, but also for a number of important

15

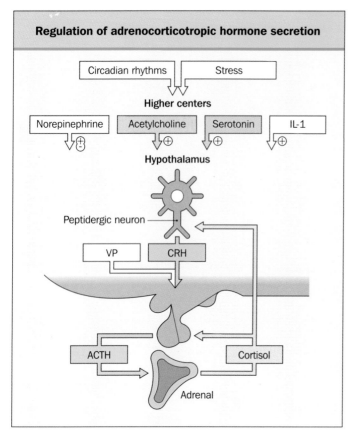

Figure 1.22 Regulation of adrenocorticotropic hormone secretion. The secretion of adrenocorticotropic hormone (ACTH) is stimulated by corticotropin-releasing hormone (CRH) and vasopressin (VP) acting synergistically and is inhibited by the feedback effects of cortisol exerted directly at the level of the pituitary. In addition, cortisol inhibits both CRH and VP secretion, thus acting on the hypothalamus as well.

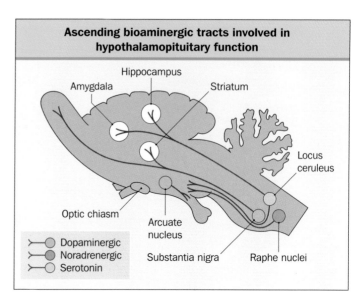

Figure 1.23 Ascending bioaminergic tracts involved in hypothalamopituitary function. An outline of the ascending bioaminergic tracts involved in hypothalamopituitary function in the rat. Dopaminergic fibers comprise one group, whose origin is in the substantia nigra in the midbrain and which project to the basal ganglia (forming part of the extrapyramidal motor system). An intrinsic tuberoinfundibular system is responsible for dopamine secretion into the hypophysial–portal vascular system, which tonically inhibits prolactin secretion. The mesolimbic dopamine system that innervates brain structures involved in affective states is not shown. Ascending fibers from the locus ceruleus bring noradrenergic influences into the hypothalamus, and fibers from the raphe nuclei carry serotoninergic signals into the hypothalamus and elsewhere. All these pathways are involved in the regulation of the anterior and posterior pituitary and, in addition, have important effects on visceral function and behavior. (Modified from Martin JB, Reichlin S, Brown GM. Clinical neuroendocrinology. Philadelphia, PA:FA Davis; 1977.)

visceral and homeostatic functions. Ascending noradrenergic fibers stimulate gonadotropin, ACTH, and GH secretion, regulate the level of alertness in the reticular activating system, and have important effects on eating and drinking behavior. The ascending serotoninergic system stimulates GH, prolactin, and ACTH secretion. Central dopaminergic, noradrenergic, and serotoninergic systems are involved in determination of affective state and may also be involved in the pathogenesis of the major psychoses. Drugs that are used in clinical psychiatry and that modulate central bioaminergic function may also influence endocrine function: for example, dopamine agonists inhibit prolactin release, and dopamine antagonists stimulate prolactin release.

Central peptidergic circuits are also important in regulating tuberohypophysial neurons. Examples of central regulatory peptidergic circuits that influence hypophysiotropic neurons are those mediated by alpha-melanocyte-stimulating hormone (α-MSH), which integrates neuroendocrine and thermal homeostasis through the melanocortin receptors, and the endogenous opioids, which influence GH secretion, the pituitary–adrenal axis, and gonadotropin secretion. Blood levels of leptin (secreted by the adipocytes) regulate the expression of TRH, thus providing the mechanism by which nutritional status can determine the set-point of pituitary–thyroid feedback control. Hypophysiotropic neurons also interact with a complex of appetite stimulatory and inhibitory peptidergic systems, such as neuropeptide Y (NPY), which display receptors for leptin. Ghrelin activates NPY neurons and stimulates appetite in addition to stimulating GH secretion. In addition, secretions of the tuberohypophysial neurons themselves interact at the hypothalamic level. Best demonstrated is somatostatin, which is capable of inhibiting the secretion of TRH and GHRH through synapses within the hypothalamus.

FURTHER READING

Dieguez C, Casanueva FF. Ghrelin: a step forward in understanding of somatotroph cell function and growth regulation. Eur J Endocrinol. 2000;142:413–7.

Engler D, Redei E, Kola I. The corticotropin-release inhibitory factor hypothesis: a review of the evidence for the existence of inhibitory as well as stimulatory hypophysiotropic regulation of adrenocorticotropin secretion and biosynthesis. Endocrine Rev. 1999;20:460–500.

Fink G. The development of the releasing factor concept. Clin Endocrinol. 1976;5:245s–60s.

Giustina A, Veldhuis JD. Pathophysiology of the neuroregulation of growth hormone secretion in experimental animals and the human. Endocrine Rev. 1998;19:717–97.

Jarry H, Heuer H, Schomburg L, Bauer K. Prolactin-releasing peptides do not stimulate prolactin release in vivo. Neuroendocrinology 2000;71:262–7.

Jessop DS. Stimulatory and inhibitory regulators of the hypothalamo-pituitary-adrenocortical axis. Clin Endocrinol Metab. 1999;13:491–501.

Knobil E. The wisdom of the body revisited. News Physiol Sci. 1999;14:1–11.

Kojima M, Hosoda H, Matsuo H, Kangawa K. Ghrelin: discovery of the natural endogenous ligand for the growth hormone secretagogue receptor. Trends in Endocrinol Metab. 2001;12:118–22.

Müller EE, Locatelli V, Cocchi D. Neuroendocrine control of growth hormone secretion. Physiological Rev. 1999;79:511–607.

Nass R, Gilrain J, Anderson S et al. High plasma growth hormone (GH) levels inhibit expression of GH secretagogue receptor messenger ribonucleic acid levels in the rat pituitary. Endocrinology 2000;141:2084–9.

Nillni EA, Sevarino KA. The biology of pro-thyrotropin-releasing hormone-derived peptides. Endocrine Rev. 1999;20:599–648.

Patel YC. Somatostatin and its receptor family. Frontiers Neuroendocrinol. 1999;20:157–98.

Reichlin S. Neuroendocrinology. In: Wilson JD, Foster DW, Kronenberg HM, Larsen PR, eds. Williams textbook of endocrinology, 9th edn. Philadelphia, PA:WB Saunders; 1998:165–248.

Reichlin S. Neuroendocrinology of infection and the innate immune system. Recent Prog Horm Res. 1999;54:133–81.

Toni R, Lechan RM. Neuroendocrine regulation of thyrotropin-releasing hormone (TRH) in the tuberoinfundibular system. J Endocrinol Invest. 1993;16:715–53.

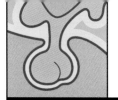

Section 1 Hypothalamus and Pituitary

Chapter 2

Control of Pituitary Hormone Secretion – Role of Pulsatility

John C Marshall

INTRODUCTION

The goal of this chapter is to examine the roles of intermittent or pulsatile hormone secretion in the integrated homeostatic unit that constitutes the hypothalamic–pituitary–target gland axes. Understanding in this field has been advanced by the ability to measure hormones in plasma at frequent intervals. These studies have shown that all pituitary hormones are secreted in an intermittent manner, and areas have been identified where changing patterns of stimulation of the pituitary by the hypothalamic neuroendocrine cells results in different pituitary responses. The hypothalamic–pituitary interface is a relatively unique signal transfer system, whereby episodic neuronal stimuli from the hypothalamus are conveyed to the pituitary for transduction and hormone secretion. Thus, minute-to-minute or hour-to-hour (short-term or ultradian) pulse mechanisms constitute the basis of long-term (circadian) rhythms of central nervous system (CNS)-initiated pituitary hormone delivery to the peripheral circulation. As an integrated unit, the hypothalamic–pituitary–target gland axis is an efficient mechanism for tuning target gland secretion. As shown in **Figure 2.1**, low concentrations of hypothalamic hormones (in the femto- (10^{-15}) to picomolar (10^{-12}) range) act on the pituitary, which responds by secreting nanomolar (10^{-9}) amounts of hormone. Pituitary hormones in turn act on target glands, which in general secrete in micromolar (10^{-6}) amounts. Thus the entire axis constitutes an amplification system to regulate concentrations of target gland hormones that are active on peripheral tissues. Homeostasis is achieved by inhibitory (negative) feedback of target hormones on higher centers, allowing fine tuning by reducing secretion of lower concentrations of trophic hormone.

As part of this mechanism, regulation of pulsatile secretion constitutes an additional mode of transferring information. Feedback at the hypothalamus can be effected by modifying the frequency of neuronal secretory bursts or by reducing the amplitude of each pulse stimulus. At the pituitary, responsiveness is modulated by changes in the amplitude of pituitary hormone release, and target gland secretions can enhance or diminish responses to a given hypothalamic signal. Thus, pulse mechanisms add another dimension to feedback control in an efficient manner. A pituitary hormone with a relatively long half-life in plasma can be released intermittently but still produce relatively constant target gland responses. The pulse stimulus mechanism also allows for a rapid enhancement of pituitary hormone secretion. An increase in the frequency or amplitude of hypothalamic stimuli can markedly enhance pituitary hormone release when

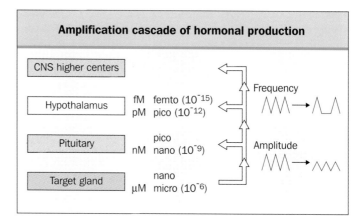

Figure 2.1 Amplification cascade of hormonal production. In most cases feedback is inhibitory and target hormones act on glands producing lower concentrations of trophic hormone, allowing fine tuning of hormone secretion. The effects of negative feedback may be mediated by a reduction in the frequency of hypothalamic signals or by reducing the amplitude of the signal or pituitary responsiveness. In certain instances, particularly in the reproductive system, feedback can be positive, whereby target hormones, such as estradiol, can augment secretion of hypothalamic peptides and enhance pituitary responsiveness.

synthesis and cellular stores are adequate. Feedback at the pituitary by target gland hormones, in general, limits the duration of enhanced responsiveness by reducing the amplitude of pituitary hormone release, restoring homeostasis to the axis.

In the pituitary, and particularly for the gonadotrope cells, intermittent stimuli are essential for optimal receptor activation and coupling to second- and third-messenger intracellular pathways. Intermittent neural stimuli allow receptor internalization, recycling, and coupling to second-messenger activation. In the gonadotrope, an intermittent signal (of the hypothalamic hormone gonadotropin-releasing hormone [GnRH]) is an absolute requirement for ongoing gonadotropin secretion and continuous stimuli effect *desensitization* with a marked reduction in luteinizing hormone (LH) and follicle stimulating hormone (FSH) release. This system is an example of mechanisms present in many cells, whereby excess hormonal stimulation results in uncoupling of receptor from second-messenger systems, forming a *protective* mechanism whereby the cell can reduce responses to incoming stimuli. In general, the intermittent pulse stimulus appears to be an important mechanism in the neuropituitary interface. Target gland responses do not appear as dependent upon pulse stimuli and in most instances continuous stimulation appears equally effective. However some examples have been identified where responses to pituitary hormones administered in intermittent or continuous manner appear to differ, and account for sexually dimorphic responses in peripheral tissues. In growth hormone (GH)-deficient rodent models, GH pulses are more effective in stimulating growth than continuous exposure, and similar observations have been made in GH-deficient children. Conversely, continuous GH-releasing hormone (GHRH) administration appears to be more efficient in reducing fat stores in rodents. GH delivery patterns to hepatic cells also modulate hepatic responses to GH. Intermittent pulses trigger rapid phosphorylation and nuclear translocation of STAT 5B, while the continuous GH exposure downregulates this signaling pathway in rodents, resulting in different levels of hepatic gene expression, specifically those coding for the P450 enzymes.

In sum, inherent patterns of intermittent neuronal discharge lead to pulsatile release of hypothalamic hormones, which are then transduced by pituitary cells to produce bursts of pituitary hormone secretion. These short-term bursts, lasting minutes, constitute the basic components of the long-term or circadian rhythms seen in mammals. Pulse stimulation of the pituitary is efficient, allowing recovery of intracellular signaling systems and some cells, such as the gonadotrope, have been adapted to allow differential responses to the same GnRH signal. Thus, pulsatile stimulation of hormone secretion can be viewed as an efficient mechanism that also allows fine-tuning of integrated feedback systems to achieve overall homeostasis.

PULSE GENERATION, PATTERNS OF SECRETION AND CLINICAL IMPLICATIONS

Pulse generation

Pulsatile secretion of pituitary hormones is achieved either by intermittent stimulation by hypothalamic-releasing hormones, by reduction in secretion of hypothalamic-inhibitory hormones or by a combination of both mechanisms. The exact mechanisms used vary for each pituitary cell type and are reviewed in Chapter 1. Generation of pulsatile GH secretion is complex and consists of intermittent stimulation by GHRH and Ghrelin, but somatotrope responsiveness is determined by the prevailing level of inhibitory influence from hypothalamic somatostatin.

In most instances, hypothalamic–trophic hormones are released from discrete hypothalamic nuclei, such as the paraventricular and arcuate nuclei. Release or inhibition of hormone secretion from these nuclei is under the influence of neurotransmitters, in turn responding to signals from higher centers (see Chapter 1).

Gonadotropin-releasing hormone neurons, however, are not located in a discrete nuclear structure. During fetal maturation, GnRH neurons originate in the olfactory placode in the upper nose and migrate through the cribriform plate of the ethmoid bone to take up residence within the hypothalamus. In most species, only some 100–200 GnRH neurons are observed and are distributed at several sites in the hypothalamus. These neurons are linked by synaptic connections to form an integrated circuit, which has an inherent oscillatory function, to form the

GnRH-pulse generator. The mechanism of pulse generation is uncertain but presumably consists of coordination of synchronous discharge of GnRH from neurons under the influence of excitatory and inhibitory neurotransmitters. In humans, the opioid peptides play a predominant role in regulating the frequency of GnRH discharge into stalk blood and subsequent pulsatile release of LH and FSH from the gonadotrope cells. In lower species, extrahypothalamic CNS structures such as the limbic system influence the pattern of GnRH secretion, but these mechanisms appear less important in primates and humans. Similarly, photoperiodicity, seasonal breeding, and pherohormones play critical roles in GnRH secretion in subhuman primates but appear to be of minor significance in humans.

The role of higher central nervous system centers
Circadian rhythms
Living organisms exhibit temporal organization with periodicities of 24 hours, which is generated by an internal timekeeping system. This circadian (approximately 1 day) rhythm is generated from two paired nuclei in the anterior hypothalamus, the suprachiasmatic nuclei, which function as the master pacemaker for all circadian rhythms. Recent studies have initiated understanding of the mechanisms involved, with recent identification of the 'clock' gene in mammals; three other genes have also been identified. The precise functions of the products of these genes are uncertain at present but the endogenous circadian rhythm is synchronized and entrained by environmental signals with light–dark and rest–activity cycles being the major synchronizing agents. Visual information is transmitted from the retina to the suprachiasmatic nuclei, which in turn influences the pineal gland and melatonin rhythmicity, with synchronizing effects on the circadian clock. The timing of sleep onset and patterns of sleep, rapid eye movement and slow-wave sleep are influenced by circadian rhythmicity. Sleep patterns in turn modulate pituitary hormone secretion, particularly GH and gonadotropin secretion during maturation, where the onset of sleep is associated with marked increases in hormone release.

The circadian patterns of pituitary hormones are shown in **Figure 2.2**. The 24-hour profiles shown result from the combined effects of circadian signals superimposed on the ultradian or pulsatile release of hypothalamic hormones and in some cases with sleep–wake cycles. Other external influences such as exercise and food intake can modify the pattern of hormone release, particularly in the case of GH. As shown in **Figure 2.2**, plasma levels of most pituitary hormones are increased from the late evening through the early hours of the morning. The magnitude of the changes varies, being relatively small for gonadotropins (25% increase at night) to two- to threefold changes for thyroid-stimulating hormone (TSH), prolactin, and adrenocorticotropic hormone (ACTH). The predominant mass of growth hormone is secreted related to the onset of slow-wave sleep and during the day levels are low, with intermittent bursts of pulse secretion associated with exercise and stress and inhibited by food intake.

Sleep–wake cycles
Sleep–wake cycles also play important roles in determining hormonal secretory patterns. Changing from day- to night-shift work results in a gradual shifting of circadian rhythms over

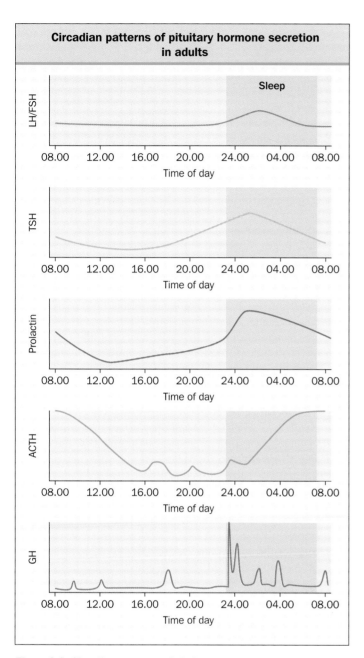

Figure 2.2 Circadian patterns of pituitary hormone secretion in adults. The overall pattern shown is of mean hormone values, which are made up of short-term pulsatile releases of pituitary trophic hormone (ultradian or circhoral). Of note, all pituitary hormones tend to have increased secretion during sleep, with values gradually falling throughout the morning and afternoon. ACTH, adrenocorticotropin-releasing hormone; FSH, follicle-stimulating hormone; GH, growth hormone; LH, luteinizing hormone; TSH, thyroid-stimulating hormone.

Stress and depressive illness

Patients suffering from clinical depression exhibit abnormalities of the circadian patterns of ACTH and cortisol secretion: the normal decline during daylight hours is impaired, and elevated ACTH and cortisol levels are seen throughout 24 hours. ACTH, prolactin, and growth hormone are also stress-responsive hormones. Acute stress, such as pain or sudden concern and anxiety, result in acute elevations of these hormones that are usually of short duration – from minutes to hours.

Clinical implications of circadian rhythms

The existence of circadian rhythms of pituitary hormones has implications for hormonal measurement and the diagnosis of pituitary disorders. For example, if excess secretion of ACTH and cortisol in Cushing's syndrome is suspected, blood should be drawn in the evening, when lower values would normally be present. Conversely, if adrenal insufficiency is suspected, plasma cortisol should be obtained at 8–9am, when levels are normally higher. In contrast, measurements of prolactin are best made later in the morning, as samples before breakfast may reveal minor elevations (to the 30–40ng/mL range) that decline slowly after the nocturnal increase. In adults, gonadotropins do not show marked changes during the day but in young men plasma testosterone levels decrease to 50% of morning values by late afternoon/evening. Thus assessment of hypogonadism is best made by measurement of testosterone between 8 and 9am.

The effects of stress should also be recognized when obtaining clinical samples. In most situations a single sample is obtained for diagnostic purposes, and multiple stressful venepunctures should be avoided to prevent obtaining transient elevations of ACTH, cortisol, prolactin, and GH. In the assessment of Cushing's syndrome, it is important to assess whether the patient is clinically depressed, as a loss of ACTH and cortisol rhythm is manifest as increased urinary free cortisol excretion. Additionally, for clinical diagnosis, it is important to recognize that the pulsatile secretion of many pituitary hormones can modify the values obtained. The amplitude of moment-to-moment pulses for most hormones is in the range of twofold changes from nadir to peak, and these variations should be taken into consideration in diagnosis, particularly when comparing measurements to previously obtained values.

MODULATION OF PULSE SECRETION OF PITUITARY HORMONES

Negative and positive feedback by target gland hormones

Intermittent stimulation of the pituitary gland by pulses of hypothalamic hormones generally elicits consistent patterns of pituitary hormone secretion. However, the amount of hormone released is dependent on the prior synthesis and storage, which in some cases are critically dependent upon the trophic action of hypothalamic-releasing hormones. In this regard, gonadotropin synthesis is dependent upon prior stimulation by GnRH, and GnRH can exert a self-priming effect on its own action. Repetitive pulses of GnRH, in the presence of estradiol, elicit LH responses of increasing amplitude over periods of 12–24 hours – the *self-priming* effect of GnRH. This action is involved in generating increased LH secretion during the midcycle ovulatory surge.

several days, and absence or poor quality of sleep can result in reduced secretion of GH and disturbance of circadian patterns. Sleep-related changes of other pituitary hormones are less marked but observations have revealed slowing of the frequency of LH (GnRH secretion) during the midfollicular phase of ovulatory cycles in women.

The major site of modulation of pituitary secretion lies at the pituitary cell, by feedback of target gland hormones that can enhance or diminish responsiveness to a given releasing-hormone stimulus. The majority of these influences are inhibitory; the selective feedback of target-gland products on pituitary trophic hormone secretion is shown in **Figure 2.3**.

In general, target gland hormones exert selective actions on their own trophic stimulus; however, some overlap occurs, particularly in the case of sex steroid hormones. Both estradiol and progesterone (after prior exposure to estradiol) can enhance the amplitude of LH responses to GnRH, and estradiol can also augment both prolactin and GH responses to trophic hormones.

Regulation of gonadotropin secretion is complex and can occur via modulation of the amplitude of the response to GnRH or alteration of the frequency and/or amplitude of the GnRH pulse stimulus. In men, testosterone acts at both the hypothalamic and pituitary levels respectively to slow GnRH pulse secretion and to reduce LH and FSH responses to GnRH. Estradiol can exert both inhibitory and stimulatory actions on pituitary responsiveness to GnRH in a time-dependent manner. In women, estradiol initially inhibits LH responses at 24–36 hours, but subsequently LH responses to each GnRH pulse are enhanced and persist for 2–3 days. This action, *positive feedback*, of estradiol is exerted on the gonadotrope cell and is important in generation of the midcycle LH surge. **Figure 2.4** (top panel) shows the biphasic effects of estradiol on pituitary responses to GnRH in a GnRH-deficient model maintained on exogenous GnRH pulse injections of constant amplitude. In contrast to its action on LH, estradiol inhibits FSH secretion by reducing release in response to GnRH. This action is seen in the late-follicular phase of ovulatory cycles, when FSH levels decline, thus limiting the number of follicles maturing and allowing development of a single preovulatory follicle.

Progesterone acts predominantly on the hypothalamus to enhance the activity of endogenous opioid peptides, which slow the frequency of pulsatile GnRH release. In **Figure 2.4** (lower two panels), progesterone given to a woman during the follicular phase results in slowing of GnRH pulse secretion to a pattern that resembles that present in the normal luteal phase. Progesterone can also exert a transient stimulatory effect on responses to GnRH in women previously exposed to estradiol, producing a transient 12–16-hour augmentation of LH and, to a lesser degree, FSH secretion. These positive and negative feedback actions of estradiol and progesterone are shown in **Figure 2.5**, in which a woman with isolated GnRH deficiency was given GnRH pulses at constant dosage and frequency for a period of 10 days.

Maturational changes

During the course of human life, the responsiveness of pituitary hormones to hypothalamic stimuli remains relatively constant, with notable exceptions in the patterns of secretion that occur at specific stages – pubertal maturation, during ovulatory cycles in women, and during aging.

Pubertal maturation

In humans and primates, the reproductive system is active during infancy and gonadotropin levels are elevated and show pulsatile changes during the first few months of life. During the subsequent decade, GnRH secretion diminishes in amplitude and frequency and gonadotropins (particularly LH) decline, resulting in an elevated FSH to LH ratio. GnRH pulses occur at slow frequency and low amplitude during childhood but a small degree of nocturnal, sleep-related augmentation occurs at this time. Studies in agonadal patients have shown increased FSH and LH values compared to normals, indicating that the steroid feedback is operative during this relatively quiescent phase of GnRH secretion. Pubertal maturation is heralded by a marked increase in the frequency, and particularly amplitude, of sleep-entrained pulsatile secretion of GnRH and gonadotropins. The enhanced LH release stimulates plasma testosterone (in boys) or estradiol (in girls) to adult values during sleep, with inhibitory feedback resulting in decreased GnRH secretion by the next morning. During this phase of increasing GnRH secretion, responses change from a prepubertal dominance of FSH

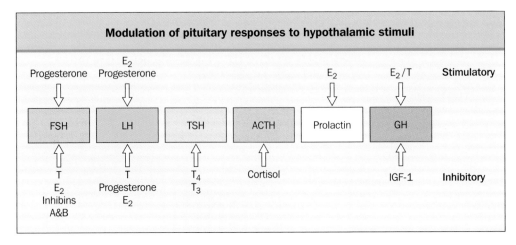

Figure 2.3 Modulation of pituitary responses to hypothalamic stimuli. Pituitary responses are modulated by target gland hormones. The majority of actions are inhibitory but, in the reproductive system, positive feedback effects of estradiol and progesterone on both follicle-stimulating hormone and luteinizing hormone are seen at the time of the midcycle surge. In addition, estrogen can induce lactotrope hyperplasia and growth hormone pulse secretion is augmented during puberty under the influence of estradiol or testosterone. ACTH, adrenocorticotropin-releasing hormone; E_2, estrogen; FSH, follicle-stimulating hormone; GH, growth hormone; IGF-1, insulin-like growth factor-1; LH, luteinizing hormone; T, testosterone; TSH, thyroid-stimulating hormone.

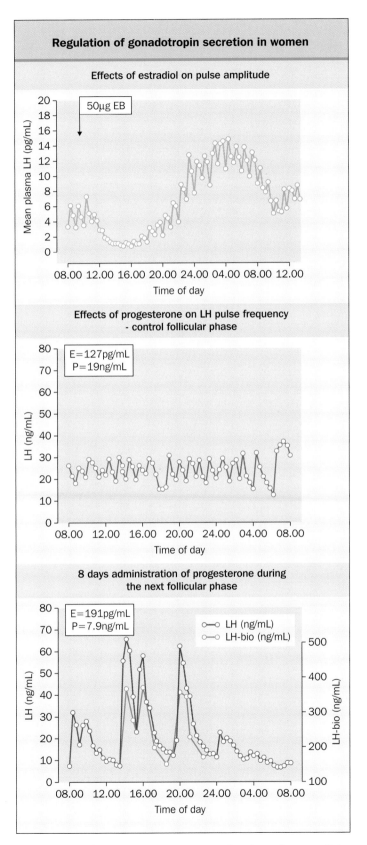

Figure 2.4 Regulation of gonadotropin secretion in women.
(Top panel) Effects of estradiol on luteinizing hormone (LH) pulse amplitude. Inhibitory and stimulatory actions of estradiol on luteinizing responses to gonadotropin-releasing hormone (GnRH). Studies were performed in ovariectomized sheep with surgical disconnection of the hypothalamus and consistent doses of GnRH given by pulse pump. After estradiol benzoate (EB), LH responses progressively diminished during the next 6–8 hours (negative feedback) but thereafter showed increasing responses to each GnRH pulse (positive feedback). (Modified with permission from Clark IJ, Cummins JT. Direct pituitary effects of estrogen and progesterone on gonadotropin secretion in the ovariectomized ewe. Neuroendocrinology 1984;39(3):267–74.) (Lower two panels) Effects of progesterone on luteinizing hormone pulse frequency. The center panel shows LH pulse patterns during a control late follicular phase and the lower panel LH profiles after 8 days' administration of progesterone during the next follicular phase. (Modified with permission from Soules MR, Steiner RA, Clifton DK, et al. Progesterone modulation of pulsatile luteinizing hormone secretion in normal women. J Clin Endocrinol Metab. 1984;58:378–83 © The Endocrine Society.)

pulse per hour during sleep, but as steroid levels rise, frequency is dampened to every 90–120min in adolescent boys. Similar changes occur in both sexes and, in girls, the initial predominance of FSH in early puberty provides the stimulus to ovarian follicular maturation. As the progressive increase in GnRH enhances LH secretion, waves of incomplete follicular development occur, ovarian steroids exert inhibitory actions to gain control of GnRH secretion, and this leads to the evolution of the cyclic events required to produce ovulatory cycles. The patterns of 24-hour LH secretion in neonates, prepubertal and early pubertal children, and adolescents/adults are shown in **Figure 2.6**.

The central mechanisms regulating these changes in GnRH secretion are unclear and the disinhibition of GnRH secretion in early puberty does not appear to be related to removal of the inhibitory actions of hypothalamic opioid peptides. In late puberty, however, the negative feedback effects of sex steroids are mediated in part via altered endogenous opioid activity.

Once established, the regular discharge of GnRH in the hypothalamus continues throughout life, but these changes can be reversed in adults by severe weight loss. In subjects with anorexia nervosa, GnRH and gonadotropin secretion revert to prepubertal patterns when bodyweight falls to less than 90% of ideal. With subsequent weight gain, the evolution of GnRH secretion follows an identical pattern to that seen in puberty, with an initial nocturnal sleep-related predominance and secretion throughout 24 hours once ideal bodyweight is approached. Thus, while the hypothalamic mechanisms regulating puberty are unknown, the process is a reversible one, particularly in situations where marked malnutrition and weight loss exist.

Pulsatile secretion of GH is also markedly enhanced during puberty, with consequent increase in IGF-1 production and skeletal growth. Enhanced GH release is in part related to the increase in gonadal steroids that occurs first during sleep and subsequently throughout 24 hours.

Ovulatory menstrual cycles
The pulsatile patterns of FSH and LH secretion show marked changes during ovulatory cycles. Patterns of LH and FSH

release to predominant LH secretion under the influence of the increasing GnRH stimulus. Subsequently, GnRH release increases during daylight hours, which reflects a diminished sensitivity of the GnRH pulse generator to the inhibitory effects of gonadal steroids. GnRH pulse frequency approximates one

Feedback actions of estradiol and progesterone on the pituitary

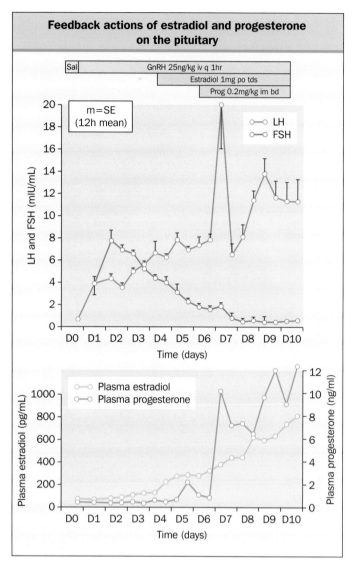

Figure 2.5 Feedback actions of estradiol and progesterone on the pituitary. Estradiol and progesterone feedback actions in a woman with hypogonadotropic hypogonadism receiving gonadotropin-releasing hormone (GnRH) pulses (25ng/kg) every hour. The initial marked increase in FSH is selectively suppressed first by endogenous and subsequently by exogenous estradiol. Plasma LH gradually rises but increases acutely after the addition of progesterone, demonstrating the positive feedback action of progesterone (prog) after prior exposure to estradiol. (Modified with permission from Nippoldt TB, Khoury S, Barkan A, Kelch RP, Marshall JC. Gonadotrophin responses to GnRH pulses in hypogonadotrophic hypogonadism: LH responsiveness is maintained in the presence of luteal phase concentrations of oestrogen and progesterone. Clin Endocrinol. 1987;26:293–301.)

Patterns of serum luteinizing hormone (LH) during pubertal maturation in females

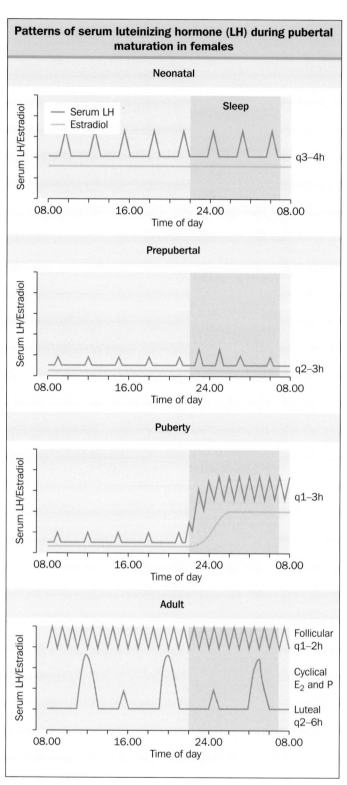

Figure 2.6 Patterns of serum luteinizing hormone (LH) during pubertal maturation in females. Data are from neonatal, prepubertal, and midpubertal girls, and adult women. The duration of sleep is shown by the bar. E$_2$, estradiol; P, progesterone. (Modified with permission from Marshall JC, Dalkin AC, Haisenleder DJ, Paul SJ, Ortolano GA, Kelch RP. Gonadotropin-releasing hormone pulses: regulators of gonadotropin synthesis and ovulatory cycles. Recent Prog Horm Res. 1991;47:155–87 © The Endocrine Society.)

secretion during the early and late follicular and early and late luteal phases of the cycle are shown in **Figure 2.7**. During the early follicular phase, GnRH pulses occur at 90–120min intervals and, as plasma estradiol and inhibin are low, GnRH releases both FSH and LH. The half-life of FSH exceeds the interval between GnRH pulses and plasma FSH levels rise, exceeding those of LH. By the midfollicular phase, the frequency of GnRH pulses increases to every 60–90min and FSH and LH induce follicular maturation, with elevation of estradiol and

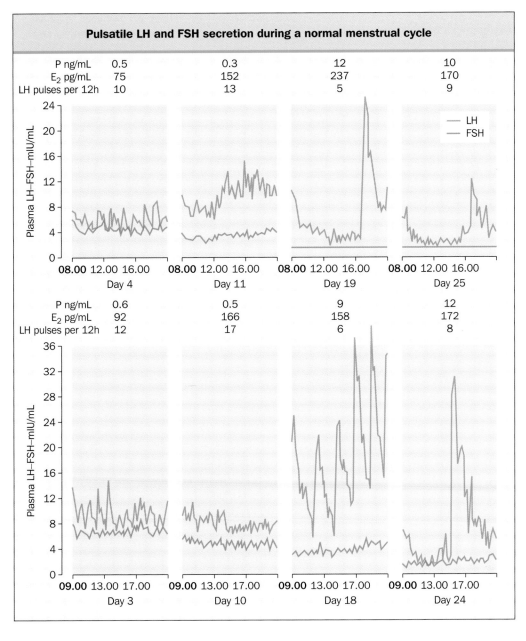

The diagrams show patterns of pulsatile luteinizing hormone (LH) and follicle-stimulating hormone (FSH) secretion during the follicular (days 3–11) and luteal (days 18–25) phases of ovulatory menstrual cycles in two women (upper and lower panel respectively). Values above the diagram for progesterone (P) and estradiol (E_2) are circulating steroid levels and the number of LH pulses per 12 hours is shown. (Modified with permission from Reame N, Sauder SE, Kelch RP, Marshall JC. Pulsatile gonadotropin secretion during the human menstrual cycle: evidence for altered frequency of gonadotropin-releasing hormone. J Clin Endocrinol Metab. 1984;59:328–37 © The Endocrine Society.)

inhibin B secretion from the maturing follicle. Estradiol and inhibin selectively inhibit FSH release, plasma FSH falls, and a single dominant follicle emerges in the ovary. GnRH pulse frequency increases further during the late follicular phase, to approximately one pulse per hour at the midcycle LH surge.

The ovulatory surge in LH is produced by a rapid GnRH pulse stimulus acting on gonadotrope cells primed by the rapid increase in plasma estradiol (positive feedback) to produce a marked transient increase in serum LH that persists for some 36 hours. Ovarian steroid production changes to favor progesterone, which assists in augmenting gonadotropin responses to GnRH. Termination of the LH surge reflects diminishing LH responses to GnRH, probably representing desensitization of LH release, together with the declining positive feedback actions as estradiol levels fall. Following ovulation, the pattern of GnRH secretion changes, as a result of progesterone increasing hypothalamic opioid activity and slowing the frequency of GnRH release. By the midluteal phase, LH pulses occur every 3–5 hours and stimulate intermittent secretion of progesterone. Estradiol, together with inhibin A from the corpus luteum, selectively inhibit FSH release, although the irregular GnRH stimulus maintains FSH synthesis.

With the death of the corpus luteum, estradiol, inhibin A, and progesterone levels fall, the last allowing increasing frequency of GnRH pulse secretion. In the absence of estradiol and inhibin A, this results in a selective increase in FSH release, which initiates the next wave of follicular development.

A diagrammatic representation of the changes in GnRH, plasma gonadotropins and ovarian steroids and peptides during ovulatory cycle is shown in **Figure 2.8**. Thus, the selective secretion of pituitary FSH and LH during ovulatory cycles reflects the effects of changing GnRH pulse stimuli, with slower frequency pulses favoring FSH and more rapid pulses favoring LH synthesis and secretion. In addition, the selective inhibitory feedback of estradiol and inhibin on FSH release, and the positive actions of ovarian steroids on LH responses, combine to produce

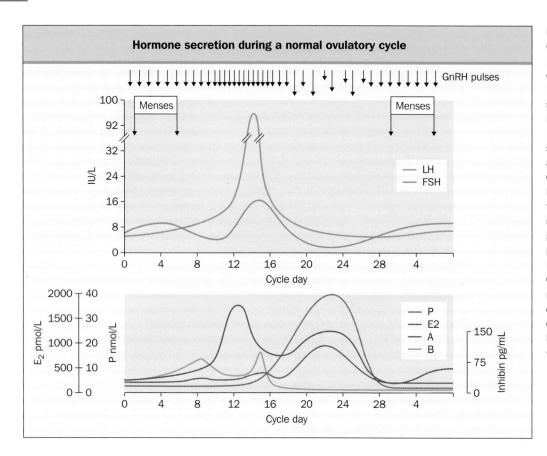

Hormone secretion during a normal ovulatory cycle

Figure 2.8 Hormone secretion during a normal ovulatory cycle. (Top panel) Hypothalamic secretion of gonadotropin-releasing hormone (GnRH), and plasma follicle-stimulating hormone (FSH) and luteinizing hormone (LH) levels. (Lower panel) Levels of ovarian steroids and inhibins A and B. The arrows above the figure indicate GnRH release, with the distance between the arrows indicating the frequency of individual pulse secretion. E_2, estradiol; P, progesterone. (Modified with permission from Marshall JC, Dalkin AC, Haisenleder DJ, Paul SJ, Ortolano GA, Kelch RP. Gonadotropin-releasing hormone pulses: regulators of gonadotropin synthesis and ovulatory cycles. Recent Prog Horm Res. 1991;47:155–87 © The Endocrine Society.)

the two essential features of an ovulatory cycle – a massive increase in LH release to produce ovulation at midcycle and the selective monotropic elevation of FSH in the late luteal to early follicular stages that initiates the next wave of follicular maturation.

Aging

Both pulsatile pituitary hormone secretion and circadian rhythmicity persist in elderly subjects but patterns are modified, with a general reduction in the amplitude of pulses and rhythm excursions. Aging is associated with a phase advance of approximately 1 hour and a marked dampening of the amplitude of circadian patterns, particularly for ACTH, cortisol, and TSH. Data from animals suggests that this reflects reduced amplitude of signals from the suprachiasmatic nuclei in older animals, but mechanisms in humans remain uncertain.

Aging is associated with significant changes in the pulsatile patterns of pituitary hormone release. Strikingly, GH secretion is markedly diminished as a function of age, with mean plasma levels of GH, and consequently insulin-like growth factor I (IGF-I), beginning to decline from their peak at midpuberty. Given the association of GH secretion with sleep and physical exercise, this may reflect increasing impairment of sleep patterns with age and a general reduction in physical activity. The consequences of reduced GH exposure include reduced lipolysis and increasing deposition of intra-abdominal fat.

Gonadotropin secretion tends to decline slightly with aging, but testis responsiveness to individual LH pulses decreases, resulting in lower plasma testosterone levels in older men. Recent evidence points increasingly to abnormalities of the orderliness of hypothalamic and pituitary hormone secretion with advancing age. More disorderly LH pulse patterns occur in older men and the patterns of pulsatile ACTH release are similarly affected. The underlying mechanisms involved in the increasingly disordered pituitary hormone secretion remain uncertain but probably reflect impaired function of the hypothalamic pulse generation systems and diminished responsiveness of pituitary and target glands.

GnRH: ONE PEPTIDE – TWO GONADOTROPINS – THE ROLE OF PULSE PATTERN

LH and FSH secretion – GnRH pulse pattern and desensitization

Within the hypothalamic–pituitary interface, the gonadotrope cell is unique in that it produces two distinct hormones, FSH and LH, regulated by a single hypothalamic hormone, GnRH. The sequential delivery of, first, FSH to induce gamete maturation, followed by LH to stimulate hormone secretion is an essential pattern for normal gonadal function, particularly in the ovary, where monthly cycles of follicular maturation are required for normal reproductive function, GnRH pulses are essential for gonadotropin synthesis, particularly that of LH, and differential secretion of LH and FSH is effected by the actions of GnRH pulse pattern and the feedback actions of gonadal steroids (**Figure 2.9**).

An intermittent GnRH pulse stimulus is an absolute requirement to maintain gonadotropin secretion. In animal models rendered GnRH-deficient, the intermittent delivery of GnRH pulses (one pulse/hour) restores secretion of LH and FSH, whereas a continuous GnRH infusion results in downregulation or

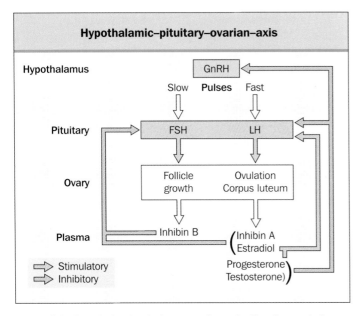

Figure 2.9 Hypothalamic–pituitary–ovarian axis. The diagram indicates the role of gonadotropin-releasing hormone (GnRH) pulse frequency and ovarian hormone feedback in the differential secretion of follicle-stimulating hormone (FSH) and luteinizing hormone (LH). Modulation of GnRH pulse secretion occurs by gonadal hormones acting on the GnRH pulse generator to slow the postpubertal pattern (one pulse per hour) of GnRH secretion. In males this is effected by testosterone and in females by progesterone following induction of hypothalamic progesterone receptors by estradiol. The final pathway in progesterone action is enhancement of endogenous hypothalamic opioid activity, which slows the GnRH pulse generator. GnRH action is modulated at the pituitary by the feedback action of gonadal hormones. In males, testosterone inhibits FSH responses to GnRH; in females, both estradiol and the inhibins A and B exert similar inhibitory actions on FSH, while estradiol and progesterone can exert transient positive actions to enhance LH secretion.

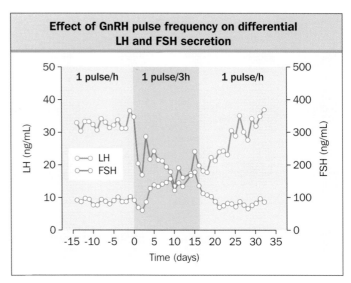

Figure 2.10 Effects of GnRH pulse frequency on differential LH and FSH secretion. In a gonadotropin-releasing hormone (GnRH)-deficient ovariectomized monkey model, one pulse per hour maintains luteinizing hormone (LH) and follicle-stimulating hormone (FSH) secretion, whereas a slower frequency of one pulse every 3 hours is inadequate to maintain plasma LH but result in increased FSH levels in plasma. (Modified with permission from Wildt L, Hausler A, Marshall G, et al. Frequency and amplitude of gonadotropin-releasing hormone stimulation and gonadotropin secretion in the rhesus monkey. Endocrinology 1981;109:376–85 © The Endocrine Society.)

desensitization of LH secretion (see Chapter 1). This latter effect of continuous GnRH stimulation is utilized clinically, where long-acting GnRH agonists effectively provide continuous stimulation of GnRH receptor at the gonadotrope and reduce LH secretion. These compounds have found extensive clinical application to reduce gonadal steroid production in the treatment of diverse disorders such as precocious puberty, endometriosis, uterine leiomyomas, and hormone-dependent cancers of the prostate and breast.

The pattern of GnRH pulse secretion can modulate differential gonadotropin secretion. In GnRH-deficient animal models a one pulse/hour GnRH stimulus maintains both LH and FSH release, while reduction in frequency to one pulse every 3 hours results in diminished LH secretion but enhanced FSH release (**Figure 2.10**). In general, secretion of LH is more dependent upon the GnRH pulse stimulus, and in GnRH-deficient subjects some FSH synthesis and secretion is maintained. As a result, GnRH pulses in GnRH-deficient patients initially result in FSH secretion, which is followed by LH release as LH synthesis is increased. These effects of GnRH pulse frequency and amplitude are essential components of the maturational changes of puberty and the sequential events dependent upon FSH and LH secretion during ovulatory cycles.

GnRH pulses and gonadotropin synthesis

The effects of GnRH pulses in large part reflect the direct actions of GnRH pulse patterns on gonadotropin subunit gene expression. LH and FSH consist of a common α subunit (shared with TSH) and specific β subunits that confer specificity of action. Differential expression of the three subunit genes is evident in mRNA concentrations in gonadotropes during the 4-day estrous cycle in rats. During metestrus (late luteal, early follicular equivalent), FSHβ mRNA alone is increased, whereas on diestrus (midfollicular phase equivalent) FSH mRNA falls while that of α and LHβ are transiently increased. On proestrus, the day of the ovulatory LH surge, LHβ mRNA increases threefold prior to the increase and is followed by a similar increase in FSHβ mRNA, which subsequently declines during estrus (luteal phase equivalent).

The increase in the β subunit mRNAs on proestrus suggests dependence on enhanced GnRH stimulation during the proestrus LH surge. Experiments in GnRH-deficient rodent models have examined the effects of GnRH pulse amplitude and frequency on differential expression of subunit genes. Changes in α, LHβ, and FSHβ mRNAs in female rats are shown in **Figure 2.11**. A wide range of pulse amplitudes increase expression of both α and FSHβ mRNAs. In contrast, LHβ mRNA is only increased by low physiologic amplitudes, and higher doses are ineffective. Similarly for FSHβ mRNA, supraphysiologic stimulation by GnRH results in absence of FSHβ gene expression. Varying frequencies of GnRH stimulation also effect differential gonadotropin synthesis. In female rats, α and LHβ mRNAs are expressed by rapid

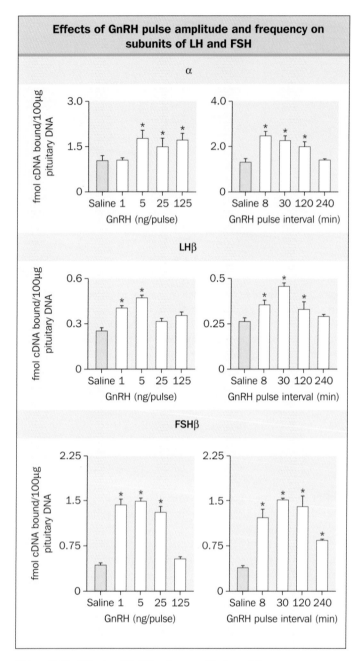

Figure 2.11 Effects of GnRH pulse amplitude and frequency on subunits of LH and FSH. The diagram illustrates the effects of gonadotropin-releasing hormone (GnRH) pulse frequency on expression of the mRNAs coding for the α and β subunits of luteinizing hormone (LH) and follicle-stimulating hormone (FSH). GnRH-deficient, testosterone-replaced, female rat models received GnRH pulses every 30min for 24 hours at the amplitude shown (left panel), or 5ng per pulse at the interval shown (right panel). Steady-state concentrations of mRNA were measured using hybridization techniques. *$p < 0.05$ vs saline control. (Modified with permission from Dalkin AC, Haisenleder DJ, Gilrain JT, Aylor K, Yasin M, Marshall JC. Gonadotropin-releasing hormone regulation of gonadotropin subunit gene expression in female rats: actions on follicle-stimulating hormone beta messenger ribonucleic acid (mRNA) involve differential expression of pituitary activin (beta-B) and follistatin mRNAs. Endocrinology 1999;140:903–8 © The Endocrine Society.)

GnRH pulse stimuli, every 8–30min, and slow frequency pulses are ineffective. For FSHβ, a wider range of pulse frequencies enhance mRNA expression and slower frequencies, every 120 and 240min, maintain increased FSHβ mRNA. Thus, alterations in the frequency and amplitude of pulsatile GnRH secretion are recognized by the gonadotrope GnRH receptor, to differentially activate intracellular signaling mechanisms, resulting in differential gene expression. The pathways involved include pulsatile increases in intracellular calcium and stimulation of the protein kinase C and mitogen-activated kinase pathways.

The actions of GnRH pulse patterns are exerted in part at the level of subunit gene transcription, and the transcription rate of the α and LHβ genes is enhanced by rapid (every 8–30min) frequencies of GnRH stimuli. Steroid hormones may play a regulatory role, and increased transcription of the LHβ gene requires the presence of testosterone. Of interest, circulating testosterone is transiently increased for a few hours immediately prior to the midcycle LH surge. GnRH pulse patterns also regulate FSHβ transcription, with intermediate and slower (120–240min) pulses selectively increasing the rate of FSHβ transcription. However, the effect on FSHβ transcription is small, suggesting the presence of other mechanisms within the gonadotrope that modulate differential expression of FSHβ mRNAs.

Intragonadotrope regulation of FSHβ mRNA expression

Both the mRNAs and proteins for the inhibin α and $β_B$ subunits are present in pituitary gonadotrope cells. Thus the gonadotrope is capable of synthesizing either inhibin B ($α β_B$ dimer) or alternatively activin B (homodimer of $β_B β_B$ subunits). The single-chain peptide follistatin is also present in pituitary gonadotrope and folliculostellate cells and follistatin binds to the $β_B$ subunit and inactivates activin. Activin is known to enhance the stability of FSHβ mRNA and may also stimulate FSHβ transcription. Thus activin may act locally (an 'autocrine action'). This hypothesis is supported by the fact that both follistatin and antibodies to activin B reduce FSH mRNA and FSH secretion.

This intragonadotrope system plays a significant role in the differential regulation of FSHβ mRNA expression. Activin stimulates follistatin expression and reduces production of the $β_B$ subunit. Inhibin and follistatin exert similar actions, reducing follistatin and increasing $β_B$ mRNAs and proteins. Thus activin secretion acts in an autocrine manner to increase FSHβ mRNA and also increases follistatin production, which in turn reduces the effectiveness of activin – constituting a self-limiting intragonadotrope mechanism to determine FSHβ mRNA concentrations. GnRH regulates expression of both follistatin and $β_B$, and the manner of the GnRH pulse stimulus determines the magnitude of gene expression. The effects of GnRH pulse amplitude and frequency on FSHβ, follistatin, and $β_B$ mRNAs are shown in **Figure 2.12**.

Thus, regulation of FSHβ mRNA expression is effected predominantly at the level of the gonadotrope cell by the actions of activin and follistatin, which are in turn regulated by the pattern of GnRH pulse stimuli. A model of the proposed intragonadotrope regulatory system is shown in **Figure 2.13**.

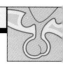

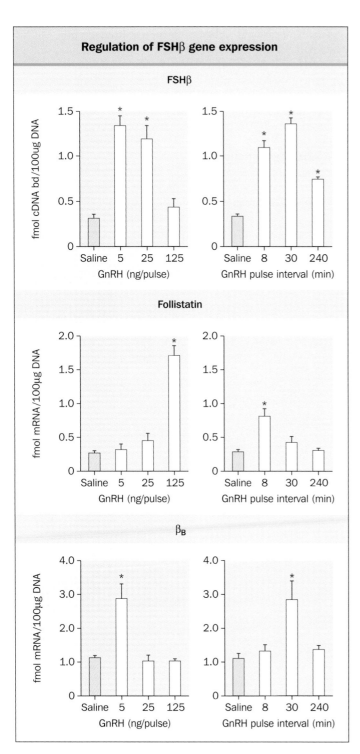

Figure 2.12 Regulation of FSHβ gene expression. Effects of pulsatile gonadotropin-releasing hormone (GnRH) given at different amplitudes (left panel) and frequency (right panel) in GnRH-deficient female rats. Pulses were given for 24 hours and the steady-state mRNA concentrations were measured either by hybridization or quantitative reverse-transcriptase–polymerase-chain reaction (RT-PCR). Low-amplitude pulses of GnRH enhance β_B expression but have no effect on follistatin, and consequently follicle-stimulating hormone beta (FSHβ) mRNA is maximally expressed. In contrast, high-amplitude GnRH pulses increase follistatin expression but are without effect on β_B, resulting in absence of FSHβ mRNA accumulation. A wide range of pulse frequencies between 8 and 240min increase FSHβ mRNA; rapid GnRH pulses increased follistatin but not β_B, and intermediate frequencies increased β_B but not follistatin. Slow-frequency pulses were without effect on follistatin and β_B and the reduced increase in FSHβ mRNA presumably reflects only the direct action of GnRH on FSHβ transcription. *$p<0.05$ vs saline control. (Modified with permission from Dalkin AC, Haisenleder DJ, Gilrain JT, Aylor K, Yasin M, Marshall JC. Gonadotropin-releasing hormone regulation of gonadotropin subunit gene expression in female rats: actions on follicle-stimulating hormone beta messenger ribonucleic acid (mRNA) involve differential expression of pituitary activin (beta-B) and follistatin mRNAs. Endocrinology 1999;140:903–8 © The Endocrine Society.)

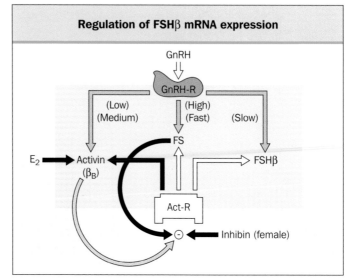

Figure 2.13 Regulation of FSHβ mRNA expression. The figure illustrates the overall scheme for the intragonadotrope regulation of follicle-stimulating hormone beta (FSHβ) gene expression by gonadotropin-releasing hormone (GnRH) pulse pattern, activin, follistatin, and peripheral inhibin. Gray arrows indicate stimulatory and black arrows inhibitory pathways. High and low refer to GnRH pulse amplitude; fast, medium and slow refer to GnRH pulse frequency. GnRH increases FSHβ mRNA, activin (β_B), and follistatin mRNAs as a function of the pattern of pulsatile stimulus. Activin is secreted by the gonadotrope and increases both FSHβ mRNA and follistatin with inhibitory effects on β_B production. As the overall effect of activin is to increase FSHβ mRNA, its effects at increasing FSHβ transcription and stabilizing FSHβ message appear to exceed its actions on follistatin. Follistatin stimulated by GnRH is secreted by the gonadotropes, binds to activin at an extracellular site, and reduces its action at the activin receptor. Plasma inhibin may act through specific inhibitory receptors or interfere with activin binding to its receptor, thus reducing the effectiveness of activin; consequently, FSHβ mRNA levels decline. Act R, activin receptor complex; E_2, estradiol; FS, follistatin; GnRH R, GnRH receptor. (Modified from Marshall JC. Regulation of gonadotropin synthesis and secretion. In: DeGroot LJ, Jameson JL, Burger H, et al, eds. Endocrinology, 4th edn. Philadelphia, PA; WB Saunders: 2000.)

CLINICAL MANIFESTATIONS OF DISORDERED PULSATILE GnRH SECRETION

Hypogonadotropic hypogonadism (isolated GnRH deficiency, Kallmann's syndrome)

This disorder consists of absent or incomplete pubertal development and can affect both sexes, but it is much more common in boys. It may occur sporadically, be inherited as X-linked autosomal dominant or recessive, and, in some cases, is associated with abnormalities of the *KAL-1* gene. This gene codes for a glycoprotein with similarities to neural adhesion molecules and may be one of the factors involved in migration of the GnRH neurons from the olfactory placode to the basal hypothalamus. In a majority of subjects, however, no genetic abnormalities have been found and the physiologic basis appears to be failure of synchronous secretion of GnRH, so that enhanced GnRH secretion at puberty does not occur or is partially arrested. Extensive studies of LH (GnRH) pulse patterns have been performed in both sexes and a variety of abnormalities of GnRH pulse pattern were observed. In a majority, LH pulse amplitude remains low and represents a prepubertal pattern, while in others pulse patterns are of irregular amplitude and frequency and lack the regular synchronous LH pulse discharge characteristic of pubertal maturation. On occasions, puberty appears to have been initiated but has been arrested and pulse patterns show evidence of some nocturnal augmentation, albeit at subnormal levels. Examples of LH pulse secretion in individuals with hypogonadotropic hypogonadism are shown in **Figure 2.14**.

While occasional subjects have impaired responses, the overwhelming majority respond briskly to pulsatile administration of GnRH, which can induce normal pubertal maturation and. if continued for periods of 1–2 years, is associated with increased sperm counts in men. In girls with this disorder, ovulation can be readily induced by pulsatile GnRH administration and ovulation achieved in over 90% after one or two cycles.

Hypothalamic amenorrhea
Hypothalamic amenorrhea, one of the most common forms of anovulation, is a diagnosis made only after exclusion of pituitary and ovarian abnormalities. While the exact etiology is unknown, conditions that often precede anovulatory cycles include marked weight loss, strenuous exercise (such as competitive gymnastics or running), psychological stress, and occasionally the prior use of oral contraceptives. In the majority of women,

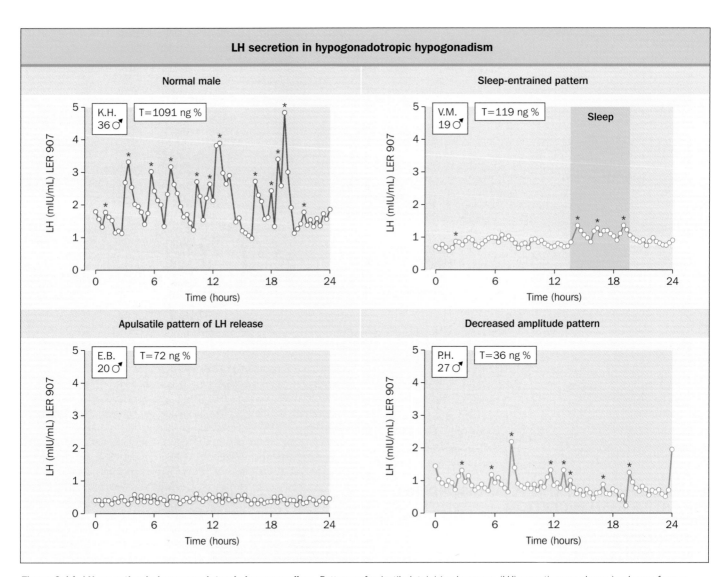

Figure 2.14 LH secretion in hypogonadotropic hypogonadism. Patterns of pulsatile luteinizing hormone (LH) secretion are shown in plasma from a normal male and three men with hypogonadotropic hypogonadism. Three different patterns of gonadotropin-releasing hormone secretion are seen – some sleep augmentation resembling early puberty (top right), low levels with no evidence of pulse secretion (bottom left), and normal frequency but reduced amplitude (bottom right). (Modified with permission from Crowley WF, Filicori M, Spratt DI, Santoro NE. The physiology of gonadotropin-releasing hormone (GnRH) secretion in men and women. Recent Prog Horm Res. 1985;41:471–531 © The Endocrine Society.)

regaining of bodyweight or reduction in competitive exercise results in return of ovulatory menses within 12 months but in some amenorrhea persists. Measurements of LH, FSH, and estradiol show low or low–normal values, prolactin is normal, and LH and FSH responsiveness to exogenous GnRH is not impaired. Studies using multiple sampling have shown that the frequency of pulsatile GnRH secretion is markedly reduced, often to one pulse every 4–5 hours, and the amplitude of LH pulses is irregular. Patterns of LH pulse secretion are variable between subjects and can vary in an individual patient over time, but overall there is consistent slow frequency of LH pulses compared to the follicular phase of a normal cycle. The slow-frequency LH pulses of irregular pattern resemble those in the normal luteal phase, suggesting that GnRH pulse secretion may be inhibited by increased hypothalamic opioid activity. This concept is supported by the results of acute infusions of naloxone, which in some 60–70% of women result in a rapid (within 1–2 hours) resumption of LH pulses at a frequency of one every 90–120min, which continue for the duration of infusion. An example of the basal LH pulse pattern and the rapid response to naloxone infusion is shown in **Figure 2.15**.

These data, together with observations that GnRH pulses given to GnRH-deficient women at slow frequencies of one every 3–4 hours do not maintain LH or induce ovulation, suggest that the basis of anovulation is the presence of a persistent slow-frequency pulsatile GnRH secretion. This does not increase LH synthesis and secretion and specifically is not adequate to produce the enhanced LH secretion required for an ovulatory midcycle surge. In some individuals, clomiphene citrate (an estrogen antagonist) can induce ovulation and examination reveals that these women have a lesser degree of impairment in GnRH pulse frequency. The rapid response of LH pulse secretion to naloxone has

suggested the use of long-acting forms such as naltrexone in efforts to induce ovulation. In many instances, naltrexone produces a transient increase in GnRH pulse frequency, and ovulation has occasionally been reported. However, this is the exception, as tachyphylaxis appears to develop and LH responses decline over time.

The variable nature of LH pulse secretion in hypothalamic amenorrhea suggests the possibility that episodes of stress may act via increased hypothalamic opioids to produce transient impairment of GnRH pulse frequency and reduce gonadotropin secretion. Such a mechanism would account for the variable patterns seen in some women over time, and could also occur as a result of stress in women with ovulatory cycles, accounting for occasional episodes of anovulation.

Hyperprolactinemia

Hyperprolactinemia from any cause will result in anovulation and amenorrhea if prolactin levels are sufficiently elevated. The magnitude of hyperprolactinemia required to inhibit reproductive function varies between individuals but, in general, when prolactin levels exceed 70–80ng/ml, anovulation ensues.

Multiple sampling has revealed that LH pulse secretion is slow and of irregular amplitude, suggesting marked disorders of hypothalamic GnRH release. When serum prolactin is suppressed by dopamine agonists in women with hyperprolactinemia, pulsatile LH release is restored to normal, with pulses occurring every 90–120min, and ovulation usually may ensue within 6 weeks. Examples of the irregular amplitude, slow-frequency (LH) GnRH pulse pattern, and the restoration of normal pulsatile secretion by bromocriptine are shown in **Figure 2.16**.

The irregular, slow-frequency GnRH pulse secretion associated with hyperprolactinemia also appears to involve increased

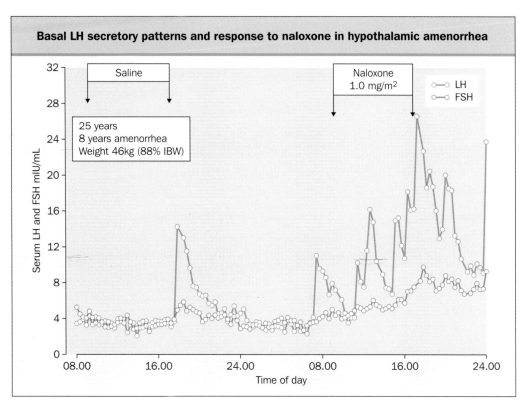

Figure 2.15 Basal LH secretory patterns and response to naloxone in hypothalamic amenorrhea. The data are from a woman with an 8-year history of amenorrhea following prior weight loss. She had regained weight to 90% of ideal 1 year before but remained amenorrheic. FSH, follicle-stimulating hormone; LH, luteinizing hormone. (Modified with permission from Koury SA, Reame NE, Kelch RP, Marshall JC. Diurnal patterns of pulsatile luteinizing hormone secretion in hypothalamic amenorrhea: reproducibility and responses to opiate blockade and an alpha 2-adrenergic agonist. J Clin Endocrinol Metab. 1987;64:755–62 © The Endocrine Society.)

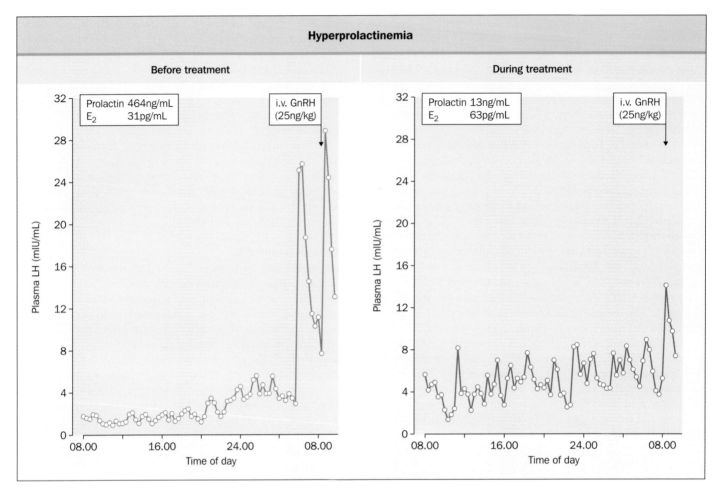

Figure 2.16 Hyperprolactinemia. Patterns of luteinizing hormone (LH) secretion in plasma and responses to exogenous gonadotropin-releasing hormone (GnRH) before and after normalization of prolactin by bromocriptine. When prolactin is elevated, the amplitude and frequency of LH pulses is highly irregular but responsiveness to exogenous GnRH is preserved (left panel). With normalization of prolactin, LH pulse patterns resemble that seen during the early to mid follicular phase of the cycle and are associated with an increase in plasma estradiol (E_2). (Modified with permission from Sauder SE, Frager M, Case GD, Kelch RP, Marshall JC. Abnormal patterns of pulsatile luteinizing hormone secretion in women and amenorrhea: responses to bromocriptine. J Clin Endocrinol Metab. 1984;59:941–8 © The Endocrine Society.)

hypothalamic opioid activity. Administration of naloxone to hyperprolactinemic women does not lower serum prolactin but is associated with a rapid increase in GnRH pulse secretion in a similar manner to that seen in hypothalamic amenorrhea. This suggests that the elevated prolactin results in increased hypothalamic opioid activity with associated inhibition of GnRH pulse secretion. Thus hyperprolactinemia, like hypothalamic amenorrhea, is associated with a persistent slow frequency of endogenous GnRH secretion, which is inadequate to maintain LH secretion and produce a midcycle LH surge.

Polycystic ovary syndrome

Polycystic ovary syndrome (PCOS) is a heterogeneous disorder of uncertain cause associated with anovulation, hirsutism, obesity, insulin resistance, and multiple cysts in the ovaries. Hyperandrogenemia is a consistent finding in PCOS, and plasma testosterone levels are at the upper limit of normal or moderately (twice normal) elevated. The excess androgen secretion is of ovarian origin and may result from a combination

of factors, including abnormal steroidogenesis, hyperinsulinemia (which augments androgen responses to LH), and increased LH stimulation of the ovaries. Plasma LH levels are elevated in over 95% of women with PCOS when measured more than 3 weeks from recent ovulation. Studies have shown that the frequency and amplitude of LH pulses are elevated, suggesting that a persistent rapid frequency of endogenous GnRH secretion underlies the increased LH secretion. An example of LH and FSH secretory patterns is shown in **Figure 2.17**.

As most women with PCOS only ovulate spontaneously on three to five occasions per year, progesterone levels remain low and the abnormally rapid GnRH/LH pulse secretion could be viewed as being secondary to anovulation and reduced progesterone feedback on the hypothalamus. Alternatively, GnRH secretion may be abnormally regulated in PCOS and constitute one manifestation of the underlying pathophysiology. In ovulatory cycles, luteal concentrations of estrogen and progesterone inhibit GnRH pulse frequency, and if hypothalamic sensitivity to these steroids was impaired, persistently increased GnRH and LH

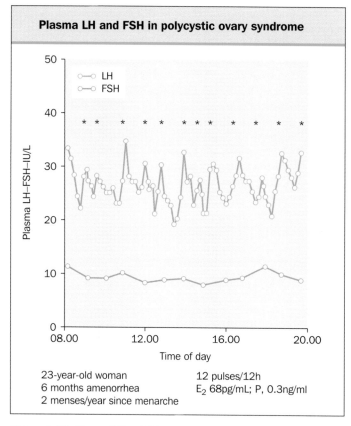

Figure 2.17 Plasma LH and FSH in polycystic ovary syndrome. Clinical details of the patient are shown. Luteinizing hormone (LH) pulses (*) occur at a frequency of approximately one pulse per hour and mean values exceed those of follicle-stimulating hormone (FSH).

secretion could result. In most women with PCOS, symptoms began soon after menarche and regular cycles are often never established. Thus if adolescents destined to develop PCOS were relatively resistant to the effects of progesterone in slowing GnRH pulse frequency, the initial small increases in progesterone in early anovulatory cycles might not slow GnRH secretion. This in turn would contribute to a relative deficiency of FSH secretion, with consequent impairment of subsequent follicular maturation. A persistent rapid GnRH pulse pattern would increase LH synthesis and secretion, leading to increased ovarian androgen production and cyst formation. Evidence to support this view has been found in studies of adolescent girls with hyperandrogenemia; in over half of these individuals LH pulse amplitude and frequency were increased. In detailed studies over 24 hours, girls with hyperandrogenemia had higher LH pulse frequency and mean LH compared to controls matched for age and similar stage of pubertal maturation.

Several studies have shown that administration of adequate amounts of exogenous progesterone given for 2–3 weeks can inhibit the amplitude and frequency of pulsatile GnRH secretion and, upon withdrawal of ovarian steroids, a transient selective increase in FSH occurs, with normal LH/FSH ratios persisting for some 10–14 days. These studies support the view that the persistent, rapid GnRH pulse stimulus may underlie the observations of increased LH and diminished FSH in plasma of women with PCOS. Evidence that sensitivity to progesterone feedback is impaired in women with PCOS is found from studies using combined oral contraceptives, where LH pulse frequency was reduced to a lesser degree than in normal ovulatory controls.

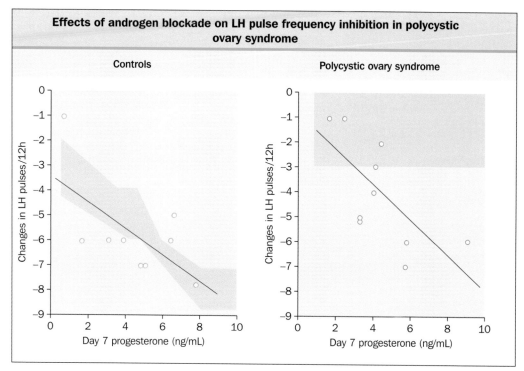

Figure 2.18 Effects of androgen blockade on LH pulse frequency inhibition in polycystic ovary syndrome. The shaded area represents the effects of exposure for 7 days to increasing plasma levels of progesterone. A progressive reduction in luteinizing hormone (LH) pulse frequency as a function of plasma progesterone is seen in controls, while progesterone levels of less than 10ng/mL were ineffective in women with polycystic ovary syndrome. Following 1 month's prior treatment with the antiandrogen flutamide (250mg bd), responses to the same protocol are shown by circles. The slope of the regression line in polycystic ovary syndrome and normal controls was not different. (Modified from Eagleson CA, Gingrich MB, Pastor CL, et al. Polycystic ovarian syndrome: evidence that flutamide restores sensitivity of the gonadotropin-releasing hormone pulse generator to inhibition by estradiol and progesterone. J Clin Endocrinol Metab. 2000;85:4047–52 © The Endocrine Society.)

Other studies have confirmed that higher plasma levels of progesterone are required to suppress GnRH in hyperandrogenemic women compared to controls, and plasma progesterone levels less than 10ng/mL are ineffective in suppressing the frequency of GnRH pulsatile release. Recent studies have cast light on the nature of this impaired sensitivity to progesterone feedback. Administration of the antiandrogen flutamide for 1 month was associated with normalization of the ability of low concentrations of progesterone to inhibit the frequency of GnRH release. The plasma levels of progesterone required to reduce GnRH pulse secretion were similar to those effective in normal women. The effects of flutamide on hypothalamic sensitivity to progesterone feedback in PCOS and normal women are shown in **Figure 2.18**.

Thus, GnRH pulse secretion in PCOS is abnormal and the anovulation in part reflects the effects of a persistent rapid frequency of GnRH stimulation of the pituitary, leading to excess LH, hyperandrogenemia, a relative deficiency of FSH in plasma, and failure of follicular maturation. The observations that blockade of androgen action can restore normal hypothalamic sensitivity to progesterone are of interest in that they indicate that a continuing presence of elevated plasma androgens is required to maintain insensitivity to progesterone feedback. This in turn suggests avenues by which the underlying abnormality of pulsatile GnRH release in PCOS may be reversed, leading to restoration of normal ovulatory cycles and a reduction in the excess androgen secretion.

FURTHER READING

Copinschi G, Spiegel K, Leproult R, et al. Pathophysiology of human circadian rhythms. In: Chadwick DJ, Goode JR, eds. Mechanisms and biological significance of pulsatile hormone secretion. Novartis Foundation Symposium 227. Chichester:John Wiley; 2000:143–63.

Dalkin AC, Marshall JC. Reproduction/fertility (inhibin/activin: regulation of fertility). In: Conn PM, Melmed S, eds. Endocrinology: basic and clinical principles. Totowa, NJ:Humana Press; 1997:405–18.

Daniels TL, Berga SL. Resistance of GnRH drive to sex steroid induced suppression in hyperandrogenemic anovulation. J Clin Endocrinol Metab. 1997;82:4179–83.

Haisenleder DJ, Dalkin AC, Marshall JC. Regulation of gonadotropin gene expression. In: Knobil E, Neill JD, eds. The physiology of reproduction, 2nd edn. New York:Raven Press; 1994:1793–832.

Marshall JC. Regulation of gonadotropin synthesis and secretion. In: DeGroot LJ, Jameson JL, Burger H, et al, eds. Endocrinology, 4th edn. Philadelphia, PA:WB Saunders; 2000.

Marshall JC, Eagleson CA. Neuroendocrine aspects of polycystic ovary syndrome. In: Dunaif A, ed. Polycystic ovary syndrome. Endocrinology & Metabolism Clinics of North America 28:2. Philadelphia, PA:WB Saunders; 1999:295–324.

Marshall JC, Kelch RP. Gonadotropin-releasing hormone – role of pulsatile secretion in the regulation of reproduction. N Engl J Med. 1986;315:1459–68.

Marshall JC, Dalkin AC, Haisenleder DJ, Paul SJ, Ortolano GA, Kelch RP. Gonadotropin-releasing hormone pulses: regulators of gonadotropin synthesis and ovulatory cycles. Recent Prog Horm Res. 1991;47:155–87.

Pastor CL, Griffin-Korf ML, Aloi JA, et al. Polycystic ovarian syndrome – evidence for reduced sensitivity of the GnRH pulse generator to inhibition by estradiol and progesterone. J Clin Endocrinol Metab. 1998;83:582–90.

Pincus SM. Orderliness of hormone release. In: Chadwick DJ, Goode JA, eds. Mechanisms and biological significance of pulsatile hormone secretion. Novartis Foundation Symposium 227. John Wiley:Chichester; 2000:82–105.

Spratt DJ, Carr DB, Merriam GR, et al. LH secretory patterns in men with idiopathic hypogonadotropic hypogonadism. In: Crowley WF, Hofler JG, eds. The episodic secretion of hormones. New York:Churchill Livingstone; 1987:257–81.

Taylor AE, McCourt B, Martin KA, et al. Determinants of abnormal gonadotropin secretion in clinically defined women with polycystic ovary syndrome. J Clin Endocrinol Metab. 1997;82:2248–55.

Urban RJ, Evans WS, Rogol AD, et al. Contemporary aspects of discrete peak-detection algorithms – the paradigm of the luteinizing hormone pulse signal in men. Endocrine Rev. 1988;9:3–37.

Veldhuis JD. Nature of altered pulsatile hormone release and neuroendocrine network signaling in human aging: clinical studies of the somatotropic, gonadotropic, corticotropic, and insulin axes. In: Chadwick DJ, Goode JA, eds. Mechanisms and biological significance of pulsatile hormone secretion. Novartis Foundation Symposium 227. John Wiley: Chichester; 2000:163–90.

Waxman DJ. Growth hormone pulse-activated STAT 5 signaling: a unique regulatory mechanism governing sexual dimorphism of liver gene expression. In: Chadwick DJ, Goode JA, eds. Mechanisms and biological significance of pulsatile hormone secretion. Novartis Foundation Symposium 227. John Wiley:Chichester; 2000:61–82.

Wu FCE, Butler GE, Kelnar CJH, et al. Patterns of pulsatile LH and FSH secretion in prepubertal boys and girls and patients with Kallmann's syndrome: a study using an ultrasensitive time resolved immunofluorometric assay. J Clin Endocrinol Metab. 1991;72:1229–37.

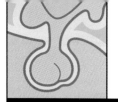

Chapter 3
Hypopituitarism – Pituitary Disease and Intrinsic Hypothalamic Disease
Ken K Y Ho and James Gibney

INTRODUCTION

Hypopituitarism is the term ascribed to deficiency of one or more hormones of the anterior or posterior pituitary gland. It results from primary pituitary pathology or from hypothalamic disease due to genetic or acquired causes. The clinical features of hypopituitarism depend on whether onset is during childhood or adulthood, which hormones are affected, and whether there are coexisting features of a pituitary or extrasellar mass lesion. The major causes of hypopituitarism are shown in **Table 3.1**.

CAUSES OF HYPOPITUITARISM

Genetic

Multiple pituitary hormone deficiencies
Major advances in the understanding of the developmental biology of the pituitary in recent years have provided insights into the molecular pathology of genetic causes of hypopituitarism. During embryonic development, the pituitary is formed by the association of neural ectodermal cells from the ventral diencephalon with ectodermal cells from the oral cavity. The former give rise to the posterior pituitary while the latter give rise to the anterior pituitary. Rathke's pouch, the primordial anterior pituitary lobe structure, originates from cells of the oral ectoderm. The formation and subsequent differentiation of Rathke's pouch into the mature pituitary gland are regulated by the actions of specific transcription factors in a spatial and temporal fashion. These include HESX-1, Prop-1 and Pit-1. Mutations in genes encoding for these transcription factors result in deficiency of one or more anterior pituitary hormones (**Table 3.2**).

HESX-1
HESX-1 is a homeobox gene that plays an important role in optic nerve and anterior pituitary development. It is expressed very early in the ectoderm, which is the precursor of Rathke's pouch. Its expression precedes that of transcription factors such as Prop-1 and Pit-1, and plays a role in pituitary cell-type differentiation. HESX-1 mutations in humans are associated with septo-optic dysplasia and growth hormone deficiency.

pit-1 and prop-1
Pit-1 (GHF-1, POU1F1) is a transcription factor found in somatotropes, lactotropes, and thyrotropes. Mutations in the gene that encodes Pit-1 result in absent growth hormone (GH) and prolactin and a variable reduction in thyroid stimulating hormone (TSH) expression. Pituitary size is typically reduced, but may be normal. A recently identified and much more prevalent mutation affects *prop-1*, a gene whose product is a prerequisite for *pit-1* expression. *Prop-1* abnormalities result in similar phenotypic abnormalities to *pit-1* mutations but with associated gonadotropin deficiency. The degree of gonadotropin deficiency is variable, even among individuals within the same family with identical mutations. Pituitary size is variable. Adrenocorticotropic hormone (ACTH) deficiency has been described but it is not known whether this is related to the underlying genetic abnormality. Overall, *pit-1* and *prop-1* mutations account for a significant number of cases of congenital multiple pituitary hormone deficiency, especially in cases when there is a family history of hypopituitarism. **Table 3.3** summarizes the endocrine manifestations of *pit-1* and *prop-1* mutations.

In some patients with combined pituitary hormone deficiency or growth hormone deficiency, an ectopic posterior pituitary is detected on magnetic resonance imaging (MRI; see Chapter 40). Posterior pituitary function is usually normal in these patients. Typically, the anterior pituitary is hypoplastic and the pituitary stalk is attenuated or absent (**Fig. 3.1**). It was initially thought that these abnormalities resulted from birth trauma, as a disproportionate number of cases were associated with breech delivery. It is now believed that the high incidence of breech presentation in these patients is secondary to abnormalities in the neuroendocrine system. This finding is not associated with *pit-1* or *prop-1* mutations.

KAL and DAX
Isolated gonadotropin deficiency is known as Kallmann's syndrome when it occurs in association with anosmia, and as idiopathic hypogonadotropic hypogonadism in the absence of anosmia. Gonadotropin-releasing hormone (GnRH) neurons originate in the olfactory placode and migrate during embryogenesis with the olfactory nerves to the hypothalamus. The KAL protein is necessary for this process to occur. The X-linked form of this disorder is due to mutations in the *KAL* gene. Associated clinical features include midline facial defects, short metacarpals, renal agenesis, and neurologic abnormalities, including sensorineural hearing loss, mirror movements, and oculomotor abnormalities. Non-X-linked forms of this disorder lack *KAL* gene abnormalities.

DAX1 is a transcription factor involved in development of pituitary gonadotrophs and the adrenal cortex. Mutations in the gene *DAX1* give rise to X-linked recessive hypogonadotropic hypogonadism and adrenal hypoplasia congenita.

Major causes of hypopituitarism		
Genetic	Multiple pituitary hormone deficiency	Mutations of: HESX-1 Pit-1 Prop-1
	Isolated pituitary hormone deficiency	Mutations of: DAX1 KAL AVP–neurophysin II GH1
		TSH-β, LH-β, FSH-β mutations
		GHRH, GnRH, TSH receptor
Neoplasms	Developmental	Craniopharyngioma
		Rathke's pouch cyst
		Arachnoid cyst
	Pituitary	Functioning
		Non-functioning
	Extrasellar	Germinoma/teratoma
		Meningioma
		Astrocytoma (including optic nerve glioma)
		Ependymoma
		Dermoid/ epidermoid cyst
	Metastatic	Renal
		Breast
Infiltrative	Granulomatous disease	Sarcoidosis
		Eosinophilic granuloma
		Tuberculosis
		Syphilis
		Wegener's granulomatosis
	Langerhans cell histiocytosis	
	Basal meningitis	
Infarction	Pituitary apoplexy	
	Sheehan's syndrome	
	Coronary artery bypass grafting	
Autoimmune	Isolated ACTH deficiency	
	Lymphocytic hypophysitis	
Radiation		
Traumatic		

Table 3.1 Major causes of hypopituitarism. ACTH, adrenocorticotropic hormone; FSH, follicle-stimulating hormone; GHRH, growth-hormone-releasing hormone; GnRH, gonadotropin-releasing hormone; LH, luteinizing hormone; TSH, thyroid-stimulating hormone.

Clinical manifestations of mutation of genes involved in pituitary development		
Transcription factor	**Function**	**Clinical presentation**
HSX-1	Optic nerve and anterior pituitary development	Septo-optic dysplasia
		GH deficiency
KAL	Migration of GnRH neurons and optic nerve	Hypogonadotropic hypogonadism, anosmia (Kallmann's syndrome)
DAX	Development of adrenal cortex and gonadotrophs	Adrenal hypoplasia congenita
		Hypogonadotropic hypogonadism
Pit-1	Development of anterior pituitary	GH deficiency
		Hypoprolactinemia
		TSH deficiency (variable)
Prop-1	Development of anterior pituitary	GH deficiency
		Hypoprolactinemia
		TSH deficiency
		LH/FSH deficiency
		ACTH deficiency (uncommon)

Table 3.2 Clinical manifestations of mutation of genes involved in pituitary development. ACTH, adrenocorticotropic hormone; FSH, follicle-stimulating hormone; GH, growth hormone; GnRH, gonadotropin-releasing hormone; LH, luteinizing hormone; TSH, thyroid-stimulating hormone.

Comparison of phenotypes produced by *pit1* and *prop1* mutations		
	pit-1	*prop-1*
Growth hormone	Absent	Low
Prolactin	Absent	Low
Thyroid-stimulating hormone	Low	Low
Luteinizing hormone, follicle-stimulating hormone	Normal	Absent
Adrenocorticotropic hormone	Normal	Low in one third
Vasopressin	Normal	Normal
Pituitary size	Small	Variable
Complex phenotype	No	No

Table 3.3 Comparison of *pit1* and *prop1* mutations.

AVP–neurophysin II

The hereditary form of diabetes insipidus, also known as familial neurohypophyseal diabetes insipidus, is autosomal dominant. It is explained by mutations in the *AVP–neurophysin II* gene, which encodes prepro-AVP–NPII, a precursor polypeptide consisting of arginine vasopressin (AVP), neurophysin II (NPII – which binds AVP), a signal peptide, and copeptin. Following synthesis in the magnocellular neurons of the supraoptic and paraventricular nuclei of the hypothalamus, processing is initiated with cleavage of the signal peptide (see Chapter 1). Subsequently, AVP, NPII, and copeptin are cloven from one another during axonal transport to the posterior pituitary. Mutations affecting both the signal peptide and NPII cause familial neurohypophyseal diabetes insipidus, which typically presents before 6 years of age.

Mutations causing isolated pituitary hormone deficiencies

Isolated growth hormone deficiency can be familial, occur in either dominant or recessive forms, and arise from mutations in the major GH gene known as the *GH1* gene. LH, FSH, TSH, and human chorionic gonadotropin (hCG) are a family of heterodimer hormones that share a common α subunit, with functional specificity residing in their β subunit. Mutations in the β subunit of LH, FSH, and TSH, resulting in deficiencies of each of these hormones, have been identified. Isolated ACTH deficiency is rarely due to a genetic defect but has been associated with a syndrome involving abnormalities of its precursor, proopiomelanocortin (POMC). Genetic defects have also been found in genes encoding hypothalamic releasing factors and their receptors. Growth-hormone-releasing hormone (GHRH) receptor deficiency has been identified in a number of kindreds worldwide. Cases of TSH and gonadotropin deficiency caused by genetic mutations in receptors of thyrotropin-releasing hormone (TRH) and GnRH have also been identified.

Tumors

Developmental

Cystic lesions that affect the sellar region include craniopharyngiomas (neoplastic) and Rathke's cleft cysts and arachnoid cysts (non-neoplastic).

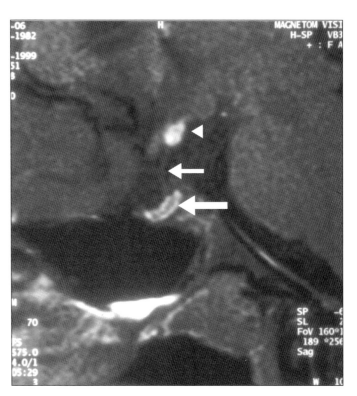

Figure 3.1 Magnetic resonance scan showing a hypoplastic anterior pituitary and an ectopic posterior pituitary gland. The posterior pituitary is identified as a high-intensity signal at the base of the hypothalamus (arrowhead). An atrophic pituitary stalk can just be seen (small arrow). This film was taken following administration of contrast, which enhances the signal of the anterior pituitary (large arrow).

Craniopharyngiomas are the most common tumor arising in the pituitary region in childhood. There is a bimodal peak in incidence at 5–14 years and again after the age of 50. It is uncertain whether they originate from ectopic embryonic remnants of the craniopharyngeal duct or arise from metaplastic squamous epithelial cells in the adenohypophysis. Tumors can be completely intrasellar, completely extrasellar, or a combination of both. There are frequently large cystic components. The cyst fluid contains cholesterol crystals and hCG secreted from the cells of the cyst wall.

Rathke's cleft cysts are cystic sellar and suprasellar lesions that originate from the remnants of Rathke's pouch and are characteristically lined by a single layer of ciliated cuboidal or columnar epithelium with goblet cells. Small asymptomatic cysts are frequently incidentally found at autopsy.

Arachnoid cysts result from herniation of the arachnoid membrane through the diaphragma sellae. They are less common than craniopharyngiomas and Rathke's cleft cysts, and typically present at a later age.

Strong clinical and radiologic similarities can make preoperative differentiation between these lesions difficult. Successful identification is usually possible histologically. Presentation is typically with headache or visual disturbance, with a large proportion having evidence of hypopituitarism at diagnosis. Diabetes insipidus may be a feature of both craniopharyngiomas and Rathke's cleft cysts. Presenting features are similar when origin is in childhood but may also include growth retardation.

Pituitary

Pituitary adenomas can arise at any time of life and may be non-functioning, or may secrete one or, less commonly, more than one anterior pituitary hormone. They are almost always benign and are thought to arise from clonal expansion of a single mutated pituitary cell. Pituitary tumors are classified as microadenomas (less than 10mm in diameter) and macroadenomas (greater than 10mm in diameter). The reported incidence of pituitary tumors ranges from 0.5 to 7.4 per 100,000 persons per year depending on age and sex, with the highest incidence occurring in women aged 15–44. Pituitary tumors, however, appear to be quite common but mostly remain undiagnosed. Autopsy studies reveal a prevalence of 10%, the majority of which are microadenomas.

Tumors that hypersecrete ACTH, GH, TSH, and prolactin result in the clinical syndromes of Cushing's disease, acromegaly, secondary hyperthyroidism, and hyperprolactinemia, respectively (**Fig. 3.2**). Most nonfunctioning tumors are of gonadotrope origin and synthesize without secreting FSH, free α or β subunits or, less commonly, LH. Clinical features are discussed below. Hyperprolactinemia due to stalk compression is present in approximately half of all cases, as is partial or complete hypopituitarism.

Extrasellar

Extrasellar tumors, which impinge on the hypothalamus, cause hypopituitarism either by damaging hypothalamic neurons regulating pituitary function or by interfering with transport of hypothalamic regulatory factors to the pituitary. The more common tumors causing hypothalamic dysfunction are detailed in **Table 3.1**. Meningiomas account for 20% of brain tumors and arise from the arachnoid. When they occur in the parasellar region they may cause third, fourth, fifth, and sixth cranial nerve deficits, as well as pituitary dysfunction. Optic nerve gliomas are a variant of astrocytoma, which lead to visual defects of varying severity in association with hypopituitarism.

Tumors arising in the pineal area include tumors of pineal cell origin (pinealomas) and, more commonly, tumors of germ-cell origin (germinomas). Germinomas may be malignant and metastasize outside the cerebrospinal fluid. Measurement of hCGβ, α-fetoprotein, and lactate dehydrogenase, which are frequently elevated in the plasma or cerebospinal fluid, is helpful in diagnosis. Production of hCG by a germinoma is a rare cause of precocious puberty. Tumors in the pineal region are the most common cause of Parinaud's syndrome (failure of upward gaze, convergence retraction nystagmus, and failure of pupillary constriction to light).

Damage to the hypothalamus or pituitary stalk causes reduced secretion of most pituitary hormones but may also cause hypersecretion of hormones normally under inhibitory control by the hypothalamus. Hyperprolactinemia frequently occurs following damage to the pituitary stalk. In children, precocious puberty caused by the loss of restraint over gonadotropin maturation may occur.

Infiltrative

Lymphocytic hypophysitis is an increasingly recognized cause of hypopituitarism. It is much more common in women, has an autoimmune basis, and typically presents in the peripartum or postpartum period. It is rare in men and postmenopausal women. It is sometimes associated with other autoimmune

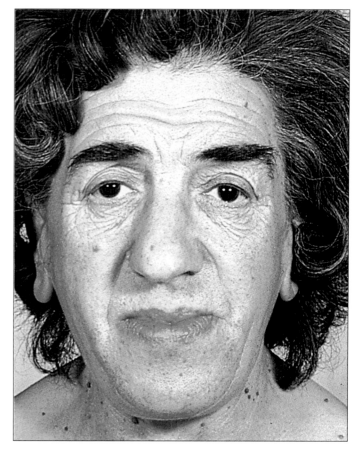

Figure 3.2 A patient with concomitant acromegaly and hypopituitarism. The presence of a GH-secreting pituitary tumor was the cause of symptoms in this patient.

disorders. Hypopituitarism, commonly isolated ACTH deficiency, can arise from either autoimmune destruction or from a local mass effect. Like Sheehan's syndrome, inability to breastfeed (because of hypoprolactinemia) is frequently the presenting complaint. MRI typically shows an enlarged pituitary gland. Biopsy is necessary to make a definitive diagnosis.

Langerhans' cell histiocytosis (previously known as histiocytosis X), is a rare proliferative histiocytic granulomatous disorder of unknown cause. Diabetes insipidus is a well-recognized and common feature of this condition but anterior pituitary dysfunction also frequently occurs.

Isolated ACTH deficiency is very rare. There is strong evidence that many cases have an autoimmune basis.

Infarction

Infarction of the already hypertrophied pituitary gland following excessive blood loss in the perinatal period is known as Sheehan's syndrome. The incidence in developed countries has fallen with improved obstetric care.

More recently, hypopituitarism resulting from infarction or hemorrhage of an undiagnosed silent pituitary tumor during coronary artery bypass grafting has been described. Several conditions predispose to this phenomenon, including heparinization and hemodynamic changes due to extracorporeal circulation that predispose to infarction. The clinical picture may present dramatically as blindness or major visual loss postoperatively.

Pituitary apoplexy is the clinical syndrome associated with pituitary hemorrhage or infarction. It usually, but not always, occurs in a pre-existing pituitary tumor and evolves over hours to days. It is characterized by a dramatic clinical picture of headache, vomiting, visual disturbance, ophthalmoplegia, and altered consciousness, and occasionally results in cure of a syndrome of hormone excess. Subclinical pituitary apoplexy refers to asymptomatic hemorrhage into a pituitary tumor.

Radiation
Anterior pituitary hormone deficiency occurs following irradiation of the pituitary gland for pituitary adenomas, nasopharyngeal tumors, and primary brain tumors, in children who had prophylactic cranial irradiation for acute lymphoblastic leukemia, or following total body irradiation for a variety of tumors and other diseases. The hypothalamus is believed to be the major site of damage. Five years following irradiation of pituitary adenomas, reported rates of pituitary dysfunction are: growth hormone deficiency 100%; gonadotropin deficiency 90%; TSH deficiency 75%; ACTH deficiency 40%. The likelihood of damage is related to total dose and is also influenced by other components of the radiotherapy schedule, such as the fraction size, number of fractions, and duration of treatment. Increased fraction size with a shorter treatment increases the risk of hypopituitarism for a given dose of radiation. Children are more sensitive to radiation damage than adults. Mild hyperprolactinemia may occur from hypothalamic damage. Posterior pituitary damage does not occur.

TRAUMATIC

Post-head-trauma hypopituitarism occurs most frequently in young males. The injury need not cause skull fracture or loss of consciousness. Incidence is probably underestimated as the head injury may have occurred years before clinical presentation. Approximately half to three quarters of reported cases have followed a road traffic accident. Anterior pituitary hormone deficiency is more common than diabetes insipidus, which occurs in about 25% of patients.

CLINICAL FEATURES OF PITUITARY LESIONS WITH HYPOPITUITARISM

The clinical features of hypopituitarism are outlined in **Table 3.4**. The manifestations depend on whether onset is during childhood or adulthood, which hormones are deficient, and whether there are concomitant features of a mass effect or of hypersecretion of hormones, including prolactin. Symptoms are frequently nonspecific and diagnosis of hypopituitarism is often delayed. In addition, the clinical features of deficiency of one hormone may make deficiency of others less apparent. For example, ACTH deficiency causes weight loss, whereas hypothyroidism and growth hormone deficiency may cause weight gain.

Pituitary mass effects
Clinical features of a mass effect include headache, visual disturbance, cranial nerve palsies, and cerebrospinal fluid rhinorrhea (**Fig. 3.3**). The classical pattern of bitemporal visual field loss due to encroachment on the optic chiasm is typically preceded by uni- or bilateral upper quadrantic field loss. Diminished visual acuity, scotomas, quadrantic defects and blindness of one or both eyes may also occur. Compression of cranial nerves leads to ophthalmoplegia and facial pain caused by compression of the trigeminal nerve. Stalk compression causes secondary hypopituitarism due to interference with delivery of hypothalamic releasing factors. Hyperprolactinemia is a frequent consequence of stalk dysfunction and may be sufficient to cause galactorrhea.

Table 3.4 Symptoms and signs of hypopituitarism.

Symptoms and signs of hypopituitarism		
Hormone deficiency	**Symptoms**	**Signs**
Adrenocorticotropic hormone	Weakness, lethargy, fatigue	Pallor
	Anorexia, weight loss, abdominal pain	Wasting
		Loss of body hair
Thyroid-stimulating hormone	Fatigue	Bradycardia
	Weight gain	Sallow complexion
	Cold intolerance	Slow-relaxing reflexes
	Constipation	
Follicle-stimulating hormone/ luteinizing hormone		
Males	Impotence, reduced libido, infertility	Fine wrinkling of skin
	Reduced muscle strength	Reduced musculature
		Small testes (childhood onset)
Females	Oligo/amenorrhea	Fine wrinkling of skin
	Dyspareunia	Breast atrophy
Growth hormone		
Adults	Reduced energy and vitality	Reduced muscle mass
	Reduced exercise tolerance	Increased fat, especially central
Children	Short stature	
Vasopressin	Polyuria/polydipsia	

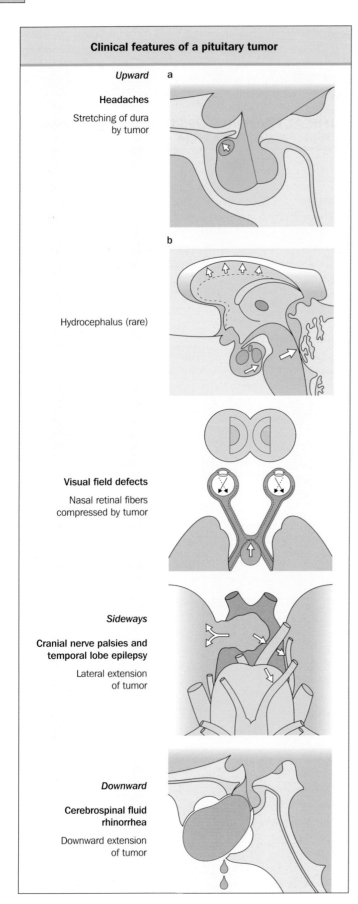

Clinical features of a pituitary tumor

Upward a

Headaches

Stretching of dura by tumor

b

Hydrocephalus (rare)

Visual field defects

Nasal retinal fibers compressed by tumor

Sideways

Cranial nerve palsies and temporal lobe epilepsy

Lateral extension of tumor

Downward

Cerebrospinal fluid rhinorrhea

Downward extension of tumor

Figure 3.3 Clinical features of a pituitary tumor. The figure illustrates the effects of local expansion of the tumor (mass effect).

Hypoadrenalism

Adrenocorticotropic hormone deficiency results in reduced production of cortisol and adrenal androgens, but not of aldosterone, which is predominantly under the control of the renin–angiotensin system. Loss of the orexigenic effect of cortisol leads to anorexia, weight loss, and gastrointestinal symptoms. Reduced androgen production contributes to loss of body hair in women and in men, when accompanied by hypogonadism (**Fig. 3.4**). In contrast to primary adrenal insufficiency, where increased ACTH has melanocyte-stimulating activity, pallor rather than skin pigmentation is found. As aldosterone production is preserved, evidence of reduced circulatory volume is less marked than with primary adrenal failure and hyperkalemia does not occur.

Hypothyroidism

The features of secondary hypothyroidism are identical to those of primary hypothyroidism and include fatigue, weight gain, cold intolerance, and constipation. There are many physical signs attributed to hypothyroidism but the most discriminating of these are bradycardia and slow-relaxing reflexes.

Hypogonadism

Hypogonadotropic hypogonadism in men results in clinical features of testosterone deficiency; reduced libido, impotence, reduced muscle and increased fat, osteoporosis, lethargy, skin thinning, fine wrinkling, reduced testicular volume and hypospermia, and hair loss (**Fig. 3.5**). In premenopausal women, hypogonadotropic hypogonadism results in amenorrhea, infertility, and estrogen deficiency, which in turn causes reduced libido, genitourinary atrophy, and osteoporosis.

Growth hormone deficiency

Growth hormone deficiency in adulthood results in a syndrome of altered body composition and dyslipidemia, reduced strength and exercise tolerance, and reduced energy levels. Linear growth retardation is the cardinal feature of childhood growth hormone deficiency and is discussed in Chapter 4.

Diabetes insipidus

Diabetes insipidus is caused by reduced secretion of vasopressin (antidiuretic hormone, ADH) by the posterior pituitary, and results in polyuria and polydipsia (see Chapter 7). Diabetes insipidus is common in tumors of the hypothalamus and extrasellar region, cranipopharyngiomas and Rathke's cleft cysts, lymphocytic hypophysitis, sarcoidosis, and Langerhans' cell histiocytosis, and following surgery or head trauma. Onset can be insidious or dramatic, e.g. following trauma or after surgery. Concurrent ACTH deficiency masks evidence of diabetes insipidus, cortisol contributing to the excretion of a water load.

Hypothalamic dysfunction

In addition to features of a pituitary mass effect and hypopituitarism, signs of hydrocephalus due to third ventricle obstruction and clinical features due to hypothalamic damage may also occur. The hypothalamus plays an important role in feeding behavior, temperature regulation, the sleep–wake cycle, memory and behavior, thirst, and autonomic nervous system function. Acute destructive processes affecting the hypothalamus

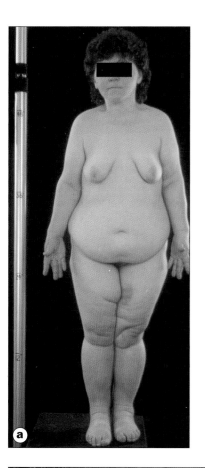

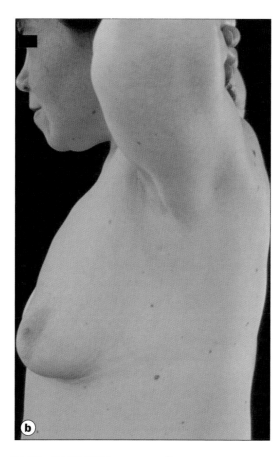

Figure 3.4 A patient with panhypopituitarism. (a) Short stature, reduced body hair and increased abdominal fat are apparent. (b) Partial breast development results from estrogen replacement. Failure of adrenal androgen production results in the absence of axillary hair.

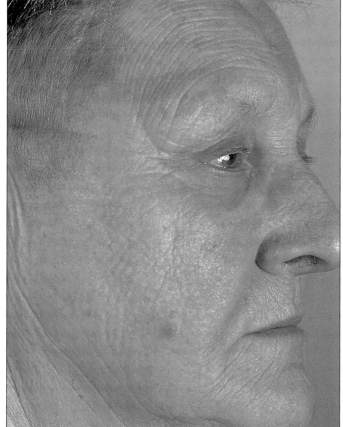

Figure 3.5 A patient with hypopituitarism. Pallor, skin wrinkling, and absence of facial hair can be clearly seen.

typically cause coma or disturbances of the autonomic nervous system, while slow-growing tumors produce dementia, disturbances of food intake (obesity or emaciation), and endocrine dysfunction. Hypothalamic obesity occurs with lesions in the vicinity of the ventromedial nucleus, which is involved in regulation of satiety (Fig. 3.6). With tumors in this area, aggressive behavior and hyperphagia may occur until the new setpoint is reached. Both hypothermia (which can be paroxysmal as a result of episodes of sweating and vasodilatation) and hyperthermia can occur. Hyperthermia results from acute pathologic processes such as hemorrhage, surgery, or infarction. Other features of hypothalamic disease are summarized in Table 3.5.

Hypopituitarism in childhood and adolescence

Infants with congenital hypopituitarism present with hypoglycemic seizures, prolonged jaundice and, if male, micropenis and undescended testes. Growth failure is often apparent by the end of the first year of life. Hypoglycemia and hypoglycemic seizures are also features of hypopituitarism early in childhood. Typically, this occurs during fasting. Body proportion is normal for age but affected individuals have a prominent calvarium, tend to be overweight in relation to height, and have prominent subcutaneous fat deposits. Delayed puberty occurs if gonadotropin deficiency is present. Failure to undergo puberty is the usual presentation of isolated hypogonadotropic hypogonadism and is difficult to distinguish from constitutionally delayed puberty.

Mortality and morbidity

A number of retrospective studies have demonstrated mortality to be doubled in patients with hypopituitarism compared to reference populations. This finding is more marked in women and

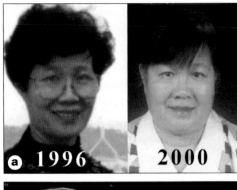
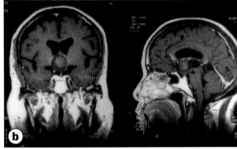

Figure 3.6 A patient with a hypothalamic tumor. (a) Presentation was with headaches and weight gain. This was found to be secondary to a large hypothalamic tumor (b).

Clinical features of hypothalamic lesions other than hypopituitarism	
Food intake	Obesity
	Hyperphagia
	Hyperglycemia (acute hypothalamic damage)
	Hypoglycemia (chronic – rare)
Temperature regulation	Hypothermia
	Paroxysmal hypothermia
	Acute hyperthermia
	Poikilothermia
	Paroxysmal hyperthermia
Sleep–wake cycle	Insomnia and agitation
	Hypersomnolent state
	Coma
Memory and behavior	Memory loss
	Dementia
	Korsakoff's syndrome
	Rage reactions
	Apathy
Thirst	Primary polydipsia
Autonomic nervous system function	Diencephalic epilepsy
	Pheochromocytoma-like syndrome

Table 3.5 Clinical features of hypothalamic lesions other than hypopituitarism.

applies even when patients who previously had Cushing's disease or acromegaly and those who have been treated with radiotherapy are excluded from analysis. The excess mortality appears to be caused by an increase in cardiovascular and cerebrovascular disease. Potential explanations include growth hormone deficiency, long-term hypogonadism, and over-replacement with glucocorticoids and thyroid hormones.

INVESTIGATION

Investigation of suspected hypopituitarism involves:
- confirming the presence and extent of hypopituitarism;
- undertaking procedures to diagnose the cause.

This review focuses on biochemical diagnosis, but high-resolution imaging plays a central role in uncovering structural causes of hypopituitarism (see Chapter 40) While MRI scanning is now the procedure of choice, computed tomography (CT) plays a complementary role, or is used exclusively in situations where MRI is contraindicated, such as when arterial clips or a pacemaker are present. In addition, CT scanning has a valuable role in defining bony anatomy in preparation for surgery.

DIAGNOSIS

Diagnosis of hypopituitarism is established by undertaking baseline and dynamic tests of pituitary function (**Table 3.6**).

Baseline assessment
Baseline assessment of pituitary function involves combined measurement from a single blood sample, of pituitary hormones and hormones produced by their respective target glands. Based on the principle of feedback regulation, hypopituitarism is present when pituitary hormones are inappropriately low in the presence of low concentrations of target gland hormones. Baseline blood testing reliably identifies hypothyroidism, hypogonadism, and severe hypoadrenalism due to pituitary insufficiency.

Dynamic testing
Dynamic testing is complementary to baseline assessment and is used to assess functional reserve in a patient with pituitary disease. Secretory stimuli are generally of two types:
- Direct – use of hypothalamic releasing hormones, e.g. TRH, GnRH, GHRH tests;
- Indirect – pharmacologic stimuli that result in endogenous release of secretagogues from the hypothalamus, e.g insulin tolerance test (ITT).

Where hypopituitarism is due to deficiency of releasing factors from the hypothalamus, the use of hypothalamic releasing factors can induce the release of anterior pituitary hormones that they regulate. Therefore, a response to a hypothalamic releasing factor does not imply normal physiologic regulation of that hormone.

Hypoadrenalism
Both baseline and dynamic tests are valuable in diagnosis of ACTH deficiency. When secondary ACTH deficiency is relatively advanced, usually in the context of a large adenoma, prolonged fatigue, and weight loss, the finding of low random cortisol and ACTH establishes the diagnosis. Where secondary hypoadrenalism is mild, basal random cortisol levels often fall within the normal circadian range. In this setting, suspicion of a reduced ACTH response to stress is confirmed by ITT. If early

Dynamic diagnostic tests of hypopituitarism

Pituitary axis	Baseline test	Finding	Dynamic test	Finding
Adrenal	ACTH	Low	ITT	Cortisol peak
	Cortisol	Low		< 550nmol/L
Thyroid	TSH	Low	TRH	Variable
	T₃, T₄	Low		
Gonads	LH, FSH	Low to normal	GnRH	Variable
	Testosterone	Low		
	Estradiol	Low		
Growth hormone	GH	Undetectable	ITT	GH peak< 5ng/mL
	IGF-1	Low to normal		

Table 3.6 Dynamic diagnostic tests of hypopituitarism. ACTH, adrenocorticotropic hormone; FSH, follicle-stimulating hormone; GH, growth hormone; GnRH, gonadotropin-releasing hormone test; IGF-1; insulin-like growth factor 1; ITT, insulin tolerance test; LH, luteinizing hormone; T3, triiodothyronine; T4, thyroxine; TRH, thyrotropin-releasing hormone test; TSH, thyroid-stimulating hormone.

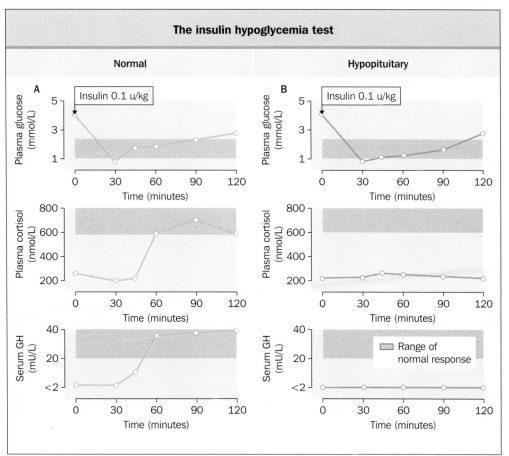

Figure 3.7 The insulin tolerance test. Plasma glucose, plasma cortisol, and serum GH levels are shown in a normal (A) and a hypopituitary (B) subject. GH levels should rise to a minimum of 20mu/L and cortisol to 550nmol/L, provided that adequate hypoglycemia is reached with blood glucose concentrations of 2.2mmol/L or more.

morning cortisol is greater than 550nmol/L, ACTH deficiency is unlikely even in response to stress, while if cortisol is less than 150nmol/L, ACTH deficiency is likely. With intermediate values, ITT is necessary. Hydrocortisone, prednisone (prednisolone), and methylprednisone all crossreact with the cortisol assay and therefore should not be administered within 24 hours of measurement of circulating cortisol.

The ITT is the gold standard for evaluation of the hypothalamo–pituitary–adrenal axis. Intravenous insulin induces hypoglycemia (blood glucose less than 2.2mmol/L) within 30–45min of injection, with a resultant increase in ACTH and cortisol as part of the counter-regulatory response. Following an adequate hypoglycemic stimulus (BSL < 2.2mmol/L), peak cortisol greater

than 550nm/L, and an increment of at least 200 nmol/L is considered an adequate response (**Fig. 3.7**).

The ITT has the advantage of allowing simultaneous assessment of growth hormone secretory capacity. It is time- and labor-intensive, however, and contraindications, including epilepsy and coronary artery disease, exist.

The short Synacthen® (Cortrosyn®, tetracosactrin) test is sometimes used as a surrogate test of ACTH deficiency on the basis that the adrenal gland will respond to an exogenous bolus of synthetic ACTH when there is a normal endogenous ACTH reserve and the gland is not atrophic. Synacthen® is a synthetic ACTH comprising the first 24 amino-acid residues of ACTH, which encompass the full biologic activity of the molecule. While it is a good test of adrenal reserve, it does not directly test pituitary ACTH reserve. In a patient with organic pituitary disease, a normal response to Synacthen does not exclude mild or recent ACTH deficiency. The test is dealt with in detail in Chapter 16.

Hypothyroidism

Secondary hypothyroidism is reliably diagnosed from TSH and thyroid hormone measurements. Despite the low thyroxine levels, baseline TSH is usually normal and rarely low. Dynamic testing using TRH has no diagnostic value for hypothyroidism but may have a role in differential diagnosis of the cause of hypothyroidism: a delayed peak is characteristic of hypothalamic dysfunction.

Hypogonadism

Baseline tests readily establish hypogonadism secondary to pituitary dysfunction in both men and women. Single measurements of LH and FSH have limited value because gonadotropin secretion is pulsatile and therefore levels fluctuate over a wide range, from low readings at the limit of assay detectability. Single random LH/FSH measurements by themselves do not distinguish gonadotropin deficiency from normal but are only meaningful with concurrent sex steroid measurement. Low gonadal steroid levels accompanied by normal or low LH/FSH levels indicate a secondary (pituitary) cause of hypogonadism.

The GnRH test has virtually no diagnostic value but may be suitable for establishing pituitary reserve in the setting of suitability for pulsatile GnRH therapy for infertility.

Growth hormone deficiency

Because there is marked fluctuation of levels throughout the day, random levels of GH are not useful for diagnosis of GH deficiency. Thus provocative tests are required. A baseline IGF-1 measurement is a specific but insensitive test of GH deficiency in patients with pituitary disease. A low IGF-1 reliably indicates GH deficiency but a normal IGF-1 does not exclude it.

A large number of dynamic tests have been used to diagnose GH deficiency, including arginine, GHRH, and clonidine. ITT is the gold standard and has been the most stringently validated (**Fig. 3.7**). Combinations of GHRH and arginine, and GHRH and GHRP-6 have also been validated and may be used if ITT is contraindicated or unacceptable. Some use administration of 1mg subcutaneous glucagon as the alternative to the ITT when the latter is contraindicated, as it normally causes ACTH/cortisol and GH secretion over the next 4 hours. However it is not as reliable as the ITT.

Diabetes insipidus

Diabetes insipidus is diagnosed by a water deprivation test followed by administration of desmopressin (see Chapter 7). The principle of the test is based on the generation of progressively concentrated urine with progressive dehydration. This does not occur in diabetes insipidus unless desmopressin is administered.

MANAGEMENT

Management of hypopituitarism involves treatment of the underlying cause and replacement of hormone deficiencies. Removal of a pituitary mass lesion may restore pituitary function. Correction of hyperprolactinemia restores gonadotrope function. In most other circumstances replacement of pituitary function is achieved either by directly replacing the deficient hormone or replacing the product(s) of their target gland(s).

Hypoadrenalism

Adrenocorticotropic hormone deficiency is corrected by glucocorticoid replacement (see Chapter 16). Available formulations include hydrocortisone, its biologic precursor cortisone acetate, and synthetic glucocorticoids such as prednisone and dexamethasone (**Table 3.7**). Previously, it was estimated that daily cortisol production was approximately 12mg/m^2 and that physiologic replacement necessitated daily doses of 30mg of hydrocortisone or 37.5mg of cortisone acetate. However, recent reappraisal of the daily physiologic secretion of cortisol in normal subjects has demonstrated that daily production is approximately 6mg/m^2. Allowing for hepatic metabolism, as part of the first-pass effect, the appropriate daily requirement is 20mg of hydrocortisone. This should be given in two divided doses. Drugs that induce mixed function oxidases (including barbiturates, rifampin (rifampicin), phenytoin, and carbamezepine) can increase metabolism of corticosteroids and thus may necessitate higher replacement doses.

Commonly used synthetic glucocorticoid preparations include prednisone and dexamethasone. These compounds have increased biologic potency as a result of increased affinity for the glucocorticoid receptor and altered metabolic clearance rates. Prednisone has a longer duration of action than hydrocortisone and may be given as a once-daily dose. Cortisone acetate should not be used as it is intrinsically inactive and has to be converted to hydrocortisone, and this occurs at various rates in different people.

The correct dose and its distribution is best judged by clinical assessment to include sense of wellbeing, energy level, postural symptoms, body weight, etc., and the measurement of circulating cortisol levels throughout the day on replacement doses (see Chapter 16)

Pharmacologic properties of commonly used glucocorticoids				
Glucocorticoid	Potency (cortisol = 1)	Tablet size (mg)	Replacement dose (mg/day)	Regimen
Hydrocortisone	1	20, 4	16–30	Twice daily
Cortisone acetate	0.8	25, 5	25–37.5	Twice daily
Prednisone, prednisolone	4	5, 1	2.5–5	Once daily
Dexamethasone	30	0.5	0.25–5	Once daily

Table 3.7 Pharmacologic properties of commonly used glucocorticoids.

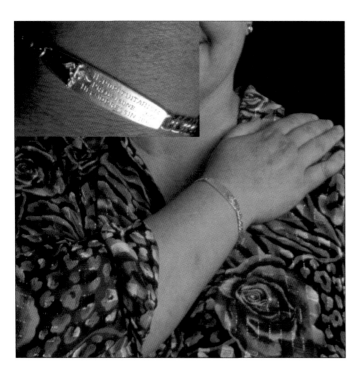

Figure 3.8 An identification bracelet worn by a patient with hypopituitarism. The bracelet details her medical condition (hypopituitarism) and her current hormone replacement regime (prednisone and desmopressin).

Education is an essential part of corticosteroid replacement. Individuals and their families must be aware of the increased cortisol requirement during stress or intercurrent illness, and of situations which require parenteral administration of glucocorticoid (see Chapter 16). Glucocorticoid-deficient individuals and their families or friends should be taught how to administer intramuscular injections. Individuals should also be strongly advised to carry a steroid card or wear some form of identification, such as a Medic-Alert bracelet, identifying them as requiring steroids in emergency situations (**Fig. 3.8**).

Mineralocorticoid replacement is not essential in hypopituitarism, unlike in primary adrenocortical failure, as regulation of mineralocorticoid is not pituitary-dependent.

Hypothyroidism

Thyroid-stimulating hormone deficiency is corrected by replacement with thyroxine (T_4). The approximate daily replacement dose in most subjects is 100μg. General principles of replacement therapy similar to those for primary hypothyroidism should be applied. Patients with pre-existing coronary heart disease should be commenced on a lower dose, e.g. 25μg/day, with the dose gradually titrated into the normal range. Treatment is monitored by measuring free or total T_4 levels, and not TSH levels. Thyroid replacement may unmask undiagnosed cortisol deficiency; hence thyroxine replacement should not be commenced without definitively ascertaining glucocorticoid reserve or commencing appropriate glucocorticoid replacement.

Hypogonadism
Men
Androgen replacement is achieved through parenteral administration as intramuscular injection, subcutaneous pellet implantation, or transdermal administration by patch or by administration of testosterone gel (**Table 3.8**).

The most common replacement therapy is the use of injectable testosterone esters, including testosterone proprionate, testosterone enanthate, testosterone cypionate, and combinations of these. These preparations have the disadvantage of requiring injections once every 3–4 weeks, and are associated with peaks and troughs of serum testosterone levels, which may lead to fluctuations in mood, libido, and energy levels.

There is no satisfactory oral formulation of testosterone for replacement therapy. Oral formulations of 17α alkyl derivatives of testosterone such as methyltestosterone and fluoxymesterone should be avoided because of potential hepatotoxicicity. Testosterone undecanoate, a commercially available oral formulation, is absorbed through the intestinal lymphatics and thus avoids hepatic metabolism and hepatotoxicity. However, it has a short half-life so that three-times-daily administration is required for sustained biologic effect. It is useful in situations where there is some residual testosterone secretion or where intramuscular injections are contraindicated or unacceptable.

Transdermal preparations of testosterone hold considerable promise as an alternative. Scrotal and nonscrotal preparations are available. Scrotal skin patches take advantage of the high

Table 3.8 Testosterone formulations for androgen replacement therapy.

Testosterone formulations for androgen replacement therapy			
Route	Formulation	Trade name	Regimen
Intramuscular	Testosterone enanthate	Primoteston – depot	250mg every 3–4 weeks
	Mixed testosterone esters	Sustanon	250mg every 3–4 weeks
Subcutaneous implant	Testosterone pellets		300–600mg every 4–6 months
Transdermal			
Patches Nonscrotal	Testosterone	Androderm	2.5mg every 24h
Scrotal	Testosterone	Testoderm	5mg every 24h
Gel	Testosterone	Androgel	5–10g every 24h
Oral	Testosterone undecanoate	Andriol	80mg every 8h
		Restandol	

Regimens for estrogen replacement			
Regimen	Estrogen	Progestogen	Notes
Combined			
Sequential	Continuous	12–14 days/4 weeks	Withdrawal bleeding
Continuous	Continuous	Continuous	Risk of breakthrough bleeding
Unopposed estrogen	Continuous	Nil	Hysterectomized women only

Table 3.9 Regimens for estrogen replacement.

absorptive capacity of the thin scrotal skin but require preparation of the scrotal skin to allow adherence of the patch. Nonscrotal patches have a number of technical drawbacks, including skin irritation. Recently, gel preparations have been developed. Subdermal testosterone implants last 4–6 months and confer significant advantages in terms of convenience and provision of stable blood concentrations of testosterone. However they require minor surgery for implantation and are occasionally extruded.

Androgen replacement by any of the above methods should be monitored by measuring serum testosterone levels. The exception is testosterone undecanoate, which needs to be monitored with circulating dihydrotestosterone measurement as it is converted by the enzyme 5α-reductase in the gut wall as it is absorbed.

Women

Estrogen replacement therapy can be administered orally or parenterally in a variety of different preparations. The addition of a progestogen such as medroxyprogesterone acetate is necessary for 12–14 days each month to prevent the development of endometrial hyperplasia and carcinomas. Progesterone can also be given continuously.

Regimen

Estrogen can be administered as part of a cyclic or a continuous regimen (**Table 3.9**). Cyclic regimens mimic the normal menstrual cycle and involve coadministration of progesterone for 12–14 consecutive days during each 4-week cycle, resulting in withdrawal menstrual bleeding.

Continuous regimens involve administration of progesterone, in combination with estrogen, throughout the cycle. These regimens have gained popularity because of the avoidance of withdrawal bleeding. However, the incidence of unacceptable withdrawal bleeding during the early months is up to 20%.

In women with an intact uterus, estrogen must always be administered with a progesterone to avoid endometrial hyperplasia and risk of carcinoma. However, in hysterectomized women, estrogen may be administered unopposed.

Route

Oral administration of estrogen can be said to be unphysiologic because of the perturbation of hepatic function during first-pass metabolism. The extent of hepatic dysfunction is dependent on the estrogen dose and formulation. Perturbations of potential clinical significance include the induction of clotting factors, development of fatty liver, and suppression of IGF-1. These effects are avoided by parenteral estrogen administration either with a patch, gel, or subcutaneous implant. Oral, but not transdermal, estradiol reduces the effectiveness of the GH–IGF-1 axis and, in women receiving concurrent GH replacement, an alternative route of administration should be considered.

Dose

Women with hypopituitarism should be placed on a regimen with the estrogen dose appropriate for physiologic replacement (similar to that for menopause), and not for oral contraception, despite the convenience of prepackaging (**Table 3.10**). Estrogen doses are higher and formulations are more potent for oral contraceptive use and increase side effects and hepatic dysfunction.

Hypopituitary women of reproductive age should be placed on a higher dose than their postmenopausal counterparts.

Follicle-stimulating hormone and LH (or, in people with hypothalamic damage only, pulsatile LH-releasing hormone) are necessary for fertility. Recombinant forms of both LH and FSH are now available. A variety of regimens have proved to be successful.

Growth hormone replacement

The importance of growth hormone replacement in adults is fully discussed in Chapter 4. GH is administered subcutaneously as a once-daily dose, at night. Replacement doses range from 0.5 to 3.2u/day (0.2–1.4mg/day) to restore circulating IGF-1 levels to the upper half of the age-related normal range, GH requirements are higher in younger individuals and in women. GH has significant interactions with cortisol, thyroid hormone, and oral estrogen. Diagnosis and treatment of growth hormone deficiency in adults are discussed in greater detail in Chapter 4.

Diabetes insipidus

The management of diabetes insipidus is discussed in Chapter 7.

Recommended estrogen doses for replacement therapy		
Route	Formulation	Regimen
Oral	17βestradiol	1–2mg/d
	Estradiol valerate	1–2mg/d
	Conjugated equine estrogen	0.3–1.25mg/d
Transdermal	17β estradiol	50–100μg/d
Implant	17β estradiol	20–100μg/4–6m

Table 3.10 Recommended estrogen doses for replacement therapy.

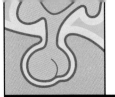

Chapter 4

Growth Hormone Deficiency in Adults

John P Monson

INTRODUCTION

Some 40 years ago, anecdotal reports of the effects of growth hormone (GH) therapy on psychological and general wellbeing in an adult with hypopituitarism provided a prophetic insight into the condition of adult GH deficiency (GHD). Limitation of supply of GH and the understandable focus on the need to treat growth failure due to GH deficiency in children precluded further work in this area until the advent of recombinant human GH in large amounts in the late 1980s. Since the publication of the first placebo-controlled trials of GH replacement in adults with GHD, there has been an accumulation of evidence supporting the existence of an adult GHD syndrome and its alleviation by GH replacement therapy. Adult-onset GHD has substantial overlap with other aspects of anterior pituitary

failure because it is most commonly the consequence of structural pituitary disease, pituitary surgery, irradiation or trauma (**Table 4.1**). Childhood-onset GHD is usually caused by a partial deficiency of growth-hormone-releasing hormone (GHRH), a condition which, possibly because of maturation of the hypothalamo–somatotroph axis, may not be evident at the time of reassessment of GH reserve when linear growth is complete. However, when childhood-onset GHD is due to structural disease or occurs as a result of irradiation, it is generally permanent. Because of the reversibility of childhood-onset GHD it is important that a detailed assessment of GH reserve be conducted at completion of linear growth. It is estimated that the prevalence of adult-onset GHD is 1 in 10 000 of the population and if adult deficiency commencing in childhood is also considered the prevalence may be nearer 3 in 10 000.

Epidemiologic studies conducted in Sweden and the UK have provided compelling evidence that adult-onset hypopituitarism is associated with premature death (standardized mortality ratios of approximately 2:1), this phenomenon being more evident in females. The Swedish observations indicated increased mortality from vascular disease, particularly cerebrovascular disease, with a similar trend in the UK. These observations have prompted the attribution of increased mortality to GHD *per se*, although this assumed that other aspects of the underlying pituitary disease were not relevant and that the replacement of glucocorticoid, thyroid and sex steroid hormones was optimal. Although the latter conclusion is open to question, the possible causal role of GHD in determining increased mortality, and particularly in predisposing to vascular disease, has been supported by the demonstration of adverse changes in a variety of cardiovascular risk factors, including lipoprotein profiles, body fat distribution, insulin sensitivity and glucose tolerance. Attempts have been made to dissect out the relative contributions of GHD, other aspects of hypopituitarism and the underlying pituitary pathology in determining mortality but such an approach is fraught with difficulty because of the very high prevalence of GHD in patients with pituitary disease. As a consequence, we are dependent on the demonstration of reversibility of adverse changes in markers of cardiovascular risk by GH replacement therapy as surrogate evidence for a causal role for GHD in mediating increased cardiovascular mortality. Further and more direct evidence for a causal role of GHD in predisposing to increased mortality will emerge from documentation of mortality rates in patients on GH enrolled into long-term surveillance studies in comparison with background mortality rates.

Causes of growth hormone deficiency		
Diagnosis	*n*	%
Non-functioning pituitary adenoma	844	30.7
ACTH-secreting pituitary adenoma	200	7.3
GH-secreting pituitary adenoma	55	2.0
Prolactin-secreting pituitary adenoma	305	11.1
Gonadotropin-secreting pituitary adenoma	11	0.4
TSH-secreting pituitary adenoma	6	0.2
Pituitary tumor – secretory status unknown	40	1.5
Craniopharyngioma	357	13.0
Surgery	25	0.9
Irradiation	54	2.0
Idiopathic	353	12.8
Trauma	55	2.0
Other	448	16.3
Total	2753	

Table 4.1 Causes of growth hormone deficiency. The table documents the cause of growth hormone deficiency in 2753 patients enrolled consecutively into KIMS (Pharmacia International Metabolic Surveillance). ACTH, adrenocorticotropic hormone; GH, growth hormone; TSH, thyroid-stimulating hormone. (Reprinted from Toogood AA, Shalet SM. Diagnosis of GHD in adults. In: Bengtsson B-Å, Monson JP, eds. GH replacement in adults – the first five years of KIMS. Oxford; Oxford PharmaGenesis: with the kind permission of Oxford PharmaGenesis Ltd © 2000.)

CAUSES OF GH DEFICIENCY

The causes of GHD in adults are indicated in **Table 4.1**, using data derived from the first 2753 patients enrolled into KIMS (Pharmacia International Metabolic Surveillance, a multinational, pharmacoepidemiologic surveillance database for adult hypopituitary patients receiving GH replacement). This population is largely composed of adult-onset hypopituitary patients but also includes a proportion of patients with childhood-onset disease who have a higher percentage prevalence of craniopharyngioma and post-irradiation GHD. Assuming a correct initial diagnosis, the reversibility of isolated, idiopathic GHD of childhood is now well established, with normal GH responses on dynamic testing being described in between 30% and 70% of subjects at completion of linear growth in various series. In contrast, isolated GHD does not arise *de novo* in adults unless accompanied by a structural lesion or radiotherapy.

It is evident that pituitary adenoma is numerically the most important cause, followed by craniopharyngioma, which combined account for 65% of cases of adult GHD. Irradiation as a primary cause refers to those instances arising as a result of primary cranial irradiation rather than those due to irradiation for pituitary adenoma or craniopharyngioma. The latter have been included under the appropriate pituitary adenoma category. The designation 'other' includes various rare causes of hypopituitarism, including lymphocytic hypophysitis, intracranial germ cell tumors, Langerhans' cell histiocytosis, and granulomatous diseases. These prevalence rates concur with experience from individual clinics and similar data have been published from several large centers.

THE DIAGNOSIS OF GH DEFICIENCY

GH is normally secreted in a pulsatile fashion, with serum measurements varying between peaks and troughs, the latter falling below the assay detection limit of conventional radioimmunoassays. Therefore, the diagnosis of GHD is dependent on the demonstration of a subnormal rise in serum GH in response to one or more dynamic stimulation tests rather than the results of single random GH levels. Options include the insulin tolerance test, glucagon test, arginine stimulation, and combinations of arginine and GHRH or GH secretagogues. Other tests such as the clonidine or exercise stimulation tests are of no value in adults. Of the various possibilities, the best validated is the insulin tolerance test, which has been demonstrated to distinguish reliably between GH responses in patients with structural pituitary disease and those of age-matched controls across the adult age range (**Fig. 4.1**). In the past, a variety of serum GH cutoff points were used to define GH deficiency. However, an international consensus (convened by the Growth Hormone Research Society) has now defined severe GHD in adults as a peak response to insulin-induced hypoglycemia of less than 9mU/L (<3ng/mL).

It is essential that the insulin tolerance test is carried out under supervision by experienced staff and should not be performed in patients with epilepsy and/or ischemic heart disease. For those patients in whom the insulin tolerance test is contraindicated, glucagon or arginine may be used and a similar serum GH cutoff is applied for the diagnosis of severe GHD. Importantly, the insulin and glucagon tests have the advantage that they simultaneously test the adequacy of ACTH reserve. Combinations of arginine and GHRH result in higher peaks of GH secretion but as yet the definition of GHD using these combinations is not clearly established.

Although increasing age is associated with a reduction in spontaneous GH secretion it has less influence on the response to dynamic testing. Severe obesity may decrease the GH response to insulin hypoglycemia to levels suggestive of GHD but this phenomenon reverses with weight loss. Because of the possibility of false-positive diagnoses of GHD, particularly in the context of obesity, it is recommended that the diagnosis should be supported by evidence of structural pituitary disease and/or the presence of additional pituitary hormone deficiencies. The latter are a particularly important adjunct in diagnosis because of the very high probability (>90%) of GHD in a patient with two or three additional pituitary trophic hormone deficiencies (**Fig. 4.2**). The conventional stipulation that a diagnosis of GHD should be confirmed by two dynamic tests is of less importance in a patient who

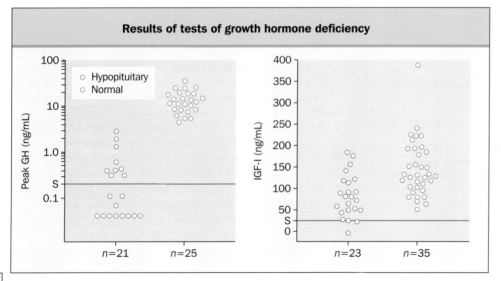

Figure 4.1 Results of tests of growth hormone deficiency. Growth hormone (GH) responses to insulin-induced hypoglycemia and baseline serum insulin-like growth factor-I (IGF-I) in patients with pituitary disorders and age-matched controls. (Modified with permission from Hoffman DM, O'Sullivan AJ, Baxter RC, Ho KY. Diagnosis of growth hormone deficiency in adults. Lancet 1994;343: 1064–8 © by The Lancet Ltd.)

Growth hormone response to insulin hypoglycemia

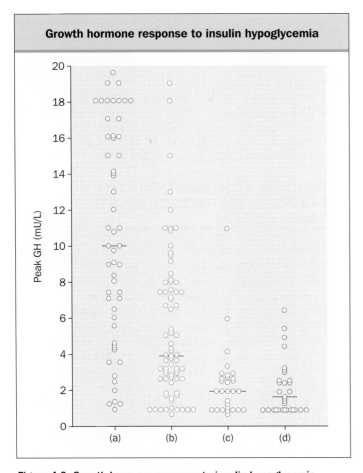

Figure 4.2 Growth hormone response to insulin hypoglycemia.
Peak serum growth hormone (GH) response to insulin hypoglycemia as a
function of numbers of additional pituitary hormone deficiencies in adult
patients with pituitary dysfunction. (a), (b), (c), and (d) indicate 0–3
additional pituitary deficiencies. (Modified with permission from
Toogood AA, Beardwell CG, Shalet SM. The severity of growth hormone
deficiency in adults with pituitary disease is related to the degree of
hypopituitarism. Clin Endocrinol. 1994;41:511–16.)

Symptoms and signs of the adult growth hormone deficiency syndrome

- Decreased energy levels
- Social isolation
- Lack of positive wellbeing
- Depressed mood
- Increased anxiety
- Increased body fat, particularly central adiposity
- Decreased muscle mass
- Decreased insulin sensitivity and increased prevalence of impaired glucose tolerance
- Increased LDL-cholesterol and Apo B. Decreased HDL-cholesterol
- Decreased bone density, associated with an increased risk of fracture
- A variable decrease in cardiac muscle mass
- Impaired cardiac function
- Decreased total and extracellular fluid volume
- Increased concentration of plasma fibrinogen and plasminogen activator inhibitor type I
- Accelerated atherogenesis

**Table 4.2 Symptoms and signs of the adult growth hormone
deficiency syndrome.** Apo B, apolipoprotein B; HDL, high-density
lipoprotein; LDL, low-density lipoprotein

CLINICAL MANIFESTATIONS OF GH DEFICIENCY

The adult GHD syndrome is characterized by a constellation
of symptoms and physical signs, which are summarized in
Table 4.2. While seemingly the most nonspecific of the clinical
features, decreased psychological wellbeing and quality of life
have proved to be the most striking subjective features of the
syndrome in the majority of patients. These have been examined using a variety of generic quality-of-life rating scales,
including the Nottingham Health Profile and the Psychological
General Well Being Schedule, and particularly significant
deficits have been documented in the domains of mood, anxiety, and social interaction. These findings are more evident in
patients with GHD of adult onset in comparison with adults
with childhood onset GHD, perhaps indicating psychological
adaptation in the latter.

Because of the heterogeneity of responses in various studies,
attempts have been made to develop quality of life instruments
that are specific for adult GHD, and of these, the Quality
of Life Assessment in Growth Hormone Deficient Adults
(QoL AGHDA) has gained wide acceptance for both baseline
assessment and longitudinal followup of patients on GH replacement. This cross-cultural, disease-specific, unidimensional, needs-
based quality of life instrument has been developed specifically
for the detection of deficits in needs achievement in areas that
had been previously demonstrated to be most commonly implicated in GHD adults. It consists of 25 questions requiring a

---

has an unequivocally abnormal GH response to a single test, combined with a pituitary lesion or previous history of radiotherapy
and/or additional endocrine deficit.

The diagnosis of GHD may also be supported by decreased
serum concentrations of the GH-dependent peptides insulin-like
growth factor-I (IGF-I), IGF binding protein 3 (IGFBP-3) and its
acid labile subunit of the ternary complex (ALS). Of these, IGF-
I is the most useful marker of GH action but its diagnostic value
for GHD is limited by the fact that approximately 30% of individuals with severe GHD will demonstrate a serum IGF-I concentration in the lower part of the age-related reference range.
Nonetheless, in the absence of other causes of a low serum
IGF-I, such as liver dysfunction or malnutrition, a low serum
IGF-I concentration provides strong confirmatory evidence for
GHD, especially if combined with other evidence of pituitary
disease and hypopituitarism.

yes/no response and the final score is obtained by summation of the 'yes' responses. The questionnaire has been shown to have excellent reliability, reproducibility, and construct validity across a range of languages. Higher numerical scores (to a maximum of 25) denote poorer quality of life.

Body composition changes, determined by quantitative computerized tomography, dual energy X-ray absorptiometry (DXA), or bioelectrical impedance methodologies, demonstrate increases in total and percentage fat mass with a predominantly central distribution that have been an invariable finding in all studies conducted to date. Importantly, they are also evident in patients who are not obese by body mass index criteria. Relatively crude, but reproducible, determination of the degree of central adiposity may also be made by calculation of the ratio of the waist to hip circumference ratio. Changes in indices of adiposity are paralleled by reductions in lean body and muscle mass, which are associated with a reduction in muscle strength and exercise tolerance evident on detailed physiologic measurement. GHD is also associated with a reduction in total body water and circulating volume. These factors, combined with a possible reduction in cardiac output, may partly explain the decrease in maximum exercise capacity and might also contribute to the deficit in subjective wellbeing. Importantly, the reduction in total body and intracellular water content may make an artifactual contribution to the decrease in lean body mass, particularly when the latter is determined by bioelectrical impedance. Reduction in insulin sensitivity and an increased prevalence of impaired glucose tolerance have been extensively documented in adult hypopituitary patients. It is postulated that the changes in body fat distribution are, at least in part, responsible for the adverse changes in insulin sensitivity.

Modest increments in median serum total cholesterol are an additional feature of adult GHD and are accounted for entirely by an increase in serum low-density lipoprotein (LDL)-cholesterol and apolipoprotein B. Median serum high-density lipoprotein (HDL)-cholesterol is slightly reduced and the overall adverse effects on lipid profiles are more striking in women. Accelerated atherogenesis, as indicated by an increment in ultrasonographically determined carotid artery intima–media thickness and fatty plaque formation, has been reported in adult-onset hypopituitarism and in adults with persisting childhood-onset GHD. Predisposition to macrovascular disease may also be exacerbated by increased plasma fibrinogen and plasminogen activator type 1.

An overall reduction in bone mineral density is well described in adult hypopituitarism and increases in fracture rates have also been reported in retrospective analyses. This relative osteopenia is accompanied by a decrease in indices of bone remodeling. Although these changes in bone metabolism are likely to be attributable to GHD, and indeed respond favorably to GH replacement, it is difficult to quantify the possible contributions of prolonged periods of untreated gonadal steroid deficiency and suboptimal replacement regimens for glucocorticoid and thyroid hormones. In contrast, adult GHD of childhood onset is associated with more profound reductions in bone mineral density. Bearing in mind the physiologic lag phase between completion of linear growth and achievement of peak bone mass, this may be a consequence of the conventional cessation of GH replacement as growth rate declines to less than 2cm/year, the latter being partly

dependent on GH action. The osteopenia of childhood-onset GHD does not necessarily imply the same degree of increased fracture risk as adult-onset osteopenia but would predict an increased risk of future osteoporosis as age-related bone loss is superimposed on a decreased peak bone mass.

Several studies have described an increase in prevalence of hypertension in adult-onset GHD. This may seem paradoxical in the context of the well-recognized antinatriuretic effects of GH but is consistent with the effects of GH in mediating the activity of nitric oxide synthase by vascular endothelium.

ADDITIONAL CONTRIBUTIONS TO THE CLINICAL FEATURES OF ADULT HYPOPITUITARISM

As indicated, it is possible that at least some of the features of adult hypopituitarism that have been attributed to GHD may be a consequence of unphysiologic replacement of glucocorticoid, gonadal steroid, and thyroid hormones. This consideration applies particularly to changes in bone mineral density and body composition. Similar regimens for hydrocortisone and thyroxine replacement as are generally used in hypopituitarism are employed in primary adrenal and thyroid failure respectively; measurements of bone density tend to be below the age-related mean in the former but are normal in the latter. Furthermore, the situation in hypopituitarism is complicated by the frequent accompaniment of gonadal steroid deficiency, which is usually of unknown duration. Nonetheless, available evidence indicates that qualitatively similar changes in bone mineral density are found in adult-onset isolated GHD as in panhypopituitarism, thus supporting a role for GHD in pathogenesis of any bone mass deficit.

The doses of glucocorticoid replacement employed in ACTH-deficient patients are similar to those used in primary adrenal failure and the latter is not associated with any change in body composition and specifically in body fat distribution. However, there are factors unique to the situation of GHD that may alter local tissue exposure to either endogenous or exogenous cortisol. The GH–IGF-I axis is known to be a determinant of the activity of the enzyme 11β-hydroxysteroid dehydrogenase type 1 (11βHSD1). This isoenzyme acts as a predominant reductase, particularly in liver and adipose tissue, increasing the net conversion of inactive cortisone to active cortisol (hydrocortisone). The activity of the enzyme is decreased by GH and, as a consequence, GHD is associated with a shift in the equilibrium set point in favor of cortisol production. It is therefore possible that the increase in central adiposity that characterizes the GHD state may be an indirect effect resulting from enhanced exposure to cortisol within adipocytes; a similar effect within hepatocytes might contribute to decreased insulin sensitivity. These phenomena would predict an increase in circulating serum cortisol in patients receiving hydrocortisone replacement but not in patients with intact ACTH reserve, in whom feedback effects would maintain normal circulating cortisol concentrations. However, because GH is also a negative determinant of circulating cortisol-binding globulin, it is not possible to directly compare serum total cortisol measurements in patients with GHD in comparison with the GH replete state.

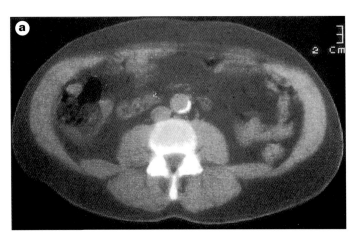
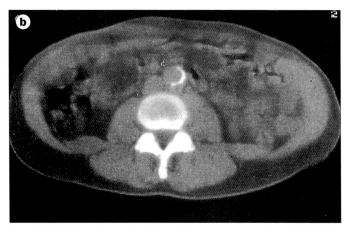

Figure 4.3 Fat distribution and growth hormone therapy. Changes in subcutaneous and intra-abdominal fat after 6 months of growth hormone replacement therapy. Computerized tomography scan of the abdomen before (a) and after (b) treatment with growth hormone demonstrates the predominant loss of 'central' as opposed to 'peripheral' fat. Fat appears black on CT image. (Courtesy of Professor B-Å Bengtsson.)

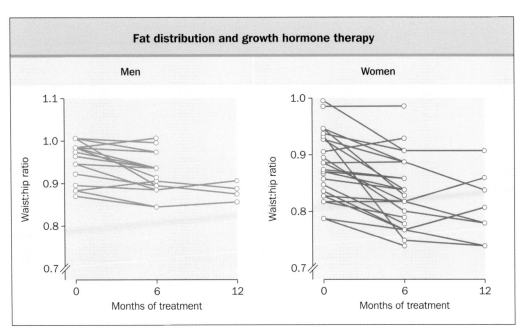

Figure 4.4 Fat distribution and growth hormone therapy. Waist:hip ratio versus months of treatment with growth hormone in men and women with growth hormone deficiency. (Modified with permission from Drake WM, Coyte D, Camacho-Hubner C, et al. Optimising growth hormone replacement therapy by dose titration in hypopituitary adults. J Clin Endocrinol Metab. 1998;83:3913–19 © The Endocrine Society.)

CLINICAL EFFICACY OF GH REPLACEMENT IN ADULT GHD

Body composition

Replacement therapy with GH results in significant reductions in total fat mass and central adiposity as determined by DXA, bioelectrical impedance, computerized tomography (**Fig. 4.3**) and waist:hip ratio (**Fig. 4.4**). While waist:hip ratio is a good indicator of baseline body fat distribution, because of simultaneous reductions in central and subcutaneous fat, it lacks sensitivity for longitudinal followup and change in waist circumference provides a more sensitive measure of improvement in central adiposity. Lean body mass increases in parallel with the change in fat mass, and total body water and circulating volume are also normalized. These beneficial effects occur within 3 months of

commencement of GH replacement and are sustained during follow up periods exceeding 2 years.

GH therapy also increases peripheral conversion of thyroxine to triiodothyronine (T_3) but this does not produce significant changes in circulating T_3 using current low dose GH replacement regimens. The set point of interconversion of cortisol and cortisone, under the influence of 11βHSD1, is also normalized. It is possible that these secondary hormonal changes may be partial mediators of the observed changes in body fat and its distribution.

Exercise performance

Improvement in exercise performance parallels the increase in lean body mass and normalization of body fluid balance. This has been examined by measurement of isometric strength, maximum oxygen uptake and maximum power output (**Fig. 4.5**). Many

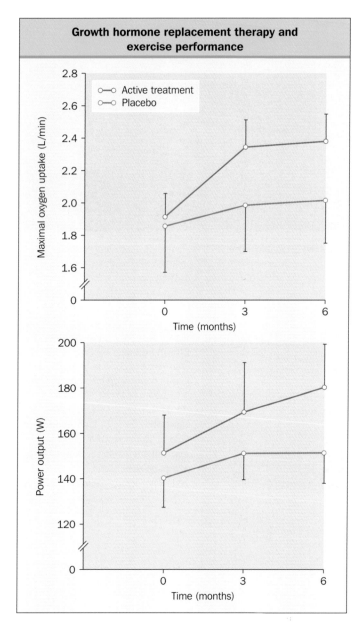

Figure 4.5 Growth hormone replacement therapy and exercise performance. Effect of 6 months of growth hormone replacement therapy on exercise performance. Maximal oxygen uptake and maximal power output were significantly impaired in adults with growth hormone deficiency but normalized following 6 months replacement therapy with growth hormone. (Modified from Cuneo RC, Salomon F, Sönksen PH. The growth hormone deficiency syndrome in adults. Clin Endocrinol. 1992;37:387–97.)

patients also report an improvement in physical activity and general vitality that overlaps with favorable changes in psychological wellbeing. The relative contributions of increased muscle mass, restoration of fluid balance, and increased wellbeing to increased physical activity remain speculative.

Psychological wellbeing and quality of life

The earliest placebo-controlled trials of GH replacement, which employed GH doses that we now know to have been excessive, suggested that approximately 50% of these patients demonstrated a significant subjective improvement and a desire

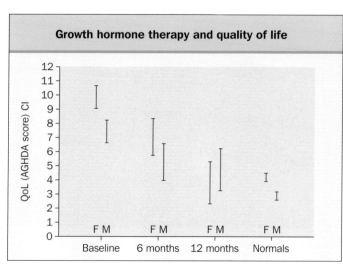

Figure 4.6 Growth hormone therapy and quality of life. Changes in the mean Quality of Life Assessment (QoL AGHDA) score in adult growth-hormone-deficient patients enrolled in the Pharmacia International Metabolic Surveillance study after 6 and 12 months of growth hormone replacement therapy compared with baseline and normal population scores from the World Health Organization Monitoring of Trends and Determinants in Cardiovascular Disease study. (Modified with permission from Bengtsson B-Å, Abs R, Bennmarker H, et al. The effects of treatment and the individual responsiveness to growth hormone (GH) replacement therapy in 665 GH-deficient adults. KIMS Study Group and the KIMS International Board. J Clin Endocrinol Metab. 1999;84:3929–35 © The Endocrine Society.)

to continue treatment long term. The most substantial benefit was evident in patients with the most severe GHD and greater perceived distress prior to commencing treatment. More recent experience has indicated a desire to continue replacement therapy in more than 80% of patients who are selected on the basis of a perceived quality of life deficit. This apparent discrepancy in efficacy of treatment is likely to be explained by two factors. First, the initial trials, by virtue of extensive exclusion criteria, may have eliminated patients who were most likely to benefit in terms of quality of life; second, the relatively high doses of GH used resulted in significant adverse effects, particularly fluid retention, which may have obscured subjective benefits. In current clinical practice, it is generally recommended that a 6-month course of GH replacement should be undertaken to assess clearly 'quality of life' benefits. These adverse effects are rarely seen with current low-dose regimens. In fact, the majority of patients will show benefit within 3 months of treatment but in a significant proportion it will be delayed until 6 months or even longer (**Fig. 4.6**). This lag phase in benefit may reflect the titration phase for achievement of optimum dose of GH replacement, which may extend beyond 3 months in women. It also provides strong evidence against a pure placebo effect in this aspect of efficacy of GH replacement.

Serum lipoproteins

GH replacement results in a significant reduction in serum total cholesterol that is most pronounced in women and persists during long-term followup (**Fig. 4.7**). This decrease in cholesterol is entirely accounted for by a reduction in LDL-cholesterol.

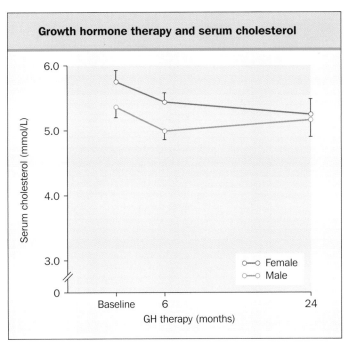

Figure 4.7 Growth hormone therapy and serum cholesterol. Changes in serum total cholesterol during 2 years of growth hormone (GH) replacement therapy in men and women with growth hormone deficiency. (Modified with permission from Florakis D, Hung V, Kaltsas G, et al. Sustained reduction in circulating cholesterol in adult hypopituitary patients given low dose titrated growth-hormone replacement therapy: a two year study. Clin Endocrinol. 2000;53:453–9.)

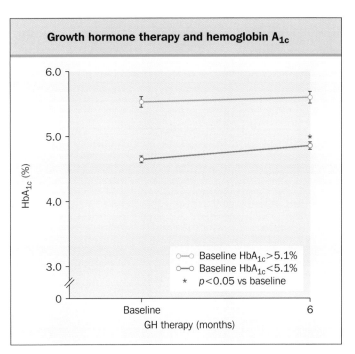

Figure 4.8 Growth hormone therapy and hemoglobin A$_{1c}$. Changes in percentage of hemoglobin (Hb)A$_{1c}$ during 6 months of growth hormone replacement therapy in adult growth-hormone-deficient patients with pretreatment percentage of HbA$_{1c}$ either above or within the reference range (<5.1%). There is no change in patients where HbA$_{1c}$ started above the normal range but a small rise, within the normal range, in patients whose pretreatment levels were within the normal range. (Modified with permission from Florakis D, Hung V, Kaltsas G, et al. Sustained reduction in circulating cholesterol in adult hypopituitary patients given low dose titrated growth hormone replacement therapy: a two year study. Clin Endocrinol. 2000;53:453–9.)

A modest increment in HDL-cholesterol is also observed but there is no significant change in serum triglyceride levels. Importantly, these reductions are greatest in those patients with pretreatment serum cholesterol levels of over 6.5mmol/L and are additive to the effects of any therapy with β-hydroxy-β-methylglutaryl-coenzyme A (HMG CoA) reductase inhibitors. Accompanying the beneficial effects of GH on LDL-cholesterol, several studies have observed modest increments in serum lipoprotein Lp(a) in patients who have otherwise demonstrated an improvement in lipoprotein profiles.

Insulin sensitivity and carbohydrate metabolism
The effect of GH replacement therapy on insulin sensitivity and glucose homeostasis is determined by the summation of the insulin-antagonistic effects of GH and its beneficial effects on central adiposity, the latter predicting an increase in insulin sensitivity. In fact, a net decrease in insulin sensitivity superimposed on the baseline state of relative insulin resistance is evident during the initial phase of GH replacement with a subsequent return to baseline sensitivity within 12 months of therapy. These phenomena are likely to explain the modest increase in plasma glucose, within the normal reference range, that is observed in many patients during GH replacement. Glycated hemoglobin (HbA$_{1c}$) also increases, albeit within the normal reference range, in patients with normal pretreatment levels but does not increase further above initial values in those patients with baseline elevation (**Fig. 4.8**). There is no evidence that GH replacement therapy results in an increased risk of

developing diabetes mellitus over and above the baseline increased prevalence but clearly continued surveillance is important. Similarly, only long-term follow up of large numbers of patients treated with GH will permit definite conclusions regarding the impact of the favorable modification of cardiovascular risk factors described above on morbidity and mortality.

Bone remodeling and bone mineral density
GH replacement results in increases in markers of bone resorption (e.g. urine or circulating deoxypyridinoline) and bone formation (e.g. osteocalcin and bone-specific alkaline phosphatase), the combination indicating an increase in bone remodeling. Bone mineral density tends to decrease by 6 months of treatment, consistent with an increase in osteoclastic activity and the bone remodeling space, but subsequently increases so that mean bone mineral density is above baseline by 18 months of GH replacement. This improvement, expressed as a standard deviation score, is sustained during long-term followup and is more pronounced in men (**Fig. 4.9**). Whether this improvement is translated into a reduction in fracture rate will only be evident during long-term followup studies.

Cardiovascular system
A hypokinetic cardiac state with reduction in left ventricular wall mass and cardiac output has been reported in adult GHD,

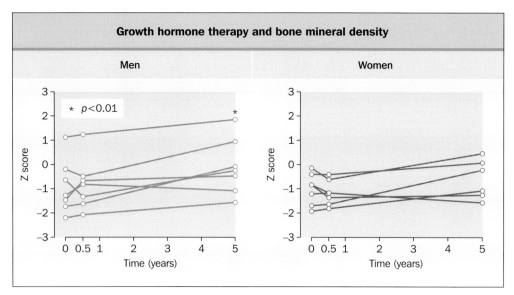

Figure 4.9 Growth hormone therapy and bone mineral density. Changes in lumbar spine bone mineral density age-related standard deviation score (Z score) during long-term growth hormone replacement therapy in men and women with growth hormone deficiency. (Modified with permission from Drake WM, Rodriguez-Arnao J, Weaver JU, et al. The influence of gender on the short and long-term effects of growth hormone replacement on bone metabolism and bone mineral density in hypopituitary adults – a 5-year study. Clin Endocrinol. 2001;54:525–32.)

particularly of childhood onset. Adult-onset GHD is also associated with increased prevalence of hypertension. While there is considerable heterogeneity in reports from different centers, most studies of GH replacement have documented an increment in left ventricular wall mass, stroke volume, fractional shortening, and improved diastolic function. Systolic and diastolic blood pressure tend to decrease in patients with baseline elevation, consistent with a reduction in peripheral vascular resistance possibly mediated by increased activity of endothelial nitric oxide synthase.

CRITERIA FOR SELECTION OF PATIENTS FOR GH REPLACEMENT

While the potential constituency for GH replacement has been clearly defined by consensus statements on diagnosis, the selection of patients for long-term treatment is less clearcut, not least because GHD does not necessarily give rise to classic symptoms or signs in all patients and the long-term effects of GH on mortality are yet to be determined. For this reason selection criteria are important and our own unit's recommendations are as follows:
- defined GHD using insulin tolerance (ITT), glucagon or arginine tests (peak GH <9mU/L (<3ng/mL)); supported by additional evidence of pituitary pathology or additional hormonal deficiencies;
- patient already receiving full supplementation of other deficient hormones as required;
- clinical symptoms or signs of GHD as follows:
  - severely decreased quality of life (QoL), as assessed using the QoL AGHDA or alternative, validated questionnaire; *and/or*
  - reduced bone density (T-score of less than –1SD), which by WHO criteria would predict a relative fracture risk of more than 2.5; *and/or*
  - reduced exercise tolerance and adverse cardiovascular risk profile.

GH DOSING

The doses used in the initial studies of GH replacement used weight- and surface-area-based dosing regimens as an extension of established pediatric practice. This approach could not take account of important differences in individual adult susceptibility to GH therapy and also resulted in excessive doses in obese patients and in men, the latter demonstrating a greater IGF-I-generating effect from a given GH dose compared with women. Subsequent studies suggest that optimum GH doses are best achieved by means of dose titration in a manner analogous to thyroid hormone replacement. Patients are commenced on 0.8IU (0.3mg) somatotropin subcutaneously once a day initially (0.4IU if known to have impairment of glucose tolerance). The dose is reviewed every 2–4 weeks according to clinical response, serum IGF-I and any side effects. Our experience has indicated a median dose requirement of 1.2IU (0.4mg) daily with a greater sensitivity to a given dose in male patients. Maintenance doses are reached significantly earlier in male patients (**Fig. 4.10**).

Because serum IGF-I may be in the lower part of the normal range in up to 30% of patients with adult-onset hypopituitarism we aim to use the minimum dose of growth hormone that will produce a serum IGF-1 level which lies between the median value and the upper limit of the age-matched normal range for the patient. This approach is empiric and is designed to minimize the risk of overtreatment with its attendant theoretical risks, which are analogous to those of acromegaly. Alternative indices of GH action, including insulin-like growth factor binding protein-3 (IGFBP-3) and acid-labile subunit (ALS), have proved to be less sensitive than IGF-I for purposes of dose titration (**Fig. 4.10**).

ADVERSE EFFECTS

The main side effects reported are arthralgia, edema, and carpal tunnel syndrome. These are believed to result from the rapid correction of the sodium and water depletion present in GHD patients. They are more frequent at the higher doses used in the

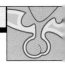

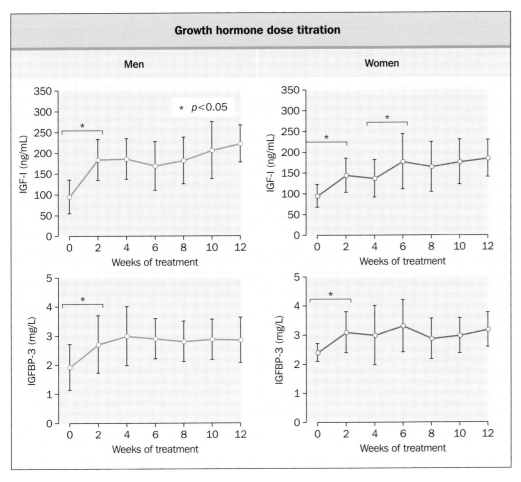

Figure 4.10 Growth hormone dose titration. Serum levels of insulin-like growth factor-I (IGF-I) and insulin-like growth factor binding protein-3 (IGFBP-3) vs weeks of treatment during growth hormone dose titration in men and women with growth hormone deficiency. (Modified with permission from Drake WM, Coyte D, Camacho-Hubner C, et al. Optimising growth hormone replacement therapy by dose titration in hypopituitary adults. J Clin Endocrinol Metab. 1998;83:3913–19 © The Endocrine Society.)

earlier studies and are uncommon when the dose is carefully titrated from a lower starting dose. Benign intracranial hypertension has been reported rarely and is less common than in pediatric practice; it is unlikely to complicate titrated dose regimens. Nevertheless, persistent severe headaches necessitate investigation. Continuing surveillance has not demonstrated an increased incidence in *de novo* neoplasia in patients on long-term GH replacement and prospective magnetic resonance imaging studies have not indicated a GH-dependent risk of pituitary tumor regrowth.

COST–BENEFIT OF GH REPLACEMENT

Cost of treating
Assuming 80% of adult-onset GHD patients require long-term treatment with GH; this equates to approximately 8 patients per 100 000 population. For a population of 1 000 000 the cost of providing a median dose to all patients can be estimated at US$410 000 on the basis of the average price in European countries. This figure might increase up to threefold if the cost of treating persisting childhood-onset GHD were included.

Cost of not treating
The main issues for consideration are reduced quality of life and burden on social services; osteoporosis, and increased fracture rate; and increased cardiovascular risk with the potential increased risk of cardiac and cerebrovascular death. The effect of GH replacement on cardiovascular morbidity will only emerge from very-long-term surveillance of treated patients, and multinational databases have been established for this purpose. GH replacement results in a reduction in LDL-cholesterol of approximately 10%. By analogy with other interventions, reducing LDL-cholesterol by 10% might cause a 30% reduction in the incidence of symptomatic coronary heart disease. Cardiac disease carries the cost of acute and long-term treatments. Prolonged GH replacement increases bone density and it seems reasonable to assume that this would reduce fracture rates and the costs of acute and long-term management. Conclusive evidence will depend on long-term clinical surveillance. Studies in Sweden show that GHD patients are more likely to be unemployed, retire early or require disability pensions. The costs to social services should therefore be included.

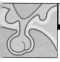
FURTHER READING

Abs R, Bengtsson B-Å, Hernberg-Ståhl E, et al. GH replacement in 1034 GH deficient adults: demographic and clinical characteristics, dosing and safety. Clin Endocrinol. 1999:50:703–13.

Bengtsson B-Å, Abs R, Bennmarker H, et al. The effects of treatment and the individual responsiveness to GH replacement therapy in 665 GH-deficient adults. J Clin Endocrinol Metab. 1999;84:3929–35.

Bülow B, Hagmar L, Mikoczy Z, Nordstrom CH, Erfurth EM. Increased cerebrovascular mortality in patients with hypopituitarism. Clin Endocrinol. 1997;46:75–81.

Capaldo B, Patti L, Oliverio U, et al. Increased arterial intima-media thickness in childhood onset growth hormone deficiency. J Clin Endocrinol Metab. 1997;82:1378–81.

Carroll PV, Christ ER, Bengtsson B-Å, et al. Growth hormone deficiency in adulthood and the effects of growth hormone replacement: a review. J Clin Endocrinol Metab. 1998;83:382–95.

Cuneo RC, Salomon F, Sönksen PH. The growth hormone deficiency syndrome in adults. Clin Endocrinol. 1992;37:387–97.

De Boer H, Blok G-J, Van der Veen EA. Clinical aspects of growth hormone deficiency in adults. Endocrine Rev. 1995;16:63–86.

Drake WM, Coyte D, Camacho-Hubner C, et al. Optimising growth hormone replacement therapy by dose titration in hypopituitary adults. J Clin Endocrinol Metab. 1998;83:3913–19.

Drake WM, Rodriguez-Arnao J, Weaver JU, et al. The influence of gender on the short and long-term effects of growth hormone replacement on bone metabolism and bone mineral density in hypopituitary adults – a 5-year study. Clin Endocrinol. 2001;54:525–32.

Florakis D, Hung V, Kaltsas G, et al. Sustained reduction in circulating cholesterol in adult hypopituitary patients given low dose titrated growth hormone replacement – a two year study. Clin Endocrinol. 2000;53:453–9.

Fowelin J, Attrall S, Lager I, Bengtsson B-Å. Effects of treatment with recombinant human growth hormone on insulin sensitivity and glucose metabolism in adults with growth hormone deficiency. Metabolism 1993;42:1443–7.

Hoffman DM, O'Sullivan AJ, Baxter RC, Ho KY. Diagnosis of growth hormone deficiency in adults. Lancet 1994;343:1064–8.

Johannsson G, Rosen T, Bosaeus I, Sjostrom L, Bengtsson B-Å. Two years of growth hormone (GH) treatment increases bone mineral content and density in hypopituitary patients with adult onset GH deficiency. J Clin Endocrinol Metab. 1996;81:2865–7.

Johansson J-O, Landin K, Tengboru L, Rosén T, Bengtsson B-Å. High fibrinogen and plasminogen activator inhibitor activity in growth hormone deficient adults. Arteriosclerosis Thrombosis 1994;14:434–7.

Markussis V, Beshyah SA, Fischer C, Sharp P, Nicolaides AN, Johnson DG. Detection of premature atherosclerosis by high resolution ultrasonography in symptom free hypopituitary adults. Lancet 1992;340:1188–92.

Olivecrona H, Ericsson S, Berglund L, Angelin B. Increased concentrations of serum lipoprotein(a) in response to growth hormone treatment Br Med J. 1993;306:1726–7.

Rahim A, Toogood AA, Shalet SM. The assessment of growth hormone status in normal young adult males using a variety of provocative agents. Clin Endocrinol. 1996;45:557–62.

Rosén T, Bengtsson B-Å. Premature mortality due to cardiovascular disease in hypopituitarism. Lancet 1990;336:285–8.

Rosén T, Bengtsson B-Å. Increased fracture frequency in adult patients with hypopituitarism and growth hormone deficiency. Eur J Endocrinol. 1997;137:240–5.

Thorner MO, Bengtsson B-Å, Ho KKY, et al. The diagnosis of growth hormone deficiency in adults: a consensus statement. J Clin Endocrinol Metab. 1998;83:379–81.

Toogood AA, Beardwell CG, Shalet SM. The severity of growth hormone deficiency in adults with pituitary disease is related to the degree of hypopituitarism. Clin Endocrinol. 1994;41:511–16.

Weaver JU, Monson JP, Noonan K, et al. The effect of low dose recombinant human growth hormone replacement on regional fat distribution, insulin sensitivity and cardiovascular risk factors in hypopituitary adults. J Clin Endocrinol Metab. 1995;80:153–9.

Weaver JU, Monson JP, Noonan K, et al. The effects of low dose recombinant human growth hormone replacement on indices of bone remodelling and bone mineral density in hypopituitary growth hormone deficient adults. Endocrinol Metab. 1996;3:55–61.

Wirén L, Bengtsson B-Å, Johannsson G. Beneficial effects of long term GH replacement therapy on quality of life in adults with GH deficiency. Clin Endocrinol. 1998;48:613–20.

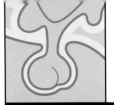

Section 1 Hypothalamus and Pituitary

Chapter 5

Acromegaly and Gigantism

John A H Wass

INTRODUCTION

Acromegaly is the clinical condition that results from prolonged, excessive circulating levels of growth hormone (GH) in adults (**Fig. 5.1**). The rare clinical counterpart of acromegaly, which occurs in younger patients before epiphyseal fusion, is called pituitary gigantism (**Fig. 5.2**).

Acromegaly was first described in 1886 by Pierre Marie, who noted 'a striking noncongenital hypertrophy of the extremities' including the face, hands, and feet. In 1891 Minkowski noted that this hypertrophy was always accompanied by an enlarged pituitary, which Tamburine in 1894 recognized as a pituitary adenoma. However, Harvey Cushing, in 1909, was the first to use the word 'hyperpituitarism' to describe the condition. This

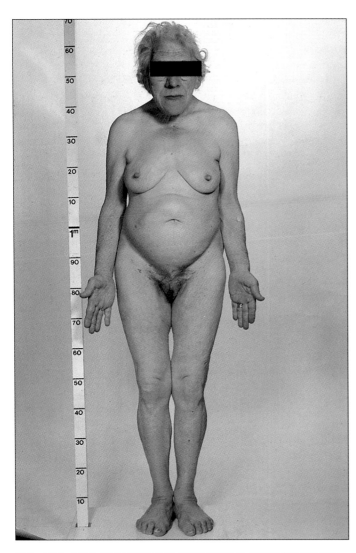

Figure 5.1 A female patient with acromegaly. The facial features have become coarse with progression of the disease.

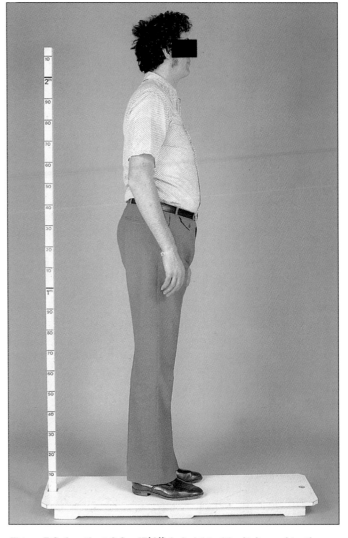

Figure 5.2 A patient 2.3m (7′6″) in height with pituitary gigantism. Gigantism is the rare, clinical counterpart of acromegaly and occurs in the young before epiphyseal fusion has taken place.

was confirmed in 1922 by Evans, who demonstrated that the parenteral injection of extracts of the anterior lobe of the pituitary gland causes true gigantism in rats, whose epiphyses never fuse, and acromegaly-like features in dogs, whose epiphyses do.

ETIOLOGY

Benign pituitary tumors are by far the most common cause of acromegaly; however, very rarely, pituitary carcinomas may be responsible (**Table 5.1**). Pituitary tumors may be associated with other endocrine adenomas (e.g. multiple endocrine neoplasia type 1), which most commonly involve the parathyroid glands, resulting in hypercalcemia.

Carcinoid tumors, usually of the pancreas or lung, may rarely be the cause of acromegaly through ectopic secretion of hypothalamic growth hormone releasing hormone (GHRH). However, instead of a pituitary tumor, these patients have somatotroph hyperplasia in the pituitary, which nevertheless may enlarge the fossa.

Histopathology of acromegaly-associated pituitary tumors

Microadenomas are rare (30%) and the tumors associated with acromegaly are more commonly intrasellar or extrasellar macroadenomas. While these tumors are usually acidophilic on conventional hematoxylin and eosin histologic staining (**Fig. 5.3**), acromegaly can also result from chromophobe adenomas. The secretion from pituitary adenomas usually consists of GH alone, but the tumor may also be of mixed cell types and 30% of patients with acromegaly are also hyperprolactinemic. Very occasionally GH and prolactin may originate from the same cell (mammosomatotropic tumor).

Growth hormone cell adenomas occur in both sparsely and densely granulated forms. The latter look very similar to normal somatotrophs and the cells stain with acid dyes, representing the eosinophil adenoma in the conventional classification. By contrast, the sparsely granulated somatotroph adenoma represents the chromophobe adenoma. Clinically, the sparsely granulated somatotroph adenomas tend to be more aggressive, the cells show less differentiation, and the tumor is more invasive.

Etiology of pituitary tumors

In some patients with acromegaly, as described previously, somatotroph hyperplasia may occur because of excessive secretion of GHRH from a hypothalamic hamartoma (a tumor-like lesion, usually present at birth, that ceases to grow when general body growth ceases), hypothalamic gangliocytoma (a tumor of mature gangliocytes), or carcinoid tumor of the lung or pancreas. However, over 99% of patients have a primary pituitary

tumor. Genetic factors may play a role in some tumors, e.g. in multiple endocrine neoplasia (MEN) syndrome type 1, where GH-secreting adenomas may constitute one of the neoplastic components (but are less common than prolactinoma).

Many receptors alter the level of intracellular cyclic nucleotides. Such receptors do not interact directly with the cyclase enzymes but work through an intermediate protein that binds guanosine 5´-triphosphate (GTP), called a GTP-binding protein or, more simply, a G-protein. Recently, a subset of GH-secreting human pituitary tumors has been discovered, which carry somatic mutations of G-protein α-chains that inhibit GTPase activity in somatotroph cells. The resulting activation of adenylate cyclase within GH-secreting adenoma cells bypasses the normal requirement of the cell to be activated by GHRH and thus it is autonomous. Such an oncogenic mutation may promote tumor growth by producing an autonomous action of proteins that normally transmit the proliferative signals initiated by extracellular factors.

DIAGNOSIS

Acromegaly is a disease of the whole organism in which everything but the central nervous system enlarges. Although the diagnosis is often made coincidentally, the patient usually presents complaining of a change in the appearance of the face, hands or whole body, headaches, sweating, goiter, or symptoms relating to renal stones. Early diagnosis is important but this depends on a high index of suspicion. It often helps to look at old photographs but a delay in diagnosis of many years may occur (**Fig. 5.4**). The condition is most frequently diagnosed in the third decade but may be found from the teenage years up until the eighth decade.

Lesions associated with excessive secretion of growth hormone (GH) and insulin-like growth factor-1		
Pituitary	Adenoma	GH-secreting adenoma
		GH and prolactin mixed adenoma
		GH- and TSH-secreting adenoma
		Carcinoma – GH-secreting
	Ectopic	GHRH-producing carcinoid, e.g. of pancreas or lung
	Hypothalamic	GHRH-producing tumors, e.g. gangliocytoma

Table 5.1 Lesions associated with excessive secretion of growth hormone and insulin-like growth factor-1. GHRH, growth-hormone-releasing hormone; TSH, thyroid-stimulating hormone.

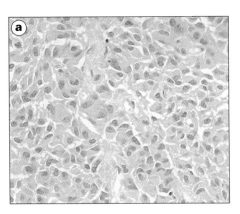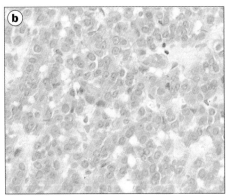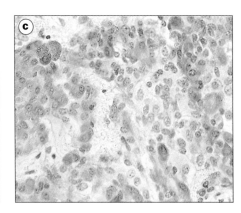

Figure 5.3 Pituitary tumor histology in acromegaly. In (a), using hematoxylin and eosin (H&E) stain, the eosinophils contain cytoplasmic red granules. The illustration shows a tumor consisting entirely of such cells. In (b), using periodic-acid–Schiff and orange G (PAS-OG) stain, the acidophils stain yellow or orange and the nuclei stain black. This stain is less subjective than H&E. In (c), an immunostain for GH in a GH-secreting tumor shows somatotrophs stained brown.

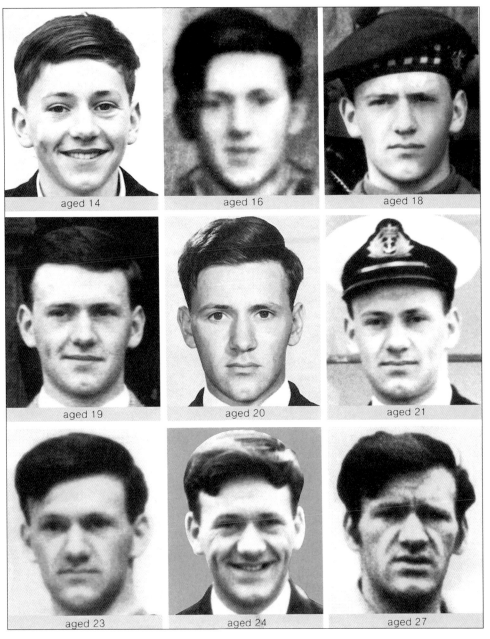

aged 14   aged 16   aged 18

aged 19   aged 20   aged 21

aged 23   aged 24   aged 27

Figure 5.4 The change in facial appearance of a patient with acromegaly taken over a 13-year period. The development of an acromegalic appearance is seen, with enlargement of the supraorbital ridges and nose, thickening of the lips and generalized coarsening of the features. (Reproduced from Wass JAH. Acromegaly. In: Belchetz PE, ed. Management of pituitary disease. London; Chapman & Hall: 1984.)

The clinical features of acromegaly		
1. GH excess	Acral enlargement	
	Skin	Increased sweating Oiliness and increased sebaceous activity
	Cardiovascular	Hypertension Ischemic heart disease Ventricular hypertrophy Cardiomyopathy
	Respiratory	Sleep apnea Kyphosis
	Alimentary	Macroglossia Visceromegaly Colonic polyps
	Neurologic	Carpal tunnel syndrome
	Musculoskeletal	Arthropathy, e.g. knee, hip, lumbar spine
	Reproductive	Amenorrhea Impotence
2. Metabolic consequences of high GH	Increased insulin resistance – diabetes mellitus (30%) Hypercalciuria Multinodular goiter Hypercalcemia (due to MEN-1)	
3. Endocrine effects of the pituitary adenoma	Co-secretion of prolactin or TSH Hypopituitarism	
4. Local tumor effects	Headache Visual field defects Cranial nerve palsy	

Table 5.2 The clinical features of acromegaly. GH, growth hormone; MEN-1, multiple endocrine neoplasia syndrome type 1; TSH, thyroid-stimulating hormone.

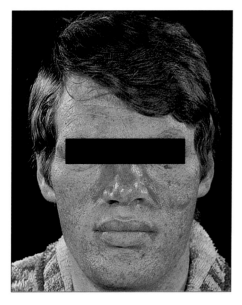

Figure 5.5 The characteristic facial features of a male patient with acromegaly.

CLINICAL FEATURES

The clinical features of acromegaly (**Table 5.2**) result from (1) oversecretion of GH, which has both clinical and metabolic sequelae, and (2) effects of the pituitary tumor, which are both local and endocrine. Several groups have noted that young patients with acromegaly tend to present with larger tumors, which appear to behave more aggressively than those that present in patients over the age of 50 years. Pituitary giants often have features of acromegaly as well as tall stature, especially when they present after the age of 16 or 17 years (see **Fig. 5.2**).

Clinical effects of growth hormone oversecretion
The typical facial appearance of a patient with acromegaly shows coarsening of the features with enlargement of the supraorbital ridges, a broad nose and also thickening of the soft tissues (**Fig. 5.5**). Sweating is excessive; sebaceous activity increases; papillomas and seborrheic warts occur; acne and hirsutism may also be present in women. Lips thicken and prognathism occurs, together with increased dental separation and macroglossia (**Fig. 5.6**). Using skull radiography (rarely performed nowadays), prognathism (where there is a loss of angle of the mandible) can be seen, as well as a thickened skull vault, enlargement of the sinuses, and, in more than 95% of patients, an abnormal and enlarged pituitary fossa (**Fig. 5.7**).

The hands also become enlarged in acromegaly and the fingers look short and fat (**Fig. 5.8**). Skin thickness and heel pad are increased, and the former is clearly visible on the dorsum of the hand (**Fig. 5.9**). Carpal tunnel syndrome often occurs because of the compression of the median nerve by soft tissue and bony overgrowth around the median nerve (see Fig 5.8). Kyphosis may be present in long-standing acromegaly or pituitary gigantism and lumbar spondylosis is common. Myopathy is frequent and, paradoxically, these patients are weak despite their muscular appearance.

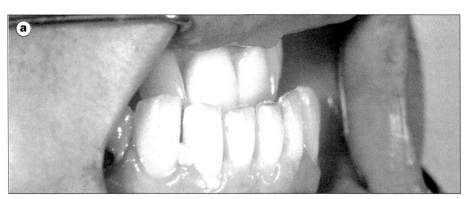

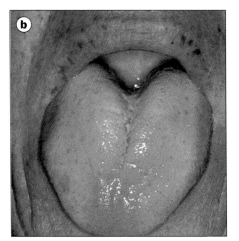
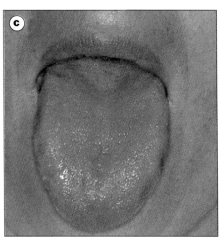

Figure 5.6 Prognathism (a) and macroglossia (b) in acromegaly. These are shown with a tongue of normal size (c) for comparison.

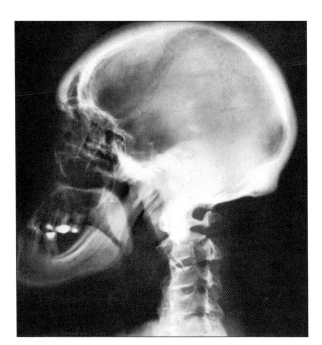

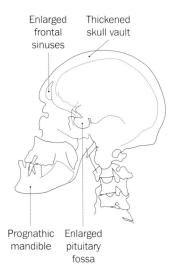

Enlarged frontal sinuses

Thickened skull vault

Prognathic mandible

Enlarged pituitary fossa

Figure 5.7 Skull radiograph of a patient with acromegaly. The enlarged pituitary fossa and sinuses, thickened skull vault, and prognathism with loss of angle of the mandible can be seen.

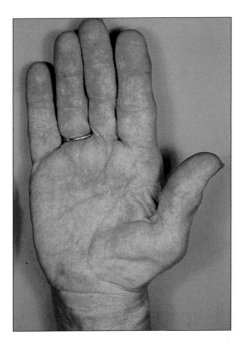

Figure 5.8 The enlarged hand of a patient with acromegaly. The hand is big and the fingers appear short because they are broad. There is thenar wasting because of longstanding compression of the median nerve in the carpal tunnel.

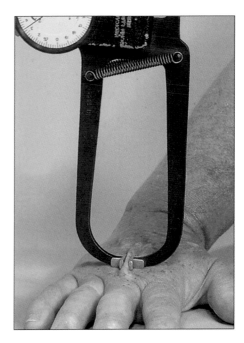

Figure 5.9 Increased skin thickness can be measured on the dorsum of the hand in acromegaly with skin fold calipers.

Radiographs of the hands show characteristic 'tufting' of the terminal phalanges. This may occur normally in heavy manual laborers but the increase in the joint spaces caused by the cartilaginous overgrowth typical of acromegaly does not (**Fig. 5.10**). Degenerative arthropathy occurs prematurely, particularly in the spine and other weightbearing joints such as the hips and knees. The joints enlarge as a result of synovial overgrowth and cartilaginous thickening. The lumbar spine may also show characteristic changes, with scalloping of the posterior vertebral margins and anterior new bone formation (**Fig. 5.11**).

Patients with acromegaly may also have cardiomegaly, related either to coronary artery disease, the incidence of which is increased in acromegaly, or to hypertension, which occurs in 35% of patients with acromegaly. In the absence of these, cardiomegaly may be related to a primary cardiomyopathy. Hypertension is usually 'essential' but may be caused by a coexistent pheochromocytoma or Conn's tumor.

Diabetes mellitus occurs in approximately 20% of patients and is secondary to insulin resistance as a consequence of raised GH levels. Hypercalcemia occurs in 5–10% of patients, usually resulting from parathyroid adenomas or hyperplasia (MEN type 1). There is also a 5% increased incidence of urinary calculi resulting from hypercalciuria, even in the absence of hypercalcemia. Hypercalciuria occurs in 80% of patients with acromegaly because GH is facultative in the synthesis of vitamin D and levels of 1,25-dihydroxycholecalciferol are raised.

Clinical effects of pituitary tumors

Patients may present with headaches caused by dural stretching. Most (>99%) have a tumor on magnetic resonance imaging (MRI; **Fig. 5.12**).

Upward extension of the pituitary tumor, when present, may cause a characteristic bitemporal field defect best found with the Goldmann perimeter. The enlarged supraorbital ridges may produce technical problems with visual field plotting; this is therefore best performed by tilting the head backwards by 20°. Lateral extension

of the tumor may cause third, fourth, and sixth cranial nerve palsies and, more rarely, temporal lobe epilepsy. Erosion into the sphenoid sinus may be associated with cerebrospinal fluid (CSF) rhinorrhea.

Hyperprolactinemia is common; females may present with amenorrhea and galactorrhea or infertility and males with low libido and impotence. Hyperprolactinemia is more commonly due to the coexistent production of prolactin by the tumor than to pituitary stalk compression by it. Stalk compression can lead to functional disconnection of the normal pituitary prolactin-secreting cells from the dopaminergic prolactin-inhibiting influence of the hypothalamus; this is then called a 'pseudoprolactinoma'. Hypopituitarism also occurs and this most frequently affects gonadotropin production. Later in the development of the disease, hypothyroidism and adrenocortical insufficiency may occur as a result of decreased thyroid-stimulating hormone (TSH) and adrenocorticotropic hormone (ACTH) reserves.

Hypopituitarism may be caused by pressure on the stalk by the tumor but is more often due to pressure of the tumor on normal pituitary tissue in the fossa. Diabetes insipidus, resulting from upward extension of the tumor into the hypothalamus, is exceedingly rare at presentation.

Growth hormone secretion in acromegaly

Basal GH levels are elevated and fluctuate widely but do not correlate well with any clinical manifestation of the disease. GH stimulates the production of insulin-like growth factor 1 (IGF-1) and levels of IGF-1 are almost always elevated in acromegaly (**Fig. 5.13**). In normal subjects, GH levels are mostly undetectable in the serum, apart from intermittent pulses of secretion, lasting approximately 90min, which occur five or six times during the day and more frequently at night. This pulsatile nature of GH secretion in normal subjects means that it may not be possible to distinguish between normality and acromegaly in some patients using basal GH concentrations; dynamic tests are therefore necessary.

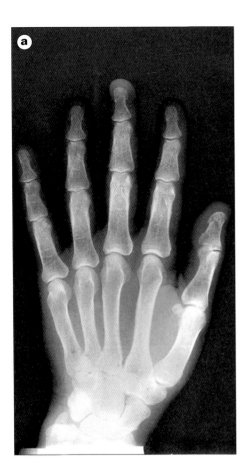

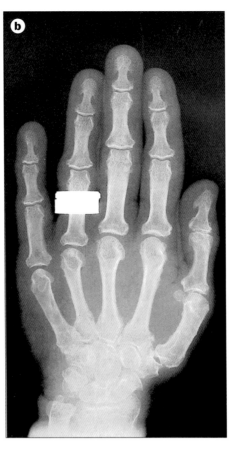

Figure 5.10 Comparison of radiographs of (a) a normal and (b) an acromegalic hand. The characteristic tufting of the terminal phalanges in the patient with acromegaly is shown, together with an increase in joint space due to cartilaginous overgrowth.

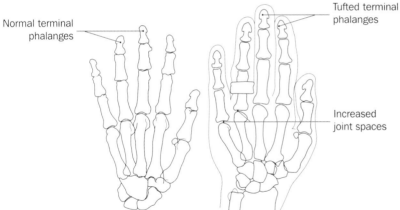

Normal terminal phalanges

Tufted terminal phalanges

Increased joint spaces

A rise in circulating glucose normally causes a suppression of GH to below 1mU/L (0.5ng/mL) but this is not the case in acromegaly (**Fig. 5.14**). Usually, only a slight or no fall in serum GH occurs in acromegaly and there may even be a paradoxical rise. This phenomenon is not specific to acromegaly and may also occur in severe hepatic or renal disease, in anorexia nervosa, in Laron's syndrome, and in patients on heroin or L-dopa. Dopamine and related drugs cause a rise in serum GH levels in normal subjects. In 1972 L-dopa was first found to cause a paradoxical suppression of GH in many patients with acromegaly; bromocriptine and cabergoline, long-acting dopamine agonists, also have this property. These effects are antagonized by haloperidol, pimozide, and metoclopramide, which are specific dopamine antagonists. The hypothalamic hormone somatostatin also decreases GH secretion in acromegaly. Unfortunately, its short half-life means that its effects wear off after a few minutes. Long-acting depot analogs of somatostatin (e.g. octreotide and lanreotide) have become available for use in the treatment of acromegaly. Normal activation of the growth hormone receptor involves binding and receptor dimerization (**Fig. 5.15**).

The investigation of a new patient with acromegaly is shown in **Table 5.3**.

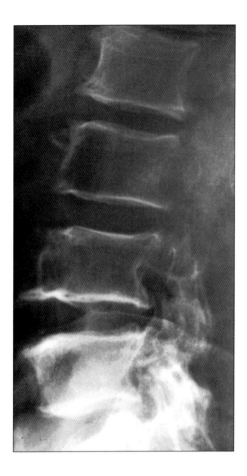

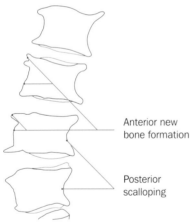

Figure 5.11 Radiographic appearance of the lumbar spine in acromegaly. Scalloping of the posterior margin of the vertebrae and anterior new bone formation are present.

Anterior new bone formation

Posterior scalloping

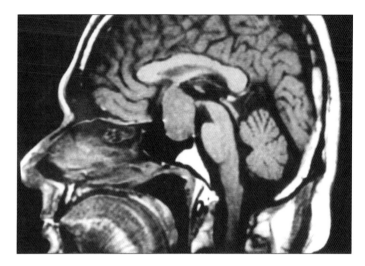

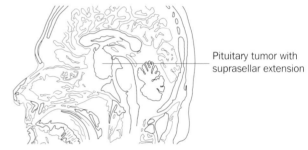

Pituitary tumor with suprasellar extension

Figure 5.12 Magnetic resonance image showing a large pituitary tumor with suprasellar extension causing acromegaly.

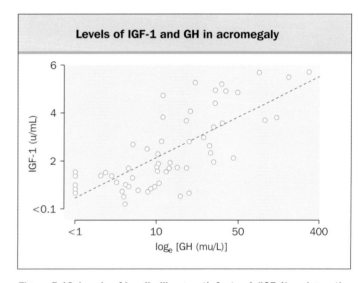

Figure 5.13 Levels of insulin-like growth factor 1 (IGF-1) and growth hormone (GH) acromegaly. The natural logarithm of serum GH concentration (mU/L) is plotted against the concentration of serum IGF-1 (u/mL), showing the relationship between them.

PROGNOSIS AND TREATMENT

Mortality is approximately doubled in acromegaly compared with the normal population (**Fig. 5.16**). The main reason for this is the presence of cardiovascular and cerebrovascular disease secondary to hypertension and diabetes mellitus. Respiratory disease also occurs with increased frequency. Early treatment is therefore recommended.

Aims of treatment should be the relief of symptoms and the reversal of the somatic changes occurring with acromegaly, together with reversal of the associated metabolic abnormalities. The ideal treatment should cause the minimum disturbance to the patient, with no side effects, particularly hypopituitarism.

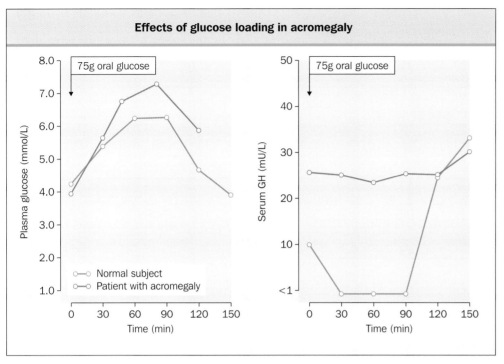

Figure 5.14 Effect of glucose loading in acromegaly. The figure shows the effects of a 75g glucose load on blood glucose and growth hormone (GH) levels in a normal subject and a patient with acromegaly. GH levels are acutely suppressed in normal subjects following a glucose load, whereas in acromegaly there is either no suppression or occasionally even a paradoxical rise. Carbohydrate tolerance is normal in both subjects.

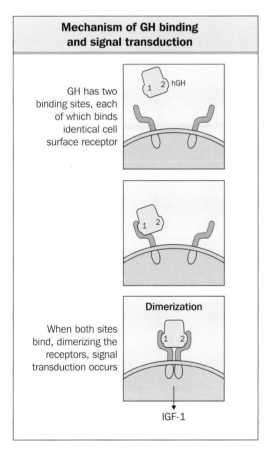

Figure 5.15 Mechanism of growth hormone (GH) binding and signal transduction. IGF-1, insulin-like growth factor 1.

Investigation of acromegaly

1. Establish diagnosis	75g OGTT Serum IGF-1
2. Establish GH levels	Mean of several serum GHs (day curve)
3. Metabolic consequences of high GH	OGTT ($\pm$HbA$_1$C) 24-hour urine calcium excretion
4. Pituitary function	Serum LH/FSH + T/E$_2$ Serum fT$_4$ + TSH Serum cortisol at 9.00 ITT for cortisol
5. Pituitary anatomy	MRI Visual fields
6. Other (coexistent) diagnoses	Serum Ca (MEN-1) Urine catecholamines (pheochromocytoma)

Table 5.3 Investigation of acromegaly. FSH, follicle-stimulating hormone; fT$_4$, free thyroxine; GH, growth hormone; IGF, insulin-like growth factor; ITT, insulin tolerance test; MEN-1, multiple endocrine neoplasia syndrome type 1; MRI, magnetic resonance imaging; OGTT, oral glucose tolerance test; T, testosterone; E$_2$, estradiol; TSH, thyroid-stimulating hormone.

Early treatment avoids the subsequent complications of diabetes mellitus, enlargement of the tumor, hypopituitarism, osteoarthritis, and cardiomyopathy.

Mortality in acromegaly is the same as normal in patients whose mean GH is 5mU/L ($\approx$ 2.5ng/mL) or less. There are few data on IGF-1, but one study showed that, if this was normal, mortality is the same as the normal population. Therefore, the biochemical aims of treatment are a mean GH through the day

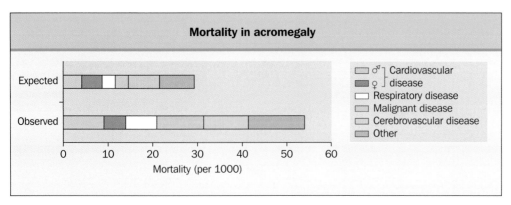

Figure 5.16 Mortality in acromegaly.
It can be seen that the observed mortality is approximately double that expected for normal patients. Significant differences are seen in cardiovascular disease in men, and in cerebrovascular and respiratory disease (Adapted from Wright AD, Hill DM, Lowy C, Russell-Fraser T. Mortality and acromegaly. Q J Med. 1970;39:1–16.).

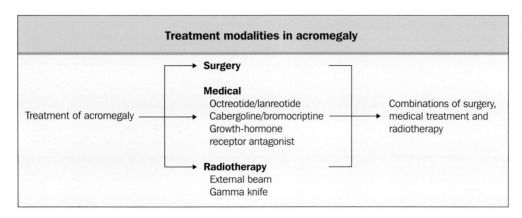

Figure 5.17 Treatment modalities in acromegaly.

of 5mU/L or less and a normal IGF-1. The treatments available fall into three groups (**Fig. 5.17**): (1) surgery, via the transsphenoidal or transfrontal route; (2) medical therapy using a long-acting somatostatin analog (e.g. octreotide or lanreotide), a GH-receptor antagonist, or a dopamine agonist (e.g. cabergoline or bromocriptine) and (3) radiotherapy using a linear accelerator, a cobalt source, or a proton beam.

Surgery

Surgery is the primary treatment for acromegaly (see Chapter 8). It most rapidly accomplishes a reduction in GH levels. The transsphenoidal route is mostly used and was the route first used by Harvey Cushing (**Fig. 5.18**). Small, medium-sized, and some large tumors, with suprasellar extensions, can be removed by this route. Removal of the latter can improve field defects once pressure on the optic chiasm is released. Cure by the transsphenoidal route is most often achieved with small tumors of under 1cm in diameter. Cure is less frequent, and postoperative hypopituitarism more frequent, with larger tumors, in part because the tumors have a tendency to infiltrate, locally, the bone and the dura (**Table 5.4**). A small proportion of tumors recur after surgery so, in any patient with GH levels that are detectable postoperatively, radiotherapy should be considered. Side effects of transsphenoidal surgery include operative bleeding, meningitis, pulmonary embolism, postoperative diabetes insipidus, hypopituitarism, and local nasal complications, but mortality is low (<1%).

A dedicated pituitary surgeon improves the outcomes of surgery. The transethmoidal approach to the sphenoid sinus is rarely

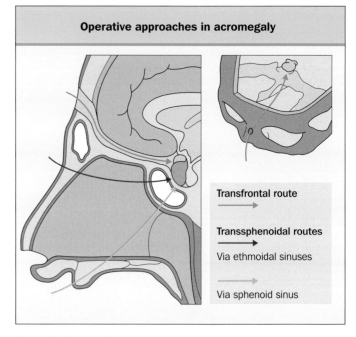

Figure 5.18 Operative approaches in acromegaly. Possible approaches are transfrontal, transsphenoidal, and transethmoidal.

used nowadays. Transfrontal surgery is occasionally necessary for very large extrasellar extensions, and these are most often seen in young patients with acromegaly presenting with rapidly growing tumors. Cure of acromegaly using this operative approach is

Table 5.4 Comparison of outcomes from transsphenoidal surgery for acromegaly

Location	Years	Cure rates (%)	Criteria for cure	Postoperative pituitary function
Newcastle, UK	1980–91	Micro 64	Nadir OGTT < 2mU/L (1.0ng/mL)	N/A
		Macro 48		
Oxford, UK	1974–95	Micro 91	OGTT < 2mU/L or mean GH < 5mU/L (2.5ng/mL)	14% deteriorated
		Macro 45		31% improved
Massachusetts, USA	1978–96	Micro 91	Normal IGF-1	17% deteriorated
		Macro 48	Random GH < 5mU/L (2.5ng/mL) or nadir GTT < 5mU/L (< 2.5ng/mL)	

Table 5.4 Comparison of outcomes from transsphenoidal surgery for acromegaly. GH, growth hormone; IGF, insulin-like growth factor; NA, not available; OGTT, oral glucose tolerance test.

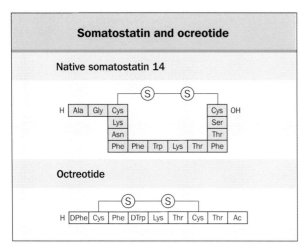

Figure 5.19 Somatostatin and octreotide. The figure illustrates the structures of native somatostatin and the long-acting somatostatin analog octreotide.

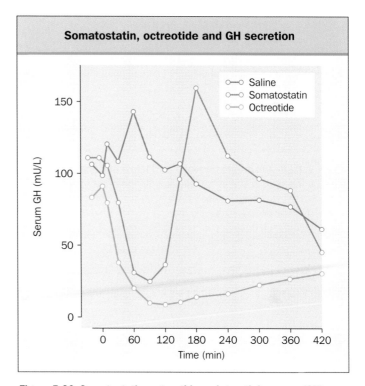

Figure 5.20 Somatostatin, octreotide and growth hormone (GH) secretion. The graph illustrates the differing effects of an intravenous infusion of octreotide, native somatostatin and saline on serum GH secretion in a patient with acromegaly.

virtually unknown, because of the difficulty in clearing the pituitary fossa of tumorous tissue, and postoperative radiotherapy is necessary. Field defects may be relieved but the morbidity of the transfrontal operative approach is higher as it involves craniotomy, frontal lobe retraction, and section of an olfactory nerve.

Medical therapy
Medical treatment of acromegaly is given using: octreotide or lanreotide, synthetic long-acting analogs of somatostatin (**Fig. 5.19**); one of the dopamine agonists, cabergoline or bromocriptine; or the GH-receptor antagonist pegvisomant.

Somatostatin analogs
Natural somatostatin, present in the hypothalamus, gastrointestinal tract, and pancreas, suppresses GH and insulin release for equal, brief periods. Octreotide has a longer duration of action on GH secretion than native somatostatin (**Fig. 5.20**) but insulin and glucagon suppression is of shorter duration than that of GH. In the majority of patients with acromegaly,

if octreotide is administered subcutaneously in doses of 300–600μg per day (100–200μg 8-hourly), GH levels are suppressed (**Fig. 5.21**) such that 50% of patients have average levels below 5mU/L. Recently, depot preparations of octreotide and other somatostatin analogs (lanreotide) have become available. These enable acromegaly to be controlled in the same proportion of patients with injections given every 4 weeks for octreotide and every 2 weeks for lanreotide. Comparison in the same patients shows that octreotide is more effective (**Table 5.5**).

Serum GH levels and octreotide therapy

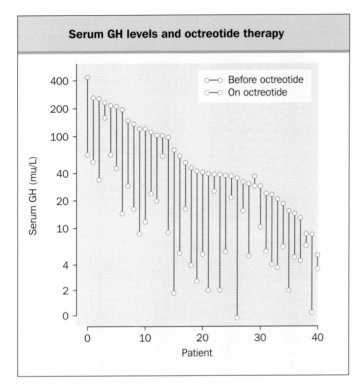

○—○ Before octreotide
○—○ On octreotide

Serum GH (mu/L)

Patient

Figure 5.21 Serum growth hormone (GH) levels and octreotide therapy. The figure illustrates the reduction in mean serum GH levels seen in patients with acromegaly receiving long-term subcutaneous octreotide therapy in doses of 150–600µg per day.

Depot octreotide and lanreotide in acromegaly

	GH <5mU/L	IGF-1 normal
Octreotide	80%	70%
Lanreotide	78%	56%

Table 5.5 Depot octreotide and lanreotide in acromegaly – within patient comparison in 10 patients.

Usually, carbohydrate tolerance does not worsen with octreotide administration, despite transient insulin suppression. Symptomatic relief is good and headaches may be dramatically reduced. At least 50% of tumors shrink in size (**Fig. 5.22**) but this is not as great in volume, nor as rapid, as the effect of bromo-criptine in prolactinoma. Side effects do occur with octreotide (**Table 5.6**). Initial diarrhea and abdominal pain usually settle with time. Gallstones have been found with increased frequency in patients on octreotide, because of a combination of factors, including gallbladder stasis, induced by octreotide, as well as biliary saturation with cholesterol. The gallstones are usually without clinical effects. Some patients have been found to have gastritis histologically, but without symptoms.

Dopamine agonists

In normal subjects, dopamine agonists raise GH levels but in patients with acromegaly, paradoxically, lower them. Cabergoline

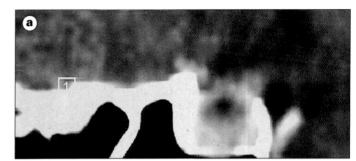

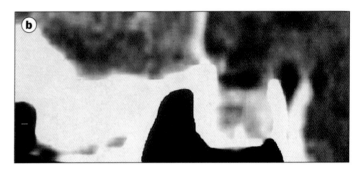

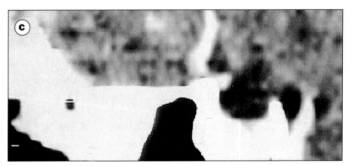

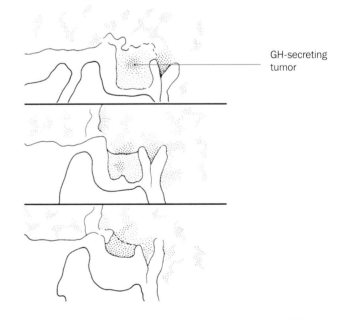

GH-secreting tumor

Figure 5.22 Effect of octreotide on tumor size in a patient with acromegaly with a pure growth-hormone-secreting tumor. Computerized tomography scans taken (a) at the commencement of treatment, (b) at 24 weeks and (c) at 43 weeks. No other treatment was given.

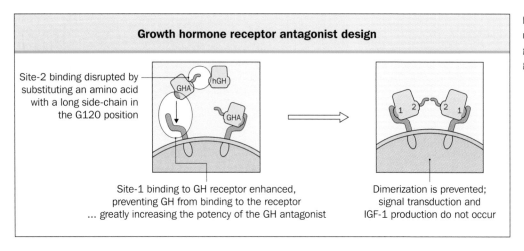

Growth hormone receptor antagonist design

Site-2 binding disrupted by substituting an amino acid with a long side-chain in the G120 position

Site-1 binding to GH receptor enhanced, preventing GH from binding to the receptor ... greatly increasing the potency of the GH antagonist

Dimerization is prevented; signal transduction and IGF-1 production do not occur

Figure 5.23 Growth-hormone-receptor antagonist design. GH, growth hormone; IGF-1, insulin-like growth factor 1.

Side effects of octreotide		
Local		Stinging
Gastroenterologic	Short term	Diarrhea
		Abdominal pain
	Long term	Gallstones
		Gastritis
Endocrinologic		Rarely, worsening of carbohydrate tolerance
		Hypoglycemia
		Dependency
Biochemical		Antibody formation

Table 5.6 Side effects of octreotide. Stinging occurring at the site of the injection is transient and may be obviated by warming the solution prior to injection. Gallstones and gastritis are usually without clinical effects.

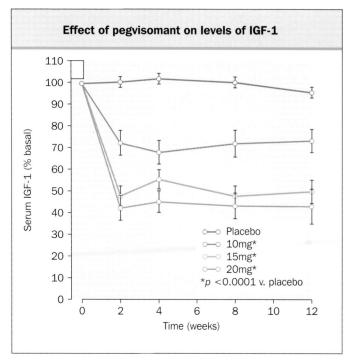

Effect of pegvisomant on levels of IGF-1

Serum IGF-1 (% basal)

Placebo
10mg*
15mg*
20mg*
*$p < 0.0001$ v. placebo

Time (weeks)

Figure 5.24 Effect of pegvisomant on levels of insulin-like growth factor 1 (IGF-1). The figure displays the serum insulin-like growth factor 1 (IGF-1) as a percentage of basal levels in 112 patients with acromegaly on daily pegvisomant or placebo. (Adapted from Trainer PJ, Drake WM, Katznelson L, et al. Treatment of acromegaly with the growth hormone-receptor antagonist pegvisomant. N Engl J Med. 2000;342:1171–7.)

and bromocriptine suppress GH levels in about 70% of patients with acromegaly but only rarely are GH levels reduced to normal.

Growth-hormone-receptor antagonists

A novel GH-receptor antagonist, pegvisomant, has recently been developed and has undergone evaluation for the treatment of acromegaly (**Figs 5.23–5.25**). The drug is a recombinant protein with a structural similarity to wild-type human growth hormone but mutations have been made at the sites of interaction with the GH receptor to leave this inactivated and unresponsive to endogenous growth hormone. Mutations at one site lead to increased affinity with the receptor compared to endogenous growth hormone and a mutation at another site prevents binding with the second growth hormone receptor and also prevents receptor dimerization. Thus irreversible binding to the growth hormone receptor leads to inhibition of signal transduction and therefore a lowering of IGF-1. Pegylation increases the drug's half life and reduces the immunogenicity. The drug has to be administered subcutaneously. IGF-1 levels fall to normal in over

90% of patients. The drug is generally well tolerated but further work is needed in this area.

Although in most patients the response of the GH level to octreotide is better than to dopamine agonists, there are occasional patients with acromegaly who respond better to the latter.

Patients who are resistant to both ocreotide and dopamine agonists usually respond to pegvisomant.

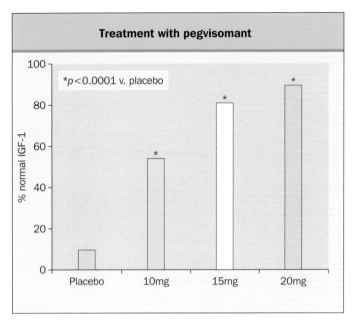

Figure 5.25 Treatment with pegvisomant. The figure shows the percentage of 112 patients with acromegaly achieving a normal age-related serum insulin-like growth factor 1 (IGF-1) on pegvisomant. (Adapted from Trainer PJ, Drake WM, Katznelson L, et al. Treatment of acromegaly with the growth hormone-receptor antagonist pegvisomant. N Engl J Med. 2000;342:1171–7.)

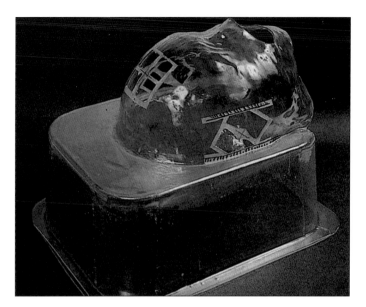

Figure 5.26 An individual head mask used to position the patient accurately during radiotherapy. Three fields are used and the daily dose of radiation should not exceed 180cGy.

Radiotherapy

Radiotherapy is an effective treatment for acromegaly but its effects are slow in onset. Although the greatest fall occurs in the first year after treatment, GH levels, if still raised, continue to fall for at least 15 years. A great deal of skill and careful planning is necessary to ensure success without complications. Best results occur using a linear accelerator and a three-field technique, which allows the largest dose of radiation to be delivered safely to the tumor; this is not the case using the simpler two-field, parallel opposed field technique. Pretreatment MRI is necessary to completely delineate the upper, lower, and lateral margins of the tumor. A dose of 4500cGy should be delivered over 25 treatment days, using five fractions per week, each fraction consisting of no more than 180cGy. Using this technique no radiation-induced neurologic damage has been recorded by the author. During treatment, an individual head mask is used to encompass and immobilize the whole of the patient's head; this improves accuracy and safety (**Fig. 5.26**).

With external pituitary irradiation using a linear accelerator, a mean fall in GH levels of 77% after 5 years has been obtained (**Fig. 5.27**) and, at the end of 10 years, 60% of patients have serum GH concentrations of less than 5mU/L (2.5ng/mL). IGF-1 values are normal in 56% at 10 years. The effect is more rapid if the initiating serum GH level prior to radiotherapy is lower. Thus, if GH levels are greater than 50mU/L (25ng/mL), the time taken for there to be a fall of the average serum GH to less than 5mU/L (2.5ng/mL) is longer: 6 years versus 4 years if pretreatment serum GH is below 50mU/L. Recurrence of tumor growth is very rare after radiotherapy – less than 1%.

Hypopituitarism occurs after external pituitary irradiation in approximately 50% of patients and may develop gradually, becoming apparent some years after treatment. Thus, it is imperative to measure pituitary function regularly after the administration of pituitary irradiation.

Gamma knife radio surgery is an effective method of delivering radiation therapy in a single session to GH secreting tumors. The data that there are suggest that pituitary hypersecretion may resolve faster with gamma knife than other forms of radiotherapy but longer term data are needed on this and the effect on pituitary function.

Choice of different treatments in acromegaly

Patients with acromegaly have either mixed GH and prolactin secreting tumors (30%) or pituitary tumors that secrete GH alone. Clinical experience suggests that there is a spectrum of disease ranging from young patients, who often have very large, aggressively behaving tumors associated with very high levels of GH, to older patients who have much smaller tumors with slower progression and lower levels of GH. Often all the available modalities of treatment are needed in a single patient (**Fig. 5.28**), particularly with aggressive tumors.

It is clear that surgery results in a rapid fall in GH levels but, equally, it is not always successful or permanent, particularly in patients with large tumors in whom there is a significant incidence of surgically induced hypopituitarism and occasional recurrence. In most cases, surgery may be performed via the transsphenoidal route.

If surgery is not curative medical treatment is advised. The first line treatment at present is long acting octreotide given after a test dose to establish response every 28 days. If there is a satisfactory response (normal IGF-1$_1$ and GH < 5mU/L) this can be continued. If not external pituitary irradiation should be recommended.

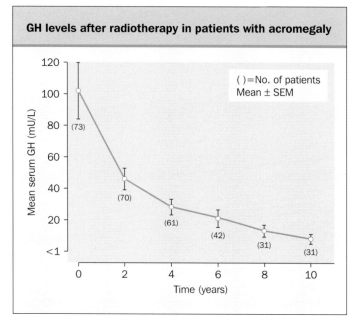

Figure 5.27 Growth hormone levels after radiotherapy in patients with acromegaly.

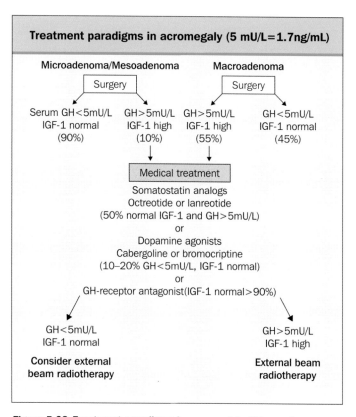

Figure 5.28 Treatment paradigms in acromegaly. GH, growth hormone; IGF-1, insulin-like growth factor 1. Mesoadenoma is an intrasellar macroadenoma.

CONCLUSIONS

Acromegaly is an insidious disease which requires a high degree of suspicion on the part of the clinician for early diagnosis to be made. This is important because of the greater mortality associated with this condition which is twice that of normal.

No treatment currently available satisfies all the requirements of an ideal therapy. Surgery, if successful, rapidly reduces GH levels to normal, but may not eradicate circulating GH and may cause hypopituitarism, particularly with large tumors. Radiotherapy is successful but takes time to act and causes hypopituitarism in a proportion of cases. Medical treatment with somatostatin analogs, dopamine agonists or the GH receptor antagonist offer the potential for the control of GH function in most patients and the latter has an exciting potential. Often, after careful judgement, all three types of treatment may be needed to reduce GH levels to normal.

FURTHER READING

Alexander L, Appleton D, Hall R, et al. Epidemiology of acromegaly in the Newcastle region. Clin Endocrinol. 1980:12:71–79.

Battershill PE, Clissold SP. Octreotide, a review of its pharmaco-dynamic properties and therapeutic potential in conditions associated with excessive peptide secretion. Drugs 1989:38:658–702.

Jones AE. Radiation oncogenesis in relation to the treatment of pituitary tumours. Clin Endocrinol. 1991:35:379–98.

Wass JAH, Laws ER, Randall RV, Sheline GE. The treatment of acromegaly. Clin Endocrin Metab. 1986:15:683–707.

Wright AD, Hill DM, Lowy C, Russell-Fraser T. Mortality and acromegaly. Q J Med. 1970:39:1–16.

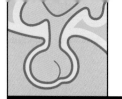

Hyperprolactinemia

Michael O Thorner

PROLACTIN SECRETION

Prolactin is secreted by the lactotroph cells of the anterior pituitary. The control of its secretion, like that of other anterior pituitary hormones, is regulated by the hypothalamus. Unlike the other anterior pituitary hormones, however, the hypothalamic influence is of tonic inhibition (**Fig. 6.1**).

The hypothalamus secretes two hypothalamic factors to control prolactin secretion: a prolactin-releasing factor (PRF) and a prolactin-release-inhibiting factor (PIF). The latter is almost certainly the catecholamine dopamine, although the possibility of the existence of noncatecholamine PIFs cannot be excluded. Additionally, γ-aminobutyric acid (GABA) may play a role as an inhibitor and there may well also be one or more PIF peptides. The nature of PRF is unclear, although it is known that thyrotropin-releasing hormone (TRH) can act as a PRF. Other candidates that may be involved in the release of prolactin include vasoactive intestinal peptide (VIP) and PHM-27, the latter being a peptide with structural homology to VIP (see Chapter 1).

CAUSES OF HYPERPROLACTINEMIA

The causes of hyperprolactinemia may be considered, in a simplified fashion, as resulting from four basic abnormalities of prolactin secretion (**Fig. 6.2**). In some patients, however, it is not possible to elucidate the cause of hyperprolactinemia.

Hypothalamic dopamine deficiency
Diseases of the hypothalamus, such as tumors, arteriovenous malformations, and inflammatory processes, might be expected to result in either diminished synthesis or release of dopamine. Furthermore, certain drugs (e.g. α-methyldopa and reserpine) are capable of depleting the central dopamine stores.

Defective transport mechanisms
Section of the pituitary stalk results in impaired transport of dopamine from the hypothalamus to the lactotrophs. Pituitary or stalk tumors with abnormal blood supplies, or their pressure effects, may interfere with the circulatory pathway from the hypothalamus down the pituitary stalk to the normal lactotrophs or a tumor, producing effective dopamine deficiency due to a functional stalk section.

Lactotroph insensitivity to dopamine
Although dopamine receptors have been found on human pituitary adenoma cells, they are often not functionally intact. Receptor sensitivity to dopamine may be diminished, which

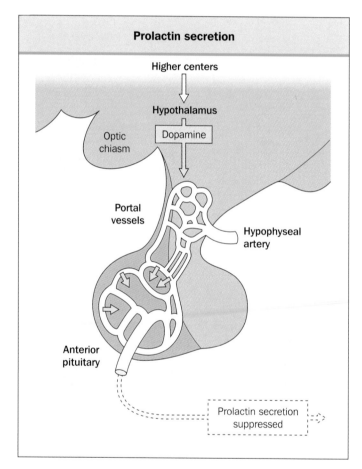

Figure 6.1 Prolactin secretion. Dopamine is formed in the hypothalamus and stored in the median eminence. It is secreted into the hypothalamohypophysial portal vessels to inhibit prolactin release tonically from pituitary lactotrophs. Any disruption of this pathway may therefore result in hyperprolactinemia.

would explain the lack of response to increased endogenous dopamine stimulation; however, an obvious response of the receptors to pharmacologic dopamine agonists makes this possibility less likely. Certain drugs act as dopamine-receptor-blocking agents, including phenothiazines (e.g. chlorpromazine), butyrophenones (haloperidol), and benzamides (metoclopramide, sulpiride, and domperidone). These drugs block the effects of endogenous dopamine and thus release lactotrophs from their hypothalamic inhibition. This sequence of events results in hyperprolactinemia.

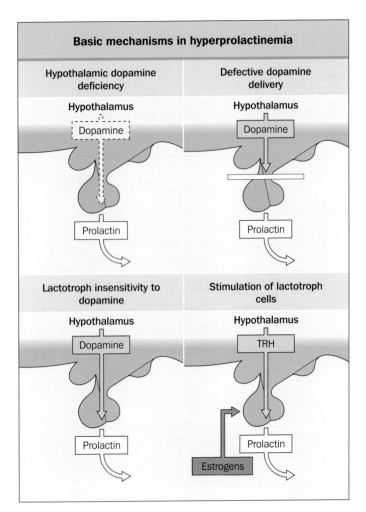

Basic mechanisms in hyperprolactinemia

Hypothalamic dopamine deficiency	Defective dopamine delivery
Hypothalamus	Hypothalamus
Dopamine	Dopamine
Prolactin	Prolactin

Lactotroph insensitivity to dopamine	Stimulation of lactotroph cells
Hypothalamus	Hypothalamus
Dopamine	TRH
Prolactin	Prolactin
	Estrogens

Figure 6.2 Basic mechanisms in hyperprolactinemia. (Top left panel) Inadequate synthesis and/or secretion of dopamine from the hypothalamus. (Top right panel) Interruption of the hypothalamo-hypophysial portal circulation. (Bottom left panel) Decreased sensitivity of the dopamine receptors. (In such cases, lactotrophs will be released from dopaminergic inhibition, thereby permitting the release of prolactin.) (Bottom right panel) Stimulation of prolactin secretion by estrogens or by excess thyrotropin-releasing hormone (TRH) in hypothyroidism.

Stimulation of lactotrophs

Hypothyroidism may be associated with hyperprolactinemia. If hypothyroidism results in increased TRH production, then TRH (which can act as a PRF) could lead to hyperprolactinemia.

Estrogens act directly at the pituitary level, causing stimulation of lactotrophs, and thus enhance prolactin secretion. Furthermore, estrogens increase the mitotic activity of lactotrophs, increasing cell numbers.

Injury to the chest wall can also lead to hyperprolactinemia. The mechanism is unclear but probably results from abnormal stimulation of the reflex associated with the rise in prolactin that is seen normally in lactating women during suckling.

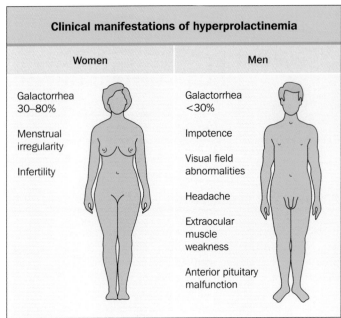

Clinical manifestations of hyperprolactinemia

Women	Men
Galactorrhea 30–80%	Galactorrhea <30%
Menstrual irregularity	Impotence
Infertility	Visual field abnormalities
	Headache
	Extraocular muscle weakness
	Anterior pituitary malfunction

Figure 6.3 Clinical manifestations of hyperprolactinemia. A variable incidence of galactorrhea is reported in different studies.

CLINICAL MANIFESTATIONS OF HYPERPROLACTINEMIA

The symptoms associated with hyperprolactinemia may be due to several factors: the direct effects of excess prolactin, such as the induction of galactorrhea or hypogonadism; the effects of the structural lesion causing the disorder (i.e. the pituitary tumor), leading to, for example, headaches, visual field defects, or external ophthalmoplegia; or associated dysfunction of secretion of other anterior pituitary hormones (**Fig. 6.3**).

The incidence of galactorrhea in hyperprolactinemic patients is between 30% and 80%, depending on the care with which the physician looks for this sign. Approximately 50% of women with galactorrhea, however, have normal prolactin and, as mentioned below, it is particularly those patients with very high prolactin levels, i.e. greater than 100ng/mL (2000mU/L), who often have no galactorrhea – thus, it is a poor marker of hyperprolactinemia. Normal prolactin levels are below 18ng/mL (360mU/L).

Women with hyperprolactinemia usually present with menstrual abnormalities – amenorrhea or oligomenorrhea – or regular cycles with infertility. Occasionally, patients may present with menorrhagia.

In contrast, men often present late in the course of the disease with symptoms of expansion of their pituitary tumor (i.e. headaches, visual defects, and external ophthalmoplegia) or symptoms from secondary adrenal or thyroid failure. These men, however, have usually been impotent for many years before their presentation.

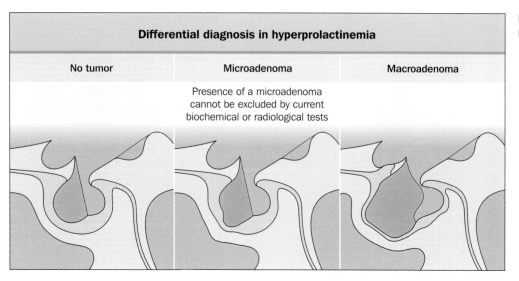

Figure 6.4 Differential diagnosis in hyperprolactinemia.

Occasionally, the syndrome may occur in prepubertal or peripubertal children, when it may present with delayed or arrested puberty or with headache and/or visual field defects.

DIFFERENTIAL DIAGNOSIS

The theoretical causes of hyperprolactinemia have already been discussed. In practice, however, it is important to exclude two causes of hyperprolactinemia: hypothyroidism and the ingestion of drugs that either deplete central dopamine or block dopamine receptors. Having excluded these two important causes, and any hypothalamic lesion, three common diagnostic possibilities remain (**Fig. 6.4**): the patient may have a micro-adenoma, a macroadenoma, or no tumor at all. If patients do not harbor an identifiable tumor, they are described as having idiopathic hyperprolactinemia.

A microadenoma is described as having a maximum diameter of up to 10mm, and a macroadenoma as having a diameter in excess of this. The normal pituitary diameter does not exceed 10mm (**Fig. 6.5**). A microadenoma is often visualized using magnetic resonance imaging (MRI) or modern computerized tomographic (CT) scanning. Usually, the serum prolactin level is below 200ng/mL (4000mU/L) in patients with microadenomas. A macroadenoma that secretes prolactin is usually associated with a serum prolactin level of more than 200ng/mL (4000mU/L). The macroadenoma is visualized with MRI or CT. If the patient has a macroadenoma and a serum prolactin level of less than 200ng/mL (4000mU/L), consideration should be given to the possibility that a nonfunctioning pituitary adenoma (pseudopro-lactinoma) is present; here, the hyperprolactinemia results from deprivation of some lactotrophs of dopaminergic inhibition. Enlargement of the pituitary fossa on a skull X-ray may represent the expansion of the fossa by the macroadenoma, but care should

be exercised to exclude the possibility of cisternal herniation (a partially empty fossa) as a cause for the enlargement. CT and MRI scans are useful (see **Fig. 6.7**) and will also demonstrate any hypothalamic pathology (see Chapter 40).

CHANGES IN THE BREAST DUE TO PROLACTIN

A woman with amenorrhea due to hyperprolactinemia does not develop the breast atrophy seen in postmenopausal women or in amenorrheic women who are gonadotropin-deficient or have primary ovarian failure. On examination, the breast is well developed and the Montgomery tubercles are hyperplastic (**Fig. 6.6**). If the breast is correctly examined, first by expressing it from the periphery towards the areola to empty milk ducts, followed by squeezing and lifting the areola (rather than the nipple itself) to empty the milk sinuses, galactorrhea can usually be found.

In patients with extremely high prolactin levels, galactorrhea may not be found. In male patients with hyperprolactinemia, there is usually no gynecomastia, but milk may be expressed from an entirely normal-sized male breast. The incidence of galactorrhea in men with hyperprolactinemia is low, however, being less than 30% (i.e. it is much less common than in women).

IMAGING OF THE PITUITARY

The anatomy of the pituitary is optimally assessed by MRI (see Chapter 40). MRI allows imaging of the optic chiasm, the cavernous sinuses, the pituitary (both the normal gland and tumors), and its stalk. In addition, aneurysms of the carotid are immediately obvious. Thus MRI allows accurate measurement of the size of the pituitary and of any tumor and its relationship to the optic chiasm and cavernous sinuses. Cisternal herniation

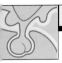

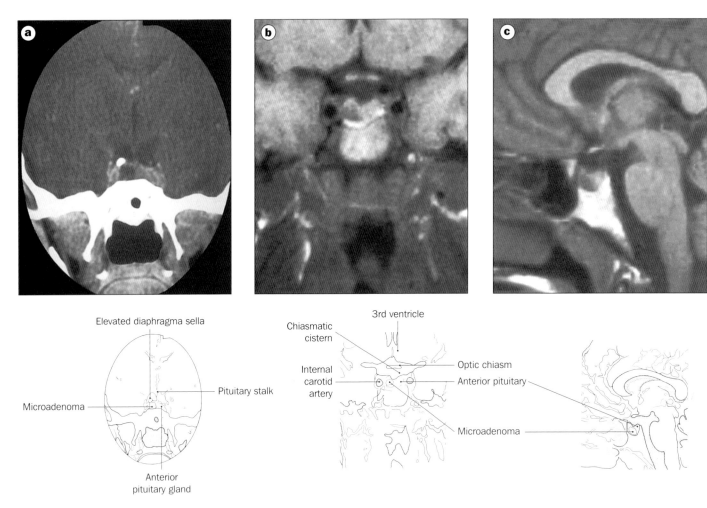

Figure 6.5 Computerized tomography (CT) and magnetic resonance imaging (MRI) scans of a microadenoma. (a) This postcontrast coronal CT scan demonstrates a 1cm mass of low density; note the elevation of the diaphragma sellae on the right side. (b) Coronal and (c) sagittal MRI scans.

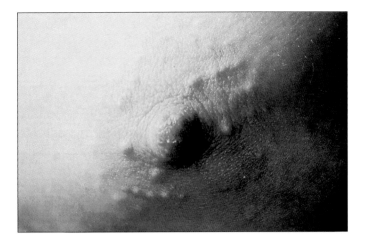

Figure 6.6 Changes in the breast due to prolactin secretion.
Prominent Montgomery tubercles are seen in the breast of a woman with hyperprolactinemia.

is also readily seen. If MRI is not available, CT scanning is also helpful but the resolution is less good and it is less satisfactory for delineating the relationship of the diaphragma sellae with the optic chiasm (**Fig. 6.7**). There is little place for skull X-ray other than for delineating bony structures.

TREATMENT OF HYPERPROLACTINEMIA

Patients with hyperprolactinemia and small pituitary tumors may be treated either by surgery, using the transsphenoidal approach, or medically, with dopamine agonist drugs. For microadenomas, the results in the hands of most experienced surgeons are similar. (In this discussion, the relative advantages of medical therapy and surgery will not be dealt with; the emphasis, reflecting our expertise, will be on medical therapy.) Pituitary surgery is discussed in detail in Chapter 8.

Bromocriptine therapy
The first dopamine agonist ergot compound to be used in clinical practice was bromocriptine, a peptide ergot.

The in vitro effects of bromocriptine
Bromocriptine has the advantage of having a long duration of action, which can be demonstrated using an *in vitro* system

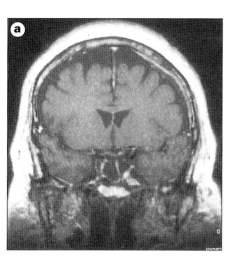

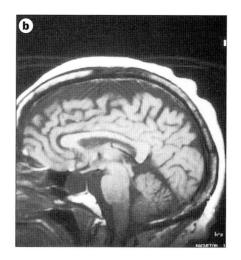

Figure 6.7 Cisternal herniation shown by magnetic resonance imaging (MRI). (a) Coronal MRI scan, which shows a deviated pituitary stalk reaching the floor of the pituitary fossa. (b) Sagittal view in the same patient.

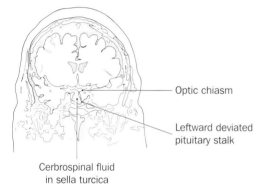

Optic chiasm

Leftward deviated pituitary stalk

Cerbrospinal fluid in sella turcica

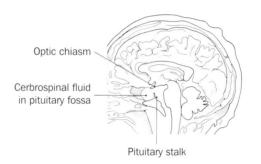

Optic chiasm

Cerbrospinal fluid in pituitary fossa

Pituitary stalk

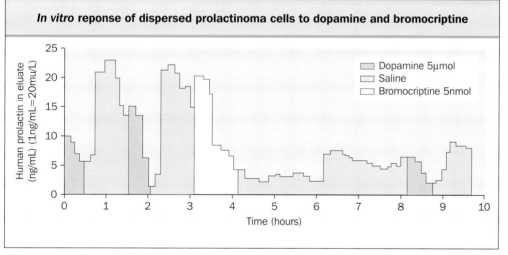

In vitro reponse of dispersed prolactinoma cells to dopamine and bromocriptine

Dopamine 5μmol
Saline
Bromocriptine 5nmol

Figure 6.8 *In vitro* response of dispersed prolactinoma cells to dopamine and bromocriptine. Both drugs suppressed prolactin secretion but, whereas prolactin secretion became maximal within 15 minutes after withdrawal of dopamine, the effect of bromocriptine was longer lasting, with prolactin levels remaining suppressed for 3 hours following withdrawal.

(Fig. 6.8). Anterior pituitary cells of a prolactinoma from a female patient were dispersed, placed in a perfusion apparatus, and perfused continuously. When the cells were exposed to dopamine, prolactin secretion was inhibited but, within 10 minutes after the withdrawal of dopamine, prolactin secretion increased, becoming maximal after approximately 15 minutes. Prolactin secretion was inhibited on exposure of the cells to bromocriptine. When the bromocriptine was withdrawn, however, prolactin secretion remained suppressed for over 3 hours.

On reexposure to dopamine, prolactin secretion was once more inhibited, recovering again on withdrawal of dopamine.

The *in vivo effects of bromocriptine*

Bromocriptine has a similar mode of action to dopamine in stimulating dopamine receptors on the prolactin-secreting pituitary cells. Stimulation of these receptors leads to inhibition of both prolactin secretion and synthesis. After a single 2.5mg dose of bromocriptine administered at 09.00h to women with

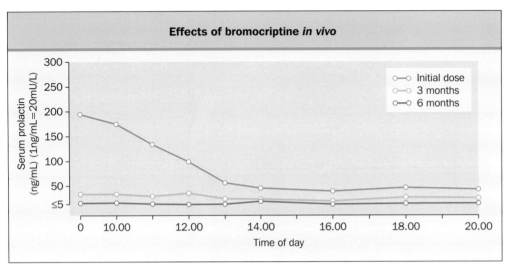

Effects of bromocriptine *in vivo*

Figure 6.9 Effects of bromocriptine *in vivo*. After a single 2.5mg dose of bromocriptine administered at 09.00h, prolactin secretion was inhibited within two hours, and reached nadir at seven hours. With chronic treatment (2.5mg three times per day) at three and six months, prolactin levels were maintained within the normal range throughout a 24-hour period.

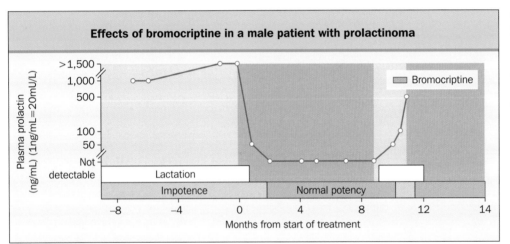

Effects of bromocriptine in a male patient with prolactinoma

Figure 6.10 Effects of bromocriptine in a male patient with prolactinoma. Normalization of serum prolactin by bromocriptine was associated with cessation of galactorrhea and with restoration of potency. On discontinuation of treatment, however, both galactorrhea and impotence returned, only to disappear after reinstitution of bromocriptine therapy.

hyperprolactinemia, prolactin secretion was inhibited within 2 hours and reached a nadir at 7 hours. When patients are treated chronically using 2.5mg three times per day, prolactin levels are maintained within the normal range, i.e. less than 20ng/mL (400mU/L), throughout a 24-hour period (**Fig. 6.9**).

Effects of bromocriptine in men

The first male patient commenced bromocriptine treatment at St Bartholomew's Hospital, London, in 1971, and his case illustrates a number of important points (**Fig. 6.10**). Initially, the prolactin levels of the patient were extremely elevated, but the administration of bromocriptine lowered them into the normal range (undetectable by bioassay); this was associated with cessation of galactorrhea. Bromocriptine therapy normalized the patient's prolactin levels and gonadal function, restoring potency. Following withdrawal of bromocriptine, hyperprolactinemia recurred, with associated galactorrhea and impotence. After restoration of bromocriptine therapy, prolactin levels rapidly returned to normal, galactorrhea ceased, and potency was restored.

Effects of bromocriptine in women

The second patient to be treated with bromocriptine was a woman with a large pituitary tumor and extremely high prolactin levels. Bromocriptine lowered her prolactin levels into the normal range, galactorrhea ceased, and menstruation returned within 1 month of starting therapy, even though the patient had been amenorrheic for several years.

The third patient had post-oral-contraceptive amenorrhea and galactorrhea associated with hyperprolactinemia. Bromocriptine therapy lowered the prolactin levels to normal and led to cessation of the patient's galactorrhea and to normal menstruation (**Fig. 6.11**).

Bromocriptine in amenorrhea

From experience of treating a large number of amenorrheic hyperprolactinemia women, the results of treating the first 58 appear to be representative of the success that can be achieved with bromocriptine therapy (**Fig. 6.12**). Within 1 month of starting therapy, a regular menstrual cycle is restored in approximately 25% of patients. Within 2 months, regular menstrual

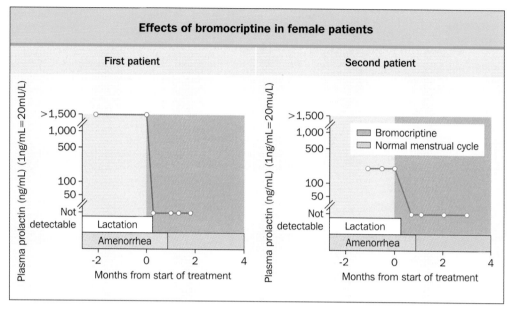

Figure 6.11 **Effects of bromocriptine in female patients.** The first female patient treated with bromocriptine had hyperprolactinemia associated with a large pituitary tumor, and the second had post-oral-contraceptive amenorrhea and galactorrhea with hyperprolactinemia. In both cases, bromocriptine therapy led to cessation of galactorrhea and the return of normal menstrual cycling.

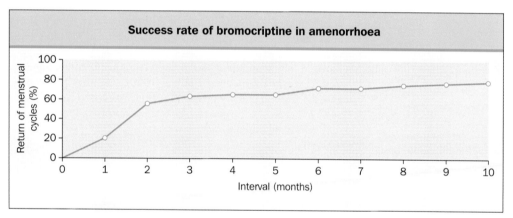

Figure 6.12 **Success rate of bromocriptine in amenorrhea.** If hyperprolactinemia is the cause of amenorrhea, the chances of restoring normal gonadal function with bromocriptine are very good. After 1 month of treatment, one woman in four will return to normal menstrual cycling; within 2 months, this number will increase to six out of 10; and after 10 months, eight out of 10 women will be menstruating normally. (Most of the remaining 20% have had pituitary surgery and irradiation therapy and are gonadotropin-deficient.)

cycling can be restored in over 60% and, within 10 months, in some 80%. Those patients who did not experience restoration of regular menstrual cycles (with only one or two exceptions) had previously undergone surgery or radiotherapy for their pituitary tumor – this rendered them gonadotropin-deficient. Thus, if hyperprolactinemia is the cause of amenorrhea, the chances of restoring normal gonadal function by medical therapy alone are extremely good, around 85%.

Long-term effects of bromocriptine
To study the long-term effects of bromocriptine on prolactin secretion, a group of patients was carefully evaluated (**Fig. 6.13**). Ten blood samples were taken from each patient before treatment; at 3, 6, and 12 months on therapy; and 2 months following drug withdrawal. All patients were treated with the same dose of bromocriptine (2.5mg three times per day). In all cases, bromocriptine lowered prolactin levels and, in nine of the 12 patients, prolactin secretion was suppressed throughout the year. After withdrawal of bromocriptine, prolactin levels rose in all patients to levels similar to those seen prior to therapy. The three patients in whom the prolactin levels were not lowered into the normal range, nevertheless, regained normal gonadal function.

Hyperprolactinemia and ovulation
Ovulation is normally associated with a dip in basal body temperature, and normal luteal function with a temperature rise. Basal body temperature is therefore a useful means of documenting ovulation. When hyperprolactinemic patients have had their prolactin levels and periods restored to normal by bromocriptine therapy, they usually demonstrate a biphasic temperature pattern. One patient had suffered from polymenorrhea for many years and was found to be hyperprolactinemic. Bromocriptine normalized her periods, and therapy was withdrawn after 1 year. During therapy, the basal body temperature chart (**Fig. 6.14**) showed a normal biphasic pattern but, following withdrawal of bromocriptine, prolactin levels rose to more than 100ng/mL (2000mU/L), galactorrhea

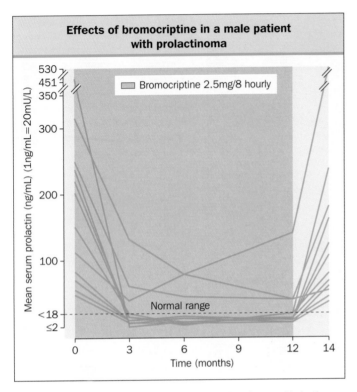

Figure 6.13 Long-term effects of bromocriptine therapy. Prolactin levels in a group of patients on long-term bromocriptine therapy were tested before therapy; after 3 months, 6 months, and 1 year of treatment (during which time all patients received bromocriptine 2.5mg three times per day); and 2 months after cessation of treatment. In all cases, prolactin remained suppressed throughout the year and, in most cases, prolactin levels were held within the normal range. Gonadal function was restored, even in patients whose prolactin levels did not return to normal.

returned, and the temperature pattern immediately became monophasic. Although the patient did not become amenorrheic, she developed irregular (presumably anovulatory) periods. Two weeks following reinstitution of therapy, the patient ovulated, demonstrating a postovulatory temperature rise. She has subsequently had a regular cycle and three successful pregnancies, each with the help of bromocriptine.

Hyperprolactinemic hypogonadism

The pathogenesis of the hypogonadal state in hyperprolactinemia is poorly understood. In men, testosterone levels may be normal or low, while in women, a hypoestrogenic state may occur, with loss of ovulation. The clinical features in hyperprolactinemic women, however, differ from those in the postmenopausal state since breast atrophy is absent and gonadotropin levels are not elevated.

Proposed explanations for the suppression of gonadal function in hyperprolactinemia include suppression of gonadotropin secretion; inhibition of positive estrogen feedback on luteinizing hormone (LH) secretion in women; an increase in adrenal androgen secretion; and blockade of the effects of gonadotropins at the gonadal level (**Fig. 6.15**). It is probable that an important mechanism is prolactin feedback at the hypothalamus, which alters secretion of gonadotropin-releasing hormone (GnRH), thus causing LH and follicle-stimulating hormone (FSH) secretion to become inappropriately low relative to gonadal steroid levels. Reduction in the normal LH pulsatility, essential for normal gonadal function, also occurs. Prolactin may interfere with LH and FSH action at the gonad, blocking progesterone synthesis, and may stimulate adrenal androgen secretion.

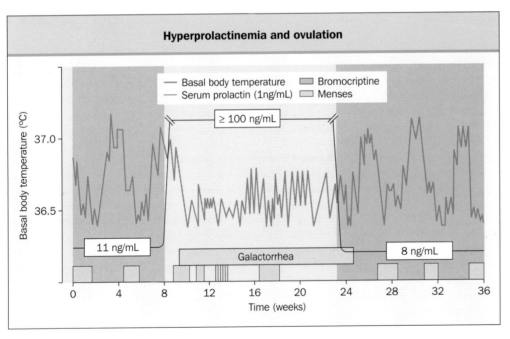

Figure 6.14 Hyperprolactinemia and ovulation. Normal ovulation and luteal function are associated with a biphasic basal body temperature. When patients have their prolactin levels and periods restored to normal with bromocriptine therapy, their temperature charts demonstrate the normal biphasic pattern. When therapy is withdrawn, the temperature chart shows a monophasic pattern, becoming biphasic again on reinstitution of bromocriptine.

Mechanisms of hyperprolactinemic hypogonadism

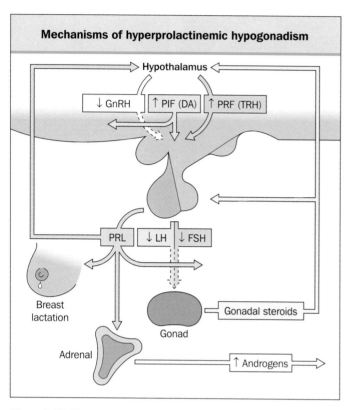

Figure 6.15 Mechanisms of hyperprolactinemic hypogonadism.
Hyperprolactinemia causes hypogonadism by several mechanisms: high prolactin (PRL) levels lead to partial suppression of gonadotropin-releasing hormone (GnRH) release, as well as loss of its pulsatility; prolactin also interferes with the action of luteinizing hormone (LH) and follicle-stimulating hormone (FSH) on the gonad, causes an increase in adrenal androgen secretion, and leads to inhibition of positive estrogen feedback on GnRH and LH secretion in women. DA, dopamine; PIF, prolactin-release-inhibiting factor; PRF, prolactin-releasing factor; TRH, thyrotropin-releasing hormone.

Visual field plots in hyperprolactinemia

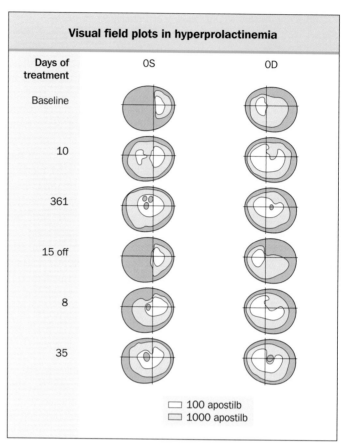

Figure 6.16 Visual field plots in hyperprolactinemia. The visual fields shown here were plotted using a Goldmann perimeter, under identical conditions, with a 0.25mm^2 object at two different light intensities: 1000 apostilb (I_4) and 100 apostilb (I_2). The black periphery indicates a normal visual field for comparison. An almost complete bitemporal hemianopia (pretherapy), which had almost disappeared after 1 year of treatment with bromocriptine, returned on cessation of therapy and began to subside after reinstitution of bromocriptine.

Reduction in size of prolactinomas

Since surgical therapy of large prolactin-secreting pituitary tumors normalizes serum prolactin levels or gonadal function in fewer than 20% of patients, particularly those with high pro-lactin levels, there is a need for another approach to the prob-lem. Three major lines of evidence suggest that medical therapy may help in the treatment of these large tumors.

- Visual field defects due to prolactinomas pressing on the optic chiasm have improved rapidly with bromocriptine therapy alone.
- Dopamine agonist therapy has been shown, by neuroradio-logic evaluation, to reduce the size of prolactinomas.
- Bromocriptine reduces DNA turnover and the mitotic index in the *in situ* pituitary of the rat.

Bromocriptine reduces pituitary tumor size in 75–80% of patients with large prolactin-secreting tumors, even with gross extrasellar extension. The type of result that can be expected is illustrated by a patient with a large prolactin-secreting tumor, who was treated with bromocriptine alone. The patient had a suprasellar extension and visual field defects. Visual field plots from this patient before and during treatment, as well as after withdrawal and reinstitution of bromocriptine therapy, are illus-trated in **Figure 6.16**. Before therapy (baseline), the patient had a bitemporal hemianopia, complete in the left eye and incom-plete in the right eye. The visual fields were greatly improved after 10 days, and only an equivocal superior bitemporal quad-rantic defect to the low intensity object was present after nearly 1 year. By 13 days after withdrawal of medical treatment, the tumor had enlarged again and the field defects recurred as an almost complete temporal hemianopia in the left eye and a par-tial temporal hemianopia in the right. Progressive improvement in visual fields was again observed over the subsequent 6 months after reintroduction of therapy.

Changes in pituitary volume during bromocriptine therapy

Figure 6.17 illustrates coronal CT head scans (postenhancement) from the patient whose visual fields are shown in **Figure 6.16**. **Figure 6.17(a)**, performed on a Delta 25 scanner, illustrates the situation before therapy; **Figure 6.17(b)** shows a scan performed on a GE 8800 scanner 2 weeks after starting bromocriptine therapy, 2.5mg three times per day. Before therapy, **Figure 6.17(a)** shows an enlargement of the pituitary fossa and an enhancing mass extending inferiorly into the sphenoid sinus, superiorly into the chiasmatic cistern, and abutting on the third ventricle. Two weeks posttreatment, **Fig. 6.17(b)** shows a marked reduction in tumor size, with regression of the suprasellar extension. The chiasmatic cistern is now largely free of tumor, apart from a finger-like process to the left of the midline. The intrasellar high density is present in the preenhancement scan and represents calcification within the tumor. Within the short space of 2 weeks, therefore, there was marked reduction in the size of the pituitary and a consequent decompression of the optic chiasm, which explains the rapid improvement in visual fields observed in this patient.

Of 16 patients with large prolactin-secreting tumors, 13 showed similar changes. The three patients in whom these changes were not observed were:

- a patient with a pituitary cyst that was associated with a small prolactinoma, but in whom the majority of the pituitary mass was the cyst;
- a patient with an extremely large tumor that was reduced in size but still remained large. The patient's serum prolactin level fell by 90% but still remained elevated at 328ng/mL (6560mU/L) at the end of 9 months of therapy, indicating relative resistance to dopamine agonists, probably because of dysfunctional or reduced numbers of dopamine receptors;
- a patient who had only been treated for 6 weeks and in whom there was as yet only equivocal evidence of reduction in the size of the tumor.

Other groups have had similar results. It seems that some 65% of macroadenomas with large extrasellar extensions may be treated with bromocriptine alone to shrink the tumors and to relieve the mass effects and the hormonal excess.

Changes in serum prolactin levels

In patients with macroadenomas, the serum prolactin levels can be readily suppressed with bromocriptine therapy. **Figure 6.18** shows serum prolactin levels throughout the day after an initial 2.5mg oral dose of bromocriptine administered at 09.00h to the patient whose visual field plots and CT scans are shown in **Figures 6.16 & 6.17**, as well as those from a patient with a similar problem. After a single dose of bromocriptine, the prolactin levels fell by approximately 90%. The mean and absolute range of prolactin levels in samples taken at the same time intervals before therapy (baseline) and during bromocriptine therapy, 7.5mg/day, are also shown in **Figure 6.18**. In the first patient, the prolactin levels were suppressed into the normal range (less than 18ng/mL, 360mU/L) and in the second patient, prolactin levels, although lowered, did not return to normal. With treatment over 1 year, however, the levels continued to fall to 78ng/mL (1560mU/L). In these patients, as with the patients with microadenomas, gonadal function is usually restored to normal. As previously noted, when therapy was withdrawn at

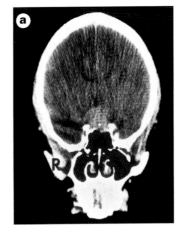
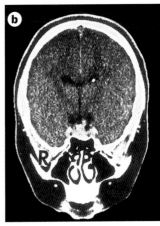

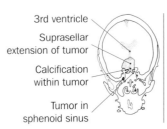
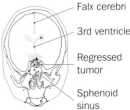

Figure 6.17 Coronal CT head scans before and during treatment with bromocriptine. (a) Scan taken before therapy shows enlargement of the pituitary fossa and an enhancing mass extending inferiorly into the sphenoid sinus, superiorly into the chiasmatic cistern, and abutting on the third ventricle. (b) Scan taken after 2 weeks of therapy shows a marked reduction in tumor size, with regression of the suprasellar extension.

1 year, visual field defects recurred in the first patient and this was associated with prolactin levels rising again to 2580ng/mL (51.6u/L) at 13 days in comparison to the pretreatment level (3940ng/mL, 78.8 u/L). However, it should be noted that, in male patients on bromocriptine, prolactin levels usually fall rapidly and easily into the normal range. If this does not occur, gonadal function may not return to normal.

Side effects

Side effects of bromocriptine therapy occur only at the start of treatment and disappear with continued therapy. There are no long-term problems associated with chronic treatment at the doses used for hyperprolactinemia – usually 7.5mg/day and rarely more than 15mg/day.

If treatment is started with full doses or increased too quickly, dizziness, nausea, and postural hypotension may occur. To avoid such effects, bromocriptine must always be taken during a meal. Administration should be started at night, with a sandwich and glass of milk, when the patient retires to bed. After taking half a tablet (1.25mg) for three nights, half a tablet is added with breakfast. After a further three days an additional half a tablet is added with lunch. At intervals of three days, additional half tablets (1.25mg increments) may be progressively added until achievement of the usual dose of one tablet (2.5mg) taken three times daily, in the middle of breakfast, lunch, and the evening meal. If side effects still occur, longer intervals and smaller increments should be used. Once established on an effective dose it is now

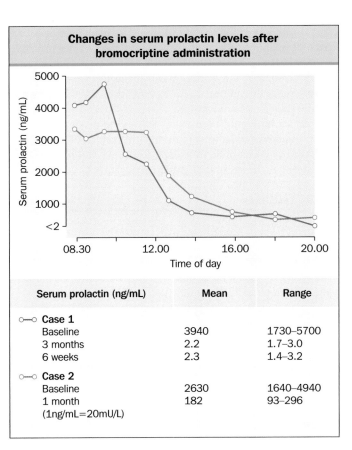

Changes in serum prolactin levels after bromocriptine administration

Serum prolactin (ng/mL)	Mean	Range
○—○ **Case 1**		
Baseline	3940	1730–5700
3 months	2.2	1.7–3.0
6 weeks	2.3	1.4–3.2
○—○ **Case 2**		
Baseline	2630	1640–4940
1 month	182	93–296
(1ng/mL=20mU/L)		

Figure 6.18 Changes in serum prolactin levels after bromocriptine administration. The effect on serum prolactin levels throughout the day of a single 2.5mg oral dose of bromocriptine at 09.00h is shown. Case 1 is the patient whose visual field chart and CT scans are shown in **Figures 6.16 & 6.17**. Case 2 is a patient with a similar problem. In patients such as these, even when prolactin levels do not come down to the normal range, gonadal function is usually restored.

established that the whole dose can be given once daily, again during the main course of a main meal. In a small proportion of patients psychosis or anxiety can be precipitated by the administration of dopamine-agonist drugs. These are usually adequately managed either by stopping the dopamine-agonist medication or lessening the dose. These symptoms are more common in parkinsonian patients, but in this group the brain is diseased and the doses used are much greater than for the indication of prolactinoma.

The only group of patients who do not suffer from such side effects if given the full dose immediately is puerperal women. They may be given bromocriptine 2.5mg two or three times daily to suppress puerperal lactation, without side effects, if treatment is started within 24 hours of delivery. The reasons for this difference are unknown.

There are several other dopamine agonists that lower serum prolactin levels and reduce tumor size to a similar extent to bromocriptine. These drugs include pergolide, lisuride, qinagolide, and cabergoline. These compounds are associated with a similar side effect profile to that observed with bromocriptine. Cabergoline has the advantage that it only needs to be taken once or twice per week and may have a reduced incidence of side effects. With the exception of bromocriptine, safety during

pregnancy has not been demonstrated. As experience with cabergoline has accumulated it appears that some patients who could not be controlled with other dopamine agonists, e.g. bromocriptine or pergolide, could be controlled by cabergoline. On occasion, the dosing may need to be increased as frequently as daily. Because of its long duration of action, the side effect profile and efficacy appear to be better than with any other dopamine agonist drug.

Pregnancy and bromocriptine
Many hyperprolactinemic women would like to become pregnant and, since the administration of bromocriptine lowers the prolactin levels and restores gonadal function, conception presents little difficulty. There are, however, several important considerations that must be recognized by both physician and patient, including the possible teratogenic sequelae of fetal exposure to bromocriptine.

There is no evidence for teratogenicity in animal studies and, in 1400 women who were taking bromocriptine when they conceived, there is no evidence of increased incidence of abortion, multiple pregnancy, or fetal abnormalities. Until these babies have lived their own complete life cycles, however, the possibility of unexpected late effects cannot be excluded.

In order to minimize fetal exposure to bromocriptine, it is suggested that patients should initially use mechanical contraception. Once three regular menstrual cycles have occurred, contraceptive precautions are discontinued. In this way, pregnancy can be suspected as soon as a menstrual period is 48 hours overdue. At that time, a serum human chorionic gonadotropin-β assay should be performed to confirm the pregnancy, and the patient should discontinue bromocriptine therapy. In this way, the fetus is exposed to bromocriptine for a theoretical maximum of 16 days.

There is little doubt that patients with pituitary tumors run a small, but significant, risk of expansion of the tumor during pregnancy. It is very difficult, however, to assess the absolute risk. With microadenomas, the incidence seems to be less than 1% and probably less than 0.5%. In patients with macroadenomas, the incidence is probably higher, perhaps between 5% and 20%. This risk is unrelated to bromocriptine therapy prior to pregnancy but may occur when fertility is induced with other drugs, including exogenous gonadotropins and clomiphene, and even when no drug therapy has been employed in patients with preexisting pituitary adenomas.

In practice, the problem of pregnancy is not great, since the vast majority of women who present with hyperprolactinemia only have microadenomas. To avoid major problems, it is extremely important that patients undergo careful endocrine, neuroradiologic, and neuro-ophthalmologic evaluation prior to treatment. If there is no suprasellar extension, and if the patient harbors only a microadenoma, then the risk of clinically significant swelling of the pituitary is extremely small; it is therefore suggested that the patient is evaluated clinically at bimonthly intervals throughout the pregnancy. If the patient has a macroadenoma and suprasellar extension, a strong case can be made for transsphenoidal decompression of the tumor prior to pregnancy. It is, however, possible even for these patients to go through pregnancy without developing visual disturbances and, furthermore, even if visual disturbances occur in one pregnancy, the problem may not recur in subsequent ones.

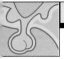

Thus, the approach to the patient with a prolactin-secreting macroadenoma who desires pregnancy can be either expectant or prophylactic. The author believes that, as the risk of swelling of the adenoma is less than 20%, it is reasonable to adopt an expectant policy. Others suggest that pituitary decompression should be performed surgically, and still others recommend that external pituitary irradiation is given. It is not clear whether external pituitary irradiation or decompression of the pituitary by surgery, or both, completely prevent symptom-generating pituitary enlargement. It should be stressed that, so far, no patient has become permanently blind following expansion of the tumor during pregnancy.

If visual field defects or headaches from tumor expansion do occur during pregnancy, a number of therapeutic options are available. Following termination of the pregnancy, either by abortion or delivery of the baby, tumors have become smaller and such symptoms and headaches have resolved in all cases. Thus, if such symptoms occur early in pregnancy, therapeutic termination may be indicated. If they occur in the eighth month of pregnancy, premature delivery of the baby may be decided upon, although, if field defects and symptoms are minor, careful observation may be all that is required. The most problematic situation arises when symptoms occur in the middle trimester. At that time, it is suggested that bromocriptine therapy is restarted and in the great majority of patients there is rapid reduction in the tumor size and further swelling is prevented. If this is unsuccessful, high-dose dexamethasone can be used to achieve the same ends. Dexamethasone also reduces the chances of fetal respiratory distress occurring should premature delivery be needed. As a last resort, transsphenoidal surgery during pregnancy can be, and has been, used to decompress the tumor. Since such complications are extremely rare, however, little data have to date been accumulated.

CONCLUSION

Dopamine-agonist therapy for hyperprolactinemia, such as with bromocriptine, leads to a reversal of the hyperprolactinemic hypogonadal state without risk of the development of pituitary insufficiency. Dopamine-agonist therapy is effective not only in patients with microadenomas but also in the majority of patients with large prolactin-secreting tumors in reducing tumor size; however, the tumor size will increase (as will prolactin levels) after withdrawal of therapy. This may give rise to problems because of compression of vital structures by the tumor.

FURTHER READING

Colao A, Di Sarno A, Sarnacchiaro F, et al. Prolactinomas resistant to standard dopamine agonists respond to chronic cabergoline treatment. J Clin Endocrinol Metab. 1997;82:876–83.

Molitch ME. Pregnancy and the hyperprolactinemic woman. N Engl J Med. 1985;312:1364–70.

Molitch ME, Elton RL, Blackwell RE, et al. Bromocriptine Study Group: bromocriptine as primary therapy for prolactin-secreting macroadenomas: results of a prospective multicenter study. J Clin Endocrinol Metab. 1985;60:698–705.

Molitch ME, Thorner MO, Wilson C. Therapeutic controversy: management of prolactinomas. J Clin Endocrinol Metab. 1996;82: 996–1000.

Thorner MO, McNeilly AS, Hagan C, Besser GM. Long-term treatment of galactorrhoea and hypogonadism with bromocriptine. Br Med J. 1974;2:419–22.

Thorner MO, Perryman RL, Rogol AD, et al. Rapid changes of prolactinoma volume after withdrawal and reinstitution of bromocriptine. J Clin Endocrinol Metab. 1981;53:480–3.

Thorner MO, Martin WH, Rogol AD, et al. Rapid regression of pituitary prolactinomas during bromocriptine treatment. J Clin Endocrinol Metab. 1980;51:438–45.

Turkalj I, Braun P, Krupp P. Surveillance of bromocriptine in pregnancy. JAMA. 1982;247:1589–91.

Vance ML, Evans WS, Thorner MO. Drugs five years later: bromocriptine. Ann Intern Med. 1984;100:78–91.

Webster J, Piscitelli G, Polli A, Ferrari CI, Ismail I, Scanlon MF. A comparison of cabergoline and bromocriptine in the treatment of hyperprolactinemic amenorrhea. Cabergoline Comparative Study Group. N Engl J Med. 1994;331:904–9.

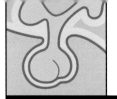

Section 1 Hypothalamus and Pituitary

Chapter 7

Posterior Pituitary

Peter H Baylis

INTRODUCTION

The pituitary is a composite gland, the anterior lobe being derived from an evagination of the stomodeal ectoderm known as Rathke's pouch while the posterior lobe is an extension of the forebrain. The weight of the adult human gland is approximately 620mg; in women 20% and in men 25% of this gland is posterior pituitary. Nervous tissue is the principal component of the posterior pituitary.

The immediate anatomic relationship of the pituitary gland with surrounding structures is seen in **Figure 7.1**. The gland lies in a bony fossa and its stalk pierces the fibrous sellar diaphragm. The lateral wall of the fossa is made up of the cavernous sinus, in which lie the siphon of the carotid artery and the cranial nerves III, IV and VI. The optic chiasm is situated immediately above the pituitary fossa, anterior to the pituitary stalk. The hypothalamus lies above the pituitary stalk and extends to the lateral walls of the third ventricle. Bounded anteriorly by the anterior commissure and posteriorly by the mammillary body, it is composed of many sets of nuclei and neuronal tracts, a number of which terminate in the median eminence.

NEURONAL TRACTS FROM THE PARAVENTRICULAR AND SUPRAOPTIC NUCLEI

Two major nuclei in the hypothalamus – the supraoptic and paraventricular nuclei – synthesize the peptides arginine vasopressin (antidiuretic hormone, AVP) and oxytocin (**Fig. 7.2**). Smaller groups of neurons that synthesize these neurohypophysial hormones are clustered in the suprachiasmatic region in some, but not all, mammals. Each neuron in these nuclei synthesizes either oxytocin or vasopressin as part of a larger precursor molecule. In the rostral (anterior) part of the supraoptic nucleus, oxytocin and vasopressin neurons are equally distributed but in the caudal part, only oxytocin neurons are found. Additionally, both hormones are present in the rostral paraventricular nucleus. In the caudal region of the paraventricular nucleus, however, the neurons close to the third ventricle contain oxytocin while those more laterally situated contain vasopressin.

At least four neuronal tracts emerge from the supraoptic and paraventricular nuclei. The main pathway terminates in the posterior pituitary to release its peptides into the systemic circulation. Both vasopressin and oxytocin are found in the zona externa of the median eminence, and the majority of fibers to this region arise from the paraventricular nucleus. From the median eminence, the peptides are secreted into the hypothalamo-pituitary portal circulation. A third tract passes to the floor of the third ventricle. It is still unknown, however, if the peptide hormones are actively secreted via this tract into the cerebrospinal fluid. The final neuronal pathway terminates in the brainstem in close proximity to the vasomotor center, and a few fibers pass down the spinal cord.

SENSORY TRACTS TO THE PARAVENTRICULAR AND SUPRAOPTIC NUCLEI

Changes in blood tonicity are recognized by osmotically sensitive cells that are situated in the circumventricular organs of the anterior hypothalamus, probably the subfornical organ and/or

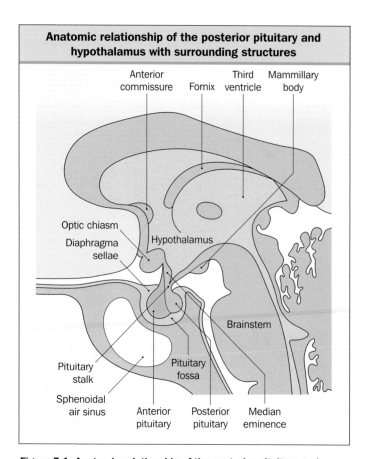

Anatomic relationship of the posterior pituitary and hypothalamus with surrounding structures

Anterior commissure

Fornix

Third ventricle

Mammillary body

Optic chiasm

Diaphragma sellae

Hypothalamus

Pituitary stalk

Pituitary fossa

Brainstem

Sphenoidal air sinus

Anterior pituitary

Posterior pituitary

Median eminence

Figure 7.1 Anatomic relationship of the posterior pituitary and hypothalamus with surrounding structures. The diagram represents a sagittal section through the pituitary and hypothalamus.

Neuronal pathways from the paraventricular and supraoptic nuclei

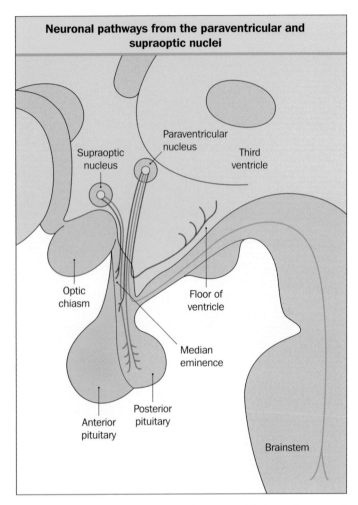

Figure 7.2 Neuronal pathways from the paraventricular and supraoptic nuclei. Neuronal tracts from the paraventricular and supraoptic nuclei connect with the posterior pituitary, the median eminence, the floor of the third ventricle, and the brainstem.

Sensory pathways to the paraventricular and supraoptic nuclei

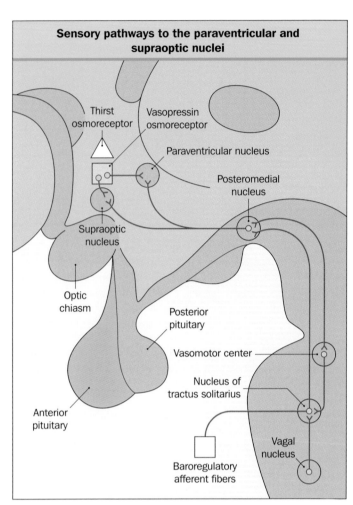

Figure 7.3 Sensory pathways to the paraventricular and supraoptic nuclei. Changes in blood tonicity are recognized by osmoreceptors in the circumventricular organs of the anterior hypothalamus. Afferent fibers connect the osmoreceptor to the neurons that synthesize vasopressin. Baroregulatory information, from afferent fibers that terminate in the brainstem nuclei, is relayed to the paraventricular and supraoptic nuclei via the posteromedial nucleus of the hypothalamus.

the organum vasculosum of the lamina terminalis. There is evidence for the existence of two distinct osmoreceptors: one controls vasopressin secretion, principally from the supraoptic nucleus; the other serves thirst appreciation (**Fig. 7.3**). Baroregulatory afferent fibers arise in low-pressure receptors that are sited in the atria of the heart and the great veins of the chest, and in high-pressure receptors that are present in the carotid body and arch of the aorta. These fibers terminate in a group of nuclei within the brainstem. They then relay in the posteromedial nucleus of the hypothalamus before ending in the paraventricular and supraoptic nuclei.

The potent stimulatory effect of severe nausea and/or vomiting on vasopressin release is probably mediated by the vagus nerve. It remains unclear whether the effects of hypoglycemia are monitored by a hypothalamic glucostat and whether an angiotensin sensor exists to appreciate changes in blood angiotensin concentration. The release of oxytocin by suckling is a neuro-hormonal reflex, the afferent fibers being carried by the vagus nerve from the breast.

ARTERIAL SUPPLY TO THE HYPOTHALAMUS AND PITUITARY GLAND

The greater part of the arterial blood supply to the hypothalamus and pituitary gland is derived from the internal carotid artery or its branches (**Fig. 7.4**). The posterior lobe is supplied by the inferior hypophysial artery and the artery of the trabecula (a branch of the superior hypophysial artery). There is no direct arterial supply to the anterior pituitary and all of its blood supply arises from the long and short hypophysial portal vessels, which drain the median eminence. Branches from the circle of Willis supply the hypothalamus, which is extremely well perfused. The paraventricular and supraoptic nuclei receive blood from branches of the suprahypophysial, anterior communicating, anterior cerebral, posterior communicating, and posterior cerebral arteries. Venous blood draining from the anterior and posterior lobes of the pituitary enters the dural, cavernous, and inferior petrosal sinuses.

CHEMISTRY OF VASOPRESSIN AND OXYTOCIN

The genes encoding vasopressin and oxytocin are tightly linked on chromosome 20p13. The structure of the neurohypophysial hormones vasopressin and oxytocin (**Fig. 7.5**) was elucidated, and their synthesis completed, by 1954. Arginine vasopressin (AVP) is the antidiuretic hormone of most mammals, although the pig family uses lysine vasopressin. Sequence analysis of the genes encoding AVP and recombinant DNA studies have confirmed the structure of the AVP precursor molecule (**Fig 7.6**). The gene consists of three exons and two introns. Genetic mutations of the precursor molecule, rarely of AVP itself, cause familial cranial diabetes insipidus (see below). The oxytocin gene is similar to the AVP gene but encodes for a precursor molecule that differs in the absence of the glycoprotein sequence. The vasopressins are basic molecules, with isoelectric points in the region of pH9–10, while oxytocin is more neutral. The ring is essential for biologic activity. Position 8 plays a key role in determining oxytocic or vasopressor characteristics. The more basic the amino acid in this position, the more vasopressor activity the molecule possesses.

Structure and activity data on a large number of analogs have facilitated the design of substances that possess desired biologic properties. An example is the synthesis of a long-acting antidiuretic molecule, 1-deamino-8-D-arginine vasopressin (desmopressin or DDAVP), which has little pressor activity but enhanced antidiuretic effect and is ideal for the treatment of cranial diabetes insipidus. Other modifications are leading to the development of vasopressin antagonists that are suitable for the treatment of disorders associated with vasopressin excess.

After secretion by exocytosis from the neurohypophysis, the peptides circulate unbound to plasma proteins. Their plasma half-life is extremely short (**Fig. 7.5**) as a result of efficient clearance by the kidney and liver (for vasopressin) and by the uterus, kidney, and liver (for oxytocin). This clearance is so rapid that changes in plasma concentration are usually a reflection of changes in secretion rather than clearance rate. In pregnancy, the plasma enzyme oxytocinase rapidly degrades both oxytocin and vasopressin.

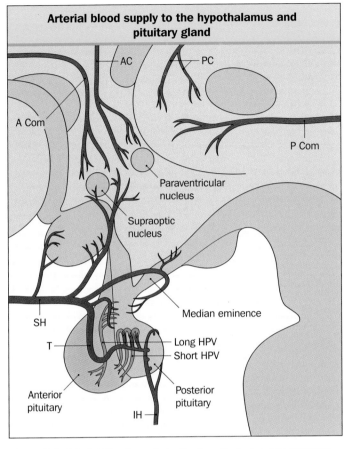

Figure 7.4 Arterial blood supply to the hypothalamus and pituitary gland. Most of the blood supply to the hypothalamus and pituitary arises from the internal carotid artery or its branches. The posterior lobe of the pituitary is supplied by the inferior hypophysial artery (IH) and the artery of the trabecula (T), while the anterior lobe is supplied indirectly via the hypophysial portal vessels (HPV). Branches from the circle of Willis supply the hypothalamus, and the paraventricular and supraoptic nuclei in particular are served by branches from the suprahypophysial (SH), the anterior communicating (A Com), the anterior cerebral (AC), the posterior communicating (P Com), and posterior cerebral (PC) arteries.

Figure 7.5 Chemical characteristics of vasopressin and oxytocin. Arginine vasopressin is the antidiuretic hormone found in most mammals. The vasopressins are basic molecules (isoelectric point, pH9–10), while oxytocins are more neutral. The more basic the amino acid in position 8, the more vasopressor activity the molecule possesses.

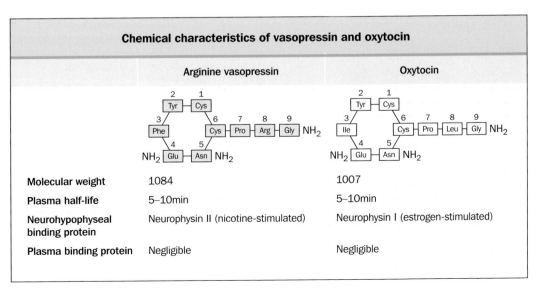

Chemical characteristics of vasopressin and oxytocin		
	Arginine vasopressin	**Oxytocin**
Molecular weight	1084	1007
Plasma half-life	5–10min	5–10min
Neurohypophyseal binding protein	Neurophysin II (nicotine-stimulated)	Neurophysin I (estrogen-stimulated)
Plasma binding protein	Negligible	Negligible

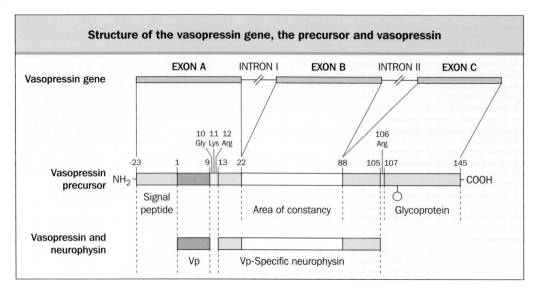

Figure 7.6 Structure of the vasopressin gene, the precursor and vasopressin. Three exons encode the precursor molecule, which comprises a signal peptide, vasopressin hormone, specific neurophysin, and a glycoprotein moiety, copeptin. (Modified with permission from Baylis PH. Vasopressin and its neurophysin In: DeGroot LJ, ed. Endocrinology, 3rd edn. Philadelphia, PA; WB Saunders: 1995.)

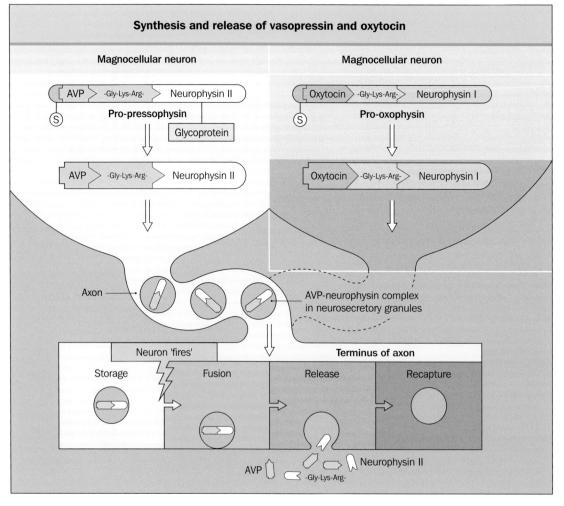

Figure 7.7 Synthesis and release of vasopressin and oxytocin. Vasopressin (AVP) and oxytocin are synthesized in the magnocellular neurons of the supraoptic and paraventricular nuclei. Each neuron synthesizes either oxytocin or vasopressin. These peptides arise from the precursor molecules pro-oxyphysin and pro-pressophysin, respectively. The neurophysin–nonapeptide groups migrate, in the form of neurosecretory granules, along the axons of the magnocellular neurons, to be stored at the ends of the neuronal tracts. When the neurons 'fire', the granules fuse with the axonal plasmalemma and each nonapeptide and its specific neurophysin are subsequently released separately. Once released, the neurophysin has no apparent physiologic function.

NEUROSECRETION OF NEUROHYPOPHYSIAL HORMONES

The principal sites of biosynthesis of vasopressin and oxytocin are the magnocellular neurons of the supraoptic and paraventricular nuclei (**Fig. 7.7**). Each neuron synthesizes either oxytocin or vasopressin as part of a larger precursor molecule (pro-oxyphysin and pro-pressophysin, respectively). Neurosecretion of neuro-hypophysial hormones is controlled by an intricate balance between stimulatory and inhibitory neurotransmitters. There are two major classes of substances, biogenic amines and peptides, which are distributed widely in the hypothalamus. The catecholamines (dopamine and norepinephrine) and acetylcholine stimulate AVP secretion, and the excitatory amino acids (glutamate and aspartate) modulate osmotically stimulated AVP mRNA and AVP secretion. Opioid peptides inhibit neuro-hypophysial hormone secretion, while interleukin-1β and angiotensin II are stimulatory. Neurophysin–nonapeptide complexes migrate, as neurosecretory granules, along the axons of the neurons from each nucleus at a rate of 1–3mm/h. The complex is then stored as granules at the end of the neuronal tracts to be released under the influence of specific stimuli. The common final pathway of these stimuli is phasic electrochemical 'firing' of the neurons themselves. The neurosecretory granules then fuse with the plasmalemma of the axon, and the nonapeptide and its specific neurophysin are released separately by exocytosis. The membrane of the granule is subsequently recaptured by micropinocytosis. Once released into the circulation, the neurophysin no longer appears to have any physiologic function. The distribution of vasopressin in neurosecretory granules within a rat neurohypophysis, demonstrated by immunocytochemical reactions that are specific for AVP, is shown in **Figure 7.8**.

FUNCTIONS OF VASOPRESSIN AND OXYTOCIN

The functions of vasopressin and oxytocin are shown diagrammatically in **Figure 7.9**. The main physiologic role of vasopressin is the reduction of free-water clearance by the kidney to produce concentrated urine. Vasopressin acts on the distal nephron to increase water permeability of the tubular cell so that solute-free water may pass along the osmotic gradient from the lumen of the nephron to the renal interstitial medulla. At supraphysiologic plasma concentrations, vasopressin contracts smooth muscle, resulting in pressor activity. Again at high concentrations, it activates liver glycogen phosphorylase to convert glycogen to glucose. Lipolysis is also increased. The secretion of vasopressin into the portal circulation of the hypothalamopituitary region, together with the secretion of corticotropin-releasing factor from the median eminence, controls the release of adrenocorticotropic hormone (ACTH) from the anterior pituitary gland. Recent studies suggest that intracerebral vasopressin influences cognitive function and behavior, and improves memory in animals. It regulates water and salt transport across the choroid plexus.

Oxytocin has no definite known role in men, although it may aid contraction of the seminal vesicles of the testis. In women, it contracts the pregnant uterus, although it is not the sole initiator of parturition. During lactation, oxytocin promotes milk ejection by contraction of smooth muscle in the breast ducts – an effect that is mediated by a neurohormonal reflex. Oxytocin also influences ovarian function. Like vasopressin, oxytocin is released from the median eminence and may affect the anterior pituitary. The response of gonadotropins to the gonadotropin-releasing hormone (GnRH) appears to be modified by oxytocin. There is tentative evidence to suggest that oxytocin increases lipolysis in the adipocyte. Oxytocin promotes maternal behavior and may affect other cerebral functions.

At pharmacologic doses, oxytocin will bind to the AVP antidiuretic renal receptor to cause increased renal water retention and concentrated urine, so that there is a danger of hyponatremia when oxytocin is delivered in high concentrations with excessive fluid (e.g. during labor).

REGULATION OF VASOPRESSIN SECRETION

The factors that regulate vasopressin secretion have been clearly defined (**Table 7.1**), the major determinant being plasma osmolality. Different solutes, however, have varying ability to stimulate vasopressin release. Sodium and mannitol appear to be the most potent solutes, while glucose has little or no effect on vasopressin secretion. Large quantities of vasopressin are released after marked hypotension, hypovolemia, and vomiting. Angiotensin II and hypoglycemia both appear to be specific

Factors regulating vasopressin release	
Osmotic regulation	**Nonosmotic regulation**
Stimulatory solutes: sodium, mannitol, urea	Hemodynamic: hypotension, hypovolemia
Nonstimulatory solutes: glucose	Nausea and/or vomiting
	Hypoglycemia
	Renin-angiotensin
	Pain, stress, emotion?

Table 7.1 Factors regulating vasopressin release.

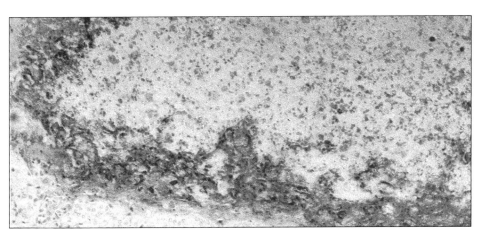

Figure 7.8 Histologic section of a rat neurohypophysis. The distribution of vasopressin in the form of neurosecretory granules is demonstrated by immunocytochemical reactions that are specific for arginine vasopressin (brown staining).

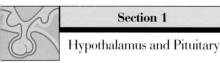

Functions of vasopressin and oxytocin

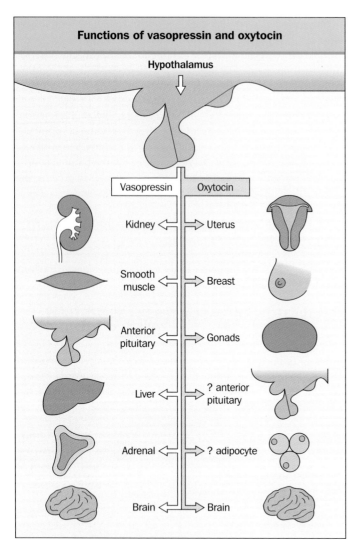

Figure 7.9 Functions of vasopressin and oxytocin. The most important function of vasopressin is the reduction of free-water clearance by the kidney. At high concentrations, it contracts smooth muscle and initiates the conversion of glycogen to glucose in the liver. Secretion of vasopressin into the hypothalamo-pituitary circulation modulates the release of adrenocorticotropic hormone from the anterior pituitary. Oxytocin aids contraction of the pregnant uterus and assists milk ejection during lactation. There is evidence that oxytocin may aid contraction of the seminal vesicles of the testis, may influence ovarian function, may have some effect in the anterior pituitary on the response of gonadotropins to gonadotropin-releasing hormone, and may also increase lipolysis in the adipocyte.

stimuli of vasopressin secretion. Although many other factors have been reported to stimulate vasopressin release (e.g. pain, stress, profound emotion), it remains controversial whether vasopressin is a true stress hormone.

FACTORS REGULATING OXYTOCIN SECRETION

The factors that control oxytocin secretion in men and in nonpregnant, nonsuckling women are unclear (**Table 7.2**). Recent studies in animals show that osmotic stimulation releases oxytocin in similar quantities to vasopressin but that the quantity of oxytocin released after hemorrhage is considerably smaller

Factors regulating oxytocin release

Physiologic regulation largely unknown
Suckling
Pregnancy and parturition
Osmotic and hemodynamic factors?

Table 7.2 Factors regulating oxytocin release.

than the quantity of vasopressin released. Oxytocin secretion appears to increase with the duration of pregnancy but the regulating factors that are involved are unknown. Suckling is a specific stimulus for oxytocin release. Plasma oxytocin concentrations rise to very high values at the end of parturition, release being stimulated by cervical dilatation (the Ferguson reflex).

OSMOREGULATION OF VASOPRESSIN SECRETION AND THIRST

Osmotic control of both vasopressin secretion and thirst are the principal factors maintaining water homeostasis in man. Slow infusion of hypertonic saline into healthy individuals causes a linear increase in plasma osmolality, which in turn stimulates vasopressin release and thirst (**Fig. 7.10**). Conversely, a fall in plasma osmolality induced by an oral water load suppresses vasopressin secretion, with plasma VP concentrations becoming undetectable, and inhibits thirst. Under normal circumstances, healthy individuals maintain their plasma osmolality within the range 282–295mosmol/kg, with plasma vasopressin concentrations varying between 0.3 and 4.0pmol/L, thus allowing the formation of maximally dilute and concentrated urine, respectively.

The relationship between plasma vasopressin (pAVP) and plasma osmolality (pOS) is linear, the average regression line being defined by the function:

$$pAVP = 0.41 \times (pOS - 284), r = 0.96, p < 0.001.$$

The slope of the line is a measure of the sensitivity of the osmoreceptor and vasopressin-releasing unit. The abscissal intercept defines the mean theoretic threshold for vasopressin release.

Using visual analog scales to assess thirst, a similar linear relationship exists between plasma osmolality (pOS) and thirst (Th), defined by the function:

$$Th = 0.30 \times (pOS - 281), r = 0.91, p < 0.001.$$

Drinking large volumes of fluid to quench thirst causes a dramatic fall in osmotically stimulated AVP concentrations and an abrupt decline in thirst analog scores, both of which occur within a few minutes of drinking and before there are significant changes in plasma osmolality. This implies a nonosmotic oropharyngeal–neurohypophysial neuronal reflex. The functional analysis of osmotically mediated vasopressin release is helpful in defining disorders of vasopressin secretion. Abnormalities in the sensitivity of the vasopressin-releasing unit and in the threshold of vasopressin secretion have been defined. Similarly, quantification of thirst has contributed to a clearer understanding of hypodipsic syndromes (see below).

Plasma osmolality, plasma vasopressin, and thirst

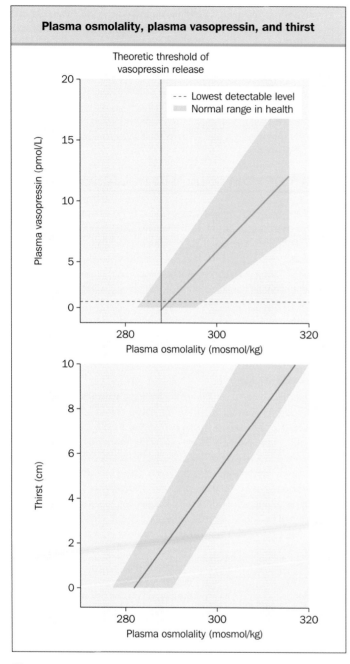

Figure 7.10 Plasma osmolality, plasma vasopressin, and thirst. (Top panel) Relationship between plasma osmolality and plasma vasopressin. (Lower panel) Relationship between plasma osmolality and thirst. Thirst is measured in arbitrary units along a linear scale. Plasma vasopressin rises in a linear fashion in response to increasing plasma osmolality. The abscissal intercept represents the theoretic threshold for vasopressin release, and the slope of the line represents the sensitivity of the osmoreceptor–vasopressin-synthesizing unit. Healthy individuals maintain their plasma osmolality within the range 282–295mosmol/kg, with plasma vasopressin concentrations varying from 0.3 to 4.0pmol/L. There is a similar progressive increase in thirst sensation with rises in plasma osmolality.

Relationship between mean arterial pressure and vasopressin release

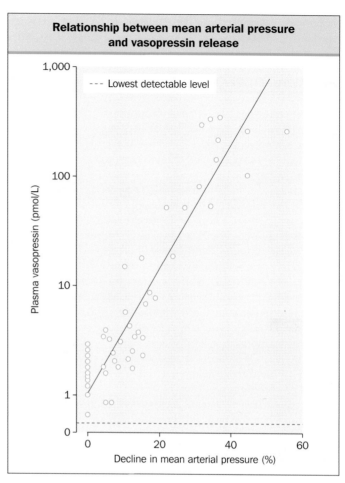

Figure 7.11 Relationship between mean arterial pressure and vasopressin release. An acute fall in blood pressure or volume causes release of vasopressin. The graph shows the exponential rise in vasopressin in response to progressive hypotension induced (in normal subjects) by infusion of the ganglion-blocking drug trimetaphan over periods ranging from 15 to 30 minutes. Blood pressure must be reduced by at least 10% before any significant rise in vasopressin secretion occurs, although a 40% reduction in blood pressure leads to plasma vasopressin concentrations of about one hundred times the normal basal level.

BAROREGULATION OF VASOPRESSIN SECRETION

An acute fall in blood pressure or blood volume causes release of vasopressin. Whether hypertension or hypervolemia affects vasopressin secretion is not known. The exponential rise in plasma vasopressin concentrations in response to progressive hypotension induced in healthy normal subjects by the infusion of the ganglion-blocking drug trimetaphan, over periods of 15–30min, is shown in **Figure 7.11**. Similar large increases in the concentration of plasma vasopressin have been demonstrated in normal humans who have been rendered hypotensive after tilting, or hypovolemic after phlebotomy. Acute severe hypovolemia and hypotension also induces intense thirst.

Minor fluctuations in blood pressure appear to have very little effect on plasma vasopressin concentration. A fall in blood pressure of 10% or more must be attained before a significant rise in

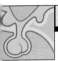

vasopressin is achieved. A 40% reduction in pressure, however, produces plasma vasopressin levels approximately 100 times greater than the normal basal concentrations.

RENAL ACTION OF VASOPRESSIN

The major physiologic function of vasopressin is the concentration of urine. AVP binds to a number of sites along the mammalian nephron, the medullary thick ascending limb of Henle's loop, the inner medullary nephron, and the collecting tubule, its major site of action.

The hormone binds to a specific receptor (V_2-receptor) on the contralateral side of the tubular cells of the distal collecting duct of the nephron. The gene for the receptor is located on the long arm of chromosome X, Xq28. The V_2-receptor is coupled to adenyl cyclase through a stimulatory G-protein, which generates cyclic adenosine monophosphate (cAMP) from adenosine triphosphate (ATP). The cAMP activates protein kinase A, which, in turn, realigns the water channel protein aquaporin-2 so that it may be inserted into the tubular luminal membrane. Aquaporin-2 is one of a family of aquaporins found throughout many membranes of mammalian cells. It is responsive specifically to the action of AVP. Tetramers of aquaporin-2 are formed prior to delivery to the tubular membrane. Human aquaporin-2 gene is located on chromosome 12.

Active insertion of water channels into the luminal membrane allows fluid to move into and across the tubular cell to the contraluminal aspect, where the fluid exits through nonsensitive AVP water-channel proteins, aquaporin-3 and aquaporin-4 (**Fig. 7.12**). The force that drives the water across the cell is an osmotic gradient generated by hypotonic luminal fluid (dilute urine) and the hypertonic renal interstitium. Thus, under the action of AVP urine is concentrated.

In addition to the AVP-sensitive water channels in the collecting tubule there is a distinct AVP-regulated urea transporter in the distal nephron. By cycling urea into the renal interstitium, urea is conserved and contributes to the osmotic gradient across the nephron, thus enhancing the concentration of urine.

As the concentration of circulating vasopressin rises there is a reduction of urine flow and an increase in urine osmolality (**Fig. 7.13**). Maximum antidiuresis occurs at plasma vasopressin concentrations of the order of 2–4pmol/L, generating a maximum urine osmolality of 800–1200mosmol/kg in humans, while maximum diuresis occurs with plasma vasopressin values less than 0.3pmol/L.

CAUSES OF POLYURIA AND POLYDIPSIA

Polyuria or diabetes insipidus can be defined by the persistent excretion of copious dilute urine (osmolality <200mosmol/kg), in excess of 2.5L/24h (40mL/kg/24h) in adults, and in infants more than 100mL/kg/24h. It is associated with increased thirst, polydipsia. One of three pathogenic mechanisms may be responsible for polyuria and polydipsia (**Fig. 7.14**), which define the three basic etiologic disorders:

- primary polydipsia.;
- cranial diabetes insipidus;
- nephrogenic diabetes insipidus.

Primary polydipsia

Primary polydipsia or dipsogenic diabetes insipidus may occur for no apparent reason but is more often related to some form of psychiatric illness. Mouth dryness caused by drugs (e.g. monoamine oxidase inhibitors) or mouth-breathing must be distinguished from true polydipsia. Occasionally, structural damage to the anterior hypothalamus due to multiple sclerosis or sarcoidosis may cause primary polydipsia (**Table 7.3**). Vasopressin secretion is normally suppressed by the low plasma osmolality in primary polydipsia but its renal action may also be impaired if excessive fluid intake is prolonged, since the solute

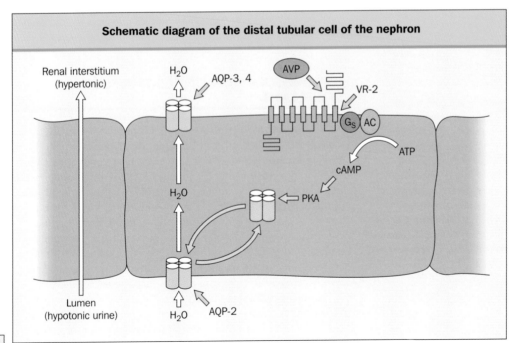

Figure 7.12 Schematic diagram of the distal tubular cell of the nephron. Vasopressin (AVP) binds to the V_2-receptor (VR-2), which generates cyclic adenosine monophosphate (cAMP). Activation of protein kinase A (PKA) aligns the water channel protein aquaporin-2 (AQP-2) into a tetramer before insertion into the luminal membrane. Solute-free water flows along the osmotic gradient formed by the hypotonic urine and the hypertonic renal interstitium. In contrast to AQP-2, aquaporin-3 and aquaporin-4 (AQP-3,4) are not AVP-sensitive. AC, adenylate cyclase; ATP, adenosine triphosphate; Gs, stimulatory G protein.

Relationship between plasma vasopressin concentration and urine osmolality

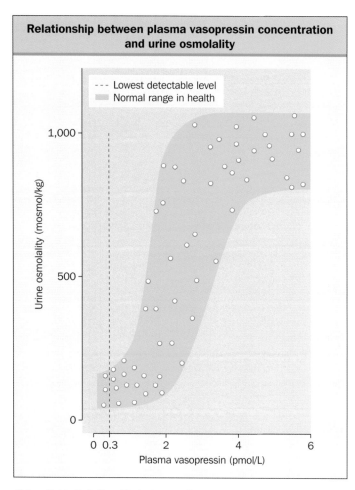

Figure 7.13 Relationship between plasma vasopressin concentration and urine osmolality. Maximum diuresis with minimal urine osmolality occurs in response to low or undetectable plasma vasopressin concentration. Maximum antidiuresis with maximal urine osmolality results from plasma vasopressin concentrations greater than 2–4pmol/L.

Causes of primary polydipsia

Causes of primary polydipsia
Associated with psychosis
Sarcoidosis
Autoimmune, multiple sclerosis
Drug-induced (lithium, tricyclic antidepressants)
Idiopathic

Table 7.3 Causes of primary polydipsia.

concentration within the renal interstitial medulla is reduced by a 'washout' effect. This leads to a reduction in the osmotic gradient across the renal tubular cell. Thus, even when there is maximum tubular permeability under the action of vasopressin, free water is unable to flow normally from the lumen to the medulla and, consequently, urinary concentrating ability is impaired. Any cause of polyuria may result in this secondary renal defect.

Causes of polyuria and polydipsia

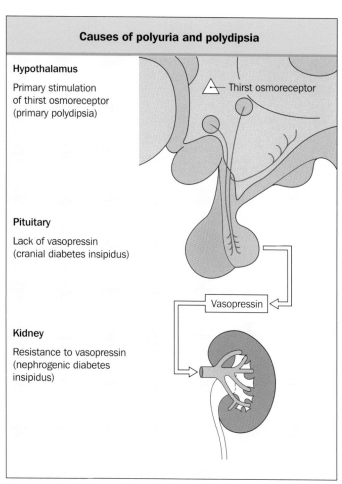

Hypothalamus

Primary stimulation of thirst osmoreceptor (primary polydipsia)

Pituitary

Lack of vasopressin (cranial diabetes insipidus)

Kidney

Resistance to vasopressin (nephrogenic diabetes insipidus)

Figure 7.14 Causes of polyuria and polydipsia. (Top) Primary polydipsia is usually related to psychiatric illness. Vasopressin secretion is suppressed by low plasma osmolality induced by the excessive water intake which, if prolonged, may also affect the kidney. (Center) Cranial diabetes insipidus is caused by a reduction or absence of vasopressin. (Bottom) In nephrogenic diabetes insipidus, there is resistance to the renal action of vasopressin, with a consequent rise in the plasma vasopressin concentration to a level that is inappropriately high relative to urine osmolality.

Nephrogenic diabetes insipidus

Acquired nephrogenic diabetes is more common than the familial form, particularly in association with the osmotic diuresis due to diabetes mellitus. Other common causes include metabolic disorders, nephrotoxic drugs and intrinsic renal disease (**Table 7.4**). The hereditary, X-linked form of nephrogenic diabetes insipidus is very rare and causes symptoms from birth. An autosomal recessive form of nephrogenic diabetes insipidus is caused by aquaporin-2 gene mutations and accounts for about 10% of familial nephrogenic diabetes insipidus.

Cranial diabetes insipidus

Cranial diabetes insipidus is an uncommon condition, with an estimated prevalence of 1:25,000 and equal gender distribution, and is characterized by an absolute or (more often) relative lack of osmoregulated vasopressin. (The causes are listed in **Table 7.5.**) The majority of patients have measurable plasma vasopressin but its concentration is inappropriately low for the concomitant plasma osmolality.

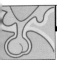

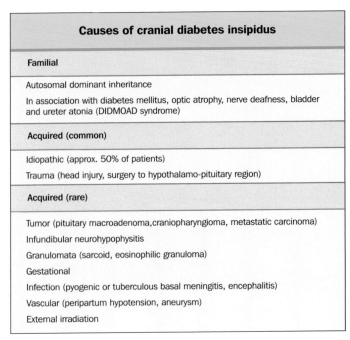

Causes of nephrogenic diabetes insipidus	
Familial	**Acquired**
X-linked recessive: V₂-receptor gene defect	Chronic renal disease
Autosomal recessive: aquaporin-2 gene defect	Metabolic disease (hypokalemia, hypercalcemia)
	Drugs (lithium, demeclocycline)
	Osmotic diuresis
	Pregnancy

Table 7.4 Causes of nephrogenic diabetes insipidus.

Causes of cranial diabetes insipidus
Familial
Autosomal dominant inheritance
In association with diabetes mellitus, optic atrophy, nerve deafness, bladder and ureter atonia (DIDMOAD syndrome)
Acquired (common)
Idiopathic (approx. 50% of patients)
Trauma (head injury, surgery to hypothalamo-pituitary region)
Acquired (rare)
Tumor (pituitary macroadenoma, craniopharyngioma, metastatic carcinoma)
Infundibular neurohypophysitis
Granulomata (sarcoid, eosinophilic granuloma)
Gestational
Infection (pyogenic or tuberculous basal meningitis, encephalitis)
Vascular (peripartum hypotension, aneurysm)
External irradiation

Table 7.5 Causes of cranial diabetes insipidus. All patients have polyuria and inappropriately low plasma vasopressin concentrations relative to their plasma osmolality. Idiopathic cranial diabetes insipidus may be due to autoimmune disease in some patients.

The familial forms of the disorder are rare. Genetic abnormalities have been identified on chromosome 20p13 in several kindreds with autosomal dominant cranial diabetes insipidus. Nucleotide deletions, missense mutations and stop codons have been found, usually in the region encoding for neurophysin or the signal peptide and very rarely for vasopressin itself (**Fig. 7.15**). The mutations interfere with the normal folding of the precursor molecule and result in abnormal processing of the prohormone. Over 43 kindreds share 31 different mutations. The onset of polyuria is usually not in the first few months of life but between the ages of 1 and 6 years. The polyuria in patients with the DIDMOAD (diabetes insipidus, diabetes mellitus, optic atrophy, and (nerve) deafness) syndrome is less profound than in those with the isolated defect. No specific cause can be found for some 30% of patients with acquired cranial diabetes insipidus, although approximately one-third of these patients may have circulating antibodies to the vasopressin-synthesizing neuron, thus suggesting an autoimmune etiology.

A pituitary tumor (or more often surgery to it) may cause cranial diabetes insipidus if there is injury to the hypothalamus or the upper part of the pituitary stalk; this accounts for a large proportion of cases. The other causes of cranial diabetes insipidus are rare.

All patients have a low or undetectable plasma vasopressin concentration in relation to their plasma osmolality. The majority of patients with cranial diabetes insipidus lose the normal hyperintense signal of the healthy posterior pituitary with T₁-weighted magnetic resonance imaging.

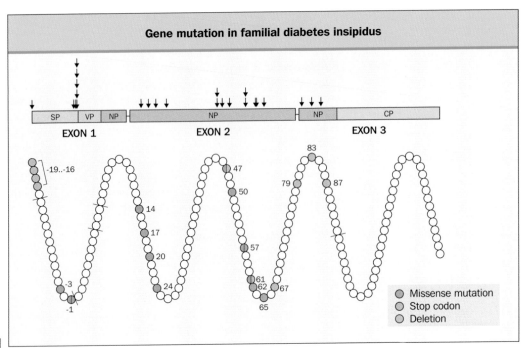

Figure 7.15 Gene mutation in familial cranial diabetes insipidus. Schematic diagram indicating the regions encoding the vasopressin precursor molecule and the primary structure of the preprohormone. The location and type of mutation in familial autosomal dominant cranial diabetes insipidus are shown. CP, copeptin; NP, neurophysin; SP, signal peptide; VP, vasopressin. (Modified with permission from Rittig S, Robertson GL, Siggard C, et al. Identification of 13 new mutations in the vasopressin-neurophysin II gene. Am J Hum Genet. 1996;58:107–17.)

Water deprivation test	
Preparation of patient	
Fluid intake encouraged during night before test	
Light breakfast, no tea, coffee, alcohol or smoking for 12 hours before test	
Dehydration test	
No fluids for 8 hours: allow only dry snacks	
Weigh patient hourly: consider stopping test if there is more than 3% loss of initial body weight	
Sample urine hourly to measure volume and osmolality	
Draw venous blood every 2 hours to measure plasma osmolality, and vasopressin if possible	
Patient to be supervised throughout test	

Table 7.6 Water deprivation test. The procedure followed in preparation of the test. In order to avoid excessive dehydration, patients must be encouraged to drink overnight before the test. They should also be closely supervised during the test to prevent clandestine drinking.

Water deprivation test
Response to exogenous vasopressin
After period of dehydration (see Table 7.6) administer desmopressin 1 µg intramuscularly
Patient allowed to eat and drink, but avoid excessive fluid intake
Sample urine at 3, 5 and 16 hours after desmopressin to measure volume and osmolality
Draw venous blood at 5 and 16 hours after desmopressin to measure osmolality
Patient to be supervised throughout test

Table 7.7 Water deprivation test. The test of response to exogenous vasopressin. This test should follow on immediately after fluid deprivation. Patients must avoid excessive fluid intake after injection of desmopressin to avoid sudden profound hyponatremia.

Interpretation of results from water deprivation test		
Urine osmolality (mosmol/kg)		**Diagnosis**
After dehydration	After desmopressin	
>750	>750	Normal
<300	>750	CDI
<300	<300	NDI
300–750	<750	Partial CDI, NDI or PP

Table 7.8 Interpretation of results from water deprivation test. Results of many polyuric patients fall into the urine osmolality ranges of 300–750mosmol/kg after dehydration and to less than 750mosmol/kg after administration of desmopressin. The test, therefore, often fails to distinguish between partial forms of cranial diabetes insipidus (CDI) and nephrogenic diabetes insipidus (NDI), and primary polydipsia (PP).

The water deprivation test

The water deprivation test has long been the 'cornerstone' for differentiating between the causes of polyuria. The protocol for a modified Dashe dehydration test, combined with an assessment of response to exogenous vasopressin, is shown in **Tables 7.6 and 7.7**. Patients with moderate or severe cranial diabetes insipidus are clearly distinguished from others by the observation of consistently hypotonic urine during fluid restriction, together with concentrated urine after the administration of exogenous vasopressin, desmopressin. Hypotonic urine following exogenous vasopressin strongly suggests nephrogenic diabetes insipidus. Interpretation of the water deprivation test is outlined in **Table 7.8**.

Difficulty is often experienced when differentiating between primary polydipsia, mild cranial diabetes insipidus and nephrogenic diabetes insipidus. This is because many polydipsic patients have a minor concentrating defect secondary to the solute loss from the renal interstitial medulla. Measurement of plasma vasopressin in response to osmotic stimulation, and the relationship of endogenous plasma vasopressin with urine osmolality after overnight dehydration, aids in the differentiation of these disorders.

The water deprivation test is difficult to perform correctly, unpleasant for the patient (who may drink surreptitiously during the test), and relies heavily on the patient's ability to empty the bladder completely. For these reasons, it is far from ideal. Furthermore, the stimulus to vasopressin secretion is a combination of hypertonicity and hypovolemia, especially towards the end of the period of dehydration.

Differentiation between the causes of polyuria

The most precise way to diagnose the three basic causes of polyuria rests on the measurement of plasma vasopressin, plasma osmolality, and urine osmolality after osmotic stimulation and/or dehydration. It can be seen in **Figure 7.16** (left panel) that, after infusion of 5% hypertonic saline, patients with cranial diabetes insipidus have values that fall to the right of the normal range, while those with primary polydipsia or nephrogenic diabetes insipidus remain in the normal range.

Nephrogenic diabetes insipidus (**Fig. 7.16**, right panel) can be readily distinguished by the inappropriately high plasma vasopressin levels in relation to the low urine osmolality attained after dehydration.

If results from a water deprivation test are equivocal (because of reduced concentrating ability secondary to chronic polyuria of any cause) and measurement of plasma vasopressin is not available, a carefully conducted therapeutic trial of desmopressin can be useful in determining the etiology of polyuria and polydipsia. A week's treatment with desmopressin will restore responsiveness of the renal tubule to endogenous vasopressin. Measurements of plasma osmolality (or sodium), urine osmolality and weight are made on a daily basis for a few days prior to administration of low-dose desmopressin (1µg intramuscularly or 20–40µg intranasally) daily for 1 week. Symptoms of patients with vasopressin deficiency (cranial diabetes insipidus) will resolve, while those with nephrogenic diabetes will remain unchanged. A patient with primary polydipsia will develop hypotonic hyponatremia (**Fig. 7.17**). A summary of the results of a low-dose therapeutic trial of desmopressin is given in **Table 7.9**.

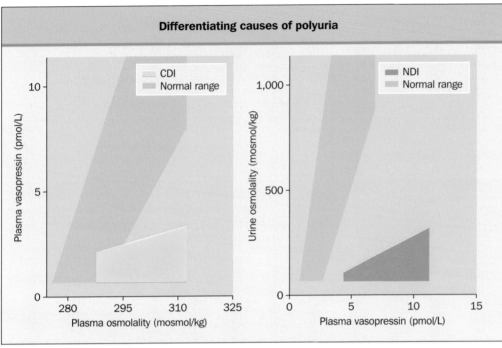

Figure 7.16 Differentiating causes of polyuria. (Left) After osmotic stimulation with 5% hypertonic saline iv, patients with cranial diabetes insipidus (CDI) exhibit values to the right of the normal range, while those with nephrogenic diabetes insipidus (NDI) and primary polydipsia will show values within the normal limits. (Right) After overnight dehydration, NDI is usually distinguishable from primary polydipsia by the inappropriately high levels of plasma vasopressin relative to urine osmolality.

Interpretation of results from therapeutic trial of low-dose desmopressin				
Symptoms	Weight	Urine osmolality	Plasma osmolality	Diagnosis
Improved	Slightly ↑	↑↑	Unchanged or ↓ slightly	Cranial diabetes insipidus
Unchanged	Unchanged	Unchanged	Unchanged	Nephrogenic diabetes insipidus
Little change	↑↑	↑↑	↓↓	Primary polydipsia (see Fig. 7.17)

Table 7.9 Interpretation of results from therapeutic trial of low-dose desmopressin.

TREATMENT OF CRANIAL DIABETES INSIPIDUS

Many patients with mild cranial diabetes insipidus (i.e. 24-hour urine volume up to 4L) decide to have no therapy and appear to remain well. These patients rely on their thirst mechanisms to maintain water homeostasis. If an untreated patient is unable to obtain fluid or loses thirst awareness (e.g. is in a coma), hypernatremia will develop and the condition can be life-threatening. Furthermore, long-standing severe cranial diabetes insipidus can lead to hydroureter and hydronephrosis, and possibly to a degree of nephrogenic diabetes insipidus due to solute 'washout' from the kidney. There are therefore arguments for treating all patients whose urinary output exceeds 4L/24h.

Desmopressin, a long-acting vasopressin analog, is the treatment of choice (**Fig. 7.18**). In comparison with the native hormone, desmopressin has greater antidiuretic potency and little (if any) pressor activity. It can be administered intranasally, as a spray or by nasal tube, parenterally, or orally (**Table 7.10**). Care must be taken to avoid overdosage, since persistent antidiuresis with continual fluid intake will eventually lead to profound hyponatremia. It is therefore wise to allow the patient to develop polyuria for a short period each week. Other than potential hyponatremia, desmopressin is remarkably free of side effects. Rarely, allergic rhinitis has occurred, caused by preservatives, not

desmopressin, in intranasal preparations. Lysine vasopressin is a poor substitute for desmopressin because its therapeutic action lasts for only 1–3 hours and it retains pressor activity.

Although use of nonhormonal drugs (**Table 7.10**) has been recommended in the past, their high incidence of significant side effects and limited antidiuretic effect have restricted their use. Chlorpropamide appears to act by increasing renal tubular sensitivity to circulating endogenous vasopressin, while carbamazepine probably increases vasopressin secretion. These drugs are suitable only for patients with partial cranial diabetes insipidus, who still secrete vasopressin but in insufficient quantities. The mechanism of action of thiazide diuretics is probably related to the reduction in extracellular sodium and decreased glomerular filtration. All these oral preparations reduce the polyuria by 25–50%.

THE SYNDROME OF INAPPROPRIATE ANTIDIURESIS

The syndrome of inappropriate antidiuresis (SIAD) is a common cause of hyponatremia (**Table 7.11**); it falls into the category of normovolemic (i.e. clinically normal extracellular volume) hyponatremia. Although total water is increased in SIAD, it is not clinically demonstrable, since water is distributed throughout intracellular and extracellular compartments. In contrast,

Diagnosis of primary polydipsia

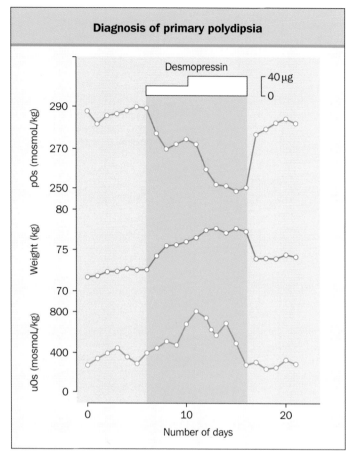

Figure 7.17 Diagnosis of primary polydipsia. The diagram shows the effect of ad libitum fluid and intranasal DDAVP (desmopressin) on plasma osmolality (pOs), weight, and urine osmolality (uOs) in a patient with primary polydipsia. Hypotonic hyponatremia is a diagnostic feature.

Structure of desmopressin

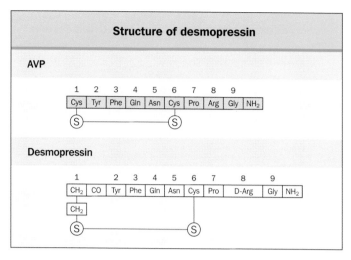

Figure 7.18 Structure of desmopressin. A schematic diagram of native vasopressin (AVP) and the synthetic antidiuretic analog DDAVP (desmopressin). The analog is deaminated at position 1, and arginine at position 8 is in the D rather than the L form.

Treatment of cranial diabetes insipidus

Vasopressin analogs		Nonhormonal oral drugs	
Desmopressin:		Chlorpropamide	250–500 mg daily
intranasal	5–100 µg daily		
intramuscular	1–4 µg daily	Carbamazepine	200–400 mg daily
oral	100–1200 µg daily	Thiazide diuretic e.g. bendrofluazide 5 mg daily	
Lysine vasopressin: intranasal	5–20 units daily		

Table 7.10 Treatment of cranial diabetes insipidus. Desmopressin is the treatment of choice.

Clinical classification of hyponatremia

Type	Hypervolemic	Normovolemic	Hypovolemic
Mechanism	Extracellular sodium content increased	Extracellular sodium content normal	Extracellular sodium content decreased
	Body water greatly increased	Body water increased	Body water slightly decreased
Examples of causes	Heart failure	SIAD	Gastrointestinal losses
	Cirrhosis	Glucocorticoid deficiency	Excessive sweating, burns
	Nephrotic syndrome	Hypothyroidism	Addison's disease
	Renal failure		Renal or cerebral salt wasting

Table 7.11 Clinical classification of hyponatremia. The three groups are distinguished by differences in extracellular volume status. The syndrome of inappropriate antidiuresis (SIAD) is the most common cause of normovolemic hyponatremia.

hypervolemic hyponatremia is recognized by features of extracellular fluid overload, e.g. dependent edema, and hypovolemic hyponatremia by signs of dehydration and hypotension. In all types of hyponatremia there is an excess of water relative to extracellular sodium, and the three categories of hyponatremia are distinguished by the extracellular sodium content. Examples of causes of the different types of hyponatremia are given in **Table 7.11**.

The cardinal features of SIAD were described by Bartter and Schwartz (**Table 7.12**). These criteria must be fulfilled before a diagnosis of SIAD can be made. The measurement of plasma vasopressin does not aid the diagnosis of SIAD because over 90% of all patients with hyponatremia, irrespective of their extracellular volume status or underlying cause, have detectable or elevated vasopressin concentrations.

Causes

Many conditions have been described in association with the cardinal manifestations of SIAD (**Table 7.13**). Four main groups of disorders emerge: neoplastic, central nervous, respiratory, and drug-related.

Features of the syndrome of inappropriate antidiuresis

Hyponatraemia and hypotonicity of plasma

Urine osmolality greater than plasma osmolality

Excessive renal excretion of sodium

Absence of volume depletion or edema-forming states

Normal renal and adrenal function

Table 7.12 Features of the syndrome of inappropriate antidiuresis. All criteria should be fulfilled before a diagnosis of syndrome of inappropriate antidiuresis (SIAD) can be made.

Causes of the syndrome of inappropriate antidiuresis

Tumours	Drugs
Carcinoma – especially of the lung	Vasopressin
Thymoma	Oxytocin
Lymphoma	Vincristine
Leukaemia	Vinblastine
Sarcoma	Cyclophosphamide
Mesothelioma	Chlorpropamide
	Carbamazepine
Respiratory disorders	Clofibrate
	Thiazide diuretics
Pneumonia	Monoamine oxidase inhibitors
Tuberculosis	Phenothiazines
Empyema	Nicotine
Pneumothorax	Selective serotonin reuptake inhibitors
Asthma	
Positive-pressure ventilation	'Ecstasy'
Central nervous system disorders	**Miscellaneous**
Meningitis	
Encephalitis	Psychosis
Head injury	Hypothyroidism
Brain abscess	Glucocorticoid deficiency
Brain tumor	Postoperative state
Subarachnoid hemorrhage	Idiopathic
Cerebral thrombosis	
Guillain-Barré syndrome	
Acute intermittent porphyria	

Table 7.13 Causes of the syndrome of inappropriate antidiuresis. The lists give a selection of the more common causes and are not comprehensive.

Types

Following extensive osmoregulatory studies of vasopressin secretion in hyponatremic patients who all fulfilled the criteria for SIAD, four patterns of vasopressin secretion emerged (**Fig. 7.19**).

The first and most common pattern (type I), accounting for approximately 40% of patients with SIAD, is characterized by excessive and erratic vasopressin secretion that is totally

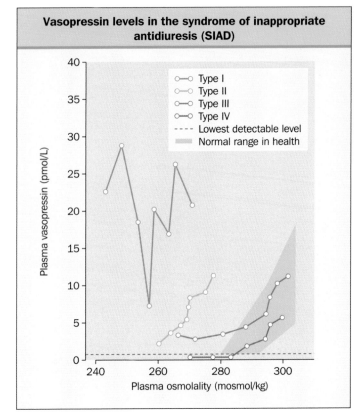

Figure 7.19 Vasopressin levels in the syndrome of inappropriate antidiuresis (SIAD). The diagram shows the vasopressin levels in the four types of SIAD. Type I accounts for some 40% of cases and is characterized by excessive and erratic vasopressin secretion unrelated to changes in plasma osmolality. Type II SIAD ('reset osmostat') is the second most common variant. Patients continue to regulate water excretion about a lowered plasma osmolality. Type III SIAD is characterized by normal osmoregulation of vasopressin except when the plasma is hypotonic, when there is constant and nonsuppressible vasopressin secretion. Type IV SIAD accounts for fewer than 10% of cases. Osmoregulation of vasopressin secretion is entirely normal and yet patients fulfill the criteria for SIAD.

unaffected by changes in plasma osmolality. Although neoplastic conditions often demonstrate this pattern, many other causes of SIAD show the same abnormality. The pathogenesis of this type of defect is unknown but several different mechanisms are possible. Ectopic production of vasopressin by neoplasms might be expected to cause random release. Rapidly fluctuating nonosmotic stimuli (e.g. hypotension) might also be responsible. Electrical instability of the neurogenic pathways that control vasopressin, or the neurohypophysis itself, is a further possible mechanism.

The type II pattern is the second most common osmoregulatory defect and has been termed the 'reset osmostat'. Patients with the type II defect continue to regulate water excretion about a lowered plasma osmolality. This pattern of vasopressin secretion is observed in patients with neoplasms, chest disease, and nervous disorders. The pathogenesis of the pattern remains unknown, but interruption of the afferent limb of the baroregulatory reflex arc that normally inhibits vasopressin secretion is one possible mechanism.

Treatment of the syndrome of inappropriate antidiuresis
Fluid restriction
500 mL/24h or less (as long as plasma remains dilute)
Drugs
Linear non-peptide V$_2$ receptor antagonist, e.g. OPC-31260
Induction of partial nephrogenic diabetes insipidus with demeclocycline or lithium
Inhibition of vasopressin release by phenytoin or oxilorphan
Induction of osmotic diuresis with oral urea
Saline infusion
Isotonic or hypertonic, to be used in emergency situation only
Infuse slowly; plasma sodium concentration should not increase more quickly than 0.5 mmol/L/h

Table 7.14 Treatment of the syndrome of inappropriate antidiuresis. Long-term fluid restriction may be inconvenient and unpleasant for the patient; drug therapy may be a more useful solution. Hypertonic saline infusion should be used only in emergencies.

The type III defect is characterized by normal and appropriate osmoregulation of the hormone, except under conditions of plasma hypotonicity when there is constant nonsuppressible vasopressin secretion. It is rarely seen in malignant disease. The abnormality may be due to a persistent 'leak' of vasopressin resulting from neurohypophysial damage, loss of inhibitory osmoregulatory neurons, or persistent nonosmotic stimulation.

Type IV is uncommon, accounting for less than 10% of all cases. Osmoregulated vasopressin secretion is entirely normal, yet patients still fulfill the criteria of SIAD. Antidiuretic hormones other than vasopressin (e.g. vasotocin) may be responsible. Alternatively, the defect may lie within the kidney.

Treatment

Asymptomatic or mild degrees of hyponatremia due to SIAD may not require specific treatment. If therapy is deemed necessary, treatment of the underlying cause of SIAD may be sufficient to correct the hyponatremia. Fluid restriction to 500mL/24h remains the mainstay of SIAD-induced hyponatremia (**Table 7.14**). In the long-term management of SIAD, fluid restriction may be inconvenient or unpleasant for the patient, so administration of drugs that inhibit the renal action of vasopressin has been advocated. Demeclocycline is preferable to lithium, since it is less toxic, but its maximum effect may take 3 weeks to achieve. Phenytoin may occasionally suppress abnormal vasopressin secretion from the pituitary. A logical therapeutic approach is the development of a V$_2$-receptor antagonist that will specifically block the antidiuretic effect of excess circulating vasopressin. No vasopressin analogs have proved to be efficacious in man but the synthetic linear nonpeptide V$_2$-receptor antagonist OPC-31260 increases renal solute-free water excretion without influencing salt excretion. Studies in patients with SIAD treated with OPC-31260 have shown substantial improvement in their hyponatremia.

Causes of chronic hypodipsic hypernatremia	
Vascular	**Granulomatous**
Anterior communicating artery aneurysm	Sarcoidosis
Intrahypothalamic bleed	Tuberculosis
Internal carotid artery ligation	Histiocytosis
Neoplastic	**Miscellaneous**
Craniopharyngioma	Head injury
Pinealoma	Toluene exposure
Metastatic lung or breast disease	Hydrocephalus

Table 7.15 Causes of chronic hypodipsic hypernatremia.

Isotonic or hypertonic saline infusion must be used with extreme caution to treat chronic hyponatremia and should be reserved for emergency situations such as associated seizures, stupor, or marked confusion. Great care should be taken to avoid rapid correction of hyponatremia, irrespective of the manner of treatment, as central pontine myelinolysis (osmotic demyelination syndrome) may ensue. The rate of increase in plasma sodium should not exceed 0.5mmol/L/h (10mmol/1/24h), and saline infusion should stop when serum sodium reaches 120–125mmol/L.

CHRONIC HYPODIPSIC SYNDROMES

Longstanding hypodipsia (reduced osmoregulated thirst appreciation) or adipsia (no thirst) lead to chronic inadequate intake of fluid, which results in hypernatremia (serum sodium >145mmol/L) and occasionally causes life-threatening hypernatremia with serum sodium in excess of 180mmol/L. There are often associated defects in osmoregulated AVP secretion. These are rare syndromes.

Causes of hypodipsia

Thirst deficiency syndromes develop as a result of pathologic processes involving the thirst osmoreceptor centers in the anterior hypothalamus. **Table 7.15** presents the more common causes. Hemorrhage from an anterior communicating artery aneurysm or its ligation is a frequent cause of hypodipsia.

Pathophysiology

Reduced fluid intake due to hypodipsia over a prolonged period causes both intra- and extracellular volume depletion, with hyperosmolar hypernatremia. Moderate hypernatremia developing slowly causes few symptoms (serum sodium <160mmol/L). More severe hypernatremia, particularly in the young or elderly, is associated with symptoms of lethargy, nausea, irritability, confusion and may progress to seizures and death.

Osmoregulatory studies have defined three types of defect (**Fig 7.20**). In type 1, patients have decreased sensitivity of both sets of osmoreceptors, resulting in partial AVP deficiency and relative hypodipsia. As there is capacity to secrete some AVP

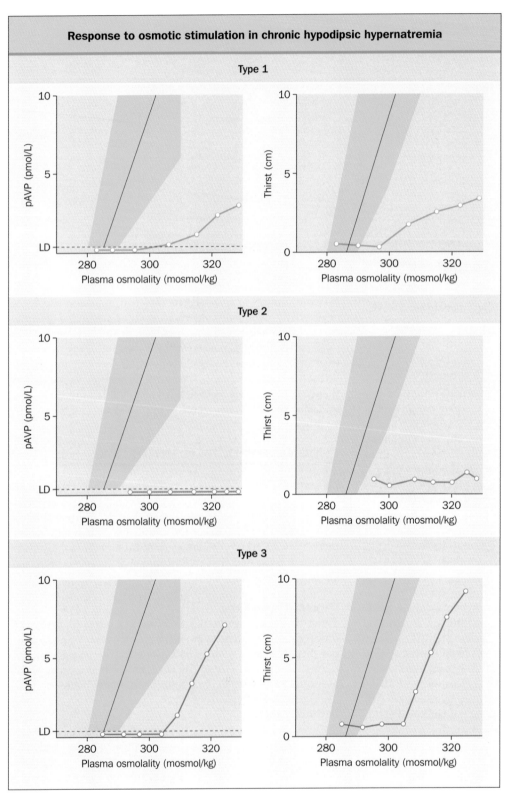

Response to osmotic stimulation in chronic hypodipsic hypernatremia

Type 1

Type 2

Type 3

Figure 7.20 Response to osmotic stimulation in chronic hypodipsic hypernatremia. The figure shows three patterns of response of vasopressin secretion and thirst appreciation (by visual analog scale) to osmotic stimulation using 5% hypertonic saline iv in patients with chronic hypodipsic hypernatremia. Type 1: reduced response. Type 2: no osmoregulation of thirst or vasopressin release. Type 3: reset osmostat to the right of normal (indicated by the shaded area). pAVP, plasma vasopressin; LD, limit of assay detection. (Modified with permission from Baylis PH, Thompson CJ. Diabetes insipidus and hyperosomolar syndromes. In: Becker KL, ed. Principles and practice of endocrinology and metabolism, 2nd edn. Philadelphia, PA; Lippincott, Williams & Wilkins: 1995.)

and appreciate thirst at high levels of plasma osmolality, patients are protected from extreme hypernatremia.

Total ablation of the osmoreceptors will cause diabetes insipidus and complete adipsia (type 2, **Fig. 7.20**). Some patients may secrete small amounts of AVP that is nonresponsive to changes in plasma osmolality; these patients usually still respond to nonosmotic stimuli of AVP secretion. Patients with type 3 have resetting of the osmotic thresholds for thirst onset and AVP release to the right of the normal distribution and have 'essential' hypernatremia. Since they continue to osmoregulate but around a higher than normal setpoint, patients do not become severely hypernatremic.

Treatment

Adequate fluid intake is the basis of treatment with partial thirst defects – hypodipsia. Complete adipsia with absent osmoregulated AVP secretion is a major management problem. These patients are at risk of severe hypernatremia. The therapeutic approach is to fix the 24h urine volume at about 2L, usually with desmopressin, and administer 2L of oral fluid plus a volume that is determined by the fluctuation in body weight from the previous day. Regular frequent (weekly) checks of serum sodium are needed to ensure that there are no wide variations in body water, and constant supervision is necessary to encourage appropriate fluid intake.

FURTHER READING

Adrogué HJ, Madias NE. Hypernatremia. N Engl J Med. 2000;342:1493–99.

Adrogué HJ, Madias NE. Hyponatremia. N Engl J Med. 2000;342:1581–89.

Arieff AI. Management of hyponatremia. Br Med J. 1993;307:305–8.

Ball SG, Vaidja B, Baylis PH. Hypothalamic adipsic syndrome: diagnosis and management. Clin Endocrinol. 1997;47:405–9.

Baylis PH, Cheetham T. Diabetes insipidus. Arch Dis Child. 1998;79:84–9.

Brownstein MJ, Russel JT, Gainer H. Synthesis, transport and release of posterior pituitary hormones. Science 1980;207:373–8.

De Bree MF. Trafficking of vasopressin and oxytocin prohormone through the regulated secretory pathway. J Neuroendocrinol. 2000;12:589–94.

Deen PM, Verdijk MA, Knoers NVAM, et al. Requirement of human renal water channel aquaporin-2 for vasopressin-dependent concentration of urine. Science 1994;264:92–5.

Ellis SJ. Severe hyponatremia: complications and treatment. Q J Med. 1995;88:905–9.

Fried LF, Palevsky PM. Hyponatremia and hypernatremia. Med Clin North Am. 1997;81:585–609.

Hansen L, Rittig S, Robertson GL. Genetic basis of familial neurohypophyseal diabetes insipidus. Trends Endocrinol Metab. 1997;8:363–72.

Mulders SB, Knoers NVAM, van Lieburg AF, et al. New mutations in the *AQP-2* gene in nephrogenic diabetes insipidus resulting in functional but misrouted water channels. J Am Soc Nephrol. 1997;8:242–8.

Pasel K, Schulz A, Timmermann K, et al. Functional characterisation of the molecular defects causing nephrogenic diabetes insipidus in eight families. J Clin Endocrinol Metab. 2000;85:1703–10.

Rittig S, Robertson GL, Siggard C, et al. Identification of 13 new mutations in the vasopressin-neurophysin II gene in 17 kindreds with familial autosomal dominant neurohypophyseal diabetes insipidus. Am J Hum Genet. 1996;58:107–17.

Robertson GL. Diabetes insipidus. Endocrinol Metab Clin North Am. 1995;24:549–72.

Saito T, Ishikawa S, Abe K, et al. Acute aquaresis by the non-peptide arginine vasopressin (AVP) antagonist OPC-31260 improved hyponatremia in patients with the syndrome of inappropriate secretion of antidiuretic hormone. J Clin Endocrinol Metab. 1997;82:1054–7.

Sterns RH, Riggs J, Schochet SS. Osmotic demyelination syndrome following correction of hyponatremia. N Engl J Med. 1986;314:1535–42.

Verbalis JHG. Adaptation to acute and chronic hyponatremia: implications for symptomatology, diagnosis and treatment. Semin Nephrol. 1998;18:3–19.

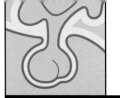

Section 1 Hypothalamus and Pituitary

Chapter 8

Pituitary Surgery

Kamal Thapar, John A Jane Jr, and Edward R Laws Jr

INTRODUCTION

The inaugural event that delivered pituitary tumors into the domain of treatable conditions was a surgical intervention performed more than a century ago. That index case, performed by FT Paul in 1892 and consisting of a transcranial temporal decompression for a pituitary tumor in a patient with acromegaly, came to represent the beginnings of pituitary surgery and firmly grounded surgery as a therapeutic cornerstone for the management of pituitary and parapituitary mass lesions. Since that time, pituitary surgery has evolved to become the treatment of choice for the majority of lesions occurring in and around the sella turcica. Medical and radiotherapeutic treatments can be used to enhance an incomplete surgical response, but surgery can enhance a suboptimal pharmacologic or radiotherapeutic effect. The concept of comprehensive multimodality therapy delivered in a multidisciplinary setting represents the best approach to many pituitary disorders.

CLINICAL PRESENTATION OF PITUITARY TUMORS

The pituitary is surrounded by many important structures (**Fig. 8.1**). Although pituitary adenomas are numerically the most significant of surgical pathologies encountered by the pituitary surgeon and are the principal subject of this chapter, it is important to acknowledge that a wide variety of other lesions can, and frequently do, manifest in the sellar region (**Table 8.1**).

Pituitary tumors typically present in one of three fashions. The most common presentation tends to be related to mass effects. Given their location at the skull base, a growing adenoma will produce a fairly predictable constellation of mass related signs and symptoms. Suprasellar extension with compression of the optic chiasm results in a characteristic bitemporal hemianopic pattern of visual loss (**Fig. 8.2**; see Chapter 3). Encroachment upon hypothalamic structures causes alterations of sleep, alertness, and behavior. Lateral extension of pituitary adenomas into the cavernous sinus occurs quite commonly. With

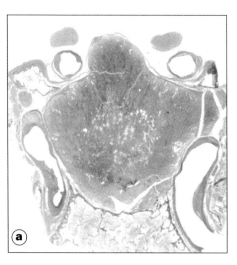

Figure 8.1 (a, b) Coronal section at the level of the cavernous sinus. (a) Whole-mount coronal section of a clinically nonfunctioning pituitary macroadenoma discovered at autopsy. Note the many pertinent anatomic structures that can be compressed by such a lesion. (b) Coronal section at the level of the cavernous sinus showing important anatomic structures in the region.

Optic nerve   Diaphragma   Optic nerve   Supraclinoid carotid artery

III cranial nerve   Pituitary tumor   Carotid artery in cavernous sinus

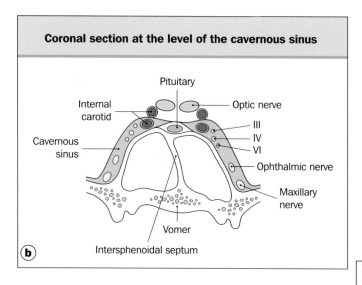

Coronal section at the level of the cavernous sinus

Pituitary
Internal carotid
Optic nerve
III
IV
VI
Cavernous sinus
Ophthalmic nerve
Maxillary nerve
Vomer
Intersphenoidal septum

Table 8.1 Differential diagnosis of a sellar mass.

Differential diagnosis of a sellar mass

Tumors of adenohypophyseal origin	Pituitary adenoma Pituitary adenoma–neuronal choristoma (pituitary adenoma–gangliocytoma) Pituitary carcinoma	
Tumors of neurohypophyseal origin	Granular cell tumor Astrocytoma of posterior lobe and/or stalk (rare)	
Tumors of nonpituitary origin	Craniopharyngioma Germ cell tumors Glioma (hypothalamic, optic nerve/chiasm, infundibulum) Meningioma Chordoma	
	Rare tumors of nonpituitary origin	Chondroma Esthesioneuroblastoma Giant cell tumor of bone Glomangioma Hemangiopericytoma Hemangioblastoma Lipoma Leiomyosarcoma Lymphoma Melanoma Myxoma Paraganglioma Postirradiation neoplasms Rhabdomyosarcoma Sarcoma (chondrosarcoma, osteosarcoma, fibrosarcoma) Schwannoma
Cysts, hamartomas and malformations	Rathke's cleft cyst Arachnoid cyst Epidermoid cyst Dermoid cyst Hypothalamic hamartoma Empty sella syndrome	
Metastatic tumors	Carcinoma Plasmacytoma Lymphoma Leukemia	
Inflammatory conditions	Pyogenic infection/abscess Granulomatous infections Mucocele Lymphocytic hypophysitis Sarcoidosis Langerhans cell histiocytosis Giant cell granuloma	
Vascular lesions	Saccular aneurysm (intracavernous carotid, supraclinoid carotid, anterior communicating artery complex, basilar artery tip) Cavernous angioma	

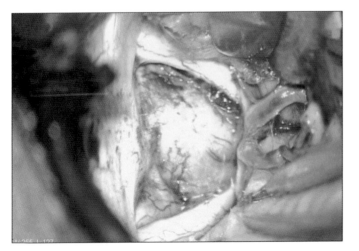

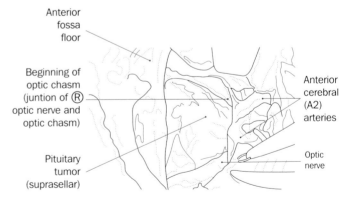

Anterior fossa floor

Beginning of optic chasm (juntion of Ⓡ optic nerve and optic chasm)

Pituitary tumor (suprasellar)

Anterior cerebral (A2) arteries

Optic nerve

Figure 8.2 Chiasmatic compression. This intraoperative photograph, taken during the transcranial resection of a pituitary adenoma (anterior interhemispheric approach) shows the compression and distortion of the optic chiasm. This patient presented with a progressive bitemporal hemianopic visual field deficit with progressive loss of visual acuity (20/400 OU).

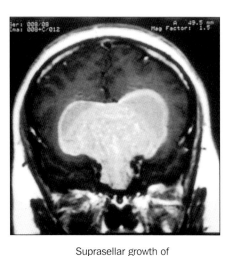

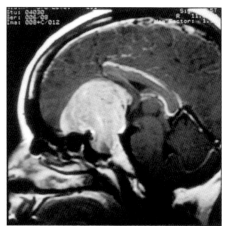

Figure 8.3 Giant pituitary adenoma with extension into the anterior, middle and posterior cranial fossa, coronal and sagittal views.

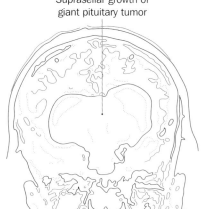

Suprasellar growth of
giant pituitary tumor

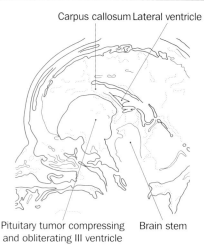

Carpus callosum Lateral ventricle

Pituitary tumor compressing   Brain stem
and obliterating III ventricle

progressive cavernous sinus invasion, transiting cranial nerves may become compressed, producing various components of a cavernous sinus syndrome. These include ptosis, anisocoria, diplopia, and facial numbness or hypoesthesia. These symptoms can mimic those of a carotid aneurysm or any type of tumor involving the cavernous sinus. Some tumors extend in other directions and, if sufficiently large, can involve the anterior, middle, and, occasionally, posterior cranial fossa, wherein they can produce a full spectrum of neurologic deficits (**Fig. 8.3**). In addition, progressive compression of the normal pituitary commonly results in hypopituitarism of varying degrees.

The second mode of presentation involves pituitary hyperfunction in the form of several characteristic hypersecretory states. Hypersecretion of prolactin, growth hormone, adrenocorticotropic hormone (ACTH), and, rarely, thyroid-stimulating hormone (TSH), luteinizing hormone (LH) or follicle-stimulating hormone (FSH) will produce their corresponding clinical phenotypes, as discussed in other chapters. An additional and diagnostically important aspect of both pituitary adenomas and other mass lesions occurring in the region is the phenomenon of functional hyperprolactinemia. It is well recognized that moderate hyperprolactinemia (<100ng/mL, 1800mU/mL) can occur with any of a variety of structural lesions involving the sellar region, and its presence should not immediately prompt a diagnosis of a prolactin-producing adenoma, although true prolactinoma can occur

in patients with this level of prolactin. This phenomenon, frequently referred to as the 'stalk section effect', is the result of compressive or destructive lesions involving the hypothalamus or pituitary stalk, placing pituitary lactotrophs in a disinhibited state with moderate hyperprolactinemia as the result, 'pseudoprolactinoma'(see Chapter 6). As a rule, prolactin levels greater than 100ng/mL are generally the result of a prolactin-producing tumor; lesser elevations may also be due to a small prolactin-producing adenoma but may be the result of any of a variety of other mass, inflammatory, or infiltrative lesions involving the parasellar region.

Thirdly, pituitary tumors may occasionally be discovered coincidentally, typically in a patient suffering from headache, sinus disease, or other nonspecific symptoms in whom routine brain imaging reveals an abnormality in the size, shape, or contents of the sella. The situation is especially common today because of the superior resolution and ready availability of magnetic resonance imaging (MRI). When carefully sought, subtle signal changes in the pituitary gland can be identified in some 10–12% or more of routine MR scans. Thus, the mere presence of a coincidental abnormality on MRI does not necessarily imply the presence of a clinically significant adenoma nor an immediate need for intervention. Instead, careful clinical and endocrinologic correlation are required for such 'coincidentalomas', especially when smaller than 1cm in diameter (**Fig. 8.4**).

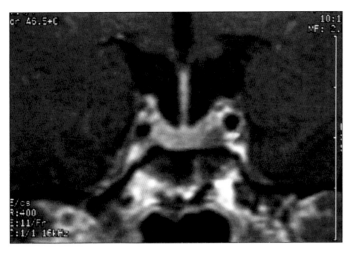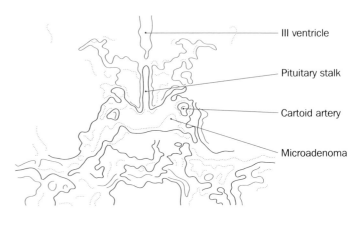

- III ventricle
- Pituitary stalk
- Cartoid artery
- Microadenoma

Figure 8.4 Incidental pituitary microadenoma. This lesion was discovered incidentally upon this imaging study, performed for chronic headaches. It was not associated with any endocrine alterations and no treatment was required.

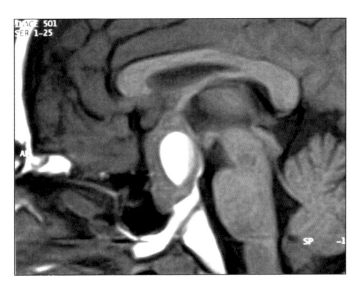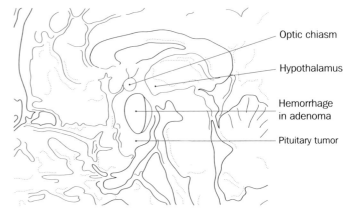

- Optic chiasm
- Hypothalamus
- Hemorrhage in adenoma
- Pituitary tumor

Figure 8.5 Hemorrhagic pituitary adenoma. Sagittal T1-weighted magnetic resonance image of a pituitary macroadenoma with high signal intensity indicating a hemorrhagic center in a patient presenting with acute headache and visual loss.

INDICATIONS FOR SURGERY

While pharmacologic treatment is appropriate for some categories of pituitary disease (e.g. prolactinomas), surgical intervention should be considered for most other symptomatic pituitary lesions. The classic surgical indications for sellar lesions include the following:

- The most urgent indication for surgical intervention relates to some instances of **pituitary apoplexy**. Patients may present with either hemorrhage into an existing pituitary tumor or acute necrosis of the tumor with subsequent swelling (**Fig. 8.5**). While some patients will improve with conservative management, using dexamethasone to suppress any surrounding edema, and a dopamine agonist if the tumor is a prolactinoma, others who do not respond will require urgent transsphenoidal surgery. In the most florid of examples, the presentation includes sudden headache, visual loss, ophthalmoplegia, altered level of consciousness, and collapse from adrenal insufficiency.

- A second clear surgical indication is **progressive mass effect** (usually visual loss) from a large macroadenoma or other sellar mass (**Fig. 8.6**). These patients should always have a serum prolactin determination because prompt and dramatic shrinkage of prolactinomas will usually occur using dopamine-agonist drugs (see Chapter 6). More often, the prolactin level will be only modestly elevated and the patient has a clinically nonfunctioning pituitary tumor or other sellar mass. Such patients will need surgical decompression.

- Among the hyperfunctioning pituitary adenomas, surgery is the treatment of choice for **Cushing's disease**, **acromegaly**, and **secondary hyperthyroidism**. In the case of Cushing's disease, medical management alone is invariably suboptimal and surgery provides the best possibility of obtaining prompt and lasting remission. In the case of somatotroph and

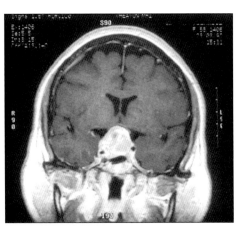

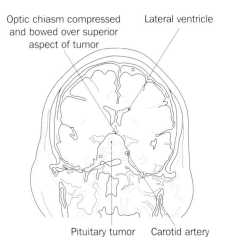

Optic chiasm compressed and bowed over superior aspect of tumor

Lateral ventricle

Pituitary tumor   Carotid artery

Figure 8.6 Chiasmatic compression. Coronal magnetic resonance image showing suprasellar extension of a clinically nonfunctioning pituitary adenoma with chiasmal compression.

thyrotroph adenomas, some latitude exists for the use of somatostatin analogs as the initial intervention; however, surgery remains the preferred, primary treatment for these conditions. For prolactinomas, however, medical therapy will be the preferred initial option (see Chapter 6).

- **Failure of prior therapy** is an increasingly common indication for surgical intervention and may occur in one of several situations. The most straightforward of these involves those patients with symptomatic recurrence in whom prior surgery resulted in a satisfactory remission; these patients frequently benefit from reoperation. Other patients will have been treated with radiotherapy and, after a favorable initial response, now present with recurrence of symptoms, in the form either of mass effect or recurrent hormonal hypersecretion. Still others will have been treated with drug therapy but the response has been suboptimal. For example, in some patients with a pseudoprolactinoma, medical therapy will normalize prolactin levels but progressive tumor growth continues. In patients with genuine prolactinomas, a suboptimal response to medical therapy may take the form of persistently elevated prolactin levels. Surgery may reduce tumor burden and lead to a more effective pharmacologic response. The same also applies to patients with acromegaly for whom somatostatin analogs were used primarily.

- A final and somewhat generic surgical indication relates to **need for a tissue diagnosis**. Although this is seldom required in the case of functioning pituitary adenomas, it may be important when the surgeon is confronted with a nonfunctioning sellar mass whose pathologic identity cannot be confirmed without histologic examination.

Contraindications to surgery

Contraindications for surgery are very few, and most are relative rather than absolute. The most important relate to the general medical condition of the patient, which, in the face of florid Cushing's disease, acromegaly, or secondary hyperthyroidism, can pose a significant anesthetic risk. In most cases, however, the medical condition of the patient can be improved and stabilized before surgery. Similarly, profound hypopituitarism can also be a temporary contraindication to surgery, although it should be fully responsive to corticosteroid and thyroid replacement.

Active sinus infection may also contraindicate the transsphenoidal approach, although this is generally responsive to appropriate antibiotic therapy. Very rarely, the MRI may reveal ectatic and tortuous carotid arteries that protrude from the region of the cavernous sinus and obstruct transsphenoidal access.

Mention should be made of the so-called 'incidentaloma', a pituitary tumor that is discovered fortuitously. Usually these otherwise clinically silent pituitary adenomas are encountered on routine imaging studies done for other reasons, occasionally after a mild head injury, or in the workup of sinus disease. If the lesion truly is asymptomatic then there is usually little reason to recommend surgical intervention and the patient can be followed closely with serial MRI scans and periodic pituitary endocrine assessment. If, however, the lesion is large enough to cause distortion of the optic chiasm, and if the patient is relatively young, one must consider the option of surgery, as most of these tumors will grow slowly over time. If the chiasm is distorted one can anticipate that the patient will ultimately require surgical removal of the lesion. This, of course, assumes that the prolactin level is normal, and factors such as the understanding and the compliance of the patient are critical when making recommendations for treatment of these benign coincidental pituitary tumors.

PRE-SURGICAL EVALUATION

The key elements include:
- establishing an endocrine diagnosis;
- establishing an anatomic diagnosis;
- surveillance for medical co-morbidities;
- evaluation of neuro-ophthalmologic status;
- selection of surgical approach;
- establishing therapeutic goals, both of the surgical procedure and of the broader program of management.

Establish an endocrine diagnosis:

Ordinarily, the history and physical examination will provide some indication as to the endocrine status of the patient. Suspicions of hormone excess and/or deficiency must then be validated by endocrine testing. These details are described elsewhere.

Radiologic classification of pituitary adenomas

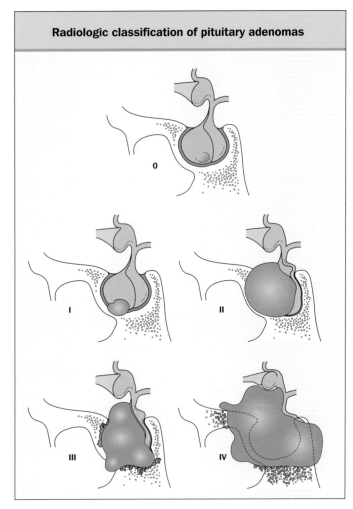

Figure 8.7 Radiologic classification of pituitary adenomas. Pituitary tumors are commonly classified on the basis of their size, invasion status, and growth patterns, as proposed by Hardy and Vezina in 1979. Tumors less than or equal to 1cm in diameter are designated microadenomas, whereas larger tumors are designated macroadenomas. Grade 0: Intrapituitary microadenoma; normal sellar appearance. Grade 1: Intrapituitary microadenoma; focal bulging of sellar wall. Grade 2: Intrasellar macroadenoma; diffusely enlarged sella; no invasion. Grade 3: Macroadenoma; localized sellar invasion and/or destruction. Grade 4: Macroadenoma; extensive sellar invasion and/or destruction. Tumors are further subclassified on the basis of their extrasellar extension, whether suprasellar or parasellar.

Establish an anatomic diagnosis:

This is provided by high-resolution, gadolinium-enhanced MR imaging, which also allows pituitary adenomas to be classified on the basis of their size, invasiveness, and growth characteristics (see Chapter 40). The Hardy classification is usually used which recognizes five different 'grades' of pituitary adenoma (**Fig. 8.7**). Tumors are first distinguished on the basis of size; those equal to or less than 10mm in diameter are designated microadenomas. Larger tumors are called macroadenomas. Microadenomas are designated grade 0 or grade I tumors, depending on whether the sellar appearance is normal or minor focal sellar changes are present, respectively. Macroadenomas causing diffuse sellar enlargement, focal destruction, and

extensive erosion of the skull base are assigned grades II, III, and IV respectively. Macroadenomas can be further subclassified according to the degree of suprasellar extension.

Magnetic resonance imaging will allow the identification of up to 70% of microadenomas, including those as small as 3mm. For macroadenomas, the merits of MR imaging lie in its capacity to identify important relationships between the tumor and surrounding neurovascular structures (**Fig. 8.8**). In this regard, the position of the carotid arteries, the status of the optic chiasm, the extent of supra- and parasellar extension, and paranasal sinus anatomy are of particular operative concern and each is well delineated by MR imaging.

Surveillance for medical co-morbidities

After anatomic and endocrine diagnoses have been established, attention is first turned to optimizing the medical and endocrine status of the patient. In all patients with a pituitary adenoma, some consideration should be given also to the possibility of multiple endocrine neoplasia type 1 (see Chapter 30). Soliciting the family history and measuring serum calcium levels is important in this regard.

Neuro-ophthalmologic evaluation

Whereas the bitemporal hemianopic defect is the classical abnormality associated with sellar tumors, a number of others can occur. Depending on the anatomic status of the chiasm (prefixed, normal, or postfixed), the size of the tumor, its precise direction of growth, and the chronicity of the process, scotomas, various monocular or other asymmetric field defects, afferent pupillary defects, impaired visual acuity, optic atrophy, and papilledema may also be observed. Assessment of visual fields and acuity on a serial basis is often necessary to document disease progression and response to intervention.

Cranial nerve palsies resulting in diplopia are infrequently caused by pituitary adenomas, including those having extension into the cavernous sinus. They can, however, be conspicuous with other histologic entities occurring in the region, particularly meningiomas or other skull-base lesions.

Choice of surgical approach

Surgical approaches to the sellar region can be broadly categorized into three basic groups: transsphenoidal approaches, conventional craniotomy, and alternative skull-base approaches (**Table 8.2**). Within each of these three groups, there is one or more standard procedure, as well as a menu of technical variations and options that allow the operation to be precisely tailored to the situation at hand. Currently, some 96% of all pituitary adenomas can be approached through one variation or another of the transsphenoidal approach. The remainder require transcranial approaches, either standard pterional or subfrontal craniotomy, or various skull-base approaches, which may be transcranial, extracranial, or a combination of the two.

The selection of surgical approach depends on a number of factors. The most important of these are:
- the size of the sella;
- its degree of mineralization;
- the size and pneumatization of the sphenoid sinus;
- the position and tortuosity of the carotid arteries;
- the presence and direction of any intracranial tumor extensions;

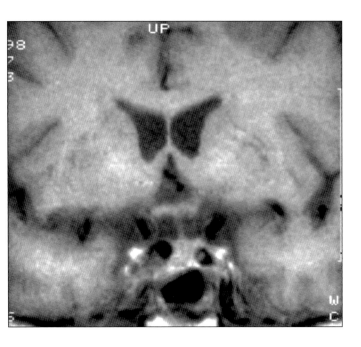

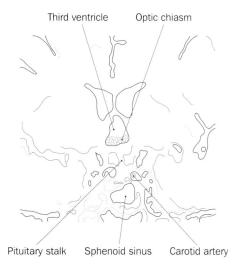

Third ventricle   Optic chiasm

Pituitary stalk   Sphenoid sinus   Carotid artery

Figure 8.8 Magnetic resonance image of a pituitary microadenoma in an acromegalic patient. The small operative corridor created by the carotid arteries on either side represents a potential operative hazard for the transsphenoidal approach.

- whether or not any uncertainty exists as to the pathology of the lesion;
- whether or not any prior therapy has been administered (surgery, drugs, or radiotherapy);
- the experience of the surgeon.

As general guidelines, a transsphenoidal approach is preferred in all but the following circumstances:

- the tumor has significant anterior extension into the anterior cranial fossa or lateral and/or posterior extension into the middle or posterior cranial fossas;
- the tumor has suprasellar extension and an hourglass configuration that is constrained by a small diaphragmatic aperture;
- when there is reason to believe that the consistency of a tumor having suprasellar extension is sufficiently fibrous to prevents its collapse and descent into the sella when resected from below;
- if there is some doubt as to the actual nature of the pathology (i.e. meningioma).

If any of these features is present, a transcranial procedure is usually preferred. The development of the extended transsphenoidal approach has now provided transsphenoidal access to a

number of lesions that would previously have been considered to be accessible by transcranial approaches only.

Occasionally, the configuration of the tumor is such that a single approach, either transsphenoidal or transcranial, would be insufficient to effect complete tumor removal. The situation is uncommon and is typically associated with dumbbell-shaped tumors having a significant intrasellar component that has grown up through and been narrowed by the diaphragmatic aperture. The suprasellar component in such cases may be inaccessible from below, whereas the infrasellar component may not be safely and readily accessible from above. Similarly, such bicompartmentalization occurs when an intrasellar component is associated with anterior, lateral, and retrosellar intracranial extensions into the anterior, middle, and posterior cranial fossa.

Establish surgical goals and an overall program of management

By the conclusion of the presurgical assessment and before embarking on a surgical intervention, some consideration should always be given to the surgical objective, particularly with respect to its role in the overall plan of care. In some instances,

Surgical approaches for pituitary tumors	
Standard transsphenoidal approaches	Endonasal submucosal transseptal transsphenoidal approach
	Endonasal submucosal septal 'pushover' approach
	Sublabial transseptal transsphenoidal approach
	Endoscopic transsphenoidal approach
Standard transcranial approaches	Pterional craniotomy
	Subfrontal craniotomy
	Subtemporal craniotomy
Alternative skull-base approaches	Cranio-orbito-zygomatic osteotomy approach
	Transbasal approach of Derome
	Extended transsphenoidal approach
	Lateral rhinotomy/paranasal approaches
	Sublabial transseptal approach with nasomaxillary osteotomy
	Transethmoidal and extended transethmoidal approaches
	Sublabial transantral approach

Table 8.2 Surgical approaches for pituitary tumors.

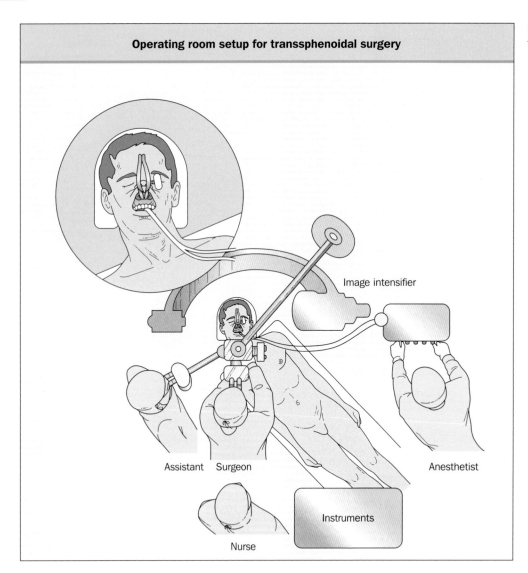

Operating room setup for transsphenoidal surgery

Image intensifier

Assistant   Surgeon

Anesthetist

Instruments

Nurse

Figure 8.9 Operating room setup for transsphenoidal surgery.

this will be straightforward. For example, in the otherwise healthy patient in whom a clinically nonfunctioning macroadenoma is compromising vision, the surgical objectives would be decompression of the optic apparatus and an attempt at gross total tumor resection. The overall plan of management would also include long-term postoperative surveillance for and treatment of hypopituitarism and possible tumor recurrence.

In other instances, however, treatment decisions will be more complicated. For example, in a patient with acromegaly having a macroadenoma whose size and invasiveness have clearly exceeded the limits of surgical resectability, the surgical objectives would be decompression of neural structures and maximal reduction of tumor burden, with the understanding that adjuvant therapy will be required. The goals would then include normalization of growth hormone/insulin-like growth factor 1 (IGF-1) levels with various forms of pharmacotherapy, consideration of radiation therapy (radiosurgery or conventional irradiation), and long-term surveillance/treatment of acromegaly-related complications (secondary neoplasms, cardiovascular disease, etc.) as discussed in Chapter 5. The surgical objectives, the alternatives of surgical management, and the potential need for additional therapy should be understood by both surgeon and patient at the outset.

TRANSSPHENOIDAL SURGERY

Ordinarily, this will imply a standard microsurgical submucosal transseptal transsphenoidal procedure. The advantages of the transsphenoidal approach are many. Most importantly, it represents the most minimally traumatic corridor of surgical access to the sella, providing direct and superior visualization of the pituitary gland and adjacent pathology. The lack of visible scars, lower morbidity and mortality as compared to transcranial procedures, the necessity of only a brief hospital stay, the relatively brief recuperative period, and the overall safety of the procedure add to the appeal of the procedure from the patient's standpoint.

Procedure

The procedure is performed under general anesthesia, with the patient placed in a semirecumbent position (**Fig. 8.9**). Anesthetic management during a transsphenoidal procedure can sometimes be difficult. This is especially true in patients with acromegaly, as the enlargement of the jaw and tongue can make airway management difficult. Jaw malocclusion, limited jaw opening, goiter, and kyphosis can further complicate the issue, sometimes necessitating awake fiberoptic intubation. Significant

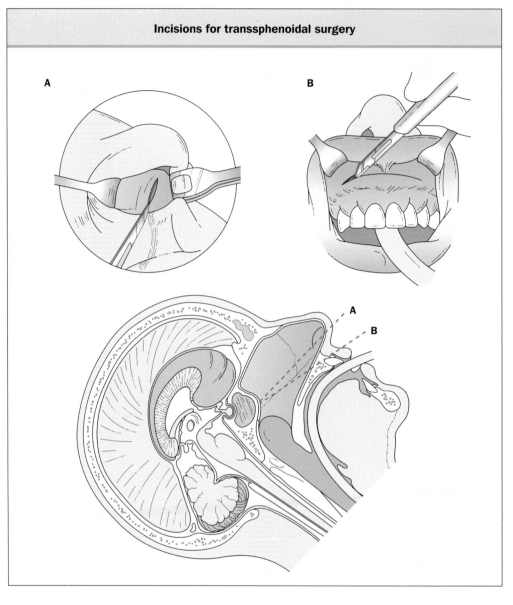

Incisions for transsphenoidal surgery

A   B

A

B

Figure 8.10 Incisions for transsphenoidal surgery. The endonasal (A) and sublabial (B) incisions are illustrated, with the direction of approach (bottom panel) afforded by each.

medical comorbidities in acromegaly and Cushing's disease further increase the demands for a safe anesthetic, and these must be anticipated and managed accordingly. Because pituitary reserve for the pituitary–adrenal axis may be impaired, it remains customary to administer exogenous corticosteroids both during surgery and in the immediate postoperative period. Antibiotic prophylaxis is usually employed.

Safe execution of the procedure requires some form of neuronavigational guidance to ensure an appropriate and safe trajectory to the sella. The standard apparatus for this has been, and continues to be, videofluoroscopy. More recently, there has been increasing reliance on computer-assisted image-guided neuronavigational systems for this purpose. Such frameless stereotactic systems afford the surgeon a far more information-rich environment in which to safely execute the transsphenoidal trajectory, and are becoming indispensable during reoperations.

After the nose and face have been cleaned with a water-based antiseptic solution, the procedure begins with preparation of the nasal mucosa. This involves the application of decongestants and

submucosal infiltration of the nasal mucosa with a dilute (1:200,000) epinephrine (adrenaline) solution. This step facilitates both submucosal dissection and hemostasis significantly.

The next major consideration is the precise route of entry into the sphenoid sinus. The three basic options are the endonasal submucosal approach, the sublabial approach, and the direct transnasal septal pushover approach. (**Fig. 8.10**). Selection of one option over the others depends on the size of the nostril, the size of the lesion, the presence of prior nasal surgery, and the preference of the surgeon. We tend to favor the basic endonasal approach in most instances. We reserve the sublabial incision for larger and more difficult lesions when a broader corridor of surgical access is required, and tend to use the transnasal septal pushover technique in the setting of prior nasal surgery or among pediatric patients.

Following a submucosal plane of dissection on one side of the septum the anterior face of the sphenoid sinus is reached (**Fig. 8.11**). The operating microscope is then introduced, the anterior wall of the sphenoid is opened, the sinus is entered, and the

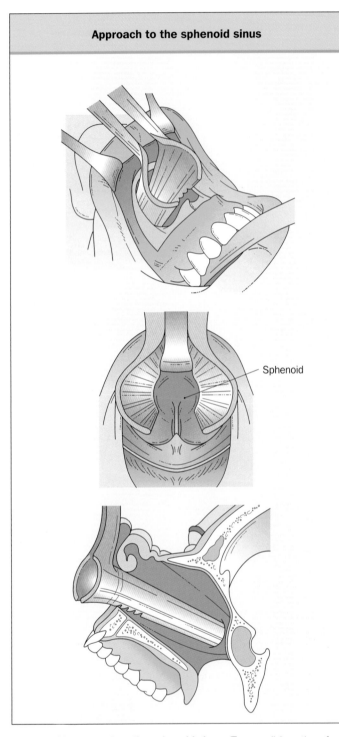

Approach to the sphenoid sinus

Sphenoid

Figure 8.11 Approach to the sphenoid sinus. (Top panel) Insertion of the transsphenoidal speculum. (Middle panel) The surgeon's view of the sphenoid. (Bottom panel) Operative approach.

removal of bone in virtually every case, extending from one cavernous sinus to the other in the lateral direction and from just short of the junction of the anterior fossa floor and sella to the clivus in the rostral–caudal direction.

Exposure within the sella proper is carried out using the operating microscope, with the magnification adjusted so that the sella fills the entire field of vision once the intrasellar portion of the operation has begun. An invasive tumor may have eroded through the anterior dura of the sella but in most cases the dura is intact. Before the dural incision is made, it is prudent to review the imaging studies once again to take note of the position of the carotid arteries, so that they are not injured upon durotomy. The site of the dural opening is selected, cauterized, and incised either in a cruciate fashion or with the excision of a dural window.

For the typical macroadenoma, the tumor is entered with a ring curette, loosened and then removed with a relatively blunt curette and forceps (**Fig. 8.12**, top panel). It is recognized that the surgeon may, on occasion, be required to follow tumor into one cavernous sinus or the other, or to deal with tumor directly involving the diaphragma. In either instance, any maneuver more forceful than gentle curetting may be a dangerous move; pulling of adherent fragments must be avoided. Decompression of the intrasellar portion of the tumor frequently permits a suprasellar extension to prolapse into view within the sella. The suprasellar extent of tumors that have an hourglass configuration created by the diaphragmatic aperture may be brought into view using forced Valsalva, jugular compression, or air instilled via a lumbar drain. Once this has been resected, the diaphragma subsequently prolapses and generally signifies that the resection is complete. Verification that no residual tumor remains is provided by direct inspection or with the help of a dental mirror, a nasopharyngoscope, or a small fiberoptic endoscope. Bleeding from the tumor bed can usually be easily controlled.

In all cases, a concerted effort is made to preserve normal pituitary tissue. In a large diffuse adenoma, normal glandular tissue usually appears as a thin membrane situated superolaterally against the sellar wall. The orange-yellow color of the gland, together with its firm consistency, usually distinguishes it from the grayish color and finely granular texture typical of the tumor.

Microadenomas necessitate a different operative strategy since it is well recognized that many will not be immediately visualized upon opening of the dura. Instead, a systematic search through a seemingly normal appearing gland is often required. We begin with a transverse glandular incision, followed by subdural dissection and mobilization of the lateral wings. If the incision in the gland is deep enough, lateral pressure usually causes the microadenoma to herniate into the operative field. Its location can, therefore, be delineated, its cavity entered, and its removal completed by use of a small ring curette and cup forceps. All suspicious tissue is removed and a biopsy specimen is occasionally obtained from the residual, and presumed normal, pituitary gland.

Some special mention is necessary of the approach to removing microadenomas in patients suffering from Cushing's disease. What is generally required is a careful and systematic dissection of the sellar contents. If a tumor is not evident upon opening the dura, or after examining all glandular surfaces, the gland must be incised and systematically explored. Subtle changes in tissue color, tissue texture, or the contour of the gland will aid in the identification of an adenoma and in distinguishing it from

mucosa within it is resected. The floor of the sella should be clearly visible. With some tumors, the floor of the sella is eroded or extraordinarily thin, so that it can be fractured with a blunt hook. If the floor of the sella is thick, a small chisel can be used to remove a square of bone. An adequate bony exposure is crucial to the success of the transsphenoidal approach, particularly when dealing with large tumors. In general, we advocate wide

Completing the surgery

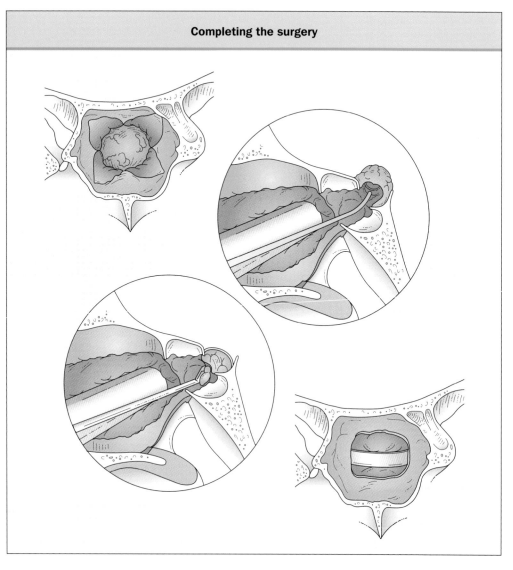

Figure 8.12 Completing the surgery.
(Top panel) Removal of the adenoma with a ring curette. (Bottom panel) At closure, the sella is packed with fat or Gelfoam and the floor is reconstructed with a stent of nasal cartilage or bone.

the normal gland. If no adenoma is found, excisional biopsies from within the substance of the gland are obtained, beginning with the central mucoid wedge. If an adenoma is not evident in the resected material, the lateral wings of the gland are carefully inspected and resected as necessary. In the adult patient in whom an adenoma cannot be identified by this stage, and for whom fertility is not an issue, a subtotal hypophysectomy is generally perfomed, leaving only a stump of residual anterior lobe tissue attached to the stalk. If careful examination of the resected tissues still fails to reveal an adenoma, both cavernous sinuses must be evaluated as well as the posterior lobe; the latter has, on rare occasion, been known to harbor a minute adenomatous nodule. Failing to see an adenoma by now, the surgeon must at least consider the possibility of a supradiaphragmatic tumor nodule. Given the additional operative risks of a diaphragmatic breach, one would not ordinarily contemplate transdiaphragmatic exploration without clear imaging evidence pointing to such a possibility.

After the tumor has been removed and hemostasis has been achieved, the sella must be carefully evaluated with regard to reconstruction and closure. We prefer not to leave dead space in

the sella. If no cerebrospinal fluid (CSF) leak has occurred, the sella is loosely packed with Gelfoam. If, however, a CSF leak has been encountered, then some form of tissue graft becomes mandatory. Reconstruction of the sellar roof can be attempted with a piece of homologous dural graft material or fascia lata; however, this step probably adds little to the security of the seal. Current practice favors simple packing of the sella with fat taken from the right lower quadrant of the abdomen. The sellar floor is then carefully reconstructed using a suitably trimmed piece of cartilage or bone (**Fig. 8.12**, lower panel). In cases where previous surgery has been performed and no bone is available, alternative materials for closure include banked bone allograft, slowly resorbable polymer stents, titanium plates, and methylmethacrylate.

In closing the nasal portion of the procedure, careful attention is paid to achieving anatomic and physiologic restoration. If an intraoperative CSF leak has occurred, the sphenoid sinus is packed with fat but, in the absence of a leak, it is left free of foreign material. The posterior septal space may be reimplanted with crushed nasal bone and cartilage. The septal flaps are reapproximated; the nasal septum is returned to its midline position. Any accessible mucosal tears are repaired with fine catgut sutures. Bilateral endonasal packs, consisting of gauze packing within the 'fingers' of a rubber glove that has been lubricated with petroleum jelly or antibiotic ointment, are placed in the nostrils. The nasal and/or gingival incisions are closed with interrupted 4–0 catgut sutures, and a gauze moustache dressing is applied.

Postoperative care

In all patients, vigilant postoperative monitoring of water and electrolyte balance is mandatory. Diuresis of varying degrees regularly occurs in the postoperative period but does not necessarily imply a diagnosis of diabetes insipidus sufficiently severe to require vasopressin. True diabetes insipidus accompanied by a brisk diuresis, defined by characteristic alterations in the serum and urine osmolalities, requires prompt fluid replacement and vasopressin in the form of desmopressin. In this situation, serum osmolality is more than 295mosmol/kg and urine osmolality less than 500mosmol/kg. When it does occur, diabetes insipidus is usually temporary.

Exogenous corticosteroids are rapidly tapered, beginning on the first postoperative day. Serum cortisol should be measured off corticosteroids and if there is any doubt as to the adequacy of ACTH levels, steroid replacement in physiologic doses (hydrocortisone 20–30mg/day) should be administered until more formal dynamic endocrine testing is undertaken.

Prophylactic antibiotics are continued until the nasal packing is removed, usually on the second postoperative day. In uncomplicated cases, the patient can be discharged from hospital by the third or fourth day. At followup, endocrine testing is performed and endocrine replacement therapy administered for any deficiencies identified, or complementary medical treatment for residual secretory excess is prescribed. Followup gadolinium-enhanced MR imaging of the sella is usually performed at approximately 3 months postoperatively and then on an annual basis as necessary. Formal visual field examinations are also performed at the 3-month visit for patients in whom preoperative visual deficits were present.

Complications of the transsphenoidal approach

Of the many virtues of the transsphenoidal approach, its safety and low complication rate are among the most important. As determined by several retrospective cumulative series, operative mortality and major morbidity rates are 0.5% and 2.2% respectively.

Operative deaths, although fortunately rare, are usually the result of intracranial hemorrhage, hypothalamic damage, or meningitis related to CSF fistulas. A wide variety of other complications can also occur with this approach (**Table 8.3**).

Hypothalamic injury

Damage to the hypothalamus may result from direct surgical injury and also from hemorrhage or ischemia provoked by the procedure. Clinical manifestations of hypothalamic damage include death, coma, diabetes insipidus, memory loss, and disturbances of vegetative functions (morbid obesity, uncontrollable hunger or thirst, and disturbances in temperature regulation). Such complications are more frequent in patients

Complications of transsphenoidal surgery	
	n
Operative mortality (30-day)	
Hypothalamic injury/hemorrhage	5
Meningitis	2
Vascular injury/occlusion	4
CSF leak/pneumocephalus, SAH/spasm, MI	1
Postoperative MI, postoperative seizure	2
Total	14 (1.0%)
Major morbidity	
Vascular occlusion/stroke/SAH/spasm	5
Visual loss (new)	11
Vascular injury (repaired)	8
Meningitis (nonfatal)	8
Sellar abscess	1
Sellar pneumatocele	1
VIth cranial nerve palsy	2
IIIrd cranial nerve palsy	1
CSF rhinorrhea	49
Total	86 (3.4%)
Lesser morbidity	
Hemorrhage (intraoperative or postoperative)	9
Postoperative psychosis	5
Nasal septal perforation	16
Sinusitis, wound infection	5
Transient cranial nerve palsy (III or IV)	5
Diabetes insipidus (usually transient)	35
Cribriform plate fracture	2
Maxillary fracture	2
Hepatitis	1
Symptomatic SIADH	37
Total	117 (4.6%)

Table 8.3 Complications of transsphenoidal surgery. The data are from the authors' series of 2562 pituitary adenomas. CSF, cerebrospinal fluid; MI, myocardial infarction; SAH, sub-arachnoid hemorrhage; SIADH, syndrome of inappropriate vasopressin secretion

with prior craniotomy or radiation. Gentle surgical techniques and avoidance of traction on the tumor capsule and pituitary stalk will minimize the occurrence of such injuries.

Visual damage

Damage to the optic nerves and chiasm can also occur from direct surgical trauma, hemorrhage, or ischemia. Fractures of bony structures at the base of the skull can damage optic nerves and can occur from misdirected placement and aggressive opening of transsphenoidal retractors. Many patients have preoperative compromise of visual function, making them more vulnerable to further damage. Assessment of the bony anatomy, careful and gentle technique, confirmation of surgical landmarks, and effective use of navigational guidance to direct the approach are the major methods of avoiding these complications. Finally, at the time of sellar reconstruction, overpacking the sella can cause chiasmal compression whereas underpacking can lead to a secondary empty sella with the late onset of visual loss due to chiasmatic prolapse.

Vascular complications

Although rare, arterial injury is a well known complication of transsphenoidal surgery and is one of the main sources of operative mortality accompanying the procedure. Virtually every transsphenoidal series includes at least one example of arterial injury, most of which have proved fatal. The intracavernous portion of the carotid tends to be the most vulnerable, followed by other components of the circle of Willis. Because the tumor may be quite adherent to arterial structures, arteries may be lacerated, perforated, avulsed, or damaged such that they develop spasm or intraluminal thrombosis. Intracranial hemorrhage, thrombotic stroke and embolic stroke, and the development of false aneurysms or carotid–cavernous fistulas are the usual sequelae of such injuries. When vascular injury is suspected, tamponade should be used to control hemorrhage and an immediate postoperative angiogram should be obtained. Again, gentle technique devoid of aggressive traction on the tumor capsule, not deviating from the midline, and repeated assessment of bony landmarks are the most effective means of avoiding these frequently devastating complications.

Cerebrospinal fluid rhinorrhea
Cerebrospinal fluid rhinorrhea and meningitis are among the most common serious complications associated with transsphenoidal surgery. They are the result of disruption of the sellar diaphragm, which is usually thinned, adherent to tumor, and susceptible to direct or traction injury. In the presence of a CSF leak, careful closure of the sella becomes a crucial part of the procedure. In the postoperative period, ready acknowledgment of a CSF leak is essential, as is early recognition of and therapy for meningitis. Postoperative CSF leaks usually manifest at the time nasal packing is removed. These are best managed by prompt transsphenoidal reexploration, identification of the leak, and resealing.

Cavernous sinus injury
Pituitary tumors involve the cavernous sinus with some regularity. In some cases, the tumor may be adherent to the medial wall of the sinus only, whereas, in other more invasive tumors, frank invasion of the sinus interstices occurs. Injury to the cavernous sinus and its contents can occur while stripping the tumor from the medial dura, in the course of following the tumor into the sinus, or with overzealous packing of sinus bleeding. The carotid artery and the sixth cranial nerve are most vulnerable to such maneuvers; the third and fourth cranial nerves are damaged less frequently.

Iatrogenic hypopituitarism
In most instances, existing pituitary function can be preserved. Among microadenomas, our recent experience indicates that loss of one or more anterior pituitary functional axis occurs in approximately 3% of cases. For macroadenomas, we have found that anterior pituitary function can be preserved in more than 95% of cases, provided that pituitary function was normal preoperatively. In contrast, in patients with established preoperative endocrine deficits, partial or complete restoration of endocrine deficits is achieved in only 16–30%. Whereas diabetes insipidus occurs temporarily in as many as one third of all patients, posterior pituitary failure is permanent in no more than 3%.

Brainstem injury
Damage to the brainstem may occur with a misdirected approach that violates the clivus or, more commonly, when a larger tumor erodes the clivus, exposing the underlying dura.

Nasal complications
Although generally less immediate and rarely fatal, complications relating to the nasofacial aspect of the procedure can be annoying and persist for some time after surgery. Imprudent use of the retractor may result in diastasis or fracture of the hard palate or the cribriform plate, the latter also being a source of CSF rhinorrhea. In the postoperative period, the mucosa of the sphenoid sinus may become infected, giving rise to a febrile sinusitis and the eventual development of a mucocele or pyocele. Inadequate hemostasis in the nasal portion of the procedure may lead to superficial wound hemorrhage and swelling. Technical errors in handling the nasal mucosa, the nasal septum, and the nasal spine may result in an external nasal deformity, which may be distressing, both cosmetically and functionally. Loss of smell can also occur, presumably as a result of damage to nerve endings in the nasal mucosa. Finally, overaggressive enlargement of the basal pyriform aperture can damage distal branches of the alveolar nerves and/or vessels, which may devitalize or desensitize the teeth and gums of the maxilla. Virtually all of these local complications can be avoided with careful nondestructive surgical technique during the exposure and meticulous reconstruction at the time of closure.

New developments in transsphenoidal surgery
Endoscopic approaches
Whereas the transsphenoidal approach has always been considered 'minimally invasive', particularly when compared to conventional transcranial approaches, the concept has been redefined in the context of endoscopic approaches to the sella. These approaches use straight and angled endoscopes either as the sole visualization tool or as a supplement to the operating microscope (the hybrid approach). Proponents of the endoscopic technique emphasize its superior and panoramic intrasellar visualization, its less traumatic nature, the avoidance of postoperative nasal packs, and shorter hospital stays. There is no question that endoscopes can improve intraoperative visualization but the cost of this is an undeniable compromise of conventional microsurgical maneuverability on the part of the surgeon. Preliminary results have been encouraging; however, additional experience and followup will be required to determine if the efficacy of this approach is comparable to standard microsurgical transsphenoidal approaches.

Other advances
An important advance during recent years has been the realization that repeat transsphenoidal surgery represents a viable option in selected patients with recurrent or persistent disease. In the past, there was a reluctance on the part of surgeons to undertake reoperations for pituitary tumors for fear of the greater technical demands and higher complication rates that accompanied reoperative transsphenoidal surgery. Today, however, experienced surgeons have become more accepting of the benefits of reoperative pituitary surgery, having developed the skills and strategies to make this a safe and reasonably effective option in selected patients. Our own experience indicates that complication rates are now only minimally higher than those of initial operations.

A final innovation has been the development of the extended transsphenoidal approach. It is a procedure that brings into the

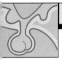

domain of transsphenoidal accessibility lesions previously thought amenable only to transcranial approaches. This category includes not only pituitary adenomas with unusual configurations but also other mass lesions with a suprasellar, retrosellar, or anterosellar disposition. This approach, which is as much a conceptual advance as it is a technical one, involves greater resection of skull base from below and permits removal of genuine intracranial pathology via the transsphenoidal route. In doing so, it pushes the limits of transsphenoidal surgery to a new and important frontier.

TRANSCRANIAL APPROACHES

Given the efficacy and safety of the transsphenoidal approach, together with its suitability for more than 96% of pituitary adenomas, transcranial approaches are infrequently required. Transcranial approaches may be necessary because of the geometry of the tumor (unusual intracranial extensions or a dumbbell-shaped tumor with a disproportionately larger suprasellar component) or when some uncertainty exists about the pathology of the lesion (i.e. meningioma). The major advantage of the craniotomy approach is that it affords the surgeon a complete view of the effect of the pituitary tumor on intracranial structures. Specifically, the optic nerves and chiasm, unusual intracranial extensions into the anterior and middle cranial fossas, and retrosellar clival extensions can all be visualized and accessed. Similarly, when sufficiently large, some suprasellar extensions involve third ventricular structures; craniotomy allows such extensions to be dealt with directly. The major limitation of the transcranial approach, however, is that the intrasellar portion of the tumor can be more difficult to remove, particularly when a prefixed chiasm also coexists.

SURGICAL RESULTS FOR SPECIFIC PITUITARY ADENOMA TYPES

Just as pituitary tumors are a pathologically, endocrinologically, and biologically heterogeneous group of lesions, so too are the results of surgery, which vary across the different pituitary tumor subtypes. Surgical outcome and considerations unique to specific adenoma subtypes are reviewed separately. It is also important to recognize that, even if a patient has a remission

following surgery, recurrence of the tumor may occur. In microadenomas causing acromegaly the recurrence rate is 8% and it is higher in macroadenomas. In microprolactinomas it is 13%, and in microadenomas causing Cushing's disease it is 12%. For macroadenomas in Cushing's disease or Nelson's syndrome the recurrence rate is more than 40%.

Prolactin-producing pituitary adenomas

The prolactinoma is the most common primary tumor of the adenohypophysis and accounts for approximately 30% of all pituitary adenomas encountered in clinical practice. Operative treatment, once the primary mode of therapy, has been replaced by dopaminergic therapy as the initial treatment of choice for most prolactinomas. In fact, the consistency with which dopamine agonists normalize prolactin levels, restore fertility, and reduce tumor mass, has supported their use as the initial therapy.

However, despite its secondary and more selective role in prolactinoma management, surgery remains an essential component of the therapeutic armamentarium against these tumors (**Table 8.4**). Occasionally, patients with prolactinomas who undergo pituitary apoplexy will need surgery. When the MRI indicates that the bulk of the tumor is composed of hemorrhagic and/or necrotic material, dopamine agonists may not provide a satisfactory reduction in tumor volume. Some clinicians believe that cystic prolactinomas are best treated surgically, but most do not agree, finding that they do respond as well as solid tumors to dopamine agonists. A small percentage of patients will be truly intolerant of the side effects of dopaminergic medication. In these situations, surgery is indicated and in some patients the tumor is resistant to dopaminergic therapy.

Resistance usually manifests in one of two ways. The first is when the prolactin levels fail to normalize. In such a situation, there is still a risk that the patient may suffer the adverse effects of hyperprolactinemia and that the tumor may continue to enlarge despite continued pharmacologic treatment. Alternatively, hyperprolactinemia may be corrected but there is little or no volumetric response and mass effects remain (**Fig. 8.13**). Included in such situations are cases of the pseudoprolactinomas – sellar masses other than genuine prolactinomas that produce hyperprolactinemia on the basis of stalk compression.

Postoperative remission and recurrence			
Clinical entity	***n***	**Remission rate (%)**	**Recurrence (%)**
Acromegaly	468	Microadenoma 72 Macroadenoma 50	8
Prolactinoma	871	Microadenoma 87 Macroadenoma 50	13
Cushing's disease	381	Microadenoma 91 Macroadenoma 56	12 (adults) 42 (children)
Nelson–Salassa syndrome	62	Microadenoma 70 Macroadenoma 40	40
Clinically nonfunctioning miscellaneous pituitary adenomas		16 (radiographic recurrence) 6 (symptomatic recurrence)	

Table 8.4 Postoperative remission and recurrence. Summary of postoperative remission and recurrence after transsphenoidal surgery for pituitary adenomas (authors' series, 1972–97, *n* = 2665).

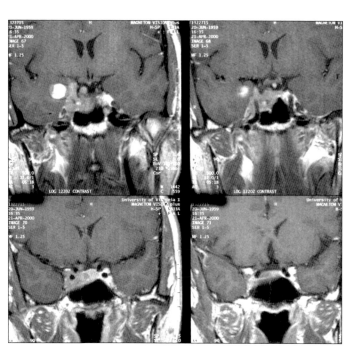

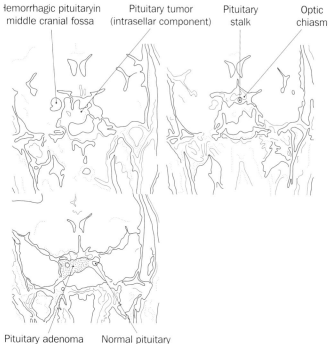

Hemorrhagic pituitaryin | Pituitary tumor | Pituitary | Optic
middle cranial fossa | (intrasellar component) | stalk | chiasm

Pituitary adenoma   Normal pituitary

Figure 8.13 Resistance to dopaminergic therapy in a prolactinoma. This patient had a long-standing prolactinoma that continued to grow despite dopaminergic therapy. It extended into the cavernous sinus, sphenoid sinus and middle cranial fossa irritating the temporal lobe and causing seizures. It was removed through a transcranial approach.

Surgery may also be indicated in the patient with a large invasive prolactinoma in whom a successful response to dopaminergic therapy can be anticipated but in whom extensive erosion of the skull base may be the source of a CSF leak when dopamine agonist therapy causes the tumor to shrink.

Curative resections, as defined by normalization of circulating prolactin levels, are achieved in only a minority of patients with macroprolactinomas. Among all prolactinomas of all sizes, immediately postoperative 'curative' resections are associated with a progressive recurrence rate over time.

Microadenomas

The rate of curative resections is highest among microadenomas, particularly when prolactin levels are less than 100ng/mL (1800mU/L). In the Mayo Clinic series involving 100 patients with prolactinomas, 32 of which met this criterion, normalization of prolactin levels was achieved in 88%. Larger tumors and/or those accompanied by higher prolactin elevations are responsible for a dramatic reduction in surgical cure rate. Among microadenomas having preoperative prolactin levels in excess of 100ng/mL (1800mU/L), a curative result was observed in only 50%. In his summary of 31 published series involving 1224 patients with microprolactinomas, Molitch calculated an overall endocrinologic cure rate of 71.2%, independent of preoperative prolactin levels.

Macroadenomas

The surgical outcome for patients with prolactin-secreting macroadenomas has proved far less encouraging. In Mayo Clinic experience, only 53% of surgically treated patients with macroadenomas experience normalization of prolactin levels. Among locally invasive macroadenomas, the surgical cure rate was further reduced to 28%. In a review of 31 published series, Molitch calculated an overall cure rate of 31.8% among 1256 macroadenomas. With patients in whom medical therapy has failed, surgery will generally relieve mass effects, even though hormonal remission is not easily achieved.

Because the degree of hyperprolactinemia reflects both the size and invasiveness of the tumor, the preoperative serum prolactin level has proved to be an especially reliable predictor of surgical outcome. As a general rule, curative resection rates drop precipitously when preoperative prolactin levels exceed 200ng/mL (3600mU/L). This has been validated by several series in which surgical cure rates varied between 74–88% when prolactin levels were below this threshold but dropped to 18–47% when they exceeded it. When the preoperative prolactin level exceeds 1000ng/mL (18,000mU/L), surgery alone seldom results in biochemical remission.

Postoperative recurrence

Ordinarily, tumor recurrence manifests endocrinologically with return of hyperprolactinemia but not necessarily with evident tumor regrowth. The reported frequency of biochemical recurrence has varied greatly, between 17% and 50% for microadenomas and 19% and 80% for macroadenomas. In the majority of 'recurrences', particularly in the setting of microprolactinomas, the relapse tends to be hormonal rather than tumor mass visible radiologically. This peculiar phenomenon of delayed recurrence of hyperprolactinemia is poorly understood and may be a variant of the 'stalk section effect'. In most instances, the hyperprolactinemia is only of a modest degree, is not always symptomatic, may spontaneously resolve, and does not necessarily warrant therapy.

Surgical issues relating to fertility and pregnancy

Prolactinomas pose three basic problems with regard to planned or established pregnancy: infertility, risk of tumor growth during pregnancy, and effects of therapy on fetal development. In that hyperplasia of normal pituitary lactotrophs is a normal physiologic response during pregnancy, it follows that a corresponding response may also occur in neoplastic lactotrophs. For microadenomas, the risk of tumor enlargement is small, symptomatic enlargement occurring in 1.6% of cases and radiologically evident enlargement occurring in 4.5%. In contrast, macroadenomas have a significantly greater propensity for pregnancy-induced growth: asymptomatic and symptomatic enlargement occur in 15.5% and 8.5% of cases respectively. Among macroadenomas that have previously undergone surgical or radiotherapeutic ablation prior to pregnancy, the risk of regrowth during pregnancy is significantly less (4.3%).

In the patient with a microprolactinoma who desires pregnancy, both bromocriptine and surgery have comparable rates of success (80–85%) in restoring fertility. In patients treated with bromocriptine, therapy is usually stopped at the first sign of pregnancy. Such patients should have careful clinical examinations throughout pregnancy to identify the very exceptional microadenoma that might enlarge. Since prolactin levels normally rise during the first trimester, they are not informative with regard to the status of the tumor.

In the patient with a macroprolactinoma who desires pregnancy, several management options exist, each of which is directed at avoiding the 15–35% risk of tumor enlargement that occurs during pregnancy. The more conservative approach begins with primary resection of the macroprolactinoma with the objective of a curative resection. Should hyperprolactinemia and ovulatory failure persist postoperatively, bromocriptine is used to restore fertility. Pregnancy in this setting will be associated with a greatly reduced risk (4.5%) of tumor expansion. A second approach involves treating the patient initially with bromocriptine to restore fertility, withdrawing therapy at the first sign of pregnancy, and carefully monitoring the patient throughout the pregnancy with serial clinical and neuroophthalmologic evaluations. Should symptomatic tumor enlargement occur, the options include urgent surgical resection or reinstitution of bromocriptine for the duration of the pregnancy. Some clinicians recommend conventional external beam radiotherapy in such patients after drug-induced tumor shrinkage has been achieved. This will prevent tumor enlargement in pregnancy; completion of the family will then be possible safely even if gonadotropin deficiency may sometimes occur several years later (see Chapter 9).

Growth hormone secreting pituitary adenomas
Acromegaly

The menu of potential treatment options for acromegaly-associated pituitary adenomas is wider than that for any other pituitary tumor. Surgical resection, radiation therapy, and medical therapy with somatostatin analogs, dopamine agonists, or growth hormone antagonists all afford the treating physician some latitude in providing a comprehensive management plan for the patient with acromegaly. Because no single form of therapy is uniformly effective, combination therapy figures prominently in the management of this disease.

Factors associated with outcome after transsphenoidal surgery for acromegaly		
Factor	Favorable outcome	Unfavorable outcome
Tumor size	Microadenoma	Macroadenoma
Invasiveness	Noninvasive	Invasive
Basal GH	<45ng/mL	>45ng/mL
Histopathology	GH only	Mixed GH–prolactin
Ultrastructure	Densely granulated	Sparsely granulated Acidophil stem-cell adenoma

Table 8.5 Factors associated with outcome after transsphenoidal surgery for acromegaly. GH, growth hormone.

For the majority of patients presenting with acromegaly, surgical resection will represent the initial treatment of choice. The efficacy of surgery will depend on a number of factors, including tumor size and invasion status, and preoperative growth hormone levels (**Table 8.5**). In the most favorable circumstances, such as those involving noninvasive intrasellar microadenomas with basal growth hormone levels less than 45ng/mL (135mU/L), surgery alone can prove curative. In other instances, such as those involving invasive macroadenomas and those with preoperative growth hormone levels in excess of 50ng/mL (150mU/L), curative resection may still represent a reasonable operative goal, although the possibility of inaccessible tumor remnants, persistent growth hormone hypersecretion, and the potential need for eventual adjuvant therapy is recognized from the outset. Finally, the least favorable situation is confronted when a tumor's size and invasiveness have clearly exceeded the limits of surgical resectability. For such tumors, surgical resection is undertaken primarily for the relief of mass effects. In achieving this, the tumor burden is also reduced, thereby possibly enhancing the effectiveness of adjuvant drug and/or radiation therapy.

Prompt regression of several symptoms can be expected postoperatively in most surgically treated patients with acromegaly. This relief occurs in all those who achieve biochemical remission, as well as those in whom growth hormone levels have been significantly reduced but not normalized. Headache frequently improves immediately. Over the next few days, this is followed by improvements in excessive sweating and paresthesias, and regression of soft-tissue swelling. Such responses tend to be the rule. Glucose intolerance also responds favorably to surgery and growth hormone levels are satisfactorily lowered. Among patients whose growth hormone levels are normalized, diabetes and/or glucose intolerance resolves in more than 80%. Significant improvements in glucose tolerance can also be expected in patients in whom surgery reduces, but fails to normalize, growth hormone levels. Hypertension tends to be considerably less responsive to surgery than the other acromegalic features.

Defining endocrinologic remission

Although it has been recognized for some time that the completeness of surgical resection must ultimately be judged on the basis of measurable endocrinologic parameters, there has been, in the past, a lack of consensus in the specific endocrinologic criteria that investigators have used to define remission or 'cure'.

It is now clear that the criteria employed to define remission in earlier series, such as reduction of basal growth hormone levels to less than 10ng/mL (30mU/L) have been too liberal. Patients thought to have been 'cured' on this basis were in fact not cured and continued to have active acromegaly and a poor prognosis. As a result, particularly during the past decade, the concept of 'cure' in acromegaly has evolved considerably. Some consensus now exists as to the minimum biochemical criteria that must underlie its definition. First, it is preferable to speak in terms of remission or 'safe level' rather than 'cure', as the long-term outcome of surgically treated somatotroph adenomas is still not definitely known and no endocrinologic criteria, however stringent, can absolutely guarantee that the patient will remain permanently free of disease. The current operational definition of endocrinologic remission in acromegaly to render the life prognosis normal requires:

- suppression of growth hormone levels to less than 1ng/mL(3mU/L) during an oral glucose tolerance test; and
- normalization of age- and gender-adjusted plasma IGF-1 levels; and
- reduction of mean serum growth hormone levels (of five values) below 1.7ng/mL (5mU/L), with a normal serum IGF-1 level.

Reported rates of endocrine remission

This is discussed in detail in Chapter 5. In spite of the varied definitions of postoperative endocrinologic remission in acromegaly used by different investigators, a large body of data does exist for evaluating the results of operative therapy for somatotroph adenomas. When surgery is used as the sole primary treatment, and in the absence of any prior therapy, overall endocrine remission can be expected in about 60–70% of patients. The remission rate among microadenomas is about 80% whereas that in macroadenomas is about 50%. The adverse effects on outcome of increasing tumor size and invasiveness are well recognized.

Tumor recurrence

The rate of recurrence in acromegaly will depend upon the stringency of the criteria with which remission was originally defined, as well as the period of followup. When strict criteria are used to define remission, a durable remission is usually achieved and recurrence is infrequent. The rate of recurrence of surgically treated acromegalic patients in whom endocrine remission had been achieved is about 8% during a 10-year followup period.

Many patients with recurrent acromegaly will be candidates for repeat surgery. The need for reoperation and its role among the alternatives of surgical management should be carefully individualized, however. Because of the tendency to group both recurrent and persistent acromegaly under the general category of 'recurrence', few data are available concerning the surgical outcomes of genuinely recurrent somatotroph adenomas, but about half the patients show secondary remission with reoperation. For tumors in which remission cannot be achieved surgically, adjuvant radiotherapy continues to be the usual next step, particularly in the presence of macroscopic or radiologically evident residual disease. Radiation therapy may involve conventional radiotherapy or gamma knife radiosurgery (discussed in Chapter 9).

Corticotroph adenomas: Cushing's disease and Nelson's syndrome

From the standpoints of both diagnosis and therapy, no type of pituitary tumor presents a greater management challenge than corticotroph adenomas. Once it has been established that the etiology for hypercortisolism is a corticotroph adenoma, surgery remains the therapy of first choice. In fact, the merits of transsphenoidal surgery are well exemplified in the treatment of corticotroph adenomas, wherein selective removal of the adenoma, cure of hypercortisolemia, and preservation of normal glandular function are all reasonable therapeutic expectations of the procedure. As most adenomas are only a few millimeters in size, together with their frequent deep location within the gland, simply finding the adenoma is the foremost operative challenge (**Fig. 8.14**). This is especially true when the tumor is not visualized on preoperative imaging studies.

The response to surgery in patients with Cushing's disease is discussed in detail in Chapter 15. The reported cure rates from large centers in patients with Cushing's disease vary from 50% to 90% depending on the definition of 'cure' or 'remission'. This is discussed in detail in Chapter 15. Cure rates in patients with macroadenomas are much lower and indeed they may be or become invasive. In our experience of some 380 patients with Cushing's disease, remission or cure can be achieved in more than 90% of microadenomas and in 60% of macroadenomas. In a recent analysis of our series, including only patients that were operated within the past decade, and with the availability of contemporary diagnostic techniques (i.e. MRI, petrosal sinus sampling), the postoperative remission rate was 89% for microadenomas. For macroadenomas and patients undergoing reoperation, a combined remission rate of 46% was recorded. Whether or not surgical cure has been achieved is generally evident by the second or third postoperative day. Morning cortisol levels should be subnormal if the procedure is to be considered curative. As a rule, a postoperative morning cortisol level that persists within the 'normal' range, even if it represents a dramatic decrease from the pretreatment level, almost always indicates incomplete removal and persistent disease.

For those patients successfully treated, regression of cushingoid features and restitution of the pituitary–adrenal axis occur within months. Patients routinely relate feelings of full rejuvenation, both physically and emotionally. Depending on the extent of glandular resection, hormone replacement may be required, although this will be a long-term requirement for only a minority of patients.

Once remission has been achieved, biochemical or radiologic recurrence is uncommon. Approximately 12% of patients can be expected to experience recurrence, although some do so many years after successful surgery.

Among patients in whom remission is not induced by surgery, radiotherapy (and in our experience radiosurgery) is the preferred next option (see Chapter 9).

Thyroid-stimulating hormone adenomas

Surgical resection, radiotherapy, and medical therapy with somatostatin analogs are all therapeutic options for thyrotroph adenomas. Surgery is the clear first choice and should be initially considered in all patients in whom a thyrotroph adenoma is suspected. Of the cases reported to date, most of which were

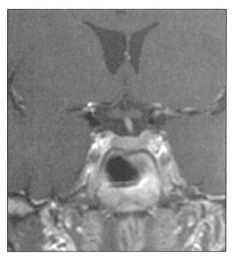
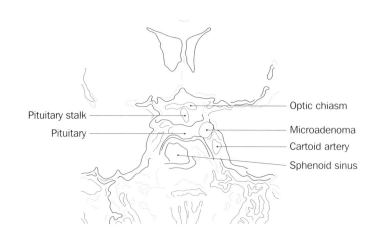

Pituitary stalk
Pituitary

Optic chiasm
Microadenoma
Cartoid artery
Sphenoid sinus

Figure 8.14 Cushing's disease. Magnetic resonance image of a patient who had had unsuccessful surgery for Cushing's disease. As is frequently the case, the magnetic resonance image is misleading. The deviation of the stalk to the left suggests a right-sided tumor, but the tumor was actually situated on the left side, adjacent to the carotid artery. This left-sided origin was suggested by preoperative petrosal sinus sampling and was confirmed intraoperatively. Removal of the tumor was followed by remission.

invasive macroadenomas, surgical remission had been achieved in about one third of all cases. Of patients in whom surgery does not induce remission, somatostatin analogs and radiation alone or in combination represent important adjuvants.

Clinically nonfunctioning pituitary tumors

Approximately one quarter of all pituitary adenomas are not associated with clinical or biochemical evidence of hormone hypersecretion. Known as clinically nonfunctioning pituitary tumors, this morphologically diverse class of lesions includes null-cell adenomas, oncocytomas, silent corticotroph adenomas, silent gonadotroph adenomas, and the rare silent somatotroph adenoma.

Surgery is the primary treatment of choice for this class of tumor. The surgical objectives involve the elimination of any mass effect, restoration of neurologic and visual function, and preservation or restoration of pituitary function. Whereas gross total removal remains an intuitive and frequently achievable surgical goal for many nonfunctioning adenomas, and should certainly be attempted to the extent that it is safely possible, it will not be a realistic expectation nor an absolute necessity for some nonfunctioning adenomas. For example, in the elderly patient in whom progressive visual loss is the only presenting feature, a radical procedure that attempts 'total' surgical resection may be less prudent than a satisfactory but less radical and less dangerous decompression. Because of the relatively slow growth of many of these tumors, symptomatic recurrence is generally a less serious and a less frequent threat than it is for most functioning adenomas.

Guided by these principles, the surgical outcome is quite satisfactory. The operative mortality is about 2%. Symptoms referable to mass effect, such as headache and cavernous sinus compression, are almost always relieved. Among all patients presenting with progressive visual field and acuity deficits, postoperative improvement occurs in about 90%, stabilization is achieved in 9%, and only 4% suffer further visual deterioration.

Preservation of pituitary function can be routinely achieved but restoration of established deficits is less likely. Permanent diabetes insipidus may be a complication in 4% of patients.

Symptomatic recurrence develops in 10–20% over 10 years. Although it was once routine practice to administer postoperative radiotherapy to all incompletely excised tumors, this has been abandoned in many centers as a routine strategy. Nowadays, radiotherapy is employed in a more selective fashion, generally being reserved for those patients in whom progression can be documented on followup scanning. For the more indolent and slow-growing lesions, where years may pass before symptomatic recurrence, repeat resection may be preferable to radiotherapy. Among the more aggressive variants, which appear destined for prompt regrowth, adjuvant radiotherapy is recommended (see Chapter 9).

SURGERY FOR LESIONS OTHER THAN PITUITARY ADENOMAS

When a patient has enlargement of the pituitary, symptoms of hypopituitarism, and impending visual loss, the offending lesion is usually a pituitary adenoma. It is important, however, for those caring for such an individual to recognize that there are a variety of other lesions that can present in a similar fashion to pituitary adenomas. These include craniopharyngioma, a Rathke's cleft cyst, meningiomas of the sella and the sellar region, germinomas, gliomas, inflammatory disorders of the pituitary such as sarcoid or hypophysitis, and the occasional patient with cancer who has a metastasis to the pituitary. Although each of these types of lesion has subtle hallmarks that produce a clinical presentation slightly different from pituitary adenoma, it is in fact impossible to make an accurate preoperative diagnosis every time. The team of physicians and surgeons treating such patients must be flexible enough to deal with a significant variety of different types of pathology, all focused in the sellar region. Transsphenoidal surgery has become highly effective for most of these lesions; however, there are certainly some craniopharyngiomas and meningiomas that are better treated using one of the craniotomy approaches. Differential diagnoses should always be kept in mind, pituitary hormonal replacement therapy should be managed with diligence and care, and employment of the basic principles outlined in this chapter will usually lead to a very satisfactory outcome.

FURTHER READING

Bradley K, Adams C, Potter C, Wheeler D, Anslow P, Burke C. An audit of selected patients with non-functioning pituitary adenoma treated by transsphenoidal surgery without irradiation. Clin Endocrinol. 1994;41:655–9.

Comtois R, Beauregard H, Somma M, Serri O, Aris-Jilwan N, Hardy J. The clinical and endocrine outcome to trans-sphenoidal microsurgery of nonsecreting pituitary adenomas. Cancer 1991;68:860–8.

Ebersold MJ, Quast LM, Laws ER Jr, Scheithauer B, Randall RV. Long-term results in transsphenoidal removal of nonfunctioning pituitary adenomas. J Neurosurg. 1986;64:713–9.

Laws ER, Thapar K. Pituitary surgery. Endocrinol Metab Clin North Am. 1999;28:119–31.

Laws ER, Fode NC, Redmond MJ. Transsphenoidal surgery following unsuccessful prior therapy: an assessment of benefits and risks in 158 patients. J Neurosurg. 1985;63:823–9.

Laws ER, Vance M, Thapar K. Pituitary surgery for the management of acromegaly. Hormone Res. 2000;53:71–5.

Massoud F, Serri O, Hardy J, Somma M, Beauregard H. Transsphenoidal adenomectomy for microprolactinomas: 10 to 20 years of follow-up. Surg Neurol. 1996;45:341–6.

Molitch M. Pregnancy in the hyperprolactinemic woman. N Engl J Med. 1985;312:1365–70.

Semple P, Laws E. Complications in a contemporary series of patients who underwent transsphenoidal surgery for Cushing's disease. J Neurosurg. 1999;91:175–9.

Serri O, Rasio E, Beauregard H, Hardy J, Somma M. Recurrence of hyperprolactinemia after selective transsphenoidal adenomectomy in women with prolactinoma. N Engl J Med. 1983;309:280–3.

Thapar K, Kovacs K. Tumors of the sellar region. In: Bigner DD, McLendon RE, Bruner JM, eds. Russell and Rubinstein's pathology of tumors of the nervous system. Baltimore, MD:Williams & Wilkins; 1998:561–677.

Trautmann JC, Laws ER. Visual status after transsphenoidal surgery at the Mayo Clinic, 1971–1982. Am J Ophthalmol. 1983;96:200–8.

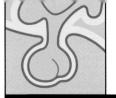

Chapter 9

Pituitary Radiotherapy

P Nicholas Plowman

PITUITARY ADENOMA

Conventionally fractionated radiotherapy has an established place in the therapy of pituitary adenomas. Some 25 years ago, recurrence rates of more than 75% were described 5 and 10 years following transcranial surgery without radiotherapy for adenomas of the pituitary. However, with the delivery of postoperative radiotherapy, the recurrence rate became less than 20% at 10 years. More modern data confirm this protection from relapse. In the case of functioning pituitary adenomas, other data have demonstrated the slow but progressive decline in the excessive circulating hormone product following radiotherapy.

Modern therapy techniques allow the safe delivery of such therapy. The usual methodology is with the patient immobilized in an individually constructed plastic mask, using three linear accelerator fields that can accurately and reproducibly be applied from both lateral positions and an antero-oblique direction. The carefully premapped pituitary tumor volume is thereby caught in the crossfire of three megavoltage X-ray portals, ensuring that it is only here that the high dose is deposited. A dose of 45Gy is delivered in 25 fractions of 1.8Gy each on weekdays over 5 weeks. The complication risks of such therapy are low. With this dose prescription, we have experienced no visual complications after more than 500 treatment courses; various degrees of hypopituitarism may occur following radiotherapy and is more common where the tumor and/or surgery has compromised pituitary function before radiotherapy. These factors make it impossible to give exact statistics on the incidence of hypopituitarism postradiation. However, in our patients with acromegaly, 25% required new endocrine replacement by 5 years after radiotherapy and that need continued to rise in the next 5 years.

Whether the incidence of late carcinogenesis after pituitary radiotherapy is as high as 1% of treated patients remains controversial: In a pooling of four published late followup studies, there were 1226 patients, among whom seven gliomas, three benign meningiomas and one parasellar fibrosarcoma were recorded. When compared to background population incidences (e.g. 3 per 1000 for glioma), it is clear that any excess is small.

With such compelling data supporting the efficacy of radiotherapy, it has been our custom for the last 25 years to recommend radiotherapy for all pituitary macroadenoma patients and those who have not been cured by surgery, as judged by their continued abnormal secretion of hormone product. That attitude has undergone some changes in the last 10 years, as a result of the increasing sophistication of magnetic resonance (MR) scanning facilities and set protocols for following up these patients, and

perhaps better surgical results using the trans-sphenoidal route. Several surgical series from the modem era have reported good results following surgery alone for macroadenomas. From the modem literature, the risk of postoperative recurrence at 5 years appears to be up to 20% and up to 44% by 10 years. Some clinicians use radiotherapy after surgery while others choose to watch and wait following surgery on the basis of the operative report and the MR scanning, but if this plan is followed it must be borne in mind that there is a risk of tumor and hormone hypersecretion recurrence so that followup must be regular, as indeed it must after radiotherapy because of the development of hypopituitarism in a significant number of patients. For secreting adenomas, the failure to achieve endocrine cure by operation and medical therapy is an indication for postoperative radiotherapy.

Attempts at predicting the recurrence potential by radiology, histology, immunohistochemical, or genetic analyses have helped the clinician in choosing which patients to recommend for radiation therapy. Invasiveness is certainly a predictor of recurrence and the presence of cavernous or sphenoid sinus invasion indicates more than a pressure effect. Adenomas infiltrating the parasellar tissues, including bone, dura, or leptomeninges, are invasive/aggressive. However, one study found that there was microscopic evidence of dural invasion in 88% of intrasellar microadenomas and 94% of those with suprasellar invasion, which suggests that too much dependence on this criterion would lead to an overestimate of the need for radiotherapy. Otherwise, routine histology (including the morphology of constituent cells) is not of great help in the definition of aggressive adenomas, and immunohistochemically detected markers probing proliferative potential are, like genetic analysis, in their infancy.

Stereotactic radiosurgery

When selecting postoperative radiotherapy, it is usual to employ conventionally fractionated radiotherapy by the technique outlined above. However, there is growing interest in the use of stereotactically delivered radiation. The improved sophistication of the planning software and accuracy of delivery of the radiation dose has made highly concentrated radiation to a small volume at any site within the cranium a reality (**Fig. 9.1**). There are three distinct methods available for such concentrated radiation therapy. The first is that effected by charged particles (e.g. protons); the other two methods are both megavoltage photon therapy methods, and small dosimetric differences may cause one of these methods to be preferred over the other in the future. In the current design of the Swedish gamma unit (Gamma Knife, Electa instruments) there are 201 fixed cobalt-60 sources, each a thin rod of 1mm diameter, the long axis of which is oriented

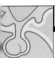

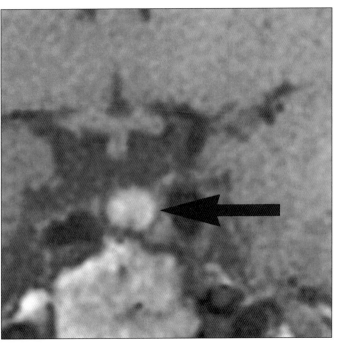

In one nonrandomized comparison involving patients with acromegaly, the benefits of conventional radiotherapy versus gamma-knife radiosurgery were assessed. There were 50 patients presenting with a mean pretreatment growth hormone of 28mIU/L and followup of 7.5 years, having been treated with conventionally fractionated radiotherapy, and these were compared with 16 patients treated radiosurgically and with a mean presenting growth hormone level of 18mIU/L and 1.4 years followup. The authors concluded that normalization of growth hormone occurred earlier with the radiosurgery therapy (70% of the radiosurgery treated patients had achieved this by 18 months) whereas the same percentage achieved this following conventional radiotherapy but took 7 years to do so. The followup in the radiosurgery group was short and this detracts from the analysis, as such focal therapy (often partial fossa radiation) risks undertreating peripheral aspects of tumor. This risk has to be balanced against the ability to create a very fast falling dose gradient at the periphery of the target, and hence spare the hypothalamus and optic chiasm.

With regard to late toxicity, the sites of concern are as for conventionally fractionated radiotherapy. The optic chiasm lies just above the fossa, is exquisitely sensitive to high single doses of radiation and is therefore very vulnerable to damage by radiosurgery. However, the physics of the radiosurgery technology ensures that the dose 'falls off' very rapidly at the perimeter of the target volume and this, together with the correct selection of cases (i.e. not selecting macroadenomas with suprasellar extension up to and displacing the chiasm), should reduce the risks to the chiasm. Whether late endocrine deficiencies and carcinogenesis are expected to be less than after conventionally fractionated therapy is still debated: on the one hand, with a partial fossa radiation technique, one might expect less late endocrinopathy and less carcinogenesis if the volume of irradiated tissues is less; on the other hand, high single-dosage radiation is more likely than conventionally fractionated therapy to cause endocrinopathy. Furthermore, it is by no means certain that second cancers, which tend to occur in the lower-dosed 'penumbral' regions around the target volume will occur perceptibly less often than after conventional therapy.

The selection of which radiation therapy modality should be chosen is currently controversial and established guidelines are required. Recognizing the excellent and durable safe results from conventionally fractionated radiotherapy in this disease, it is conventional to use this rather than stereotactic technology as the primary radiation therapy technology. In our own department 20 of the first 21 patients accepted on to its radiosurgery program had persistent or relapsed pituitary adenoma after previous conventional radiotherapy – mainly disease in the cavernous sinus, a site that is well treated by focal radiation, whereas it is difficult for the surgeon to access and radically resect tumor from this area lateral to the fossa (**Fig. 9.2**). This is still our preferred strategy of used radiotherapy for relapsed focal disease within the fossa; however, we now consider highly focal disease within the fossa for radical radiosurgery as first-line therapy if attempted curative trans-sphenoidal surgery is contraindicated. The subject of optimal radiation therapy for pituitary adenoma will continue to breathe controversy well into the future.

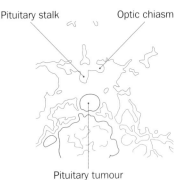

Pituitary stalk Optic chiasm

Pituitary tumour

Figure 9.1 Coronal magnetic resonance scan of small discrete pituitary adenoma. If surgery is not curative, the optimal radiation therapy method for such a tumor is controversial. While stereotactic radiosurgery at first seems ideal for such a well-demarcated and small lesion, well away from the chiasm, is it too focal for a case that surgery has failed to cure and would it jeopardize subsequent conventional radiotherapy, for which longterm experience is better?

along the radius of a hemisphere (the helmet into which the patient's head fits for therapy). The center point (or isocenter) of this hemisphere is the point at which the stereotactic coordinates of mapped intracranial target are centered. Different apertured collimators (4, 8, 14, or 18mm in diameter), all radially pointing at the isocenter, allow the 201 cobalt sources to concentrate their emissions on the target. The linear accelerator methodology again maps the intracranial target stereotactically, giving it three-dimensional coordinates and placing it at the isocenter of the beam. However, here it is a single beam of X-rays that arcs around the isocenter such that only the target is receiving the primary ionizing radiation beam during the whole arc. Several noncoplanar arcs allow a therapeutic dose to be built up on the target, with a sharp fall-off in dose at the perimeter similar to that achieved by the gamma unit methodology. The planning software has acquired the nickname 'x-knife'. The overall term used for such concentrated radiation therapy, usually delivered as a single dose, is 'radiosurgery'.

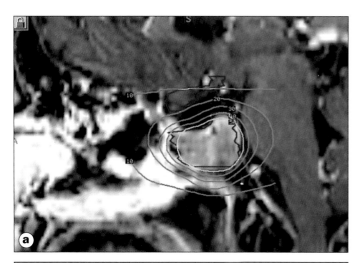

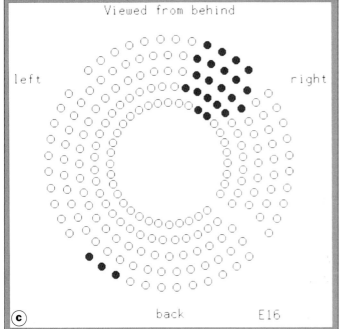

CRANIOPHARYNGIOMA

Craniopharyngioma constitutes 8% of all childhood tumors and 2% of adult tumors of the central nervous system (CNS) – with a median age of presentation of 8 years and two thirds of patients presenting before the age of 20 years. Grossly, craniopharyngiomas are cystic, solid, or partly both, not obviously encapsulated and not separated by leptomeninges from the brain parenchyma. Indeed, invasion into the brain, particularly the infundibulum, median eminence, and other areas of the hypothalamus, make radical resection potentially hazardous as it is difficult to define surgical planes between tumor and critical central nervous system. Thus, while all authorities agree that surgical excision is the optimal primary initial management, there is persisting controversy as to whether radical resection should be attempted because of its significant risk of morbidity. However, without radical resection, the regrowth rate of subtotally resected tumors is high. In a pooled series of 111 subtotally resected craniopharyngioma patients, Amacher found that 75% regrew, requiring further treatment. In a San Francisco series,

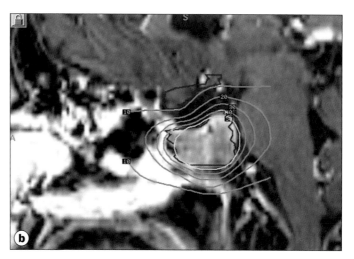

Figure 9.2 Sagittal magnetic resonance scans of pituitary adenoma with superimposed Gamma Knife isodosimetry. (a) Standard isodosimetry, with the 50% isodose well encompassing the target/tumor; the optic chiasm is outlined in purple and the 20% isodose is seen to just 'touch' this structure. (b) The added facility of blocking portals facing the chiasm has been employed – the blocking pattern is shown in (c). This has the added advantage of reduction to the 10% isodose to the chiasm – see isodoses in (b). This is particularly important when the patient is being re-treated, having received conventional radiotherapy in the past.

the surgeons considered that they had achieved complete excision in only 10% of 74 consecutive craniopharyngioma patients. Thus, it is clear that safe complete excision is both difficult to achieve and difficult to forecast even at the end of the operation. In patients with incomplete tumor excision, fewer than half survive for 10 years and 50–75% have recurrent disease within 2–5 years in the absence of radiotherapy.

Accumulating data heavily support the practice of postoperative radiotherapy. Heideman and his colleagues pooled the survival rate from various series to obtain the following results: 'total resection', 58–100% and 24–100%; subtotal excision, 37–71% and 31–52%; and subtotal excision and postoperative radiotherapy, 69–95% and 62–84%, at 5 and 10 years respectively. Additionally, neuropsychologic function was better preserved in the combined treatment group. The case for postoperative radiotherapy appears, therefore, to be overwhelming. There has been interest in the use of stereotactic radiosurgery for this disease, which is clearly a well-demarcated volume of benign tumor in the brain of usually young patients. The use of such focal radiation technology at first seems compelling (**Fig. 9.3**). However, the optic chiasm usually lies within the treatment volume and is likely to receive the full dose of this single high-dose radiation therapy technique, and complications are likely.

The problem of recurrent cystic craniopharyngioma is an occasional but very difficult one for clinicians interested in this disease. Beta-ionizing radiation has been shown *in vivo* and in tissue culture *in vitro* to destroy the epithelial lining of craniopharyngioma cysts. Early Scandinavian work established that instillation of a β-emitting isotope into fluid within the cyst of a craniopharyngioma resulted in reduction in fluid accumulation from cyst wall secretion and in tumor volume. We recently

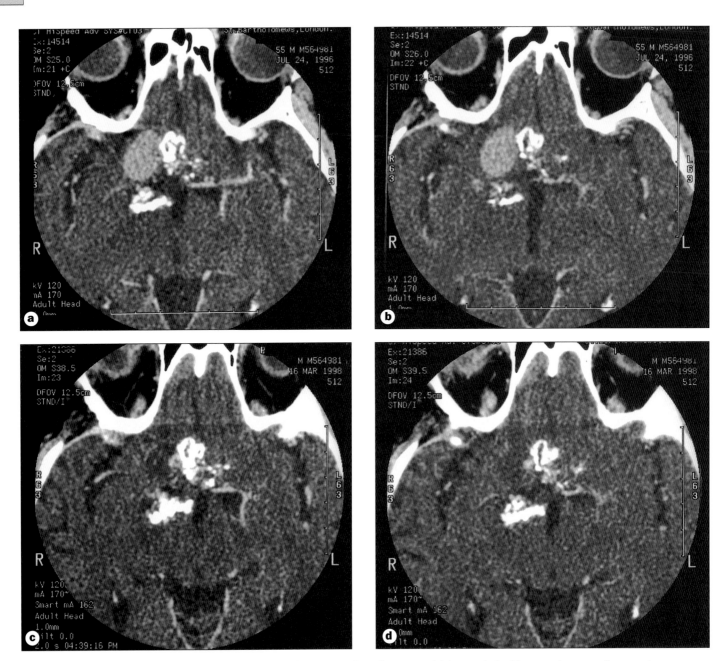

Figure 9.3 Treatment of recurrent craniopharyngioma with stereotactic radiosurgery. Axial computerized tomography scans of recurrent craniopharyngioma before (a, b) and after (c, d) stereotactic radiosurgery, demonstrating the complete response of this solid recurrence.

collated the published experience since that time. From a total of 149 cysts treated, 121 either reduced in size, stopped re-filling, or were obliterated. Our own experience to date is with nine cases and we have used yttrium-90 colloidal solution to deliver the dose to the secreting epithelium of the cyst of 200Gy (**Fig. 9.4**). At present, stereotactic delivered radiation therapy is more appropriate for solid craniopharyngiomas and intracystic instillation of isotopes for cystic disease.

LANGERHANS CELL HISTIOCYTOSIS (LCH)

Formerly called histiocytosis X, Langerhans cell histiocytosis (LCH) is a disease characterized by the aggressive infiltration of

tissues by Langerhans cells (a unique subset of macrophages); in up to 15% of childhood cases (the commonest age group), diabetes insipidus caused by LCH affecting the posterior pituitary and hypothalamus occurs. Medical therapy (corticosteroids and chemotherapy with agents such as vinca alkaloids or etoposide, or immunotherapy with cyclosporin) is used, particularly where there is multisystem disease. Low-dose radiotherapy (say, 1200–1500cGy in eight to 10 fractions) to this brain region may be useful in limiting the diabetes insipidus and anterior pituitary deficiency due to hypothalamic involvement where this is the dominant problem. Whenever cytotoxic chemotherapy or radiotherapy is to be used for apparently benign disease, the pretreatment counseling has to be thorough.

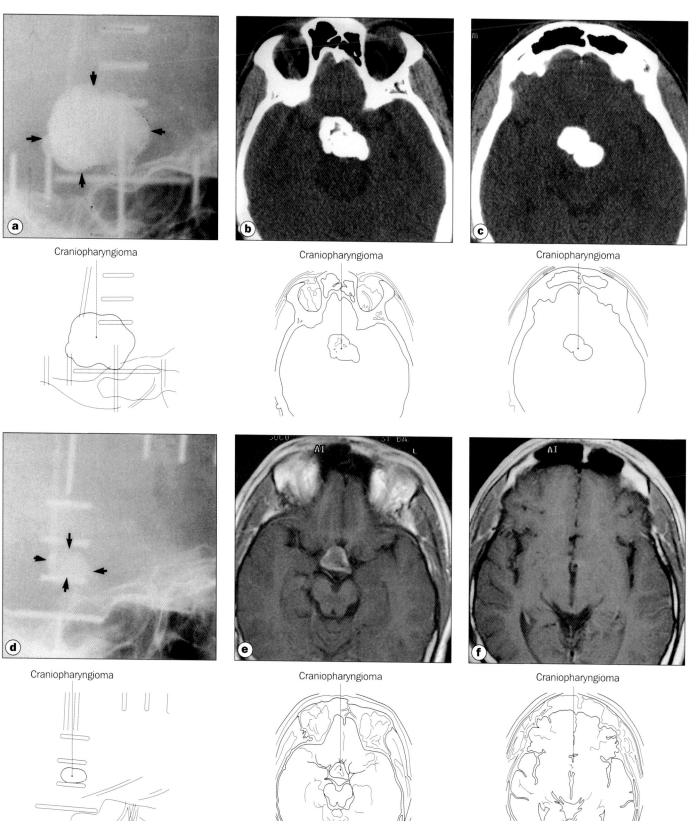

Figure 9.4 Treatment of recurrent cystic craniopharyngioma by intracystic instillation of radioactive isotopes. Recurrent cystic craniopharyngioma before (a–c) and after (d–f) intracystic instillation of yttrium-90 colloidal solution, demonstrating a good response to intracystic instillation of contrast on plain lateral skull films (a, d; lesion arrowed), computerized tomography (b, c) and magnetic resonance imaging (e, f).

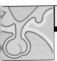

NEUROSARCOIDOSIS

When sarcoidosis affects the nervous system, the sites of predisposition for lesions are the hypothalamus, pituitary, and third ventricle, as well as the cranial nerves (most frequently the facial and optic nerves) as part of a basal meningitis. Diabetes insipidus occurs in 33% of patients with neurosarcoidosis and other features of hypothalamo-pituitary dysfunction frequently accompany this, e.g. somnolence/sleep disorder, weight gain, impotence/hypogonadism, amenorrhea, and panhypopituiarism. The hypothalamus is the usual site of first involvement in this region but the anterior pituitary itself may be affected, although its involvement by itself (i.e. without diabetes insipidus) is rare. Imaging may demonstrate 'space-occupying' granulomas or thickened basal meninges. The cerebrospinal fluid may show a raised lymphocyte count and protein as well as angiotensin-converting enzyme levels but, importantly, may also be normal.

Corticosteroid treatment in high dosage (e.g. prednisolone at 80mg per day) may be useful therapy in the acute labile phase; those patients demonstrating only partial response may need longer-term maintenance. Isolated reports of response to low-dose radiotherapy justify the inclusion of the problem here.

SUPRASELLAR GERM CELL TUMORS

Primary intracranial germ cell tumors (IGCTs) are rare and most commonly occur in the first two decades of life. The incidence varies geographically; thus, although they account for 4–10% of all childhood brain tumors in Japan, the comparable figure in the West is 0.2–2%. The annual incidence in the USA is 40 per year.

IGCTs are histologically a heterogenous group of tumors and their clinical presentation also differs according to their site of origin. Germinomatous germ cell tumors or germinomas – the homologue of seminoma – are the most exquisitely chemo- and radiosensitive; nongerminomatous germ cell tumors, comprising choriocarcinoma, teratoma, and embryonal sinus (yolk sac) tumor and embryonal carcinoma have a poorer overall response to therapy and a worse prognosis. Human chorionic gonadotropin-beta (hCGβ) may be produced by germinomas in small amounts but is secreted by choriocarcinoma elements of nongerminomatous germ cell tumors in large amounts. We described how, when paired measurements are taken in secreting IGCTs, the CSU:blood ratio of hCG shows a 10:1 ratio. Alphafetoprotein is secreted by yolk sac elements of nongerminomatous germ cell tumors. Detection of these markers in the serum or cerebrospinal fluid is diagnostically and prognostically useful. IGCTs most commonly occur in the pineal and then the suprasellar regions; less commonly they occur in other midline brain sites. Synchronous IGCTs occurring at pineal and suprasellar locations is a well-recognized phenomenon (**Fig. 9.5**). Whereas there is a definite male preponderance in the incidence of pineal IGCTs, this sex inequality is not found in suprasellar IGCTs, where there is either an equal sex incidence or even a slight female preponderance. In our small experience, dual-site primaries did show a male preponderance.

Suprasellar IGCTs represent 30% of all IGCTs, are most commonly germinomatous germ cell tumors and present with diabetes insipidus, visual failure, and hypopituitarism – indeed, in our own series of 10 cases, diabetes insipidus was invariably present at presentation. Modest hyperprolactinemia due to stalk disruption was also very common. There was a high incidence of

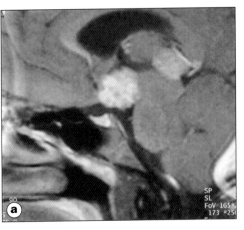
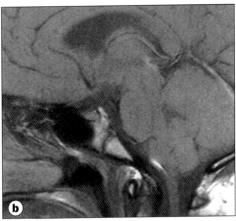

Figure 9.5 Treatment of intracranial germ cell tumors by chemoradiotherapy. Sagittal magnetic resonance scans of a dual-site intracranial germ cell tumor before (a) and after (b) chemoradiotherapy, demonstrating a complete imaging response (also reflected in normalization of markers).

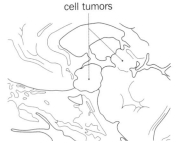

Intracranial germ cell tumors

abnormalities of thirst, which, in combination with diabetes insipidus, led to some serious abnormalities in fluid balance – compounded when platinum-based chemotherapy was used (for which pre- and posthydration is mandatory). Weight loss due to anorexia was also a feature.

Diagnosis is nowadays based on MR imaging demonstrating a midline mass (also positive on 2-deoxy-glucose positron emission tomography, unlike benign tumors of these regions) and either diagnostic levels of cerebrospinal fluid/serum markers (hCGβ, alphafetoprotein) and/or biopsy.

Curative therapy occurs with chemoradiotherapy (**Fig. 9.5**). Traditionally, the results of radiotherapy for this disease have been good but more recently it has been appreciated that there are differing cure rates within the IGCT spectrum. The prognosis for germinomatous germ cell tumors appears excellent, whereas it is poor for alphafetoprotein/hCG-secreting non-germinomatous germ cell tumors. Clinical trials have been conducted of systemic chemotherapy for such patients and found to be useful. The current view is that initial chemotherapy followed by radiotherapy appears to be the best practice.

OTHER CONDITIONS

Secondary cancer (metastatic deposits) occurs with a preferential disposition in the posterior pituitary and hypothalamus; bronchus and breast primary carcinomas are common sites of origin. Radiotherapy is the treatment of choice.

Meningiomas of the sphenoid ridge and cavernous sinus commonly spread across the fossa, as do clivus chordomas, chondrosarcomas, plasmacytomas, and lymphomas. They may present with pituitary endocrinopathy. Other conditions include the advanced nasopharyngeal carcinoma that has infiltrated through the skull base and other skull-base tumors. Radiotherapy has an important role in the management of all these conditions.

FURTHER READING

Bejar J, Kerby G, Ziegker D, Festoff B. Treatment of CNS sarcoidosis with radiotherapy. Ann Neurol. 1985;18:258–60.

Blackburn TPD, Doughty D, Plowman PN. Stereotactic intracavity therapy of recurrent cystic craniopharyngioma by instillation of 90-yttrium. Br J Neurosurg. 1999; 13:359–65.

Brada M, Rajan B, Traish D, et al. The long-term efficacy of conservative surgery and radiotherapy for pituitary adenoma. Clin Endocrinol. 1993;38:571–578l

Ciccarelli EC, Orsello SM, Plowman PN, Besser GM, Wass JAH. Prolonged lowering of growth hormone after radiotherapy in acromegalic patients followed over 15 years. Adv Biosci. 1988;69:269–72.

Heideman RL, Packer RJ, Albright LA, Freeman CR, Rorke LB. Tumors of the central nervous system. In: Pizzo PA, Poplak DG, eds. Principles and practice of pediatric oncology. Philadelphia, PA:Lippincott-Raven; 1997:633–97.

Landolt AM, Haller D, Lomax N, et al. Stereotactic radiosurgery for recurrent surgically treated acromegaly: a comparison with fractionated radiotherapy. J Neurosurg. 1998;88:1002–8.

Plowman PN, Kingston JE, Sebag-Montefiore DSM, Doughty D. Clinical efficacy of perceived CNS friendly chemoradiotherapy for primary intracranial germ cell tumors. Clin Oncol. 1997;9:48–53.

Plowman PN. Pituitary radiotherapy – when, who and how? Clin Endocrinol. 1999;51:265–71.

Sano K. The so-called intracranial germ cell tumors: are they really of germ cell origin? Br J Neurosurg. 1995;9:391–401.

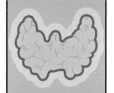

Chapter 10 — Thyroid Physiology

John T Dunn and Ann D Dunn

STRUCTURE

The thyroid is a butterfly-shaped gland consisting of two lateral lobes joined by an isthmus, situated slightly below the thyroid cartilage in the anterior neck. Its size varies greatly, especially with iodine nutrition. In the USA, with a relatively high iodine intake, the average adult thyroid usually has a volume of less than 10ml, whereas thyroids in Europe are larger, reflecting borderline iodine deficiency. Microscopically the thyroid contains numerous follicles, each composed of columnar cells grouped around a central lumen. The latter is filled with stored thyroglobulin (Tg) to make a gelatinous material called colloid. In thyroid hyperplasia the thyrocytes become more columnar and the lumen smaller, reflecting accelerated hormone synthesis and release.

BASIC THYROID PHYSIOLOGY

The thyroid's only clearly established function is to produce the hormones thyroxine (T_4) and triiodothyronine (T_3; Fig. 10.1). The parafollicular cells of the thyroid make thyrocalcitonin, a useful marker for medullary cancer but of uncertain function in normal humans. While 90% or more of secreted thyroid hormone is T_4, its action at target tissues occurs after its deiodination to T_3.

Effective thyroid hormone synthesis depends on three factors: *iodine*, the essential raw material; proper *cell machinery*; and *control elements*, particularly thyroid-stimulating hormone (TSH).

Iodine

Iodine may be ingested in a variety of chemical forms, but most is converted to iodide (I^-) in the gut and promptly absorbed into the circulation. It is then either excreted by the kidney or concentrated by the thyroid. Other tissues concentrating iodine are the salivary glands, choroid plexus, and breast, the latter being essential to the nutrition of the nursing infant.

Cell machinery

The sodium/iodide symporter (NIS) located in the thyroidal basal membrane governs iodide uptake (Fig. 10.2 & Table 10.1). This protein of 65kDa spans the membrane, with the amino terminus outside and the carboxyl terminus within. It cotransports

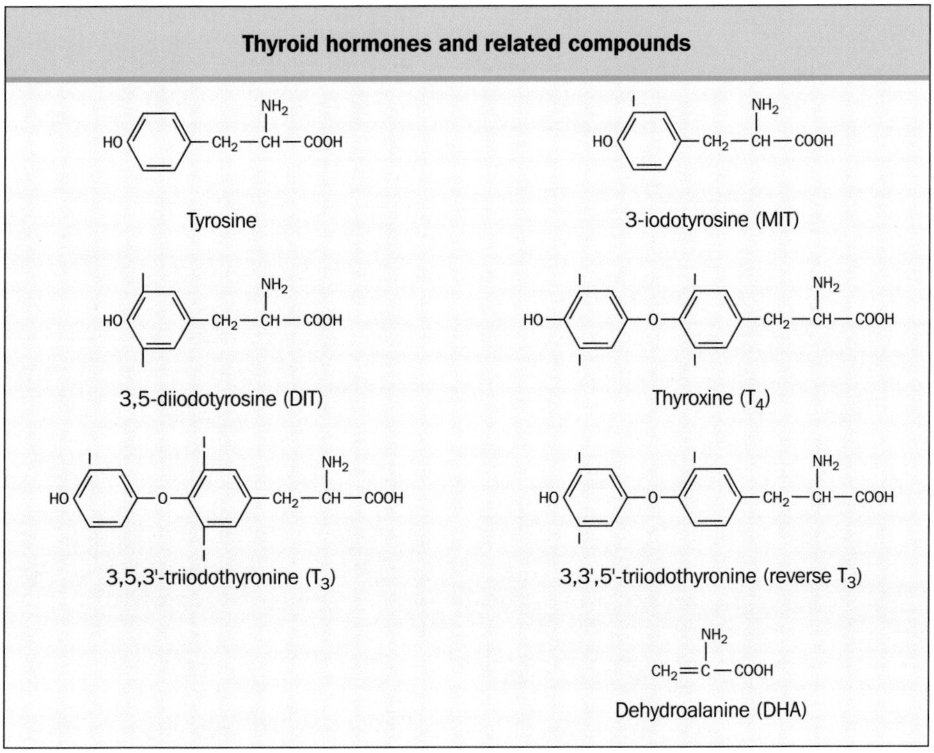

Figure 10.1 Thyroid hormones and related compounds.

Thyroid hormones and related compounds

Tyrosine

3-iodotyrosine (MIT)

3,5-diiodotyrosine (DIT)

Thyroxine (T_4)

3,5,3'-triiodothyronine (T_3)

3,3',5'-triiodothyronine (reverse T_3)

Dehydroalanine (DHA)

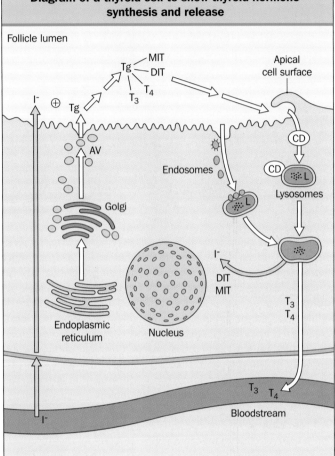

Diagram of a thyroid cell to show thyroid hormone synthesis and release

Follicle lumen

Figure 10.2 Diagram of a thyroid cell to show thyroid hormone synthesis and release. Tg, thyroglobulin.

Once in the thyroid cell, iodide migrates to the apical membrane, where it meets Tg. This 660kDa glycoprotein is synthesized by the thyroid's endoplasmic reticulum, and its glycosylation is completed in the Golgi apparatus. Molecular chaperones exert quality control to ensure that only properly folded Tg molecules reach the apical membrane. Another key protein is thyroperoxidase (TPO), a 103kDa enzyme having 44% homology with myeloperoxidase. Both Tg and TPO are antigenic in autoimmune thyroid disease and provide useful serum markers.

Thyroid hormone forms at the apical membrane in a complex series of reactions involving iodide, Tg, TPO, and hydrogen peroxide (**Fig. 10.3**). Hydrogen peroxide production requires calcium, nicotinamide adenine dinucleotide phosphate (NADPH), and NADPH oxidase, the latter poorly characterized. Iodide is oxidized by H_2O_2 and TPO, and then attaches to tyrosyl residues within the peptide chains of Tg, to form 3-monoiodotyrosine (MIT) or 3,5-diiodotyrosine (DIT). Next, two DIT molecules, still part of Tg, couple to form T_4, combining the diiodophenyl group of the donor DIT with the acceptor DIT by a diphenyl ether link (**Fig. 10.1**). This process leaves dehydroalanine at the site of the DIT donor within the Tg molecule. Some T_3 is formed by a similar coupling of donor MIT with acceptor DIT. The favored acceptor for T_4 formation is Tyr_5 of Tg's polypeptide chain, very close to the N terminus; its likely donor is Tyr_{130}. Other important acceptors are Tyr_{2553}, about 200 residues from Tg's C terminus, and Tyr_{2746}, three residues from the C terminus; this latter position favors T_3 synthesis in some species.

After hormone synthesis is complete, the Tg is stored extracellularly in the lumen of the thyroid follicle. Normally, about one-third of its iodine is in T_4 and T_3 and the remainder in DIT and MIT. Most of the colloid in the follicular lumen consists of Tg. This provides a useful mechanism for storage of both iodine and thyroid hormone, to be called upon when needed. Immunostaining for Tg can help microscopic identification of thyroid-derived tissue, as in metastatic differentiated thyroid cancer.

Release of thyroid hormone usually begins with formation of endocytotic vesicles followed by Tg digestion with endosomal and lysosomal enzymes. The major proteolytic enzymes are the endopeptidases cathepsins C, B, and L, and several exopeptidases.

Na^+ and I^- ions into the cell. The thyroid:circulation gradient can reach 100:1, varying widely with iodide supply and thyroid activity. The process is energy-dependent, requires O_2, and is stimulated by TSH.

Some key players in hormone synthesis and release

	Location	Function	Features
Thyroid transcription factors (TTF)	Genes	Transcribe genes for Tg, TPO, TSH receptor	Several TTFs shared by Tg, TPO, TSHr
TSH receptor (TSHr)	Basal membrane	Mediate TSH effects	85kDa glycoprotein, homology to other hormone receptors
Na/I symporter	Basal membrane	I^- transport into cell	65kDa transmembrane protein
Thyroglobulin (Tg)	Cell, follicular lumen	Matrix for hormone formation	660kDa glycoprotein, made in endoplasmic reticulum
Molecular chaperones	Endoplasmic reticulum	Quality control of Tg	Several identified; ↑ activity against defective proteins
Thyroperoxidase (TPO)	Apical membrane	Catalyze I^- oxidation, iodotyrosine coupling	103kDa glycoprotein, antigenic in autoimmune thyroid disease
H_2O_2	Apical membrane	Substrate for TPO	Generated by NADPH, Ca^{2+}
Pendrin	Apical membrane	Cl^-/I^- transporter	Mutations produce Pendred's syndrome
Cathepsins C, D, L	Lysosomes	Digest Tg	Proteolytic enzymes, some specificity to Tg cleavage
Thyroid iodotyrosine deiodinase	Cytoplasm	Deiodinate DIT and MIT	Flavoprotein, NADPH-dependent
5'-iodothyronine deiodinase	Basal membrane	Deiodinate T_4 to T_3	Same as 5'-deiodinase type I in liver, muscle, etc.

Table 10.1 Some key players in hormone synthesis and release. DIT, 3,5-diiodotyrosine; MIT, 3-monoiodotyrosine; NADPH, nicotinamide adenine dinucleotide phosphate; T_3, triiodothyronine; T_4, thyroxine; TSH, thyroid-stimulating hormone.

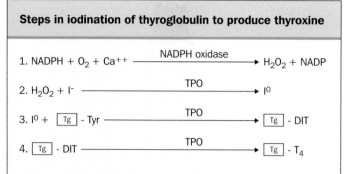

Steps in iodination of thyroglobulin to produce thyroxine

1. $NADPH + O_2 + Ca^{++} \xrightarrow{\text{NADPH oxidase}} H_2O_2 + NADP$

2. $H_2O_2 + I^- \xrightarrow{\text{TPO}} I^0$

3. $I^0 + \boxed{Tg} \text{-Tyr} \xrightarrow{\text{TPO}} \boxed{Tg} \text{-DIT}$

4. $\boxed{Tg} \text{-DIT} \xrightarrow{\text{TPO}} \boxed{Tg} \text{-}T_4$

Figure 10.3 Steps in iodination of thyroglobulin to produce thyroxine. DIT, 3,5-diiodotyrosine; NADP, nicotinamide adenine dinucleotide phosphate; NADPH, NADP (reduced form); TPO, thyroperoxidase.

Their action releases free T_4 and T_3 into the circulation (**Fig. 10.2**). Thyroglobulin's DIT and MIT are not usually released but instead are deiodinated by an iodotyrosine deiodinase, and their iodide re-enters the intrathyroidal pool. This can be an important mechanism for iodine conservation.

Control elements

Thyroid-stimulating hormone is the major modulator of thyroid hormone physiology (**Table 10.2**). Its influence appears at most steps in thyroid hormone synthesis and release. It acts through the TSH receptor (TSHr), a 85kDa member of the G-protein-coupled receptor family, located at the basal membrane, to sequentially stimulate adenyl cyclase, cyclic adenosine mono-phosphate (cAMP) production and target gene response. Antibodies to TSHr in autoimmune thyroid disease can either stimulate or block the TSHr, to produce hyper- or hypo-thyroidism, respectively.

The earliest cellular effect of TSH is increased breakdown of Tg to release stored thyroid hormone. In addition, TSH increases

thyroidal uptake of iodine and thyroid hormone synthesis, by simulating production of NIS, TPO, Tg, and H_2O_2. It also favors production of T_3 relative to T_4, shifts the priority of iodization among Tg's tyrosyl residues, and accelerates action of specific proteases. These various steps and effects are related. Overall, TSH stimulation increases the synthesis and release of thyroid hormones and favors production of T_3 relative to that of T_4. In turn, TSH secretion responds to circulating T_4 and T_3 and to TSH-releasing hormone (TRH) from the hypothalamus, to provide optimal hormone delivery to target tissues (**Fig. 10.4**).

Hormone metabolism

Once released from the thyroid gland, T_4 and T_3 bind to specific transport proteins, all synthesized in the liver. Thyroxine-binding globulin (TBG) has high affinity for both hormones and carries about 60–70% of the total secreted. Transthyretin (TTR; previously called T_4-binding prealbumin) carries about 15% but has lower affinity and dissociates more rapidly to deliver free hormone to tissues. Transthyretin also transports vitamin A. Albumin carries most of the remainder of the thyroid hormone, and its binding is relatively nonspecific. Serum lipoproteins also bind a small amount of thyroid hormone, especially high-density lipoprotein. Normally, about 0.1% of the total T_4 is free. This is the form accessible to target tissues, and is in equilibrium with bound hormone.

Hormone action

Most of T_4's action at the tissue level is through its conversion to T_3, the metabolically active form of the hormone (**Table 10.3**). Two selenium-containing deiodinases exist. Type 1 occurs principally in the thyroid, kidney, liver, and muscle; its action increases in hyperthyroidism, decreases in hypothyroidism, and is inhibited by thiouracils. Type 2 is found mainly in the central nervous system, pituitary, and brown adipose tissue. It is influenced by iopanoic acid but not much by thiouracils. Its activity decreases in hyperthyroidism and increases in hypothyroidism. A third deiodinase (5-deiodinase) removes iodine from the inner

Some actions of thyroid-stimulating hormone on thyroid

Action	Effect
↑ Sodium/iodide symporter synthesis	↑ I⁻ uptake
↑ thyroperoxidase synthesis	↑ thyroglobulin iodination and hormonogenesis
↑ thyroglobulin synthesis	Enhance hormonogenesis
↑ NADPH oxidase	↑ H_2O_2 generation, promote hormonogenesis
↑ iodine-associated thyroglobulin cleavage	May prepare thyroglobulin for proteolysis
Alter sites of hormone synthesis	↑ T_3/T_4 ratio in thyroglobulin
↑ activity of cathepsins B and L	↑ thyroglobulin proteolysis
Colloid droplet formation	↑ thyroglobulin resorption into cell
↑ T_4 deiodination to T_3	↑ T_3 release from thyroid

Table 10.2 Some actions of thyroid-stimulating hormone on thyroid. NADPH, nicotinamide adenine dinucleotide phosphate; T_3, triiodothyronine; T_4, thyroxine.

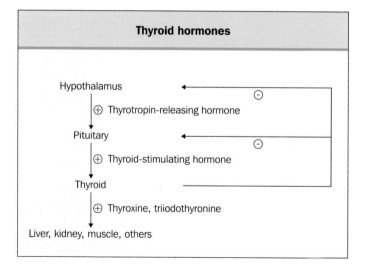

Figure 10.4 Thyroid hormones. The figure shows the glands in control of hormone delivery and their hormones.

Steps in thyroid hormone action		
Step	Location	Description
T_4 conversion to T_3	Liver, muscle, etc.	Type I 5'-deiodinase action
	Pituitary, CNS	Type II 5'-deiodinase action
T_3 interaction with thyroid hormone receptor	Cell nucleus	Receptors similar to those for steroids, retinoic acid, others
Receptor binding to thyroid hormone response element	Gene	Receptor recognition, to modify gene translation
Gene expression	Cytoplasm	Modulate protein synthesis

Table 10.3 Steps in thyroid hormone action. T_3, triiodothyronine; T_4, thyroxine.

ring of T_4 and T_3, and is responsible for the production of reverse T_3 (rT_3), which is metabolically inert. Patients with chronic non-thyroidal illness or the 'euthyroid sick syndrome' typically have decreased serum T_3 concentrations and increased rT_3.

In the target cell, T_3 interacts with specific nuclear receptors; these act in turn on thyroid hormone response elements to regulate gene expression for key proteins. Examples are growth hormone, myosin heavy chain, TSH, liver enzymes associated with lipogenesis, myosin, and unidentified genes in brain.

CLINICAL CONSIDERATIONS

Assessment of thyroid status

Both static and functional tests are available. Immunoassays exist for total T_4, total T_3, free T_4, free T_3, and reverse T_3. **Table 10.4** summarizes normal ranges, although each may vary slightly in different assays. The serum total T_4 reflects the 99.9% of serum

T_4 bound to carrier proteins and has been one of the most widely used tests to assess thyroid function. However, the serum *free* T_4 is much more relevant, because it represents the fraction that is actually available to tissues for hormone action. The free T_4 is normally in equilibrium with the total. Alterations in binding proteins affect this ratio. For example, TBG increases during euthyroid pregnancy or estrogen exposure, elevating the total T_4, but the free T_4 remains normal. Alterations in binding protein can be recognized by an additional test, the T_3 resin uptake. Several techniques exist for its measurement but most express results as percentage binding: a low value accompanies an increase in binding proteins and a high value the opposite. Thus, in the euthyroid individual with increased binding protein (e.g. pregnancy or other estrogen exposure), the serum total T_4 is elevated, the T_3 resin uptake is low, and the TSH and free T_4 are normal. Similarly, in conditions of decreased binding proteins (e.g. malnutrition, nephrosis), the euthyroid individual has a low serum total T_4 but a high T_3 resin uptake. Multiplying the total T_4 by the resin uptake provides a 'free T_4 index', sometimes used to indicate the serum free T_4. Better, the free T_4 can be measured directly in newer assays, which are gradually replacing the combination of total T_4 and T_3 resin uptake.

The thyroid secretes much more T_4 than T_3, but T_3 binds less tightly to carrier proteins. In hyperthyroidism, both serum T_4 and T_3 are typically elevated but the T_3 increase is frequently earlier and more pronounced. This difference may be particularly striking in toxic nodular goiter, probably reflecting increased production of T_3 relative to that of T_4 in the thyroid. Lowering of the serum T_3 often nonspecifically accompanies chronic or severe illness, and may be complemented by an increase in serum reverse T_3, although the latter measurement is not often necessary for clinical use.

Table 10.4 Tests for assessing thyroid status. T_3, triiodothyronine; T_4, thyroxine.

Tests for assessing thyroid status		
	Normal range	Clinical use
Serum		
Total T_4 (µg/dL)	4.5–11.0	Measures circulating hormone; ↑ in hyper, ↓ in hypo
Total T_3 (ng/dL)	60–180	
Free T_4 (ng/dL)	0.6–1.8	
Free T_3 (pg/dL)	0.2–0.5	
Reverse T_3 (ng/dL)	15–45	↑ in euthyroid sick
T_3 resin uptake (%)	25–35	Reflects hormone binding to serum proteins
Thyroid-stimulating hormone (mU/L)	0.5–6.0	Pituitary response to circulating T_4 & T_3; ↑ hypo, ↓ hyper
Thyroglobulin (µg/L)	5–50*	↑ in hyperplasia, ↑ in papillary and follicular cancer
Thyroperoxidase antibodies (Iu/mL)	<2	↑ in autoimmune thyroid disease
Thyroglobulin antibodies (Iu/mL)	<2	
Thyroid-receptor-stimulating antibodies		↑ in Graves' hyperthyroidism
Thyrocalcitonin (pg/L)	≤ 4	↑ in medullary thyroid cancer
Urine		
Urine iodine concentration (µg/L)	100–200	Measures iodine nutrition
Isotopes		
24h radioiodine uptake (%)	8–20	↑ in hyperthyroidism, iodine deficiency; ↓ in subacute thyroiditis
* Normal range given only as example; these tests vary considerably in different assay systems and the range established for each laboratory must be respected.		

The single most useful test of thyroid function is the serum TSH. It reflects the pituitary's perception of whether circulating thyroid hormone levels are appropriate. Thus, the earliest laboratory sign of primary hypothyroidism is usually an elevation in serum TSH, and the earliest for hyperthyroidism is a low TSH. In this sense, the TSH is a dynamic indicator, in contrast to the serum thyroid hormone levels as static markers. A caveat, of course, is that the serum TSH level alone will not detect the few percentage of all hypothyroid cases that arise from pituitary failure. Usually this secondary hypothyroidism is apparent from other clinical features but initially should be considered by measuring serum thyroid hormone levels as well.

The other tests in **Table 10.4** have more special application. Antibodies to TPO and to Tg are useful in establishing autoimmune thyroid disease when that diagnosis is in doubt but do not correlate well with thyroid function. Assays for thyroid binding proteins are available when the question of abnormal binding proteins needs addressing.

The normal thyroid secretes some Tg, and this is often increased nonspecifically in conditions associated with thyroid hyperplasia. Many differentiated cancers (papillary and follicular) also secrete Tg, reflecting their primitive urge to behave like normal thyroid tissue. In patients who have had thyroid ablation with surgery and radioiodine for thyroid cancer, persistence of detectable serum Tg makes the continued presence of thyroid cancer likely. Thus, the serum Tg is the most useful laboratory test for following patients who have been treated for differentiated thyroid cancer, and is more sensitive and less cumbersome than repetitive scanning with radioiodine. Tg sensitivity increases when the patient's TSH is elevated, either from hormone replacement withdrawal or by stimulation with recombinant TSH.

The serum calcitonin is a good marker for medullary carcinoma, which arises from the thyroid parafollicular cells. This cancer is frequently a difficult cytologic and histologic diagnosis, so serum calcitonin is a useful test in patients with a greater than ordinary risk of medullary carcinoma (e.g. MEN II syndrome, some solitary nodules in the upper part of the thyroid). The serum CEA, although nonspecific, is also usually elevated in medullary cancer.

The thyroid can be assessed by imaging, discussed more extensively in Chapter 42. Ultrasonography is especially useful for judging overall thyroid volume and architecture, and the size and character of individual nodules. Simple, inexpensive instruments are rapidly becoming an indispensable part of thyroid practice. Imaging with radioactive iodine (^{123}I, ^{131}I) or its surrogates (e.g. technetium-99, ^{99m}Tc) shows the uptake of iodine by the thyroid overall and in individual parts (e.g. nodules). Normal values for uptake depend heavily on dietary iodine, being higher with decreased iodine availability. Succeeding chapters discuss clinical use of the radioactive iodine uptake more extensively.

Many factors affect the body's ability to maintain euthyroidism. These can be broadly classified as genetic alterations, iodine nutrition, and various other extrinsic influences. The latter involve drugs and other agents directed (intentionally or not) at the thyroid, as well as other endocrine influences; they are discussed elsewhere in this book. This chapter comments on some genetic factors and on iodine nutrition.

Genetic alterations

Thyroid hormone synthesis, transport, and utilization involve many different proteins. Defects can potentially occur at most levels and many have been documented. When the thyroid confronts inefficient hormone production resulting from impaired genes, it can adapt by increasing its size to provide more cell activity and increased production of the required amount of hormone. Subjects with alterations in binding proteins can adapt by altering the ratio of bound to free hormone, thus providing adequate free hormone to the tissue. These various circumstances lead to a thyroid system that, although heterogeneous from considerable genetic variation that produces varying degrees of thyroid efficiency and occasionally goiter, still leaves the subject otherwise fairly intact. Severe defects at critical metabolic points produce significant clinical disease, usually goiter or hypothyroidism. The rapid expansion of molecular genetics is identifying many new associations between specific genes and clinical thyroid disorders. **Table 10.5** gives some examples, and there are many others.

Defects exist at most of the steps in thyroid hormone synthesis. With the discovery and characterization of each of the major proteins, NIS, TPO, and Tg (**Table 10.5**), the defects can be localized to specific mutations. Most of these genetic disorders have goiter as a consequence. More severe cases also have

Thyroid disorders arising from altered genes			
Function	Defective gene	Consequence	Mechanism
Iodide transport	NIS	Goiter, hypothyroidism	↓ I⁻ concentration in thyroid
Iodide organification	Pendrin	Goiter, deafness	↓ hormone formation
	Tg, TPO	Goiter, hypothyroidism	↓ hormone formation
Iodotyrosine deiodination	Thyroidal deiodinase (?)	Goiter, hypothyroidism, iodine deficiency	↓ intrathyroidal conservation of I⁻ from MIT and DIT
Serum hormone binding	TBG, TTR	↑ ratio fT_4:TT_4, usually euthyroid	↓ serum total T_4
	Albumin	↓ ratio fT_4:TT_4, usually euthyroid	↑ serum total T_4
Hormone action	Thyroid hormone receptor β	↑ serum T_4, ↑ or normal TSH, varying clinical features	Tissue resistance to T_4 action

Table 10.5 Thyroid disorders arising from altered genes. DIT, 3,5-diiodotyrosine; fT_4, free thyroxine; MIT, 3-monoiodotyrosine; NIS, sodium/iodide symporter; T_4, thyroxine; TBG, thyroxine-binding globulin; Tg, thyroglobulin; TPO, thyroperoxidase; TSH, thyroid-stimulating hormone; TT_4, bound thyroxine; TTR, transthyretin.

hypothyroidism and occasionally even cretinism. Iodine deficiency, which occurs in much of the world, can be a confounding cofactor because it adds an additional stress on a defective thyroid that may already be working at full capacity.

Abnormalities in protein binding usually have no adverse effects, except to initially puzzle the clinician reviewing routine tests of serum thyroid hormones. For example, a subject with deficient TBG binding has a low total T_4 level, and a high T_3 resin uptake, but the free T_4 is normal because the ratio of free to bound T_4 has been increased and so tissues get the right amount of hormone. Binding proteins increase physiologically in pregnancy and decrease with impaired liver function or malnutrition; these changes alter the total T_4 and T_3 resin uptake, but the free T_4 and TSH remain normal in the euthyroid subject. Familial dysalbuminemic hyperthyroxinemia involves an abnormal serum albumin that binds thyroid hormone more tightly, thus keeping more in the bound form; to compensate, the ratio of free to bound T_4 is lowered accordingly, and tissues receive the appropriate amount of free T_4.

The thyroid hormone resistance syndrome may also cause confusion because it alters the usual relationship between serum T_4 and TSH. Extensive work has characterized many mutations, most in the thyroid hormone receptor β gene. Clinical expression is quite varied. Because the pituitary as well as other tissues is resistant to thyroid hormone action, TSH remains normal or elevated despite a high serum T_4.

The synthesis of T_4 involves TPO, Tg, and other proteins, and many defects in these and other factors have been recognized. Pendred's syndrome is a special case, characterized by defective iodide organification, goiter, and congenital deafness from cochlear and endolymph defects. The thyroidal disorder has recently been traced to a molecular defect in pendrin, a protein associated with iodide transport at the apical membrane. As more is learned about thyroid proteins and their role in hormone formation, many more defects and their association with disease will be uncovered.

Iodine malnutrition

Because iodine is an essential component of the thyroid hormones, its deficiency carries the risk of hypothyroidism. Iodine deficiency is one of the world's most prevalent endocrine problems, with about one-third of the global population at risk (**Table 10.6**). Seawater is a good source, but iodine's distribution over the earth's surface is uneven; many inland areas, particularly those associated with high mountains or frequent flooding, are deprived. The clinical consequences are those from other causes of hypothyroidism, often complicated by additional nutritional and socioeconomic deficits. **Table 10.7** lists the effects both on the individual and on the community – the iodine deficiency disorders. Obviously, the two overlap considerably, but it is important to recognize that this deficiency has major consequences for the community as well as for its individual members. The priority list in **Table 10.7** is quite arbitrary. It is meant to emphasize the current reasons for prompt correction of iodine deficiency; for example, some of the most extreme consequences, like cretinism, are already disappearing as partial improvement in iodine nutrition occurs, while small but widespread intelligence impairment poses a greater overall threat.

The most apparent feature is goiter, as the thyroid threatened by hypothyroidism enlarges in its struggle to produce more thyroid hormone (**Fig. 10.5**). If the adaptation is successful, the individual is clinically euthyroid but with a goiter and, possibly, subtle departures from euthyroidism. In more severe deficiency the subject is hypothyroid. The most troubling consequence of iodine deficiency during development is irreversible mental retardation, from inadequate thyroid hormone at a critical point in central nervous system development during fetal and early postnatal life; thyroid hormone is particularly important for myelination of the central nervous system. Other consequences are deaf mutism, gait disturbances, decreased child survival, and reproductive failure. The most severe form is cretinism, defined as severe mental retardation with varying degrees of deaf mutism, neuromuscular disorder, and short stature (**Fig. 10.6**).

The public health dimensions of this problem are staggering because all people living in areas of deficiency risk these consequences, including some degree of mental impairment and goiter. One meta-analysis reports average loss of 13.5 IQ points in individuals living in iodine-deficient regions. Consequences to the thyroid alone cost Germany an estimated annual US$1 billion.

The iodine-deficiency disorders are more prevalent among remote, isolated, poor communities. They can be completely corrected by adequate provision of iodine, and massive international efforts led by the International Council for the Control of Iodine Deficiency Disorders, the World Health Organization, and UNICEF have produced remarkable progress since 1990. **Table 10.6** summarizes current status. Iodized salt is the main corrective vehicle, although other forms of iodine delivery such as iodized vegetable oil, iodized water, and iodine tablets are occasionally used. Vigorous efforts to achieve adequate iodine in areas that are still deficient continue, but sustaining progress and ensuring *optimal* iodine nutrition now claim equal attention.

Iodine deficiency status by region								
	Africa	Americas	EMRO	Europe	South-east Asia	West Pacific	Total	%
Countries with iodine deficiency	44	19	17	32	9	9	**130**	
Population with goiter (millions)	124	39	152	130	172	124	**740**	13
Population at risk (millions)	295	196	348	275	599	513	**2225**	38
Household iodized salt consumption (%)	63	90	66	27	70	76	**68**	

Table 10.6 Iodine deficiency status by region. EMRO, Eastern Mediterranean region. Data from WHO, in IDD Newsletter. 1999;15:18.

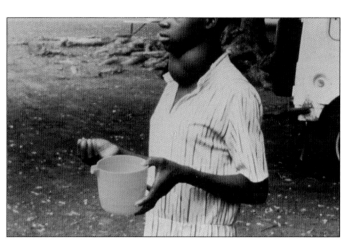

Figure 10.5 Young African woman with large goiter.

Consequences of iodine deficiency	
Individual	**Community**
Decreased child survival	Increased child mortality
Mental retardation	Poor educability
Reproductive impairment	Impaired economic productivity
Hypothyroidism	Increased health costs
Deaf mutism	
Cretinism	
Neurologic deficits	
Goiter	
Late hyperthyroidism	

Table 10.7 Consequences of iodine deficiency. The effects are listed in approximate order of health significance for individual and community. The overlap between the categories and the arbitrariness of the ranking are acknowledged.

Experience in a number of countries shows that initially successful programs may later founder on the rocks of complacency and monitoring lapses. The key to sustainability is regular monitoring of iodine nutrition. Population intakes of iodine fluctuate widely and unpredictably, probably related to changes in food processing and dietary habits. For example, in the USA iodine intake decreased by over 50% between the 1970s and the 1990s.

An optimal iodine intake is about 150µg/day for adults. Slightly lower values apply for children and higher amounts during pregnancy and lactation. Iodine concentration in urine is the preferred indicator for iodine nutrition (**Table 10.8**) because over 90% of ingested iodine eventually appears there. Other useful indicators are thyroid volume, preferably by ultrasound, incidence of transient hypothyroidism on neonatal TSH screening, and serum Tg. Serum T_4, T_3, and TSH (except in newborns) are less valuable because they overlap with normals

Sources of iodine vary widely among cultures and individuals. In Western countries, dairy products, fish, and meat are major contributors. Iodine is added to many products for commercial reasons. Examples are iodate for bread conditioning, iodine as a skin disinfectant, iodine from kelp as a 'health food', iodinated oils as radiocontrast media, and iodine-containing medicines such as

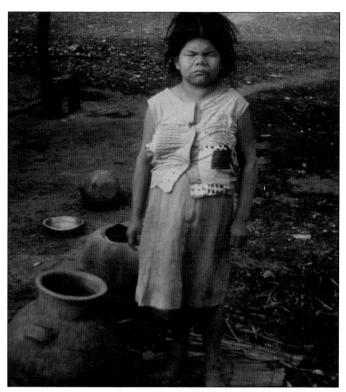

Figure 10.6 Iodine-deficient cretin, from the Andes; mental retardation, deaf mutism, short stature.

amiodarone. Most people can tolerate high doses of iodine without apparent ill effect, although they are accompanied by slight changes in thyroid hormone levels. People with underlying autoimmune disease, or a tendency towards it, are frequently quite sensitive to iodine, and amounts over 1mg/day may paradoxically produce goiter and hypothyroidism. Individuals from a previously iodine-deficient area, particularly older subjects with autonomous nodules, can develop hyperthyroidism even with modest increases in dietary iodine, and this is to be expected as an inevitable part of most prophylaxis programs. Also, epidemiologic studies show that populations with higher mean iodine intakes tend to have a higher frequency of autoimmune thyroid disease, and possibly of papillary thyroid cancer as well.

Iodine treatment for hyperthyroidism

Excess iodine saturates the thyroperoxidase enzyme, hindering thyroxine formation on Tg. Iodine also inhibits the release of hormones from the thyroid, partly by reducing the activities of key proteolytic enzymes and also by slowing colloid droplet formation. These effects make iodine, as Lugol's solution or saturated solution of potassium iodide, useful for treating autoimmune hyperthyroidism. It acts earlier than do thionamides because it lowers hormone release as well as synthesis; however, many patients escape from its block, occasionally within a few days. For several decades in the early 20th century, iodine was the only medicine available for controlling hyperthyroidism of Graves' disease in preparation for thyroidectomy, and it greatly reduced perioperative morbidity, particularly the risks associated with anesthesia in patients with uncorrected hyperthyroidism.

Classification of community iodine nutrition status				
	Features	Approx. daily iodine intake* (adults; µg/day)	Urinary iodine concentration (µg/L)	Urgency for correction
Severe deficiency	Cretinism, goiter, hypothyroidism	< 30	< 20	Emergency
Moderate deficiency	Goiter, hypothyroidism	30–74	20–49	Urgent
Mild deficiency	Goiter	75–149	50–99	Important
Optimal intake	Euthyroid; no complications	150–300	100–199	None
More than adequate intake	Possible: ↑ autoimmune disease, ↑ iodine-induced hyperthyroidism	300–450	200–300	Watch closely
Excess	↑ autoimmune disease, probable iodine-induced hyperthyroidism, possible ↑ papillary cancer	> 450	> 300	Important
* Daily intake is calculated from iodine in casual urine samples in adults, about 1.5L urine per day.				

Table 10.8 Classification of community iodine nutrition status. Nutrition status is classified by median urinary iodine excretion to establish degree of malnutrition and the urgency for its correction.

FURTHER READING

Delange F. The disorders induced by iodine deficiency. Thyroid 1994;4:107–128.

Dunn JT, Dunn AD. Thyroglobulin: chemistry, biosynthesis, and proteolysis. In: Braverman LE, Utiger RD, eds. Werner & Ingbar's the thyroid, 8th edn. Philadelphia, PA:Lippincott Williams & Wilkins; 2000:91–104.

Dunn JT. Biosynthesis and secretion of thyroid hormones. In: DeGroot LJ, Jameson JL, eds. Endocrinology, 4th edn. Philadelphia, PA:WB Saunders 2000:1290–300.

Dunn JT. Seven deadly sins in confronting endemic iodine deficiency and how to avoid them. J Clin Endocrinol Metab. 1996;81:1332–5.

Jameson JL. Mechanisms of thyroid hormone action. In: DeGroot LJ, Jameson JL, eds. Endocrinology, 4th edn. Philadelphia, PA:WB Saunders 2000:1327–44.

Kim PS, Arvan P. Endocrinopathies in the family of endoplasmic reticulum (ER) storage diseases: disorders of protein trafficking and the role of ER molecular chaperones. Endocrinol Rev. 1998;19:173–202.

Medeiros-Neto G, Stanbury JB. Inherited disorders of the thyroid system. Boca Raton, FL:CRC Press; 1994.

St Germain DL, Galton VA. The deiodinase family of selenoproteins. Thyroid 1997;7:655–68.

Schussler GC. The thyroxine-binding proteins. Thyroid 2000;10:141–9.

Spitzweg C, Heufelder AR, Morris JC. Thyroid iodine transport. Thyroid 2000;10:321–30.

Stanbury JB, ed. The damaged brain of iodine deficiency. New York:Cognizant Communication Corp.; 1994.

Taurog AM. Hormone synthesis: thyroid iodine metabolism. In: Braverman LE, Utiger RD, eds. Werner & Ingbar's the thyroid, 8th edn. Philadelphia, PA:Lippincott Williams & Wilkins; 2000:61–85.

WHO/ICCIDD/UNICEF. Assessment of the iodine deficiency disorders and monitoring their elimination (in press; summary in IDD Newsletter 1999;15:33–9).

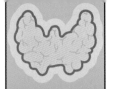

Chapter 11

Hypothyroidism

Grace Kim and Terry F Davies

INTRODUCTION

History

It was as recent as the late 1800s that scientists began to understand the importance of the thyroid gland and only then were the consequences of removal of the thyroid recorded in post-thyroidectomized patients. At that time, thyroid gland extract from sheep was given to patients to treat 'myxedema', first by George Murray in Newcastle upon Tyne, UK, and this proved so successful that thyroid extract was prescribed for a variety of nonspecific symptoms as a panacea for illhealth. Fortunately, more than a century since the discovery of the actions of the thyroid hormones, we now understand that hypothyroidism is the consequence of a variety of specific diseases that present with similar symptoms and signs (**Fig. 11.1**). Today, the diagnosis of primary hypothyroidism, with the highly sensitive thyrotropin assays, is straightforward and its treatment is safe and effective with synthetic thyroxine.

Types of hypothyroidism

The classification of hypothyroidism is summarized in **Table 11.1**. For normal thyroid hormone production, the hypothalamic–pituitary–thyroid axis must be intact, with appropriate positive and negative control via feedback loops. (**Fig. 11.2**) Alterations in the signaling peptides and hormones and their targets can lead to hypothyroidism. However, failure of the thyroid gland itself is the most common cause, accounting for up to 95% of cases. This is termed primary hypothyroidism, while the term secondary hypothyroidism is reserved for rare cases of either pituitary or hypothalamic insufficiency. Furthermore, thyroid failure may be severe or mild and the mild form is often confusingly referred to as 'subclinical' hypothyroidism.

Overview of causes of hypothyroidism

The causes of primary hypothyroidism are summarized in **Table 11.2**. Worldwide, the most common cause of hypothyroidism is iodine deficiency, which remains an international problem in large areas of Africa and Asia. In iodine-sufficient areas such as much of Europe and the USA, the most common cause of thyroid failure, which affects 2–10% of the population, is autoimmune thyroid disease.

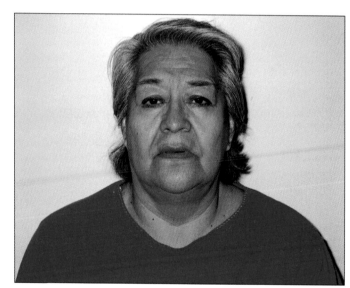

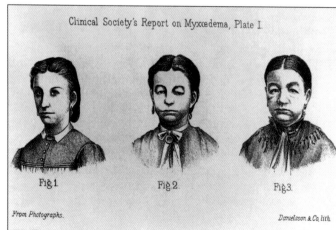

Figure 11.1 Clinical appearance of myxedema. (a) Myxedematous face of a 58-year-old female. (b) Change in the appearance of an untreated hypothyroid female over an 11-year period. (From Ord DR. Clinical Society of London Report on Myxoedema. Medico-Chirurgical Transactions 1888:1:xi.)

	Definition of hypothyroidism		
	Common		Rare
Variable	Primary		Secondary
	Clinical	Subclinical (mild)	
Symptoms	Present	Absent or mild	Present
TSH	++	+	Inappropriately low or normal
Free T₄ or T₄/TBG	Low	Normal	Low

Table 11.1 Definition of hypothyroidism. T_4, thyroxine; TBG, thyroxine-binding globulin; +, increased.

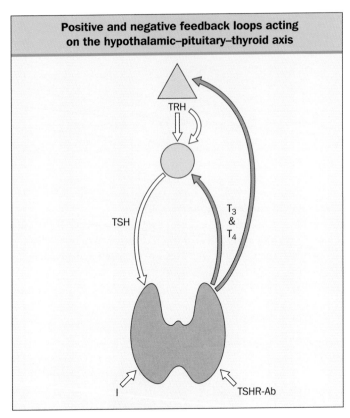

Positive and negative feedback loops acting on the hypothalamic–pituitary–thyroid axis

Figure 11.2 Positive and negative feedback loops acting on the hypothalamic–pituitary–thyroid axis. I, iodine; T$_3$, triiodothyronine; T$_4$, thyroxine; TRH, thyrotropin-releasing hormone; TSH, thyroid-stimulating hormone (thyrotropin); TSHR-Ab, antibodies to the thyroid-stimulating hormone receptor. (Modified from Hall R, Smith BR, Mukhtar ED. Thyroid stimulators in health and disease. Clin Endocrinol (Oxf). 1975;4:213–30, with permission from Blackwell Science Ltd.)

Causes of hypothyroidism

Causes of primary hypothyroidism.		
Congenital	Athyreosis	
	Dyshormonogenesis	
	Thyroid hormone resistance	
	TSH-receptor defect	
Acquired	Iodine deficiency	
	Autoimmune thyroid disease	
	Iatrogenic	Post-thyroidectomy
		Radioactive iodine treatment
		Thyroid irradiation
		Medications/goitrogens
Transient	Subacute thyroiditis (de Quervain's)	
	Silent thyroiditis	
	Post-partum thyroiditis (Hashimoto's)	
	Transient neonatal hypothyroidism	
Causes of secondary hypothyroidism		
Pituitary	Tumor	
	Infectious disease	
	Infiltrating disease	
	Vascular insufficiency	
	Empty sella syndrome	
	Iatrogenic	
Hypothalamic	Tumor	
	Infectious disease	
	Infiltrating disease	
	TRH deficiency	
	Iatrogenic	

Table 11.2 Causes of hypothyroidism. TSH, thyroid-stimulating hormone.

CAUSES

Congenital hypothyroidism

In iodine-sufficient regions of the world, congenital hypothyroidism occurs in approximately 1 in 4000 births and is one of the most common causes of preventable mental retardation. Up to 85% of congenital primary hypothyroidism is sporadic, while less than 15% is familial. The prevalence of secondary hypothyroidism in the newborn ranges between 1:25,000 and 1:100,000 and only rarely is this an isolated defect. Thus most programs screen for primary hypothyroidism by checking thyroxine (T$_4$) levels postpartum, which is cheap, with subsequent TSH assays only in those with a T$_4$ level below the 10th percentile. This screening is currently mandatory in the USA, Canada, Europe, Japan, and Australia.

The most common sporadic cause of congenital primary hypothyroidism is thyroid dysgenesis, either athyreosis or associated with an ectopically located thyroid. This happens when there is developmental failure of the thyroid gland resulting in either the complete absence of the gland or a small ectopic gland that is unable to produce sufficient thyroid hormone. The causes of thyroid dysgenesis are unknown. However, there are differences in the prevalence among various ethnic groups. In the USA, Latinos are most affected, followed by Whites, while African Americans are the least affected. There is also a 2:1 female preponderance, which is unexplained. These observations have led investigators to suspect a genetic contribution to the development of thyroid dysgenesis.

The most common hereditary causes of hypothyroidism are inborn errors of thyroxine synthesis. They account for approximately 10% of all cases of congenital hypothyroidism. Hereditary defects have been found in many different steps of thyroid hormone synthesis, secretion, and action. In addition, sodium/iodide symporter mutations, mutations in the enzyme thyroid peroxidase (TPO), thyroglobulin gene mutations, deiodinase defects, and even thyroid-stimulating hormone (TSH) receptor mutations have all been observed.

Acquired hypothyroidism

Acquired primary hypothyroidism can be viewed as any mechanism that renders the thyroid gland unable to produce adequate amounts of thyroid hormone. Lack of substrate, such as iodine deficiency, lack of sufficient thyroid tissue, such as after surgery, and destruction via autoimmune attack, external irradiation, and radioactive iodine are all well-recognized causes **(Figs 11.3 & 11.4)**.

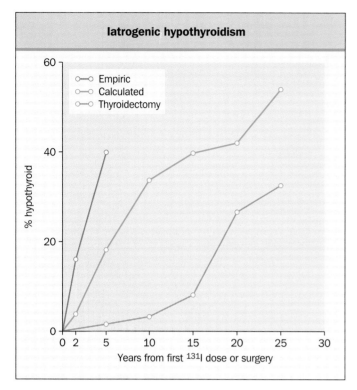

Figure 11.3 Iatrogenic hypothyroidism. Risk of hypothyroidism over time after radioactive iodine given by empiric dose (red) or calculated dose (green), and after sub-total thyroidectomy (blue). (Modified from Franklyn JA, et al. Long-term follow-up of treatment of thyrotoxicosis by three different methods. Clin Endocrinol (Oxf). 1991;34:71–76, with permission from Blackwell Science Ltd.)

Iodine deficiency

Iodine deficiency remains common in many parts of the world. The sea remains one of earth's main iodine reserves and foods from the sea are rich in iodine. In contrast, fresh water and soil vary greatly in iodine content depending upon location. Years of

Excretion in iodine deficiency

Iodine deficient state	Urinary iodine excretion (µg/L)
Normal	100–200
Mild	50–99
Moderate	20–49
Severe	<20

Table 11.3 Excretion in iodine deficiency.

rain and floods can leach iodine from the soil and water and foods grown in such areas are low in iodine. People in such areas become iodine-deficient unless their food is imported or iodine is supplemented. This problem is particularly pronounced in mountainous regions of the world such as the Andes and Himalayas, and the World Health Organization has an active program to promote iodine supplementation. However, a recent World Health Organization estimate places over 1.6 billion people still at risk for iodine deficiency in the world.

The average thyroid gland needs to trap 60µg of iodine per day to maintain normal function, and urinary iodine excretion is 100–200µg/L (**Table 11.3**). Depending on the degree, the manifestations of iodine deficiency can be highly variable. It may manifest as a simple goiter, with maintenance of euthyroidism by TSH-induced compensatory hyperplasia of the gland, or hypothyroidism may ensue when the thyroid gland is no longer able to compensate for the deficiency. In areas of severe iodine deficiency, mental retardation and delays in growth and development can be seen in children as a result of their own nutritional deficiency as well as the endemic cretinism that occurs in infants born to mothers with severe iodine deficiency.

There seem to be two distinct, although not mutually exclusive, forms of cretinism. Neurologic and myxedematous cretinism differ in their clinical presentation as well as the presence or absence of hypothyroidism in the infant. Neurologic cretinism

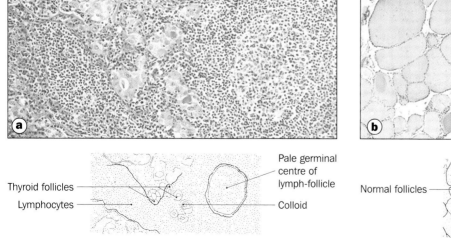

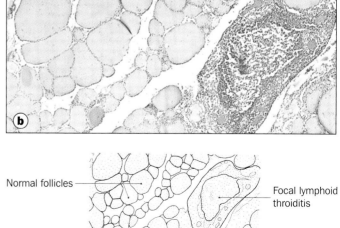

Figure 11.4 Autoimmune thyroid disease. (a) Histologic appearance of the thyroid in a patient with Hashimoto's thyroiditis. The parenchyma (compromising colloid-containing follicles) is almost totally replaced by oxyphil cells (Ashkenazy cell change). On the right of the field, a lymph follicle containing a large, pale, germinal center can be seen. Hematoxylin–eosin stain. (b) Focal lymphoid thyroiditis. In this condition, most of the thyroid follicles are normal but focal lymphoid infiltration is seen. The lymphocytes lie separately in a diffuse mass.

manifests with severe sensorimotor defects and mental retardation not associated with neonatal hypothyroidism. Myxedematous cretinism manifests with severe stunted growth and psychomotor retardation. The exact mechanism of the development of cretinism is unknown. Why some develop neurologic cretinism and some develop myxedematous cretinism is also unclear. Dietary differences have been implicated but not proved. Nevertheless, both forms of cretinism have been successfully treated in populations supplemented with iodine. Iodine supplementation via pills or injections has proved to be a cheap and effective measure in preventing these diseases in many studies throughout the world.

Chronic autoimmune thyroiditis

Autoimmune thyroid disease (AITD), in iodine-sufficient countries, is the most common cause of chronic hypothyroidism. Like other autoimmune diseases, these diseases are much more common in females. Across all ages, females generally have five to 10 times more autoimmune thyroid disease than males. AITD develops in a variety of forms, ranging from autoimmune destruction of the gland (Hashimoto's disease) to thyroid hyperfunction, which is seen in Graves' disease along with many extrathyroidal manifestations including eye disease (Graves' ophthalmopathy) and skin involvement (localized or pretibial myxedema). Indeed, hypothyroidism may be the endpoint of both Hashimoto's and Graves' diseases. In addition, both eye disease and skin disease are occasionally seen with Hashimoto's disease in the absence of any history of hyperthyroidism (**Fig. 11.5**).

Autoimmune thyroiditis (Hashimoto's disease) is associated with the presence of increased titers of autoantibodies to the enzyme thyroid peroxidase and to thyroglobulin (**Table 11.4**). Some 10–15% of patients also have detectable antibodies to the TSH receptor. Thyroid peroxidase antibodies, and less commonly thyroglobulin antibodies, may fix complement and effect thyroid-cell killing by lysis. TSH-receptor antibodies may act as TSH antagonists and may contribute to thyroid cell blockade. However, thyroid-antigen-specific T cells appear to be the main event in AITD, with widespread thyroid cell apoptosis causing Hashimoto's thyroiditis. Indeed, the degree of cell death may be so great that sufficient thyroid hormones are released to cause a transient hyperthyroidism. Hence, patients may present with a characteristically firm, goitrous form of the disease with massive lymphocytic infiltration (as originally described by Hashimoto) or,

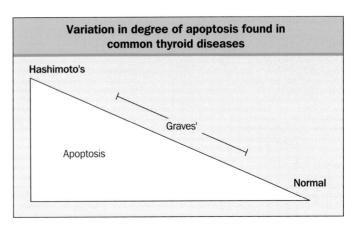

Figure 11.5 Variation in degree of apoptosis found in common thyroid diseases. (Modified from Palazzo FF, et al. Death of the autoimmune thyrocyte: is it pushed or does it jump. Thyroid 2000;10:561–72, with permission from Mary Ann Liebert, Inc.)

following widespread cell destruction, they may have an atrophic form with no thyroid to feel.

Some risk factors for autoimmune thyroiditis

The risk of developing overt hypothyroidism is dependent on many factors, including age, sex, pregnancy, stress, degree of TSH elevation, and the presence of thyroid autoantibodies. Females have a five- to 10-fold higher incidence of hypothyroidism than males and this difference becomes exaggerated with age. The degree of TSH elevation at presentation and the presence of thyroid autoantibodies are independent risk factors and when present together more than double the risk of developing overt hypothyroidism (**Table 11.5**). In fact, having both these risk factors gives a person a 4–5% annual incidence of developing overt hypothyroidism.

Transient hypothyroidism

Thyroiditis is the main cause of transient hypothyroidism. Thyroiditis is a general term referring to inflammation of the thyroid and thyroid cell destruction, usually due to apoptosis. There are many different causes, including infection, autoimmunity, and trauma. Infections usually cause transient hypothyroidism but some permanent hypothyroidism can ensue depending on the degree of thyroid damage.

Table 11.4 Classification of thyroiditis.
ESR, erythrocyte sedimentation rate.

Classification of thyroiditis

	Etiology	Pain	ESR	Thyroid antibodies	% resolved at 1 year
Acute	Bacterial, fungal	++++	High	–	100
Subacute	Viral	+++	High	–	95
Postpartum	Autoimmune	–	Normal, or may be increased	+++	80
Chronic	Autoimmune	–	Normal, or may be increased	+++	0

Epidemiology of hypothyroidism (from the Whickham survey)		Women	Men
Prevalence (per 1000 persons)	Overt hypothyroidism	18	1
	Elevated TSH (>6mU/L)	75	28
	Thyroid autoantibodies*	133	36
Incidence (per 1000 person/year)	Spontaneous overt hypothyroidism	3.5	0.6
Risk of overt hypothyroidism (over 19 years from baseline risk)	Elevated TSH	8-fold	44-fold
	Thyroid autoantibodies*	8-fold	25-fold
	Elevated TSH + thyroid autoantibodies*	38-fold	173-fold

* Thyroid peroxidase and/or thyroglobulin antibody positivity, depending on assay technique.

Table 11.5 Epidemiology of hypothyroidism (from the Whickham survey). TSH, thyroid-stimulating hormone

Acute thyroiditis

Acute painful thyroiditis is caused by a bacterial or fungal infection, usually from bacteremia or local infection that has extended into the thyroid bed. The patients are usually toxic and treatment is aimed at treating the underlying infection. Broad-spectrum antibiotics and drainage of any collection are indicated.

Subacute (de Quervain's) thyroiditis

Subacute thyroiditis is thought to be caused by viral infection. Many different viruses have been associated in case reports, including Coxsackie and mumps virus. However, no single agent has been consistently implicated. In clinical practice, patients can usually recall a recent viral infection with flu-like symptoms that preceded the thyroid complaints. Interestingly, beyond the environmental factors, there seems to be an additional genetic predisposition for subacute thyroiditis. The majority of sufferers are women and it has been estimated that more than 80% are human lymphocyte antigen (HLA)-Bw35-positive. Hence, once again there are environmental triggers that induce disease in a susceptible host.

The course of subacute thyroiditis is predictable, although not all phases may be clinically apparent. There are four recognized stages.

- **Stage 1** is the actual inflammation and destruction of the thyroid follicular cells causing pain and tenderness. This results in the outpouring of preformed hormones from the gland and the patient may be thyrotoxic. The degree of thyrotoxicosis is usually mild to moderate although it is highly variable. The apoptosed thyroid cells are unable to take up and concentrate iodine and thus radioiodine uptake is usually suppressed to less than 5%. This phase may last between 1 and 3 months.
- **Stage 2** is a euthyroid phase, which is often short-lived, lasting between 1 and 2 weeks. This phase results from the clearing of the high levels of T_4 from the body once the massive cell destruction has slowed.
- **Stage 3** is the hypothyroid phase, in which follicular cells begin to recover and regenerate but are unable to produce adequate amounts of thyroxine. This can last up to several months and treatment with thyroxine may be indicated. Occasionally, this phase may be clinically silent, particularly if the thyroid damage has been minimal. Thus stage 1 or the

hyperthyroid phase may be the only clinical manifestations in some patients.
- **Stage 4.** Finally, complete recovery is the rule in subacute thyroiditis and Stage 4 represents permanent euthyroidism. More than 95% of all patients regain normal thyroid function, with a minority requiring some thyroxine supplementation after 1 year.

Subacute thyroiditis can be suspected with a history of recent upper respiratory infections or flu-like symptoms and with a very painful thyroid upon examination. Radioiodine uptake is classically less than 1% and other helpful findings are an elevated erythrocyte sedimentation rate and elevated serum thyroglobulin. Thyroid autoantibodies are generally negative or at low titer but can be transiently positive or increased in some patients. Radioiodine or technetium uptake may be valuable in differentiating thyroiditis from Graves' disease in the hyperthyroid phase. Histopathology shows granulomatous changes with giant cells, although a biopsy is rarely indicated.

Treatment is aimed at controlling the symptoms. Beta-blockers can be used to ameliorate the adrenergic symptoms during the hyperthyroid phase but therapy with antithyroid medications or radioactive iodine ablation is contraindicated. Nonsteroidal antiinflammatory drugs and glucocorticoids in severe cases can help relieve pain. Thyroxine replacement may be indicated in patients with symptomatic or severe hypothyroidism but the clinician should anticipate recovery in most patients and attempt tapering of the dose.

Postpartum thyroiditis

Postpartum thyroiditis is a variant of autoimmune thyroiditis. As the immunosuppressive state of pregnancy ends with delivery of the fetus, exacerbation of autoimmune thyroid disease is commonly seen in the postpartum period. Painless postpartum thyroiditis occurs in 5–9% of unselected women and in up to 50% of women with positive thyroid antibodies. The clinical stages are similar to those of subacute thyroiditis but complete resolution does not occur in all patients.

The hyperthyroid stage occurs 2–4 months postpartum and may be the only presentation in up to 40% of all women. Although hyperthyroidism is usually mild, because it is normally painless it must be distinguished from Graves' disease (which also tends to exacerbate, recur, or present for the first time in the postpartum period). The distinction is important as treatment and long-term prognosis differ. The hypothyroid phase follows a short euthyroid phase and may be the initial presentation in up to 35% of postpartum patients. Although much talked about, fewer than 25% of patients with postpartum thyroiditis present with both hyper- and hypothyroid phases.

Thyroid antibodies are invariably present in postpartum thyroiditis. The erythrocyte sedimentation rate is normal and permanent hypothyroidism is not uncommon. Up to 20% of patients require thyroxine supplementation at 3 years and 50% at 7–9 years.

Painless (silent) thyroiditis

The complex nomenclature used in thyroiditis has made this entity confusing for many clinicians. Painless (or silent) thyroiditis refers to thyroiditis without pain. The term does not infer a cause. The etiology may be a rare painless presentation of subacute thyroiditis or, more probably, a transient variant of autoimmune thyroiditis, i.e. Hashimoto's. This variant is different from the typical Hashimoto's disease presentation in that it may completely resolve.

Transient congenital hypothyroidism

This is another, although uncommon, cause of transient hypothyroidism. This accounts for approximately 5% of cases of congenital hypothyroidism. Infants born to mothers with autoimmune thyroid disease are at risk but only in the presence of high titers of TSH-receptor-blocking antibodies. Pathophysiologically, there is blocking of the infant's TSH receptor by maternal IgG antibodies that have crossed the placenta. The hypothyroid phase lasts until the newborn is able to clear the blocking immunoglobulins; typically between 3 and 6 months. The pediatrician should be made aware of the mother's autoimmune thyroid disease at the time of delivery and careful followup of the newborn's thyroid function is warranted. Treatment, if indicated, should be prompt and aggressive. All pregnant women with AITD or a history of AITD should have their serum checked for TSH-receptor antibodies.

DIAGNOSIS

Because primary hypothyroidism is so much more common than other causes, the measurement of an increased serum concentration of thyrotropin should always be the first laboratory value obtained when hypothyroidism is suspected. The combination of an elevated TSH and low total or free thyroxine level is diagnostic. Triiodothyronine (T_3) has no role in the assessment of hypothyroidism since it is often normal and may be decreased by many other factors. Anyone with secondary hypothyroidism would have a reduced T_4 measurement in the presence of a low or normal TSH. TSH by itself is insufficient in evaluating central disease as an intact feedback loop cannot be assumed.

The diagnosis of hypothyroidism, especially that of primary hypothyroidism, is straightforward with the availability of today's sensitive third-generation TSH assays. Eliciting the cause of hypothyroidism can be more challenging. A careful history can be invaluable. Any history of radiation exposure, surgery to the neck, radioactive iodine therapy, recent viral illness, recent pregnancy,

Examples of drugs that cause hypothyroidism

Thiourea (propylthiouracil and methimazole)

Lithium

Iodine-containing drugs/agents (amiodarone/iv radiological contrast media)

Alpha-interferon and other cytokines

Table 11.6 Examples of drugs that cause hypothyroidism

Signs and symptoms of hypothyroidism

Symptoms	Signs
Weakness	Lethargy
Voice change	Hoarseness
Weight gain	Slow speech
Edema	Periorbital edema
Myalgia	Dry, flaky skin
Cold intolerance	Alopecia
Constipation	Bradycardia
Dry skin	Effusions
Hair loss	Delayed relaxation of deep tendon reflexes
Menorrhagia	
Depression	
Impaired memory	

Table 11.7 Signs and symptoms of hypothyroidism.

medications, or unusual diet can be uncovered (**Table 11.6**) The presence of other autoimmune diseases in the patient or a family member is pertinent history that should not be missed. The physical examination can reveal the presence or the absence of a goiter. If present, the characteristics of the goiter in terms of its size, diffuseness, consistency, and pain can be helpful in elucidating the etiology. Finally, the next test is for the presence of thyroid antibodies. Having thyroglobulin antibodies and/or thyroperoxidase antibodies suggests autoimmune thyroid disease, particularly if the levels are high.

There is rarely any role for radiologic studies or tissue biopsies in the evaluation of hypothyroidism. However, ultrasonography can be helpful in gathering additional data such as size, echogenicity, presence or absence of nodules.

CLINICAL MANIFESTATIONS

The symptoms of hypothyroidism can be subtle or flagrant. (**Table 11.7**) The lack of specificity in the symptoms of hypothyroidism may be difficult to differentiate from many other conditions.

Skin and appendages

The classic description of 'myxedematous' or 'nonpitting edema' is caused by the accumulation of mucopolysaccharides and thickening of the dermal layer. There is enlargement of the tongue and laryngeal soft tissue, leading to the change in voice. There is decreased sebaceous and sweat-gland secretion, leading to dry skin and dry hair. Hair and nail growth is slow and is of dry or brittle quality.

Cardiovascular

There is decreased inotropic and chronotropic drive with the lack of thyroid hormone effects on the heart. Decreased overall cardiac output and bradycardia can be observed. Initially, there is decreased oxygen demand from the peripheral tissues of the hypothyroid individual and the oxygen supply can be matched by the compromised cardiovascular system when at rest. However, upon exercise or other stress factors requiring more oxygen delivery, cardiac performance is likely to be inadequate to meet the metabolic needs. Chronic severe hypothyroidism can lead to cardiomegaly with decreased ventricular function. An electrocardiogram usually shows bradycardia and low voltage as a result of pericardial effusion. Serum creatine kinase can be significantly elevated. Cholesterol, including both low-density and high-density lipoprotein, has been classically shown to be elevated in hypothyroid patients.

Pulmonary

A decrease in the ventilatory drive, as well as changes in the respiratory muscles, may lead to hypercapnia and hypoxemia. Exudative pleural effusions also can be present in severe hypothyroidism.

Renal

Decreased renal blood flow and glomerular filtration rate contribute to delayed and overall decreased water excretion, which can manifest as mild hyponatremia.

Gastrointestinal

Delayed peristalsis and bowel-wall thickening lead to distention and constipation. In persons with autoimmune hypothyroidism, autoimmune pernicious anemia can coexist in up to 10% of patients. This can lead to vitamin B_{12} deficiency, which may exacerbate the neurologic features.

Musculoskeletal

Lack of thyroid hormone effects on the skeletal system during normal growth can lead to delayed and abnormal epiphyseal ossification, especially at the hip, and impaired linear growth. As measured by bone markers, there seems to be decreased bone turnover. Hypothyroidism also affects growth by decreasing levels of the effector hormone of growth hormone, insulin-like growth factor (IGF)-1. Inflammation and infiltration of the muscle tissue can cause diffuse myalgias.

Neuropsychiatric

Lack of thyroid hormone during neurologic development leads to decreased cerebral perfusion, myelination, and cortical development (see congenital hypothyroidism, above). In the adult population all aspects of cognitive as well as psychomotor function are retarded. Lack of concentration and memory is common. In addition, peripheral nerves can be infiltrated with glycosaminoglycans, leading to edema and delayed conduction. There is typically a delay in the relaxation phase of tendon reflexes, which is characteristic. Depression and lack of drive and motivation are common. The carpal tunnel syndrome is a common feature and is often a feature at presentation.

Reproductive

In children, lack of thyroid hormone can lead to delayed puberty. In adults, the most common menstrual disturbance is oligomenorrhea and menorrhagia. In severe cases, decreased ovulation and reduced fertility has been observed. Hypothyroidism in men may cause oligospermia and erectile dysfunction. Reversible hyperprolactinemia may result from the thyroxine deficiency.

SUBCLINICAL HYPOTHYROIDISM

In multiple population-based studies, the most common thyroid function abnormality found is subclinical or mild hypothyroidism. The prevalence in the general population ranges between 7% and 11% among women and from 2–3% among men. This figure dramatically increases with age, with a prevalence above 17% in women over the age of 65. Besides being at risk for the development of overt hypothyroidism, the long-term consequence of subclinical hypothyroidism is now better defined and involves hypercholesterolemia and decreased cardiac function. However, to date, there have been no large randomized prospective trials demonstrating that thyroxine replacement in subclinical hypothyroidism decreases morbidity and mortality. The few blinded studies in which subjects with subclinical hypothyroidism were treated reported that they felt improved with thyroxine rather than placebo and there was an improvement in a variety of cardiac parameters (Table 11.8).

Effects of subclinical (mild) hypothyroidism as compared to normal subjects			
	Subclinical		Subclinical after treatment
Serum cholesterol	Increased		Improved*
Vital capacity	Reduced		Improved
	At rest	Exercise	
Left ventricular ejection fraction†	Normal	reduced	Improved

* Not yet evidence-based.
† Levels of thyroid-stimulating hormone above 10 in most studies.

Table 11.8 Effects of subclinical (mild) hypothyroidism as compared to normal subjects.

These trial subjects had TSH levels above 10μU/L but those patients in the 5–10μU/L range have not been studied extensively. However, it has been shown that the higher the TSH, the more likely the patient is to progress to overt hypothyroidism.

Most interest has been generated in terms of cardiovascular consequence of mild hypothyroidism. In recent years, there have been epidemiologic data and small studies that associated lower cardiac performance and higher lipid levels in persons with mild hypothyroidism and a clear linear relationship between total serum cholesterol and TSH. It is accepted that overt hypothyroidism is a risk for hypercholesterolemia but recent surveys have demonstrated that subjects with subclinical hypothyroidism also have higher cholesterol than those with normal TSH levels.

There is no 'Wilson's syndrome', which has been erroneously defined as low body temperature and multiple other nonspecific symptoms with normal thyroid function tests. Proponents advocate treatment with T_3. This is not a disease nor an entity warranting treatment because diagnosis of thyroid function by body temperature is unreliable. T_3 prescriptions may be inconsistent with normal physiology and pose potential danger to patients with heart disease. Only anecdotal reports exist to support this treatment. (Note: the 'Wilson's syndrome' website is a fee-for-service site, see www.thyroid.org/annonc.wilson.htm.)

DIFFERENTIAL DIAGNOSIS

The differential diagnosis of the symptoms of hypothyroidism can be multiple. However, after finding low T_4 and an elevated TSH in a patient there can very little doubt as to the diagnosis. Two entities commonly encountered in the hospital, although not in the outpatient setting, can be confused with true thyroid disease. The clinical presentation of depression can be similar to hypothyroidism and an acute episode can affect the thyroid axis in many ways. Classically, there is a blunted TSH response to TRH stimulation. Furthermore, a transient decrease in T_4 levels may be seen. In patients with severe medical illness, abnormal thyroid function tests can be commonly confused with hypothyroidism. In acute illness, T_4 may be depressed, followed by elevation of TSH when the patient begins to recover. In both these cases, unless the degree of thyroid test abnormalities is severe, it is best to retest the patient when he or she is clinically improved.

TREATMENT

Treatment of hypothyroidism is safe and efficient with synthetic thyroxine (**Table 11.9**). The goal of replacement should be to normalize the TSH, although this can take many months in patients with long-standing hypothyroidism. The severity and duration of hypothyroidism as well as the age and medical condition of the patient should be assessed upon the initiation of replacement. The starting dose of thyroxine can be full if hypothyroidism is sudden, i.e. after total thyroidectomy, or gradually increased. In most adults, it is prudent to start at 75–100μg per day and adjust gradually by monitoring TSH. Lower doses such as 50–75μg per day can be used when treating subclinical or mild hypothyroidism or the elderly. Although thyroid hormone need is dependent on weight, justifying the common method of estimating requirements (1.6μg/kg/day), 80–90% of adults are euthyroid on a daily dose between 100μg and 200μg (**Fig. 11.6**).

If secondary hypothyroidism is suspected, a full pituitary workup is indicated. Particular attention must be paid to the adrenal status of the patient before initiating thyroxine replacement because increased metabolism caused by thyroid hormones can precipitate an adrenal crisis in an adrenally insufficient patient. If the patient is adrenally insufficient, glucocorticoids must be replaced prior to thyroxine therapy.

There are some conditions that may increase or decrease requirements. One important state is pregnancy. In addition, growing infants and children may have different dose requirements (**Table 11.10**). Decreased absorption, caused either by intrinsic bowel pathology or by medications such as bile acid resins or iron, can also lead to increased dose requirements. Anticonvulsant medication such as phenytoin and phenobarbital can also increase T_4 and T_3 metabolism, requiring increased dose also.

Controversies in T_4 replacement
Subclinical hypothyroidism
Treatment of subclinical hypothyroidism in the elderly or cardiac patients is unclear. On one hand, evidence points to lower cholesterol and improved cardiac function in patients with normal TSH and the rate of conversion from subclinical to overt hypothyroidism is higher in the elderly as compared to the general population. But on the other hand, in a minority of patients with ischemic heart disease there is a risk of worsening angina and/or arrhythmias with T_4 treatment. Therefore, the risks and the benefit of treatment in these patients should be individualized.

Different commercial brands
There is a variety of commercially available preparations of thyroxine and controversy regarding the dose accuracy among the different brands exists. For example, whether 100μg of T_4 from one brand equals 100μg from another is a frequently asked question among clinicians. What is recognized is that, within the same brand, the doses are consistent and reliable. Therefore,

Thyroid hormone replacement in hypothyroidism		
Oral compounds	Half life	Indication
Thyroxine (T_4)	6–7 days	Hypothyroidism or subclinical hypothyroidism
Triiodothyronine (T_3)	1–2 days	None
Combination ($T_4 + T_3$)		Patients dissatisfied with thyroxine alone
Desiccated thyroid ($T_4 + T_3$)		None
Thyroglobulin	2–3 days	None

Table 11.9 Thyroid hormone replacement in hypothyroidism.

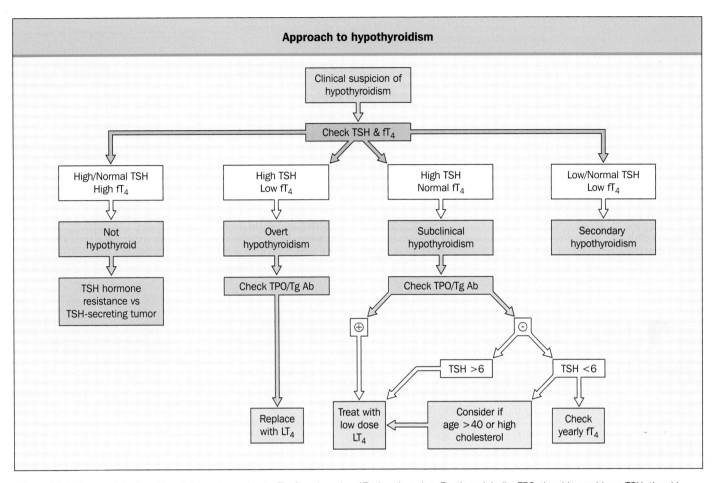

Figure 11.6 Approach to hypothyroidism. Ab, antibody; fT$_4$, free thyroxine; LT$_4$, levothyroxine; Tg, thyroglobulin; TPO, thyroid peroxidase; TSH, thyroid-stimulating hormone.

Special cases in thyroxine replacement	
Newborn	Aggressive and prompt replacement should be instituted as soon as possible. Goal is to achieve normal T$_4$ as soon as possible and a starting dose of 10–15µg/kg of thyroxine has been shown to safely achieve this in about 1 week. T$_4$ should be monitored every 2 weeks for the first few months and then monthly. Inadequate dosage and delayed initiation of replacement have been shown to have long-term consequences, with delayed development and low IQ scores.
Pregnancy	Pregnant women with hypothyroidism should have aggressive T$_4$ replacement. Increased requirements should be anticipated and T$_4$ doses should be raised before TSH levels starts to rise. The average dose requirement is 50–60% increase from baseline. Monitoring with free T$_4$ and TSH (as increased thyroxine-binding globulin of pregnancy can mislead total T$_4$ values) should be carried out every 2–3 months. It has long been known that hypothyroidism during pregnancy can cause malformations, growth retardation, and neurologic deficits. However, a recent study has associated lower IQ scores of children born to mothers with even mildly elevated TSH levels.
Elderly/cardiac disease	Thyroxine should be replaced slowly in hypothyroid elderly and cardiac patients. Starting dose should be 25µg per day, titrated to full dose over a few months. Signs and symptoms of cardiac decompensation should be monitored carefully.
Myxedema coma	Although rare these days, myxedema coma is one of the few indications for intravenous thyroxine. Patient suspected with myxedema coma should have blood taken for cortisol, TSH, and thyroxine measurement and should then be treated empirically for adrenal insufficiency and hypothyroidism. Giving thyroxine to adrenally insufficient patients can elicit an adrenal crisis. They should be given hydrocortisone 100mg iv every 8 hours and thyroxine 200–300µg, followed by 100µg daily. Steroids can be tapered over the next few days.

Table 11.10 Special cases in thyroxine replacement. T$_3$, triiodothyronine; T$_4$, thyroxine; TSH, thyroid-stimulating hormone.

it is our recommendation and that of the American Thyroid Association that a patient is loyal to one brand, regardless of which, and is monitored by TSH if there is a switch in preparation.

T_3 use

The accepted thyroid hormone for replacement is T_4. Taking advantage of its long half-life and the additional regulated step of peripheral conversion to T_3, the biologically active hormone, makes this a safe and effective drug. However, it is known that, normally, around 10% of the hormone produced by the thyroid is T_3. Thus not all of the T_3 circulating is from peripheral conversion. Furthermore, there are recent data showing that giving T_3 to hypothyroid patients in conjunction with T_4 not only made them feel better but also enabled them to perform better in standardized tests of psychomotor abilities, memory, and concentration. Because information such as long-term safety issues, the correct ratio of T_3 and T_4, and morbidity and mortality differences comparing T_4 alone to T_3 and T_4 are unavailable, it is premature to accept T_3 use as a standard. More studies are awaited.

Triiodothyronine has also been shown, mostly in psychiatric literature, to be beneficial in hastening recovery time and improving efficacy of antidepressant medications in patients with major depression. However, most of these studies were performed with older antidepressants (tricyclics) that are no longer used as first-line therapy. Furthermore, most studies did not elucidate the thyroid status of the patients. There are few studies with serotonin reuptake inhibitors and it is therefore difficult to advocate T_3 use in patients with major depression at this time.

COMPLICATIONS

Depending on when during life a patient is hypothyroid, clinical outcomes vary. The degree of deficit seems to correlate with the degree of hypothyroidism at all stages. Severe hypothyroidism during gestation can lead to malformations, growth retardation and neurologic deficits, which are usually irreversible. During infancy and early childhood, hypothyroidism can result in decreased linear growth and inadequate brain maturation, leading to low IQ performance and psychomotor development (**Table 11.10**). Fully developed adults usually manifest with classic hypothyroid symptoms that usually reverse with treatment.

Myxedema coma

Hypothyroidism can cause death from myxedema coma. Susceptible patients are those with longstanding, severe hypothyroidism who face a precipitating factor such as infection, a cardiovascular event, or overmedication with sedating agents, usually phenothiazines with their propensity to lower the already reduced body temperature. Two cardinal features are severe hypothermia (<80°F) and loss of consciousness. Diagnosis is imperative, as high doses of thyroid hormone can be dangerous. Severe illness can not only be clinically similar to myxedema coma but can alter thyroid function tests by lowering both TSH and T_4, thus confusing the picture. As with severe illness, lack of TSH elevation could also imply secondary hypothyroidism in the patient.

There are many protocols to treat myxedema coma. It is debated whether to use T_4 alone or T_3. Because T_3 has quicker onset and severe illness can inhibit the conversion of T_4 to T_3,

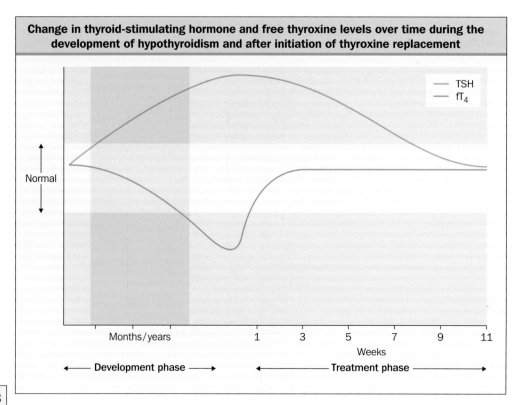

Change in thyroid-stimulating hormone and free thyroxine levels over time during the development of hypothyroidism and after initiation of thyroxine replacement

Figure 11.7 **Change in thyroid-stimulating hormone and free thyroxine levels over time during the development of hypothyroidism and after initiation of thyroxine replacement.** fT$_4$, free thyroxine; TSH, thyroid-stimulating hormone.

some have advocated the use of T_3 in conjunction with T_4. Regardless of therapy, this entity portends a mortality of more than 60% and supportive care in an intensive care unit as well as thyroid hormone and corticosteroid replacement is warranted.

CLINICAL OUTCOME

Treatment of hypothyroidism can be highly satisfying as patients respond quickly and completely. Synthetic thyroxine is safe and close monitoring is feasible with highly sensitive thyrotropin assays. Except for the severe hypothyroidism encountered during gestation and early childhood, most clinical manifestations of hypothyroidism are completely reversed with thyroxine replacement. In the past there has been overzealous thyroid replacement by clinicians driving TSH levels to below normal. This is disadvantageous, particularly with respect to osteoporosis in postmenopausal women and atrial fibrillation in the elderly. A normal TSH is the goal in primary hypothyroidism and normal T_4 is the goal in secondary hypothyroidism.

The clinical outcome of treating overt hypothyroidism is straightforward. However, there is emerging evidence that subclinical mild hypothyroidism may have negative health consequences. It remains to be seen whether treating this entity has long-term benefits, although the limited data thus far seems to suggest that it does. This question is an important one that needs to be answered as this is the most common thyroid function abnormality found in the general population and could have important implications for screening and healthcare policy (**Fig. 11.7**).

FURTHER READING

Arem R, Patsch W. Lipoprotein and apolipoprotein levels in subclinical hypothyroidism. Effects of levothyroxine therapy. Arch Intern Med. 1990;150:2097–100.

Bunevicius R, Kazanavicius G, Zalinkevicius, Prange AR. Effects of thyroxine as compared with thyroxine plus triiodothyronine in patients with hypothyroidism. N Engl J Med. 1999;340:424–9.

Canaris GJ, Manowitz NR, Mayor G, Ridgway C. The Colorado Thyroid Disease Prevalence Study. Arch Intern Med. 2000;160:526–33.

Davies TF, 1999 The thyroid immunology of the postpartum period. Thyroid 1999;9:675–84.

Cooper DS, Halpern R, Wood LC, Levin AA, Ridgeway EC. L-Thyroxine therapy in subclinical hypothyroidism. A double-blinded, placebo-controlled trial. Ann Intern Med. 1984;101:18–24.

Franklyn JA, Daykin J, Drolc Z, Farmer M, Sheppard MC. Long-term follow-up of treatment of thyrotoxicosis by three different methods. Clin Endocrinol. 1991;34:71–6.

Hak AE, Pols HAP, Visser TJ, Drexhage HA, Hofman A, Witteman JCAM. Subclinical hypothyroidism is an independent risk factor for atherosclerosis and myocardial infarction in elderly women: the Rotterdam Study. Ann Intern Med. 2000;132:270–8.

Jackson I. The thyroid axis and depression. Thyroid 1998;8:951–6.

Kahaley G. Cardiovascular and atherogenic aspects of subclinical hypothyroidism. Thyroid 2000;10:665–79.

LeFranchie S. Congenital hypothyroidism: etiologies, diagnosis and management. Thyroid 1999;9:735–40.

Palazzo FF, Hammond LJ, Mirakian R, Goode AW. Death of the auto-immune thyrocyte: is it pushed or does it jump? Thyroid 2000;10:567.

Ridgeway EC, Cooper DS, Walker H, Rodbard D, Maloof FM. Peripheral responses to thyroid hormone before and after L-thyroxine therapy in patients with subclinical hypothyroidism. J Clin Endocrinol Metab. 1981;53:1238–42.

Rovet JF. Congenital hypothyroidism: long-term outcome. Thyroid 1999;9:741–8.

Stagnaro-Green A. Recognizing, understanding and treating post-partum. thyroiditis. Endocrinol Metab Clin North Am. 2000;29: 417–30.

Surks MI, Sievert R. Drugs and thyroid function. N Engl J Med. 1995;333:1688–94.

Toft AD. Thyroxine therapy. N Engl J Med. 1994 331:174–80.

Vanderpump MPJ, Tunbridge WMG, French JM, et al. The incidence of thyroid disorders in the community: a 20-year follow-up of the Whickham Survey. Clin Endocrinol. 1995;43:55–68.

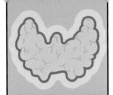

Chapter

12

Thyroid Nodular Disease and Carcinoma of the Thyroid

James A Fagin and Yancey R Holmes

INTRODUCTION

Clinically apparent thyroid nodules are present in about 4–7% of the general population. They are more common in women, and their prevalence increases with age. When sought for by high-resolution ultrasonography, unsuspected thyroid nodules are found in up to 44% of women and 20% of men. The frequency of nodularity is even higher in autopsy studies. Approximately 90% of solitary thyroid nodules are benign, and the clinical challenge is to identify those few that are caused by thyroid cancer.

Thyroid nodules may be the only abnormality in an otherwise normal gland. However, about half of seemingly solitary nodules prove to be the dominant lesion arising within a multinodular gland. In most cases multinodular goiters (MNG) first manifest as a diffuse thyroid enlargement, which then progresses to a multinodular stage through development of foci of autonomously growing and/or functioning cells. MNG may develop as a consequence of iodine deficiency (endemic MNG), which is now quite infrequent in Western industrialized countries, or as a sporadic abnormality in iodine-sufficient populations. Rarely, MNG may occur in families with genetic predisposition, or in individuals exposed to goitrogens. In most cases the cause of MNG is unknown, although it is believed that many patients may harbor subtle defects in thyroid hormone biosynthesis, resulting in compensatory thyroid-stimulating hormone (TSH)-driven thyroid hyperplasia. Of the nodules that develop later in the course of the disease, some are hyperplastic but many are clonal neoplasms. Most of the latter are benign adenomas and only a minority will prove to be thyroid cancers. In general, nodules within multinodular glands are less likely to be malignant than solitary lesions.

The incidence of papillary thyroid cancer has been increasing in industrialized nations (**Fig. 12.1**). The higher incidence can be

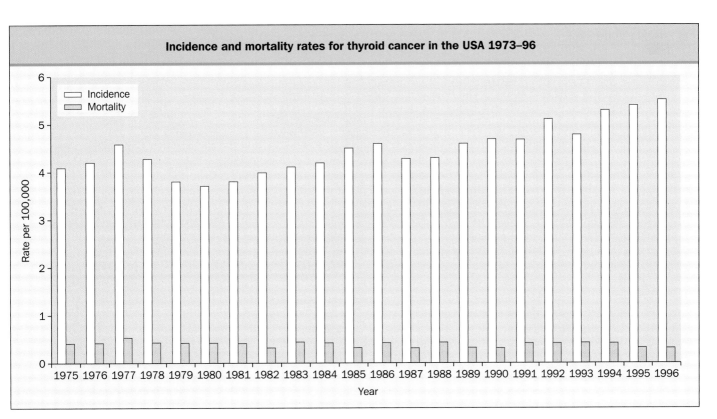

Figure 12.1 Incidence and mortality rates for thyroid cancer in the USA 1973–96 (Source: SEER Cancer Registry).

Classification of thyroid tumors
Tumors of follicular cells
Papillary carcinoma
Papillary microcarcinoma
Follicular variant
Diffuse sclerosing variant
Solid cell variant
Tall cell variant
Follicular neoplasms
Follicular adenoma
Follicular carcinoma
Oncocytic (Hurthle cell) neoplasms
Oncocytic adenoma
Oncocytic carcinoma
Poorly differentiated carcinoma
Undifferentiated (anaplastic) carcinoma
Tumors of parafollicular C-cells
Medullary thyroid carcinoma
Malignant lymphomas
Rare tumors
Sarcomas

Table 12.1 Classification of thyroid tumors.

attributed in part to earlier diagnosis. However, this alone does not account for the higher frequency of thyroid cancer. In the USA, administration of external radiation for benign conditions of the head and neck in children, a practice continued until the 1960s, may have played a role.

CLASSIFICATION AND PATHOLOGY OF THYROID TUMORS

More than 90% of thyroid neoplasms are primary tumors arising from follicular cells (**Table 12.1**). Papillary carcinomas are the most common form of thyroid malignancy (about 80%) in populations exposed to sufficient iodine in their diets. Various pathologic variants of papillary carcinomas have been described, which vary depending on the architecture of the tumor tissue but have in common the typical papillary cell with its characteristic nuclear morphology (**Fig. 12.2**). Cervical lymph node metastases are common. Although there is no well-established benign precursor for papillary carcinoma, recent molecular genetic studies indicate that papillary 'microcarcinomas' (lesions less than 1cm), which are found commonly in the general population, may represent early stages of the disease. Transition from microscopic to overt papillary carcinoma is likely to be a very low probability event. Follicular adenomas are benign, relatively common thyroid neoplasms. The majority of thyroid adenomas do not undergo malignant transformation, but when they do they give rise to follicular carcinomas, which represent between 5% and 10% of thyroid cancers (**Fig. 12.3**). The prevalence of follicular carcinoma is higher in iodine-deficient regions. Oncocytic or Hurthle cell adenomas and carcinomas are considered to be variants of follicular neoplasms, although this has recently been questioned based on molecular genetic data. Oncocytic cells are characterized by abundant, granular eosinophilic cytoplasm. Papillary, follicular and to a lesser extent oncocytic cell carcinomas usually retain

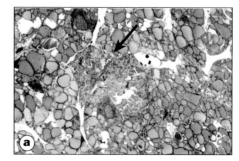

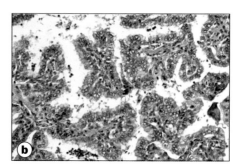

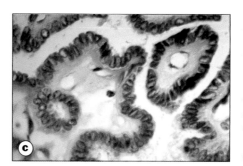

Figure 12.2 Papillary thyroid carcinoma. (a) Microscopic papillary carcinomas (arrow) are often incidental findings. Although they may represent a precursor lesion, further progression is very unusual. (b) Low-power magnification shows the typical architectural feature of papillary carcinoma, consisting of a single layer of overlapping epithelial cells surrounding a fibrovascular core. (c) At high power, the characteristic cellular appearance of papillary carcinoma cells is noted. Hypochromatic nuclei with a ground-glass appearance are typical. Nuclei often contain pseudoinclusions, and linear grooves giving a coffee-bean-like appearance. (Courtesy of Dr Paul Biddinger, University of Cincinnati.)

partial differentiation, including the ability to trap iodide, and synthesize thyroglobulin. By contrast, poorly differentiated and undifferentiated or anaplastic carcinomas are exceedingly rare, and lose all thyroid-specific function (**Fig. 12.4**). Cancers may also arise from other cell types within the thyroid. The most significant are medullary thyroid carcinomas (MTCs), which originate from parafollicular C cells and represent up to 10% of all thyroid malignancies. These are discussed in a separate section at the end of this chapter. Primary thyroid lymphomas and sarcomas are also exceedingly rare.

PATHOGENESIS OF THYROID NEOPLASMS

Exposure to ionizing radiation during childhood increases the relative risk for both benign thyroid nodules and thyroid papillary carcinomas. Risk of cancer is also increased in patients with a history of benign nodular disease. Most thyroid neoplasms derived from follicular cells are sporadic, although genetic predisposition may play a role in a minority of cases (**Table 12.2**). Thus, the genetic defects involved in follicular cell tumor initiation and progression are somatic (i.e. acquired after birth). Several of these have been identified and are associated with specific tumor phenotypes (**Fig. 12.5**).

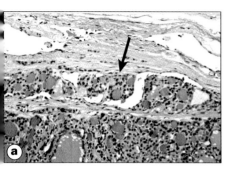

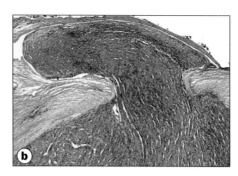

Figure 12.3 Follicular carcinoma. The distinction between follicular adenoma and carcinoma is based on the presence of either vascular invasion (a), or infiltration of the capsule (b).

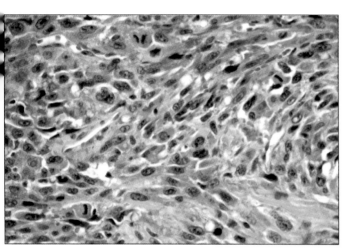

Figure 12.4 Undifferentiated or anaplastic carcinoma. These aggressive cancers usually result in total effacement of the gland. Giant, squamoid or sarcomatoid cells may be present, with pleomorphic nuclei and multinucleated cells.

CLINICAL MANIFESTATIONS

Thyroid nodules are usually asymptomatic and are discovered as a visible or palpable neck mass by the physician or patient. Few patients complain of dysphagia, hoarseness, or rapid tumor growth, symptoms that increase the likelihood of cancer. Pain is infrequent and suggests subacute thyroiditis or spontaneous bleeding into a preexisting nodule. The risk of cancer is higher in children, males, and older patients. Patients receiving external radiation during childhood for benign conditions such as thymic or tonsillar enlargement, acne, or tinea capitis are at greater risk for thyroid cancer. Although the practice of administering radiation for benign conditions has ceased, the risk persists several decades after exposure. Also at risk are patients treated with high doses of radiation for Hodgkin's disease, children exposed to internal radiation by radioiodines, such as those living in areas contaminated by fallout from the Chernobyl nuclear accident, and atomic bomb survivors. Radiation exposure is associated specifically with papillary thyroid carcinomas.

Nodules greater than 1.5cm can usually be palpated if they are located close to the surface of the gland. Most are of soft or firm consistency. Physical characteristics of the nodule are not usually helpful in differential diagnosis, as most cancers are found within lesions that are clinically indistinguishable from benign tumors. However, presence of a hard nodule, fixation to adjacent structures, vocal cord paralysis, and palpable enlargement of regional lymph nodes are highly suspicious of malignancy. Large nodules (>1.5cm) from multinodular goiters can be malignant and should be evaluated in the same manner as solitary nodules. Increasingly, thyroid nodules are discovered incidentally during carotid ultrasonography, neck computer tomography (CT), or magnetic resonance imaging (MRI) studies.

Inherited cancer syndromes associated with thyroid cancer		
Syndrome	Chromosomal localization	Gene
Familial adenomatous polyposis	5q21–22	APC
Cowden's syndrome	10q23.3	PTEN
Peutz–Jeghers syndrome?	19p13.3	STK11/LKB1
Ataxia–telangiectasia?	11q22–23	AT
Familial nonmedullary thyroid cancer		
PTC–RCC	1q21	?
PTC–oxyphilia	19p13.2	?
PTC–multinodular goiter	14q31	?
Familial clear-cell RCC–PTC	t(3;8)(p14.2;q24.1)	?

Table 12.2 Inherited cancer syndromes associated with thyroid cancer. Most papillary and follicular thyroid cancers are sporadic. However, thyroid cancers are more common in certain inherited cancer syndromes. Familial clusters of thyroid cancer have been noted and in several kindreds the genetic locus conferring susceptibility has been mapped. PTC, papillary thyroid cancer; RCC, renal cell carcinoma.

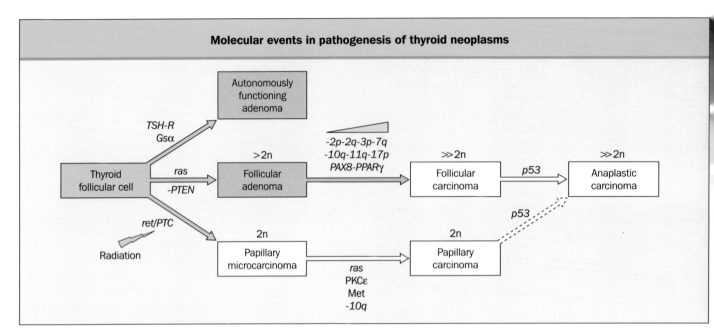

Molecular events in pathogenesis of thyroid neoplasms

Figure 12.5 Molecular events in pathogenesis of thyroid neoplasms. The nature of the tumor-initiating oncogenic hit is critical in determining the phenotype of the tumor. Activating mutations of the thyroid-stimulating hormone receptor (TSH-R) or of Gsα are responsible for most autonomously functioning (hot) thyroid adenomas. These rarely become malignant. Rearrangements of the *RET* tyrosine kinase receptor gene, leading to aberrant expression of a constitutively activated form of RET (RET/PTC), are the key events in initiation of papillary thyroid carcinomas, particularly after exposure to radiation. Further accumulation of other genetic (*ras*) or epigenetic (increased expression of Met, loss of protein kinase Cε – PKCε) abnormalities results in tumor progression. By contrast, activating mutations of *ras* are associated with initiation of follicular neoplasms. These tumors are often aneuploid (>2n), and progress to follicular carcinomas through additional genetic changes (chromosomal losses, *PAX8–PPARγ* rearrangements). Loss of function of *PTEN*, a tumor suppressor gene with tyrosine phosphatase activity, is also common in follicular neoplasms. Inactivating mutations of *p53* are associated with transformation to anaplastic carcinomas and complete loss of differentiated function. Italic lettering indicates genetic mutations; Roman lettering indicates epigenetic changes.

LABORATORY EVALUATION

Fine needle aspiration (FNA) biopsy is the initial procedure of choice in the evaluation of a thyroid nodule. This is also the case for nodules discovered incidentally as a consequence of imaging studies of the neck. Solitary nodules greater than 1cm should be biopsied. Cytologic evaluation of the aspirate indicates whether the nodule is benign (i.e. features consistent with colloid nodules, thyroiditis, or benign cysts; **Fig. 12.6**), suspicious (hypercellular follicular lesions, Hurthle cell changes without lymphocytic infiltration; **Fig. 12.7**), or malignant (**Fig. 12.8**). When the smear does not contain at least five or six groups of well-preserved cells, the aspirate is considered unsatisfactory or nondiagnostic. In this event, a repeat aspirate may be diagnostic in about 50% of cases. The false-negative rate for a benign cytologic diagnosis is about 5%, whereas false-positive tests are seen in about 1% of aspirates classified as malignant. Classification of aspirates as indeterminate or suspicious stems from the inability to distinguish benign follicular or Hurthle cell adenomas from their malignant counterparts (i.e. follicular or Hurthle cell carcinomas) on the basis of their cytologic appearance. About 25% of all aspirates fall into this category, and 10–15% of these ultimately prove to be malignant (**Table 12.3**). The likelihood of cancer is considerably diminished in autonomously functioning nodules, which are also follicular

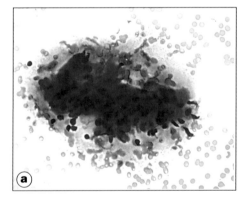

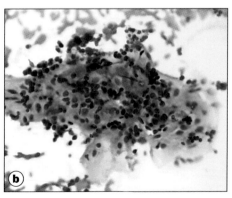

Figure 12.6 Adenomatoid nodule from patient with a multinodular goiter. Many of these are hyperplastic lesions. Cells may be polymorphous, but nuclei are usually no larger than 10–15μm. Presence of abundant colloid, shown by either Diff–Quik stain (a) or Papanicolaou stain (b), is characteristic. (Courtesy of Dr Rawia Yassin and Dr Anna Gomez, University of Cincinnati.)

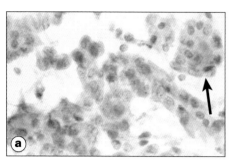

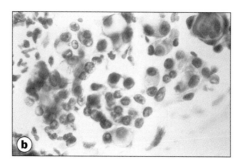

Figure 12.7 Suspicious fine needle aspiration biopsy specimen. (a) Aspirate of a follicular adenoma. Enlarged follicular cells are often arranged in rosettes or microfollicles. Cells are enlarged and nuclei have chromatin of variable density. (b) Aspirate of follicular carcinoma. Cellular characteristics are undistinguishable from a benign adenoma.

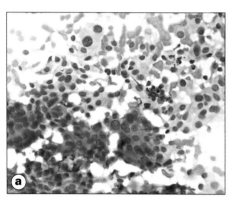

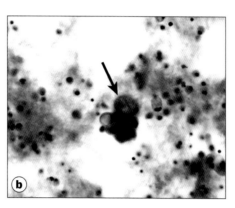

Figure 12.8 Cytologic aspirate of papillary thyroid carcinomas. (a) Example of cytologic aspirate with characteristic clusters of overlapping neoplastic cells. Nuclei vary in size, shape, and chromatin density, and intranuclear inclusions are typical. (b) Suspicious aspirate for papillary thyroid carcinoma. Note the variability in cell size and cytoplasmic volume, along with increased density of nuclear chromatin and presence of intranuclear inclusions (arrow).

neoplasms and thus can give rise to suspicious aspirates. It is therefore prudent to perform radionuclide scans and exclude hyperthyroidism in patients with suspicious or indeterminate cytology. Aspirates from patients with MTCs are often not diagnostic, particularly if not followed by immunostaining for calcitonin. For clarity, the diagnosis and management of MTC will be discussed in a separate section.

Thyroid function should be assessed routinely in patients with thyroid nodules. Patients with lymphocytic (Hashimoto's) thyroiditis may present occasionally with regional thyroid enlargement giving the appearance of a discrete thyroid nodule. Determination of antithyroid antibodies is helpful in these cases. Patients confirmed to be thyrotoxic should have a radionuclide scan with ^{131}I, ^{99m}Tc-pertechnetate or ^{123}I to determine whether the nodule is 'hot' (i.e. incorporates higher levels of the isotope than the surrounding gland). This is caused by autonomously functioning thyroid nodules, which are most often benign. Alternatively, hyperthyroidism may be associated with diffusely increased thyroid uptake, with the nodule appearing as a hypofunctioning ('cold') lesion; this infrequent eventuality is of concern, as thyroid cancers may run an aggressive course in patients with Graves' disease. In this case, the nodule should be evaluated carefully by fine-needle aspiration biopsy (see below). Other than in these specific settings, radionuclide scanning is not of value in the primary diagnostic screening of thyroid nodules (**Fig. 12.9**).

Similarly, high-resolution ultrasonography is not recommended in the initial evaluation of a thyroid nodule, as it does not help to distinguish benign from malignant tumors. Furthermore, as this technique allows imaging of lesions of 1–2mm in size, its use in screening could result in inappropriate evaluation of subclinical conditions. Occasionally, ultrasound-guided FNA biopsy is indicated to assess nodules that are difficult to palpate or embedded deeply within the gland. It is also useful when conventional FNA

Fine-needle aspiration biopsy of thyroid nodules	
Result	Percentage
Benign	57
Malignant	3
Indeterminate	24
Nondiagnostic	16

Table 12.3 Fine-needle aspiration biopsy of thyroid nodules. These are the results in a large series of patients (16,576 specimens) from the University of Catania and the Mayo Clinic. (Adapted from Giuffrida D, Gharib H. Controversies in the management of cold, hot, and occult thyroid nodules. Am J Med. 1995;99:642, with permission from Excerpta Medica, Inc.)

has failed to provide a diagnostic specimen, and to help direct the biopsy needle to the solid component of cystic nodules. In patients with cystic lesions, aspiration decreases the size of the nodule, and cures many of them. There is a place for ultrasonography in the management of patients with presumed benign nodular disease when palpation is not sufficient to track lesion size during prolonged followup, as discussed below.

MANAGEMENT OF PATIENTS WITH THYROID NODULES

About 60–70% of patients will prove to have a benign thyroid aspirate, in many cases corresponding to adenomatoid or hyperplastic colloid nodules. These patients are best managed expectantly, by monitoring changes in nodule size over time. Nodules

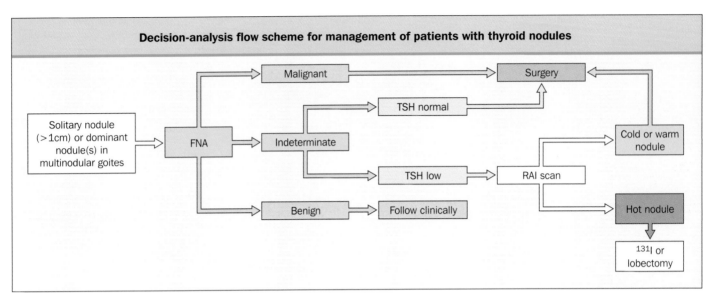

Figure 12.9 Decision-analysis flow scheme for management of patients with thyroid nodules. FNA, fine-needle aspiration biopsy; RAI, radioactive iodine; TSH, thyroid-stimulating hormone. (Modified from Mazzaferri EL. Management of a solitary thyroid nodule. N Engl J Med. 1993;328:553–9 © 1993 Massachusetts Medical Society. All rights reserved.)

showing significant growth during the observation period should be rebiopsied. As cells from colloid adenomas are thought to retain responsiveness to TSH, some physicians treat these patients with L-thyroxine to suppress TSH levels below the normal range, and hence reduce the size of the nodule. (Note: a *suppressive* dose of thyroid hormone is one that reduces TSH to levels below the normal range, as opposed to a *replacement* dose, in which TSH levels are maintained within the normal range.) The use of suppressive doses of thyroid hormone for benign nodules is controversial. Short-term treatment (about 6 months) with L-thyroxine was formerly advocated to help identify those nodules most likely to be malignant, based on their failure to decrease in size when TSH levels were low. However, the good predictive power of FNA cytology, and the fact that many benign nodules do not shrink with L-thyroxine suppressive therapy, has largely outmoded this practice. Long-term TSH-suppressive therapy to prevent growth of benign nodules is also of uncertain efficacy. It is unknown whether this practice decreases the likelihood that benign tumors will become malignant over time, a rare occurrence in these nodules. Furthermore, supraphysiologic doses of thyroid hormone may be associated with osteopenia and cardiac arrhythmias, and should therefore be avoided in postmenopausal women and older patients. In summary, suppressive therapy with thyroid hormone is usually not indicated for benign nodules, which are best followed by clinical observation (with or without ultrasonography) over time. Suppressive therapy should be restricted to selected patients with large nodules, particularly if they cause symptoms (i.e. dysphagia, stridor), or are cosmetically disfiguring, and to prevent recurrence of nodules in irradiated patients previously treated with partial thyroidectomy.

Patients with suspicious or indeterminate aspirates should be referred for surgery, as the possibility of malignancy cannot be excluded. Another circumstance in which surgery is advisable is for clinically significant nodules in which FNA biopsy has been repeatedly nondiagnostic. Cysts that are greater than 4cm in size,

or that recur after drainage, may also require surgery. Nodules from patients with a history of radiation exposure have a higher likelihood of being malignant (about 30%) and therefore merit closer surveillance and a lower threshold for surgical referral. In solitary nodules from irradiated patients, FNA biopsy with multiple sampling of the lesion is appropriate. If the patient has multiple nodules, particularly if many of them are greater than 1cm in size, FNA sampling becomes more cumbersome, and these patients should be treated with a near-total thyroidectomy. Treatment with suppressive doses of thyroid hormone prevents recurrence of nodules in patients who have had only part of the thyroid removed.

PROGNOSTIC FACTORS

Long-term cure rates for differentiated thyroid cancer are high. However, in some patients the disease can run an insidious course punctuated by local recurrences, development of distant metastases, mainly to lung and bone, and, in a minority of cases, death. Disease prognosis can be assessed on the basis of certain clinical and pathologic features at the time of presentation. The major prognostic variables for thyroid cancer are age at diagnosis, tumor extent, and histologic type. The risk of recurrence and death rises with age, particularly after the age of 40 years, perhaps because tumors present at a more advanced stage and have more aggressive properties in older patients. Extent of the disease is a critical prognostic factor, assessed by tumor size, multifocality, extrathyroidal invasion, and presence of lymph node or distant metastases. Papillary carcinomas have a better prognosis than follicular carcinomas, in part because the latter present at an older age and tend to metastasize at a distance. Poorly differentiated and anaplastic carcinomas carry a particularly poor prognosis. In addition, male gender and the DNA-ploidy of the tumors may also provide prognostic information (**Table 12.4**). Molecular genetic markers are not yet of proven value.

Prognostic factors for poor survival in differentiated thyroid cancer		
Patient features	Older age	
	Male	
Tumor features	Histology	Papillary variants: tall-cell, columnar-cell
		Follicular: widely invasive, poorly differentiated
	Tumor extent	Larger tumor size
		Extension of tumor beyond the thyroid capsule
		Distant metastases
		Others: multifocality, lymph node metastasis (if large, multiple, bilateral, or in the mediastinum)
	Aneuploidy	
Treatment	Incomplete resection	
	No administration of an ablative dose of ^{131}I	
Elevated serum thyroglobulin level more than 3 months after surgery		

Table 12.4 Prognostic factors for poor survival in differentiated thyroid cancer. (With permission from Schlumberger M, Pacini F. Thyroid cancer. Paris:Editions Nucleon; 1992)

Several scoring systems have been devised for disease staging, which differ in the relative weight they assign each variable. The purpose of staging is to increase predictive power in order to guide long-term therapy. As all staging methods appear to perform equally well, we describe in detail only the one developed at the Ohio State University (**Table 12.5**). Other commonly used prognostic systems include the TNM classification developed by the International Union Against Cancer, and those of the Mayo Clinic (AMES/MACIS), the University of Chicago, and the Institut Gustav Roussy (IGR). As described below, the extent of surgery and type of postoperative therapy also influence long-term prognosis.

TREATMENT OF THYROID CANCER

Surgery

Patients with malignant or suspicious cytopathologic aspirates are treated surgically. Additional preoperative evaluation may include a calcitonin level when the cytopathologic diagnosis is equivocal and/or suspicious for MTC. Patients with hoarseness should have their vocal cords examined by direct or indirect laryngoscopy. Occasionally, ultrasonography may be helpful to determine presence and/or extent of lymph node involvement.

The type of surgery will depend in part on the extent of tumor as determined by visual and gross pathologic inspection of the nodule at the time of surgery, evidence of regional lymph node enlargement, and histologic examination of the frozen section of the tumor. A total or near-total thyroidectomy is the procedure of choice in most cases with a firm preoperative diagnosis of differentiated (i.e. papillary or follicular) thyroid carcinoma. A near-total thyroidectomy involves resection of the entire affected lobe, the isthmus, and all but the upper pole of the contralateral lobe, while leaving the posterior capsule intact. In this situation the small remnant of thyroid tissue (usually less than 2g) can be destroyed later with radioactive iodine. Total thyroidectomy is reserved for patients with larger tumors, bilateral lobar involvement, extensive bilateral lymph node metastases, or extrathyroidal tumor extension. The risk of permanent hypoparathyroidism and recurrent laryngeal nerve palsy is greater with more extensive thyroid surgery, although it should be low in experienced hands.

Some controversy about the appropriate extent of surgery still remains, because most patients have an excellent prognosis regardless of the surgical modality. Thus, some surgeons believe that a hemithyroidectomy (removal of the affected lobe and isthmus) may be sufficient, particularly for patients with relatively small malignant nodules (<1.5cm) and no evidence of regional lymph node involvement. The advantage of a more limited thyroid resection is a lower rate of postsurgical complications. However, several groups have reported higher recurrence rates with lobectomy than with near-total or total thyroidectomy, even for small tumors. This is probably because papillary carcinomas are multicentric and bilateral in a significant proportion of cases.

Ohio State University staging system of differentiated thyroid cancer				
Variables	Stage I	Stage II	Stage III	Stage IV
Tumor size (cm)	<1.5	1.5–4.4	≥ 4.5	Any size
Cervical metastases	No	Yes*	Yes/No	Yes/No
Multiple thyroid tumors (>3), any size	No	Yes*	Yes/No	Yes/No
Local tumor invasion	No	No	Yes	Yes/No
Distant metastases	No	No	No	Yes

* Includes tumors <1.5cm with cervical metastases and palpable tumors of uncertain size confined to the thyroid gland; any tumor that fulfills one of the three criteria for size, cervical metastases, or multiple intrathyroidal tumors is considered to be stage II.

Table 12.5 Ohio State University staging system of differentiated thyroid cancer. (Modified with permission from Mazzaferri E. Thyroid cancer: impact of therapeutic modalities on prognosis. In: Fagin JA, ed. Thyroid cancer. Boston, MA:Kluwer Academic Publishers; 1998.)

There is no justification for lobectomy for patients presenting with stage II tumors or above, as mortality rates are higher.

Lymph node involvement is found in 35–65% of papillary thyroid carcinomas and is usually ipsilateral. By contrast, follicular carcinomas have a lower frequency of lymph node involvement. As the prognostic impact of lymph node metastases on survival is still controversial, there is no firm consensus on the appropriate extent of lymph node surgery. Most advocate sampling and removal of enlarged cervical lymph nodes only, whereas others routinely perform central compartment node dissection and removal *en bloc*.

In patients referred to surgery for a suspicious or indeterminate nodule, removal of the affected thyroid lobe and isthmus (hemithyroidectomy) is appropriate if the frozen section is consistent with a benign lesion. However, the resolution of frozen section histopathology is not sufficient to provide a conclusive diagnosis, particularly in follicular neoplasms. Occasionally, the final histopathology may reveal evidence of microscopic invasion of the tumor capsule (minimally invasive follicular carcinoma, see **Fig. 12.3**), or allow better observation of nuclear changes consistent with a papillary carcinoma. In this event, a completion thyroidectomy is performed at a later date. Incidental discovery of a papillary microcarcinoma within a lobe removed for a benign nodule is not in itself an absolute indication for second-stage removal of the contralateral lobe, providing the patient has no documented history of radiation exposure.

Radioiodine

The purpose of postoperative administration of radioactive iodine (^{131}I) in patients with differentiated thyroid cancer is to destroy remnants of normal thyroid tissue. Even after a total thyroidectomy, almost all patients will have at least a small amount of residual tissue left in place. The rationale for postoperative radioablation is that this may diminish the risk of recurrences by eliminating small foci of thyroid cancer cells that may remain. In addition, rendering patients completely athyrotic enables the use of diagnostic radioiodine whole-body scans and plasma thyroglobulin levels to monitor for disease recurrence. However, the appropriate indications for postoperative radioiodine therapy are controversial, particularly when there is no known residual disease (i.e. prophylactic radioablation). This therapy is not necessary in patients with papillary thyroid cancers less than 1.5cm in size, as the evidence that ablation improves long-term outcome is not compelling. There is disagreement on whether prophylactic radioiodine ablation decreases recurrences and mortality in patients with larger tumors, capsular or extrathyroidal extension, or extensive lymph node metastases (particularly bilateral), although in most centers this is considered an acceptable indication, particularly in patients with other negative prognostic indicators. There is no question that postoperative radioablation should be administered to patients with incompletely resected tumors, or with known distant metastases.

Postoperative ^{131}I therapy is usually performed approximately 6 weeks after surgery. Thyroid hormone replacement should be withdrawn in sufficient time to allow endogenous TSH levels to rise above 30mU/L, to stimulate iodine uptake by the remnant thyroid tissue. This is usually achieved by treating patients with triiodothyronine 1μg/kg/day for 4 weeks, and then stopping the medication for 2 weeks. Patients are instructed to avoid iodine-containing drugs, food, or hair dyes (e.g. henna) after surgery, and to follow a strict low-iodine diet for 1 week prior to therapy. Most groups do not perform a diagnostic whole-body scan prior to postoperative ablation, as the presence of a thyroid remnant is the norm and the diagnostic ^{131}I dose can potentially diminish the effectiveness of the therapeutic dose through cell 'stunning'.

The dose of ^{131}I used for ablation varies between centers. Some advocate using arbitrary standard doses, which vary from 30–100mCi (1.1–3.7Gbq). The lower amount is chosen to diminish radiation exposure and because of practical considerations, as in many countries 30mCi is the maximum allowable dose that can be given without mandatory hospitalization. Others choose higher doses because of the better potential for eradicating malignant cells, and to maximize efficiency of thyroid remnant ablation. Alternatively, a dosimetry technique has been developed to individualize the amount of ^{131}I needed to deliver 300Gy to the thyroid bed (believed to be the appropriate dose for ablation) while exposing the bone marrow to less than 2Gy. This technique is efficacious, but more cumbersome and costly, and is performed in only a few centers. Some 3–5 days after the therapeutic dose, it is advisable to perform a whole-body scan, which can occasionally reveal sites of uptake outside the thyroid bed consistent with regional or distant metastases, which may alter staging, prognosis, and future therapy. The place of adjuvant external radiotherapy in the initial management of patients with locally invasive differentiated thyroid cancer is controversial.

After the initial therapy, patients are treated with L-thyroxine to suppress TSH levels below the normal range (to about 0.1mU/L in third-generation assays) to minimize any potential stimulation of thyroid cell growth. In those patients receiving radioablation, whole-body scanning with ^{131}I is repeated 6 months after the treatment dose to monitor the appropriateness of thyroid destruction and presence of residual or metastatic disease. Traditionally this has been done after discontinuing thyroid hormone, to allow TSH levels to rise (**Fig. 12.10**, left panel). Recently, recombinant human TSH (rhTSH) has been approved for whole-body scanning of thyroid cancer patients. Patients are administered two injections of TSH on the week of the study, followed by ^{131}I scanning and measurement of TSH-stimulated serum thyroglobulin (Tg) levels (**Fig. 12.10**, right panel). This allows patients to remain on thyroid hormone throughout the testing period, and avoid the unpleasant symptoms of hypothyroidism. When both ^{131}I scanning and Tg levels are considered, rhTSH testing has a comparable sensitivity to thyroid hormone withdrawal in detecting persistent uptake in the thyroid bed or in thyroid cancer metastases.

The appropriate place for rhTSH versus conventional thyroid hormone withdrawal scanning in the management of thyroid cancer is still being defined. When the presence of a normal thyroid remnant and/or residual or metastatic disease is anticipated (e.g. following total thyroidectomy, known residual disease in the neck, imaging evidence of local or distant metastases, or high serum Tg in spite of TSH suppression), ^{131}I scanning should be performed after withdrawal of thyroid hormone, as radioiodine therapy can then be instituted without additional delay (**Fig. 12.11**). As measurement of serum Tg is needed to maximize sensitivity of scanning after rhTSH, this approach is best avoided if patients have antithyroglobulin antibodies, which invalidate the result of Tg radioimmunoassays. Scanning with rhTSH may

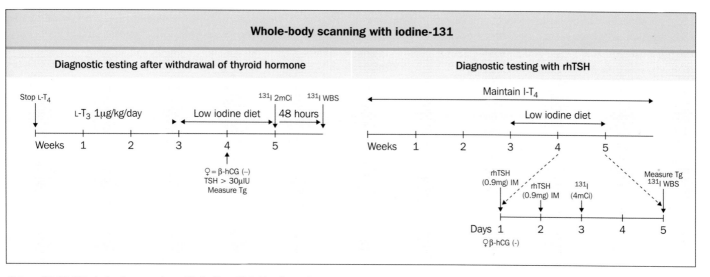

Figure 12.10 Whole-body scanning with iodine-131. The figure illustrates protocols for diagnostic whole body ^{131}I scan in followup of patients with differentiated thyroid cancer. hCG, human chorionic gonadotropin; rhTSH, recombinant human thyroid-stimulating hormone; T$_3$, triiodothyronine; T$_4$, thyroxine; Tg, thyroglobulin; TSH, thyroid-stimulating hormone; WBS, whole-body scan.

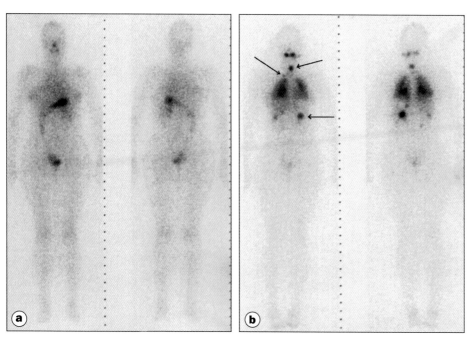

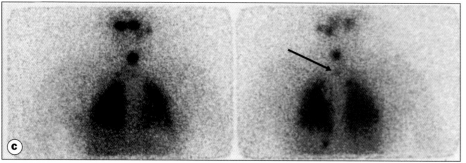

Figure 12.11 Whole body ^{131}I scan. (a) Whole-body scan 1 day after treatment with 179mCi of ^{131}I for recurrent metastatic papillary carcinoma. Uptake is initially seen only in the nasopharyngeal, salivary, and gastrointestinal tissues. (b) Whole-body scan 1 week after treatment now shows marked diffuse uptake in the lungs with locally recurring disease at the base of the neck (arrows) and right supraclavicular region (arrow). A metastatic lesion is also seen in the superior region of the left kidney (arrow). (c) A close-up image of the 7-day posttreatment scan also suggests the presence of mediastinal disease (arrow).

prove of particular value in the subsequent followup of patients who have already had a negative whole-body scan. Diagnostic testing with rhTSH should also be considered for patients with neuropsychiatric or medical conditions in which transient hypothyroidism could be particularly disabling or dangerous.

Although rhTSH is expensive, it should be used for ^{131}I therapy in patients with hypopituitarism, or with functioning thyroid cancer metastases if they cannot mount an appropriate endogenous TSH rise after thyroid hormone depletion. rhTSH may prove be of particular value in ^{131}I therapy of patients with thyroid cancer metastases close to vital structures (e.g. brain, paraspinal), which may be susceptible to significant growth with more prolonged exposure to TSH.

The frequency with which diagnostic testing is repeated in the follow-up of thyroid cancer patients varies according to the initial stage at presentation, the outcome of the initial ^{131}I therapy, and the presence or not of measurable serum thyroglobulin when patients are either on or off suppressive thyroid hormone therapy. Testing is usually repeated every 6–12 months until the patient has two successive negative ^{131}I scans. If the patient also has negative Tg levels when TSH levels are maximal, it is reasonable to defer further testing for 3–5 years. Additional imaging studies to detect local recurrence or metastatic disease are warranted at regular intervals, particularly in patients who originally presented with advanced disease (i.e. stage 2 or more). To this end, high-resolution ultrasonography, CT, or MRI of the neck, CT of the chest and bone scintigraphy may be helpful.

Residual or metastatic disease that concentrates radioiodine should be treated with therapeutic doses of [131]I. Most centers use empiric doses ranging between 75mCi and 200mCi. Others advocate the use of dosimetry to establish a dose that will deliver 80Gy to each tumor deposit, which is needed to obtain predictable tumoricidal effects.

Short-term side effects of radioiodine therapy include headaches, nausea, vomiting, epigastric pain, and salivary gland inflammation due to trapping of radioiodine. These side effects are usually mild and are seen particularly with higher radiation doses. Radioiodine may induce acute edema in brain or spinal metastases, which may be prevented by prophylactic administration of dexamethasone and/or mannitol. Acute radiation pneumonitis may occur in patients with extensive pulmonary metastases, although this is rare. Bone marrow depression usually

peaks by 6 weeks, is also dose-dependent, and is minimized when the maximum dose to whole blood is less than 2Gy.

The long-term effects of ^{131}I therapy include increased incidence of leukemia, particularly when cumulative lifetime doses exceed 800mCi and the interval between doses is less than 1 year. Prevalence of permanent cytopenia is low and seen only in patients with a very high lifetime dosage. There may be a small increase in incidence of certain solid cancers, particularly of the bladder, salivary glands, and breast. In men, transient spermatogenic depression may be seen with high ^{131}I doses but permanent gonadal failure is rare. Fertility in women does not appear to be significantly affected by [131]I. When pregnancies begin more than 1 year after radioiodine therapy, the incidence of birth defects is not increased.

When residual disease is amenable to surgical resection, this should always be attempted. Surgery or external radiotherapy should also be considered when the tumor deposits have low or absent iodine uptake, or for bone metastases, as these do not usually respond to [131]I. Patients with local or metastatic disease unresponsive to internal or external radiation do not usually benefit from chemotherapy, although treatment with doxorubicin may be of marginal benefit in a small proportion of cases. Many patients with disseminated thyroid cancer may remain asymptomatic for months or years and enjoy a good quality of life.

Surgical cure rates for undifferentiated or anaplastic carcinomas are very low, and the goal of postoperative care is to achieve local control of the disease through external radiotherapy and to give palliative care. Multimodality approaches incorporating radiation and chemotherapy have at best a marginal impact on patient survival.

MEDULLARY THYROID CARCINOMA

Medullary thyroid carcinomas originate from calcitonin-secreting parafollicular C cells and represent 5–10% of all thyroid cancers. About 25% of MTCs are hereditary, either as part of multiple endocrine neoplasia type 2 (MEN 2) or of familial MTC (FMTC; **Fig. 12.12**). Germline mutations of the *RET* proto-oncogene confer predisposition to all hereditary forms of MTC, through an autosomal dominant mode of transmission. The genetic and clinical characteristics of the MEN syndromes are discussed in Chapter 34.

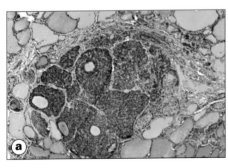
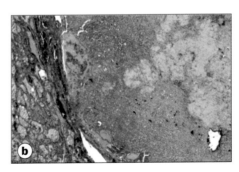
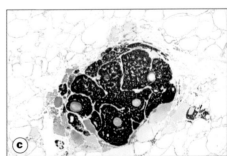

Figure 12.12 Medullary thyroid carcinoma. (a) Photomicrograph of hematoxylin–eosin-stained section of a medullary thyroid carcinoma. Medullary thyroid carcinomas usually have well-defined boundaries and are arranged as rounded nests of cells. (b) Amyloid deposits are seen in up to 80% of cases and may be a favorable indicator. (c) Definitive diagnosis is confirmed by demonstrating calcitonin immunoreactivity.

Medullary thyroid carcinoma		
Syndrome	**Associated conditions**	**Predominant forms of mutant RET (codon)**
Familial medullary thyroid carcinoma	None	609>61>618>620>768>V804M>891
Multiple endocrine neoplasia type 2A	Hyperparathyroidism	634>618>620>611>609>790>V804L
	Pheochromocytoma	
Multiple endocrine neoplasia type 2A and cutaneous lichen amyloidosis	Hyperparathyroidism	634
	Pheochromocytoma	
	Cutaneous lichen amyloidosis	
Multiple endocrine neoplasia type 2A and Hirschsprung's disease	Hyperparathyroidism	609, 618, 620
	Pheochromocytoma	
	Hirschsprung's disease	
Multiple endocrine neoplasia type 2B	Pheochromocytoma	918>>883>922
	Ganglioneuromas	
	Marfanoid habitus	

Table 12.6 Medullary thyroid carcinoma. Genotype–phenotype correlations in familial syndromes of medullary thyroid carcinoma. See also Chapter 34.

Pathogenesis

Hereditary MTCs are associated with activating point mutations of *RET*. The RET proto-oncogene is a plasma membrane tyrosine kinase receptor involved in the regulation of growth, survival, differentiation, and migration of cells of neural crest origin. The mutations in *RET* that are involved in generation of MTC code for constitutively active receptors in which one of the key regulatory functions that control their activation has been subverted. The different clinical variants of MEN 2 and FMTC are preferentially associated with distinct point mutations of *RET* (**Table 12.6**). Germline mutations of *RET* are found in 97–100% of unrelated MEN 2A families, 95% of MEN 2B families, and 88% of FMTC kindreds. About 2.5–7% of patients presenting with an apparently sporadic MTC carry a germline *RET* mutation. Moreover, 25–75% of genuinely sporadic MTCs have acquired a somatic activating mutation of *RET*. The key role of the RET oncogene in pathogenesis of MTC is strongly substantiated by evidence that transgenic mice in which mutant RET is expressed under control of a calcitonin promoter develop C-cell hyperplasia and MTC.

Pathology

Sporadic MTCs usually present as a single lesion, with well-defined boundaries. They are often located in the upper third of the thyroid lobe, may be encapsulated, and consist of rounded nests of cells separated by thin fibrovascular stroma. Most commonly, MTC cells are oval or spindle-shaped, although they may have a wide range of appearances. Stromal amyloid is seen in 80% of cases (**Fig. 12.12**). The vast majority show immunoreactivity to calcitonin, as well as carcinoembryogenic antigen and a variety of neuroendocrine markers. In hereditary MTC, tumors are often multicentric, bilateral, and surrounded by regions of C-cell hyperplasia, the precursor lesion for MTC. In thyroid glands removed prophylactically from carriers of germline *RET* mutations, C-cell hyperplasia may be the only abnormality observed. Rarely, nests of hyperplastic C cells may be seen in the peritumoral regions surrounding a sporadic MTC.

Clinical manifestations

Sporadic or previously unrecognized familial MTC usually presents as one or more palpable thyroid nodules. Patients with sporadic MTC are usually in the fourth or fifth decade of life. Although nodules are usually painless, they may be associated with pain, dysphagia, and hoarseness. Lymph node metastases are detected at diagnosis in more than 50% of cases. Patients may also present with symptoms arising from distant metastases, most commonly in lung, liver, bone, and brain. A small proportion of patients complain of flushing, which may be alcohol-induced. Patients with large tumors or widespread metastatic disease may have secretory diarrhea. A syndrome of hypercortisolism due to ectopic secretion of corticotropin by the tumor's C cells may be seen. Index cases with MEN 2A may also present with symptoms associated with hyperparathyroidism or pheochromocytoma. A careful family history focused on possible manifestations of the MEN 2A or 2B syndromes must be obtained in all patients. Increasingly, many patients with familial forms of MTC are asymptomatic at presentation and are detected by genetic screening studies.

Laboratory evaluation

The thyroid mass is usually solid, and coarse calcification may be seen within the nodule on plain X-rays of the neck. Patients with sporadic MTC will usually have a FNA thyroid biopsy as the first diagnostic test. Cytologic smears are usually markedly cellular, but quite variable in appearance. Often the aspirate is reported as containing atypical cells, or as 'suspicious' for malignancy (**Fig. 12.13**). A firm diagnosis of MTC may not be made unless immunocytochemical staining for calcitonin is also performed. Almost all patients with a palpable mass will have high basal serum calcitonin levels. If none of the features of the patient's clinical presentation or cytopathology are suggestive of MTC, and calcitonin levels are not determined, the diagnosis may not be made until after the surgery is completed. This presents a significant problem, as the appropriate surgery for MTC differs from that used for most tumors of thyroid follicular

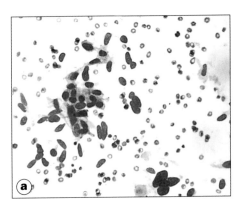
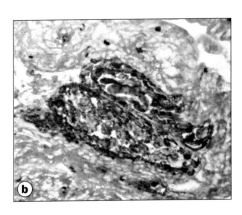

Figure 12.13 The cytopathology of medullary thyroid cancer is highly variable. (a) A mixture of loosely associated spindle-shaped and rounded cells is noted, with nearly invisible nucleoli. (b) Calcitonin immunostaining should be performed when the condition is suspected, as it confirms the diagnosis.

cells, highlighting the need for accurate preoperative diagnosis. However, the diagnostic accuracy and cost-effectiveness of screening all patients with thyroid nodules for MTC by determining plasma basal calcitonin levels has not been established conclusively, and this is not performed by most practitioners. When a diagnosis of sporadic or familial MTC is suspected on the basis of cytopathology and serum calcitonin levels, screening for pheochromocytoma should be performed prior to surgery.

Patients at risk for hereditary forms of MTC are now identified by genetic testing, as discussed in Chapter 34. The availability of molecular diagnostic tools to screen for mutations of *RET* has dramatically changed the management of this disease. Mutational analysis of the most common MEN 2 *RET* mutations is performed in several laboratories around the world, and genetic testing deeply influences the management of patients at risk for hereditary MTC. This is feasible because the mutations are restricted to fairly discrete regions of the gene. Mutation of a single codon, 634, is found in more than 80% of all hereditary MTC. When mutations of five other codons (609, 611, 618, 620, and 918) are included, a molecular defect can be identified for more than 95% of all hereditary MTC. Moreover, these mutations are clustered in three relatively small exons (10, 11, and 16), which simplifies genetic screening strategies and diminishes cost.

Mutations are commonly screened by amplifying the target exon with the polymerase chain reaction and then sequencing the resulting DNA product. Patients presenting with an apparently sporadic MTC should also be tested for germline *RET* mutations, which are found in up to 7% of cases. As discussed in Chapter 34, the nature of the germline *RET* mutation has important prognostic implications and influences the timing of surgery.

Treatment

The goal of treatment is total surgical removal of the cancerous tissue from the neck. This is attempted by total thyroidectomy and bilateral central compartment lymph node dissection and removal *en bloc*. Dissection of the anterosuperior mediastinum is indicated if there is evidence of disease. It may be appropriate to minimize the extent of neck surgery in patients with widespread distant metastases, as determined by preoperative staging. Postoperative serum levels of calcitonin and carcinoembryonic antigen provide a useful test for residual disease, which is found in about 70% of cases of patients presenting with a neck mass. Sensitivity of postoperative screening for persistent MTC

is increased by determining pentagastrin-stimulated calcitonin levels. Those with persistently undetectable calcitonin levels are considered free of disease, and no longer need regular imaging followup studies. In those patients with continued elevation of calcitonin, efforts should be made to localize the tumor deposits by ultrasonography, CT or MRI scanning of the neck, CT of the chest, CT or ultrasound exam of the liver, or bone scintigraphy. Reintervention is indicated if regional lymph node metastases are detected, in the absence of distant metastases.

It is controversial whether selective venous sampling should be performed to localize disease in patients with no abnormal imaging findings. Adjuvant external radiotherapy is advocated by some for patients at high risk of local regional relapse. Although MTC is not particularly radiosensitive, local control may be improved by radiotherapy in about 20% of patients with gross inoperable residual or recurrent disease. Palliative external radiotherapy may help to control symptoms associated with distant metastases.

Prophylactic thyroidectomy should be performed in patients at risk for familial MTC. MEN 2B *RET* carriers should have a total thyroidectomy during infancy, whereas in MEN 2A, surgery should be performed before the age of 6 years. Pentagastrin stimulation testing may be value in *RET* carriers from FMTC pedigrees with variable penetrance to determine the need and timing for surgery.

Prognosis

The 10-year survival of sporadic MTC is 65%. Negative prognostic variables are extent of disease at diagnosis, older age, and male sex. Long-term survival of patients receiving prophylactic thyroidectomy for hereditary forms of MTC is greater than 90%.

THYROID LYMPHOMAS

Primary thyroid lymphomas represent about 2% of cancers of the thyroid gland. They are a disease of the elderly, and usually present as a rapidly enlarging neck mass. They are more common in women, and often arise in glands with chronic autoimmune thyroiditis. The majority are classified as mucosa-associated lymphoid tissue lymphomas (MALT-L), and arise from B cells. Patients frequently complain of local compression symptoms. The thyroid mass is often hard and fixed to surrounding tissue, and lymph node involvement is common. Thyroid FNA biopsy reveals lymphoid cells, which cannot easily be distinguished from infiltrating cells from a gland affected by chronic thyroiditis. Imaging and biochemical studies are performed to determine extent of the disease outside the neck. The majority of thyroid lymphomas are confined to the thyroid and cervical lymph nodes, with a small proportion involving the stomach or abdominal cavity. Usually, complete surgical removal is not possible, and this should only be attempted with small tumors. In the majority, an open thyroid biopsy to confirm the diagnosis is sufficient. MALT-L thyroid lymphomas show an excellent response to combined therapy with external radiotherapy and chemotherapy with CHOP (cyclophosphamide, doxorubicin, vincristine, and prednisone), with a cause-specific mortality of less than 10%.

FURTHER READING

Brierley J, Maxon HR. Radioiodine and external radiation therapy in the management of thyroid cancer. In: Fagin JA, ed. Thyroid cancer. Boston, MA:Kluwer Academic Publishers; 1998:285–318.

Fagin JA. Molecular genetics of tumors of thyroid follicular cells. In: Braverman LE, Utiger RD. The thyroid. A fundamental and clinical text. Philadelphia, PA:Lippincott Williams & Wilkins; 2000:886–98.

Grebe SK, Hay ID. Follicular cell-derived thyroid carcinomas. Cancer Treat Res. 1997;89:91–140.

Hoff AO, Cote GJ, Gagel RF. Multiple endocrine neoplasias. Annu Rev Physiol. 2000;62:377–411.

Ladenson PW. The role of recombinant thyrotropin in management of patients with thyroid cancer. Thyroid Today 2000;23(2):1–11.

Mazzaferri EL. Thyroid cancer. In: Becker KL, ed. Principles and practice of endocrinology and metabolism, 2nd edn. Philadelphia, PA:JB Lippincott; 1995:354–65.

Peplinski GR, Wells SA. Surgical management of thyroid cancer. In: Fagin JA, ed. Thyroid cancer. Boston, MA:Kluwer Academic Publishers; 1998:233–54.

Puxeddu E, Fagin JA. Genetic markers in thyroid neoplasia. Endocrinol Metab Clin North Am. 2001;30:493–513.

Schlumberger M. Papillary and follicular thyroid carcinoma. N Engl J Med. 1998;338:297–306.

Schlumberger M, Pacini F. Thyroid tumors. Paris:Editions Nucleon; 1999;85–167; 267–307.

Singer PA, Cooper DS, Daniels DG, et al. Treatment guidelines for patients with thyroid nodules and well differentiated thyroid cancer. Arch Intern Med. 1996;156:2165–22.

Wartofsky L, Sherman SI, Gopal J, Schlumberger M, Hay ID. The use of radioactive iodine in patients with papillary and follicular thyroid cancer. J Clin Endocrinol Metab. 1998;83:4195–203.

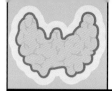

Section 2 Thyroid

Chapter 13

Hyperthyroidism and Graves' Disease

Anthony P Weetman

INTRODUCTION

Thyrotoxicosis is the clinical state produced by excessive circulating thyroid hormones. Hyperthyroidism exists when thyrotoxicosis is the result of thyroid overactivity. Although most types of thyrotoxicosis are due to hyperthyroidism, thyrotoxicosis can also be caused by destruction of thyroid tissue, leading to release of an excess of stored thyroid hormones, and by ingestion of too much thyroid hormone.

Causes of thyrotoxicosis

As well as grouping thyrotoxicosis into disorders with and without hyperthyroidism, it is useful to think of primary and secondary causes (**Table 13.1**). Around 70% of all cases of thyrotoxicosis are due to Graves' disease, with toxic multinodular goiter and toxic adenoma accounting for around 25% of the remainder. Unusual causes are considered after these major types of hyperthyroidism.

Causes of thyrotoxicosis	
Primary hyperthyroidism	**Graves' disease**
	Toxic multinodular goiter
	Toxic adenoma
	Drugs: iodine excess (Jod–Basedow phenomenon), lithium
	Thyroid carcinoma or functioning metastases
	Activating mutation of the TSH receptor
	Activating mutation of the $G_{s\alpha}$ protein (McCune–Albright syndrome)
	Struma ovarii (ectopic thyroid tissue)
Thyrotoxicosis without hyperthyroidism	**Ingestion of excess thyroid hormone (thyrotoxicosis factitia)**
	Subacute (viral or de Quervain's) thyroiditis
	Silent thyroiditis
	Other causes of thyroid destruction: amiodarone, iodine-131 or external irradiation, infarction of an adenoma
Secondary hyperthyroidism	TSH-secreting pituitary tumor
	Chorionic-gonadotrophin-secreting tumors
	Gestational thyrotoxicosis (due to chorionic gonadotrophin in first trimester)
	Thyroid hormone resistance (usually euthyroid)

Table 13.1 Causes of thyrotoxicosis. Common causes are shown in bold. TSH, thyroid-stimulating hormone.

GRAVES' DISEASE

The prevalence of Graves' disease in Caucasians and Asians is around 1–2%, with a lower prevalence in black Africans. Women are five to 10 times more commonly affected than men and the mean age of onset is 40–60 years but Graves' disease can occur at the extremes of life. The condition is caused by autoantibodies against the thyroid-stimulating hormone (TSH) receptor, which bind to regions of the receptor overlapping the TSH-binding site, thus stimulating thyroid cell division (leading to goiter) and thyroid hormone secretion in an unregulated fashion (**Fig. 13.1**). Most patients also have evidence of auto-immunity to other thyroid autoantigens, such as antibodies against the intrathyroidal enzyme thyroid peroxidase, or to thyroglobulin, and infiltration of the thyroid gland with lymphocytes (**Fig. 13.2**). These concurrent autoimmune phenomena account for unusual presentations of Graves' disease in which there is fluctuation between hyperthyroidism and hypothyroidism, and for the development of hypothyroidism in some patients successfully treated with antithyroid drugs.

In common with most autoimmune disorders, Graves' disease is the result of the interaction of a number of genetic and

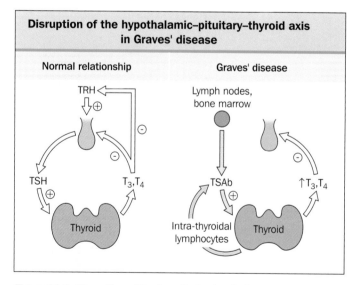

Figure 13.1 Disruption of the hypothalamic–pituitary–thyroid axis in Graves' disease. (Left panel) Normal relationship between hypothalamus, pituitary and thyroid. (Right panel) Graves' disease, with production of thyroid stimulating antibodies (TSAb). T_3, triiodothyronine; T_4, thyroxine; TRH, thyrotropin-releasing hormone; TSH, thyroid-stimulating hormone.

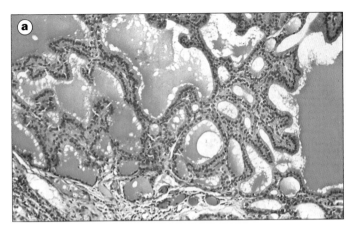

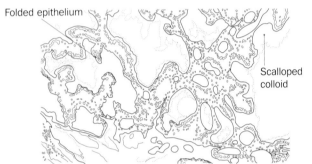

Folded epithelium

Scalloped colloid

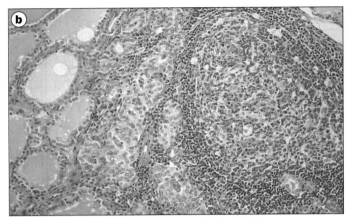

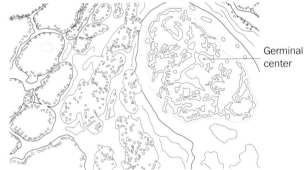

Germinal center

Figure 13.2 Histology of thyroid tissue in Graves' disease. (a) Thyroid follicles showing tall, folded columnar epithelium and scalloping of the colloid. (b) Lymphoid infiltration, with a germinal center to the right. (c) High-power view showing lymphocytic and plasma cell infiltration.

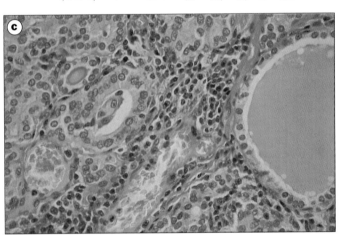

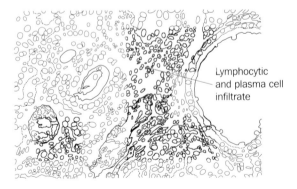

Lymphocytic and plasma cell infiltrate

polymorphisms in the gene encoding the T cell regulatory molecule CTLA-4. Stress, in the form of adverse life effects, smoking, and increased iodide intake, are probable risk factors, but additional unknown environmental agents are also likely to be involved. Because of a shared genetic susceptibility, many other autoimmune disorders occur at increased frequency in either Graves' patients or their families (**Table 13.2**).

Around 50% of Graves' patients have clinical signs of ophthalmopathy (**Fig. 13.3**) and most of the remainder have subclinical evidence of involvement in the form of extraocular muscle enlargement on orbital imaging. Conversely, around 90% of patients presenting with clinical ophthalmopathy have Graves' disease; 5% have autoimmune hypothyroidism, and 5% are euthyroid – but usually these patients have positive thyroid antibodies or a goiter. The term thyroid-associated ophthalmopathy has been introduced to cover all such forms of ophthalmopathy, even in the absence of Graves' disease. The cause of the ophthalmopathy is unknown. The most likely explanation is an autoimmune response against an orbital autoantigen shared by the thyroid (**Fig. 13.4**). This autoimmune response leads to fibroblast activation, extraocular muscle edema, and later fibrosis. Similar events involving dermal fibroblasts may underlie thyroid dermopathy.

Diagnosis

There are two steps to making the diagnosis of Graves' disease; confirming the presence of thyrotoxicosis biochemically and then establishing the etiology (**Fig. 13.5**). An undetectable TSH

environmental susceptibility factors, which affect the processes of immunoregulation and allow autoimmune responses against the TSH receptor to emerge. There is a well established association with certain human lymphocyte antigen (HLA) alleles, particularly the HLA-DR3 specificity in Caucasians; several non-HLA loci are also likely to contribute to susceptibility, including

Autoimmune disorders associated with Graves' disease

Type 1 diabetes mellitus

Addison's disease

Pernicious anemia

Vitiligo

Alopecia areata

Myasthenia gravis

Celiac disease, dermatitis herpetiformis

Premature ovarian failure

Idiopathic thrombocytopenic purpura

Chronic active hepatitis, primary biliary cirrhosis

Systemic lupus erythematosus, rheumatoid arthritis

Table 13.2 Autoimmune disorders associated with Graves' disease.

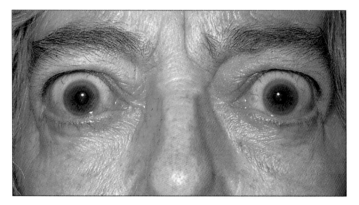

Figure 13.3 Thyroid-associated ophthalmopathy in Graves' disease. There is bilateral upper eyelid retraction, mild proptosis, and periorbital edema.

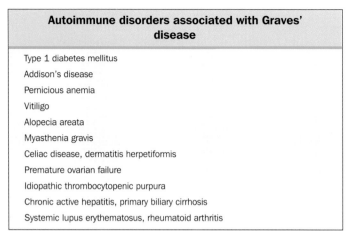

Figure 13.4 Pathogenic mechanisms in thyroid-associated ophthalmopathy. IL-1, interleukin-1; TNF, tumor necrosis factor; γ-IFN, gamma-interferon.

Causes of a low or undetectable TSH level

Lowered TSH	Free thyroid hormone levels
Overt thyrotoxicosis	↑
Subclinical thyrotoxicosis	N
Recently treated hyperthyroidism	N
Thyroid-associated ophthalmopathy without Graves' disease	N
Excessive thyroxine treatment	N or ↑
Nonthyroid illness (sick euthyroid syndrome)	↓ or N
First trimester of pregnancy	N or ↑
Pituitary or hypothalamic disease	N or ↓
Anorexia nervosa	N or ↓
Dopamine, somatostatin (acute effect)	N
Glucocorticoids	N
↑ = raised; ↓ = lowered, N = normal	

Table 13.3 Causes of a low or undetectable TSH level.

by sensitive immunoradiometric assay is a useful screening test for thyrotoxicosis, but a low or undetectable TSH level is not always due to thyrotoxicosis (**Table 13.3**). Thyrotoxicosis is confirmed by the presence of an elevated free thyroxine (T_4) level. Total T_4 levels give the same information but cannot be interpreted in the presence of thyroid hormone binding protein abnormalities, and therefore routine use of free hormone assays is preferable. At the beginning of most episodes of hyperthyroidism, T_3 but not T_4 is elevated (T_3-toxicosis) and therefore if the TSH level is suppressed but free T_4 levels are normal, free T_3 should be measured.

The diagnosis of Graves' disease in a patient with thyrotoxicosis is often based on clinical features (**Fig. 13.5**). The presence of a diffuse goiter with signs of ophthalmopathy or thyroid dermopathy confirms the diagnosis. Measuring the TSH-receptor antibodies that cause Graves' disease is the most definitive way to establish the diagnosis, but assays for TSH-receptor antibodies are not always routinely available and are not necessary in most cases. Antibodies to thyroid peroxidase or thyroglobulin are found in around 80% of Graves' patients, are easily measured and can be used as a surrogate to establish the autoimmune basis for the disease. In cases of doubt, and to rule out destructive thyroiditis (see below), radionuclide (^{99m}Tc, ^{123}I or ^{131}I) uptake studies are

useful, together with a thyroid scan. In Graves' disease, the isotope uptake is increased and there is diffuse thyroid enlargement (**Fig. 13.6**).

Around 10% of patients with ophthalmopathy have unilateral signs and, particularly when the patient is euthyroid, this raises the possibility of an alternative diagnosis (**Table 13.4**). Orbital computerized tomography (CT) or magnetic resonance imaging (MRI) is useful to confirm Graves' ophthalmopathy, recognized by the presence of enlargement in multiple extraocular muscles, with tendon sparing (**Fig. 13.7**). Other techniques for assessing ophthalmopathy include measuring MR T2 relaxation time and ^{111}In-octreotide scanning but these assessments require further evaluation. All patients with moderate to severe ophthalmopathy should have formal ophthalmologic evaluation (**Table 13.5**).

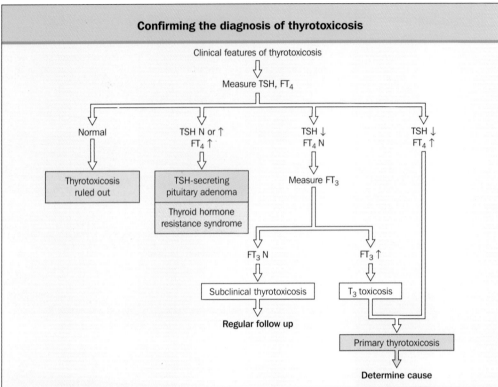

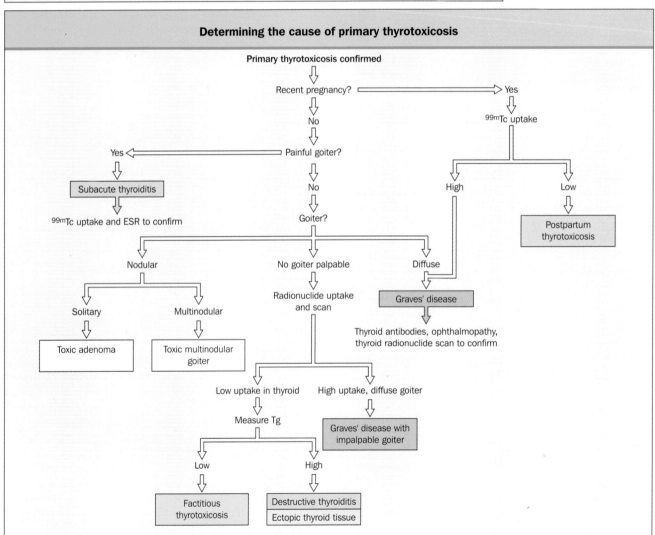

Figure 13.5 Flow charts for the investigation of suspected thyrotoxicosis. (Top panel) Confirming the diagnosis of thyrotoxicosis. (Bottom panel) Determining the cause of primary thyrotoxicosis. ESR, erythrocyte sedimentation rate; FT_4, free thyroxine; FT_3, free triiodothyronine; ↑, increased; ↓, decreased; N, normal; ^{99m}Tc, technetium-99m; Tg, thyroglobulin; TSH, thyroid-stimulating hormone.

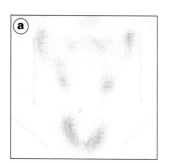
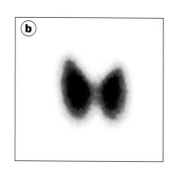
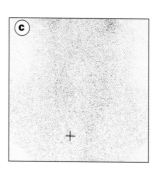

Figure 13.6 Technetium-99m thyroid scans. (a) Normal. (b) Graves' disease, showing enlarged thyroid with increased uptake. (c) Low, patchy uptake in destructive thyroiditis.

Differential diagnosis of Graves' ophthalmopathy	
Unilateral or bilateral proptosis	Orbital myositis or pseudotumor
	Arteriovenous malformation
	Neoplasia (e.g. lymphoma, glioma, metastasis)
	Granulomatous disease (e.g. sarcoidosis, Wegener's granulomatosis)
	Amyloidosis
Unilateral or bilateral proptosis	Infection
	Severe myopia or shallow orbits (e.g. Crouzon's syndrome)
	Cushing's syndrome
	Cirrhosis

Table 13.4 Differential diagnosis of Graves' ophthalmopathy.

Clinical manifestations

The signs and symptoms comprise those found in any cause of thyrotoxicosis and those specific for Graves' disease (**Table 13.6**). Thyrotoxic manifestations depend on the severity and duration of disease, and the age of the patient. While weight loss despite increased appetite is typical, with increasing age, weight loss becomes more frequent, accompanied by poor rather than increased appetite; atrial fibrillation occurs in up to a quarter of patients older than 50. Irritability and heat intolerance are less frequent in the elderly and may be associated with proptosis rather than exophthalmos. Apathetic thyrotoxicosis, mimicking depression, is another, less common type of presentation in the elderly. Decompensation of thyrotoxicosis, secondary to thyroid damage or to an intercurrent illness, may occur rarely, leading to thyrotoxic crisis (see below). Nonspecific biochemical abnormalities in thyrotoxicosis include abnormal liver function tests, elevated ferritin and sex-hormone-binding globulin, hypercalciuria, hypercalcemia, and hyperglycemia.

A diffuse goiter is clinically evident in most young patients but may be evident in only three quarters of the elderly. The main symptoms and signs of ophthalmopathy are listed in **Table 13.5**; these are more common in smokers, probably accounting for the higher frequency of ophthalmopathy in men and the elderly. Asians have a lower frequency of eye signs than western Caucasians. The commonest sign is lid retraction or lag, caused partly by sympathetic overactivity and partly by the ophthalmopathy autoimmune process (**Fig. 13.3**). Periorbital edema is another common feature (**Fig. 13.8**). A third of patients have proptosis, and diplopia, typically on upward and outward gaze, occurs in up to 10% (**Fig. 13.9**). Visual failure may be due to optic nerve compression by swollen extraocular muscles at the apex of the orbit (**Fig. 13.10**) or, less commonly, may be caused by corneal damage secondary to severe proptosis or chemosis, resulting in inability to protect the cornea (**Fig. 13.11**). The earliest signs of optic neuropathy are loss of color vision and a constriction of visual fields. Papilledema is present in rare patients.

Although the pretibial area is the most commonly affected by localized myxedema (**Fig. 13.12**), skin changes can occur at other sites, especially after trauma. In recognition of this, the term thyroid dermopathy is preferable to the older term, pretibial myxedema. The lesions are indurated, nonpitting and have no features of acute inflammation. Dermopathy occurs in around 1% of Graves' patients, almost always in the presence of moderate or severe ophthalmopathy. Thyroid acropachy (**Fig. 13.13**) is indistinguishable clinically from other forms of clubbing and is closely associated with dermopathy but less common.

Main signs and symptoms of thyroid-associated ophthalmopathy		
	Assessment	Approximate frequency (%)*
Lid lag, lid retraction	Measure lid fissure width	50
Grittiness, discomfort, excessive tearing, retrobulbar pain, periorbital edema	Self-assessment score by patient; activity score by clinician	40
Proptosis (or exophthalmos)	Exophthalmometry or CT/ MRI-based measurement	30
Extraocular muscle dysfunction (especially diplopia looking up and out)	Hess chart or similar; CT/MRI scan can be used to measure muscle size	10
Corneal involvement, resulting in exposure keratitis	Rose Bengal or fluorescein staining	<5
Loss of sight through optic nerve compression	Visual acuity and fields, color vision; CT/MRI scan	<1

* In patients with Graves' disease.
Patients often have multiple signs and, in 5–10%, signs are unilateral.

Table 13.5 Main signs and symptoms of thyroid-associated ophthalmopathy. CT, computerized tomography; MRI, magnetic resonance imaging.

Symptoms and signs of thyrotoxicosis	
Common to any cause of thyrotoxicosis	
Symptoms	Hyperactivity, irritability, altered mood, insomnia
	Heat intolerance, increased sweating
	Palpitations
	Fatigue, weakness
	Weight loss with increased appetite (occasional weight gain)
	Diarrhea, steatorrhea
	Polyuria
	Oligomenorrhea, amenorrhea, loss of libido
Signs	Sinus tachycardia, atrial fibrillation in the elderly
	Fine tremor, hyper-reflexia
	Warm, moist skin
	Goiter (character depends on cause)
	Palmar erythema, onycholysis, pruritus, urticaria, diffuse pigmentation
	Diffuse alopecia
	Muscle weakness and wasting, proximal myopathy
	Eyelid retraction or lag
	Gynecomastia
	Rarely: chorea, periodic paralysis (in Asian men), psychosis, high-output heart failure, thyrotoxic crisis
Specific for Graves' disease	
Ophthalmopathy (Table 13.5)	
Thyroid dermopathy	
Lymphoid hyperplasia (lymph nodes, thymus, spleen)	
Thyroid acropachy	
Associated autoimmune disease (Table 13.2)	

Table 13.6 Symptoms and signs of thyrotoxicosis.

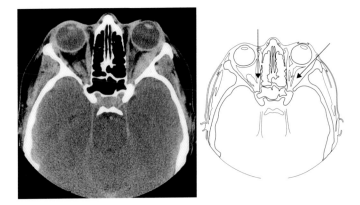

Figure 13.7 Computerized tomography scan showing enlarged extraocular muscles with tendon sparing in thyroid-associated ophthalmopathy.

Differential diagnosis

Thyrotoxicosis has a wide differential diagnosis that includes any cause of weight loss; the increase in appetite usual with Graves' disease is a useful clue. It is sometimes difficult to

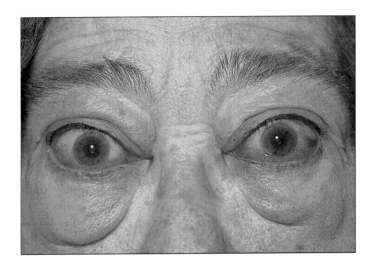

Figure 13.8 Periorbital edema in thyroid-associated ophthalmopathy.

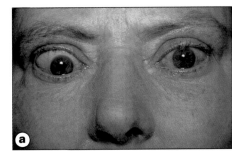
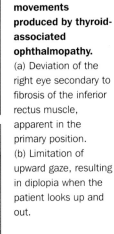
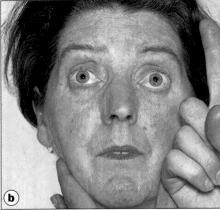

Figure 13.9 Abnormal eye movements produced by thyroid-associated ophthalmopathy.
(a) Deviation of the right eye secondary to fibrosis of the inferior rectus muscle, apparent in the primary position. (b) Limitation of upward gaze, resulting in diplopia when the patient looks up and out.

distinguish an anxiety state from thyrotoxicosis, but the palms are typically cool rather than warm in anxiety. Pheochromocytoma may also be suspected initially if palpitations and tremor are prominent. In the elderly, nonspecific tiredness and the presentation of apathetic thyrotoxicosis may be confused with depression.

Graves' disease is readily excluded in any differential diagnosis by simple testing, most easily by demonstrating a normal TSH level. A strategy for distinguishing Graves' disease from other causes of thyrotoxicosis is shown in **Figure 13.5**. Destructive thyroiditis, particularly in the postpartum period (see below), is the cause of thyrotoxicosis most often confused with Graves' disease, as thyroid peroxidase antibodies and a diffuse goiter

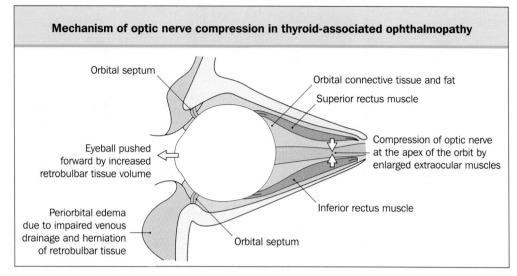

Mechanism of optic nerve compression in thyroid-associated ophthalmopathy

Orbital septum

Orbital connective tissue and fat

Superior rectus muscle

Eyeball pushed forward by increased retrobulbar tissue volume

Compression of optic nerve at the apex of the orbit by enlarged extraocular muscles

Periorbital edema due to impaired venous drainage and herniation of retrobulbar tissue

Inferior rectus muscle

Orbital septum

Figure 13.10 Mechanism of optic nerve compression in thyroid-associated ophthalmopathy. The edematous extraocular muscles and increased volume of the retrobulbar connective tissue and fat compress the optic nerve at the orbital apex. The same increase in tissue volume is responsible for proptosis, the severity of which is limited by the restriction provided by the orbital septum. A tight septum results in minimal proptosis but increases the risk of optic nerve compression, because the retrobulbar pressure is higher.

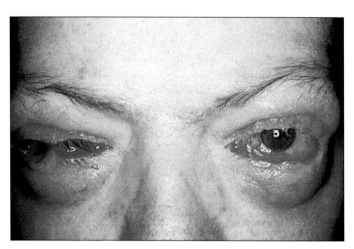

Figure 13.11 Severe chemosis and periorbital edema in congestive ophthalmopathy. Inability to cover the cornea may cause corneal damage. A suture has been inserted on the right hand side to prevent this (tarsorrhaphy) but surgical orbital decompression is now the preferred management.

occur in both conditions. Symptoms persisting longer than 2 months strongly suggest Graves' disease rather than a destructive thyroiditis and the diagnosis can be confirmed by demonstrating a diffuse, high radionuclide uptake (**Fig. 13.6**). This test can be performed safely in lactating women by using ^{99m}Tc and discontinuing breast feeding for 24 hours. The differential diagnosis of ophthalmopathy is shown in **Table 13.4**. Orbital imaging is used to distinguish between these conditions if the diagnosis is unclear on clinical grounds.

Treatment

There is considerable regional variation in the treatment recommended for Graves' disease at initial presentation and if it recurs. Antithyroid drugs (**Fig. 13.14**) reduce thyroid hormone synthesis in all types of hyperthyroidism but only cure Graves' disease, probably because the drugs have an immunomodulatory action, leading to a reduction in thyroid-stimulating antibodies, in addition to their biochemical effect of inhibiting the function of thyroid peroxidase. Even so, the success of treatment in the long-term is modest, with only 40–50% of patients remaining in remission 10 years or more after stopping antithyroid drugs. To improve this cure rate, and achieve definitive control of hyperthyroidism, radioiodine (^{131}I) is used increasingly as first-line treatment for Graves' disease, especially in the elderly. Radioiodine is also widely used to treat recurrence after antithyroid drugs, with surgery or indefinite antithyroid drug treatment being alternatives. In practice, an antithyroid drug is a reasonable choice for an initial episode of Graves' disease in patients under 50 years old, and radioiodine is usually recommended for patients over this age, as the adverse effects of hyperthyroidism are more serious, and for those with a recurrence. Surgery is usually reserved for those who are unwilling to have radioiodine.

Antithyroid drugs

There is little to choose between the three main antithyroid drugs (carbimazole, methimazole, and propylthiouracil) in the routine management of Graves' disease, although the additional ability of propylthiouracil to block T_4 to T_3 conversion may be useful in very severe thyrotoxicosis and thyrotoxic crisis. As the drugs usually take 2–3 weeks to control symptoms, propranolol 20–80mg three times a day can be added initially to block the sympathetic manifestations of thyrotoxicosis, but is not always needed. Antithyroid drugs can be administered by two equally effective methods, titration and block-replacement, to avoid hypothyroidism as treatment continues. In the titration regimen, the starting dose of antithyroid drug is gradually reduced to maintain euthyroidism and treatment is continued for 18–24 months. In the block-replace regimen a high dose of drug is used (carbimazole or methimazole 40mg daily or propylthiouracil 150mg three times daily) and thyroxine, 100μg daily, is added after 3–6 weeks. The dose of thyroxine is adjusted to maintain euthyroidism and treatment is continued for 6 months.

Outcome cannot be readily predicted but remission rates are highest in those with the least severe thyrotoxicosis and the smallest goiters. A low iodine intake is also associated with an increased remission rate. Relapses are most common in the year after stopping treatment, and patients should be reviewed every

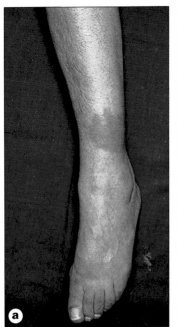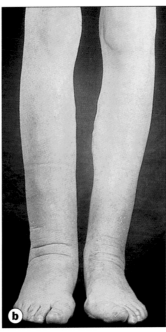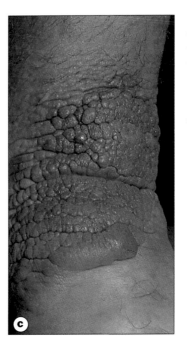

Figure 13.12 Thyroid dermopathy. (a) Localized plaque on the outer aspect of the skin. (b) Sheet-like involvement of the lower leg, with coarse skin, thickened hair, and nonpitting edema. (c) Horny form over shin and dorsum of the foot.

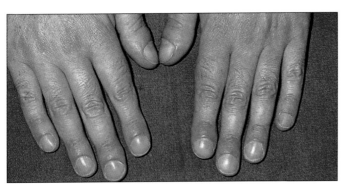

Figure 13.13 Thyroid acropachy. This is most marked in the index fingers and thumbs.

2–3 months during this period. Thereafter, annual followup is needed to check for recurrence or the emergence of hypothyroidism. Antithyroid drugs are the treatment of choice for Graves' disease in pregnancy but should be given only by the titration regimen (see below).

The side effects of antithyroid drugs (Table 13.7) most often occur during the first 3 months of treatment. If a rash occurs, one drug can be substituted for another, but if serious side effects such as agranulocytosis occur, all antithyroid drugs should be stopped. Patients must be given a warning sheet about side effects at the start of treatment, telling them in particular to stop medication and seek an urgent white cell count if a sore throat, fever, mouth ulcers, or other signs of infection develop.

There are few alternatives to the thionamide class of drugs. Potassium perchlorate and lithium both lower thyroid hormone secretion but are difficult to use, with serious side effects including, with perchlorate, a high frequency of agranulocytosis. The long-term outcome in terms of remission is unknown with these drugs but is unlikely to be satisfactory. Cholestyramine impairs the enterohepatic circulation of thyroid hormones and can be

used acutely to lower thyroid hormone levels, in combination with antithyroid drugs, more rapidly than with antithyroid drugs alone. Anticoagulation with warfarin (or use of aspirin if warfarin is contraindicated) should be considered in all patients in atrial fibrillation. Around half of such patients will return to sinus rhythm when euthyroid and cardioversion should be attempted in the remainder when they are euthyroid. In high-output heart failure due to thyrotoxicosis, rhythm control is essential and cautious use of beta blockers may be required to achieve this. If digoxin is indicated to control atrial fibrillation, higher doses than normal are needed in thyrotoxicosis, because of more rapid clearance of the drug while the patient is thyrotoxic.

Radioiodine

A wide range of dosage schedules for radioiodine have been employed, most easily classified as those based on radionuclide tracer studies to determine dosimetry, those based on clinical assessment of goiter size and the severity of hyperthyroidism, and the administration of a single, usually high (or ablation) dose of radioiodine. Accurate dosimetry calculations were often used in the past in the forlorn hope that a dose of radioiodine could be given that achieved euthyroidism without hypothyroidism. It is now obvious that a low rate of hypothyroidism is accompanied by an unacceptably high rate of recurrent hyperthyroidism and that hypothyroidism continues to occur indefinitely after radioiodine. Moreover, dosimetry measurements are inconvenient for the patient and wasteful of resources. The use of a single high dose of radioiodine to ablate the thyroid is based on the precept that hypothyroidism is inevitable, so that a high rate of early hypothyroidism is acceptable if more patients are reliably cured of the hyperthyroidism with a single radioiodine treatment. In fact, only two thirds of patients treated with a dose of 600MBq (16.2mCi) of ^{131}I are hypothyroid after a year, and a few patients still require a second dose. This approach therefore does not offer the predictability that makes it theoretically attractive.

Figure 13.14 Antithyroid drugs.

Antithyroid drugs			
Drug	Formula	Usual starting dose	Inhibitor of thyroxine deiodination?
Propylthiouracil	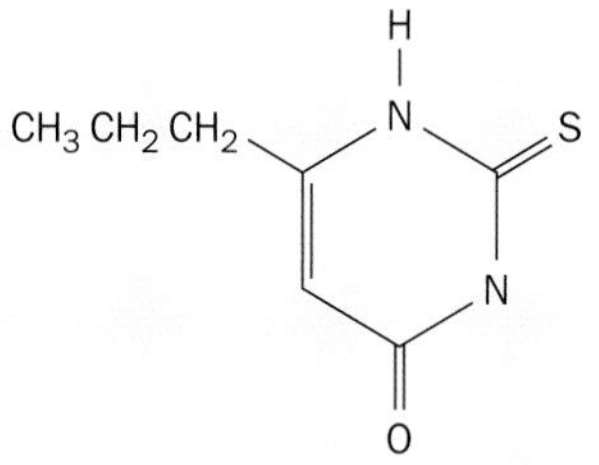	100–200mg three times daily	Yes
Carbimazole	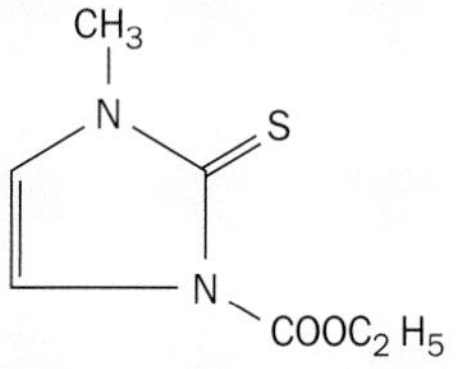	20mg two or three times daily	No
Methimazole (active metabolite of carbimazole)	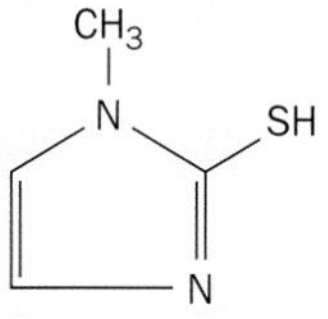	15–30mg twice daily	No

Side effects of antithyroid drugs	
Common	Rash
	Urticaria
	Arthralgia
	Fever and malaise
Uncommon	Gastrointestinal symptoms
	Abnormal taste and smell
	Arthritis
	Agranulocytosis*
Very rare	Thrombocytopenia
	Aplastic anemia
	Hepatitis
	Lupus-like syndrome, vasculitis
	Hypoglycemia (the insulin autoimmune syndrome)

* All patients must be warned, before treatment commences, to seek medical advice and stop medication if features suggesting agranulocytosis (fever, mouth ulcers, sore throat) develop.

Table 13.7 Side effects of antithyroid drugs.

Many centers now use simple clinical assessment to establish the required radioiodine dose. For example, in a patient with a small goiter, 200MBq (5.4mCi) of ^{131}I is given, with a large goiter 400MBq (10.8mCi) and for severe or completed hyperthyroidism (e.g. associated with heart failure) 600MBq (16.2mCi). Local iodine intake is an important determinant of the dose, less radioiodine being needed when dietary iodine is low. Conversely, pharmacologic iodine overload, usually due to certain contrast media, skin sterilizing solutions for surgery, or amiodarone, will prevent successful radioiodine treatment. Using this type of empiric dosage calculation, around 5–20% of patients will require a second dose of radioiodine. Hypothyroidism occurs in 10–20% within a year and then continues at a rate of 5–10% per year.

Outcome is also influenced by antithyroid drugs given before or after radioiodine. It is usual to stop antithyroid drugs several days before administration of radioiodine but the radioprotective effect of propylthiouracil may last for several weeks after stopping the drug. Patients with mild hyperthyroidism do not require antithyroid drugs before radioiodine, and can be managed symptomatically with beta-blockers. Patients who are elderly or have severe hyperthyroidism should be given a short course of antithyroid drugs to minimize the risk of thyrotoxic crisis (see below), e.g. carbimazole 20mg twice a day for 4 weeks. Antithyroid drugs are not usually needed after radioiodine but in patients with cardiac or other complications it may be helpful to maintain euthyroidism by resuming treatment with an antithyroid drug several days after radioiodine. If this is thought necessary, a higher than usual dose of radioiodine should be given to overcome the radioprotective effect of drug. The efficacy of radioiodine is enhanced by concurrent administration of lithium, which blocks the release of organic iodide (and hence radioiodine) from the gland. This effect may be useful in patients with very large goiters, who are often resistant to conventional doses of radioiodine.

Patients should be followed up every 2–3 months in the year after treatment. Hyperthyroidism within the first few months should be treated with beta-blockers or antithyroid drugs; a second dose of radioiodine should only be given 4–6 months after the first, as control of hyperthyroidism is slow. Hypothyroidism during this time may be temporary, caused by cytoplasmic rather

Time period (days) after administration of iodine-131 during which patients should take precautions				
	Dose of iodine-131 (MBq)			
	200	**400**	**600**	**800**
Avoid public transport	0	0	1	2
Remain off work	0	0	1	2
Avoid places of entertainment, or close contact with other people; remain off work if this entails close contact with others	1	5	9	12
Avoid close contact with pregnant women and children or radiosensitive work	14	21	24	27

Table 13.8 Time period (days) after administration of iodine-131 during which patients should take precautions. (Modified with permission from Guidelines: The use of radioiodine in the management of hyperthyroidism. Radioiodine Audit Sub-committee and Research Office, Royal College of Physicians of London, 1995, p. 16.)

than nuclear radiation damage. After a year, euthyroid patients should have an annual check of thyroid function and receive instructions about the symptoms of hypothyroidism that may appear in the period between blood tests.

Apart from hypothyroidism, radioiodine has few side effects. Pregnancy and breast feeding are absolute contraindications but there are no teratogenic effects if pregnancy is delayed for at least 4 months after treatment. Simple precautions are necessary with regard to radioprotection (**Table 13.8**). Rarely, an acute thyroiditis or sialadenitis may occur in the first few days after treatment. This settles spontaneously but may require nonsteroidal antiinflammatory drugs or even corticosteroids temporarily. Ophthalmopathy worsens or appears in up to 15% of Graves' patients treated with radioiodine, especially in smokers. Many prefer to avoid radioiodine in those patients with severe eye disease, or at least defer its use by giving antithyroid drugs until the eye signs are stable. An alternative is to give a 3-month tapering course of prednisolone, starting at 40mg daily at the time of radioiodine treatment, in those with moderate or severe eye disease. This prevents any worsening of ophthalmopathy but means that many patients receive steroids unnecessarily.

Overall mortality from cancer after radioiodine is not increased, but the mortality rate for thyroid and other individual cancers is higher than normal. It is unclear whether this is an effect of radioiodine or an association between Graves' disease and these malignancies, particularly as there is some evidence that thyroid cancer is more aggressive in Graves' disease because of the stimulatory action of thyroid-stimulating antibodies. However, this theoretic risk of malignancy makes many endocrinologists hesitant about using radioiodine in children and adolescents, unless there are no suitable alternatives.

Surgery

The surgical treatment of Graves' disease is subtotal or near-total thyroidectomy, the latter being preferable when performed by an experienced surgeon, as complication rates (except hypothyroidism) are not increased but the risk of recurrence is considerably reduced. The best centers produce cure in over 98% of

patients. The only absolute indication for surgery in Graves' disease is the coexistence of a thyroid nodule whose nature is uncertain and excision is required to exclude malignancy. However, surgery may be preferred by patients who cannot follow instructions about radioprotection, who wish to avoid any uncertainty of cure after a single dose of radioiodine, or who want rapid removal of an unsightly goiter.

Euthyroidism should be restored by antithyroid drug treatment prior to surgery to reduce the risk of thyrotoxic storm. Many surgeons also give stable iodine (e.g. Lugol's iodine three drops three times daily or potassium iodide capsules 60mg three times daily) for 7–10 days prior to surgery; this temporarily blocks thyroid hormone synthesis. Thyroidectomy has no adverse effect on ophthalmopathy. Apart from the possible complications of any surgical operation, subtotal or near-total thyroidectomy is associated with the risk of laryngeal edema secondary to hemorrhage, recurrent laryngeal nerve damage and hypoparathyroidism. The latter two may be transient and permanent hypocalcemia is easily treated with alfacalcidol. These complications occur in fewer than 1% of cases.

Graves' disease in pregnancy

Because of the high fetal loss and complications such as premature closure of the cranial sutures associated with neonatal thyrotoxicosis, women with Graves' disease should ideally defer pregnancy until their hyperthyroidism has been definitively treated. When Graves' disease occurs during pregnancy an antithyroid drug should be given in the smallest dose, titrated as necessary, to maintain maternal free T_4 levels in the upper half of, or just above, the reference range. The block-replace regimen should be avoided as this may result in fetal hypothyroidism, goiter, and impaired neurologic development. Although propylthiouracil probably crosses the placenta less well than methimazole, because it is more strongly protein-bound, there is actually little to choose between antithyroid drugs in terms of their effect on fetal thyroid function. There is continuing concern over an association between methimazole and carbimazole use and the development of fetal aplasia cutis and choanal atresia. Any connection must be very weak but many prefer to use propylthiouracil during pregnancy to avoid any suspicion of these adverse effects arising.

Maternal thyroid-stimulating antibody levels decline naturally during pregnancy and this usually induces remission of Graves' disease in the last trimester. Antithyroid drugs can usually be stopped at this time, but the woman is at increased risk of recurrence 2–6 months after delivery, and followup should be arranged with this in mind. Breast-feeding is safe with low doses of carbimazole (less than 20mg daily). Periodic checks of neonatal thyroid function should be performed when the mother is taking higher doses. Propylthiouracil is hardly excreted in milk and may be preferable for this reason in lactating women; daily doses of 400mg are not associated with effects on the baby.

Neonatal thyrotoxicosis is caused by the transplacental transfer of thyroid-stimulating antibodies from mother to baby and predictably occurs when there are very high levels of these antibodies in the mother's circulation during the last third of pregnancy. Fortunately it complicates only around 1% of Graves' pregnancies. The diagnosis is suggested by poor intrauterine growth and persistent fetal tachycardia. Measurement of TSH-receptor antibodies in the mother at the beginning of the third trimester is useful to predict those pregnancies at risk, and is particularly useful in women still taking antithyroid drugs at this time, as these cross the placenta and may mask signs of fetal hyperthyroidism. Treatment of the mother with an antithyroid drug during the last trimester is needed if there is fetal hyperthyroidism, otherwise the baby will have low birthweight, craniosynostosis, and impaired neurologic development. The effectiveness of intrauterine treatment can be monitored by measuring fetal free T_4 levels after cordocentesis if needed. Thyroid function should be assessed urgently at birth in all babies born to mothers with Graves' disease, and reassessed around 5 days after birth if the mother was taking antithyroid drugs at delivery. Neonatal thyrotoxicosis requires treatment of the baby with a careful titrated dose of antithyroid drug until the maternal antibodies disappear, usually 3 months after birth.

Thyroid-associated ophthalmopathy

Most patients with ophthalmopathy have only mild or moderate symptoms and signs. Reassurance, an explanation of the natural history of the eye disease and meticulous control of thyroid function are usually all that is necessary in such cases, although other simple measures such as lubricating eye drops and ointment may also be needed (Table 13.9).

Severe ophthalmopathy, with congestive changes anteriorly, threatening the cornea, worsening diplopia or optic nerve compression, demands more active intervention. First-line medical treatment consists of corticosteroids, which are often needed initially at high dosage, e.g. prednisolone 60–80mg daily. Some prefer to use daily intravenous boluses of 0.5–1g methylprednisolone initially, and then convert to oral steroids. Treatment should be tailed off slowly, over at least 3 months, to prevent recurrence. Even so, only around two thirds of patients fully improve, and often at the expense of major side effects. Orbital radiotherapy (usually 20Gy as 10 fractions over 2 weeks) is as effective as glucocorticoids but works more slowly and therefore cannot be relied on in those with optic neuropathy. Combined steroids and radiotherapy are therefore used in some centers.

Cyclosporin A may be added to steroids to improve outcome when steroids alone have failed, and azathioprine has been used as a steroid-sparing agent in those with cushingoid side effects. The place of other medical treatments is unclear and more work is needed in this area, particularly the development of safe and specific immunologic therapy.

When medical therapy is unsuccessful and vision is threatened, the only remedy is orbital decompression (Fig. 13.15). A number of surgical approaches have been used to achieve this, usually depending on the specialty of the surgeon doing the operation (ophthalmology, otorhinolaryngology, or neurosurgery). All give good results in expert hands but often with worsening of diplopia as a side effect, because the extraocular muscles prolapse into the space created by removal of part of the orbital wall. However, further surgery, once the eye disease is stable, can substantially correct this by recession or other techniques, and this rehabilitative surgery is also helpful for the more common type of strabismus occurring as a result of the ophthalmopathy disease process, where prisms have been tried and found inadequate. Eyelid surgery is indicated in patients with cosmetic problems, once the eye disease is stable (Fig. 13.16).

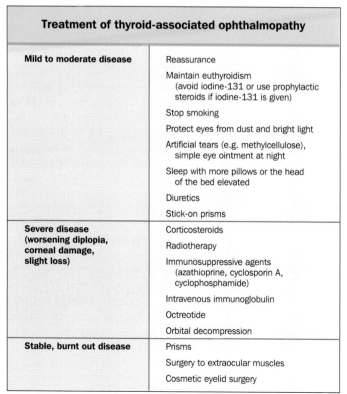

Treatment of thyroid-associated ophthalmopathy	
Mild to moderate disease	Reassurance
	Maintain euthyroidism (avoid iodine-131 or use prophylactic steroids if iodine-131 is given)
	Stop smoking
	Protect eyes from dust and bright light
	Artificial tears (e.g. methylcellulose), simple eye ointment at night
	Sleep with more pillows or the head of the bed elevated
	Diuretics
	Stick-on prisms
Severe disease (worsening diplopia, corneal damage, slight loss)	Corticosteroids
	Radiotherapy
	Immunosuppressive agents (azathioprine, cyclosporin A, cyclophosphamide)
	Intravenous immunoglobulin
	Octreotide
	Orbital decompression
Stable, burnt out disease	Prisms
	Surgery to extraocular muscles
	Cosmetic eyelid surgery

Table 13.9 Treatment of thyroid-associated ophthalmopathy.

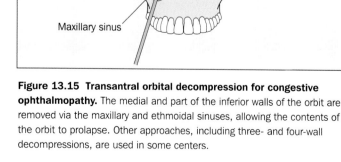

Figure 13.15 Transantral orbital decompression for congestive ophthalmopathy. The medial and part of the inferior walls of the orbit are removed via the maxillary and ethmoidal sinuses, allowing the contents of the orbit to prolapse. Other approaches, including three- and four-wall decompressions, are used in some centers.

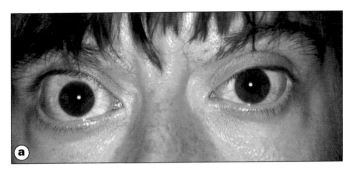

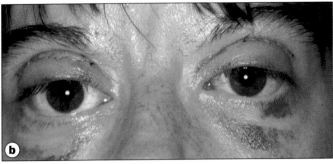

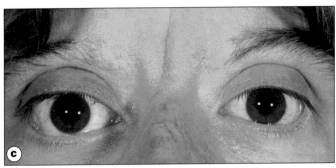

Figure 13.16 Outcome after surgical correction for lid retraction due to thyroid associated ophthalmopathy. (a) Presurgery. (b) Immediately after surgery. (c) Final result. (Courtesy of Professor I Rennie.)

Thyroid dermopathy

This is usually left untreated and can regress spontaneously. Surgery should be avoided as trauma may exacerbate the condition. When the skin lesions cause problems, e.g. with wearing shoes, potent topical corticosteroids can be used under an occlusive dressing. Octreotide, given in the conventional manner, may also improve dermopathy.

Complications

Thyrotoxic crisis or thyroid storm is a rare, life-threatening exacerbation of hyperthyroidism of any cause. There is usually a precipitating cause (**Table 13.10**). The severity of the clinical changes bear little relation to the circulating thyroid hormone levels, and the underlying mechanisms are unknown, although a rapid change in free thyroid hormone levels caused by saturation of binding sites on circulating transport proteins has been postulated. As well as the features of hyperthyroidism and marked fever and tachycardia, there can be vomiting, diarrhea, jaundice, delirium, seizures, and coma. Even with treatment, mortality is around 30% due to heart failure, arrhythmia, or hyperthermia.

Thyrotoxic crisis		
Precipitating causes	Thyroid damage	Surgery, radioiodine, or palpation of goiter in untreated or partially treated patients
	Severe illness	Nonthyroidal surgery, systemic infection, stroke, pulmonary embolus, diabetic ketoacidosis
	Parturition	
Treatment summary	Propylthiouracil 300mg 4-hourly by nasogastric tube or per rectum	
	Stable iodine (e.g. Lugol's iodine 8 drops 6-hourly) or ipodate 0.5g 12-hourly, starting 1 hour after propylthiouracil	
	Dexamethasone 2mg 6-hourly	
	Propranolol 40mg 4-hourly	
	External cooling	
	Intravenous fluids (caution in heart failure)	
	Treat precipitating cause	

Table 13.10 Thyrotoxic crisis.

Treatment has three elements: reduction of thyroid hormone secretion, supportive therapy, and treatment of any underlying disorder (**Table 13.10**). Propylthiouracil should be given, starting with 600mg and then 300mg every 4–6 hours. Rectal administration is used if a nasogastric tube cannot be placed. One hour later, stable iodine is given to further block thyroid hormone production; the delay is necessary to allow propylthiouracil to prevent excess iodine being incorporated in thyroid hormone synthesis. Ipodate 0.5g orally every 12 hours, or Lugol's iodine 5–8 drops or potassium iodide 60mg every 6 hours, can be used. Propranolol is also given orally (40–60mg 4-hourly) or intravenously (2mg 4-hourly).

Clinical outcomes

The natural history of Graves' disease is now impossible to determine. Temporary remission may occur in up to 20% of patients treated with beta-blockers alone, but the likelihood of permanent, spontaneous recovery is likely to be much less than this. Hypothyroidism develops in around 15% of those whose Graves' disease remains in remission 10–15 years after antithyroid drug treatment is stopped. This probably reflects the natural history of the autoimmune disorder rather than any effect of the drugs themselves. Historical data indicate a mortality rate of up to 30% in untreated Graves' disease and a slight increase in the mortality rate is still evident even after successful radioiodine treatment, as a result of cardiovascular disease, fracture of the femur, and thyrotoxic crisis.

Thyroid-associated ophthalmopathy typically runs a course in which there is worsening over 6–18 months, followed by a period of stabilization or, in up to two thirds with mild eye disease, improvement. Soft tissue changes are the most likely to improve, whereas longstanding diplopia secondary to fibrosis is unlikely to change. However, the course of ophthalmopathy in individual patients cannot be predicted reliably as there are many exceptions to this pattern and the orbital disease follows a natural history that

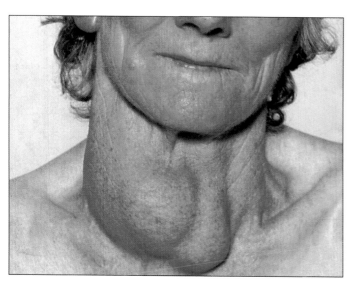

Figure 13.17 A large multinodular goiter with a dominant nodule in the right lobe.

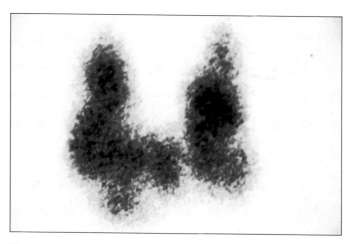

Figure 13.18 Technetium-99m thyroid scan of a multinodular goiter.

is largely independent of thyroid status, although more severe eye disease occurs in those patients who do not maintain euthyroidism.

TOXIC MULTINODULAR GOITER

Goiter occurs in around 5% of the population in iodine-sufficient areas, and is four times more common in women. Over half of goiters in adolescents disappear but many of the remainder change character from diffuse enlargement to multinodularity, and a proportion of these individuals subsequently develop hyperthyroidism (**Fig. 13.17**). The rate of progression to hyperthyroidism increases with age and iodine intake. The etiology of toxic multinodular goiter is unknown but it is likely that several factors contribute, including previous exposure to goitrogens, a low iodine intake in early life and genetic susceptibility.

Toxic multinodular goiter is the second most common cause of hyperthyroidism and the commonest cause in patients over 60 years old. Histologically there are unencapsulated, colloid-rich nodules, follicular hyperplasia and, in some cases, encapsulated adenomas. The nodules have varying degrees of function and this gives the characteristic pattern of 'hot' and 'cold' areas on radionuclide scans of the thyroid (**Fig. 13.18**). Some cold nodules are due to hemorrhage, fibrosis, and cyst formation rather than nonfunctional thyroid tissue.

Diagnosis

The confirmation of biochemical hyperthyroidism follows the same strategy as for Graves' disease (**Fig. 13.5**). A low or undetectable TSH and elevated free thyroid hormone concentrations establish that a clinically obvious, multinodular goiter is indeed toxic and nothing further by way of investigation is required. In some patients with a goiter that is difficult to palpate, Graves' disease is excluded by the absence of clinical features such as ophthalmopathy and negative thyroid antibodies. In cases of doubt, a radionuclide scintiscan will confirm the diagnosis (**Fig. 13.18**). Because thyroid autonomy becomes established slowly, many elderly patients with multinodular goiter are

investigated at a stage when the TSH level is low but the free thyroid hormone serum concentrations are normal, a state called subclinical hyperthyroidism (**Table 13.3**). Repeat testing should be performed 2–3 months later to establish whether there is any progression to overt hyperthyroidism, indicated by raised free T_3 levels. In the absence of progression, thyroid function should be checked at least annually, as such patients are clearly at risk of developing overt hyperthyroidism at an unpredictable time in the future.

Clinical manifestations

The features are those of any cause of thyrotoxicosis (**Table 13.6**). Sometimes it is the presence of the goiter that provokes biochemical testing and leads to the diagnosis of clinically unsuspected, mild thyrotoxicosis. The goiter can be of any size and may be asymmetric. Any retrosternal extension masks the true size of the thyroid (**Fig. 13.19**). Large goiters may produce local symptoms, such as neck discomfort, dysphagia, or stridor.

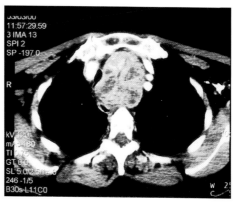

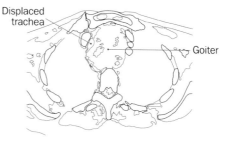

Displaced trachea

Goiter

Figure 13.19 Computerized tomography scan of the upper thorax showing retrosternal extension of a multinodular goiter, causing tracheal displacement and compression.

Treatment

Antithyroid drugs will control hyperthyroidism but not produce a cure. Radioiodine is therefore usually the treatment of choice, given at a larger dose (600–800MBq [16.2–21.6mCi]) that is typically given for Graves' disease, because there is uneven distribution of the isotope. In the very frail, or if incontinence poses a problem for the safe disposal of radioiodine-contaminated urine, indefinite treatment with an antithyroid drug can be used instead of radioiodine. If there is a retrosternal goiter, surgery may be preferable to radioiodine, as this can deal rapidly with any local compressive symptoms and allows histologic diagnosis of any suspicious intrathoracic nodules that are obviously not accessible to fine needle aspiration biopsy.

TOXIC ADENOMA

A solitary, hyperfunctioning nodule in the thyroid is the third most common cause of hyperthyroidism, accounting for around 5% of cases in areas of adequate iodine intake. In over half of all true toxic adenomas there is an activating mutation in the genes encoding the TSH receptor or the associated $G_{s\alpha}$ protein. The diagnosis is made by demonstrating a single thyroid nodule with radionuclide uptake in excess of the surrounding tissue in a patient with biochemically confirmed thyrotoxicosis. Usually there is little or no uptake in the remainder of the thyroid because production of excessive thyroid hormone by the autonomous nodule has suppressed the TSH necessary for stimulating the function of normal thyroid tissue (**Fig. 13.20**). For this reason, radioiodine is particularly effective treatment, as it is concentrated by the nodule but not the surrounding tissue, and the rate of subsequent hypothyroidism is therefore low. Surgical excision of the nodule is equally effective and is preferable for patients aged less than 20 years. Large nodules (>5cm) are more difficult to treat with radioiodine and surgery is also indicated in such patients.

JOD–BASEDOW PHENOMENON

The term Jod–Basedow is used to describe iodide-induced hyperthyroidism, which is more common in subjects with pre-existing thyroid disease, such as those with a nodular goiter, but can also occur in individuals with an apparently normal thyroid. It should be suspected in any patient presenting with hyperthyroidism after exposure to excessive iodide, although the source of the iodide excess may be difficult to identify (e.g. some contrast media). Typically, the free T_4 is greatly elevated in contrast to the free T_3 level. The condition is more common in iodide-deficient areas where nodular goiter is frequent. It is difficult to treat because of the large stores of preformed thyroid hormone in the gland, and may require treatment with corticosteroids and perchlorate along with antithyroid drugs.

DESTRUCTIVE THYROIDITIS

Thyrotoxicosis without hyperthyroidism can be caused by acute destruction of thyroid tissue, resulting in leakage of stored thyroid hormone from the colloid. The commonest causes are subacute (de Quervain's or viral) thyroiditis and silent thyroiditis. The latter is a transient autoimmune disorder that most

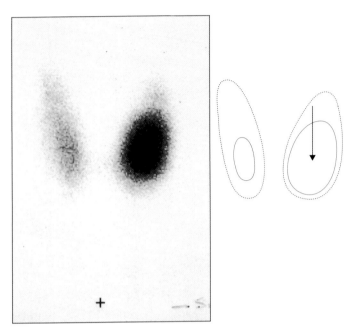

Figure 13.20 Technetium-99m thyroid scan of a toxic adenoma in the left lobe of the thyroid (arrow).

typically occurs as postpartum thyroiditis during the months after delivery in a woman who has preexisting autoimmune thyroiditis. Further details of the clinical features of these conditions are given in Chapter 11. The typical course of destructive thyroiditis is shown in **Figure 13.21**. Because the thyrotoxic phase is limited by the amount of hormone stored in the thyroid, the duration of this phase is usually around 3–8 weeks. The presence of thyrotoxicosis for more than 2 months virtually rules out these conditions. For those patients with symptoms of lesser duration, the main differential diagnosis is Graves' disease. A number of simple tests can be used to distinguish between these conditions (**Table 13.11**). It is important to make the correct diagnosis, as antithyroid drug treatment is useless in destructive thyroiditis; beta-blockers are all that is required to ameliorate symptoms until spontaneous recovery occurs.

AMIODARONE-INDUCED THYROTOXICOSIS

Amiodarone is an increasingly used antiarrhythmic agent that has diverse and, at first sight, paradoxical effects on thyroid function (**Table 13.12**). In all patients, there is partial inhibition of thyroid hormone deiodination, leading to a rise in circulating total and free T_4 levels and a modest reduction in total and free T_3 levels. As a result, free T_4 levels tend to be in the upper half or above the usual reference range and free T_3 levels in the lower half of the reference range. TSH levels show a small acute rise but thereafter return to normal. If only free T_4 levels are assessed in a patient on amiodarone, there is the potential for thyrotoxicosis to be suspected biochemically, while free T_3 levels at the upper limit of the reference range may represent a significantly increased level of T_3 that could mistakenly be assumed to be normal in a patient with true thyrotoxicosis.

In addition to these changes, which may confuse the unwary, amiodarone can cause hypothyroidism (Chapter 11) and two types of thyrotoxicosis. In type 1 amiodarone-induced

Differentiation of destructive thyroiditis from Graves' disease

	Graves' disease	Subacute thyroiditis	Silent/ postpartum thyroiditis
Ophthalmopathy present	Yes	No	No
Symptom duration >2 months	Yes	No	No
Tender goiter	No	Yes	No
Raised ESR/CRP	No	Yes	No
Technetium-99m uptake	High	Low	Low*

* Lactating women should stop breast feeding for 24 hours after a typical tracer dose of technetium-99m.

Table 13.11 Differentiation of destructive thyroiditis from Graves' disease. CRP, C-reactive protein; ESR, erythrocyte sedimentation ratio.

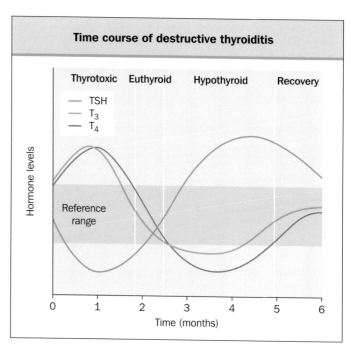

Figure 13.21 Time course of destructive thyroiditis. TSH, thyroid-stimulating hormone; T_3, triiodothyroxine; T_4, thyroxine.

thyrotoxicosis there is precipitation of incipient hyperthyroidism, usually due to Graves' disease or toxic multinodular goiter, by the high iodine load: each 200mg amiodarone tablet contains 75mg of iodine, 6mg of which is free. Essentially, this is an example of the Jod–Basedow phenomenon. By contrast, there is destructive thyroiditis with release of stored thyroid hormones in type 2 amiodarone-induced thyrotoxicosis, the consequence of lyso-somal activation by the drug (a similar mechanism is also responsible for amiodarone-induced lung damage). There is an associated intrathyroidal inflammatory response, primarily comprising macrophages. The two types of thyrotoxicosis can be distinguished by color-flow Doppler studies and circulating IL-6 levels but mixed forms occur that can make a clear-cut diagnosis impossible. Although thyroid function tests should routinely be performed in amiodarone-treated patients, this is primarily to pick up the slow emergence of hypothyroidism: thyrotoxicosis is usually of abrupt onset and difficult to predict unless there is a history of previous Graves' disease or multinodular goiter.

Treatment can be problematic. Discontinuing amiodarone is recommended but may not be possible on clinical grounds and is not guaranteed to reverse the thyrotoxicosis; in any case, the 40-day half-life of the drug means that any benefit is greatly delayed. The high intake of stable iodine generally prevents the immediate use of radioiodine, which would of course only help in the type 1 condition. Antithyroid drugs are less effective than usual, because of the state of iodine excess, but can be tried at high dosage, particularly when type 1 thyrotoxicosis is present. Their efficacy is greatly increased by adding prednisolone 40–60mg and this approach is particularly effective for type 2 thyrotoxicosis. In resistant cases, potassium perchlorate, 1g daily in divided doses, is often effective, as it reduces thyroidal iodine content. Failing that, urgent thyroidectomy should be considered in severe cases.

RARER CAUSES OF THYROTOXICOSIS

Even deliberate overtreatment with T_4, to suppress TSH levels in thyroid cancer (Chapter 12), is rarely associated with features of thyrotoxicosis unless greatly excessive doses are given, because there is regulation of T_3 release at the tissue level of T_4 deiodination. Occasional patients take thyroxine surreptitiously

Amiodarone effects on thyroid function

All patients

	Acute effect (up to 3 months)	After 3 months
T_4	↑	High N/↑
T_3	↓	Low N/↓
TSH	↑	N
rT_3	↑	↑

Specific long-term problems

	Frequency	Risk factor	Possible mechanism
Hypothyroidism	13% HID area 6% LID area	TPO Ab	Persistent block in thyroid hormone synthesis due to iodine
Thyrotoxicosis	2% HID area 12% LID area	Preexisting subclinical hyperthyroidism (type 1)	Jod–Basedow phenomenon (type 1); destructive thyroiditis (type 2)

↑ = increased; ↓ = decreased; N, normal

Table 13.12 Amiodarone effects on thyroid function. HID, high iodine diet; LID, low iodine diet; rT_3, reverse triiodothyronine; T_3, triiodothyronine, T_4, thyroxine; TPO Ab, thyroid peroxidase antibodies; TSH, thyroid-stimulating hormone.

to lose weight or boost energy, so-called *thyrotoxicosis factitia*. The diagnosis is suggested by a very high free T_4 level relative to the T_3 level; hyperthyroidism due to the Jod–Basedow phenomenon is the other typical cause of this biochemical picture. The demonstration of a low rather than high serum thyroglobulin level distinguishes thyrotoxicosis factitia from all other types of thyrotoxicosis.

Human chorionic gonadotrophin (hCG) weakly stimulates the TSH receptor and, when levels are extremely high, during the first trimester of pregnancy in some women, and more often in trophoblastic malignancies, this effect can cause hyperthyroidism. It is likely that differences in the glycosylation of hCG and its metabolism determine the ability of hCG to stimulate the thyroid, as there is variation in thyroid status between individuals with similar elevations of hCG. In 1–2% of normal pregnancies this effect of hCG may produce a modest elevation of free thyroid hormones with a suppressed TSH, a state termed *gestational hyperthyroidism*, which is usually transient and asymptomatic. However, some patients do experience symptoms, particularly hyperemesis gravidarum; around 50% of such women have evidence of hyperthyroidism. Treatment is usually supportive, particularly with intravenous fluids, as spontaneous resolution typically occurs within 1–2 weeks. Use of an antithyroid drug is logical in severe cases, but this can be stopped after 14 weeks, once Graves' disease has been excluded, as hCG levels are declining at this stage of pregnancy.

TSH-secreting pituitary adenomas (thyrotropinomas) are the rarest type of anterior pituitary tumor, especially those secreting a combination of growth hormone and TSH. Clinically, these tumors generally present with mild to moderate thyrotoxicosis, a diffuse goiter and local features of the tumor, which is often large (**Fig. 13.22**). In contrast to other types of thyrotoxicosis (**Table 13.1**), the TSH is normal or elevated. The only other condition to cause elevated thyroid hormone levels with a normal or elevated TSH is *thyroid hormone resistance syndrome*, the result of mutation in one allele of the β thyroid hormone receptor gene. Thyrotoxic features are unusual in this syndrome and this explains

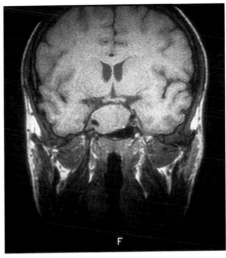

Figure 13.22 Thyroid-stimulating-hormone-secreting pituitary adenoma. These are usually large tumors, as in this case with lateral and small suprasellar extensions.

the normal levels of ferritin, sex-hormone-binding globulin, and liver enzymes, which are usually elevated in patients with hyperthyroidism, including those cases arising from a TSH-secreting pituitary tumor. The differentiation of the two conditions can be made readily by measuring α subunit levels (elevated in TSH-secreting pituitary tumors) and demonstrating the tumor by CT or MRI imaging. Direct mutational analysis of the thyroid hormone receptor gene confirms a resistance syndrome, which is an autosomal dominant condition. Treatment of a TSH-secreting pituitary tumor follows conventional lines (Chapter 3), hyperthyroidism prior to surgery being controlled by an antithyroid drug or octreotide. Thyroid hormone resistance syndrome does not usually require treatment; ill-advised attempts to normalize thyroid hormone levels cause hypothyroidism. Thyrotoxic symptoms may respond to beta-blockers; rarely triac, a thyroid hormone analog, may be needed to lower TSH secretion.

FURTHER READING

Bartalena L, Pinchera A, Marcocci C. Management of Graves' ophthalmopathy: reality and perspectives. Endocrine Rev. 2000;21:168–99.

Beck-Peccoz P, Brucker-Davis F, Persani L, Smallridge RC, Weintraub BD. Thyrotropin-secreting pituitary tumors. Endocrine Rev. 1996;17:610–38.

Brix TH, Kyvik KO, Hegedüs L. What is the evidence of genetic factors in the etiology of Graves' disease? A brief review. Thyroid 1998;8:727–32.

Burch HB, Wartofsky L. Graves' ophthalmopathy: Current concepts regarding pathogenesis and management. Endocrine Rev. 1993;14:747–93.

Davies TF ed. Newer aspects of clinical Graves' disease. Baillière's Clin Endocrinol Metab. 1997;11:431–601.

Hermus AR, Huysmans DA. Treatment of benign nodular thyroid disease. N Engl J Med. 1998;338:1438–47.

Koutras DA. Subclinical hyperthyroidism. Thyroid 1999;9:311–5.

Mourits MP, van Kempen-Harteveld ML, García MB, Koppeschaar HPF, Tick L, Terwee CB. Radiotherapy for Graves' orbitopathy: Randomised placebo-controlled study. Lancet 2000;355:1505–9.

Newman CM, Price A, Wyn-Davies D, Gray T, Weetman AP. Amiodarone and the thyroid: a practical guide to the management of thyroid dysfunction induced by amiodarone therapy. Heart 1998;79:121–7.

Rapoport B, Chazenbalk GD, Jaume JC, McLachlan SM. The thyrotropin (TSH) receptor: interaction with TSH and autoantibodies. Endocrine Rev. 1998;19:673–716.

Rivkees SA, Sklar C, Freemark M. The management of Graves' disease in children, with special emphasis on radioiodine treatment. J Clin Endocrinol Metab. 1998;83:3767–76.

Radioiodine Audit Subcommittee of the Royal College of Physicians Committee on Diabetes and Endocrinology and Research Unit of the Royal College of Physicians. Guidelines: The use of radioiodine in the management of hyperthyroidism. London:Royal College of Physicians of London; 1995.

Tonacchera M, Vitto P, Agretti P, et al. Functioning and non-functioning thyroid adenomas involve different molecular pathogenetic mechanisms. J Clin Endocrinol Metab. 1999;84:4155–8.

Vanderpump MP, Ahlquist JA, Franklyn JA, Clayton RN. Consensus statement for good practice and audit measures in the management of hypothyroidism and hyperthyroidism. Br Med J. 1996;313:539–44.

Weetman AP. Graves' disease. N Engl J Med. 2000; 343:1236–48.

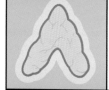

Section 3 Adrenal

Chapter 14

Adrenal Cortex Physiology

D Lynn Loriaux and Vivian H T James

INTRODUCTION

The human adrenal glands are paired structures, situated at the upper pole of each kidney. Each gland is shaped roughly like a cocked hat, is highly vascularized, and weighs approximately 4–5g in a normal healthy adult. The outer cortex, comprising 90% of the gland, surrounds the central medulla. The cortex is a zonated structure (**Fig. 14.1**) and is covered by a thin capsule, below which isolated groups of glomerulosa cells are found. Most of the cortex is made up of the zona fasciculata and the zona reticularis, the latter adjoining the medulla. The blood supply is derived from the inferior phrenic artery, the aorta, and the renal arteries, and is largely subcapsular. The venous circulation within the gland is complex and is thought to play an important role in regulating steroid synthesis. The central vein from the right adrenal is short and enters the inferior vena cava directly, whereas that from the left adrenal drains into the left renal vein.

HORMONE PRODUCTION IN THE GLOMERULOSA CELLS

The adrenal cortex produces three major types of steroid hormone: mineralocorticoids, glucocorticoids, and androgens. The source of the mineralocorticoids (aldosterone and, in part, deoxycorticosterone) is the zona glomerulosa. The major factor controlling aldosterone secretion is angiotensin, but increased plasma potassium concentration is also an efficient aldosterone-stimulating agent (**Fig. 14.2**). The role of corticotropin (adreno-corticotropic hormone, ACTH) is less clear; it is more effective in salt-depleted subjects than in those with normal salt balance, and is probably relatively unimportant in the normal situation. There is also evidence of the existence of other factors, as yet unknown.

Angiotensin I is formed from angiotensinogen substrate by the action of renin. Renin synthesis occurs in the juxtaglomerular cells of the kidney and is released in response to changes in tubular sodium concentration, renal arteriolar blood pressure, and stimulation via sympathetic nerves. The decapeptide angiotensin is converted into the octapeptide angiotensin II by a converting enzyme (angiotensin converting enzyme: ACE); this conversion takes place primarily, but not exclusively, in the lungs. The heptapeptide angiotensin III is also formed and can stimulate aldosterone secretion, although a physiologic role for it has not yet been established.

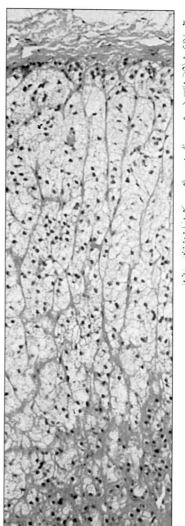

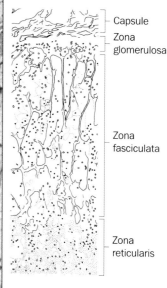

- Capsule
- Zona glomerulosa
- Zona fasciculata
- Zona reticularis

Figure 14.1 Histologic section of an adrenal gland. The medulla represents 10% of the gland, while the remaining 90% is made up of cortical tissue – the zonae glomerulosa, fasciculata, and reticularis. The whole gland is surrounded by a fibrous capsule below which the zona glomerulosa cells appear only focally. Hematoxylin–eosin stain, magnification × 250.

HORMONE PRODUCTION IN THE FASCICULATA AND RETICULARIS CELLS

Cortisol and the adrenal androgens are derived from the fasciculata and reticularis cells. The only known important control mechanism is by means of ACTH (**Fig. 14.3**). This anterior pituitary hormone regulates adrenocortical growth; it also

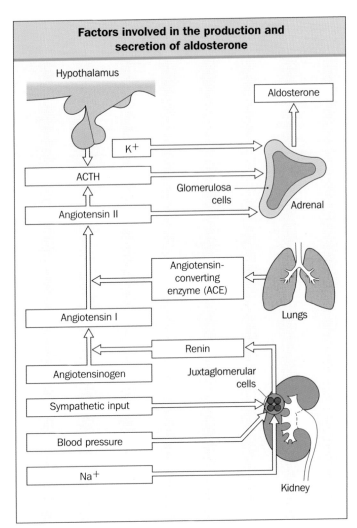

Figure 14.2 Factors involved in the production and secretion of aldosterone. The major factor influencing aldosterone secretion is angiotensin, although an increased plasma potassium concentration also contributes. Renin output, in turn, is regulated by sympathetic tone, blood pressure, and tubular sodium concentration. ACTH, adrenocorticotropic hormone.

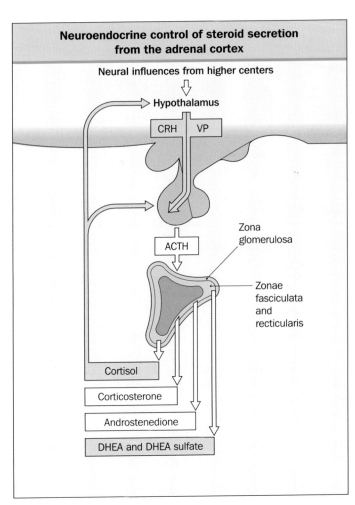

Figure 14.3 Neuroendocrine control of steroid secretion from the adrenal cortex. Negative feedback in the hypothalamus and pituitary operates through cortisol and, to a minor extent, through corticosterone. Thus, high cortisol levels suppress adrenocorticotropic hormone (ACTH) output, whereas low cortisol levels stimulate ACTH production by increasing the release of corticotropin-releasing hormone (CRH) and also by increasing the sensitivity of ACTH to CRH.

mediates the rate at which steroid biosynthesis occurs. Other fragments of the ACTH precursor, pro-opiomelanocortin, may also have a trophic effect on the adrenal, and vasopressin (VP, antidiuretic hormone) may act synergistically with ACTH to stimulate steroid biosynthesis.

The effect of ACTH is rapid, occurring within a few minutes. The release of ACTH, leading to the secretion of cortisol and androgen, occurs episodically throughout the 24-hour cycle in a circadian pattern. ACTH release occurs in response to low circulating levels of cortisol (as in Addison's disease) and is inhibited by high circulating levels of cortisol or synthetic glucocorticoids (as in corticosteroid therapy). This negative feedback occurs at *both* hypothalamic and pituitary sites. ACTH is also released in response to stress (such as trauma, surgery, anxiety, and emotional disturbance).

MECHANISM OF ACTION OF ADRENOCORTICOTROPIC HORMONE

Adrenocorticotropic hormone acts on the adrenal gland by binding to a specific receptor in the membrane of the cell (**Fig. 14.4**). This results in the stimulation of the membrane-bound adenylate cyclase enzyme, leading to rapid production of intracellular cyclic adenosine monophosphate (cAMP), a mechanism that may also involve calcium entry into the cell. Other cyclic nucleotides such as cyclic guanosine monophosphate (guanylic acid, cGMP) may also be important. cAMP, in turn, activates a protein kinase (by dissociating an active subunit), which then stimulates a number of protein-phosphorylation processes using adenosine triphosphate. The role of the phosphoproteins that are formed is to enhance the reaction converting cholesterol

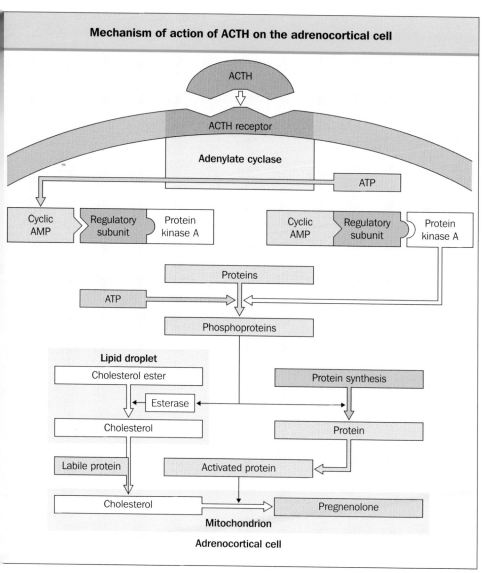

Figure 14.4 Mechanism of action of ACTH on the adrenocortical cell. The adrenocorticotropic hormone receptor is linked to the adenylate cyclase membrane enzyme system, which is responsible for cyclic adenosine monophosphate (cAMP) production. This 'second messenger' triggers the intracellular events that are responsible for steroid production and secretion. Pregnenolone is subsequently converted to other corticosteroids (see Figs 14.6 and 14.12). ACTH, adrenocorticotropic hormone; ATP, adenosine triphosphate.

into pregnenolone. This reaction can be inhibited by cyclohexamide, indicating that new protein synthesis is necessary for the process. At least one such protein, steroid acute regulatory (STAR) protein, a unique 37kDa phosphoprotein, has been well characterized. STAR enters the mitochondria, is cleared to a 30kDa form, and acts on the outer mitochondrial membrane to enhance the conversion of cholesterol to pregnenolone. This pregnenolone is the substrate for steroid hormone biosynthesis.

Angiotensin II binds to specific high-affinity sites in the plasma membrane of the adrenal glomerulosa cell. Unlike ACTH, cAMP does not appear to be a 'second messenger' in aldosterone biosynthesis. Sensitivity to angiotensin is increased by sodium deficiency, with the formation of more angiotensin receptors and an increase in binding affinity. The major pathway involved in the biosynthesis of aldosterone is probably as shown in **Figure 14.5**, although others almost certainly exist and may be important in particular conditions.

Cortisol and androgens are synthesized from cholesterol, which is mainly derived from circulating cholesterol esters, although intracellular cholesterol biosynthesis also occurs (**Fig. 14.6**). Low-density lipoprotein (LDL) is an important source of cholesterol, particularly during ACTH stimulation.

Specific enzymes and cofactors are required for glucocorticoid and androgen biosynthesis. These enzymes are located either in the smooth endoplasmic reticulum or in the mitochondria within each cell. Movement of substrate between these organelles is therefore necessary, and this mechanism of intracellular transport may require specific steroid-binding proteins. Thus, intracellular feedback effects of intermediates in the earlier biosynthetic steps may be of importance in regulating cholesterol biosynthesis.

Hydroxylation steps in the biosynthesis of adrenal steroids (**Fig. 14.7**) require nicotinamide adenine dinucleotide phosphate (NADPH), molecular oxygen, and an enzyme complex. The complex consists of a flavoprotein dehydrogenase, a nonhem

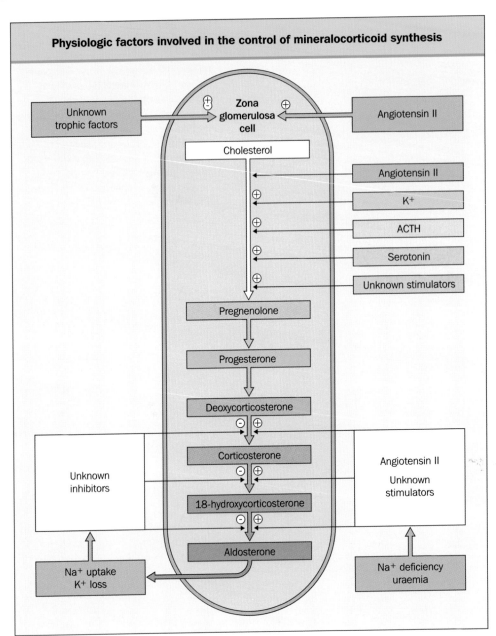

Physiologic factors involved in the control of mineralocorticoid synthesis

Figure 14.5 Physiologic factors involved in the control of mineralocorticoid synthesis. Angiotensin II appears to be the major stimulus of mineralocorticoid synthesis and secretion. Other factors play a minor role. ACTH, adrenocorticotropic hormone.

iron-containing protein (adrenodoxin), and cytochrome P450 (so called since a characteristic spectrophotometric absorption band is observed when it complexes with carbon monoxide). This oxidase system is essentially similar for 11β-, 20,22-, 17α and 18-hydroxylation, and it appears that specificity is achieved through differences in the respective P450 cytochromes. Hydroxylation is mediated by the introduction of one electron into the electron transport chain, with the introduction of one atom of oxygen into the steroid. The remaining oxygen atom combines with hydrogen to form water. This system is known as a 'mixed-function oxidase'.

Biosynthesis of the adrenocortical steroids is thus effected by the interaction of the various steroid hydroxylases: $P450_{scc}$, $P450_{C21}$, $P450_{C21}$, $P450_{C17\alpha}$ and $P450_{C11\beta}$. In addition, 3β-hydroxysteroid dehydrogenase isomerase is required to change the structure in ring A to the important 4-ene-3-one configuration. $P450_{C21}$ appears to be capable only of effecting hydroxylation at C21 (e.g. of 17-hydroxyprogesterone to 11-deoxycortisol), whereas other hydroxylases are multifunctional. Thus, $P450_{scc}$ effects hydroxylation at C20 and C22, and also acts as a 20,22 lyase. $P450_{C17\alpha}$ mediates hydroxylation at C17α and also acts as a 17,20 lyase. This enzyme is absent from the zona glomerulosa cells, which

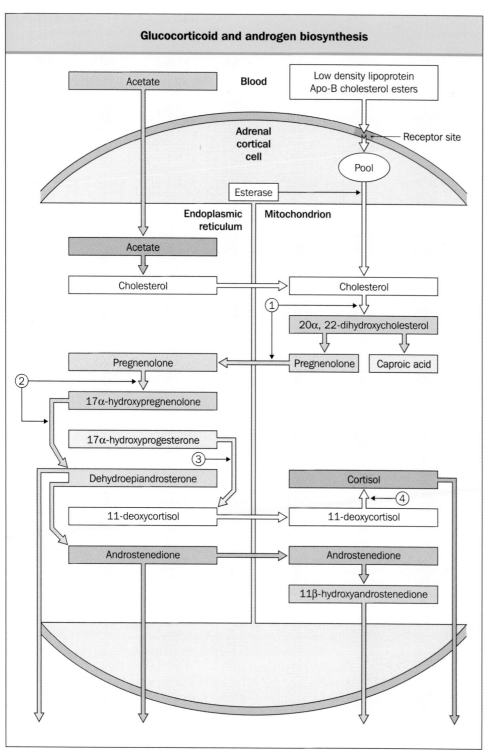

Figure 14.6 Glucocorticoid and androgen biosynthesis. An adrenocortical cell showing the intracellular organelles in which biosynthesis of glucocorticoid and androgen occurs from a cholesterol precursor. Low-density lipoprotein is the major cholesterol-transport lipoprotein in human blood, and most of this cholesterol is located in the central core and is esterified. The core is surrounded by a small amount of free cholesterol, phospholipids, and a protein known as apolipoprotein B (Apo B). This is specifically bound to the cell-surface receptor site. It is this mechanism that is postulated as the major route of cholesterol entry to the adrenocortical cells. The sites of action of the cytochrome P450 enzymes that are involved in steroidogenesis are shown: ¿, $P450_{scc}$ (cholesterol side-chain cleavage); ≠, $P450_{C17\alpha}$ (17α-hydroxylation); ¬, $P450_{C21}$ (21-hydroxylation); √, $P450_{C11\beta}$ (11β-hydroxylation).

limits the steroidogenic capacity of the cells to mineralocorti-coid production. $P450_{C11\beta}$ causes hydroxylation at C11, C18, and C19, and can also act in some species as an aromatase.

Molecular biologic techniques have been employed with considerable effect to widen our knowledge of the structure of the steroid hydroxylase genes and of the mechanism of action of ACTH. Human $P450_{scc}$, $P450_{C17\alpha}$, and $P450_{C21}$ are encoded by a single mRNA species, some 2kb in length. Bovine $P450_{C11\beta}$ is encoded by three mRNAs, with the smallest being 4.3kb in length. Exposure of adrenocortical cells to ACTH (or cAMP) causes the accumulation of all four P450 steroidogenic enzymes, as well as of adrenodoxin and adrenodoxin reductase. Chronic exposure to ACTH involves transcription of the genes for steroid hydroxylases. The structure of the genes has now been elucidated: $P450_{C11\beta}$ contains nine exons and is located on chromosome 15; $P450_{C17\alpha}$ also contains nine exons and is located on

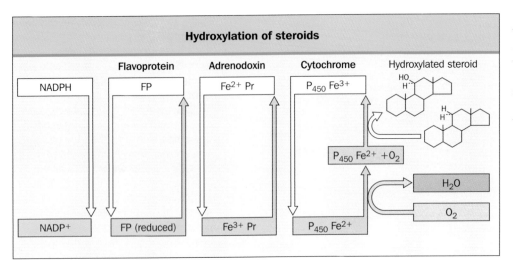

Figure 14.7 Hydroxylation of steroids. The role of nicotinamide adenine dinucleotide phosphate (NADPH), a flavoprotein, and cytochrome P$_{450}$ in the hydroxylation of steroids. All hydroxylation steps share this common pathway. Fe PR, nonhem iron-containing protein; FP, flavoprotein.

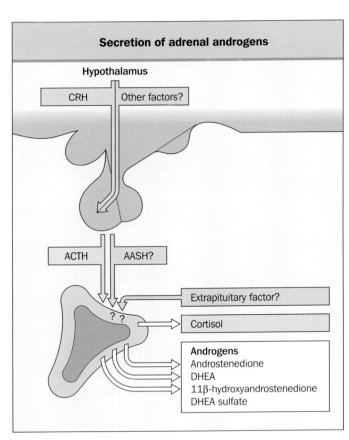

Figure 14.8 Secretion of adrenal androgens. The diagram shows the possible control mechanisms involved. Although adrenocorticotropic hormone (ACTH) seems to be an important physiologic regulator of adrenal androgen production, there is evidence supporting the existence of another separate hormone, adrenal androgen-stimulating hormone (AASH – as yet unidentified), which stimulates dehydroepiandrosterone (DHEA)-sulfate production. CRH, corticotropin-releasing hormone.

chromosome 8. There are possibly two gene products of $P450_{C11\beta}$, one that uses 11-deoxycortisol as a substrate to produce cortisol, and the other involved in the final synthesis of aldosterone. The $P450_{C17\alpha}$ gene is on chromosome 10 and contains eight exons; and

the $P450_{C21}$ gene contains 10 exons and is closely united to a pseudogene on chromosome 6 in the histocompatibility leukocyte antigen locus.

The steroid hydroxylases represent three gene families in the P450 superfamily. It seems likely that these genes have evolved from a common progenitor, several hundred million years ago, into distinct steroid hydroxylase gene families that now catalyze specific reactions.

CONTROL OF ANDROGEN SECRETION

The main 'adrenal androgens' are androstenedione, dehydroepiandrosterone (DHEA), 11-hydroxyandrostenedione, and DHEA sulfate, some of which are 'prohormones' of testosterone. The possible control mechanisms involved in the secretion of these androgens are shown in **Figure 14.8**. Although ACTH is capable of stimulating adrenal androgen secretion, there are several well-documented situations in which secretion of cortisol and 'adrenal androgens' is dissociated.

In addition, the secretion of 'adrenal androgens' has a 'lifelong' pattern of high secretion in infancy, falling to very low levels in childhood, rising again in the preadolescent years, and 'peaking' in early adulthood (adrenarche) followed by a progressive fall into senescence. These dramatic changes are not associated with measurable changes in ACTH secretion. These findings have led to the concept of an additional factor, adrenal androgen-stimulating hormone (AASH – as yet undefined), which can specifically stimulate adrenal androgen secretion. Prolactin has been invoked as such a factor, since hyperprolactinemia is associated with increased production of DHEA sulfate in the rat and in some patients, but this appears to be only a pathologic phenomenon. Other largely discredited agents are growth hormone, estrogen, and gonadotropins. It is possible that nonACTH peptides that are derived from the precursor of ACTH may be involved, but this is still to be established.

CIRCADIAN VARIATION

Adrenocorticotropic hormone is secreted episodically throughout a 24-hour period. There are between seven and 13 episodes,

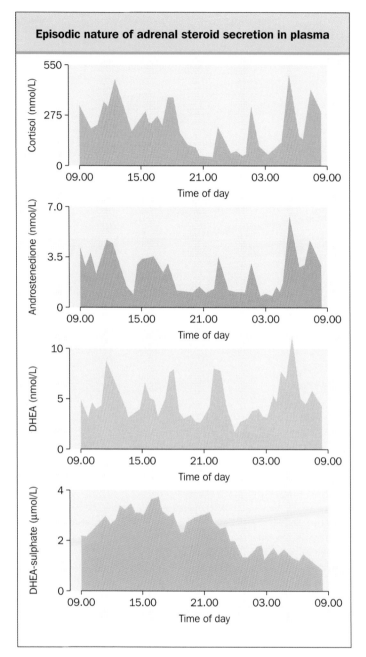

Figure 14.9 Episodic nature of adrenal steroid secretion in plasma.
DHEA, dehydroepiandrosterone.

such as that which occurs after travel across time zones, and 5–7 days (1 day/hour of time change) are required to complete the shift. Alterations of circadian rhythm also occur in disease states that short-circuit the hypothalamus, such as Cushing's syndrome. It is also 'phase advanced' in most cases of depressive illness.

Aldosterone is also secreted episodically, and the pattern closely resembles that for cortisol (**Fig. 14.10**). The mechanism and purpose of the episodic release of aldosterone, however, are unknown. The release of aldosterone is not caused by ACTH release, since aldosterone secretion continues to follow an episodic pattern of release in the absence of ACTH, nor is it due to changes in plasma potassium or sodium levels. Furthermore, it is not entirely established whether the periodicity is caused by changes in angiotensin. Whatever mechanism is involved, it is apparently closely coordinated with that which causes ACTH release. As with cortisol, the pattern appears to be disrupted by disease.

Stress also causes the release of ACTH and other pituitary hormones (such as growth hormone and prolactin). Chronic stress (anxiety or trauma) produces prolonged elevation of ACTH levels and thus an increase in cortisol secretion. In the investigation of patients with suspected hypopituitarism, it is clinically advantageous to be able to provoke ACTH release by producing controlled hypoglycemia. The integrity of the hypothalamic–pituitary–adrenal axis may thus be examined by measuring the plasma concentration of cortisol (**Fig. 14.11**) and, if necessary, of other pituitary hormones that are released by stress, e.g. prolactin and growth hormone.

BIOSYNTHESIS OF STEROID HORMONES

The overall scheme of biosynthesis of steroid hormones is shown in **Figure 14.12**. Although the pathways are common to the various steroids shown, specificity is achieved by specific receptors for ACTH or angiotensin, and also by the location of specific enzyme systems. Thus, the glomerulosa cells lack 17-hydroxylase and do not participate in the synthesis of cortisol or androgens, for which this enzyme is essential. Conversely, fasciculata and reticularis cells lack the enzyme 18-hydroxylase and cannot synthesize aldosterone. All cells can produce deoxycorticosterone, however, since the proximal pathway is common to both of these enzyme systems.

Steroid production

At normal plasma concentrations, approximately 90% of cortisol is bound to the specific binding protein – corticosteroid-binding globulin (CBG). The average production rate of cortisol is 12–15mg/m^2/day. More stringent measurements using deuterated cortisol infusions consistently reduce the accepted production rate by about half. Cortisol is metabolized rapidly, mainly by the liver, and has a plasma half-life of approximately 2 hours; the metabolic clearance rate is 200L/day. The major metabolites are formed by reduction of the double bond and ketone groups to produce tetrahydrocortisol, tetrahydrocortisone, cortol, and cortolone (**Fig. 14.13**). These are excreted into the urine in conjugation with glucuronic acid and

most of which occur during the second half of the normal sleep period and which are largely reproducible from one 24-hour period to another. Since cortisol and all of the 'adrenal androgens' are responsive to ACTH, there are also episodic changes in the peripheral plasma levels of these steroid hormones throughout the day (DHEA sulfate does not appear to respond, but this is because of its very long plasma half life of about 9 hours) (**Fig. 14.9**). It is not known what factors cause this pattern of ACTH release, and the physiologic advantage, if any, is also not clear. The 'rhythm generator' is located in the hypothalamus. The rhythm is shifted by an alteration in the sleep–wake pattern,

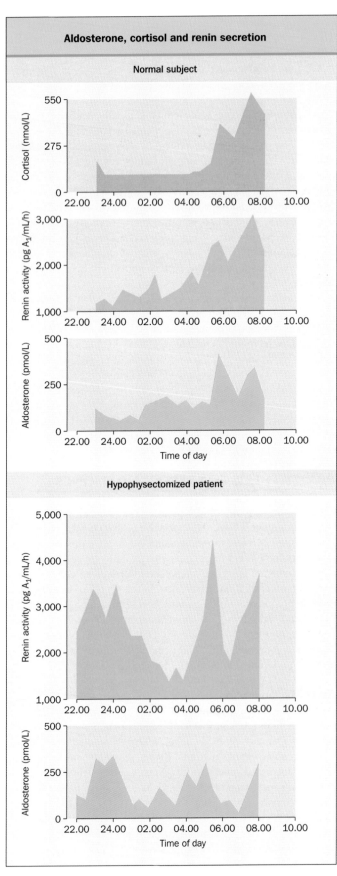

Aldosterone, cortisol and renin secretion

Normal subject

Hypophysectomized patient

Figure 14.10 Aldosterone, cortisol, and renin secretion. The mechanism behind these closely coordinated patterns in serum levels over time is unclear.

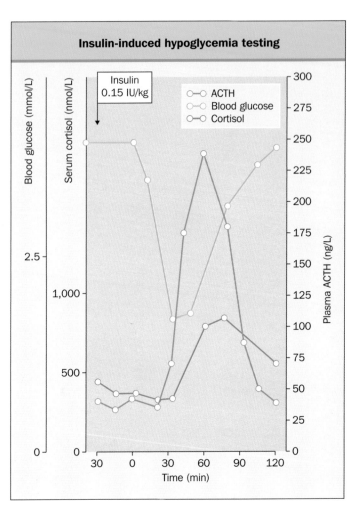

Insulin-induced hypoglycemia testing

Figure 14.11 Insulin-induced hypoglycemia testing. This demonstrates the changes in blood glucose, and in adrenocorticotropic hormone (ACTH) and cortisol secretion, induced by the intravenous administration of 0.15IU/kg soluble insulin. Insulin-induced hypoglycemia testing reveals the integrity of the entire hypothalamic-pituitary-adrenal axis.

account for approximately 60–70% of the total cortisol produced. Estimation of these steroids in a 24-hour urine sample thus provides an estimate of the secretion rate of cortisol. A small amount of cortisol (up to 50μg/day) is excreted unchanged and represents the unbound cortisol in plasma that is filtered through the kidney.

The average secretion rate of aldosterone is 100–200μg (**Fig. 14.14**). It is only weakly bound to plasma proteins and thus has a relatively short half-life (20min) and a high metabolic clearance rate (1500L/d). Both the liver and kidney are sites of metabolic clearance and only a small percentage of aldosterone is excreted unchanged in the urine. A measurement of plasma aldosterone levels, or an estimation of the levels of the metabolite 18-glucuronoside, is commonly used in clinical situations. Diet, posture, and time of day affect aldosterone secretion and must be adequately controlled to permit interpretation of results.

The major androgens produced by the adrenal cortex are DHEA sulfate, androstenedione, DHEA, 11-hydroxyandrostenedione, and small amounts of testosterone (**Fig. 14.15**).

Biosynthesis of glucocorticoids, mineralocorticoids and adrenal androgens

Cholesterol

Pregnenolone

3–5

17

Progesterone

17-hydroxypregnenolone

Dehydroepiandrosterone

21

17

Deoxycorticosterone

3–5

17-hydroxyprogesterone

Androstenedione

11

21

Corticosterone

11-deoxycortisol (substance 'S')

18

11

Aldosterone

Cortisol

Cortisone

3–5	3β-hydroxydehydrogenase, Δ5-isomerase		17	17α-hydroxylase
11	11β-hydroxylase		18	18-hydroxylase
21	21-hydroxylase			

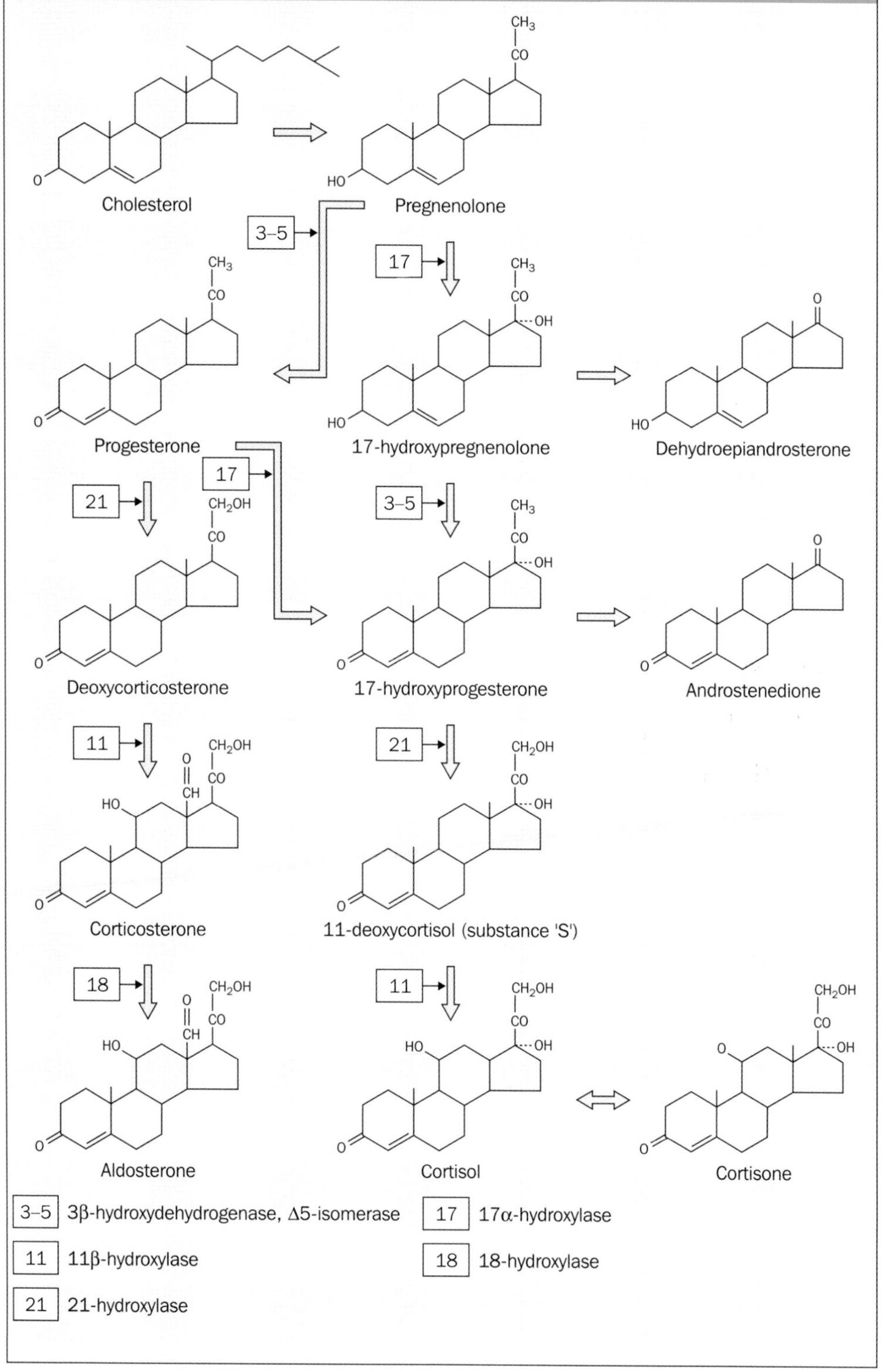

Figure 14.12 Biosynthesis of glucocorticoids, mineralocorticoids, and adrenal androgens. The pathways and the enzymes involved in the synthesis of glucocorticoids, mineralocorticoids, and adrenal androgens from a cholesterol precursor are illustrated. Deficiency of any of the enzymes may occur, leading to different forms of congenital adrenal hyperplasia. Deficiency of 21-hydroxylase is the most common, resulting in virilization, *in utero* or later, with variable degrees of adrenal insufficiency.

Androstenedione and testosterone are also secreted by the ovary and the testis, and a small amount of DHEA arises from the ovary. Androgen metabolism is therefore complex because of these dual sources and also because androgens undergo extensive interconversion and metabolism. The major metabolic pathway proceeds via the reduction of ring A, and the resulting metabolites are conjugated and excreted into the urine as sulfates and glucuronosides. Formerly, the conjugated urinary metabolites DHEA, etiocholanolone, and androsterone were measured collectively as 'urinary 17-oxosteroids' (17-ketosteroids). Although this assay

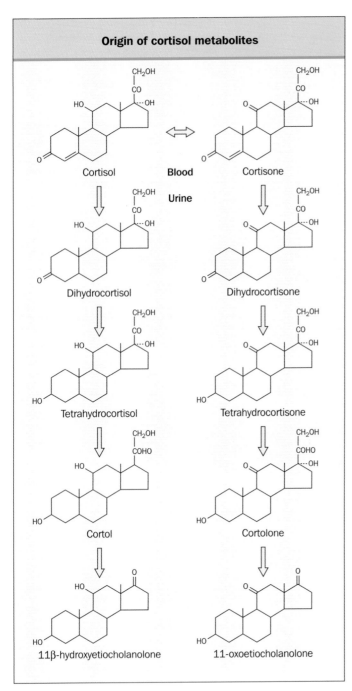

Origin of cortisol metabolites

Cortisol — Blood — Cortisone

Urine

Dihydrocortisol — Dihydrocortisone

Tetrahydrocortisol — Tetrahydrocortisone

Cortol — Cortolone

11β-hydroxyetiocholanolone — 11-oxoetiocholanolone

Figure 14.13 Origin of cortisol metabolites.

has been used extensively in the past, it is now little employed because of the difficulty of interpretation. Currently, clinical investigations of androgen metabolism are predominantly based on the measurement of plasma androgen levels rather than urinary excretion products. The peripheral interconversion of androgens has important physiologic consequences. Androstenedione is a major precursor of testosterone and, in the female, is a major source of

this hormone. It is also converted to estrone and, in older women, when ovarian secretion of estrogen is less important, the production of estrone from androstenedione contributes significantly to the total production of estrogen.

Inhibitors of steroid biosynthesis

Steroid biosynthesis can be blocked by a number of compounds that inhibit the activity of one or more of the enzyme systems involved in the pathway. These agents have been found to have clinical use in the investigation of pituitary–adrenal function, as an adjunct to the treatment of Cushing's syndrome, and as a method of reducing estrogen synthesis in the treatment of women with breast cancer.

Metyrapone acts by interfering with the cytochrome P450 system and mainly affects 11β- hydroxylation. This causes a relative increase in the production of the immediate precursor steroid, 11-deoxycortisol, with a concomitant decrease in cortisol synthesis. These actions have been exploited in the development of a test of pituitary–adrenal function that has been used clinically. In a subject with intact pituitary–adrenal function, following administration of metyrapone, a fall in cortisol production is seen, with a subsequent fall in plasma cortisol levels (**Fig. 14.16**). This causes a compensatory release of ACTH for as long as the drug is administered. ACTH, acting on the adrenal cortex, accelerates the early stages of steroid biosynthesis and therefore increases the production of all of the steroids up to the step that is blocked by metyrapone. The increased production of 11-deoxycortisol can be measured directly in the blood, or by measuring the metabolite tetrahydro-11-deoxycortisol in urine, where it appears as a 17-hydroxy-corticosteroid. A patient with hypothalamic, pituitary, or adrenal insufficiency will show a diminished or absent response.

Aminoglutethimide also interferes with several of the biosynthetic steps involved in steroid biosynthesis, exerting its effects on the C20-, C22, 11β, 18-, 19-, and 21-hydroxylases, and also on aromatase. Since it inhibits biosynthesis early in the pathway, it is useful as a blocking agent when alleviating the effects of excessive steroid production, as in the treatment of patients with Cushing's syndrome resulting from adrenal carcinoma. The action of aminoglutethimide on aromatase is useful in the treatment of breast cancer, since it inhibits peripheral formation of estrogens; however, it has now been superseded for this purpose by more selective aromatase inhibitors such as 4-hydroxyandrostenedione, which do not cause the problem of cortisol deficiency (as seen with aminoglutethimide).

Ketoconazole, an antifungal drug, inhibits several cytochrome-P450-dependent enzymes, including 11β-hydroxylase, thus interfering with cortisol synthesis (an unwanted effect in most cases). It is, however, being used increasingly to treat Cushing's syndrome, precocious puberty, and prostatic carcinoma.

Trilostane inhibits steroid hormone synthesis by acting on 3β-hydroxysteroid dehydrogenase; it has been used to reduce cortisol and aldosterone production in the treatment of Cushing's syndrome and Conn's syndrome, respectively, but its action is weak.

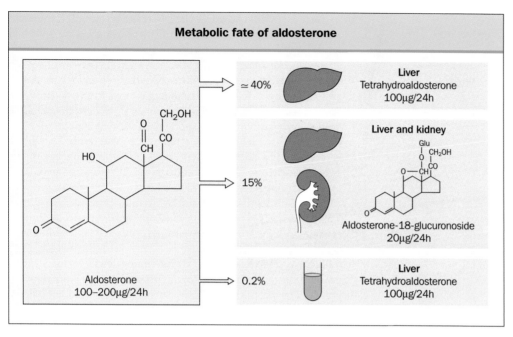

Figure 14.14 Metabolic fate of aldosterone. Only 0.2% of the daily amount of aldosterone that is produced is directly excreted in the urine, while approximately 40% is converted to tetrahydroaldosterone within the liver. The remaining aldosterone is converted into many other metabolites.

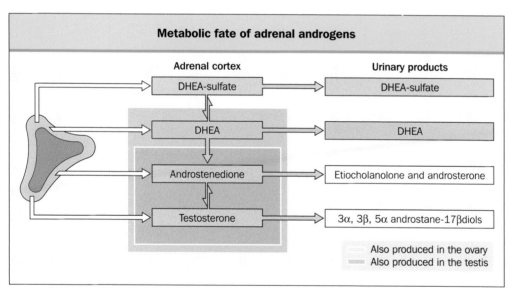

Figure 14.15 Metabolic fate of adrenal androgens. Dehydroepiandrosterone (DHEA), DHEA-sulfate, etiocholanolone, androsterone, and the androstanediols are all excreted in the urine.

METABOLIC ERRORS

The major pathways of steroid biosynthesis within the human adrenal cortex (see **Fig. 14.12**) emphasize the crucial dependence upon the availability of specific enzyme systems. Given the vital role that adrenocortical steroids play in human metabolism, it is not surprising that even a partial deficiency in the activity of these enzymes produces serious metabolic disturbance. Clinical syndromes corresponding to deficiencies of each of the enzymes that are involved have been described and are referred to as different forms of congenital adrenal hyperplasia. (See Chapter 38.)

The most common group of disorders of the type are due to C21-hydroxylase deficiency. This results in an inability to produce cortisol and in an increase in ACTH levels, which leads to adrenocortical hyperplasia and excessive production of androgens.

This in turn results in virilization of the external genitalia in the female fetus, and precocious pseudopuberty in male infants. If the deficiency extends to the zona glomerulosa $P450_{C21}$, deficiency of aldosterone production with salt loss will also occur. This can result in adrenocortical deficiency or crisis, neonatally or later in life. In this disorder, the substrate for the defective enzyme is 17-hydroxyprogesterone (see **Fig. 14.12**), and synthesis of this steroid, and its plasma levels, will increase.

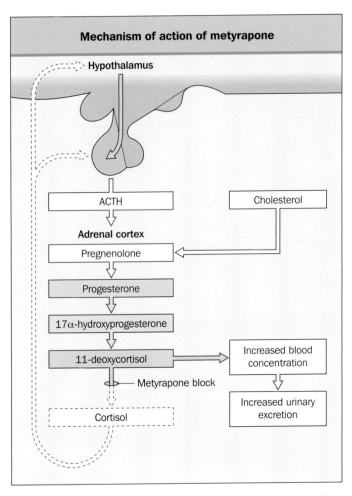

Mechanism of action of metyrapone

Hypothalamus

ACTH

Cholesterol

Adrenal cortex

Pregnenolone

Progesterone

17α-hydroxyprogesterone

11-deoxycortisol

Increased blood concentration

Metyrapone block

Increased urinary excretion

Cortisol

Figure 14.16 Mechanism of action of metyrapone. Metyrapone will cause an increase in the production of deoxycortisol and of its urinary metabolites, providing that the function of the hypothalamus, pituitary and adrenal is intact.

Deficiency of 11-hydroxylase is relatively less common and results in inadequate production of cortisol, an increase in ACTH levels, and an increase in the production of the precursor steroids 11-deoxycortisol and deoxycorticosterone. The latter is a powerful mineralocorticoid and produces hypertension and salt retention.

Deficiency of P450$_{scc}$ results in a serious disorder, since the biosynthesis of all the steroid hormones is prevented, leading to lipid accumulation in the gland (lipoid adrenal hyperplasia) and disorders of sexual differentiation in the male fetus. The defect is rare, and few patients survive early infancy. Deficiency of 17-hydroxylase is also rare, but it does occur. It results in a decreased synthesis of cortisol (see **Fig. 14.12**), an overproduction of ACTH, and decreasing secretion of androgens because of the lyase deficiency. The primary clinical manifestations are hypertension, failure to progress through puberty, and ambiguous genitalia in the male.

Hydroxysteroid-isomerase deficiency leads to inadequate production of cortisol, mineralocorticoids, and androgens; an inadequate production of the latter causes mild ambiguity of the male external genitalia. Excess secretion of 5α-androgens causes mild virilization of the female fetus. Cortisol and aldosterone deficiencies lead to salt losing crises.

FURTHER READING

Beato M. Gene regulation by steroid hormones. Cell 1989;56:335–44.

Brown MS, Kovanen PT, Goldstein JL. Receptor-mediated uptake of lipoprotein-cholesterol and its utilization for steroid synthesis in the adrenal cortex. Recent Prog Horm Res. 1979;35:215–57.

Dallman MF, Akana SF, Cascio CS, et al. Regulation of ACTH secretion. Recent Prog Horm Res. 1987;43:113–74.

James VHT. Comprehensive endocrinology: The adrenal gland. New York: Raven Press; 1992.

Lieberman S, Prasad VVK. Heterox notions on pathways of steroidogenesis. Endocr Rev. 1990;11:469–93.

Makin HJL. Biochemistry of steroid hormones, 2nd edn. Oxford: Blackwell Scientific Publications; 1984.

Miller WM. Molecular biology of steroid hormone synthesis. Endocr Rev. 1988;9:295–318.

Moore CCD, Miller WL. The role of transcriptional regulation in steroid hormone biosynthesis. J Steroid Biochem Mol Biol. 1991;40:517–25.

Muller J. Regulation of aldosterone biosynthesis. Berlin: Springer; 1988.

Parker LN. Adrenal androgens in clinical medicine. San Diego: Academic Press; 1989.

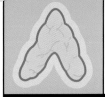

Cushing's Syndrome

Peter J Trainer and G Michael Besser

INTRODUCTION

Cushing's syndrome is the associated symptoms and signs that result from long-term inappropriate elevation of free (non-protein-bound) circulating glucocorticoid levels. It has an incidence of approximately 30:1,000,000. Historical references attribute to Cushing's syndrome a 50% 5-year mortality but with earlier diagnosis and modern treatment the outlook has improved greatly. However it remains a physically and psychologically disabling condition with high morbidity. The syndrome as described by Harvey Cushing in 1912 and the images reproduced in many textbook are of patients with florid Cushing's but the reality is that the disease is being suspected and investigated much earlier now by the astute physician in patients attending diabetes, hypertension, osteoporosis, psychiatric, and gynecologic clinics to name but a few. The challenge in the diagnosis of Cushing's syndrome remains as great as ever but has evolved with refinements in diagnostic tests that allow diagnosis much earlier in its natural history.

ETIOLOGY

In most large series of patients with endogenous Cushing's syndrome, approximately 80% are adrenocorticotropic hormone (ACTH)-dependent and 20% ACTH-independent, i.e. primarily adrenal in origin (**Table 15.1**). An ACTH-secreting pituitary adenoma (corticotropinoma) is present in 80% of patients with ACTH-dependent Cushing's syndrome and this clinical entity is referred to as Cushing's disease because this is the variety of Cushing's syndrome he first described; the other 20% have non-pituitary tumors that secrete ACTH 'ectopically', most commonly bronchial in origin although many other sources are recognized (**Table 15.2**). Pituitary corticotroph hyperplasia is extremely rare and the demonstration of the frequent monoclonal origin of corticotropinomas indicates that Cushing's disease is a primary pituitary disease rather than a consequence of hypothalamic overstimulation. The ectopic ACTH syndrome originally described was almost exclusively the consequence of overt, rapidly growing, highly malignant small (oat)-cell carcinomas of the lung. In recent years the occult ectopic ACTH syndrome has been more commonly recognized due to small carcinoid tumors and represents a major diagnostic challenge as the clinical features and biochemical abnormalities often closely imitate those of Cushing's disease.

Etiology of Cushing's syndrome

	n	%
Cushing's disease	274	67
Ectopic ACTH	44	11
Adrenal adenoma	60	14
Adrenal carcinoma	30	7
Nodular adrenocortical hyperplasia	5	1

Table 15.1 Etiology of Cushing's syndrome. These are the causes of Cushing's syndrome in 413 patients seen at St Bartholomew's Hospital between 1969 and 2001.

Etiology of ectopic ACTH syndrome

	n	%
Bronchial carcinoid tumor	11	30
Small-cell lung cancer	2	5
Medullary thyroid carcinoma	1	3
Pancreatic carcinoid tumor	12	33
Thymic carcinoid tumor	2	5
Disseminated carcinoid tumor	1	3
Pancreatic carcinoma	1	3
Colonic carcinoma	1	3
Pheochromocytoma	1	3
Gallbladder carcinoma	1	3
Source never found	3	9

Table 15.2 Etiology of ectopic ACTH syndrome. The table lists the tumors causing clinical Cushing's syndrome in 36 patients seen at St Bartholomew's Hospital between 1969 and 2001.

Non-ACTH-dependent Cushing's syndrome is due to corticosteroid administration or primary adrenocortical tumors. Some 60% of these adrenal tumors are benign adenomas, the remainder carcinomas. The latter group is characterized by large size, capsular or vascular invasion and infiltration of surrounding tissues, and dissemination, usually to the liver and peritoneum. Distinguishing between the two types may be difficult. Any tumor above 6cm in diameter (approximately 100g) or one that secretes more than one class of steroid in significant amounts, typically androgens in addition to cortisol, must be regarded as potentially malignant.

Adrenal nodules commonly develop in the hyperplastic adrenal cortex in patients with ACTH-dependent Cushing's syndrome, but distinct from that is the syndrome of ACTH-independent adrenal nodular hyperplasia. This accounts for approximately 1% of cases of Cushing's syndrome and in turn can be subdivided into micro- and macronodular. The etiology of bilateral nodular adrenal hyperplasia is ill-understood but individual case reports have associated aberrant expression of gastric inhibitory peptide, vasopressin, and β-adrenergic receptors in the glands, which can weigh 500g (normal adrenal weight <7g) in this condition. Micronodular hyperplasia accounts for less than 1% of cases of Cushing's syndrome and is of uncertain etiology. It may occur in patients with longstanding Cushing's disease when adrenal nodules become autonomous. Carney's complex is a rare, autosomal-dominant cause of non-ACTH-dependent Cushing's syndrome in which the adrenal glands contain multiple, deeply pigmented nodules. Other components of this syndrome may include cardiac myxomas, pigmented skin lesions, peripheral nerve tumors, and endocrine disorders.

DIAGNOSIS

Clinical features

Depression, serious illness, cancer, and the polycystic ovary syndrome may all be associated with disturbed dynamics of the pituitary adrenal axis, which can result in a failure of dexamethasone to suppress cortisol secretion normally and elevate urinary free cortisol excretion, but these patients do not have Cushing's syndrome and do not develop its clinical characteristics. Clinical examination and elucidation of the clinical features

Major clinical features in Cushing's syndrome
Weight gain
Central obesity
'Moon face' with purplish plethora
Muscular weakness, especially proximal backache and vertebral collapse
Malaise
Agitated depression and/or psychosis
Hirsutism
Purple striae
Acne
Skin-thinning
Bruising
Nocturia/polyuria
Decreased libido and impotence in males
Oligomenorrhea or amenorrhea in females
Hypertension
Diabetes mellitus or impaired glucose tolerance
Infection

Table 15.3 Major clinical features in Cushing's syndrome. Patients with Cushing's syndrome gain weight but suffer muscular disability, malaise, and depression. In addition, they are susceptible to various skin disorders such as acne and bruising; decreased fertility and libido may also be present.

of Cushing's syndrome is a prerequisite for making the diagnosis (**Table 15.3, Figs 15.1 & 15.2**). The most common presenting complaints are often rather nonspecific: weight gain, fatigue, and depression. Agitated depression, which may be severe, or psychosis are characteristic in patients with any cause of Cushing's syndrome. Skin thinning, particularly of the shins or

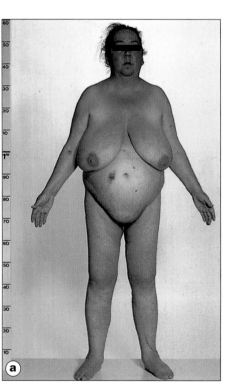
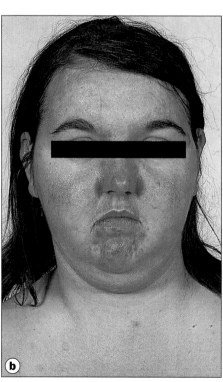

Figure 15.1 Clinical appearance of Cushing's syndrome. (a) Typical clinical appearance of a patient with Cushing's syndrome. Central obesity with proximal muscle wasting can be seen. (b) Typical 'moon face' appearance of a patient with Cushing's syndrome. A plethoric face with acne and hirsutism is characteristic and there is evidence of temporal hair recession.

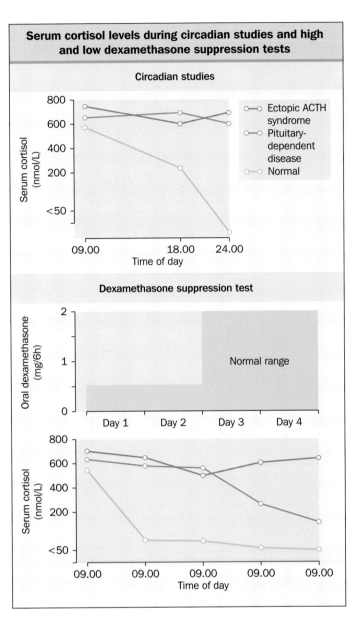

Serum cortisol levels during circadian studies and high and low dexamethasone suppression tests

Circadian studies

○○ Ectopic ACTH syndrome
○○ Pituitary-dependent disease
○○ Normal

Dexamethasone suppression test

Normal range

Figure 15.6 Serum cortisol levels during circadian studies and high and low dexamethasone suppression tests. In a healthy individual, the serum cortisol level falls naturally during the day, and administration of a low dose of oral dexamethasone (0.5mg 6-hourly) will lead to suppression of cortisol levels below 50nmol/L. No fall occurs in patients with ectopic adrenocorticotropic hormone (ACTH) syndrome, even with high doses of dexamethasone. This contrasts with the responses seen in patients with pituitary-dependent disease in whom inadequate suppression after low-dose administration of dexamethasone, and at least 50% suppression after administration of a high dose of dexamethasone (2mg 6-hourly) are characteristic. A serum cortisol of 50nmol/l=2µg/dL.

Low-dose dexamethasone suppression test

The purpose of the dexamethasone suppression test (DST) is to demonstrate the impaired feedback regulation of the pituitary–adrenal axis in Cushing's syndrome of any cause. When originally described in 1960 the dexamethasone suppression test relied on measurement of urinary steroid metabolite (17-hydroxycorticosteroids) but, not withstanding the refinements

in urinary cortisol and metabolite assays, measurement of serum cortisol is easier and of greater diagnostic accuracy. Several variations of the dexamethasone suppression test for the diagnosis of Cushing's syndrome have been described but in our experience the only reliable test is the full 48-hour low-dose dexamethasone test. The overnight 1mg DST is acknowledged to be of less diagnostic value because of the large number of false positives. However it is often argued by its proponents that it is more convenient and easier to perform than the 48-hour low-dose DST and can be performed on outpatients. In our experience, with adequate written instructions the low-dose DST can be performed reliably without hospitalization of the patient and unequivocally results in fewer false positives. The supposed advantage of the overnight DST is often negated by the necessity of proceeding to the latter in investigation in patients who fail to suppress. The 48-hour DST can be undertaken as an outpatient and entails the patient taking 0.5mg of dexamethasone at precisely 6-hour intervals for 48 hours (eight doses) with measurement of serum cortisol at 09.00h before and at 48 hours, i.e. 6 hours after the last dose of dexamethasone. In normal individuals, the serum cortisol at 48 hours will be under 50nmol/L(< 2µg/dL,) with higher values being strongly suggestive of Cushing's syndrome (**Fig. 15.6**). False-positive results can be caused by failure to take the dexamethasone as prescribed or by accelerated hepatic metabolism of dexamethasone, usually as a consequence of hepatic enzyme induction by drugs such as phenytoin, carbamazepine, phenobarbital (phenobarbitone), or rifampicin. With these exceptions, 98% of patients with Cushing's syndrome fail to suppress normally. In moderate or severe depression, resistance to normal dexamethasone suppression may occur and this may cause diagnostic confusion, as agitated depression is a typical feature of Cushing's syndrome. Suppressibility returns with successful treatment of primary depression.

Some alcoholic patients not only may look somewhat cushingoid but may also show failure of circadian rhythmicity or dexamethasone suppressibility of circulating cortisol; however, these return within a few days when alcohol consumption is stopped.

On occasion, and despite meticulous investigation, it is not possible to make the diagnosis with confidence, particularly in patients with cyclical Cushing's syndrome. Often these patients have mild disease and may be left untreated for a while and reinvestigated at an appropriate interval, such as 6 months.

Differential diagnosis

It is of crucial importance to prove unequivocally the diagnosis of Cushing's syndrome before proceeding to establish the precise etiology. An important consideration when assessing the diagnostic sensitivity of individual test is the pretest probability. This is particularly pertinent in women with ACTH-dependent Cushing's syndrome, as a pituitary adenoma is 10 times more likely than an ectopic source of ACTH secretion (**Table 15.2**). Thus, the pretest probability of the cause being Cushing's disease in a woman is 90%.

Basal sampling

Measurement of 09.00h plasma ACTH differentiates primary adrenal disease from ACTH-driven cortisol secretion. In patients in whom the plasma ACTH concentration is undetectable, adrenal computerized tomography (CT) or magnetic resonance imaging (MRI) will usually reveal a unilateral tumor, although occasionally bilateral nodular hyperplasia is encountered.

Plasma ACTH levels (**Fig. 15.7**) can be within the normal range for 09.00h in patients with ACTH-dependent Cushing's syndrome, in particular in those with pituitary disease, but there is no circadian rhythm and the ACTH levels are maintained at this level throughout the 24 hours, increasing the 24-hour production of cortisol. There is considerable overlap between plasma ACTH levels in the ectopic ACTH syndrome and Cushing's disease, although levels tend to be higher in the former group.

Hypokalemic alkalosis is present in 100% of patients with the ectopic ACTH secretion. Care must be taken when drawing blood as only slight hemolysis can mask hypokalemia, although, when available, a raised serum bicarbonate is a surrogate marker. Hypokalemia occurs as a result of saturation of the 11β-HSD type 2 enzyme and consequent binding of cortisol to renal mineralocorticoid receptors. Hypokalemia is much less common in Cushing's disease (about 10%) and alerts the physician to an increased likelihood of the occult ectopic ACTH syndrome, although hypokalemia is truly only a marker of the severity of hypercortisolemia. Diabetes mellitus is also uniformly found as an accompaniment of the ectopic ACTH syndrome but is less common in other forms of Cushing's syndrome, although this is again indicative of disease severity rather than any mechanism unique to the ectopic ACTH syndrome.

High-dose dexamethasone suppression test

The principle of this test (see Fig. 15.6) is that, although there is resistance to the normal negative feedback effects of increased circulating corticosteroid levels in all causes of Cushing's syndrome, in pituitary-dependent Cushing's disease some negative feedback effects will be seen if the corticosteroid levels are high enough. The test is performed in an identical manner to the low-dose DST except that a dose of 2mg is administered every 6 hours. A dose of 8mg of dexamethasone is about 10–15 times the normal physiologic replacement dose of glucocorticoid. It can, rarely, precipitate psychosis and may also worsen hypokalemia and diabetes mellitus, and requires inpatient supervision. A fall of over 50% in serum cortisol from basal values before dexamethasone is indicative of pituitary-dependent Cushing's disease in a patient with proven Cushing's syndrome. False positives occur in less than 10% and there is a similar incidence of false negatives. The high-dose DST can be performed in immediate succession to a low-dose DST, the baseline of the low-dose DST being used to define the response to both tests (**Fig. 15.6**).

The metyrapone test was described in 1959, before plasma ACTH could be measured routinely or the adrenals imaged, for the differentiation of pituitary from adrenal causes of Cushing's syndrome. Metyrapone blocks cortisol synthesis and therefore induces a rise in ACTH in patients with Cushing's disease – but also sometimes in patients with ectopic ACTH secretion, as well as pituitary disease. Thus the metyrapone test is more often confusing than enlightening in the investigation of ACTH-dependent Cushing's syndrome and it should no longer be used.

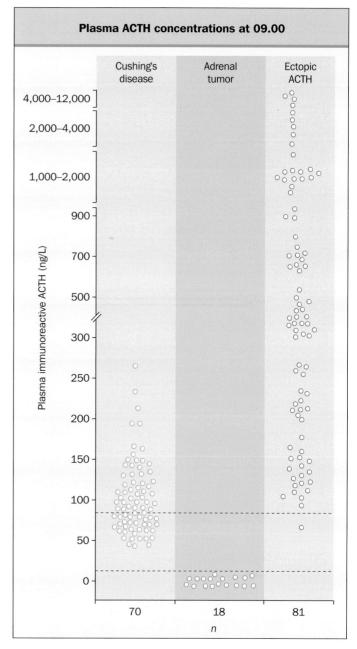

Figure 15.7 Plasma adrenocorticotropic hormone (ACTH) concentrations at 09.00h. Each point on the graph represents one patient. Patients with adrenal tumors have subnormal levels of ACTH. Those with the ectopic ACTH syndrome tend to have higher levels than those with pituitary-dependent disease, although a considerable overlap exists. The shaded area represents the normal range at 09.00h.

Corticotropin-releasing hormone and desmopressin tests

Pituitary ACTH secretion is regulated principally by two hypothalamic secretagogues: corticotropin-releasing hormone (CRH) and arginine–vasopressin (AVP). CRH was identified and sequenced in 1981, and is available for clinical practice as either the ovine or human sequence, which are equally bioactive but differ by 7 amino acid residues. Ovine CRH is the preferred form in North America, while in Europe the majority of the experience is with human CRH: available evidence indicates that they are of equal value in the investigation of Cushing's syndrome. AVP sensitizes the corticotroph to CRH but also has some intrinsic ACTH-releasing activity of its own. Synthetic CRH stimulates ACTH secretion in normal subjects and patients with Cushing's disease but it is rare to see a response in a patient with the ectopic ACTH syndrome. The CRH test is of no value in the preliminary establishment of a diagnosis of Cushing's syndrome but is a powerful discriminator (85%) between pituitary and ectopic ACTH secretion. A dose of 100μg of either human or ovine CRH is given intravenously and plasma cortisol and ACTH are measured every 15min for 120min. Approximately 75% of patients with Cushing's disease respond characteristically to CRH, defined as an increase in serum cortisol of at least 12%, but it is usually prompt and excessive. However, occasionally a response in the ectopic ACTH syndrome is seen. Some investigators administer CRH after dexamethasone dosing and maintain that there is a better differentiation between Cushing's disease and normality, but this is not generally agreed.

Arginine–vasopressin has been used in the differential diagnosis of ACTH-dependent Cushing's syndrome but is limited by a high false-negative rate and gastrointestinal side effects. The arginine–vasopressin analog desmopressin (DDAVP) stimulates ACTH secretion in patients with pituitary-dependent Cushing's disease but rarely in healthy subjects or patients with the ectopic ACTH syndrome. Testing with DDAVP alone is inferior to CRH in distinguishing between ectopic and pituitary ACTH secretion but the combined simultaneous intravenous administration of CRH (100μg) and DDAVP (10μg) is even better than either test performed alone. An increase in serum cortisol of 37% or above is indicative of Cushing's disease.

Although each of the dynamic tests has limited specificity and is of finite value in isolation, the cumulative data from both high-dose dexamethasone testing and CRH/DDAVP testing will differentiate between pituitary and ectopic causes of Cushing's syndrome in the great majority of cases.

Inferior petrosal sinus sampling

Inferior petrosal sinus sampling (**Fig. 15.8**) is the test of greatest diagnostic specificity and sensitivity in the differentiation of ACTH-dependent Cushing's syndrome but relies on access to specialist facilities and a skilled radiologist and can, rarely, result in major complications such as cerebrovascular accident and death. The venous drainage of the pituitary is into the cavernous sinuses, which principally drain into the inferior petrosal sinuses and then into the internal jugular veins: an ACTH gradient between these sinuses and a peripheral vein is indicative of the pituitary as the source of ACTH secretion. Two catheters are inserted into the right femoral vein and guided through the venous system into the internal jugular veins and into the right and left inferior petrosal sinuses. Heparinization of patients is recommended once the catheters are *in situ*. Basal ACTH samples are drawn simultaneously from both catheters and a peripheral vein, and then an intravenous injection of 100μg of CRH is administered. Blood is sampled for plasma ACTH levels at 5, 10 and 15min. Peripheral blood samples are also taken simultaneously. A central to peripheral ACTH ratio of greater than 2 in our assay and more than 3 in other series is indicative of pituitary ACTH secretion. An important proviso is that the

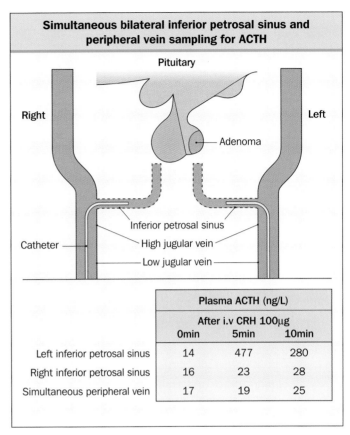

Figure 15.8 Simultaneous bilateral inferior petrosal sinus and peripheral vein sampling for adrenocorticotropic hormone (ACTH). The positions from which samples are obtained are shown. The diagnosis of Cushing's disease is established by an ACTH ratio of over 3 between one side and the other and usually indicates the side of the tumor.

patient must have been demonstrated already to have ACTH-dependent Cushing's syndrome as a ACTH secretion is always pituitary-derived in healthy individuals!

Large series have reported the results of inferior petrosal sinus sampling to be approaching 100% sensitive and specific in the diagnosis of pituitary-dependent Cushing's disease. A plasma ACTH between the two inferior petrosal sinuses of more than 1.4 is of some limited value in localizing ACTH-secreting adenomas within the pituitary gland, but must be interpreted with caution and in conjunction with pituitary imaging (**Fig. 15.8**).

Radiology

Magnetic resonance imaging is the modality of choice for the pituitary and with the availability of improved machines allowing faster image acquisition, the potential for movement artifact is reduced and image resolution is improved. MRI of the pituitary demonstrates adenomas in 50–70% of patients with Cushing's disease but the position is confused by the presence of pituitary coincidentalomas, i.e. lesions present on scanning of the pituitary but not functionally significant, in 10% of normal adults. The significance of a pituitary adenoma must always be judged in the light of a knowledge of the biochemistry. The larger an adenoma the more likely it is to significant. The majority of corticotroph microadenomas are hypointense on MRI and fail to enhance with gadolinium contrast medium (**Fig. 15.9**).

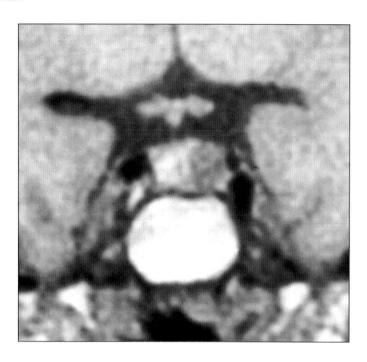

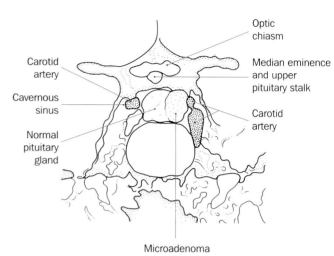

Figure 15.9 Magnetic resonance imaging of the pituitary in Cushing's disease (coronal plane). A right-sided pituitary tumor can be seen.

However, precontrast images are essential, since in approximately 5% of pituitary microadenomas the tumor will take up the gadolinium contrast medium, giving an isointense signal, so they cannot then be seen postcontrast.

In patients with suspected ectopic ACTH secretion, chest and abdominal high-resolution CT scanning should be performed at 1cm overlapping slices. The refinements in imaging techniques mean that whole-body venous sampling to identify a source of ACTH is no longer of value in the majority of patients with ectopic ACTH secretion.

Radioactive iodocholesterol adrenal scintigraphy provides insight into the function, rather than the anatomy, of the adrenal glands and related masses. However in an era of sophisticated biochemistry and high resolution CT and MR imaging, scintigraphy rarely provides additional information.

Octreoscanning

The somatostatin analog octreotide, labeled with radioactive indium, can identify carcinoid lesions of 5mm and above, and may be a useful adjunct as it provides both information on localization and function of an identified ectopic source of ACTH secretion. However it rarely if ever identifies lesions not visible on high-quality CT scanning (see Fig. 41.16).

TREATMENT

Establishing the differential diagnosis of the precise cause is fundamental to the optimal management of Cushing's syndrome, as it permits specific therapy, such as pituitary microsurgery or removal of an ectopic source of ACTH.

Surgery

Trans-sphenoidal hypophysectomy

Trans-sphenoidal microadenectomy (see Chapter 8) is the treatment of choice for Cushing's disease, with potential for cure of the syndrome with retention of normal pituitary function.

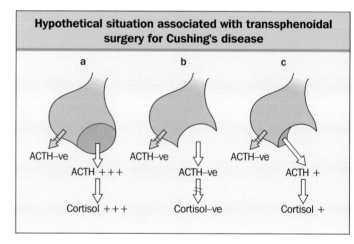

Figure 15.10 Hypothetical situation associated with transsphenoidal surgery for Cushing's disease. (a) Preoperative state. (b) Postoperative 'cure': all tumor removed, ACTH secretion is suppressed from the normal gland and serum cortisol is undetectable. (c) Some tumor remains and cortisol secretion is detectable. +++, secretion above normal; +, secretion detectable; – secretion suppressed; shaded area, ACTH-secretion tumor. (Redrawn from Trainer PJ, et al. Trans-sphenoidal resection in Cushing's disease: undetectable serum cortisol as the definition of successful treatment. Clin Endocrinol (Oxf). 1993;38:73–8.)

Hypersecretion of ACTH by a corticotropinoma results in suppression of ACTH release from the surrounding healthy pituitary and complete excision of the tumor will therefore result in prolonged ACTH deficiency and hypoadrenalism. A postoperative serum cortisol level of less than 50nmol/L (2μg/dL) has been shown to predict long-term 'cure' (**Fig. 15.10**).

In experienced hands at least 50% of patients will be rendered hypoadrenal and cured by pituitary surgery. An additional 30% will have most of the tumor removed, leading to a reduction in ACTH secretion with cortisol production rates being normalized over 24 hours. However, in these patients the normal circadian rhythm of secretion remains absent because of residual tumor; the signs and symptoms may resolve but this must be considered a state of remission rather than cure, and relapse is common in such patients. Thus in different series between 50% and 80% of patients are reported as 'cured' depending on the criteria used – whether cortisol production is simply normalized or rendered hypoadrenal. The latter definition is the more stringent. A normalized cortisol production rate is indicated by a serum cortisol, averaged from five samples taken through one day, of between 150 and 300nmol/L.

The commonest complication of pituitary surgery is hypopituitarism, including diabetes insipidus; the latter is usually transient. The more extensive the surgery the greater the risk of hypopituitarism but of paramount importance is achieving a 'cure'. In a younger, fitter patient who desires fertility, initial surgery may be more selective, with the understanding that repeat surgery may be necessary. In the older, frailer patient in whom the anesthetic risk is greater, a more radical first operation may be indicated. Detailed postoperative assessment of pituitary function, including growth hormone, is mandatory in all patients. Growth hormone replacement therapy is particularly important in patients who have had Cushing's syndrome and are left with growth hormone deficiency, since this will help to restore normal muscle function and bone density much faster.

Pituitary radiotherapy

In patients in whom pituitary surgery has not been completely successful or is contraindicated, carefully planned radiotherapy via three fields at a dose of 4500cGy in 25 fractions is safe and effective (see Chapter 9). Correctly performed the only side-effect encountered is hypopituitarism in a proportion of patients. Alternatively stereotactic radiation may be used, which can be given as a single fraction. Cortisol secretion rates are normal in 80% of patients 4 years after treatment and medical therapy is required in the interim. The dose of medical therapy required diminishes as the radiotherapy reduces ACTH drive.

Bilateral adrenalectomy

Bilateral adrenalectomy should cure all patients with ACTH-dependent Cushing's syndrome, irrespective of the etiology. It used to be the routine management option before modern pituitary surgery and continues to have an occasional place in the management of patients with ACTH-dependent Cushing's syndrome. In pituitary-dependent disease, bilateral adrenalectomy should be considered only after failed pituitary surgery, or following pituitary radiotherapy (which may itself follow unsuccessful pituitary surgery) if hypercortisolemia cannot be satisfactorily controlled medically. Bilateral adrenalectomy may be indicated in patients with severe ectopic ACTH syndrome when it is not possible to excise the tumor fully, or in patients where the source of ACTH secretion cannot be identified and if the hypercortisolemia cannot be controlled medically. A major disadvantage of bilateral adrenalectomy is the necessity for lifelong glucocorticoid and mineralocorticoid replacement therapy and consequent risk of life-threatening hypoadrenal crisis. In patients with Cushing's disease the principal other long-term complication of bilateral adrenalectomy is Nelson's syndrome: hyperpigmentation in association with a enlargement of the

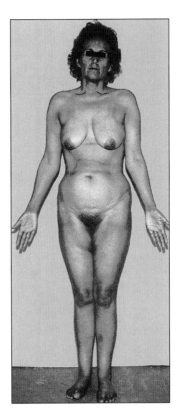

Figure 15.11 Appearance of a patient with Nelson's syndrome. The gross pigmentation that occurs in this syndrome is best seen on the flexural surfaces of the body.

pituitary tumor. The hyperpigmentation is disturbing for the patient, but of greater concern is the morbidity and mortality consequent upon a expanding infiltrative pituitary tumor. Nelson's syndrome occurs in about 40% of patients undergoing bilateral adrenalectomy for Cushing's disease, but prophylactic pituitary radiotherapy alters the natural history either by preventing, or at least delaying, the development of Nelson's syndrome and if given at the time of adrenalectomy is believed to reduce the prevalence dramatically (**Fig. 15.11**).

Early published series of bilateral adrenalectomy reported high morbidity and mortality rates of up to 15% but, with meticulous preoperative care, control of hypercortisolemia with drugs, and modern anesthetic and surgical techniques, morbidity should be low and mortality rates around 1%. The less invasive nature of laparoscopic adrenalectomy permits more rapid postoperative mobilization and more rapid discharge from hospital but the patient still requires careful preoperative preparation, the operating time is longer and care is required to ensure all adrenal tissue is excised

Unilateral adrenalectomy

Unilateral adrenalectomy will cure an adenoma and debulking of tumor mass even in the presence of metastases will improve the prognosis of adrenal carcinoma. Local radiotherapy and the adrenolytic agent mitotane (o,p'DDD) is used in the management of metastatic adrenal carcinoma but the prognosis remains bleak. Routine chemotherapy is of little use for patients with carcinoma of the adrenal cortex.

Unilateral adrenalectomy may result in long-term remission in patients with Cushing's disease providing pituitary radiotherapy is given at the same time. This may be preferred to bilateral adrenalectomy in patients who fail to respond to other modes of treatment.

Medical therapy

Medical therapy is used to lower cortisol secretion under specific circumstances such as in preparation for surgery, in those not cured by or not fit enough for surgery, while waiting for radiotherapy to be effective, and when the patient's physical or psychiatric state at presentation requires rapid control of circulating cortisol levels. Very occasionally, detailed investigation fails to establish the source of ACTH secretion and medical treatment is then needed to control hypercortisolemia so that the patient can be reinvestigated after an appropriate interval. The only drugs that consistently control cortisol secretion are those directed at inhibiting it. Drugs directed at the hypothalamus or pituitary are generally ineffective, but dopamine agonists such as bromocriptine may be occasionally of value in lowering pituitary ACTH levels.

Metyrapone and ketoconazole are the clinically most useful as they are both effective blockers of cortisol synthesis and well-tolerated. Aminoglutethimide is limited by side effects and its limited efficacy. Etomidate is an intravenous anesthetic agent and, in common with ketoconazole, is an imidazole compound that inhibits cortisol synthesis by acting on cytochrome P450 enzymes. In emergencies when oral therapy cannot be used, subhypnotic doses (up to 3.5mg/h) of etomidate, administered as a continuous intravenous infusion, can control hypercortisolemia, although it is most effective in nonpituitary ACTH-dependent causes of Cushing's syndrome.

Metyrapone lowers serum cortisol within 2 hours of the first dose, which is an advantage in controlling hypercortisolemia, but if treatment is not closely supervised adrenocortical insufficiency can occur. The dose of metyrapone is titrated up until the mean serum cortisol obtained from five samples through the day is in the range 150–300nmol/L, with the required dose varying in the range 750–4000mg daily in three divided doses. Other than hypoadrenalism, the principal side effect is hirsutism in women secondary to an accumulation of androgenic cortisol precursors. The cortisol precursor 11-deoxycortisol accumulates in high concentrations in blood. Some cortisol immunoassays detect this precursor at high concentrations. This can result in spuriously elevated apparent cortisol levels and hypoadrenalism can be missed.

Ketoconazole has a slower onset of action but has the advantage of lowering circulating androgens. The required dose varies between 600 and 1200mg per day. Occasionally, disturbance of liver function tests complicates therapy and abdominal pain can be a problem in some patients. Metyrapone and ketoconazole inhibit cortisol synthesis at different stages of steroidogenesis and are thereby highly effective in inhibiting cortisol and androgen secretion when used together.

Mitotane destroys adrenocortical cells and, in doses up to 12g per day, is used to manage (at least temporarily) patients with carcinoma of the adrenal cortex. However, doses up to 3g are usually well-tolerated and it can be used to help in the control of benign causes of Cushing's syndrome that are otherwise difficult to manage. It has a slow onset of action and can offer long-term control of cortisol secretion. Hypercholesterolemia uniformly accompanies mitotane therapy but is reversible with HMG-CoA reductase inhibitors such as simvastatin.

RECOVERY FROM SUCCESSFUL THERAPY FOR CUSHING'S DISEASE

Following successful surgery for Cushing's disease, the patient will need appropriate glucocorticoid replacement therapy. The patient has been habituated to excessive glucocorticoid levels and may feel unwell even when adequately replaced. Patients often complain of lethargy, muscle and joint pains, and general asthenia. It is important that this is explained to patients before surgery and that they are warned that these symptoms may persist for as long as a year following successful surgery. It is often helpful to tell patients that the longer it takes before the replacement therapy can be stopped the greater the chance that they will be permanently cured.

SUMMARY

The diagnosis of Cushing's syndrome relies on a combination of detailed clinical examination and a systematic approach to the biochemical and radiologic investigation. The initial step is confirmation of the diagnosis, followed by establishment of the precise etiology. Proceeding to the second step without definitively substantiating the diagnosis of Cushing's syndrome may lead to an inappropriate diagnosis of pituitary-dependent Cushing's disease; in pseudo-Cushing's syndrome the pituitary is always the source of ACTH. Successful treatment is dependent on the correct diagnosis but before undertaking surgery, or in cases where the precise etiology cannot be established or treatment is not curative, ketoconazole and/or metyrapone should be used to control cortisol production.

FURTHER READING

Crapo L. Cushing's syndrome: a review of diagnostic tests. Metabolism 1979;28:955–77.

Faiman C. The etiology and management of Cushing's syndrome. In: Anderson DC, Winter JSD, eds. Adrenal cortex. London:Butterworth's International Medical Reviews; l985:154–68.

Howlett TA, Rees LH, Besser GM. Cushing's syndrome. Clin Endocrinol Metabol. 1985;14:911–45.

Krieger DT. Physiopathology of Cushing's disease. Endocrine Rev. 1983;4:22–43.

Nelson DH. Cushing's syndrome. In: De Groot LJ, ed. Endocrinology. Philadelphia, PA:WB Saunders; 1989.

Newell-Price JD, Trainer PJ, Besser GM, Grossman A. The diagnosis and differential diagnosis of Cushing's syndrome and pseudo-Cushing's states. Endocrine Rev. 1998;19:647–72.

Ross EJ, Linch DC. Cushing's syndrome – killing disease: discriminatory values of signs and symptoms aiding early diagnosis. Lancet 1982;2:646–9.

Trainer PJ, Besser GM. The diagnosis and differential diagnosis of Cushing's syndrome. Clin Endocrinol. 1991;34:317–30.

Trainer PJ, Besser GM. Cushing's syndrome: therapy directed at the adrenal glands. Endocrinol Metab Clin North Am. 1994:23;571–84.

Trainer PJ, Lawrie HS, Verheist J, et al. Transsphenoidal resection in Cushing's disease: undetectable serum cortisol as the definition of successful treatment. Clin Endocrinol. 1993;38:73–8.

Verhelst TA, Trainer PJ, Howlett TA, et al. Short and long-term responses to metyrapone in the medical management of 9l patients with Cushing's syndrome. Clin Endocrinol. 1991;35:169–78.

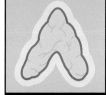

Section 3 Adrenal

Chapter 16 Addison's Disease

Peter J Trainer and G Michael Besser

INTRODUCTION

In 1855 Thomas Addison described the symptoms associated with the fatal consequences of destruction of the adrenal glands. In the intervening years we have come to understand much of the physiology underpinning his original observations and effective treatment is available, but the diagnosis continues to be delayed or missed; sadly, from time to time, patients still die unnecessarily from this condition.

The adrenal glands are essentially pyramidal in shape and sit on top of the kidneys and just below the diaphragm, each being perfused by three arteries. Each gland weighs approximately 5g, of which 4g is the cortex and 1g the medulla, the former being of mesodermal origin while the later is derived by migration of cells from the neural crest and is ectodermal in origin. The cortex comprises three histologically distinct components and is responsible for steroid hormone synthesis. The cleavage of the six-carbon fragment from the cholesterol side-chain, within mitochondria, gives rise to pregnenolone, which is the precursor for all synthesis of corticosteroids, and over 50 distinct steroid hormones are synthesized in the adrenal cortex. The zona vesiculata and zona reticularis of the inner cortex are responsible for glucocorticoid synthesis and secretion, in humans principally cortisol, under the influence of adrenocorticotropic hormone (ACTH). Under basal, unstressed conditions, the cortisol reproduction rate in an adult is approximately 10mg/day. The outer zona glomerulosa is responsible for the synthesis and secretion of aldosterone, the main mineralocorticoid in humans, and is under the regulation of the renin–angiotensin system. Although cortisol and aldosterone are the principal adrenal steroids in humans, the importance of the adrenal glands as a source of androgens in women is emerging (see below). In men the contribution of the adrenals to total androgen production is tiny in comparison with that of the testes.

The adrenal medulla, under the modulation of preganglionic cholinergic neurons, secretes three distinct catecholamines: epinephrine (adrenaline), norepinephrine (noradrenaline) and dopamine (see Fig. 18.1). Catecholamine release by noradrenergic neurons of the sympathetic nervous system is responsible for many of the systemic manifestations of catecholamine action, with only 2% of circulating norepinephrine being adrenal in origin. The adrenal enzyme phenylethanolamine-N-methyl transferase is responsible for the final step in epinephrine synthesis, namely the conversion of norepinephrine to epinephrine. The function of this enzyme requires the high concentrations of cortisol found in the adrenal medulla and hence plasma epinephrine is exclusively adrenal in origin.

CLINICAL MANIFESTATIONS OF ADRENOCORTICAL INSUFFICIENCY

Hypoadrenalism can occur either as primary disease due to destruction of the adrenal glands or as secondary to hypothalamic–pituitary disease and ACTH deficiency (Fig. 16.1). In primary adrenal failure aldosterone production is deficient; in contrast, in ACTH-deficient states, mineralocorticoid secretion is essentially normal, since renin is the dominant controller rather than ACTH. As a consequence of this distinction the metabolic complications of primary adrenal failure are greater.

Many of the symptoms of adrenal failure are of low specificity for the diagnosis and relatively common in the general population and therefore the diagnosis may be delayed for months or even years, particularly as it is usually of insidious onset. Fatigue is uniform in patients with adrenal failure, with anorexia, nausea, diarrhea, and weight loss being extremely common. Ill-defined epigastric or other abdominal pains and muscle aches are present in many patients and the first presentation may be to a gastroenterologist or rheumatologist. Postural hypotension is often a later manifestation and is more common in primary adrenal failure. Supine hypotension is an advanced feature and may presage impending adrenal crisis. The severity of symptoms can fluctuate as the failing glands may manage to maintain adequate basal cortisol production in the unstressed state but are unable to increase production at times of intercurrent illness, such as influenza. What would normally be a trivial illness is associated with an exacerbation of the symptoms of adrenal failure and delayed recovery. In primary adrenal failure the rising ACTH levels are responsible for the excessive pigmentation, typically of the pressure points, skin creases, genitalia, recent scars, buccal mucosa, and sun-exposed areas and this again can fluctuate, with scars often becoming darker during concurrent illnesses when pituitary ACTH secretion is maximal (Figs 16.2–16.4). Women may report loss of axillary hair through adrenal androgen deficiency.

Such pigmentation may precede frank adrenocortical insufficiency, sometimes for years, as adrenal reserve slowly declines, but circulating cortisol levels are maintained for a while under the increased ACTH drive. In primary adrenal failure there may be evidence of other organ-specific autoimmune diseases, such as vitiligo (Fig. 16.5), pernicious anemia, diabetes mellitus, or primary thyroid failure (Table 16.1); the association is often referred to as autoimmune polyglandular deficiency type II (or Schmidt's syndrome).

Adrenocorticotropic hormone is normally the last hormone to become deficient in patients with progressive pituitary disease;

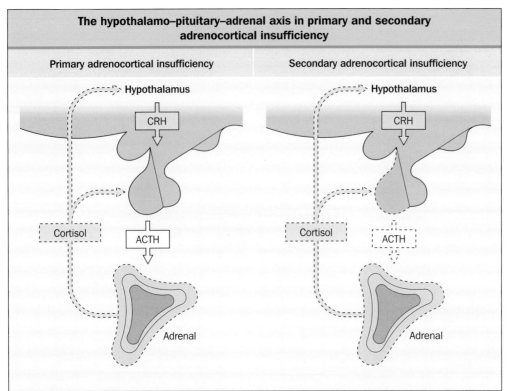

The hypothalamo–pituitary–adrenal axis in primary and secondary adrenocortical insufficiency	
Primary adrenocortical insufficiency	**Secondary adrenocortical insufficiency**

Figure 16.1 The hypothalamo–pituitary–adrenal axis in primary and secondary adrenocortical insufficiency. In primary adrenocortical insufficiency, circulating adrenocorticotropic hormone (ACTH) levels are elevated because of the negative feedback effects of low circulating cortisol. In secondary adrenocortical insufficiency, low circulating ACTH levels result from either hypothalamic or pituitary disease; as a consequence, cortisol levels are low. In secondary adrenocortical failure, aldosterone secretion is maintained as its principal controller is renin.

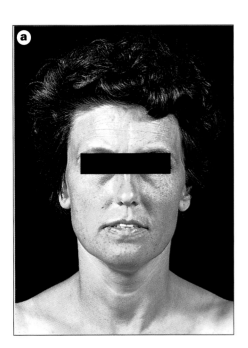

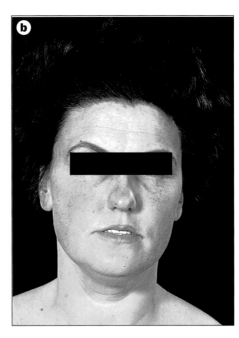

Figure 16.2 A patient with Addison's disease. (a) Before treatment. Note that the face is thin and pigmented. (b) During glucocorticoid replacement therapy.

therefore, the clinical consequences of other deficiencies may be manifest, plus additional evidence of pituitary disease such as hypersecretion or tumor pressure effects. Secondary (pituitary) adrenocortical insufficiency is similar but usually milder than primary insufficiency under unstressed conditions, except that the pigmentation does not occur, as ACTH levels are low. Aldosterone secretion is maintained in secondary adrenocortical insufficiency as it is dependent on the secretion of renin rather than ACTH for its control. The rare diagnosis of isolated ACTH deficiency is discussed elsewhere.

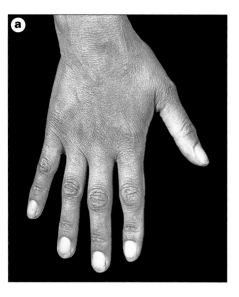 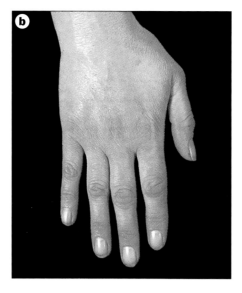

Figure 16.3 Pigmentation of the dorsal surface of the hands in a patient with Addison's disease. (a) Before treatment. (b) During glucocorticoid therapy; the normal hand color is now restored.

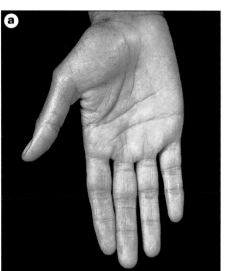 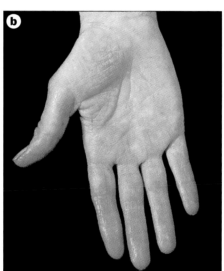

Figure 16.4 Pigmentation of the palmar creases of the hands in a patient with Addison's disease. Pigmentation in Addison's disease commonly occurs in areas exposed to light and pressure. It is unusually seen in the skin creases, as shown in (a). (b) During treatment, the normal color returns.

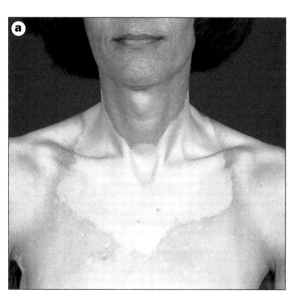 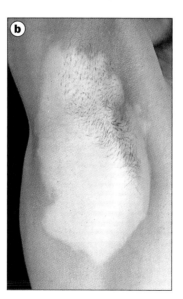

Figure 16.5 Vitiligo in a patient with Addison's disease. Depigmentation can be seen on the neck and chest (a) and in the axillary region (b). Increased pigmentation can be seen surrounding the areas of depigmentation.

Causes of primary adrenocortical failure		
Autoimmune		
Infection	Tuberculosis	
	Fungal infection	Histoplasmosis
		Blastomycosis
		Coccidioidomycosis
		Cryptococcosis
		Paracoccidoidomycosis
	Acquired immune deficiency syndrome (AIDS)	
	Cytomegalovirus	
Congenital or hereditary	Congenital adrenal hyperplasia	
	StAR mutations lipoid adrenal hyperplasia (cholesterol 20,22 desmolase defect)	
	DAX1 mutations	
	Adrenal cysts	
	ACTH-receptor gene mutations	
	Allgrove's syndrome (Triple A syndrome)	
	Adrenoleukodystrophy	
	Adrenomyeloneuropathy	
Drugs inhibiting cortisol synthesis	Aminoglutethimide	
	Metyrapone	
	o,p'DDD	
	Ketoconazole	
	Suramin	
	Etomidate	
Drugs increasing cortisol clearance	Barbiturates	
	Phenytoin	
	Rifampicin	
Other	Hemorrhage	Infection (Waterhouse–Friderichsen syndrome)
		Neisseria meningitides
		Haemophilus influenzae
		Pseudomonas aeruginosa
		Escherichia coli
		Streptococcus pneumoniae
		Anticoagulant therapy
	Metastatic tumor (commonly lung)	
	Amyloidosis	
	Hemochromatosis	
	Sarcoidosis	
	Bilateral adrenalectomy	

Table 16.1 Causes of primary adrenocortical failure. ACTH, adrenocorticotropic hormone; StAR, steroidogenic acute regulatory protein.

LABORATORY FINDINGS

In adrenocortical failure the blood count is often abnormal with a normocytic normochromic anemia, although if associated with vitamin B_{12} deficiency or hypothyroidism a macrocytosis may be encountered. A relative lymphocytosis is seen with glucocorticoid deficiency and eosinophilia is very common.

Hyponatremia is common in both primary and secondary adrenal failure, with hyperkalemia being essentially restricted to primary adrenal failure due particularly to the associated aldosterone deficiency. The patient will be hypovolemic with an elevated serum urea and possibly prerenal renal failure with an evaluated serum creatinine and mild metabolic acidosis. The hypovolemia causes a state of appropriate vasopressin secretion and the consequent water retention contributes to the hyponatremia, which is common to both primary and secondary adrenal insufficiency, although the abnormalities are more distinct in the former. Hypercalcemia is occasionally encountered. Plasma glucose is usually in the low–normal range, although occasionally hypoglycemia is encountered in patients with longstanding glucocorticoid deficiency (with consequential hepatic glycogen store deficiency) at times of decompensation associated vomiting or fasting; it is particularly common after excessive ethanol consumption, in children, and in isolated ACTH deficiency.

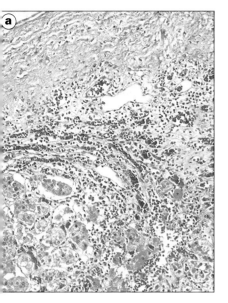

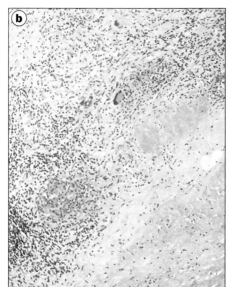

Figure 16.6 Histologic appearances of Addison's disease. The postmortem histology is shown of (a) autoimmune adrenalitis and (b) tuberculous adrenalitis in patients who died of Addison's disease. (a) The adrenal capsule is markedly thickened and the surviving cortex consists of scattered hypertrophied adrenocortical cells that are heavily infiltrated with lymphocytes. Hematoxylin–eosin stain, magnification × 120. (b) Pink-staining amorphous, caseous necrosis can be seen in addition to tuberculous granulation tissue and a Langerhans' giant cell. Hematoxylin–eosin stain, magnification × 80. (Courtesy of Professor I Doniach.)

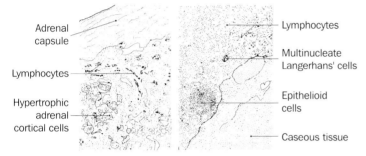

THYROID FUNCTION TESTS

Abnormalities of thyroid function tests are common at diagnosis of hypoadrenalism of any etiology. In the acutely unwell patient, thyroid function tests in keeping with the sick euthyroid syndrome may be encountered (see Chapter 10) with a low total and free thyroxine (T_4) and triiodothyronine (T_3), low normal thyroid-stimulating hormone (TSH) and, if measured, raised reverse T_3.

The more challenging abnormality is the patient with a low T_4 and T_3 and raised TSH. Autoimmune primary adrenal failure is common in patients with autoimmune adrenal failure. However, identical thyroid function tests can be encountered in patients as a secondary phenomenon to untreated primary adrenal failure; this corrects with hydrocortisone replacement therapy. The mechanism of these changes is ill-understood but has major clinical indications for patient care. Failure to appreciate that such thyroid function tests may be the result of hypoadrenalism rather than thyroid disease can result in unnecessary and potentially dangerous thyroxine therapy. In a patient with untreated cortisol deficiency, instigation of thyroxine will increase the metabolic rate and exacerbate the adrenal failure. For this reason, serum cortisol should be checked prior to starting thyroxine therapy in patients with apparent autoimmune thyroid failure.

ACUTE ADRENAL INSUFFICIENCY

This is often precipitated in an individual with borderline adrenal reserve by intercurrent illness, trauma, or surgery. The patient is weak, anorexic, and often nauseated and vomiting. Abdominal pain is frequently present and the patient is clinically dehydrated, hypovolemic, and hypotensive with the blood pressure falling further with an upright posture. Low-grade pyrexia and hyperpigmentation may be present. The electrolyte abnormalities described are likely to be present and the hypovolemic shock will respond poorly to fluid replacement in the absence of corticosteroid administration. The possibility of adrenal insufficiency should be considered in any patient with unexplained hypovolemic shock and in particular should be borne in mind in any patient who has taken exogenous glucocorticoids within the last year.

THE ETIOLOGY OF ADRENOCORTICAL FAILURE

Primary adrenal failure

Worldwide, tuberculosis of the adrenal glands remains the commonest cause of adrenal insufficiency (**Table 16.1, Fig. 16.6**), often presenting many years after the initial diagnosis, by which stage the caseating granulomas have been replaced by calcification, such that the glands have gone from being initially large to being small and calcified.

In the developed world, autoimmune adrenal destruction is responsible for more than 80% of cases (**Fig. 16.6**) and often occurs in the context of two distinct polyglandular deficiency syndromes. Autoimmune polyendocrinopathy syndrome type 1 (APS1) is a rare, autosomal-recessive disorder. The first manifestation is neonatal-onset mucocutaneous candidiasis with subsequent development of hypoparathyroidism and adrenal failure. In addition to the defining triad of features, other autoimmune conditions are associated: pernicious anemia, hypothyroidism, vitiligo, insulin-dependent diabetes mellitus, autoimmune hepatitis, celiac disease, and primary gonadal failure. The gene responsible for APS1 has been identified as *AIRE* (autoimmune regulator), with frame shift and nonsense mutations being found in affected individuals.

APS2 is far more common than type 1 and is defined by autoimmune thyroid disease and insulin-dependent diabetes mellitus plus, rather variably, adrenal failure, pernicious anemia, and primary gonadal failure. No single gene is responsible but strong associations with human leukocyte antigen (HLA) haplotypes DRB1, DQA1, and DQB1 are found. Adrenocortical autoantibodies are present in between 50% and 90% of patients with autoimmune adrenal failure. However, these antibodies are not responsible for adrenal destruction but are more probably markers of the autoimmune process, with the damage being the result of cell-mediated immunity.

Globally, fungal infection continues to be an important cause of adrenal insufficiency, with essentially all fungi being capable of destroying the adrenals with the exception of *Candida albicans*. Histoplasmosis is common in North America, with blastomycosis being the more prevalent in South America. Fungal infection is a particular problem in the immunocompromised and as such is encountered in patients with advanced human immunodeficiency virus (HIV) disease, particularly cryptococcosis. HIV adrenalitis and adrenal insufficiency are increasingly recognized, but without superadded infection. In common with tuberculosis, the glands are initially enlarged but progressively shrink, fibrose, and calcify. In primary fungal infections the glands may remain large because of a periadrenalitis.

Bilateral adrenal hemorrhage was described many years ago as the Waterhouse–Friderichsen syndrome in the context of septicemia, especially with meningococcal and pneumococcal infections. It is now recognized as occurring in other conditions associated with impaired coagulation, in particular during treatment with warfarin and heparin.

The adrenal glands are extremely vascular, receiving approximately 11% of cardiac output. Therefore the adrenals are a common site of tumor metastasis, but bilateral adrenal destruction by metastases sufficient to cause clinical insufficiency is rare.

Adrenoleukodystrophy (ALD) and adrenomyeloneuropathy can be regarded as different phenotypes of the same illness and are due to defects in the same enzyme. The defect is impaired metabolic degradation of very long chain fatty acid (VLCFA) in the peroxisomal system. The accumulation of VLCFA in the white matter of the central nervous system results in demyelination. ALD is an X-linked recessive disorder with very variable manifestations. The major clinical problems are in males and consist of hypoadrenalism and central nervous system demyelination, often producing dementia. The condition is in the differential diagnosis of multiple sclerosis, with progression of the neurologic manifestations being variable. Female heterozygote carriers may develop neurologic symptoms such as spastic paraparesis but the features are often milder and more slowly progressive than in affected males and adrenocortical failure is not characteristic. Treatment of the hypoadrenalism is standard but there is no satisfactory treatment of the underlying metabolic defect. Attempts to arrest or delay the accumulation of VLCFA by dietary modification have been disappointing.

Cortisol deficiency of variable severity is a feature of congenital adrenal hyperplasia (see Chapter 24). In classical 21-hydroxylase deficiency the presentation of hypoadrenalism takes the form of a salt-losing crisis at approximately 1 week of age. Cortisol deficiency and salt wasting are also encountered in congenital adrenal hyperplasia resulting from defects in the enzymes 11β-hydroxylase, 3β-hydroxysteroid dehydrogenase, or 17α-hydroxlase.

Congenital lipoid adrenal hyperplasia is a severe form of congenital adrenal hyperplasia. All affected individuals have a female phenotype and presentation is in the neonatal period with salt-wasting crises. All steroid production in the adrenals and gonads is impaired as a consequence of mutations in the steroidogenic acute regulatory protein (StAR) gene and consequential failure to convert cholesterol to pregnenolone.

Congenital adrenal hypoplasia is an X-linked autosomal recessive condition presenting in boys with childhood adrenocortical insufficiency and a failure to enter or progress through puberty because of hypogonadotropic hypogonadism. It is caused by mutations of the steroidogenesis gene *DAX1* (see Chapter 3).

Other single-gene disorders associated with neonatal adrenal insufficiency include the ACTH resistance disorders caused by mutations either of the melanocortin receptor type 2 (MC2-R) or the triple A syndrome, both of which are of autosomal recessive inheritance. The latter ill-understood syndrome is characterized by ACTH resistance, achalasia and alacrima. The single gene responsible for this disease has now been identified.

Secondary adrenal failure

Hypopituitarism of any etiology may result in ACTH and cortisol deficiency, although not aldosterone deficiency. In hypopituitarism, ACTH is usually the last pituitary hormone to be affected and other evidence of pituitary disease and hypopituitarism should therefore be sought.

The syndrome of isolated ACTH deficiency is a rare and ill-understood condition of uncertain etiology, with the peak age of presentation between 40 and 50 years of age. The presentation and symptoms at diagnosis are much as with other causes of secondary hypoadrenalism, except that hypoglycemia is found in 50% of patients at diagnosis. Symptoms are often nonspecific and unclear - prolonged lethargy, tiredness, depression – and their significance is often missed The majority of cases are probably a consequence of lymphocytic hypophysitis and, in keeping with this, an ACTH response to exogenous CRH is rarely seen. Very rare reports of patients with hypothalamic and pro-opiomelanocortin processing defects exist.

Exogenous glucocorticoid therapy given by any route can result in hypothalamic–pituitary suppression and ACTH deficiency, and may persist for up to 2 months following discontinuation of treatment but occasionally longer. The patient is particularly at risk of hypoadrenalism if glucocorticoid therapy is stopped

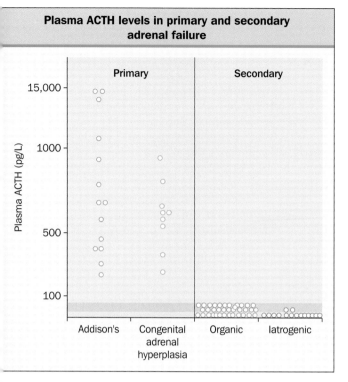

Figure 16.7 Plasma adrenocorticotropic hormone (ACTH) levels in primary and secondary adrenal failure.

abruptly; this can result in the paradoxical situation of a patient looking cushingoid but being cortisol-deficient. In patients on low-dose glucocorticoid therapy or within 2 months of discontinuing it, the unstressed, basal cortisol production rate may be normal but, if confronted with a physiologically stressful event, may not increase as required and hypoadrenalism can occur.

DIAGNOSIS

The acutely unwell patient

The commonest reason for failure to diagnose adrenal disease is failure to consider the diagnosis. Once this step has been taken, confirmation of the diagnosis is usually straightforward. Since the presenting symptoms may be nebulous, the diagnosis should be considered in any acutely unwell patient with unexplained hypovolemic features. In the acutely unwell patient a random serum cortisol of less than 100nmol/L (3.5µg/dL) is diagnostic and, if accompanied by a plasma ACTH of more than 100pmol/L, is indicative of primary adrenal failure (**Fig. 16.7**). If the diagnosis is considered, once basal diagnostic bloods have been drawn, treatment should be initiated without delay. Once the patient has recovered from the acute illness, and if doubt persists, the diagnosis can be confirmed by more detailed investigations, performed as described below. No patient ever died from a single dose of hydrocortisone; many have died for want of a dose of hydrocortisone! In the conscious patient a history of exogenous glucocorticoid therapy should be sought, be it in the form of tablets, creams, or inhalers, and the unconscious patient should be searched for evidence of a steroid card or similar indicator of exogenous glucocorticoid therapy.

Elective diagnosis
ACTH testing

The cortisol stimulating activity of ACTH lies in the N-terminal 1-24 sequence of amino acids, and the use of 250mg of soluble synthetic $ACTH_{(1-24)}$ (Synacthen®, Cortrosyn®, tetracosactrin) is the gold standard for the diagnosis of primary adrenal failure. The test (**Fig. 16.8**) should be performed at 09.00h when circulating cortisol levels are high, since the normal range of responses was estimated at this time and this improves the interpretation of the baseline plasma cortisol and ACTH values. Then cortisol is measured at 30 and 60min after the intramuscular administration of 250µg of $ACTH_{(1-24)}$. The maximal serum cortisol response is normally seen at 30min and, if more than 500nmol/L (18µg/dL), effectively excludes a diagnosis of primary adrenal failure. The interpretation of suboptimal responses is aided by reference to the baseline plasma ACTH, which will be elevated in primary adrenal failure. Any form of exogenous glucocorticoid – oral, transdermal, inhaled, or intranasal – may result in a suboptimal response but will be associated with secondary adrenocortical failure, ACTH deficiency, and a low circulating ACTH level.

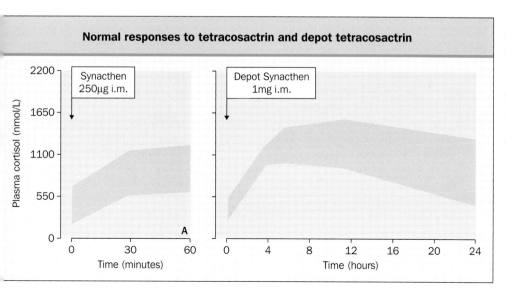

Figure 16.8 Normal responses to tetracosactrin and depot tetracosactrin. Tetracosactrin (Synacthen®, Cortrosyn®) is administered intramuscularly in doses of 250µg, whereas depot tetracosactrin is given in doses of 1mg (27.5nmol/dL cortisol; 1µg/dL). Tetracosactrin is a form of synthetic ACTH.

The 250μg ACTH test can be used for the diagnosis of secondary adrenal failure as well, but the supraphysiologic dose of ACTH may induce cortisol responses in patients with pituitary disease and partial ACTH deficiency. For this reason there is interest in the use of a more physiologic 1μg ACTH test. Although this still results in supraphysiologic plasma ACTH levels, the risks of missing hypopituitarism are diminished, although the limitation of this test is the frequently inadequate cortisol response in patients with a normal hypothalamic–pituitary–adrenal axis, thereby necessitating the use of a further test, such as an insulin tolerance test. A peak plasma cortisol of more than 600nmol/L (22μg/dL) excludes ACTH deficiency but a lower response in a patient with suspected pituitary disease necessitates further investigation with an insulin tolerance test.

No commercial 1μg ACTH preparation is available, thus necessitating dilution of 250μg ACTH ampoules and, in conjunction with problems of ACTH adhesion to plastic tubing and syringes, this means that the dose of ACTH administered is variable.

A zinc-absorbed depot preparation of $ACTH_{(1-24)}$ (Synacthen Depot® or Cortrosyn Depot®), administered intramuscularly, can be used to differentiate primary adrenal failure from adrenal atrophy due to ACTH deficiency if ACTH assays are not available. A dose of 1mg is administered at 09.00h and serum cortisol is measured half-hourly for 2 hours and then at 4, 6, 8, 12 and 24 hours. No response is anticipated in patients with primary adrenal disease, while in patients with ACTH deficiency an increment in cortisol is seen, maximal at 12–24 hours; occasionally it is necessary to administer 1mg of depot ACTH for 3 days before a significant rise is seen. The response in the first hour after 1mg of depot ACTH is essentially the same as is seen with 250μg soluble $ACTH_{(1-24)}$.

Serum cortisol measurement

There are several important variables that need to be considered when interpreting serum cortisol measurements. Significant interassay differences in cortisol assays are seen and therefore all cutoff values are approximations rather than absolute and need validation for specific assays in different laboratories. Some 90% of serum cortisol is bound to cortisol-binding globulin (CBG) and is therefore inactive, and anything that alters CBG will alter measured serum cortisol without altering the bioactive, free cortisol concentrations. Elevated serum estrogen levels, either caused by exogenous therapy, such as oral contraceptive pill or hormone replacement therapy, or as seen during pregnancy, result in an elevated CBG level and spuriously high serum cortisol level, thus masking a diagnosis of hypoadrenalism. Patients should discontinue oral estrogens, when feasible, for 6 weeks prior to pituitary function testing. Similarly, in patients with hypoproteinemia, e.g. the nephrotic syndrome, serum cortisol may be misleadingly low and adrenal failure can be diagnosed erroneously. CBG levels tend to be low in active acromegaly.

In patients with suspected primary adrenal failure already established on replacement therapy and in need of further investigation, it is important to ensure that the glucocorticoid replacement therapy does not interfere with cortisol measurement following $ACTH_{(1-24)}$ administration. Prednisolone and prednisone crossreact with many commercial cortisol assays and, along

with hydrocortisone, must be discontinued 24 hours before $ACTH_{(1-24)}$ administration. To avoid precipitating hypoadrenalism, it may be necessary to cover a patient with dexamethasone, which does not crossreact, during depot $ACTH_{(1-24)}$ tests (see below).

In patients with insidious adrenal destruction, e.g. secondary to tuberculosis or histoplasmosis, or autoimmune adrenalitis, ACTH levels may be high for prolonged periods while total cortisol levels remain normal. The patient will be pigmented but otherwise symptom-free (just suntanned and looking inappropriately healthy!) during this phase of compensated adrenocortical insufficiency, until stressed by intercurrent illness.

In primary adrenal disease the zona glomerulosa is destroyed and there is aldosterone deficiency; a high plasma renin activity with an inappropriately low aldosterone is therefore further evidence of primary adrenal failure and is not seen in patients with ACTH deficiency. Care must be taken when measuring plasma renin activity, as estrogen therapy interferes with some assay methodologies.

Establishing the etiology of primary adrenal failure

In the developed world, as already discussed, autoimmune adrenal failure accounts for 80% of new cases of primary adrenal failure. In such patients events of adrenal antibodies should be sought. In direct support of an autoimmune etiology is the presence of other organ-specific endocrine disease, such as hypothyroidism, diabetes mellitus, primary ovarian failure, or vitiligo. If there is any history to suggest tuberculosis, fungal infection or immunocompromise, then evidence of the relevant infection should be sought.

Contrast-enhanced computerized tomography provides the best-resolution images of the adrenal glands and should be performed in any patient in whom there is doubt as to the etiology of adrenal failure. A good history and examination for the other features is crucial to the diagnosis of the various hereditary forms of adrenal failure, although it must be recognized that adrenal failure may be the first presentation and neurologic decompensation may develop only after the patient is established on replacement therapy.

TREATMENT

Emergency treatment

In the acutely unwell patient with suspected hypoadrenalism, the basal bloods (discussed above) should be obtained as described above and hydrocortisone administered immediately. A dose of 100mg of hydrocortisone intramuscularly every 6 hours will provide adequate serum cortisol concentrations and, because of the mineralocorticoid activity of high levels of hydrocortisone, will also correct mineralocorticoid deficiency. Alternatively, hydrocortisone can be administered as an intravenous infusion at 3–4mg/hour, but the risk of this is that any interruption to the infusion will result in rapid decompensation. Intravenous bolus hydrocortisone should not be used as it is cleared rapidly. Hydrocortisone has the advantage over other synthetic glucocorticoids that it can be measured in plasma to ensure that adequate circulating concentrations (500–700nmol/L; 18–25μg/dL) are achieved and, as indicated above, mineralocorticoid therapy is unnecessary during high-dose parenteral hydrocortisone replacement therapy.

Long-term replacement therapy

The aim of replacement therapy is to reproduce the circadian rhythm of cortisol in the unstressed patient while educating the patient to ensure an appropriate response to any intercurrent illness or physiologic stressful events such as surgery. Cortisol (called hydrocortisone when used as a pharmaceutical preparation) is the obvious glucocorticoid to use in patients with adrenal failure as it is the true replacement for the deficient glucocorticoid. Moreover, plasma levels can be readily measured and the dose thus titrated to achieve, as near as possible, a normal circadian rhythm of plasma cortisol.

Cortisone acetate, historically a popular form of replacement therapy, requires enzymatic activation in the liver by the enzyme 11β-hydroxysteroid dehydrogenase type 1 and any factors modulating activity of the enzyme will alter circulating cortisol levels. Further, the conversion of cortisol to hydrocortisone may be slow in some patients so that cortisol levels remain low for several hours after cortisol administration. Oral hydrocortisone is speedily absorbed, especially if the patient is fasting, and is thus a more satisfactory replacement therapy.

Potent synthetic glucocorticoids such as dexamethasone and prednisolone have long half-lives and cannot be measured routinely in plasma. Greater potential for overtreatment therefore exists. These glucocorticoids lack mineralocorticoid activity, which is an advantage when used at pharmacologic doses for inflammatory conditions but a potential disadvantage in patients with adrenal failure.

In recent years there has been a move to use a lower total daily dose of hydrocortisone and to divide it into three daily doses rather than two. Ideally, in a compliant patient, the first dose should be taken first thing in the morning on awakening, fasting before rising, to ensure rapid absorption, with the second dose prior to the midday meal and the last dose prior to the evening meal, no later than 18.00h. A common dosing regimen is a first of dose 10mg with the second and third doses being 5mg. However this is entirely dependent on the plasma cortisol levels achieved and patient's wellbeing. The appropriateness of a dosing regimen can be assessed by multiple serum cortisol measurement during a single day, with dose adjustment based on serum levels and patient symptomatology.

Aldosterone replacement therapy is provided as fludrocortisone administered usually twice daily by mouth. The dose of fludrocortisone should be titrated against plasma renin activity. With the vogue for low salt diets it is important to ensure an adequate dietary salt intake, particularly in hot weather.

A usual dose of fludrocortisone is 0.1mg twice daily. The dose is adjusted to maintain a normal lying plasma renin level. Renin levels are elevated if mineral corticoid replacement is inadequate and suppressed if it is excessive.

In healthy women, the adrenal glands are the principal source of androgens, particularly dehydroepiandrosterone (DHEA), and deficiency in women with adrenocortical failure is alleged to effect wellbeing adversely. Recent evidence from studies of oral DHEA replacement therapy (50mg/day) in women with primary adrenal disease suggests that it may improve general wellbeing and physical, mental, and sexual satisfaction. Further work is required to define the role and optimal means of delivering androgen replacement therapy in women with hypoadrenalism.

Patients need to be educated to double the dose of hydrocortisone when unwell and if for any reason, e.g. diarrhea or vomiting, they are unable to take the medication orally they must ensure they receive it intramuscularly. Written instructions should be provided about hydrocortisone replacement therapy and a vial of hydrocortisone plus needle and syringe for self-administration. A steroid card must be carried at all times and patients should be encouraged to become members of a reference agency such as the MedicAlert Foundation (9 Hanover Street, London W1R 9HF, UK) and wear a bracelet or necklace indicating their therapy. There are patient support groups in many countries, which provide valuable advice and other counseling and patients should be encouraged to join such a group (see Chapter 43.5).

In summary, great advances have been made in our understanding of the mechanisms underlying some of the rare, single-gene causes of hypoadrenalism, but the majority of patients worldwide continue to develop hypoadrenalism as a consequence of infection or autoimmune destruction. Death from hypoadrenalism is, virtually always, avoidable. Once the diagnosis is suspected, investigation need not delay treatment and confirmation of the diagnosis is rarely difficult. In addition to the instigation of long-term replacement therapy, patient education is crucial to prevent hypoadrenal crisis at times of intercurrent illness.

FURTHER READING

Bondy PK. Disorders of the adrenal cortex. In: Wilson JD, Foster DW, eds. Williams textbook of endocrinology, 7th edn. WB Saunders: Philadelphia; 1985:816–90.

Gilkes JJH, Rees LH, Besser GM. Plasma immunoreactive corticotrophin and lipotrophin in Cushing's syndrome and Addison's disease. Br Med J. 1977;1:966–98.

Hornsby PH. The regulation of adrenocortical function by control of growth and structure. In: Anderson DC, Winter JSD, eds. Adrenal cortex. Butterworth's International Medical Reviews: London; 1985:1–31.

Irvine WJ, Toft AD, Feek CM. Addison's disease. In: James VHT, ed. Comprehensive endocrinology: The Adrenal gland. Raven Press: New York; 1979:131–64.

Takahashi H, Teranishi Y, Nakanishi S, Numa S. Isolation and structural organisation of the human corticotropin-beta-lipotropin gene. FEBS Letters 1981;135:97–102.

Whitfeld PL, Seeburg PH, Shine J. The human pro-opiomelancortin gene: organisation, sequence and interspersion with repetitive DNA. DNA 1982;1:133–43.

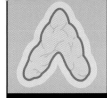

Chapter 17

Adrenal Cortex: Renin–Angiotensin System in Adrenocortical Hypertension

Paul M Stewart

INTRODUCTION

Hypertension affects 10–25% of the population and is an important risk factor for cardiovascular, cerebrovascular, and renal diseases. In the majority of cases, no underlying cause for the patient's raised blood pressure is apparent and they are labeled as having 'essential' hypertension. However, in approximately 5% of patients an underlying cause can be identified. Once coarctation of the aorta, acromegaly, hyperparathyroidism, estrogen-induced hypertension, and pheochromocytomas have been excluded, the cause is invariably underlying renal disease or mineralocorticoid-based hypertension (**Table 17.1**). These diagnoses are important to make because the hypertension may be reversible with surgery or appropriate medical therapy. In addition, within the last 5 years, the genetic basis for several novel forms of mineralocorticoid hypertension has been elucidated and this has raised new questions as to the prevalence of mineralocorticoid-based hypertension in patients with 'essential' hypertension. Such cases provide a fascinating insight into the underlying basis of hypertension and this may have important implications for others with 'essential' hypertension.

The basis for these forms of hypertension requires an understanding of the renin–angiotensin–aldosterone system. What are these secondary forms of hypertension, and how are they diagnosed and treated appropriately?

THE RENIN–ANGIOTENSIN–ALDOSTERONE SYSTEM

Adrenal corticosteroids have been classified as either mineralocorticoids or glucocorticoids. Both classes of hormone are secreted from the adrenal cortex, glucocorticoids in relatively high amounts (cortisol 10–20mg/day) from the zona fasciculata under the control of adrenocorticotropin (ACTH; Chapters 15, 16) and mineralocorticoids in low amounts (aldosterone 100–150µg/day) from the zona glomerulosa. In normal physiology, aldosterone secretion is under the principal control of the renin–angiotensin system in a classic endocrine negative feedback loop. Renin is a proteolytic enzyme that is synthesized and stored by specialized cells in the wall of the afferent arteriole situated in the glomerulus of the kidney. These cells are anatomically and functionally associated with the cells in the wall of the distal convoluted tubules (the 'macula densa'), and the whole structure is known as the juxtaglomerular apparatus. The release of renin activates a cascade system (**Fig. 17.1**) in which renin cleaves a leucine–valine bond in the liver-derived CC2-globulin prohormone angiotensinogen to form the decapeptide

Differential diagnosis of renal and mineralocorticoid-based hypertension	
Cause	**Offending mineralocorticoid**

Renal hypertension
Renovascular hypertension
  (atheroma, fibromuscular dysplasia)
Renal parenchymatous disease
Primary reninism (juxtaglomerular tumor,
  "ectopic" renin)
	Activation of renin–
	angiotensin–
	aldosterone axis

Primary aldosteronism
  Aldosterone-producing adenoma (APA)
  Bilateral idiopathic hyperplasia (IHA)
  Glucocorticoid-suppressible
    hyperaldosteronism (GSH)
  Adrenal carcinoma
	Aldosterone

Congenital adrenal hyperplasia
  11β-hydroxylase deficiency
  17α-hydroxylase deficiency
	Deoxycorticosterone

Glucocorticoid receptor resistance
  Glucocorticoid receptor mutations
  Metyrapone, RU486 ingestion
	Deoxycorticosterone

Deoxycorticosterone- secreting adrenal tumor	Deoxycorticosterone
Liddle's syndrome	None

11β-hydroxysteroid
  dehydrogenase deficiency
  Apparent mineralocorticoid excess
  Licorice and carbenoxolone
    ingestion
Ectopic adrenocorticotropin syndrome
	Cortisol

Table 17.1 Differential diagnosis of renal and mineralocorticoid-based hypertension.

angiotensin I. This is subsequently converted by angiotensin-converting enzyme (ACE) to the octapeptide angiotensin II. ACE is a dipeptidyl carboxypeptidase that is found in high concentrations in the pulmonary circulation; it is, however, also present in the systemic vasculature and the kidney. Angiotensin II is a potent vasoconstrictor and can thus elevate blood pressure but it also stimulates aldosterone secretion directly, leading to the retention of sodium and loss of potassium. The major

Factors involved in the production and secretion of aldosterone

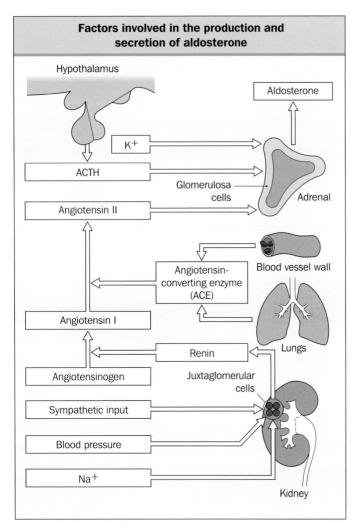

Figure 17.1 The renin–angiotensin–aldosterone axis. Following release, renin converts angiotensinogen to angiotensin I which is subsequently converted to angiotensin II by angiotensin-converting enzyme (ACE). Angiotensin II raises blood pressure through its vasoconstrictor action and in addition directly stimulates aldosterone secretion from the zona glomerulosa of the adrenal cortex. ACTH, adrenocorticotropic hormone.

trigger for renin release is a decrease in perfusion pressure, and this may result from hemorrhage, hypotension, or a reduction in the extracellular fluid volume after sodium depletion. Negative feedback control of aldosterone secretion is ensured: increased renin secretion increases angiotensin II and aldosterone levels, which will raise blood pressure and result in sodium retention and volume expansion; in turn this will switch off renin secretion, maintaining homeostasis.

Although angiotensin II is the principal secretagogue, aldosterone secretion is also regulated by ACTH and potassium. Although acute administration of ACTH stimulates aldosterone secretion, chronic ACTH excess is associated with normal or even low levels of aldosterone. Elevation of circulating potassium can directly stimulate the zona glomerulosa, while hypokalemia may inhibit aldosterone synthesis.

The primary effect of aldosterone is to increase the resorption of sodium by the distal convoluted tubule of the kidney, in exchange for potassium and hydrogen ions through the interaction of aldosterone with the mineralocorticoid receptor (MR) and induction of the basolateral sodium–potassium ATPase pump and the apical sodium channel. Therefore, if aldosterone levels are persistently elevated, hypokalemia and alkalosis will ensue.

The MR, however, is nonselective *in vitro*. Paradoxically, cortisol and aldosterone have the same intrinsic affinity for this receptor, raising the question as to how aldosterone is the preferred mineralocorticoid *in vivo*. This selectivity is achieved at a prereceptor level through the expression of an enzyme, 11β hydroxysteroid dehydrogenase type 2 (11β-HSD2), which efficiently converts cortisol to its intrinsically inactive metabolite, cortisone, allowing aldosterone to occupy the MR. Inhibition of 11β-HSD2 results in the glucocorticoid cortisol, acting as a potent mineralocorticoid.

RENAL HYPERTENSION

Renal hypertension constitutes the commonest cause of secondary hypertension, although its true incidence is difficult to define. The causes can most readily be divided into renovascular or renal parenchymatous disease (**Table 17.2**). The hallmark of renal-based hypertension is increased renin secretion with activation of the renin–angiotensin–aldosterone system (**Fig. 17.2**). Primary reninism is rare, with less than 50 cases reported in the literature.

The two most common causes of renal artery stenosis are atheromatous plaques and fibromuscular hyperplasia. Atheromatous stenoses may be unilateral or bilateral, are most frequently found in the proximal third of the renal artery, frequently at its origin, and present in middle-aged and elderly patients. They are common and occur in the context of generalized atheromatous disease elsewhere (coronary and carotid arteries).

Renal causes of hypertension

Renal parenchymatous	Renovascular
Acute and chronic glomerulonephritis	Coarctation of the aorta
Chronic pyelonephritis – especially if calculi or obstruction with hydronephrosis	Renal artery stenosis e.g. with fibromuscular hyperplasia, atheromatous plaque, congenital
Polycystic disease	Malignant or accelerated-phase hypertension
Interstitial nephritis, e.g. with gout, hypercalcemia, or excessive analgesics (analgesic nephropathy)	**Primary reninism**
Amyloidosis	Reninomas (juxtaglomerular tumors)
Connective tissue disease, e.g. with polyarteritis, systemic lupus erythematosus, and diabetes mellitus	Some Wilm's tumors
	Ectopic renin secretion

Table 17.2 Renal causes of hypertension. These can be classified into renovascular hypertension, renal parenchymatous disease, and primary reninism. Of these, renovascular hypertension is the most common.

Sequence of events in secondary hyperaldosteronism

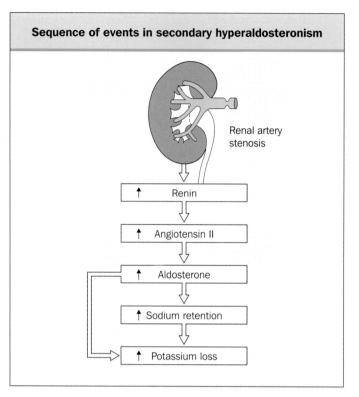

Figure 17.2 Sequence of events in secondary hyperaldosteronism.
In secondary hyperaldosteronism, circulating renin levels are elevated as a consequence of renal artery stenosis, renal hypoperfusion, or volume depletion. High renin levels, in turn, lead to increased angiotensin II levels and hyperaldosteronism, with concomitant sodium retention and potassium wastage.

Diagnosis of renal artery stenosis: captopril renogram

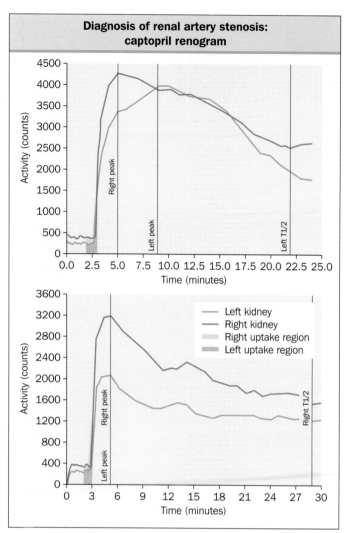

Figure 17.3 Diagnosis of renal artery stenosis: captopril renogram.
Renal blood flow is shown (top panel) before captopril, and (bottom panel) after captopril. Captopril renogram demonstrating fall in glomerular filtration rate (GFR) 1 hour after the administration of 25mg captopril orally. The fall in GFR after angiotensin-converting enzyme (ACE) inhibition in the lower panel indicates the probability of left sided renal artery stenosis.

In contrast, fibromuscular hyperplasia involves the middle and distal thirds of the renal artery and is the most common cause of renal artery stenosis in young patients.

Renovascular hypertension may be suggested by finding a renal artery bruit. This is best heard over the long muscles of the back at the level of L1 or in the epigastrium. In most patients, however, there are no specific clinical clues and it is important to stress that the presence of a renal vascular lesion does not necessarily imply a functional effect. Nevertheless the diagnosis should be considered:

- in patients developing hypertension at extremes of age (before 30 and after 60 years);
- in patients with accelerated-phase or malignant hypertension;
- in hypertensive patients with unexplained deterioration in renal function;
- in hypertensive patients with unexplained sudden-onset pulmonary edema.

Hypertension follows reduced arterial perfusion to the kidney and activation of the renin–angiotensin–aldosterone axis. The raised renal perfusion pressure in the nonstenotic kidney induces a natriuresis that partially offsets the effect of the vascular stenosis but equally prevents restoration of pressure to the stenotic kidney. As a result, angiotensin-II-dependent hypertension

is maintained. Furthermore in this situation, glomerular filtration rate in the stenotic kidney is critically dependent upon angiotensin-II-mediated glomerular efferent arteriolar tone. This observation forms the basis for a diagnostic test in patients with suspected renal artery stenosis, the 'captopril renogram'. Removal of angiotensin II from the stenotic kidney following ACE inhibition with captopril results in a marked fall in glomerular filtration rate on the affected side (**Fig. 17.3**). False-positive results are reported but a normal captopril renogram virtually excludes a functionally significant renovascular lesion. Other diagnostic tests include duplex ultrasonography, magnetic resonance angiography (**Fig. 17.4**) and spiral CT angiography.

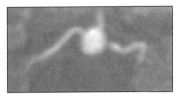
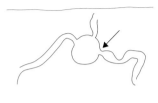

Figure 17.4 Magnetic resonance angiography showing the presence of renal artery stenosis (arrow).

Treatment for renal artery stenosis comprises:

- medical therapy, which is effective in 75–80% of cases – ACE inhibitors are particularly effective but renal function may deteriorate and should be monitored closely;
- transluminal angioplasty, in which expansion of a balloon on the end of a catheter opens up the narrowed area (**Fig. 17.5**);
- surgical reconstruction;
- renal artery stenting via a catheter, using a rigid coil to hold the artery open after dilatation.

Re-stenosis rates following simple angioplasty and revascularization are high and renal artery stenting is probably the invasive procedure of choice, particularly for atheromatous disease. There continues to be debate over medical versus invasive therapy but recent data indicate renal protection following stenting compared to medical therapy alone. Controlled trials are under way to evaluate this in more detail and also to assess blood pressure control.

Renal parenchymal disease may cause hypertension because of a combination of loss of functional nephrons (and a reduction in ability to excrete salt) together with stimulation of renin secretion due to intrarenal vascular disruption and fibrosis.

Juxtaglomerular cell tumors may cause hypertension and hypokalemia because of autonomous renin secretion. Ectopic renin-secreting tumors have also been reported notably in patients with lung carcinoma and tumors of the urogenital tract.

MINERALOCORTICOID EXCESS

In contrast to renal hypertension, mineralocorticoid-based hypertension classically describes hypertension caused by increased sodium and water retention by the kidney and expansion of the extracellular fluid compartment, and results in suppression of endogenous plasma renin activity. Unlike the majority of cases of secondary aldosteronism, which arise either in the setting of reduced oncotic pressure (nephrosis, cirrhosis) or in patients with cardiac failure, edema is not a feature of primary aldosteronism, probably because of renal compensatory mechanisms, which result in a secondary natriuresis ('escape' phenomenon). Nevertheless, in the short term, intravascular volume is reset at a higher level and this leads to increased cardiac output and blood pressure. In the chronic state hypervolemia cannot be consistently demonstrated and other mechanisms may be equally important in raising blood pressure. Mineralocorticoid receptors have been characterized in the vasculature and heart, and, depending upon the activity of local

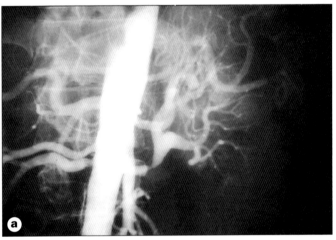
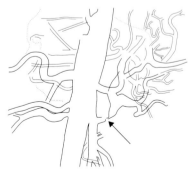
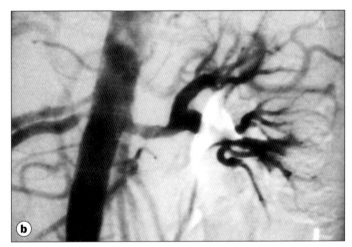
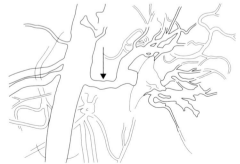

Figure 17.5 Atheromatous renal artery stenosis. Contrast radiography showing the renal artery (a) before and (b) following transluminal angioplasty. The arrows show the site of the stenosis before (a) and after (b) angioplasty.

11β-HSD, either glucocorticoids or mineralocorticoids may induce cardiac fibrosis and increase vascular tone by potentiating catecholamine and angiotensin-II-induced vasoconstriction, or by inhibiting endothelial relaxation. Mineralocorticoids can also modulate blood pressure centrally, independent of changes in renal electrolyte transport or vascular reactivity.

DIFFERENTIAL DIAGNOSIS OF MINERALOCORTICOID HYPERTENSION

Primary aldosteronism

First described by Conn in 1955, this is the commonest cause of mineralocorticoid hypertension. Prevalence rates of 0.5–2% have been widely reported in the literature in unselected patients with 'essential' hypertension, but many of these studies relied on detecting hypokalemia and, in the light of recent observations, will have underestimated true prevalence rates. By contrast, studies suggesting much higher prevalence rates of 5–12% in hypertensive populations have been conducted in specialist centers and are therefore subject to selection bias.

Symptoms are often absent or nonspecific but include tiredness, muscle weakness, thirst, polyuria, and nocturia resulting from the hypokalemia. Spontaneous hypokalemia (<3.5mmol/L) is rare in untreated hypertension; when found in a patient on diuretics these should be withdrawn, potassium stores replenished, and remeasured 2 weeks later. Despite this, it is now accepted that up to 40% of patients with surgically confirmed primary aldosteronism will have normal serum potassium concentrations.

In approximately two thirds of cases, primary aldosteronism occurs as a result of a small (0.5–2cm), solitary, aldosterone-producing adenoma of the adrenal, which is commoner in women than men (M:F ratio 1:3). One third of cases are caused by idiopathic bilateral adrenal hyperplasia (**Figs 17.6 & 17.7**) and the remaining few (<2%) by glucocorticoid suppressible hyperaldosteronism or aldosterone-secreting carcinomas. The etiology of aldosterone-producing adenoma is unknown, although rarely it may have a genetic basis and can occur as a component of multiple endocrine neoplasia type 1.

Diagnosis

Primary aldosteronism is confirmed by demonstrating subnormal supine and erect plasma renin and an elevated plasma aldosterone concentration in a patient off all antihypertensive treatment for at least 3 weeks. However, primary aldosteronism may also occur with suppressed plasma renin and normal aldosterone levels and some investigators advocate measures of urinary aldosterone secretion over a 24-hour period or salt suppression studies to further confirm the diagnosis. If severe hypertension prevents complete cessation of antihypertensive therapy during this diagnostic period, alpha-blockers such as prazosin or doxazosin interfere least with the renin–angiotensin–aldosterone axis. A single measurement of the ratio of plasma renin activity to plasma aldosterone concentration may be a sensitive screening test, even in patients still taking antihypertensive medication, but, depending upon the assays used and population salt intake, this requires validation in each center.

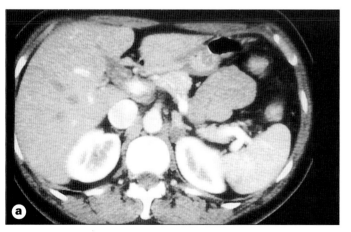

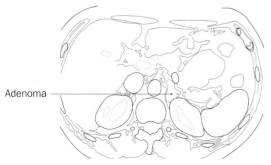

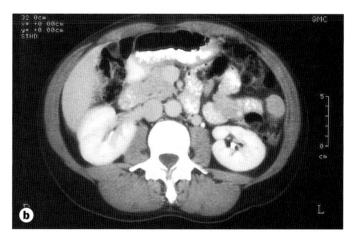

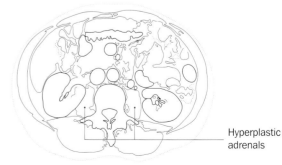

Figure 17.6 Adrenal computerized tomography (CT) in primary aldosteronism. CT scans demonstrating (a) the presence of a solitary, small, left-sided aldosterone-producing adenoma in a middle-aged woman with hypertension and hypokalemia and (b) bilateral hyperplasia in a patient with idiopathic hyperplasia of the adrenal cortex.

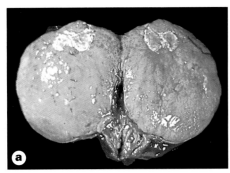

Figure 17.7 Primary hyperaldosteronism. (a) Adrenal adenoma removed from a patient with primary hyperaldosteronism (Conn's syndrome). The canary-yellow color of the adenoma is typical. (b) Nodular hyperplasia associated with Conn's syndrome. Bilateral hyperplasia occurs in approximately 30% of patients with primary hyperaldosteronism.

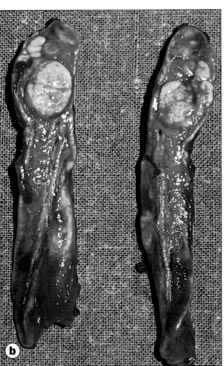

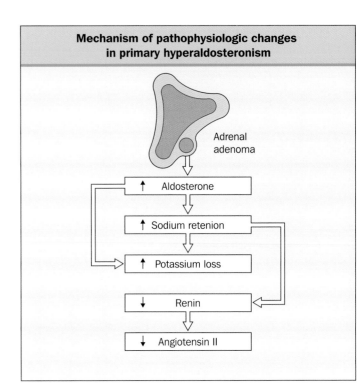

Figure 17.8 Mechanism of pathophysiologic changes in primary hyperaldosteronism. The autonomous production and release of aldosterone from the tumor leads to excessive sodium retention and potassium wasting; these occur largely as a result of the effects of aldosterone on the distal tube of the kidney. Renin release from the kidney is therefore inhibited and this leads to a fall in circulating levels of angiotensin II.

The distinction between adenomatous and idiopathic hyperaldosteronism and glucocorticoid-suppressible hypertension (GSH) is facilitated through the understanding of the differential control of aldosterone secretion in each condition. The adenoma is an autonomous source of aldosterone secretion, which is not regulated by angiotensin II; ACTH assumes more importance in the control of aldosterone secretion by adenomas. In contrast, the zona glomerulosa in hyperaldosteronism due to idiopathic hyperplasia is more sensitive to angiotensin II than normal. Finally, in glucocorticoid-suppressible hypertension the secretion of aldosterone secretion and its intermediary metabolites (18-OH and oxo-metabolites of cortisol and corticosterone) are under the control of ACTH.

The optimal methods of establishing the differential diagnosis of primary aldosterone are controversial but initially can be undertaken as an outpatient, 4-hour 'posture study' as illustrated in **Figure 17.9**, measuring the response of aldosterone to the erect posture (marked with idiopathic hyperplasia, absent in adenomas), to ACTH (absent with hyperplasia, increased with adenomas, exaggerated in GSH), and 18-hydroxy or 18-oxo-cortisol/corticosterone in the plasma or urine. This study can only be interpreted if the renin level is seen to rise on adopting the erect posture and cortisol to fall between 08.00h and 12.00h (reflecting the underlying circadian ACTH secretion).

Adrenal computerized tomography (CT) or magnetic resonance imaging (MRI) should not be performed until a biochemical diagnosis has been made because of the high incidence of nonfunctioning adrenal nodules ('incidentalomas'). Thereafter, a CT or MRI scan should be the first localization procedure; CT has a better spatial resolution and may be more sensitive in detecting small adrenal adenomas (see **Fig. 17.6**). Adrenal scanning using radiolabeled iodocholesterol is used in some centers. Invasive adrenal vein cannulation may be required to make a diagnosis or to assist in the lateralization of a lesion if the posture and/or imaging studies are inconclusive. In particular, angiotensin-II-responsive adenomas have been reported, and this may explain why the overall accuracy of posture studies in primary aldosteronism is only 70–80%. Although technically difficult and not without risk, the demonstration of an aldosterone ratio in one adrenal vein compared to another of more than 10:1 remains the most sensitive diagnostic test. Simultaneous cortisol measurements are needed to confirm that the adrenal vein has been cannulated and, when expressed as an aldosterone:cortisol ratio, improves diagnostic accuracy.

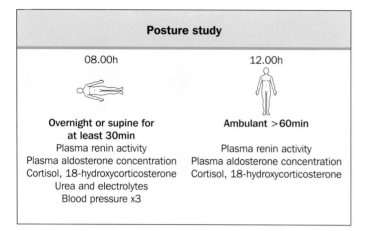

Figure 17.9 Day case investigation of a patient suspected of having primary aldosteronism. Supine and erect plasma renin activity, plasma aldosterone concentration, cortisol, 18-hydroxycorticosterone, electrolytes, and blood pressure are measured as shown. The posture study is only valid if there is a rise in plasma renin activity on adopting the erect posture and a fall in cortisol concentrations between 08.00 and 12.00 (reflecting a circadian fall in adrenocorticotropic hormone levels).

Treatment

One reason for establishing a definitive diagnosis is that the treatment is surgical excision in the case of aldosteronoma but strictly medical for patients with adrenal hyperplasia or aldosteronism, who are not suitable for surgery or decline operation. Such patients should be treated with amiloride, starting with a dose of 5–10mg/day and increasing to 30mg/day depending upon blood pressure, urea, and electrolyte responses. Spironolactone is as effective but in high doses frequently causes painful gynecomastia and menstrual irregularity. In patients with adenomas, normokalemia is restored postoperatively in 100% of cases and blood pressure falls to normal values in 70%. Laparoscopic adrenalectomy is the surgical treatment of choice as this has reduced morbidity compared to an open adrenalectomy. Pre- and perioperative management should involve the coordinated management of surgeon and endocrinologist. Aldosterone secretion from the contralateral normal adrenal gland may be suppressed and hypoaldosteronism postoperatively should be anticipated and treated appropriately by increasing sodium intake and/or transient fludrocortisone therapy.

Monogenic hypertension

The causes of monogenic hypertension are summarized in **Figure 17.10**.

Congenital adrenal hyperplasias

Biglieri and colleagues have described a syndrome of deficient 17α-hydroxylase in the adrenals and gonads impairing steroidogenesis. The resultant low levels of cortisol, acting via the negative feedback mechanism, stimulate ACTH release, with consequent bilateral hyperplasia and excessive secretion of corticosterone and deoxycorticosterone. These, in turn, cause sodium retention, potassium loss, hypertension, and a hypokalemic alkalosis. The absence of normal androgen secretion in men causes male pseudohermaphroditism, while defective

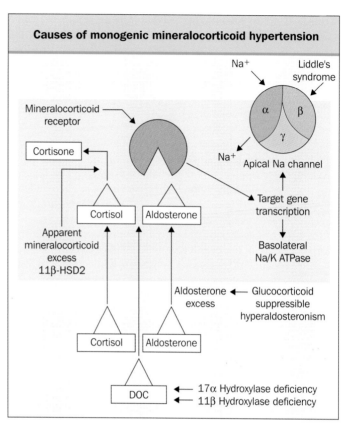

Figure 17.10 Causes of monogenic mineralocorticoid hypertension. A schematic diagram shows an epithelial cell in the distal colon or distal nephron. In normal physiology aldosterone interacts with the mineralocorticoid receptor to stimulate sodium reabsorption via induction of the apical Na channel and serosal Na/K ATPase pump. In patients with 17α-hydroxylase or 11β-hydroxylase deficiency, the mineralocorticoid receptor is stimulated by excessive concentrations of 11-deoxycorticosterone (DOC). Glucocorticoid-suppressible hyperaldosteronism is a cause of aldosterone excess because of of a chimeric, 11β-hydroxylase/aldosterone synthase gene, within the adrenal cortex. The syndrome of apparent mineralocorticoid excess comes about because cortisol cannot be inactivated to cortisone by the type 2 isoform of 11β-hydroxysteroid dehydrogenase (11β-HSD2); cortisol can then act as a potent mineralocorticoid. Liddle's syndrome occurs because of constitutively active mutations in the β and γ subunits of the apical Na channel.

estrogen secretion in women results in primary amenorrhea. Renin levels are also suppressed. Replacement therapy with glucocorticoids rapidly suppresses ACTH levels and corticosterone and deoxycorticosterone levels, and results in correction of the hypertension and electrolyte abnormalities.

In congenital 11β-hydroxylase deficiency, defective cortisol secretion leads to a secondary elevation of ACTH and bilateral adrenal hyperplasia. In addition, there are high circulating levels of precursor products 11-deoxycortisol and deoxycorticosterone. Hypertension ensues, as does virilism as a result of elevated androgen levels derived from the cortical precursors. The process can be reversed by glucocorticoid replacement therapy. A similar process is thought to explain the hypertension seen in patients with familial glucocorticoid resistance due to mutations in the glucocorticoid receptor gene.

Glucocorticoid-suppressible hyperaldosteronism

Glucocorticoid-suppressible hyperaldosteronism was first reported in 1966 and is an autosomal dominant form of low-renin hypertension characterized by aldosterone excess under the control of ACTH rather the normal principal secretagogue, angiotensin II. There are two important consequences of this: first, there is dysregulation of aldosterone secretion because of loss of the negative feedback loop (aldosterone does not suppress ACTH secretion). Second, the exogenous administration of a glucocorticoid such as dexamethasone, by decreasing ACTH secretion, results in suppression of aldosterone secretion and can be used therapeutically. Long-term glucocorticoid therapy leads to reactivation and normal regulation of the renin–angiotensin–aldosterone axis. A further characteristic of GSH is the secretion of large quantities of 18-OH and 18-oxo corticosterone/cortisol metabolites, again under the control of ACTH, and, while there is some overlap with levels seen in patients with aldosteronomas, these provide a diagnostic marker for the condition.

The molecular basis for GSH was described by Lifton and colleagues following the cloning and characterization of the two final enzymes in cortisol and aldosterone synthesis, 11β-hydroxylase and aldosterone synthase respectively. 11β-hydroxylase converts 11-deoxycortisol to cortisol in the zona fasciculata and aldosterone synthase corticosterone to aldosterone through an enzymatic step involving 11β-hydroxylation and 18-hydroxylation and oxidation. These enzymes are encoded by two genes, CYP11β1 and CYP11β2, lying in tandem on chromosome 8. Despite the similarity in the coding sequences of 11β-hydroxylase and aldosterone synthase (>95%), their 5′ sequences differ, permitting regulation of 11β-hydroxylase by ACTH through cAMP and aldosterone synthase by angiotensin II through intracellular Ca^{2+}, thereby establishing functional zonation of the adrenal cortex. In GSH a hybrid gene is formed at meiosis from unequal crossover of the CYP11β1 and CYP11β2 genes and this contains proximal components of CYP11β1 and distal components of CYP11β2. So long as the breakpoint of the hybrid gene is in or 5′ to exon IV of the CYP11β1 gene, the product of this gene can synthesize aldosterone but is now under the control of ACTH (**Fig. 17.11**). The chimeric gene can be detected by Southern blotting or by long polymerase chain reaction providing a screening test for GSH and the facility for prenatal diagnosis.

Following such advances, numerous kindreds have been reported with GSH. Studies on larger cohorts indicate that potassium may be normal in up to 50% of cases and there exists a poor correlation between genotype and phenotype (potassium, blood pressure) both between and within families. Severe mineralocorticoid excess has been reported in some affected cases of GSH but in other members of the same family the gene defect has caused no abnormal phenotype. Patients with GSH are more susceptible to cerebrovascular hemorrhage.

Liddle's syndrome

In 1963, Grant Liddle described a family with multiple siblings affected by early-onset hypertension and hypokalemia associated with low renin and low aldosterone levels. The condition responded well to inhibitors of epithelial sodium transport such as triamterene, but not to mineralocorticoid-receptor antagonists such as spironolactone, and a generalized defect in sodium

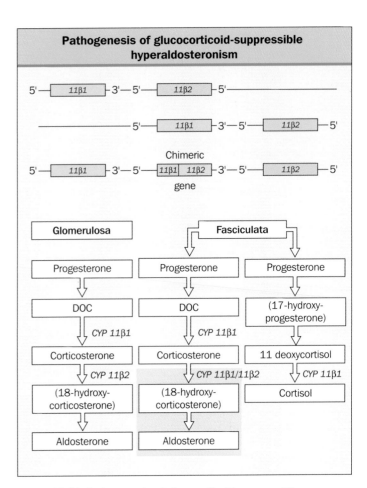

Figure 17.11 Pathogenesis of glucocorticoid-suppressible hyperaldosteronism. A chimeric *11β1/11β2* gene arises from unequal cross-over at meiosis. This results in the expression of an enzyme in the zona fasciculata that can synthesize aldosterone (possessing the 3′ sequences of *11β2*) but is under the regulatory control of ACTH (possessing the 5′ sequences of *11β1*).

transport was identified. Furthermore, renal transplantation resulted in normalization of blood pressure and potassium, arguing against a circulating mineralocorticoid.

Mineralocorticoid-dependent epithelial sodium transport requires the activation of the apical sodium channel in renal epithelial cells. Three subunits of this channel, α, β, and γ, have been cloned and characterized. Full sodium conductance requires the concerted action of an α/β or α/γ subunit and cannot be sustained by any subunit in isolation. The genes encoding the β + γ subunits lie in close proximity on chromosome 16 and mutations in these have been described in kindreds affected with Liddle's syndrome. In each case these cause deletions of the C-terminus part of the protein (45–75aa), producing a sodium channel that is persistently active. The mechanism underlying this is uncertain but may involve the induction of synthesis of new sodium channels.

Liddle's syndrome is inherited as an autosomal dominant trait and several other kindreds have been reported following the description of the genetic basis for the condition. As is the case with GSH, potassium has been reported to be normal in several cases.

Syndrome of apparent mineralocorticoid excess and licorice ingestion

The syndrome of apparent mineralocorticoid excess (AME) was first described in detail by Ulick and New in the late 1970s. This is an autosomal recessive form of low-renin, low-aldosterone hypertension in which cortisol acts as a potent mineralocorticoid.

The condition can be diagnosed from a 24-hour urine collection analyzed for cortisol metabolites using gas chromatography. Affected cases have a characteristic increase in urinary cortisol compared to cortisone metabolites (tetrahydrocortisol/tetrahydrocortisone ratio or urinary free cortisol/urinary free cortisone ratio). Serum cortisol levels are unhelpful because, although patients with AME have a prolonged plasma cortisol half-life, a reduction in cortisol secretion rate mediated by the negative feedback mechanism ensures normal circulating concentrations. This defect in cortisol metabolism occurs because of loss of 11β-hydroxysteroid dehydrogenase (11β-HSD) activity.

Two isozymes of 11β-HSD catalyze the interconversion of hormonally active cortisol to inactive cortisone. 11β-HSD1 is predominantly found in the liver, adipose tissue, and gonad and acts principally as an oxo-reductase, generating cortisol from cortisone. However, it is the 11β-HSD2 isoform, acting as an efficient dehydrogenase inactivating cortisol to cortisone, and expressed in the mineralocorticoid target tissues, kidney, colon, and salivary gland, that is more important in modulating corticosteroid control of blood pressure. Aldosterone gains access to the mineralocorticoid receptor *in vivo* only when 11β-HSD2 activity is intact and cortisol can be inactivated by conversion to cortisone at a prereceptor level. Homozygous inactivating mutations in the human 11β-HSD2 gene have been identified in patients with AME and result in cortisol-mediated, mineralocorticoid hypertension. The condition is inherited as an autosomal recessive trait and the majority of heterozygotes have a normal phenotype. Milder forms of AME have been described and there appears to be a close correlation between genotype and phenotype. Spironolactone or amiloride (often in higher doses than those used to treat primary aldosteronism) can be used therapeutically, as can dexamethasone, which suppresses endogenous cortisol secretion but itself is not a good substrate for 11β-HSD2.

Licorice has been recognized to be associated with a mineralocorticoid excess state since the late 1940s, when Reevers, a Dutch physician, used a licorice preparation, 'succus liquoritiae', to treat patients with dyspepsia. This was the origin of the antiulcer drug carbenoxolone, which also resulted in mineralocorticoid side effects in up to 50% cases. The active 'mineralocorticoids' in both cases are glycyrrhizic acid and its hydrolytic product, glycyrrhetinic acid, which themselves have little inherent mineralocorticoid activity but cause hypertension and hypokalemia by inhibiting 11β-HSD2. Such patients will also have an increase in the urinary ratio of cortisol to cortisone metabolites (THF+allo-THF/THE), although not to the same degree as patients with AME.

Blood pressure is elevated in 75% of patients with Cushing's syndrome and, while the pathogenesis of this multifactorial, cortisol acts as a mineralocorticoid in some patients. In ectopic ACTH syndrome, for example, the high cortisol secretion rate overwhelms renal 11β-HSD2 so that cortisol accumulates in the mineralocorticoid sensitive renal tissues and activates the

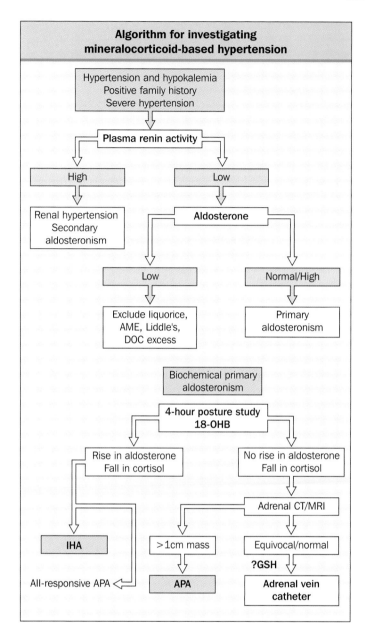

Figure 17.12 Algorithm for investigating mineralocorticoid-based hypertension. In practice, the posture study (see **Fig. 17.9**) can be included when the initial biochemical confirmation studies are performed. The clinician should consult the local endocrinology laboratory for reference ranges for plasma renin activity and aldosterone concentrations (top panel). If available, assays for 18-hydroxycortisol or 18-hydroxycorticosterone (18-OHB) are valuable in establishing the differential diagnosis. Adrenal imaging should be undertaken only when biochemical confirmation of primary aldosteronism has been confirmed, and should be interpreted together with the results of the posture study and 18-OHB data (lower panel). Adrenocorticotropin stimulation tests and dexamethasone suppression studies may be helpful in diagnosing glucocorticoid-suppressible hyperaldosteronism (GSH) and this can be confirmed by genetic analysis. Adrenal vein catheterization remains the most accurate diagnostic test in difficult cases and may also be used to assist lateralization of a functioning adrenal lesion. AII, angiotensin II; AME, syndrome of apparent mineralocorticoid excess; APA, aldosterone-producing adenoma; CT, computerized tomography; DOC, 11-deoxycorticosterone; IHA, idiopathic hyperplasia of the adrenal cortex; MRI, magnetic resonance imaging.

mineralocorticoid receptor. This is also observed in some patients with pituitary-dependent Cushing's syndrome and may explain the hypertension and hypokalemia in these cases.

These unusual causes of mineralocorticoid hypertension raise new questions as to the role of adrenal steroids in wider populations of patients with hypertension. Defects in the activities of 11β-hydroxylase and 11β-HSD have been reported in patients with 'essential hypertension' but have not consistently been associated with mineralocorticoid excess. Endogenous circulating inhibitors of 11β-HSD2 have also been described, so-called 'glycyrrhetinic-acid-like factors' or GALFs. Levels are higher in pregnancy and some studies, but not others, report increased levels in patients with hypertension. At present, however, the identity of such GALFs is unknown. In addition, GSH, Liddle's syndrome, and AME have provided the molecular geneticist with invaluable candidate genes in the analysis of the genetic basis for 'essential' hypertension. Reports are already appearing demonstrating either association or linkage of hypertension with polymorphisms in these genes in subgroups of patients with hypertension. Larger, more powerful studies are now required.

WHO SHOULD WE SUSPECT AS HAVING MINERALOCORTICOID-BASED HYPERTENSION?

All hypertensive patients should have serum electrolytes measured and those with hypokalemia must be investigated (**Fig. 17.12**). Because hypokalemia may be absent in many cases of proven mineralocorticoid hypertension, patients with severe hypertension (e.g. those on triple antihypertensive therapy) and those with a family history of hypertension or cerebrovascular disease should also be screened. At present the incidence of primary aldosteronism, glucocorticoid-suppressible hypertension, Liddle's syndrome, and apparent mineralocorticoid excess in unselected (i.e. community- rather than hospital-based) populations of 'essential' hypertensives is unknown. Until this is defined, one cannot be more dogmatic in deciding who should and should not be screened for mineralocorticoid-based hypertension. In the interim, like many disease processes, these diagnoses will not be made unless they are considered. Wherever possible the elucidation of the underlying basis of a patient's hypertension should be sought so that appropriate therapy can be targeted to the patient.

FURTHER READING

Edwards CRW, Stewart PM, Burt D, et al. Localisation of 11β-hydroxysteroid dehydrogenase-tissue specific protector of the mineralocorticoid receptor. Lancet 1988;2:986–9.

Funder JW, Pearce PT, Smith R, Smith AI. Mineralocorticoid action: target tissue specificity is enzyme, not receptor, mediated. Science 1988;242:583–5.

Gordon RD, Stowasser M, Klemm SA, Tunny TJ. High incidence of primary aldosteronism in 199 patients referred with hypertension. Clin Exp Pharmacol Physiol. 1994;21:315–8.

Young WF. Primary aldosteronism: update on diagnosis and treatment. Endocrinologist 1997;7:213–21.

Gittler RD, Fajans SS. Primary aldosteronism (Conn's syndrome). J Clin Endocrinol Metab.1995;80:3438–41.

McKenna TJ, Sequeira SJ, Heffernan A, Chambers J, Cunningham S. Diagnosis under random conditions of all disorders of the renin–angiotensin–aldosterone axis, including primary aldosteronism. J Clin Endocrinol Metab. 1991;73:952–7.

Gagner M, Pomp A, Heniford BT, Pharand D, Lacroix A. Laparoscopic adrenalectomy: lessons learned from 100 consecutive procedures. Ann Surg. 1997;226:238–46.

Rich GM, Ulick S, Cook S, Wang JZ, Lifton R, Dluhy RG. Glucocorticoid-remediable aldosteronism in a large kindred: clinical spectrum and diagnosis using a characteristic biochemical phenotype. Ann Intern Med. 1992;116:813–20.

Gomez-Sanchez CE, Montgomery M, Ganguly A, et al. Elevated urinary excretion of 18-oxocortisol in glucocorticoid-suppressible hyperaldosteronism. J Clin Endocrinol Metab. 1984;59:1022–4.

Lifton RP, Dluhy RG, Powers M, et al. A chimaeric 11β-hydroxylase/aldosterone synthase gene causes glucocorticoid-remediable hyperaldosteronism and human hypertension. Nature 1992;365:262–5.

Botero-Valez M, Curtis JJ, Warnock DG. Brief report: Liddle's syndrome revisited – a disorder of sodium reabsorption in the distal tubule. N Engl J Med. 1994;330:178–81.

Shimkets RA, Warnock DG, Bositis CM, et al. Liddle's syndrome: heritable human hypertension caused by mutations in the β-subunit of the epithelial sodium channel. Cell 1994;79:407–14.

Stewart PM, Corrie JET, Shackleton CHL, Edwards CRW. Syndrome of apparent mineralocorticoid excess: a defect in the cortisol–cortisone shuttle. J Clin Invest. 1988;82:340–9.

Stewart PM, Wallace AM, Valentino R, Burt D, Shackleton CHL, Edwards CRW. Mineralocorticoid activity of liquorice: 11β-hydroxysteroid dehydrogenase comes of age. Lancet 1987;1:1208–10.

Stewart PM, Walker BR, Holder GI, O'Halloran D, Shackleton CHL. 11-β hydroxysteroid dehydrogenase activity in Cushing's syndrome: explaining the mineralocorticoid excess state of the ectopic ACTH syndrome. J Clin Endocrinol Metab. 1995;80:3617–20.

Yanase T, Simpson ER, Waterman MR. 17α-hydroxylase/17,20 lyase deficiency: from clinical investigation to molecular definition. Endocrinol Rev. 1991;12:91–108.

White PC, Curnow KM, Pascoe L. Disorders of steroid 11β-hydroxylase isozymes. Endocrinol Rev. 1994;15:421–38.

White PC, Mune T, Agarwal AK. 11β-hydroxysteroid dehydrogenase and the syndrome of apparent mineralocorticoid excess. Endocrinol Rev. 1997;18:135–56.

Junor BJ, Briggs, JD, Moss JG. Effect of renal artery stenting on progression of renovascular renal failure. Lancet 1997;349:1133–6.

Corvol P, Pinet F, Plouin PF, Bruneval P, Menard J. Renin-secreting tumors. Endocrinol Metab Clin North Am. 1994;23:255–70.

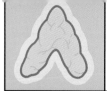

Section 3 Adrenal

Chapter 18

Adrenal Medulla: Physiology and Pathology

Ashley B Grossman and Gregory Kaltsas

PHYSIOLOGY

The adrenal medulla and the sympathetic nervous system constitute the anatomic and physiologic unit that is referred to as the *sympatho-adrenomedullary system*. Descending pathways from the hypothalamus, pons, and medulla synapse with preganglionic sympathetic neurons in the spinal cord; preganglionic cholinergic neurons in turn innervate the adrenal medulla directly or synapse in paravertebral ganglia with postganglionic sympathetic neurons. The latter give rise to sympathetic nerves, which are distributed to the viscera and blood vessels.

Embryology

The adrenal medulla is composed of cells derived from the neural crest (sympathogonia); these cells subsequently differentiate into neuroblasts (sympathoblasts), which become sympathetic and other autonomic ganglion cells, and pheochromoblasts, which become pheochromocytes or mature chromaffin cells. Those pheochromocytes destined to form the adrenal medulla are then enveloped by the mesenchymal primitive adrenal cortex. Pheochromocytes also collect on both sides of the aorta to form the paraganglia, of which the organ of Zuckerkandl (found in front of the aorta and below the inferior mesenteric artery) is prominent in fetal life. This accessory tissue usually degenerates within the first 2 years of life but may persist and give rise to hormonally active tumors. Pheochromocytes are also found scattered throughout the abdominal sympathetic plexuses as well as in other parts of the sympathetic nervous system, and may be the site of subsequent tumor formation.

Gross and microscopic anatomy

The adrenal medulla occupies a central position in the widest part of the gland, with only small portions extending into the narrower parts. It constitutes approximately 10% of the weight of the gland and there is no clear anatomic demarcation between cortex and medulla. The adrenal medulla is composed of chromaffin cells, which are large ovoid columnar cells arranged in clumps or cords around blood vessels. Their name is derived from the observation that their granules turn brown (*pheo-*) when stained with chromic acid; the color is due to the oxidation of the catecholamines, the main secretory products of the gland, to melanin. Ultrastructurally, they contain numerous small electron-dense organelles called chromaffin vesicles, 100–300nm in diameter, in which the main catecholamines, epinephrine (adrenaline) and norepinephrine (noradrenaline), are stored. In humans, epinephrine accounts for 85% of the adrenomedullary catecholamine store but, as with the sympathetic nerve endings, a variety of noncatecholamine mediators have also been identified.

Nerve and blood supply

The adrenal medulla has a dual blood supply: portal blood flows in the corticomedullary sinuses (having previously drained the adrenal cortex) and arterial blood from the adrenal medullary arteries. Epinephrine-secreting cells may receive a disproportionate part of their supply from the portal source, where they are exposed to the secretion of cortisol from the adrenocortical cells; cortisol is necessary for the induction of the enzyme phenylethanolamine-*N*-methyltransferase (PNMT), which converts norepinephrine to epinephrine. Medullary capillaries, which are fenestrated and thus allow free diffusion and release of catecholamines, coalesce to form a single adrenal vein, which usually drains directly into the inferior vena cava on the right and into the renal vein on the left. The cells of the adrenal medulla are innervated by preganglionic fibers of the sympathetic nervous system, which release acetylcholine and enkephalins at the synapses, leading to the release of catecholamines into the circulation. The major portion of this innervation is from the greater splanchnic nerve (T5–9).

Hormones of the adrenal medulla

The catecholamines (dopamine, norepinephrine, and epinephrine), widely distributed biogenic amines that include the 3,4-dihydrophenyl group, are the main secretory products of the adrenal medulla and serve multiple physiologic roles. Epinephrine is predominantly found in sympathetic neurons, the adrenal medulla and the central nervous system (CNS), where it acts as a neurotransmitter. Norepinephrine is the neurotransmitter for most sympathetic postganglionic fibers and in certain tracts in the CNS, while dopamine is the predominant neurotransmitter in the extrapyramidal system and several mesocortical and mesolimbic neuronal pathways. Dopamine is also found in specialized mast cells and enterochromaffin cells.

Biosynthesis

The major pathway for the biosynthesis of catecholamines is identical in both the adrenal medulla and sympathetic neurons (**Fig. 18.1**). The ultimate source of catecholamines is the amino acid tyrosine, which may be derived from dietary sources or is synthesized from phenylalanine in the liver. Tyrosine hydroxylase catalyzes the conversion of tyrosine to dihydroxyphenylalanine (dopa), which is the rate-limiting enzyme for the regulation of

Pathway of catecholamine synthesis in the adrenal medulla

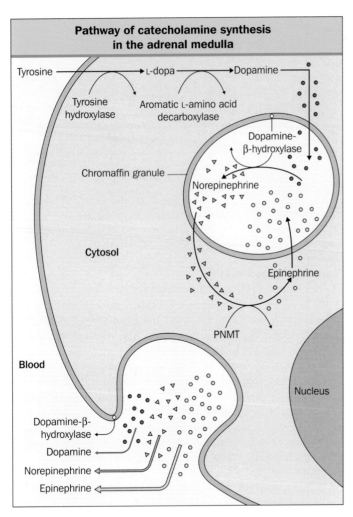

Figure 18.1 Pathway of catecholamine synthesis in the adrenal medulla. PNMT, phenylethanolamine-*N*-methyltransferase. (Modified with permission from Feldman JM. Diagnosis and management of pheochromocytoma. Hosp Pract. 1989;24:175–98 © 1989 The McGraw-Hill Companies, Inc. Original illustration by Ilil Arbel.)

catecholamine synthesis. The relatively nonspecific enzyme aromatic L-amino acid decarboxylase (ALAAD/dopa decarboxylase) catalyzes the decarboxylation of dopa to dopamine; unlike the other reactions of catecholamine biosynthesis, which are limited to the sympathetic nerve endings and the adrenal medulla, decarboxylation of circulating dopa occurs in a variety of tissues, with the local production of dopamine. Indeed, much of the dopamine secreted in the urine appears to originate from the decarboxylation of dopa in the kidneys. Dopamine is then converted to norepinephrine by dopamine-β-hydroxylase (DBH); this enzyme does not exist in tissues outside the neuron or the adrenal medulla. In the adrenal medulla, norepinephrine is methylated to form epinephrine, the reaction being catalyzed by PNMT, which is also found in small neurons in the CNS where epinephrine is used as a neurotransmitter; norepinephrine leaves the granules and after methylation re-enters different granules. Catecholamine biosynthesis is coupled to secretion, so that the stores of norepinephrine remain relatively constant; however, in the adrenal medulla it is still possible to deplete stores with prolonged hypoglycemia.

Catecholamine storage and release

The processes of catecholamine storage and release are similar in the sympathetic nerve endings and the adrenal medulla. In the adrenal medulla, where conversion to epinephrine occurs through the action of PNMT in the cytoplasm, norepinephrine leaves the storage vesicle and epinephrine is taken up. The chromaffin granules contain catecholamines and ATP in a 4:1 ratio, plus lipids, calcium, magnesium, and water-soluble proteins called chromogranins; a higher catecholamine-to-ATP ratio is found in granules isolated from patients with catecholamine-producing tumors. Chromogranin is the most abundant molecule in the chromaffin granule and has been demonstrated in a variety of polypeptide-secreting endocrine cells, including the parathyroids, anterior pituitary, thyroid (parafollicular or C cells), and pancreatic islet cells. In addition to catecholamines, the granules contain small neuropeptides, including opioid peptides, met- and leu-enkephalins, neurotensin, neuropeptide Y, galanin, and somatostatin. On stimulation of the adrenal medulla, the catecholamines are released into the extracellular space adjacent to a capillary and carried to distant sites of action, while with neurotransmission they are released locally into the synaptic space: this is achieved by exocytosis, whereby vesicle contents are discharged when the vesicle membrane and the limiting membrane of the cell fuse (**Fig. 18.2**). This requires an acetylcholine-induced action potential, which in turn causes an influx of calcium. Along with catecholamines, the other major soluble components (adenosine triphosphate (ATP), chromogranins, and enkephalins) are also released from the chromaffin granules, including free DBH but not membrane-bound DBH.

During stimulation of sympathetic neurons, only a small fraction of the catecholamines released binds to postganglionic receptors. A fraction is metabolized, while some enters the circulation; the majority is, however, actively transported across the preganglionic neuronal membrane by an energy- and sodium-dependent specific mechanism (type 1 uptake). Type 1 uptake serves at least two important physiologic functions: (1) recapture of locally released norepinephrine, which conserves the transmitter and serves to maintain the constancy of norepinephrine stores despite variations in nerve activity; (2) uptake of circulating or locally released amines inactivates these amines by intraneuronal storage or metabolism. However, this mechanism plays a less important role in the inactivation of circulating catecholamines as it is energy-dependent and saturable.

Measurement of plasma catecholamines is one index by which sympathoadrenal activity may be estimated. Under basal conditions, the major circulating catecholamine is norepinephrine, with 95% of this representing spillover from peripheral sympathetic nerve endings, the remainder being secreted directly by the adrenal medulla. Epinephrine, which reflects the true secretory product of the adrenal medulla, circulates at much lower levels but levels can increase markedly (up to 20-fold) in states of stress. Dopamine circulates in a predominantly conjugated form as a glucuronide or sulfate, only about 1% being free dopamine.

The metabolism and inactivation of catecholamines

The plasma half-life of catecholamines is short (between 1 and 2min) because of rapid enzymatic degradation or cellular uptake. The principal pathways for the metabolism of catecholamines include 3-O-methylation and oxidative deamination, facilitated

Release of catecholamines from the adrenal medulla

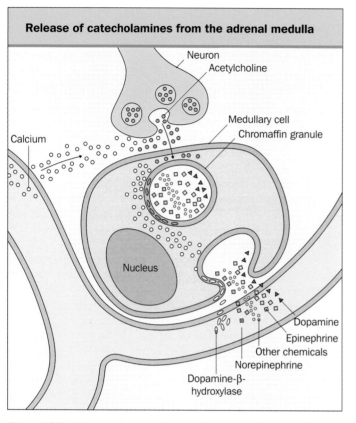

Figure 18.2 Release of catecholamines from the adrenal medulla.
(Modified with permission from Benowitz NL. Diagnosis and management
of pheochromocytoma. Hosp Prac. 1990;25:163–77 © 1990
The McGraw-Hill Companies, Inc. Original illustration by Ilil Arbel.)

The metabolic fate of catecholamines

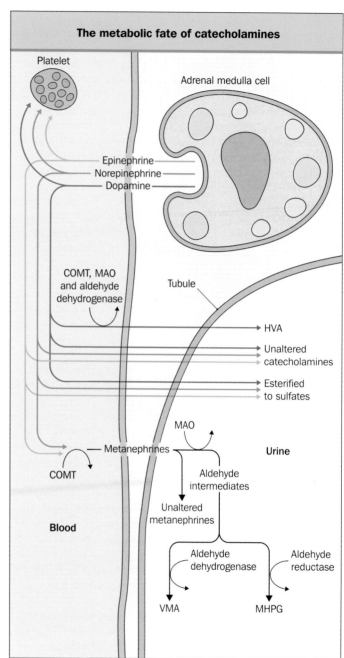

Figure 18.3 The metabolic fate of catecholamines. COMT, catechol-
O-methyl transferase; HVA, homovanillic acid; MAO, monoamine oxidase;
MHPG, 3-methoxy-4-hydroxy-phenylglycol; VMA, vanillylmandelic acid.
(Modified with permission from Feldman JM. Diagnosis and management
of pheochromocytoma. Hosp Pract. 1989;24:175–98 © 1989
The McGraw-Hill Companies, Inc. Original illustration by Ilil Arbel.)

by catechol-O-methyl transferase (COMT) and monoamine
oxidase (MAO) activity, and conjugation with sulfate and
glucuronide; the later process is saturable and not specific for
catecholamines (**Fig. 18.3**).

Norepinephrine is converted to normetanephrine, epinephrine
to metanephrine, and dopamine to 3-methoxytyramine, predominantly extraneuronally (uptake 2), by COMT. As noted above, the
uptake of norepinephrine by presynaptic neurons (type 1 uptake),
where it is either destroyed by MAO or reused in the synaptic
vesicles, plays a relatively minor role in the inactivation of circulating catecholamines. Normetanephrine and metanephrine are
converted to 3-methoxy-4-hydroxymandelic acid (vanillylmandelic acid, VMA) by MAO and aldehyde oxidase.

An alternative sequence of reaction is that in which norepinephrine and epinephrine are converted to 3,4-dihydroxyman-
delaldehyde by MAO, then to 3,4-dihydromandelic acid by
aldehyde oxidase, and finally to VMA by COMT. An additional
pathway is that in which COMT and aldehyde dehydrogenase
act on 3,4-dihydromandelaldehyde to yield 3-methoxy-4-
hydroxyphenylacetic acid (homovanillic acid, HVA) rather than
VMA. COMT is predominantly an extraneuronal enzyme and
acts on circulating catecholamines as well as on the locally
released norepinephrine; it is the most important enzyme in the
metabolism of circulating amines.

Approximately 70% of circulating epinephrine is methoxylated
and about 24% is also deaminated. Catecholamines may also be
conjugated to sulfates or glucuronide; the urine excretion of these

conjugates exceeds that of free catecholamines severalfold. All
these metabolites are biologically inactive, but their excretion
rates provide indices of sympatho-adrenomedullary function.

The physiologic actions of catecholamines

The effects of catecholamines are mediated by binding to specific cell-surface receptors. Pharmacologic studies have led to
the recognition of three major types of receptor: α_1 and α_2, β_1

and β_2, and dopamine 1 and 2. The adrenergic receptors are transmembrane proteins with an extracellular amino terminus and an intracellular carboxyl terminus. These receptors are termed G proteins because they bind guanosine 5´ triphosphate (nucleotides) and have seven hydrophobic regions that span the cell membrane; these proteins are activated by receptor ligand interaction. Although these regions exhibit significant amino-acid homology, differences in the fifth and sixth segments determine whether the receptor is coupled to the stimulatory (G_s) or inhibitory (G_i) guanyl-nucleotide binding proteins. Binding of catecholamines to the receptor initiates a series of intracellular changes: with β_1 and β_2 receptors on the cell membrane, adenylate cyclase mediates a rise in intracellular cyclic adenosine monophosphate (cAMP), leading to protein kinase activation; α_1 receptors mediate calcium influx while α_2 receptors are linked to an inhibitory guanine nucleotide regulatory protein and thus inhibit adenylate cyclase. Dopamine type 1 receptors mediate adenylate cyclase activation while type 2 inhibits it. Receptors may also be controlled by means of down-regulation; in homologous desensitization, binding of specific agonist leads to phosphorylation of specific amino-acids by a β-adrenoceptor kinase (βARK), which in turn allows an arrestin to bind and hence inactivate the receptor. Other receptors can also cause heterologous desensitization, while receptor internalization decreases the total receptor pool. All may be involved in the termination of activity of the adrenoceptor.

The effects of catecholamines are highly diverse, reflecting the wide distribution of adrenergic receptors. Norepinephrine is a potent agonist at α_1 and β_1 receptors, whereas the predominant effect of epinephrine is on β_1 and β_2 receptors with relatively weak actions at α receptors. Dopamine receptors are widespread within the autonomic system and are physiologically important in vascular regulation in the renal and mesenteric beds; they are also found in the autonomic and basal ganglia. The cardiovascular effects of adrenoceptors include mediation of positive inotropism and chronotropism on the heart (β_1-receptors), vasoconstriction by α-receptors and vasodilatation by β_2-receptors. Norepinephrine leads to generalized vasoconstriction and diastolic and systolic hypertension, leading to reflex bradycardia. Epinephrine, which has a more marked β_2-agonist effect, causes vasodilatation, diastolic hypotension, systolic hypertension, tachycardia, and increased cardiac output. Dopamine in low concentrations dilates renal and mesenteric vascular beds, and in addition increases cardiac output with increased systolic blood pressure, with little effect on diastolic pressure.

The metabolic effects of adrenoceptor stimulation include stimulation of glycogenolysis, gluconeogenesis, lipolysis, hepatic ketogenesis, increased thermogenesis (probably by a novel β_3-adrenoceptor), amino-acid release from muscle, and induction of hypokalemia and hypophosphatemia, which may result from increased cellular uptake of potassium and inorganic phosphate. Smooth muscle relaxation in the bronchi and uterus is β_2-mediated. Other involuntary muscle actions are mydriasis (α-receptor) and a reduction in gastrointestinal motility (β_1-receptor). Catecholamines modulate hormone secretion, stimulating glucagon, growth hormone, and renin. Insulin secretion is stimulated by β_2-agonists and suppressed by α_2-agonists. Dopamine in the hypothalamus suppresses prolactin secretion from pituitary lactotrophs (see Chapters 1 & 6).

PATHOLOGY – CATECHOLAMINE-PRODUCING TUMORS (PHEOCHROMOCYTOMAS AND PARAGANGLIOMAS)

Introduction

Pheochromocytomas are tumors that arise from the adrenal medulla, while those arising in extra-adrenal tissues are called paragangliomas. The most frequent sites of paragangliomas include the superior para-aortic region (46%), the inferior para-aortic region (29%), the urinary bladder (10%), the thorax (10%), the head and neck (3%), and the pelvis (2%). Occasionally, the tumors may be nonsecretory. The term catecholamine-secreting tumors will be used to refer to both pheochromocytomas and paragangliomas. Primitive and usually highly malignant tumors of this system include neuroblastomas and ganglioneuroblastomas.

The incidence of pheochromocytomas among hypertensive patients has been estimated to be in the range from 0.1% to 1%. Pheochromocytomas occur with equal frequency in both sexes with an estimated incidence of about 1–2 cases per million, and although they can be found at all ages they are most commonly diagnosed in the third or fourth decade. However, the incidence of pheochromocytomas increases continuously with advancing age for both men and women, while a significant number (>50%) are found at autopsy, having escaped diagnosis in life. The mean age of such patients is 66 years, compared with 48 years for those with symptomatic disease. In one study of 54 patients found to have pheochromocytomas at autopsy, only 13 (24%) had had the tumor correctly diagnosed during life.

Generally, the occurrence of pheochromocytoma obeys the *rough rule of 10:* about 10% are malignant, 10% are familial, 10% are not associated with hypertension, 10% are extra-adrenal (of these about 10% are extra-abdominal), 10% are bilateral and 10% occur in children. With early accurate diagnosis and appropriate management, almost all benign tumors should be surgically curable.

Causes

Pheochromocytomas are sporadic in approximately 90% of cases and inherited in at least 10%. Inherited tumors, either alone or more commonly in association with other endocrine tumors, are often bilateral or even multiple, and arise from hyperplastic adrenomedullary tissue. They include familial pheochromocytomas, presenting as an isolated trait with an autosomal dominant mode of inheritance, and the autosomal dominant multiple endocrine neoplasia syndromes (MEN). In the MEN 2A and 2B syndromes there is a 40% prevalence of pheochromocytomas. Oncogenic mechanisms have been linked to tumor *RET* proto-oncogene missense point mutations on chromosome 10 (10q11.2). *RET* encodes a tyrosine kinase receptor and has an extracellular calcium-binding domain with a cysteine-rich region proximal to the transmembrane domain. At least six germline mutations in these cysteine-rich regions have been associated with MEN type 2A. *Neurofibromatosis type 1*, also an autosomal dominant condition, is associated with pheochromocytomas in 1% and is due to loss of function of a tumor-suppressor gene. The *Von Hippel–Lindau syndrome* (VHL), another autosomal dominant disorder associated with loss of function of a tumor suppressor gene located on chromosome 3p25–26, is associated with pheochromocytomas in 15%. More than 75 VHL germline mutations have been identified. Pheochromocytomas may be the only manifestation in about 25% of carriers of the MEN 2A mutation.

Pathology and biology

Pheochromocytomas are often solitary, usually less than 10cm in diameter, the cut surface showing areas of hemorrhage and necrosis with the rest of the adrenal usually displaced and compressed. Microscopically, large pleomorphic chromaffin cells are present with nuclear atypia and mitoses; they contain sheets of homogeneous cells that are frequently basophilic because of their neurosecretory granules containing catecholamines, chromogranin A, and other secretory substances. However, conventional histologic analysis fails to discriminate between benign and malignant tumors: even capsular invasion and vascular penetration are not proof of malignancy.

Diagnosis

Once the diagnosis of a catecholamine-secreting tumor is clinically suspected the principal diagnostic considerations are twofold: to prove autonomous catecholamine secretion and then to demonstrate the source. Diagnosis is made biochemically by the demonstration of inappropriately high circulating or urinary free catecholamines.

Common clinical symptoms/signs suggestive of a catecholamine-producing tumor include: unusually labile blood pressure; paroxysms of tachycardia and hypertension; episodes of headache (80%); excess sweating (71%); palpitations (64%) and pallor; accelerated hypertension; hypermetabolism and weight loss; impaired carbohydrate tolerance; pressor responses to anesthetic, antihypertensive or sympathomimetic drugs; and the presence of a suprarenal or midline abdominal mass.

Biochemical diagnosis

In most patients with pheochromocytomas the synthesis, storage, or metabolism of catecholamines is deranged, and measurement of catecholamines and their metabolites in urine or blood forms the cornerstone of the diagnosis, as most affected persons will have abnormal values.

Clinical manifestations

Patients with pheochromocytomas present with a diversity of symptoms that have been attributed to the excessive catecholamine release as well as to a variety of other co-secreted active metabolic substances. However, the clinical correlates of pheochromocytoma and the catecholamine content or secretion are variable, and typically there is a lack of correlation between the height of blood pressure and plasma catecholamine concentration. Pheochromocytomas produce a number of vasoactive substances (dopa, calcitonin-gene-related peptide, vasoactive intestinal peptide, adrenomedullin, met-enkephalin, atrial natriuretic peptide, neuropeptide Y, etc.) that might influence vascular responsiveness. Furthermore, chronic exposure to high circulating levels of catecholamines does not produce the hemodynamic characteristics of acute administration, and this may explain the clinical observation that some patients can be completely asymptomatic despite harboring an actively catecholamine-secreting tumor. In addition, the hypertension found in such patients may be directly related to sympathetic activity,

as norepinephrine release from sympathetic postganglionic neurons may be upregulated by circulating catecholamines. Therefore, any reflex or direct stimulus to the sympathetic nervous system can release excessive amounts of catecholamines into the synaptic cleft and produce a hypertensive crisis. This may account for the observation that spontaneously evoked crises in blood pressure can occur without detectable increases in plasma catecholamines, while conversely blood pressure may be normal despite high circulating levels of catecholamines.

Cardiovascular manifestations

An elevation in mean blood pressure is the most consistent manifestation of secretory pheochromocytomas and paragangliomas. The hypertension is sustained in about half of patients, paroxysmal in about a third and absent in approximately one fifth. Use of 24-hour ambulatory blood pressure monitoring has demonstrated that most patients have paroxysms, only some of which are symptomatic; however, characteristically all patients lack the normal nocturnal reduction in blood pressure. Hypertension is characteristically resistant to conventional treatment, particularly β-adrenoceptor blockade, which actually exacerbates hypertension because of unopposed α-adrenergic stimulation. Hypertensive crises with malignant hypertension or in association with induction of anesthesia, hypertensive encephalopathy, hypertension with severe headache and sweating, paroxysmal episodes of spells suggestive of seizures, and anxiety attacks or hyperventilation, should all evoke suspicion of an underlying catecholamine-producing tumor. Severe hypertension may be associated with sudden left ventricular failure, dysrhythmias, and circulatory collapse. The classic triad of severe headache, sweating, and palpitations carries a high degree of specificity (94%) and sensitivity (91%) for pheochromocytoma in the hypertensive population. The absence of all three symptoms renders the diagnosis highly unlikely.

Myocardial infarction is often diagnosed in such patients, based on either 'myocarditis', presumably a catecholamine cardiomyopathy, or coronary spasm. Cerebral infarction can result from enhanced coagulopathy or vasospasm, while intracranial hemorrhage can be the result of severe arterial hypertension. Dilated cardiomyopathy with mural thrombus is an occasional cause of brain emboli. Some patients may initially be hypotensive or in shock, particularly patients with pure epinephrine-producing tumors, since epinephrine induces peripheral vasodilatation. Bleeding into the tumor is a common occurrence and may cause abdominal discomfort. Hemorrhagic necrosis of the tumor may present as an acute surgical abdomen associated with marked hypertension followed by hypotension and even shock and sudden death. Other recognized manifestations include neurogenic pulmonary edema, heat intolerance, weight loss, and unexplained pyrexia. Constipation, occasionally mimicking pseudo-obstruction and paralytic ileus, has also been reported.

Pheochromocytoma crisis

This is a consequence of abrupt catecholamine release with or without other contained biologically active peptides. Crises tend to have a characteristic and reproducible pattern for each individual, although their severity and duration is variable. Typically, two or more symptoms occur synchronously with a sudden onset and a peak severity occurring within minutes to several hours, most crises lasting 15–60min. Headache (in 80%), often throbbing, associated with a feeling of intense malaise and impending doom, is characteristic. Sweating, palpitations, a feeling of apprehension with discomfort in the chest or abdomen, and pallor may occur. Flushing is uncommon.

Blood pressure may rise alarmingly, either with reflex brady-cardia (secondary to norepinephrine secretion) or tachycardia (epinephrine secretion). Precipitants include movements that disturb the abdominal viscera, lifting, straining and bending, as well as certain drugs and radiographic contrast media. Often, however, no precipitant is identifiable.

Metabolically there may be glucose intolerance secondary to catecholamine-induced suppression of insulin release or inhibition of hepatic or muscle uptake of glucose. Other humoral syndromes encountered are hypercalcemia due to ectopic production of parathormone (PTH) or PTH-related peptide (PTHrP), diarrhea resulting from associated production of vaso-active intestinal peptide (VIP), and severe hypokalemic alkalosis caused by ectopic ACTH production. Increased metabolic rate may also cause heat intolerance and weight loss or lack of weight gain (in children).

Malignant catecholamine-producing tumors

The incidence of malignancy is about 10%. The most common metastatic sites are the skeleton (>50%), liver (50%), and lung (30%). The most significant prognostic factors that predict a malignant course are the size of the tumor and local extension at the time of surgery. An older age and an absence of familial syn-dromes are considered to be favorable factors. Although it has been suggested that aneuploid and tetraploid tumors often appear to have a poorer prognosis than diploid ones, the predic-tive value of ploidy for malignancy is low. Until more reliable indicators of malignancy are identified and validated, lifelong clinical and biochemical followup of patients who have had pheochromocytomas remains essential, particularly as meta-static dissemination, the only real proof of malignancy, may become manifest extremely late in the clinical course.

Familial syndromes

MEN type 2A (pheochromocytomas with hyperparathyroidism and medullary carcinoma of the thyroid) and *type 2A* (pheochromocytoma, medullary carcinoma of the thyroid, mucosal neuromas, thickened corneal nerves, a marfanoid habi-tus, and intestinal ganglioneuromatosis) are associated with pheochromocytomas in approximately 40% of carriers. *Von Hippe–Lindau* syndrome (hemangioblastoma of the central nervous system, retinal angiomas, renal cysts and carcinomas, pancreatic cysts, and epidymal cystadenoma) carries about 15% incidence of pheochromocytoma. *Neurofibromatosis type 1* is associated with pheochromocytomas in up to 1% of cases. Additional catecholamine-secreting tumor-related neurocuta-neous syndromes include ataxia–telangiectasia, tuberous sclero-sis, and the Sturge–Weber syndrome. Other known associations that do not appear to have a familial basis are Carney's triad (adrenal paragangliomas, gastric epithelioid leiomyosarcomas, and pulmonary chordomas), cholelithiasis, and renal artery stenosis.

Patients who should be screened for catecholamine-producing tumors
Young patient with hypertension
Hypertensive patients with:
Atypical myocardial infarction, cerebrovascular accident, arrhythmias, renal failure
Unexplained weight loss
Seizures
Orthostatic hypotension
Unexplained shock
Family history of pheochromocytoma or medullary thyroid carcinoma
Neurofibromatosis or other neurocutaneous syndromes, mucosal neuromas
Hyperglycemia
Cardiomyopathy
Marked lability of blood pressure
Family history of pheochromocytoma
Shock or pressor responses to:
Induction of anesthesia and surgery
Parturition
Invasive procedures
Antihypertensive drugs
Radiologic evidence of an adrenal mass

Table 18.1 Patients who should be screened for catecholamine-producing tumors.

Differential diagnosis

Table 18.1 gives a suggested list of patients in whom the diagno-sis of a pheochromocytoma should be considered, while **Table 18.2** provides a differential diagnosis of conditions that can mimic catecholamine-producing tumors.

Diagnostic procedures

Biochemical

Measurement of catecholamine and metabolites

Once a catecholamine-producing tumor is suspected, biochemi-cal tests, based on catecholamine metabolism, can establish the diagnosis in more than 95% of cases. In patients with pheo-chromocytomas the synthesis, storage, and metabolism of cate-cholamines is deranged; in general, the activities of the enzymes involved in catecholamine synthesis are markedly enchanced whereas those involved in catecholamine metabolism are reduced. Thus, excessive amounts of newly synthesized cate-cholamines cannot be stored or degraded and are released into the circulation. In general, the pattern of plasma catecholamine secretion shows predominantly norepinephrine secretion in catecholamine-secreting tumors, but epinephrine can (very rarely) be dominant, while dopamine excess suggests malignancy (**Fig. 18.4**).

In healthy individuals, endogenous catecholamine metabolism is mediated initially by neuronal MAO and subsequently by COMT in the circulation; the end product of this accounting for 90% of urinary catecholamines and their metabolites being VMA. By contrast, intravenously infused catecholamines are metabolized primarily by COMT, which results in greater

Differential diagnosis of conditions with catecholamine-induced-like symptoms	
Endocrine	Thyrotoxicosis
	Primary hypogonadism (menopausal symptoms)
	Medullary thyroid carcinoma
	Hypoglycemia
	Carbohydrate intolerance
Cardiovascular	Labile or sustained essential hypertension
	Pulmonary edema, myocarditis
	Syncope, orthostatic hypotension
	Paroxysmal cardiac arrhythmias
	Renovascular disease
Neurologic/psychologic	Autonomic neuropathy
	Diencephalic epilepsy
	Migraine headache
	Cerebrovascular ischemia
	Anxiety, panic attacks, somatization disorder
	Hyperventilation
Pharmacologic	Withdrawal of adrenergic inhibitor
	Treatment with monoamine-oxidase inhibitors, tyramine, or sympathomimetic drugs
	Drugs (cocaine, LSD, PCP, monoamine-oxidase inhibitors and sympathomimetic amines)
	Alcoholism
	Vancomycin ('red man syndrome')
Miscellaneous	Mastocytosis
	Carcinoid syndrome
	Recurrent idiopathic anaphylaxis
	Eclampsia
	Hypertensive crises associated with paraplegia, tabes dorsalis, lead poisoning, acute porphyria

Table 18.2 Differential diagnosis of conditions with catecholamine-induced-like symptoms.

urinary excretion of normetanephrine and metanephrine. Catecholamine metabolism in pheochromocytomas generally follows the infusion model; there is a proportionally greater increase in metanephrine and free catecholamine concentrations rather than VMA levels.

The size of the tumor is also an important determinant of the relative amount of catecholamine excretory product, as occasionally bulky tumors containing large amounts of MAO are associated with high levels of metanephrine and VMA but normal free catecholamine concentrations. This is particularly important as small tumors (<50g) have been shown to have rapid turnover rates and release free unmetabolized catecholamines and have more symptoms and higher catecholamine levels in the plasma. On the other hand, patients with large tumors may metabolize most of the secreted catecholamines, have fewer symptoms and relatively lower circulating free catecholamines, but high urinary catecholamine metabolites.

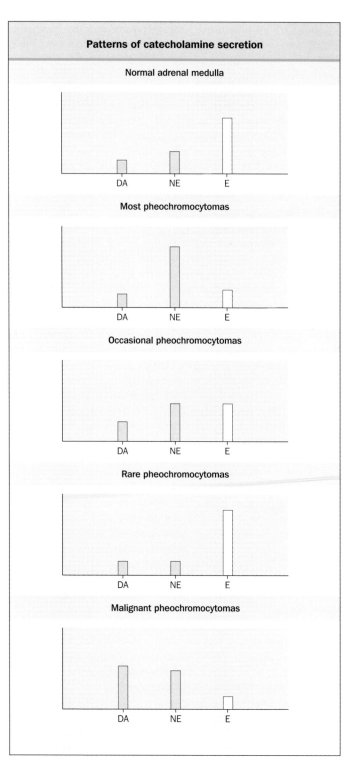

Figure 18.4 Patterns of catecholamine secretion. The patterns in different patient groups are reflected in 24-hour urine catecholamine levels. Most pheochromocytomas are predominantly norepinephrine-secreting, but pure epinephrine secretors have rarely been identified. Dopamine excess is often an indicator of malignancy. DA, dopamine; NE, norepinephrine; E, epinephrine. (Modified with permission from Feldman JM. Diagnosis and management of pheochromocytoma. Hosp Pract 1989;24:175–98 © 1989 The McGraw-Hill Companies, Inc. Original illustration by Albert Miller.)

Assays for 24-hour urinary metanephrines and free (unconjugated) catecholamines are more sensitive than VMA (see **Table 18.4**). The false-negative rate of 35% for VMA renders this test unreliable for clinical testing, particularly as a high-vanilla diet (bananas, coffee, ice-cream, etc.) can produce false-positive results. Urinary metanephrine measurement has a sensitivity of 80–85%, which may rise to 95% if the urine-to-creatinine ratio is used. However, urinary free catecholamine measurement is now favored for the diagnosis of pheochromocytomas. As 24-hour urine collections are occasionally difficult to obtain, evaluation of random urine samples or overnight urine collections has been suggested but with some compromise in sensitivity.

In a symptomatic patient, the sensitivity approaches 100%, with a specificity greater than 95% with two or more samples. Catecholamine and metabolite excretion may also be influenced by such variables as renal function, urine flow, and pH; in patients with renal failure, results may be difficult to interpret, particularly with a creatinine clearance less than 40mL/min. Currently, most laboratories measure catecholamines by high-pressure liquid chromatography with electrochemical detection or gas-chromatograph methods, and previous problems associated with fluorometric analysis (e.g. false-positive results caused by α-methyldopa or other drugs with high native fluorescence) are irrelevant. Occasionally, disproportionately high urinary VMA to catecholamine levels may imply malignancy, while elevated dopamine levels have been found in 64% of patients with malignant lesions. Levels above the normal range may be seen in patients with acute debilitating non-endocrine illness. These patients may be discriminated from those with true catecholamine-producing tumors by post-suppression plasma catecholamine levels (see below).

If results of urine studies are equivocal and pheochromocytoma is strongly suggested clinically, plasma catecholamines should be measured. Basal concentrations of plasma catecholamines are usually several times higher in patients with pheochromocytomas than others, if hypertensive when the sample is obtained, even when normal variations due to postural change, exercise, or emotional arousal are taken into consideration; plasma catecholamine levels are also affected by smoking, diuretics, and renal insufficiency. Plasma catecholamines are well above the normal range when sampled during a pheochromocytoma crisis, where diagnostic sensitivity and specificity are greatest compared to urinary catecholamine metabolites. The presence of normal levels in a hypertensive patient reduces the probability of a pheochromocytoma as the cause of that hypertensive episode. Because 99% of plasma dopamine is conjugated, measurement of free dopamine in plasma may fail to reveal excessive dopamine secretion. Greater dependence is therefore placed on urinary dopamine assays for the diagnosis of dopamine-secreting tumors.

Certain medications are capable of producing 'false-positive' results (**Table 18.3**). Labetalol is the most commonly used anti-hypertensive medication that interferes with metanephrine and catecholamine assays, and its use should be discontinued for 4–7 days before assay. Tricyclic antidepressants, antidopaminergic agents (such as sulpiride and metoclopramide), and naloxone also frequently interfere with the interpretation of urine collections, and such treatment should be tapered and discontinued 2 weeks before any hormonal measurements. In addition, false-negative results may be obtained from tumors with an episodic mode of

Medications that increase catecholamine levels and/or their metabolites
Tricyclic antidepressants
Monoamine-oxidase-inhibitor therapy and concomitant consumption of cheese, or wine; or concomitant monoamine-oxidase inhibitor and sympathomimetic–amine therapy (episodic hypertension)
Labetalol
Levodopa
Drugs containing catecholamines (decongestants)
Amphetamines, buspirone, and most psychoactive agents (mainly tricyclic antidepressants)
Sotalol
Methyldopa
Withdrawal from clonidine
Ethanol
Benzodiazepines

Table 18.3 Medications that increase catecholamine levels and/or their metabolites.

catecholamine secretion if collections of catecholamines or metabolites are obtained when the tumor is not hormonally active. Serum chromogranin has been suggested as an alternative to the previously mentioned tests in the diagnosis of pheochromocytomas, particularly as it is not influenced by drugs used in the treatment of pheochromocytomas. However, although it is a sensitive test in confirming the diagnosis of a pheochromocytoma, it has a poor diagnostic specificity in excluding the disease. Furthermore, its diagnostic sensitivity is also influenced by creatinine clearance.

Pharmacologic testing

Several factors, including diseases, anxiety, drugs, and essential hypertension, can cause moderate elevations of plasma catecholamines. Failure of catecholamines to suppress after 200μg of clonidine, an α_2-adrenoreceptor agonist, given orally is suggestive of a tumor with 97% sensitivity and a false-positive rate of only 1.5% in essential hypertension. A provocative test may be employed when the clinical suspicion is high but the catecholamine production is only marginally elevated. Glucagon, 1–2mg iv, is widely used as it has fewest side effects with adequate α/β-adrenoceptor blockade. A positive test requires a clear increase, at least threefold, in plasma catecholamines 1–3min following drug administration; a simultaneous increase in blood pressure is desirable but not essential. The glucagon test has high specificity (100%) but low sensitivity (81%). When the glucagon and clonidine tests are both negative, a diagnosis of a pheochromocytoma is highly unlikely. However, in practice, stimulation tests have occasionally failed to identify patients with catecholamine-producing tumors in a large series from the Mayo Clinic.

A summary of the performance of some of the common biochemical tests is given in **Table 18.4**.

Trial of phenoxybenzamine

In the occasional patient in whom the biochemical and radiologic tests are inconclusive, therapy with phenoxybenzamine over a period of 1–2 months can be given to observe the effects

Table 18.4 Sensitivity and specificity of common biochemical tests in the diagnosis of catecholamine-secreting tumors.

Sensitivity and specificity of common biochemical tests in the diagnosis of catecholamine-secreting tumors				
Measurement	Normal range	If measurement greater than:	Sensitivity (%)	Specificity (%)
Urinary metanephrines	<5μmol/24h	9μmol/24h	79	93
Urinary VMA	<35μmol/24h	55μmol/24h	42	100
Urinary free norepinephrine	<290nmol/24h	720nmol/24h	95	95
Urinary free epinephrine	<90nmol/24h	200nmol/24h	95	95
Plasma norepinephrine	0.3–2.8nmol/L	5nmol/L	94	97
Plasma epinephrine	0.1–0.52nmol/L	1.5nmol/L	90	90

on the nature and frequency of the attacks and on the blood pressure. A good response indicates the need for re-evaluation of the patient.

Localization imaging of catecholamine-producing tumors
Computerized tomography/magnetic resonance imaging
About 98% of catecholamine-secreting tumors are located in the abdomen, with the majority arising from the adrenal gland. At present CT and MR scanning offer the most reliable methods for preoperative localization of catecholamine-producing tumors, as they can identify lesions as small as 5mm.

CT scanning is very accurate in the detection of adrenal pheochromocytomas, with a sensitivity ranging from 93% to 100%, but it lacks in specificity in failing to distinguish between pheochromocytoma, adrenal adenomas, and myelolipomas. In sporadic cases pheochromocytomas usually do not present until they are large (average size 5cm in diameter); lesions are often smaller in patients with MEN or VHL, presumably because these tumors are often specifically sought even in the absence of symptoms. On unenhanced scans they are usually of homogeneous density similar to the liver, discrete, rounded, or oval masses. Occasionally, they may contain central low-attenuation areas representing necrosis and may become cystic; calcification, although a well recorded feature, is infrequent. The tumors usually enhance markedly following intravenous injection of contrast medium (**Figs 18.5–18.7**). Intravenous injection of ionic contrast

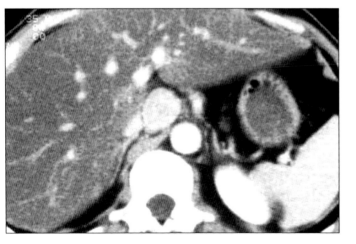

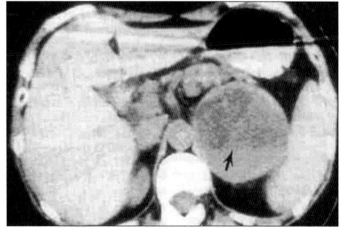

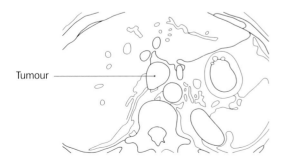

Figure 18.5 Paraganglioma. Computerized tomography scan showing a small tumor lying anterior to and separate from the right adrenal; this proved to be a paraganglioma. (Reproduced with permission from Besser M, Thorner MO. Atlas of endocrine imaging. London;Mosby: 1993.)

Figure 18.6 Pheochromocytoma. Unenhanced computerized tomography scan showing a large left pheochromocytoma with a fluid level (arrow). (Reproduced with permission from Francis IR, Korobkin M. Pheochromocytoma. Radiol Clin North Am 1996;34:1101–11.)

231

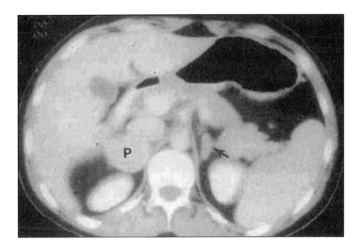

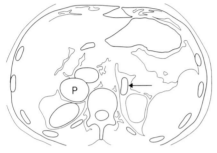

Figure 18.7 A marginally enlarged left adrenal (arrow) in a patient with MEN2. Surgical biopsy of the gland confirmed adrenal medullary hyperplasia. In our experience these lesions can often be identified at venous catheterization. P, small right-sided pheochromocytoma. (Reproduced with permission from Francis IR, Korobkin M. Pheochromocytoma. Radiol Clin North Am. 1996;34:1101–11.)

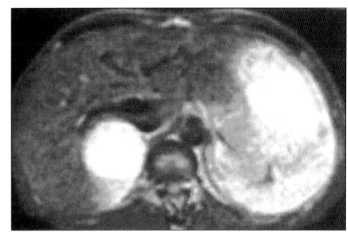

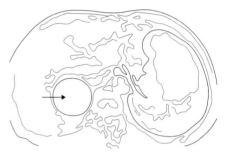

Figure 18.8 T2-weighted MRI of a right adrenal pheochromocytoma (arrow). (Reproduced with permission from Besser M, Thorner MO. Atlas of endocrine imaging. London;Mosby: 1993.)

medium can precipitate crises in inadequately alpha-blocked patients, although this does not seem to be the case with the newly developed nonionic contrast media. On MRI T1-weighted images, pheochromocytomas show similar low signal intensity to the liver, but are markedly hyperintense on T2-weighted images, with almost 100% sensitivity (**Figs 18.8–18.10**). Several studies have shown that MRI is equivalent to CT in diagnosing adrenal pheochromocytomas but more accurate in detecting extra-adrenal tumors, while it is clearly the modality of choice in pregnancy. MRI has the advantage of an absence of ionizing radiation, good multiplanar display and evaluation of vascular extension; by using the newer technique of chemical shift, it can potentially distinguish between adrenocortical adenomas, metastatic tumors, and pheochromocytoma. Thus, MR may in time replace CT as the predominant radiologic modality in displaying adrenal pheochromocytomas.

Radionuclide imaging

Sympathoadrenal imaging is performed with ^{131}I-meta-iodo-benzylguanidine (MIBG) or ^{123}I-MIBG, a catecholamine (norepinephrine) analog that utilizes the amine precursor uptake mechanism and may thus be incorporated into vesicles or neurosecretory granules in the cytoplasm. Typically, 0.5mCi of ^{131}I-mIBG or 5mCi of ^{123}I-MIBG is injected into the patient, after blocking the thyroid uptake of free radioiodine with potassium

iodides. Gamma images are then obtained using either a high-energy (^{131}I) or low-energy collimator (^{123}I) interfaced with a computer. Posterior and anterior images are obtained of the whole body 24–72 hours later, with additional views obtained in selected cases as needed. Very small lesions can be safely and conventionally located by this method. The sensitivity of the technique in detecting functioning catecholamine-producing tumors is slightly less than 90%, although the specificity can exceed 90%. MIBG imaging is particularly useful for the detection of extra-adrenal and metastatic disease because, unlike CT or MRI, it is inherently a whole-body imaging technique (**Figs 18.11 & 18.12**). Scintigraphy with radiolabeled octreotide (^{111}In-pentetreotide), an analog of somatostatin, has been shown to be as sensitive although less specific than MIBG in the detection of catecholamine-producing tumors. Both these radionuclides may exert a complementary role in the diagnosis of such tumors; furthermore, scintigraphy with ^{111}In-pentetreotide may occasionally reveal ^{123}I-MIBG-negative lesions or a differential location of uptake, which may have therapeutic implications. When the above methods fail to localize a lesion, positron emission tomography performed after the administration of [2,18]F-fludro-2-deoxy-D-glycose (the accumulation of which reflects tumor activity) or imaging with ^{11}C-hydroxyephedrine have correctly localized tumors in rare cases.

A helpful imaging algorithm is to perform ^{123}I-MIBG scintigraphy in all patients with biochemically proven catecholamine-producing tumors. On detection of a lesion, MR imaging of the region is obtained for detailed anatomic localization prior to

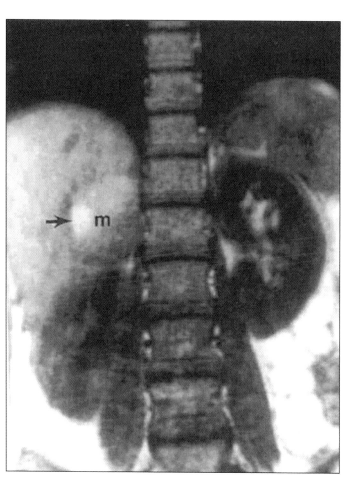

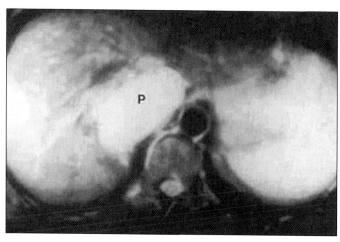

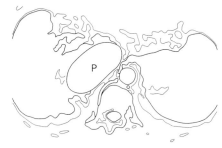

Figure 18.10 T2-weighted MRI (fast spin echo) showing hyperintense right adrenal pheochromocytoma (P) on axial imaging. (Reproduced with permission from Francis IR, Korobkin M. Pheochromocytoma. Radiol Clin North Am. 1996;34:1101–11.)

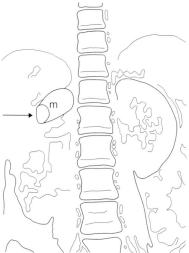

Figure 18.9 T2-weighted MRI (fast spin echo) showing hyperintense right adrenal pheochromocytoma (m) on coronal imaging. (Reproduced with permission from Francis IR, Korobkin M. Pheochromocytoma. Radiol Clin North Am. 1996;34:1101–11.)

surgical removal. If ^{123}I-MIBG is negative and a catecholamine-secreting tumor is still highly suspected, MR imaging of the neck, chest, abdomen, and pelvis should be obtained as ^{123}I-MIBG scintigraphy has a 10% false-negative rate.

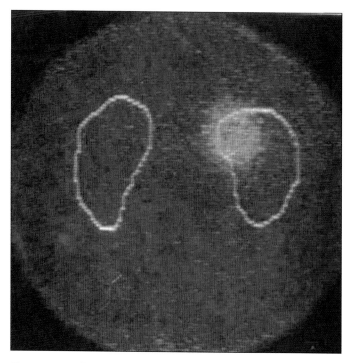

Figure 18.11 ^{123}I-MIBG scan of a left adrenal pheochromocytoma with superimposed renal outlines. (Reproduced with permission from Hall R, Evered DC. Colour atlas of endocrinology, 2nd edn. London;Wolfe Medical: 1990.)

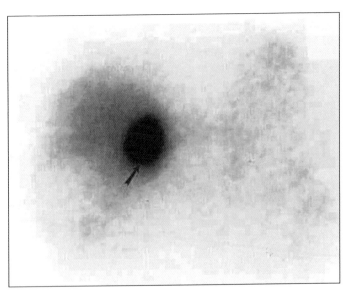

Figure 18.12 Anterior abdominal view on ^{123}I-MIBG scan (72 hours postinjection) of a right adrenal pheochromocytoma (arrow).

Venous sampling

Venous sampling can be a useful complementary investigation to the previous imaging modalities when there is high clinical and/or biochemical suspicion of a catecholamine-secreting tumor with negative imaging studies (particularly if ^{123}I-MIBG is negative), to confirm bilateral lesions, or when a suspicious mass warrants further clarification; it should always be performed under previous α- and β-adrenoceptor blockade. Although there is no established normal range for adrenal venous catecholamine concentrations, effluent plasma epinephrine:norepinephrine ratios are normally between 4 and 10 under normal conditions; this ratio is reversed when adrenomedullary pathology is present, and certainly a ratio of less than 1 in adrenal effluent blood (confirmed by simultaneous cortisol estimation) is highly suspicious of intra-adrenal pathology. In addition, whole-body venous catheterization and sampling has been shown to be successful in identifying extra-adrenal pheochromocytomas. However, the results may be misleading in cases with periodic hormonal secretion.

Diagnosis in familial syndromes

Measurement of 24-hour urinary levels of metanephrine, epinephrine, and norepinephrine, combined with selective use of thin-section contrast-enchanced CT or MR imaging, and imaging dity ^{123}I-MIBG, provides the optimal screening for asymptomatic patients at risk of developing MEN2- or VHL-associated pheochromocytomas. Urinary catecholamines and metanephrine should be measured yearly in asymptomatic potential or proven MEN2 and VHL gene carriers and, if abnormal, CT or MR is performed. The presumed symptomatic patient with normal urinary studies and no abnormality on MR scanning or ^{123}I-MIBG presents a difficult therapeutic dilemma. In such cases, venous sampling may confirm adrenal medullary pathology.

Screening for catecholamine producing tumors

In addition to screening patients with typical clinical manifestations, assays for catecholamines and their metabolites can be used to screen other patients at high risk (**Tables 18.1 & 18.4**). When the presence of an undetected catecholamine-producing tumor is particularly dangerous, as in pregnancy or prior to surgery, screening should be considered even when clinical manifestations are minor or atypical.

Treatment

Surgical

Surgical resection is the treatment of choice for isolated unilateral catecholamine-producing tumors and should always be carried out as an elective procedure after careful preoperative preparation. The resection of these tumors has great potential for intraoperative and postoperative complications because of excessive release of catecholamines and the metabolic and hemodynamic effects associated with the removal of the catecholamine excess. Major factors responsible for the reduction in the operative risks are blood-pressure control and close monitoring of fluid balance.

For blood-pressure control, preoperative treatment with the mixed α_1/α_2 noncompetitive adrenoceptor antagonist phenoxybenzamine is initiated, starting at a dose of 10mg orally every 12 hours and gradually building up to 10–20mg four times daily. This agent causes noncompetitive α-adrenergic blockade and permits expansion of the intravascular volume while also reducing intraoperative pressor episodes. After the first few doses of the α-antagonist, the β_1/β_2-antagonist propranolol is given orally in a dose of 40mg three times a day to avoid reflex tachycardia. The fall in intravascular tone may cause substantial postural hypotension; hemodilation occurs after use, with a fall in hematocrit, and it may be necessary to transfuse the patient preoperatively. There are advantages to giving this regimen over several weeks to establish effective blockade before surgery.

Criteria considered to suggest an adequate preoperative preparation include a supine arterial blood pressure not exceeding 140/90mmHg; initial orthostatic hypotension should gradually diminish with adequate volume expansion. However, despite adequate alpha-blockade, total elimination of cardiovascular disturbances is seldom achieved and significant elevations of blood pressure should be anticipated during manipulation of the tumor. This can be minimized by the preoperative administration of iv phenoxybenzamine 0.5mg/kg in 250mL 5% dextrose, over 2 hours, daily for three successive days before surgery, to ensure that as many α-adrenoreceptors as possibly are irreversibly blocked before surgery. Even so, given the large number of vasoconstrictor peptides that may be released by pheochromocytomas (neuropeptide Y, endothelin, etc.), it is not surprising that the pressor episodes cannot be fully blocked with adrenoreceptor blockade alone.

Newer selective α_1-antagonists such as terazocin and doxazocin, which block only postsynaptic α_1-adrenoreceptors and do not produce reflex tachycardia, can be used as an alternative to phenoxybenzamine, although we have little experience with their use in this situation. Labetalol, a combined α- and β-adrenergic blocker, has also been used at doses of 800–1600mg/day but can precipitate a hypertensive crisis and interfere with the measurement of plasma catecholamines. It is a weak α-adrenoceptor blocker and also interferes with MIBG scintigraphy. Similarly, calcium-channel blockers have been successfully used in controlling blood pressure, not by directly affecting catecholamine

Medical management of pheochromocytoma	
Therapeutic target	Medical therapy
Control of blood pressure	Alpha-blockers (phenoxybenzamine, terazocin)
	Calcium channel blockers
	Metyrosine
Treatment of hypertensive crisis	Phentolamine
	Sodium nitroprusside
Management of arrhythmias	Beta-blockers (propranolol, esmolol)
Prevention of postsurgical hypotension	Adequately long preoperative alpha- and beta-blockade
	Volume replacement
	Pressor agents (norepinephrine, phenylephrine)

Table 18.5 Medical management of pheochromocytoma.

synthesis but by decreasing epinephrine-mediated transmembrane calcium influx in vascular smooth muscle. They can be used as an adjunct to alpha-blockade treatment in high-risk patients partially controlled on alpha-blockers or where these drugs are contraindicated. An outline of the medical management is given in **Table 18.5**.

Both diazepam and barbiturates may be used safely as sedatives for premedication, while enflurane and isoflurane are the anesthetics of choice. Meticulous continuous intraoperative monitoring is required as unexpected surges of blood pressure may be encountered, as well as sudden tachyarrhythmias, which are best managed with the administration of a short-acting cardioselective beta-blocker such as esmolol, or with lidocaine. Although hypertensive episodes can be treated with intermittent intravenous injections of phentolamine, this drug can cause repeated cycles of hyper- or hypotension; nitroprusside is used instead, which provides a shorter and more controllable mode of action (**Fig. 18.13**).

Laparoscopic adrenalectomy is being increasingly used for benign, sporadic, intra-adrenal catecholamine-secreting tumors. Postoperative recovery times are greatly shortened, compared with open surgery. With the conventional technique many approaches are available, which vary according to pathology, diameter of the adrenal mass, location of the lesion, and patient morphology. Bilateral pheochromocytomas can also be removed laparoscopically. The surgeon operating laparoscopically must be prepared to proceed to open surgery immmediately should complications ensue. During conventional surgery, most surgeons prefer an anterior transabdominal approach, usually with bilateral subcostal incisions, because both adrenals and other abdominal sites may need to be examined. This allows exploration of the adrenals, sympathetic ganglia, bladder, and other pelvic structures. Pheochromocytomas are vascular tumors that vary in size, commonly containing cystic or hemorrhagic areas, with a median weight of 100g (range 1g to kilograms). Any catecholamine-producing tumor found should be regarded as potentially malignant and accordingly removed with the capsule intact. Posterior and flank incisions may occasionally be preferable for removal of larger tumors.

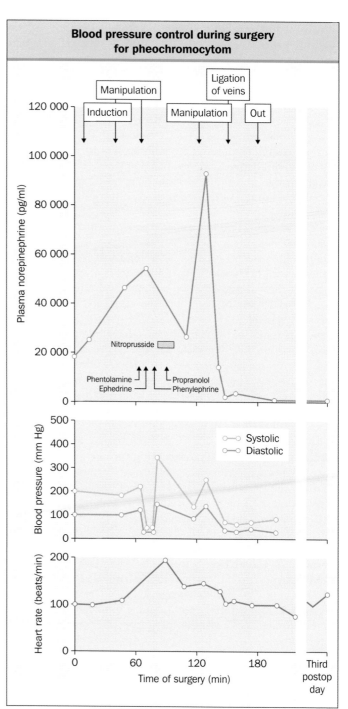

Figure 18.13 Blood pressure control during surgery for pheochromocytoma. Changes in catecholamine levels (top panel), arterial blood pressure (center panel) and pulse rate (bottom panel) in a patient with a large adrenal pheochromocytoma undergoing surgical manipulation. (Modified with permission from Feldman JM. Diagnosis and management of pheochromocytoma. Hosp Pract. 1989;24:175–98 © 1989 The McGraw-Hill Companies, Inc. Original illustration by Albert Miller.)

Following surgery, and after restoration of blood pressure, regulation of the circulating volume may take days to become normal; this is partly caused by the insensitivity of adrenergically innervated vasculature to relatively normal levels of catecholamines because of previous downregulation of adrenoreceptors.

Plasma and urinary catecholamines may take days to weeks to fully normalize. The longer the postoperative preparation with α- and β-adrenergic blockade the more rapidly volume dynamics are normalized postoperatively.

Treatment of hypertensive crisis

During the crisis of a catecholamine-producing tumor, sodium nitroprusside should be used at a dose of 0.5–10µg/kg/min through continuous intravenous infusion in order to obtain gradual and controlled reduction in blood pressure; phentolamine is an alternative but with the limitations mentioned previously. Nifedipine has also been used with some success.

Treatment of pheochromocytomas in patients with familial syndromes

Controversy exists regarding the optimal management of patients with MEN and VHL. On the basis of the observation that only 50% of patients have bilateral involvement at diagnosis, adrenalectomy of the neoplastic gland and monitoring of the contralateral has been advocated. However, many patients develop a tumor in the contralateral adrenal requiring reoperation. An alternative approach, because of potential bilaterality and risk of second operation, is bilateral adrenalectomy as the initial procedure, with replacement for hypoadrenalism. Our current policy is to consider a venous catheter study and only advise bilateral adrenalectomy if there is clear imaging or biochemical evidence of bilaterality.

Malignant catecholamine-secreting tumors

For patients with inoperable, malignant, recurrent or multicentric pheochromocytomas, long-term medical therapy is the treatment of choice, particularly as prolonged survival in patients with frankly malignant tumors has been described. Phenoxybenzamine can be given orally at doses that fully control symptoms, although this may be limited by side effects; doses up to 120mg have occasionally been used. Alternatively, α-methyl-paratyrosine, which inhibits tyrosine hydroxylase, the rate-limiting enzyme in catecholamine biosynthesis, has been used to decrease catecholamine production from the tumor itself. Although the drug can decrease circulating catecholamines by nearly 80%, control of blood pressure may be incomplete and serious adverse effects have been reported; however, it may be used as a dose-sparing adjunct to the alpha-blockers.

Targeted radiotherapy with radionuclides has been effective in treating such tumors because of the localization of a beta-emitting radionuclide, either within the tumor cell or in its proximity, compared to nontarget cells. ^{131}I-MIBG, based on a positive ^{123}I-MIBG uptake, has been used in this setting for the treatment of malignant pheochromocytomas, paragangliomas, and neuroblastomas. Although ^{131}I-MIBG dosage regimens have not been clearly established, doses totaling up to 1000mCi have been employed, giving doses at 6-monthly intervals. The overall consensus is that, although complete responses have been observed in only a minority of cases, partial responses are common, and in most cases clinically useful hormonal and symptomatic responses may be obtained. Therapy with somatostatin analogs radiolabeled with beta-emitters such as yttrium-90, may also become applicable in the future, particularly in patients who show complementary uptake with ^{123}I-MIBG and ^{111}In-pentetreotide scintigraphy; in such patients therapy with both labeled radionuclides might be feasible.

Cytotoxic chemotherapy, using a combination of cyclophosphamide, vincristine, and dacarbazine, has been shown to produce a complete or partial response rate of 57% in tumor bulk with a biochemical response rate of 80%; however, experience is limited. External beam therapy with doses of 3000–5000cGy provides useful palliation in cases of skeletal deposits but less so if deposits are in soft tissues. Clinically useful reductions in tumor bulk have been described with the embolization of inoperable or metastatic lesions. The feasibility of this approach is operator-dependent, while the vascular supply of the tumor must be readily accessible and the patient adequately blocked.

Complications

Surgical treatment

With complete surgical removal of the tumor the majority of patients are rendered normotensive. A transient form of hypertension may also be found, reflecting fluid shifts and autonomic instability from persistently high catecholamine levels in adrenergic neurons rather than residual tumor; as these stores become depleted, blood pressure normalizes. With removal of the tumor, blood pressure may also fall significantly; this is less likely to occur if attention has been paid to intravenous adrenergic blockaded volume repletion prior to surgery. Persistence of hypotension may be caused by hemorrhage, sudden increases in venous capacitance, or residual effects of preoperative alpha-blockade. Another occasional postoperative problem is hypoglycemia, which is usually temporary and rarely severe. When bilateral tumors are found and both adrenals are removed, adrenocortical corticosteroid replacement therapy is required. Following laparoscopic adrenalectomy many patients are ambulatory by the evening of the procedure, and most leave hospital by the third postoperative day.

Clinical outcomes

Sporadic catecholamine-secreting tumors

With complete surgical removal, 70% of patients become normotensive; a further 30% remain hypertensive, probably reflecting underlying essential hypertension or end-organ damage (renovascular hypertension). Increased levels of catecholamines or metabolites postoperatively indicate the presence of residual tumor, a second primary lesion, or occult metastases. As the routine use of MIBG has shown that the presence of metastatic or multicentric tumors is more common than previously suspected, we recommend lifelong biochemical (with urinary catecholamines) and clinical followup to detect early recurrence. The 5-year survival for the patients followed in the Mayo clinic was 96% but after apparent curative surgery 5–10% showed local recurrence.

Malignant catecholamine-secreting tumors

The 5-year survival of patients with malignant metastasized pheochromocytomas is around 44% but some patients have survived up to 20 years. However, a recent series has shown a poor overall survival and response to current treatment modalities. If at the time of initial resection there are no gross histopathologic features of malignancy, the probability that the tumor will ultimately prove to be malignant is in the region of 8–9%. Previous experience suggests that, in patients with any type of neuroendocrine tumor showing ^{123}I-MIBG uptake, therapy with ^{131}I-MIBG may improve overall survival.

FURTHER READING

Bouloux PMG, Fakeeh M. Investigation of phaeochromocytoma. Clin Endocrinol (Oxf). 1995;43:657–64.

Bravo EL. Evolving concepts in the pathophysiology, diagnosis and treatment of pheochromocytoma. Endocrinol Rev. 1994;15:356–68.

Bravo EL, Gifford RW. Pheochromocytoma. Endocrinol Metab Clin North Am. 1993;22:329–41.

Chew, S.L., Reznek RH, Sheaves R, et al. The diagnosis of bilateral phaeochromocytomas in Von Hippel–Lindau disease by adrenal vein sampling. Q J Med. 1994;87:49–54.

Fonseca V, Bouloux PM. Pheochromocytoma and paraganglioma. Baillière's Clin Endocrinol Metab. 1993;7:509–50.

Gagner M. Laparoscopic adrenalectomy. Surg Clin North Am. 1996;76:523–37.

Goldstein RE, O'Neil JA, Holcomb GW, et al. Clinical experience over 48 years with pheochromocytoma. Ann Surg. 1999;229:755–66.

Jarrott B, Luis WJ. Abnormalities in enzymes involved in catecholamine synthesis and catabolism in pheochromocytoma. Clin Sci Molec Med. 1977;53:529–35.

Mukherjee JJ, Peppercorn PD, Reznek RH, et al. CT imaging of pheochromocytoma: effect of non-ionic contrast medium on circulating catecholamine levels. Radiology 1996;202:227–31.

Nativ O, Grant CS, Sheps, SG, et al. The clinical significance of nuclear DNA ploidy pattern in 184 patients with pheochromocytoma. Cancer 1992;69:2683–7.

Neumann HPH, Berger DP, Sigmund G, et al. Pheochromocytomas, multiple endocrine neoplasia type 2, and von Hippel–Lindau disease. N Engl J Med. 1993;329:1531–8.

Newbould EC, Ross GA, Dacie JE, Bouloux PMG, Besser GM, Grossman A. The use of venous catheterisation in the diagnosis and localisation of bilateral phaeochromocytoma. Clin Endocrinol (Oxf). 1991;35:55–9.

Pomares FJ, Canas R, Rodriguez JM et al. Differences between sporadic and multiple endocrine neoplasia type 2A phaeochromocytoma. Clin Endocrinol (Oxf). 1998;48:195–200.

Reznek RH, Amstrong P. The adrenal gland. Clin Endocrinol (Oxf). 1994;40:561–76.

Roberts NB, Dutton J, McClelland P, Bone JM. Urinary catecholamine excretion in relation to renal function. Ann Clin Biochem. 1999;36:587–91.

Ross GA, Newbould EC, Grossman A, Perrett D. Analysis of urinary and plasma catecholamines using a single LC–EC system. J Pharmacol Biomed. Anal. 1990;8:1039–43.

Shapiro B, Fig LM. Management of pheochromocytoma. Endocrinol Metab Clin North Am. 1989;18:443–81.

Sutton MG, Sheps GS, Lie JT. Prevalence of clinically unsuspected pheochromocytoma. Review of a 50-year autopsy series. Mayo Clin Proc. 1981;56:354–60.

Young WF Jr. Pheochromocytoma and primary aldosteronism: diagnostic approaches. Endocrinol Metab Clin North Am. 1997;26:801–13.

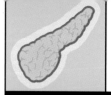

Section 4 Control of Blood Glucose and its Disturbance

Chapter 19 Physiologic Mechanisms in Homeostatic Control of Glucose

Simon J Fisher and C Ronald Kahn

GLUCOSE HOMEOSTASIS

Regulation of blood glucose control

Plasma glucose concentrations are tightly controlled by a balance between actions of hormones, enzymes, and substrates that act to either raise or lower blood glucose levels. In normal individuals, this balance exists such that, despite periods of feeding and fasting, blood glucose concentrations are normally kept in a narrow range between 70mg/dL and 120mg/dL (4–7mmol/L; **Fig. 19.1**). Since glucose is the primary fuel for the central nervous system (CNS) under most physiologic conditions, its constant supply at sufficient levels is critical for normal CNS functioning. Low blood sugar limits glucose utilization, which can result in seizures, coma, and even brain death under conditions of severe hypoglycemia. Likewise, prevention of hyperglycemia is important to avoid the loss of calories that would occur through glycosuria if glucose concentrations exceeded the renal threshold (about 180mg/dL, 10.5mmol/L). Additionally, prevention of hyperglycemia limits fetal mortality and morbidity in patients with gestational diabetes and prevents common complications associated with uncontrolled diabetes.

Plasma glucose concentrations are determined by the net balance between glucose released into the circulation and glucose uptake from the plasma. In the fed condition, glucose is absorbed from the gastrointestinal tract into the plasma but, during postabsorptive conditions, plasma glucose is primarily derived from the liver. Glucose uptake from the plasma can be divided into those tissues where glucose uptake or utilization is regulated by insulin, such as muscle, fat and liver, and those in which insulin has no apparent role in stimulating glucose uptake, such as brain and kidney.

Although blood glucose levels can be affected by many physiologic and pathologic signals, normal regulation of glucose levels depends largely on only three factors: the ability of the pancreatic β cell to secrete insulin both acutely and in a sustained fashion; the ability of insulin to inhibit hepatic glucose production and promote glucose utilization (i.e. insulin sensitivity); and the ability of glucose to enter cells in the absence of insulin (termed glucose sensitivity or glucose effectiveness; **Table 19.1**).

Absorptive and post-absorptive regulation of glucose

Blood glucose is derived from absorbed carbohydrate for the first 3–4 hours after glucose ingestion. During this period, plasma levels of glucose and insulin are elevated while glucagon levels are suppressed. The absorbed glucose provides the metabolic needs of the brain and serves to replete glycogen stores in liver and muscle. Although skeletal muscle is approximately

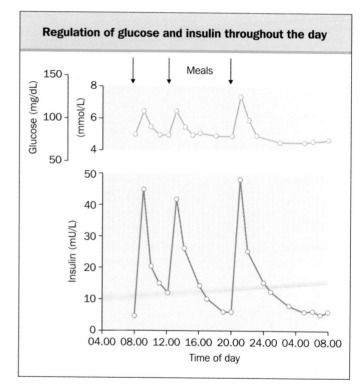

Figure 19.1 Regulation of glucose and insulin throughout the day.
Note that increased plasma glucose levels following meals are limited by the marked increases in plasma insulin.

40% of the body mass, it is estimated to account for more than 80% of glucose disposal at high insulin concentrations or after an oral glucose load. Thus skeletal muscle plays a critical role in both insulin-dependent and non-insulin-dependent glucose disposal. Skeletal muscle insulin resistance is the earliest detectable lesion in the prediabetic state and is therefore thought to a key contributor in the pathogenesis of type 2 diabetes. Transgenic mice in which the insulin-sensitive glucose transporter (GLUT4) was deleted specifically in muscle developed impaired glucose tolerance; however, somewhat surprisingly, mice that lacked skeletal muscle insulin receptors were not hyperglycemic and did not develop diabetes. Thus the extent to which skeletal muscle insulin resistance contributes to type 2 diabetes may be a function of exactly where in the intracellular insulin action signaling pathway the defect lies and how an additional defect in insulin action or secretion accompanies this early abnormality.

Table 19.1 Metabolic actions of insulin.

Metabolic actions of insulin

	Action	Tissue
Carbohydrate metabolism		
Glucose transport	Increase	Muscle, adipose tissue
Glycolysis	Increase	Muscle, adipose tissue
Glycogen synthesis	Increase	Liver, adipose tissue, muscle
Glycogen degradation	Decrease	Liver, adipose tissue, muscle
Gluconeogenesis	Decrease	Liver
Lipid metabolism		
Lipolysis	Decrease	Adipose tissue
Triglyceride and fatty acid synthesis	Increase	Liver, adipose tissue
Very low density lipoprotein synthesis	Increase	Liver
Lipoprotein lipase activity	Increase	Adipose tissue
Fatty acid oxidation	Decrease	Muscle, liver
Cholesterol formation	Increase	Liver
Protein metabolism		
Amino acid transport	Increase	Muscle, liver, adipose tissue
Protein synthesis	Increase	Muscle, liver, adipose tissue
Protein degradation	Decrease	Muscle
Urea synthesis	Decrease	Muscle

The postabsorptive phase from 4–24 hours after a meal is characterized by decreasing insulin and glucose levels back to baseline values with an increase in glucagon to base levels. These signals switch the liver from a consumer of glucose to the primary producer of glucose. Initially, hepatic glucose production consists primarily of glycogenolysis. After 12–48 hours of starvation, a further fall in insulin and rise in glucagon enhances the hepatic gluconeogenesis, which replaces glycogenolysis (in the setting of depleted glycogen stores) as the primary contributor to hepatic glucose production (**Fig. 19.2**).

Under these fasted conditions, 80% of glucose uptake is non-insulin-mediated and the majority is taken up by the central nervous system (**Fig. 19.3**). Other tissues that depend on anaerobic glycolysis, such as red and white blood cells, also contribute to non-insulin-mediated glucose utilization. In the setting of starvation and decreased insulin levels, pyruvate dehydrogenase activity is decreased and this limits glucose oxidation, thereby promoting release of lactate, pyruvate, and alanine, which can serve as substrates for gluconeogenesis. This pathway, referred to as the Cori cycle, is one of the body's adaptations to conserve protein and maintain substrate flux for gluconeogenesis, thus ensuring a constant glucose supply to the brain (**Fig. 19.4**).

Altered glucose homeostasis in the diabetic state

The genetic and environmental factors that contribute to the causes and complications of both type 1 and type 2 diabetes are the subject of other chapters in this book; however, it is worthwhile considering how each of these forms of diabetes contribute to alterations in glucose homeostasis.

The development of type 1 diabetes is the culmination of autoimmune destruction of the pancreatic β cell. This destruction results in severe, and sometimes complete, insulin deficiency. In the absence of insulin, fasting hyperglycemia is due primarily to

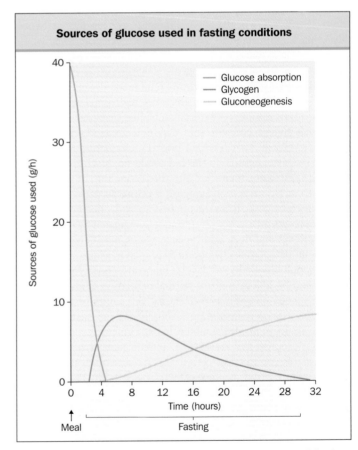

Figure 19.2 Sources of glucose used in fasting conditions. Following a meal, plasma glucose is derived from absorbed carbohydrate. Beyond 3–4 hours after a meal, the breakdown of glycogen provides glucose for tissue metabolic needs. As fasting continues and glycogen stores wane, gluconeogenesis surpasses glycogenolysis as a source for glucose.

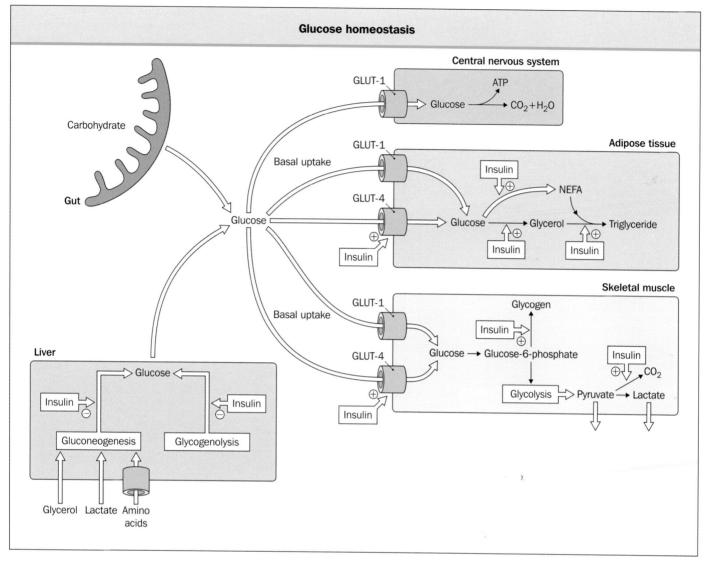

Figure 19.3 Glucose homeostasis. Plasma glucose is derived from carbohydrate absorption in the alimentary tract and hepatic glucose released from the sum processes of gluconeogenesis and glycogenolysis. In the basal state, the majority of glucose utilization occurs in the central nervous system. Under insulin-stimulated conditions, an insulin-induced recruitment of glucose transporters allows for increased glucose uptake and metabolism in adipose tissue and muscle. ATP, adenosine triphosphate; GLUT1, GLUT4, glucose transporter 1, 4; NEFA, non-esterified fatty acids.

an unrestrained increase in hepatic glucose output (**Fig. 19.5**). Levels of gluconeogenic precursors are also elevated to supply the necessary fuel to support increased rates of gluconeogenesis. The resulting chronic hyperglycemia also causes a degree of insulin resistance because of 'glucose toxicity' (see below) that further complicates the metabolic picture. Hyperglycemia itself leads to increased glucose uptake by a mass-action effect, although this does not correct the defects in glucose oxidation and metabolism that occur in the absence of insulin. Additionally, insulin deficiency results in unrestrained lipolysis and increased ketogenesis that can lead to diabetic ketoacidosis.

Type 2 diabetes is caused by a complex interaction between insulin resistance in skeletal muscle, adipose tissue, and the liver and a relative failure of the β cell to appropriately increase insulin secretion in response to increased glucose levels (**Fig. 19.6**). Insulin resistance in patients with type 2 diabetes is defined by defects in insulin-stimulated glucose transport, glycogen synthesis, and glucose oxidation. The β-cell failure is characterized

by loss of pulsatility and blunted response to increases in plasma glucose levels and gut-derived incretins (hormones that normally augment insulin secretion). The relative insulin deficiency and insulin resistance together contribute to both fasting and postprandial hyperglycemia. In the basal state, many studies suggest that increased gluconeogenesis contributes to the increased hepatic glucose production and fasting hyperglycemia. In response to a meal, however, the loss of first-phase insulin release caused by the β-cell failure, which is characteristic of the type 2 diabetic state, results in a failure to suppress hepatic glucose production and postprandial hyperglycemia. Enough insulin is present in patients with type 2 diabetes to prevent uncontrolled lipolysis and ketogenesis. Therefore, except under conditions of extreme stress, patients with type 2 diabetes generally do not become ketoacidotic. They may, however, develop a hyperosmolar state characterized by polyuria, polydipsia, profound dehydration, and possibly cardiovascular compromise and thrombotic events.

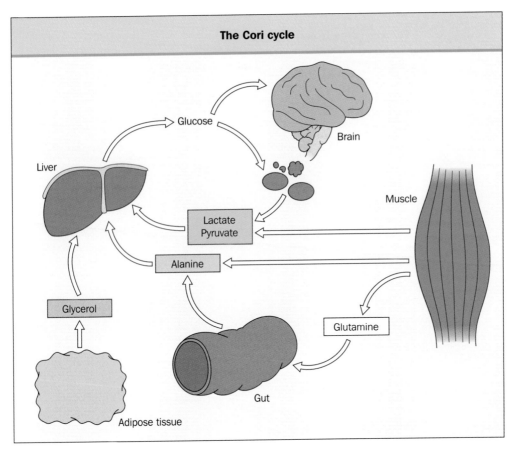

Figure 19.4 The Cori cycle.
Gluconeogenic precursors such as alanine, pyruvate, glycerol, and lactate are products of glucose metabolism in muscle, adipose tissue, blood cells, and the gut. These gluconeogenic precursors are synthesized back into glucose in the liver.

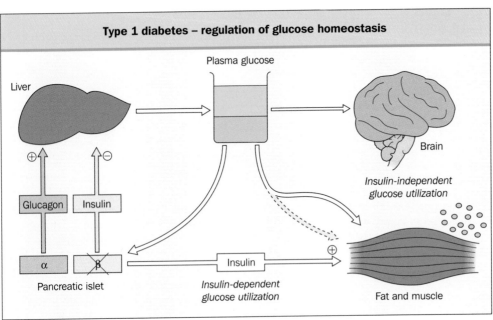

Figure 19.5 Type 1 diabetes – regulation of glucose homeostasis.
Autoimmune destruction of the pancreatic β cell results in insulin deficiency. In the absence of insulin, unrestrained hepatic glucose production and decreased glucose utilization contribute to hyperglycemia.

REGULATION AND MECHANISM OF INSULIN SECRETION

Islet cell morphology

The pancreas contributes to glucose homeostasis as both an exocrine and an endocrine organ. The endocrine portion of the pancreas constitutes about 2–3% of the total gland mass divided into approximately 1 million small endocrine glands, the islets of Langerhans. The islets are scattered throughout the exocrine parenchyma of the pancreas but are most dense in the tail region. At least four different cell types within the islets have been identified, based on histology (**Table 19.2**). The α, β, δ, and PP cells produce and secrete hormones and substrates and are located at the periphery of the islets and along the blood

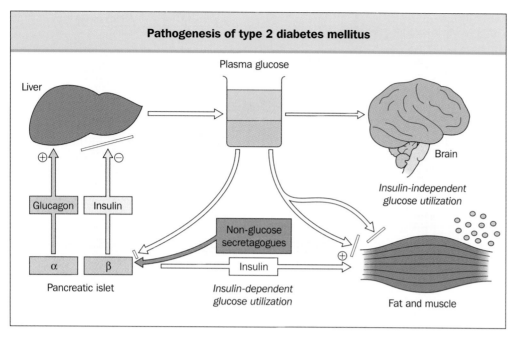

Pathogenesis of type 2 diabetes mellitus

Figure 19.6 **Pathogenesis of type 2 diabetes mellitus.** Insulin resistance in muscle, fat, and liver, coupled with an impaired pancreatic β-cell response, results in hyperglycemia.

Table 19.2 **Characteristics of islet cell morphology.** GLP, glucagon-like peptide.

Characteristics of islet cell morphology

Cell type	α (alpha)	β (beta)	δ (delta)	PP
Location within islet	Cortex	Medulla	Cortex	Cortex
Peptide products	Glucagon, GLP-1, GLP-2	Insulin, proinsulin, C-peptide, amylin	Somatostatin	Pancreatic polypeptide
Percentage of total	5–10	60–80	15–20	5–10

supply. The most numerous islet cell types are the β cells, which produce insulin. As outlined below, the β cells have secretory granules that release insulin into the circulation in response to rising plasma glucose levels.

Islets are richly vascularized and, although they constitute only 2% of islet mass, they receive 10–15% of pancreatic blood flow. Blood from afferent arterioles flows first into the core of the islet to supply the β-cell-rich medulla and carry insulin 'downstream' to the α, δ, and PP cells to influence their activity (the mnemonic BAD has been used to describe this pattern of flow).

Alpha and δ cells may additionally effect intrapancreatic β-cell insulin secretion via paracrine effects or by means of transfer of small ions and molecules through gap junctions in order to allow synchronized or amplified β-cell responses. The islets are also richly innervated by parasympathetic cholinergic fibers from the vagus, sympathetic adrenergic fibers from the celiac ganglion, and certain peptidergic nerves (vasoactive intestinal peptide, gastric-releasing polypeptide, galanin, neuropeptide-Y-releasing) that are important in regulating islet cell secretion (**Table 19.3**).

Insulin biosynthesis and secretion

The islet β cell synthesizes and stores insulin in secretory granules for release into the circulation in response to specific stimuli. The production of insulin is initiated by transcription of the gene encoding preproinsulin (the precursor of insulin), located on the short arm of chromosome 11. The primary gene transcript is spliced in the β-cell nucleus to remove sequences encoding introns. Once processed, the 600-nucleotide messenger RNA for preproinsulin is moved to the cytosol, where it becomes associated with ribosomes in the rough endoplasmic reticulum (RER). In the RER, the mRNA is translated into *preproinsulin* which has a 23-amino-acid leader sequence necessary to facilitate entry of the preproinsulin molecule into the lumen of the RER (**Fig. 19.7**).

Preproinsulin has a very short half-life, as this leader sequence is cleaved to form proinsulin. Proinsulin is transported in microvesicles from the RER to the Golgi apparatus, where it is packaged in secretory granules. Proinsulin is composed of an A chain (21 amino acid residues) and a B chain (30 amino acids) joined by the C-peptide (30–35 amino acids) in humans. Proinsulin is converted to insulin by cleavage of the C-peptide segment by the sequential action of two endopeptidases (prohormones convertase 2 and 3) and carboxypeptidase H.

Budding of selective clathrin-coated regions of the Golgi apparatus allows for the formation of secretory granules. In the secretory granule, the low pH environment allows insulin to co-precipitate with zinc ions to form small crystals. The mechanism by which granules are shuttled to the plasma membrane is complex and involves both regulated and constitutively active pathways. Evidence suggests that microtubules and/or

Major acute regulators of insulin secretion		
	Increase insulin secretion	**Decrease insulin secretion**
Islet hormones	Glucagon	Insulin
		Somatostatin
Metabolites	Glucose	
	Amino acids	
	Fatty acids	
Neural signals	β-adrenergic	α-adrenergic
	Acetylcholine	Galanin
	Vasoactive intestinal peptide	Neuropeptide Y
	Gastric-releasing polypeptide	
Gastrointestinal hormones	Gastrin	
	Cholecystokinin	
	Gastric inhibitory peptide	
	Secretin	
	Glucagon-like peptide-1	

Table 19.3 Major acute regulators of insulin secretion.

microfilaments are involved to provide a measure of directional movement. In the regulated pathway, appropriate stimuli signal for the granule sac to fuse with the plasma membrane and extrude insulin and C-peptide from the cell. A reservoir of granules close to the plasma membrane may appear to be most readily secreted and provide the rapid first-phase release of insulin that is seen in response to glucose stimulation.

Regulation of β-cell function

Under physiologic conditions, the most important determinant of insulin secretion is the blood glucose concentration, although numerous other endocrine, metabolic, or neuronal pathways play physiologic roles in the fine-tuning of insulin secretion. The β cell is exquisitely sensitive to changes in plasma glucose within the physiologic range and can quickly release insulin in response to a rise in glucose. The characteristic dose–response curve is determined by the activity of the enzyme glucokinase (GK), which acts as a 'glucose sensor' to link insulin secretion with the ambient glucose level (**Fig. 19.8**).

The intracellular signaling pathways that allows for stimulus–secretion coupling within the β cell have been extensively studied. Briefly, metabolism of glucose within the β cell generates adenosine triphosphate (ATP) via glycolysis and the Krebs cycle. The rise in ATP or ATP/adenosine diphosphate (ADP) ratio leads to closure of ATP-sensitive potassium channels and depolarization of the β cell. This process opens voltage-mediated calcium channels. The subsequent influx of ionized calcium mediates granule translocation and fusion with the plasma membrane and the exocytosis of insulin into the circulation (**Fig. 19.9**). The actual intracellular signaling pathway mediating insulin secretion is far more complex and may involve signaling via cyclic adenosine monophosphate (cAMP), calcium-dependent regulatory proteins, calmodulin, protein kinase C, inositol triphosphate, diacylglycerol, and arachidonic acid.

INSULIN ACTION

Once released into the circulation, insulin acts on multiple tissues to produce its wide range of effects, which include regulation of glucose, regulation of lipid, and protein metabolism. Insulin's actions at the cellular level can be categorized into three groups based on the time course of their occurrence. The *immediate effect* of insulin occurs within seconds after insulin binding and involves a cascade of covalent modifications (phosphorylation and dephosphorylation) of pre-existing enzymes to lower blood glucose levels. The *intermediate effects* of insulin involve the induction of genes and expression of proteins such as GK and pyruvate kinase, which can be detected within 5–60 minutes but reach a maximum in 3–6 hours after insulin stimulation. The *long-term effects* of insulin in stimulating DNA synthesis, cell proliferation, and cell differentiation require hours to days to be manifest. These rapid, intermediate, and long-term effects of insulin may not share a single common mechanistic pathway but may result from diverging and converging pathways initiated by the insulin receptor (**Figs 19.10, 19.11**).

Insulin receptor

The insulin receptor is a large transmembrane glycoprotein complex whose function is to bind insulin and generate a transmembrane signal to initiate its intracellular actions. Chemically, the receptor consists of two α subunits and two β subunits linked by disulfide bonds to create a β–α–α–β heterotetramer. The α subunit contains the insulin-binding site and is entirely extracellular. The β subunit has an extracellular, transmembrane, and intracellular domain and is responsible for signal transduction through tyrosine kinase activation in its intracellular portion. Thus, insulin binding to the α subunit leads to a conformational change in the receptor that stimulates the kinase activity of the β subunit. The insulin receptor kinase, like other

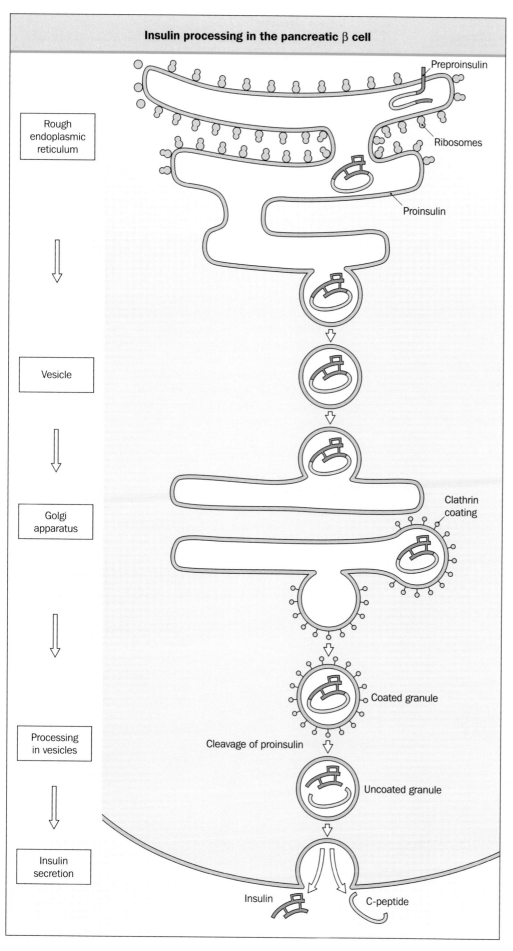

Insulin processing in the pancreatic β cell

Rough endoplasmic reticulum

Vesicle

Golgi apparatus

Processing in vesicles

Insulin secretion

Preproinsulin

Ribosomes

Proinsulin

Clathrin coating

Coated granule

Cleavage of proinsulin

Uncoated granule

Insulin

C-peptide

Figure 19.7 Insulin processing in the pancreatic β cell. Proinsulin is synthesized in the rough endoplasmic reticulum and then processed in the Golgi apparatus and within secretory vesicles to release insulin and C-peptide.

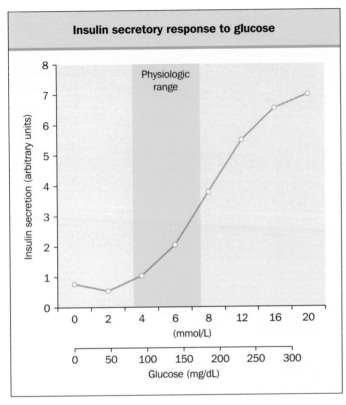

Figure 19.8 Insulin secretory response to glucose. With an increase of plasma glucose levels, the physiologic response of the pancreatic β cell is to increase insulin secretion.

Insulin signaling

At least nine intracellular substrates of the insulin receptor have been identified. These IRS proteins contain between one and 20 tyrosine phosphorylation sites. Once phosphorylated, these sites serve a special function in signal transduction by acting as intracellular 'docking sites' for downstream proteins in the insulin action network (**Fig. 19.11**). Most of these proteins contain specialized regions that recognize the phosphorylated tyrosines called SH2 (Src-homology) domains.

SH2 domain proteins that bind to IRS proteins fall into several categories. Some are adapters, i.e. they relay the signal by additional protein–protein interactions. The best-known examples of adapter proteins that interact with IRSs to propagate insulin receptor signaling are the regulatory subunit of phosphatidylinositol 3-kinase (PI3-kinase) and Grb2. PI3-kinase is a lipid-modifying enzyme that consists of a regulatory subunit (p85) and a catalytic subunit (p110). When the regulatory subunit binds to the phosphorylated IRS proteins, the lipid kinase in the catalytic subunit phosphorylates phosphatidylinositols (found in cellular membrane) on the 3-position to produce PI3-phosphates. PI3-kinase signaling is responsible for most of the metabolic actions of insulin, including antilipolysis, increased glucose transport, activation of glycogen synthase, and stimulation of protein and DNA synthesis. Another well characterized SH2-adapter protein is Grb2, which docks to tyrosine-phosphorylated IRSs and activates the Ras–MAP kinase pathway, which is essential in signaling the mitogenic pathway. Other proteins that bind to IRS proteins include enzymes such as SHP2 (a phosphotyrosine phosphatase) and SERCA1 and 2 (calcium-dependent ATPases).

GLUCOSE UTILIZATION

Insulin acts to lower blood sugar levels by increasing glucose uptake in muscle and fat. An impaired ability of insulin to stimulate glucose uptake is the criterion used clinically to determine the extent of decreased insulin sensitivity in insulin-resistant states such as obesity, impaired glucose tolerance, and type 2 diabetes.

growth factor receptor kinases, catalyzes the transfer of phosphate groups from ATP to tyrosine residues of proteins. The first protein phosphorylated by the insulin receptor is the insulin receptor itself. Thus, autophosphorylation of the receptor β subunit further activates the receptor kinase, allowing it to phosphorylate intracellular insulin receptor substrate (IRS) proteins.

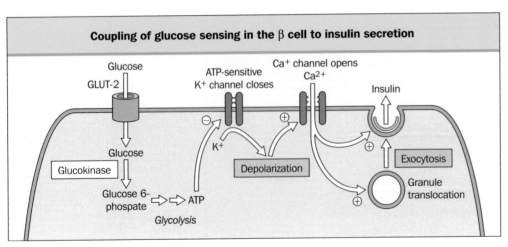

Figure 19.9 Coupling of glucose sensing in the β cell to insulin secretion. Glucose metabolism in the pancreatic β cell results in its depolarization. The subsequent rise in intracellular calcium ions allows for exocytosis of insulin into the bloodstream. ATP, adenosine triphosphate; GLUT2, glucose transporter protein 2.

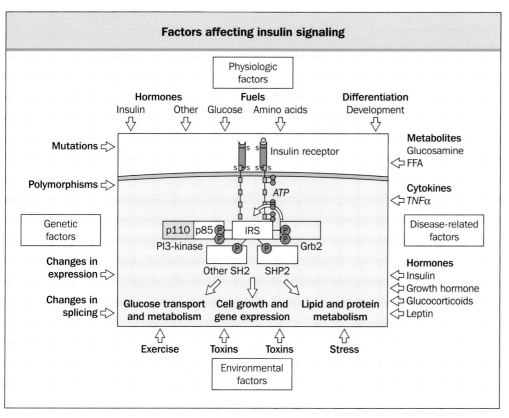

Figure 19.10 Factors affecting insulin signaling. Genetic, physiologic, environmental and disease related factors contribute to alteration in insulin signaling. ATP, adenosine triphosphate; FFA, free fatty acids; IRS, insulin receptor substrate; TNFα, tumor necrosis factor α.

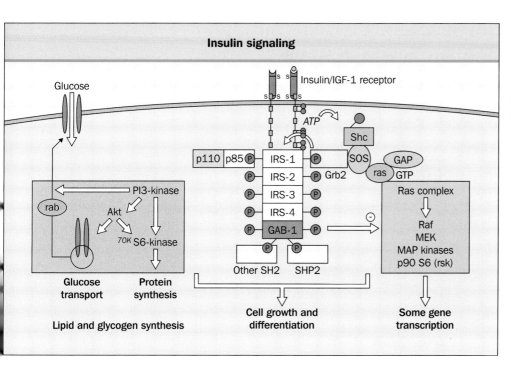

Figure 19.11 Insulin signaling. Diverse pathways of insulin signaling can regulate gene transcription, cell growth, differentiation, and metabolism. ATP, adenosine triphosphate; GTP, guanosine triphosphate; IGF-1, insulin-like growth factor 1; IRS, insulin receptor substrate protein; PI, phosphatidylinositol.

Glucose transport and phosphorylation

Under physiologic conditions, the rate-limiting step of glucose utilization in muscle and fat is glucose transport. Glucose transport is a passive process facilitated by a family of glucose transporter (GLUT) proteins expressed in different tissues (**Table 19.4**). Insulin induces glucose entry into muscle and adipose tissue by stimulating translocation of the insulin-responsive transporter (GLUT-4) from an intracellular pool to the cell membrane (**Fig. 19.12**). This translocation results in an increase in the number of GLUT-4 transporters at the plasma membrane and thus increases glucose uptake by these facilitative transporters across the cell membrane. It has also been suggested that insulin increases the activity of glucose transporters, once translated to the plasma membrane, although this is less clear.

Table 19.4 Family of glucose transporters.

Family of glucose transporters		
Glucose transporter	Tissue	Role
GLUT1	Erythrocytes, endothelium, adipocytes, blood–brain barrier	Widely distributed, mediates basal glucose transport and non-insulin mediated glucose uptake (NIMGU)
GLUT2	Islet β cells, hepatocytes	Low affinity, acts as 'glucose sensor'
GLUT3	Neurons, intestine, heart	Hypoglycemia increases expression in brain
GLUT4	Skeletal muscle, cardiac muscle, adipocytes	Mainly intracellular in basal state, translocated to the plasma membrane in response to insulin or exercise
GLUT5	Skeletal muscle, heart, intestine, adipocyte	Fructose transporter
GLUT7	Hepatocyte endoplasmic reticulum	Final pathway for hepatic glucose production, releasing glucose derived from glucose 6-phosphate into cytosol

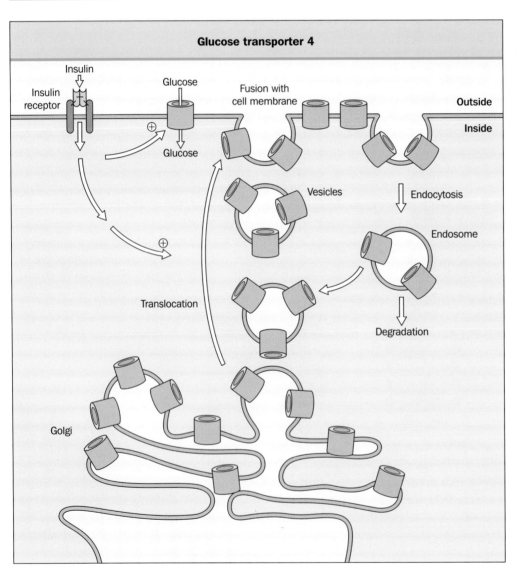

Figure 19.12 Glucose transporter 4. Insulin signaling results in the translocation and fusion of the insulin-responsive glucose transporter (GLUT4) to the plasma membrane, allowing for the increase in facilitative transport of glucose.

In muscles of patients with type 2 diabetes there appears to be a normal amount of GLUT4 protein. This suggests that there is an impairment in the recruitment of GLUT4 to the plasma membrane in response to insulin, leading to the decreased insulin-stimulated glucose uptake characteristic of this condition.

In addition to increasing glucose uptake in muscle and fat, insulin acts to stimulate metabolism and storage of glucose by stimulating glucose oxidation and glycogen synthesis. Thus, despite insulin-induced increase in glucose uptake, insulin acts to maintain low intracellular glucose and glucose 6-phosphate concentrations, allowing for a net influx of glucose along its extracellular-to-intracellular gradient. Insulin, at least at pharmacologic levels, also acts as a vasodilator, which can increase glucose delivery and glucose uptake in skeletal muscle. Similarly, during exercise, increased skeletal muscle blood flow may increase glucose uptake independently of GLUT4 recruitment to the plasma membrane. Since insulin suppresses lipolysis and reduces plasma free fatty acid (FFA) levels, insulin may act indirectly to increase glucose uptake by the glucose–fatty acid cycle (Randle cycle). The glucose–FFA cycle proposes that increased FFA supply and oxidation in the muscle generates acetyl-coenzyme-A, which feeds back to limit key enzymes necessary for glucose oxidation (pyruvate dehydrogenase), glycolysis (phosphofructokinase), and glucose transport (hexokinase). In addition to this metabolic pathway, there is evidence that high FFA levels may directly cause insulin resistance by downregulating key enzymes in the insulin-signaling cascade.

Glucose can also enter the cell through a facilitated diffusion pathway involving another member of the glucose transporter family, GLUT1, which is independent of insulin stimulation (see **Fig. 19.3**). Thus, independent of insulin action, hyperglycemia *per se* increases glucose utilization by a 'mass effect' as long as intracellular glucose is metabolized. This mass effect can compensate for defective glucose clearance in insulin-resistant states. Hyperglycemia-induced increase in glucose uptake is somewhat regulated, however, by at least two other processes. First, hyperglycemia downregulates glucose transporter availability at the plasma membrane, thus limiting excessive glucose uptake by muscle. Secondly, excessive glucose entry into muscle leads to an intracellular accumulation of glucose 6-phosphate, which allosterically inhibits hexokinase, resulting in increased intracellular glucose levels, and decreases the gradient necessary for glucose entry into muscle.

The role of hexokinase in overall glucose utilization by muscle should not be underestimated. Hexokinase II rapidly phosphorylates glucose that has entered the muscle to glucose 6-phosphate for metabolism and storage. Insulin acts to increase the rate of transcription of hexokinase II, thus increasing the level of this enzyme. Decreased expression of hexokinase II is found in patients with type 2 diabetes and may be reversed in part by insulin administration.

The endocrine signals for glucose uptake and metabolism in the liver are more complex. In contrast to muscle and fat, the liver lacks GLUT4 and thus insulin has a minimal effect on stimulating glucose uptake into the liver. However, insulin does facilitate hepatic glucose uptake by activating glycogen synthase and enhances glucose uptake by decreasing intrahepatic glucose 6-phosphate levels. It is only under conditions of increased portal vein glucose delivery (such as after an oral glucose load) that the liver demonstrates a marked increase in glucose uptake. This portal-artery glucose gradient across the liver that signals for hepatic glucose uptake may be mediated by the autonomic nervous system via hepatic afferent nerves that sense portal glucose levels.

The liver and the pancreatic β cell express a unique glucose transporter, GLUT2. GLUT2 is a high-capacity, low-affinity transporter that resides primarily in the plasma membrane and thus does not require insulin for translocation. GLUT2 in the liver and β cell is often expressed in parallel with a specialized form

of hexokinase, GK, and together they may function as a 'glucose sensor' (see **Fig. 19.9**). GK acts in the liver and β cell to phosphorylate glucose to glucose 6-phosphate. In the liver, GK activity is mainly regulated by the changes in the amount of protein rather than phosphorylation. Therefore, acute changes in glucose flux through GLUT2 and GK are regulated by glucose supply rather than changes in enzyme activities. Chronically, on the other hand, insulin promotes GK gene expression to increase glucose phosphorylation and metabolism while counter-regulatory hormones such as glucagon and catecholamines inhibit GK gene expression. In the chronic absence of insulin, such as occurs in diabetes and in liver-specific GK knockout mice, GK level and activity are significantly reduced, resulting in an impaired ability to synthesize glycogen. Mutations in GK have been linked to an uncommon form of type II diabetes, maturity-onset diabetes of the young, demonstrating the importance of glucose phosphorylation and metabolism with glucose sensing in the β cell.

Glycolysis

In the fed state, glycolysis (the metabolic breakdown of glucose) is mediated via increased flux through the key regulatory enzyme 6-phosphofructokinase. The activity of this enzyme is potently activated by the metabolite fructose-2,6-bisphosphate. This metabolite is a key to intracellular signaling production that can switch a cell between modes of gluconeogenesis and glycolysis in the liver. Fructose-2,6-bisphosphate is generated by the phosphorylation of fructose 6-phosphate by the enzyme 6-phosphofructo-2-kinase/fructose 2,6-bisphosphatase. This is a remarkable bidirectional enzyme that acts as a cellular switch. For example, under conditions of feeding and rising insulin levels, it is dephosphorylated, enhancing its kinase activity and resulting in the formation of the fructose-2,6-bisphosphate product. Increased fructose-2,6-bisphosphate levels promote glycolysis and restrict gluconeogenesis by activating 6-phosphofructokinase and suppressing fructose-1,6-bisphosphatase activity, respectively (**Fig. 19.13**). The converse is true during starvation. A rise in glucagon is seen, which acts on the liver, via a cAMP-dependent kinase, to phosphorylate 6-phosphofructo-2-kinase/fructose-2,6-bisphosphatase, enhancing relative phosphatase activity and decreasing fructose-2,6-bisphosphate levels. This limits glycolysis and promotes gluconeogenesis by diminishing 6-phosphofructokinase activity and increasing fructose-1,6-bisphosphatase activity.

Glycogen synthesis

Under conditions of increased glucose uptake into muscle, the insulin-induced increase in glycogen synthesis is quantitatively more important than the increase in glucose oxidation. Thus with increasing levels of insulin, the increased glucose entry into muscle is preferentially shunted toward glucose storage. Glycogen synthesis in the liver after a meal occurs via an indirect pathway, since glycogen is derived not directly from glucose but rather by three carbon precursors. When muscle glycogen is fully replete, glucose entry will be diverted through glycolysis to lactate and three carbon gluconeogenic precursors, which are used to restore glycogen stores in the liver.

The rate-limiting step in the formation of glycogen is the coordinated stimulation of glycogen synthase activity and decreases in phosphorylase activity that allows for net glycogen formation

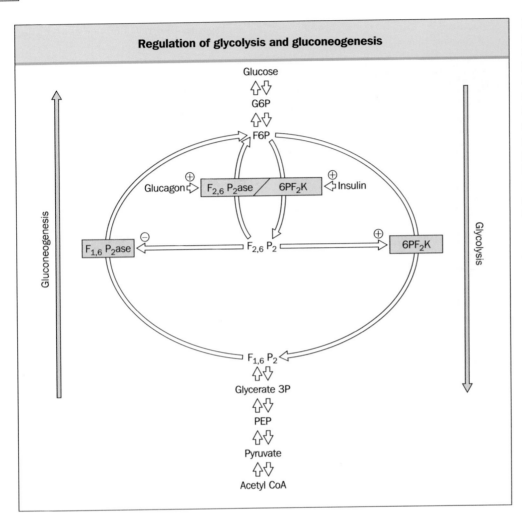

Regulation of glycolysis and gluconeogenesis

Figure 19.13 Regulation of glycolysis and gluconeogenesis. Depending on feeding or fasting, the liver switches between glycolysis and gluconeogenesis. One primary metabolic switch relies on the metabolite fructose-2,6-bisphosphate ($F_{2,6}P_2$). Under conditions of feeding and rising insulin levels, 6-phosphofructo-2-kinase ($6PF_2K$) phosphorylates fructose-6-phosphate to increase $F_{2,6}P_2$. An increase in $F_{2,6}P_2$ promotes glycolysis and restricts gluconeogenesis by activating 6-PFK and suppressing fructose-1,6-bisphosphatase activity, respectively. It is interesting that the converse is true during starvation. During starvation, a rise in glucagon acts to phosphorylate $6PF_2K/F_{2,6}P_2$, enhancing its relative phosphatase activity and decreasing $F_{2,6}P_2$ levels to limit glycolysis and promote gluconeogenesis.

(Fig. 19.14). Insulin signaling through phosphatidylinositol 3-kinase results in the activation of an enzyme called AKT, which in turn inactivates glycogen synthase kinase-3. An insulin-induced decrease in glycogen synthase kinase-3 activity results in an increase in glycogen synthase phosphatase activity, which results in a net dephosphorylation (activation) of glycogen synthase to promote glycogen synthesis. A defect in insulin-induced glycogen synthesis is a hallmark of insulin-resistant states, including type 2 diabetes mellitus. Although the gene for glycogen synthase has been proposed as a 'diabetogene', analysis of the coding regions of glycogen synthase in type 2 diabetes mellitus has yielded negative results to date. Defects in insulin stimulation of glycogen synthase in insulin-resistant states are therefore probably caused by defects in insulin signaling.

GLUCOSE PRODUCTION

Glucose production is the sum processes of glycogen breakdown (glycogenolysis) and new glucose formation (gluconeogenesis) from amino acids, lactate, pyruvate, and glycerol. As noted above, in the fasted state, the liver is primarily responsible for the maintenance of normal blood glucose levels. This unique role is due to the presence of the enzyme complex glucose-6-phosphatase (not present in muscle or fat), which dephosphorylates glucose 6-phosphate to glucose for release into the circulation. The kidney also possesses glucose-6-phosphatase and may contribute 5–10% of glucose production after an overnight fast, or more during prolonged periods of starvation or insulin deficiency.

In the fed state, elevated insulin levels suppress endogenous hepatic glucose production. Therefore, the physiologic rise in blood glucose after a carbohydrate-containing meal results from an increased rate of glucose appearance in the plasma from the splanchnic bed exceeding glucose disposal in both insulin-dependent and insulin-independent tissues.

In the postabsorptive state, as gut-derived carbohydrates decrease, blood glucose levels are maintained within the normal range by an increase in hepatic glucose production. This increased hepatic glucose production occurs via two mechanisms. In the early postabsorptive period (3–6 hours after glucose ingestion), glucose production from the liver is primarily determined by glycogenolysis (see **Fig. 19.2**). After an overnight fast, as liver glycogen stores are used up, hepatic glucose production rates are maintained because the rate of gluconeogenesis increases and begins to replace glycogenolysis as the major provider of glucose. In patients with type 2 diabetes, increased rates of gluconeogenesis lead to elevated rates of hepatic glucose production, resulting in the fasting hyperglycemia that is diagnostic of this condition.

Glycogenolysis

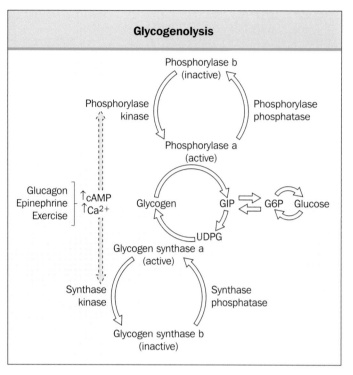

Figure 19.14 Glycogenolysis. Glucagon, epinephrine (adrenaline), and exercise signal for an intracellular signal cascade resulting in net glycogen breakdown. This pathway involves the activation of phosphorylase kinase and then glycogen phosphorylase, while also acting on glycogen synthase kinase to inhibit glycogen synthase a. Glycogen breakdown is the coordinated effects of activation (phosphorylation) of glycogen phosphorylase and inactivation (phosphorylation) of glycogen synthase. G1P, glucose 1-phosphate; G6P, glucose 6-phosphate; UDPG, uridinediphosphoglucose.

Glycogenolysis

Net glycogen breakdown occurs in the early postabsorptive period or under conditions of stress, when counter-regulatory hormones are activated. The neurohormonal stimulation of hepatic glycogenolysis is primarily mediated by glucagon, epinephrine (adrenaline), and norepinephrine (noradrenaline) while it is inhibited by insulin. In muscle, glycogenolysis is also stimulated by mechanical contraction. These counter-regulatory hormones and signals trigger an intracellular signal cascade that results in net glycogen breakdown to glucose for metabolism. The final reaction in glycogen breakdown is the activation (phosphorylation) of glycogen phosphorylase and the inactivation (phosphorylation) of glycogen synthase (**Fig. 19.14**). Briefly, when glucagon binds to its receptor it activates G proteins, stimulating the formation of cAMP under the influence of adenylate cyclase. An increase in cAMP activates the cAMP-dependent protein kinase phosphorylation cascade. The net result of this kinase pathway is the activation of phosphorylase kinase and then glycogen phosphorylase while also inhibiting glycogen synthase a (**Fig. 19.14**). The resulting activation of glycogenolysis and simultaneous inhibition of glycogen synthesis results in the net degradation of glycogen.

The situation is more complex than illustrated because glycogen synthase can be phosphorylated at more than nine sites and at least 10 protein kinases may be involved. Another mechanism by which glycogen phosphorylase is activated is by an increase in intracellular calcium ions, such as occurs during exercise. Increased ionized calcium binds to calmodulin, which activates phosphorylase b kinase. Epinephrine can also raise intracellular calcium levels via activation of phospholipase C to generate inositol triphosphate, which liberates intracellular calcium stores to activate phosphorylase kinase.

The cascade signal, although complex, has the advantage of signal amplification and allows for influence of opposing enzymes in related pathways. For example, insulin signaling through phosphatidyl inositol 3-kinase affects downstream targets, PDK-1, PKB/Akt, GSK-3. Additionally, insulin signaling activates glycogen-associated protein phosphatase-1 (PP-1), which dephosphorylates three key enzymes (glycogen synthase, phosphorylase kinase, and glycogen phosphorylase,) all resulting in net glycogen storage. In such a manner, insulin action promotes glycogen formation and therefore antagonizes the effects of glucagon and the catecholamines.

Gluconeogenesis

Gluconeogenesis contributes between 30% and 70% of hepatic glucose production after overnight fast. Hepatic gluconeogenesis involves glucose formation from pyruvate using many of the same enzymes involved in glycolytic pathway. The key regulatory sites are unique enzymes that catalyze reactions and determine the direction of carbon flux. The key enzymes committed to gluconeogenesis are phosphoenol pyruvate carboxykinase, fructose 1,6-bisphosphatase, and glucose-6-phosphatase. Under conditions of insulin deficiency/resistance and glucagon excess, such as occurs in type 1 and type 2 diabetes, increased expression and activity of these enzymes, and increased carbon fluxes, contribute to increased rates of gluconeogenesis, hepatic glucose production, and hyperglycemia.

There are several sources for the carbons needed to generate new glucose. Lactate (from muscle, red blood cells, and other tissues) comprises 50% of the substrate for hepatic gluconeogenesis. Lactate generated as the product of glycolysis is released by muscle and converted into glycogen in the liver via the Cori cycle (see **Fig. 19.4**). The primary amino acids used for gluconeogenesis are alanine and glutamine. In a similar fashion, during starvation or insulin deficiency there is an increased release of alanine into the circulation that serves as substrate for hepatic gluconeogenesis. Finally, lipolysis of triacylglycerol from adipocyte stores releases glycerol into the plasma that serves as triose phosphates for hepatic gluconeogenesis.

Regulation of hepatic glucose production

Insulin acts to suppress glucose production both via direct mechanisms (e.g. action on hepatocyte) and indirect mechanisms (e.g. through metabolic actions in peripheral tissues such as muscle, fat, pancreas, etc.; **Fig. 19.15**).

Evidence for direct hepatic actions of insulin came from many *in vitro* studies on perfused livers or isolated hepatocytes, which have shown that insulin acts directly on the hepatocyte to change hepatic enzyme activities through effects following insulin binding to its cell surface receptor. Insulin has been shown to exert its inhibitory effects on gluconeogenic and glycogenolytic enzymes via a rapid cascade of covalent modification (i.e. phosphorylation

Direct and indirect effects of insulin to suppress glucose production

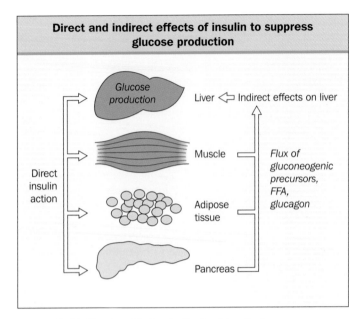

Figure 19.15 Direct and indirect effects of insulin to suppress glucose production. In addition to direct actions of insulin on the liver, insulin suppresses the flux of gluconeogenic precursors (alanine, pyruvate, lactate, glycerol) and energy substrates (free fatty acids, FFA), and suppresses glucagon secretion from the pancreatic α cell. These extrahepatic actions of insulin constitute an indirect mechanism by which insulin suppresses glucose released from the liver.

Regulation of hepatic glucose output

	Stimulatory	Inhibitory
Neuroendocrine	Glucagon	Insulin
	Epinephrine (adrenaline)	
	Norepinephrine (noradrenaline)	
	Cortisol	
	Growth hormone	
Substrates	Hypoglycemia	Hyperglycemia
		↓ Gluconeogenic substrates
		↓ Free fatty acids

Table 19.5 Regulation of hepatic glucose output.

dinucleotide (NADH) and acetyl-CoA, which promote gluconeogenesis. Thus insulin's effect to restrict FFA supply to the liver may limit gluconeogenesis.

Since up to 75% of glucose production is regulated by glucagon under basal conditions, even small changes in glucagon levels may play a significant role in regulating glucose production. Some of insulin's action to indirectly reduce glucose production may be mediated through the suppression of glucagon secretion from the pancreatic α cell (**Table 19.5**).

EXERCISE

During moderate exercise, at intensities of 50–80% of $\dot{V}_{O_{2max}}$, blood sugar levels are maintained in the normal range by a complex neurohormonal and substrate regulation. There is an increase in glucose utilization during exercise. Muscle contraction results in a translocation of glucose transporter (GLUT4) to the plasma membrane of the muscle, to facilitate glucose uptake. Although insulin induces GLUT4, translocation via its intracellular signaling cascade involves activation of phosphatidylinositol 3-kinase; these pathways are not activated by muscle contraction. The exact mechanism of exercise-induced translocation of GLUT4 to the plasma membrane to increase glucose utilization is not known; there has been recent evidence that a 5´ adenosine monophosphate (AMP)-activated protein kinase (AMPK) may be involved.

The increased glucose utilization during exercise is precisely matched by increased hepatic glucose production. During exercise there is a fall in insulin and rise in glucagon levels, which act on the liver to increase glycogenolysis and gluconeogenesis. Initially, glycogenolysis provides the glucose necessary to keep blood sugar levels within the normal range but, during prolonged exercise, gluconeogenesis predominates. During low- to moderate-intensity exercise, fatty acid oxidation is the primary fuel for the exercising muscle. The fall in insulin levels allows for an increased rate of lipolysis releasing free fatty acids from adipocyte stores into the circulation to be taken up by the muscle. The intracellular metabolism of glucose can vary markedly between the liver and muscle during exercise. In the muscle there is increased glycolysis and glucose oxidation to provide the necessary ATP for contraction. In contrast, glycolysis and oxidation in the liver is reduced because most of the substrate flux is towards gluconeogenesis.

and dephosphorylation) of pre-existing enzymes. In this manner, insulin acts to activate certain enzymes (i.e. pyruvate dehydrogenase, acetyl CoA carboxylase, and glycogen synthase) and inactivates other enzymes (i.e. glycogen phosphorylase and phosphorylase kinase). As suggested above, insulin also acts in a slower fashion by regulating gene expression of gluconeogenic and glycogenolytic enzymes via stimulation of gene transcription (i.e. pyruvate kinase, GK, and 6-phosphofructo-2-kinase/fructose-2,6-bisphosphatase) or inhibition of gene transcription (i.e. phosphoenolpyruvate carboxykinase and fructose 1,6-bisphosphatase).

Insulin may also act indirectly in suppressing glucose production *in vivo* through actions on extrahepatic tissues. Because supraphysiologic insulin concentrations are needed to directly suppress glucose production with *in vitro* studies of perfused livers or hepatocytes, it is thought that, *in vivo*, the liver may not be directly responsive to physiologic insulin concentrations and therefore indirect actions of insulin in regulating glucose production may be important.

One way by which insulin may be indirectly inhibitory is by limiting gluconeogenic precursor supply to the liver. By decreasing protein catabolism and increasing amino acid uptake in muscle and promoting intracellular glucose oxidation and glycogenesis, insulin acts peripherally to decrease gluconeogenic substrate supply (i.e. alanine, pyruvate, lactate) to the liver. Insulin also inhibits lipolysis and stimulates FFA uptake and re-esterification, thus reducing plasma FFA and glycerol concentrations. Although the carbons from FFA oxidation in the hepatocytes are not directly incorporated into glucose during gluconeogenesis, FFA oxidation provides energy in the form of nicotinamide adenine

During intense exercise (85–100% $\dot{V}O_{2max}$), blood sugars actually rise. At this higher intensity, the high release of catecholamines markedly augments glycogenolysis resulting in up to 10-fold increase in hepatic glucose production. During this period, when hepatic glucose production exceeds glucose utilization, there is an increase in blood glucose levels but these promptly return to normal in the postexercise period.

Long-term exercise training enhances insulin sensitivity and glucose disposal. Training is associated with increased insulin binding to muscle and increased insulin receptor and GLUT4 glucose transporter content in muscle, suggesting that exercise can increase insulin sensitivity at receptor and postreceptor levels.

PHARMACOLOGIC THERAPY FOR DIABETES

When diet and exercise fail to control glycemia in patients with type 2 diabetes, pharmacologic therapy is usually initiated. Oral hypoglycemic agents, insulin, or a combination of these may be employed. Oral agents include the insulin secretogogues, metformin, an α-glucosidase inhibitor, and the thiazolidinediones.

Sulfonylureas have represented the key class of agents for the treatment of type 2 diabetes for the past 50 years. Sulfonylureas increase β-cell sensitivity to glucose by closing ATP-sensitive potassium channels and depolarizing the cell membrane. The resultant influx of calcium stimulates insulin secretion. Nonsulfonyurea insulin secretogogues in the meglitinide class (repaglinide and nateglinide) bind to a different site on β-cell ATP-sensitive potassium channels. These agents are rapidly absorbed and enhance insulin secretion within 30–60 minutes, and therefore act quicker than the sulfonylureas. Major clinical problems with these insulin secretagogue agents include the loss of effectiveness over time, weight gain, and hypoglycemia.

The biguanide metformin can reduce plasma glucose concentrations by 25%. Despite over 25 years of use, its exact mechanism of action is unclear although may be related to AMP-kinase avtivation. In patients with type 2 diabetes, metformin acts primarily on the liver by inhibiting gluconeogenesis and decreasing hepatic glucose production. Some studies suggest that metformin may also augment peripheral glucose disposal, but this effect appears to be minor. The major adverse effects of metformin are gastrointestinal discomfort and the risk of lactic acidosis.

The thiazolidinediones represent a new class of antihyperglycemic agents that directly decrease insulin resistance and enhance insulin action in skeletal muscle, liver, and adipose tissue. Thiazolidinediones interact with nuclear receptors called peroxisome proliferator activated receptor-gamma (PPAR-γ) to effect transcription of genes that mediate insulin sensitivity. Receptors for PPAR-γ are expressed mainly in fat, suggesting this as the primary site of their action. Hepatotoxicity is a rare side effect, but more common side effects include back pain, fatigue, headache, high blood sugar, respiratory tract infections, sinus inflammation, and swelling.

The antihyperglycemic effects of the α-glucosidase inhibitor acarbose are based on its ability to delay carbohydrate digestion. This delayed absorption significantly decreases the postprandial rise in plasma glucose after a mixed carbohydrate load. In some individuals, acarbose can decrease glycated hemoglobin (HbA_{1c}) by 1–2%, especially those with large postprandial glucose excursions. The major side effects include flatulence and diarrhea related to carbohydrate malabsorption but low starting doses and slow titration minimize these effects.

Since these oral hypoglycemic agents have different mechanisms of action and work at different tissue sites, combination therapy of two or more agents has been advocated when monotherapy fails to control hyperglycemia (**Fig. 19.16**). Additionally, oral hypoglycemic agents have been used in combination with insulin therapy because, with better glucose control, these agents have an insulin-sparing effect.

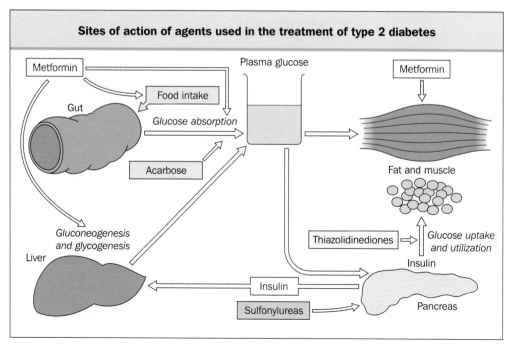

Figure 19.16 Sites of action of agents used in the treatment of type 2 diabetes.

FURTHER READING

Bonner-Weir S. Anatomy of the islet of Langerhans. In: Samols E, ed. The endocrine pancreas. New York:Raven Press; 1991:15–27.

Cherrington AD. Control of glucose uptake and release by the liver in vivo. Banting Lecture 1997. Diabetes 1999;48:1198–214.

Hattersley AT, Turner RC, Permutt MA, et al. Linkage of type 2 diabetes to the glucokinase gene. Lancet 1992;340:54–5.

Kahn CR. Insulin signaling and the molecular mechanisms of insulin resistance. In: Imura H, Kasuga M, Nakao K, ed. Common diseases – genetic and pathogenetic aspects of multifactorial diseases. Uehara Memorial Foundation Symposium 1999. New York:Elsevier; 1999:61–77.

Orci L, Ravazzola M, Storch MJ, Anderson RG, Vassalli JD, Perelet A. Proteolytic maturation of insulin is a post-Golgi event which occurs in acidifying clathrin-coated secretory vesicles. Cell 1987;49:865–8.

Pessin JE, Saltiel AR. Signaling pathways in insulin action: molecular targets of insulin resistance. J Clin Invest. 2000;106:165–9.

Rossetti L, Giaccari A, DeFronzo RA. Glucose toxicity. Diabetes Care 1990;13:620–30.

Rothman DL, Magnusson I, Katz LD, Shulman RG, Shulman GI. Quantification of hepatic glycogenolysis and gluconeogenesis in fasting humans with 13C NMR. Science 1991;254:573–6.

Shepherd PR, Kahn BB. Glucose transporters and insulin action – implications for insulin resistance and diabetes mellitus. N Engl J Med. 1999;341:240–6.

Summers SA, Yin VP, Whiteman EL, et al. Signaling pathways mediating insulin-stimulated glucose transport. Ann NY Acad Sci. 1999;892:169–86.

Taylor SI, Accili D, Imai Y. Insulin resistance or insulin deficiency: which is the primary cause of NIDDM? Diabetes 1994;43:735–40.

Vranic M. Banting Lecture: glucose turnover. A key to the understanding the pathogenesis of diabetes (indirect effects of insulin). Diabetes 1992;41:1188–206.

Yki-Jarviven H. Pathogenesis of non-insulin-dependent diabetes mellitus. Lancet 1994;343:91–5.

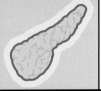

Chapter	Hypoglycemia and Insulinomas
20	Robert F Gagel

INTRODUCTION

Glucose provides an important energy source for normal cellular physiology and is particularly important for neurons within the central and peripheral nervous system. To maintain the serum glucose concentration within the optimal and narrow physiologic range, the human species has evolved a number of sophisticated regulatory mechanisms. Particularly important for this chapter are those that function to prevent hypoglycemia, a low and nonphysiologic plasma glucose concentration that, if allowed to persist, will lead to reduced cellular function, damage, and death. Neurons are particularly sensitive to hypoglycemia, because they cannot utilize short-chain fatty acids as an energy source. To prevent hypoglycemia and neuronal dysfunction, any fall in the plasma glucose concentration below the normal results in prompt activation of several counterregulatory mechanisms designed to increase glucose production (**Fig. 20.1**). Hypoglycemia associated with treatment of diabetes mellitus (iatrogenic hypoglycemia) will not be discussed in this chapter.

CAUSES

To understand these counterregulatory mechanisms, it is useful to briefly review the physiologic events that occur during the fed and fasting state. In a simple model, energy requirements and glucose availability could be provided by a continuous ingestion of food. However, during evolution food was inconstant, resulting in the need for development of nutrient storage and retrieval mechanisms. Thus during the fed state, nutrients are processed to produce a storage pool of fat, protein, and glycogen to be used during periods of prolonged fasting. The transition between the fed and fasting state begins 4–6 hours following a meal and, in contemporary societies where multiple meals are consumed, the only significant period of fasting occurs during sleep.

During the transition from fed to fasting, certain regulatory processes are activated. These include mobilization of hepatic glycogen stores and synthesis of glucose from lactate/pyruvate, amino acids, and glycerol. Enzymatic cleavage of glycogen provides most of the glucose during the first 10 hours of fasting. As

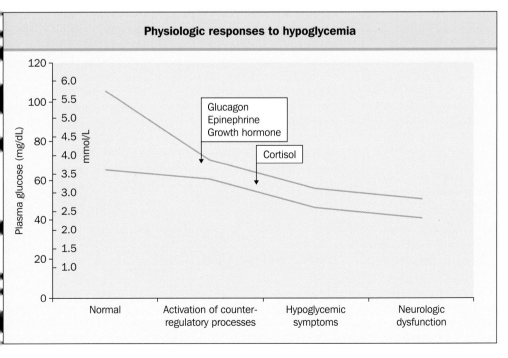

Figure 20.1 Physiologic responses to hypoglycemia. As the plasma glucose falls glucagon, epinephrine (adrenaline), growth hormone, and cortisol are released. A further reduction in the plasma glucose concentration leads to hypoglycemic symptoms and neurologic dysfunction.

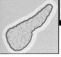

Processes that contribute to gluconeogenesis and whose perturbation may cause hypoglycemia	
Production and enzymatic cleavage of glycogen	
Gluconeogenesis	
Hydrolysis of triglycerides to long chain fatty acid and glycerol	
Adequate storage pools of glycogen, protein, and fat	
Hormonal processes that regulate gluconeogenesis	Insulin
	Glucagon
	Catecholamines (epinephrine and norepinephrine)
	Growth hormone
	Cortisol

Table 20.1 Processes that contribute to gluconeogenesis and whose perturbation may cause hypoglycemia.

glycogen stores become depleted, gluconeogenesis (synthesis of glucose from precursor substances) becomes the main source of glucose production and will continue as long as substrate is available. Gluconeogenesis occurs predominantly in the liver, but other organs such as the kidney also contribute to this process. Continuation of the fasting or hypoglycemic state will eventually lead to hydrolysis of triglycerides and production of fatty acids and glycerol. Fatty acids are converted to acetoacetic acid and β-hydroxybutyric acid, energy substrates for both neurons and peripheral tissues; glycerol is converted to glucose.

The hormonal cues for initiation of these counterregulatory processes include a lowering of the plasma insulin concentration and an increase in the plasma concentrations of epinephrine (adrenaline), growth hormone, glucagon, and cortisol. It is difficult to identify one of these as the most important; all contribute to the increased hepatic and renal glucose production and lipolysis that reverse hypoglycemia. Most importantly for the clinician seeking a cause of hypoglycemia, perturbation of glucose production caused either by a primary defect in gluconeogenesis, its hormonal regulation, or pharmacologic effects on these processes is an important cause of hypoglycemia during the fasting period (**Table 20.1**).

The other broad mechanism for causing hypoglycemia is to increase glucose uptake by cells, thereby reducing plasma glucose. This is a process that is directly controlled by insulin. There are a variety of mechanisms for enhancing glucose uptake that will be discussed in this chapter. In most cases the development of hypoglycemia is a combination of decreased glucogenesis and increased cellular uptake of glucose.

CLINICAL MANIFESTATIONS

The initial manifestations of hypoglycemia include increased tremulousness, palpitations, hypertension, anxiety, sweating, and hunger, most of which are caused by increased epinephrine release from the adrenal medulla (**Fig. 20.1**). In most individuals, prompt intake of glucose or carbohydrate will lead to an immediate reversal of these symptoms. Indeed, the clinical separation of hypoglycemia from anxiety disorders or symptoms caused by other disorders such as pheochromocytoma (which may present with similar symptoms) is the reversal of the process following ingestion of carbohydrate. If the hypoglycemic symptoms are not addressed by food intake, there is the possibility of progression to neuroglycopenic symptoms, so

named because they result from disordered neuronal function caused by glucose deficiency. These symptoms can include disordered mentation and confusion, drowsiness, dizziness, visual effects such as blurring or spots, and dysarthria (**Fig. 20.1**). In the absence of food intake or a reversal of the hypoglycemia by counterregulatory mechanisms, this condition can progress to loss of consciousness, other neurologic manifestations including a 'stroke-like' clinical syndrome, seizures, and death. Hypoglycemia should be considered in the differential diagnosis of any neurologic syndrome of acute onset; treatment with intravenous glucose will generally result in prompt reversal of the neurologic deficit.

In the evaluation of a patient for hypoglycemia it is important to keep in mind that hypoglycemia is a clinical syndrome characterized by a low plasma glucose concentration, the appropriate clinical features outlined in the paragraphs above, and reversal of symptoms when glucose is administered (Whipple's triad). Hypoglycemia is generally defined as a plasma glucose concentration lower than 55mg/dL (3mmol/L) but multiple studies document the fact that normal human subjects may routinely have glucose values between 50 and 60mg/dL (2.8–3.4mmol/L) without symptomatology. Thus a patient with a plasma glucose of 55mg/dL (3mmol/L,) who presents with vague and nonreproducible symptoms not relieved by glucose administration is more likely to have an anxiety disorder than true hypoglycemia. This patient will probably benefit from appropriate anxiolytic therapy more than from evaluation or treatment for hypoglycemia. It is also important to be aware that the ambient glucose concentration can impact on the level of symptomatology. For example, diabetics with poor control may develop hypoglycemic symptoms at glucose concentrations considered normal or even elevated. Similarly, repetitive periods of hypoglycemia, such as are seen in patients with insulin-secreting islet cell tumors, may lead to a condition of 'unawareness' of hypoglycemia.

DIFFERENTIAL DIAGNOSIS

Hypoglycemic disorders are most commonly separated into those that occur during the immediate *postprandial* period and those associated with *fasting*. Not only is there a physiologic basis for the separation into these two categories but the history provided by the patient and the diagnostic evaluation of an individual patient follow directly from this categorization. It is therefore important to take a careful history noting the relationship of symptomatology to meals. If this history cannot be provided, it is important to request the patient to keep a diary for a week or two to document any relationship of symptoms to meals. During the initial categorization the clinician should also consider the diagnosis of artifactual hypoglycemia, a laboratory artifact most commonly caused by delayed separation of blood cells from plasma or in conditions such as leukemia or polycythemia where cellular glucose utilization is increased.

Postprandial hypoglycemia

Development of symptoms suggestive of hypoglycemia following ingestion of food is perhaps the most common reason for hypoglycemic referral. In these patients there should be a reproducible history of hypoglycemic symptoms within 1–5 hours following ingestion of a meal. Patients with documented hypoglycemia fit into several different types: those who have an exaggerated release of insulin caused by rapid gastric emptying; those who develop early hypoglycemia with apparent normal gastric emptying; children with leucine sensitivity, fructose intolerance, or galactosemia; and those who have a delayed onset of hypoglycemia, most commonly associated with early diabetes mellitus (**Table 20.2**). Rarely, patients with insulinoma will develop postprandial hypoglycemia.

Hypoglycemia caused by rapid gastric emptying occurs in patients who have had prior gastric surgery (gastrectomy, pyloroplasty with vagotomy, or gastrojejunostomy). Rapid glucose absorption stimulates an exaggerated release of insulin, causing hypoglycemia, either directly or through glucagon-like peptide release.

Individuals who develop hypoglycemia with normal gastric emptying are the most difficult to categorize. These individuals are frequently thin, young, and somewhat anxious patients who develop hypoglycemic symptoms within 1–2 hours after food ingestion. In general there is no evidence for an exaggerated release of insulin. Several different mechanisms have been invoked in an attempt to explain this clinical syndrome, including inappropriate secretion of the insulin secretagogue glucagon-like peptide-1, exaggerated insulin release caused by heightened autonomic nervous activity, or functional early gastric emptying. None of these explanations is completely satisfactory. Fortunately, symptomatology rarely persists long-term in these individuals and the symptoms are generally responsive to reassurance that there is no serious problem and smaller, more frequent meals.

Hypoglycemia associated with early-onset type 2 diabetes mellitus is characterized by the onset of delayed postprandial hypoglycemia, most commonly 3–4 hours following food ingestion. The apparent cause in these patients is a delay of insulin secretion. The peak plasma insulin concentration occurs as the plasma glucose is falling, driving the glucose concentration below normal.

Fasting hypoglycemia

The least frequent but most challenging causes of hypoglycemia occur during the fasting period, most commonly more than 6 hours following food ingestion. These are categorized as: clinical conditions associated with decreased production or increased utilization of glucose (**Table 20.3**). In the evaluation of fasting hypoglycemia, the clinical context becomes important. For example, in hospitalized ill patients with no prior history of

Causes of postprandial hypoglycemia	
Accelerated gastric emptying causing hyperinsulinism	Most commonly associated with prior gastrointestinal surgery
Idiopathic	Thin, anxious patients
	Generally no identifiable abnormality of insulin secretion
Leucine sensitivity	
Hereditary fructose intolerance	
Galactosemia	
Early diabetes mellitus (Type 2)	
Insulinoma	

Table 20.2 Causes of postprandial hypoglycemia.

hypoglycemia, the search for a cause will revolve around acute medical or pharmacologic events causing decreased production or increased utilization of glucose. In contrast, in adult patients in the outpatient setting, pharmacologic causes, endocrine deficiency or excess, or neoplastic disorders become more likely. In the newborn period or early childhood, genetic causes of hypoglycemia should be considered.

Decreased glucose production

Alcohol may cause hypoglycemia in adult patients by inhibition of gluconeogenesis, an effect mediated by acetaldehyde inhibition of nicotinamide–adenine dinucleotide production, resulting in decreased entry of glucose precursors into the gluconeogenic pathway. In adults, alcohol alone is insufficient for hypoglycemia. It must be combined with a period of fasting that is long enough to deplete hepatic glycogen stores (usually during an alcoholic binge period, when caloric intake is diminished or absent). Children are much more susceptible to the effects of alcohol. In one report approximately 3% of children who accidentally ingested alcohol were found to have symptomatic hypoglycemia. Alcohol may also inhibit growth hormone, cortisol, and catecholamine responses to hypoglycemia and there is some evidence that these effects may be more important in childhood.

Beta-adrenergic antagonists can cause hypoglycemia, particularly in diabetic patients. The presumed mechanism is inhibition of the epinephrine-mediated response to hypoglycemia. Salicylates in large doses (>4g/day) can cause hypoglycemia in pediatric patients by unknown mechanisms.

Renal and hepatic disorders may be associated with decreased gluconeogenesis. In general, symptomatic hypoglycemia is observed only in patients with extensive hepatic or renal disease when combined with poor nutritional status. Extensive hepatic metastasis may also reduce glycogen storage and gluconeogenesis.

Several types of infectious process cause hypoglycemia. Sepsis-associated hypoglycemia appears to be caused by a combination of decreased hepatic and renal glucose production combined with increased glucose utilization. The mechanism of hypoglycemia in sepsis is unclear, although there is evidence that cytokines inhibit gluconeogenesis and stimulate insulin release from the β cell. Hypoglycemia may also be seen in malaria, an effect thought to be related to the combined effect of quinine on insulin release and the aforementioned effects of sepsis on glucose metabolism.

Causes of fasting hypoglycemia			
Decreased glucose production	Drug-induced	Alcohol	
		β-adrenergic antagonists	
		Salicylates	
	↓ Hepatic glucose synthesis	Hepatocellular disease	
		Uremia	
		Replacement of the liver by metastatic tumor	
	↓ Renal glucose synthesis	Uremia	
		Decreased renal mass in chronic renal failure	
	Hormonal deficiency	Pituitary insufficiency leading to growth hormone or cortisol deficiency	
		Glucagon deficiency	
		Addison's disease	
		Epinephrine	
	Genetic causes	Glycogen synthetase	
		Glucose-6-phosphatase	
		Liver phosphorylase	
		Pyruvate carboxylase	
		Phosphoenolpyruvate carboxykinase	
		Fructose-1,6-bisphosphatase	
Increased glucose utilization	Drugs	Pentamidine	
		Quinine	
		Sulfonylureas	
		Exogenous insulin administration	
	Genetic disorders	Recessive forms	Inactivating mutations of the sulfonylurea receptor or $K_{IR}6.2$
		Dominant forms	Mutations of glutamate dehydrogenase
			Other forms of leucine-induced hypoglycemia
			Glucokinase (Val455Met) mutation
	Neoplastic disorders	Insulin-producing tumors	
		IGF-2-producing tumors	
		Other tumors	
	Autoimmune	Insulin antibodies	
		Insulin receptor antibodies	

Table 20.3 Causes of fasting hypoglycemia. IGF, insulin-like growth factor.

An important component of the counterregulatory pathway is hormonal activation of gluconeogenesis (**Fig. 20.1**). Deficiency of cortisol, growth hormone, catecholamines, or glucagon can cause or contribute to the development of hypoglycemia. However, more commonly single hormone deficiency produces hypoglycemia only when combined with another cause of hypoglycemia. For example, insulin-dependent diabetic patients with diminished growth hormone, cortisol, or glucagon release or those with autonomic neuropathy (leading to decreased catecholamine release) frequently mount an insufficient gluconeogenic or glycogenolytic response to hypoglycemia. The clinical conditions of Addison's disease and hypopituitarism may have hypoglycemia as a presenting complaint, although these patients do not generally develop hypoglycemia until they are chronically ill with muscle wasting and poor nutritional status.

There are several genetic causes of hypoglycemia caused by decreased glucose production, which are listed in **Table 20.3**.

Increased glucose utilization

Pharmacologic agents that cause hypoglycemia by increasing glucose utilization mediate their effects by increasing the plasma concentrations of insulin. The most common cause is hypoglycemia associated with insulin use for treatment of diabetes mellitus. Sulfonylureas, which stimulate insulin release, are another common cause of hypoglycemia. Surreptitious use of insulin or sulfonylureas is uncommon but should always be considered in the differential diagnosis of fasting hypoglycemia. Pentamidine, a drug used to treat *Pneumocystis carinii* pneumonia, is toxic to the β cell, resulting in degranulation and insulin release. In 10–15% of cases the toxicity to the β cell is great enough for the initial hypoglycemia to be followed by diabetes mellitus. Quinine, used in the treatment of malaria, may contribute to the hypoglycemia associated with malaria by stimulation of insulin release.

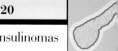

The SUR/K$_{IR}$6.2 functions as a K–ATP channel

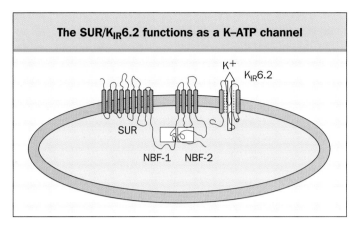

Figure 20.2 The SUR/K$_{IR}$6.2 functions as a K–ATP channel. The inward potassium rectifier K$_{IR}$6.2 complexes with the sulfonylurea receptor (SUR), a member of the ABC transporter family, to form an adenosine triphosphate (ATP)-sensitive K$^+$ channel. Activity of this channel is modified by binding of sulfonylureas to the SUR (closes the channel) or diazoxide (opens the channel). Inactivating mutations of *SUR* or *K$_{IR}$6.2* result in closure of the channel and K$^+$-mediated depolarization the cell, leading to calcium entry and insulin release.

During the past 5 years there has been considerable progress in the identification of genetic abnormalities that cause fasting hypoglycemia. Persistent hyperinsulinemic hypoglycemia of infancy (PHHI) is an autosomal-recessive condition in which affected children have unregulated production and release of insulin that causes profound and life-threatening hypoglycemia. The causative gene for this disorder was mapped to chromosome 11p by several groups and the subsequent recognition that a putative receptor for sulfonylureas (termed the sulfonylurea receptor or SUR) mapped to this same locus led to the identification of inactivating mutations of *SUR*. It was subsequently learned that SUR is a member of a multi-component transporter system that includes a small inward rectifier of potassium (K$_{IR}$6.2); inactivating mutations of *K$_{IR}$6.2* also cause PHHI (**Fig. 20.2**).

To understand how defects in SUR and K$_{IR}$6.2 cause excessive insulin secretion and hypoglycemia, it is helpful to review normal mechanisms involved in insulin secretion. An increase in the plasma glucose concentration results in increased transport of glucose into the β cell via the GLUT 2 transporter (**Fig. 20.3**, top left panel). The glucose is subsequently phosphorylated by glucokinase and serves as a substrate to increase plasma ATP concentrations. An increased ATP/ADP (adenosine diphosphate) ratio causes diminished channel activity of SUR/K$_{IR}$6.2, leading to K$^+$ accumulation, depolarization of the cell, calcium entry from the extracellular fluid, and insulin secretion. Sulfonylureas cause increased insulin secretion by binding to SUR and causing closure of the channel; diazoxide interaction with SUR causes channel opening (**Fig. 20.3**, top left panel). It is this effect of diazoxide that makes it useful for treatment of certain conditions associated with increased insulin production. Inactivation of either SUR or K$_{IR}$6.2 results in closure of the channel, increased depolarization, and excessive insulin secretion.

Children with PHHI generally have a normal pregnancy and delivery. Frequently the clinical state of these children is characterized by poor feeding, hypotonia, cyanosis, seizures, and sudden death if the hypoglycemia is not detected. Prolonged hypoglycemia

may lead to mental retardation and some children develop cardiomyopathy. The diagnosis is generally confirmed by the presence of hypoglycemia and an inappropriately high plasma insulin concentration. Other diagnostic features include the requirement for a glucose infusion rate greater than 15mg/kg/min (normal is less than 5mg/kg/min), the absence of ketone bodies, and a rise in the glucose concentration following glucagon, excluding a defect in glycogenolysis. There is a variable pancreatic histology in PHHI with a spectrum ranging from normal appearing to hyperplasia of the islet cells (commonly termed nesidioblastosis). In general, mutations of *SUR* or *K$_{IR}$6.2* cause increased insulin secretion; hyperplasia of the islet cells is an uncommon finding.

Heterozygous loss of a portion of maternal chromosome 11p15, an event that occurs somatically, has been found in focal adenomatous hyperplasia of β cells. These results suggest that there is a maternal gene in this region, probably other than *SUR* or *K$_{IR}$6.2* (which map there also), which is lost through a somatic mechanism. The presumption is that the paternal allele of this gene is silenced, leading to a functional loss of heterozygosity, or alternatively there exists the possibility of a heterozygous mutation of the paternal *SUR* or *K$_{IR}$6.2* allele, which is manifested only when the maternal allele is lost. In a French series, all 10 patients with focal adenomatous hyperplasia had 11p15 loss of heterozygosity, making this a compelling possibility.

A second genetic defect that has been shown to cause hyperinsulinemic hypoglycemia is a heterozygous mutation of the glucokinase gene that lowers the affinity of enzyme for glucose. The net effect of this mutation is to activate glucokinase at lower glucose concentrations (**Fig. 20.3**, bottom left panel). Unlike PHHI, where prolonged fasting will result in a further decrease of the plasma glucose concentration, the plasma glucose concentration remains at a low but stable level in the reported patients.

A third genetic defect that leads to insulin secretion is an activating mutation of the glutamate dehydrogenase (GDH) gene (**Fig. 20.3**, bottom right panel). Activating mutations of *GDH* result in enhanced conversion of glutamate to α-ketoglutarate, which increases the ATP/ADP ratio, closes the SUR/K$_{IR}$6.2 channel, and causes increased insulin secretion by the β cell. There is increased NH$_4^+$ production, particularly in the liver, as a result of the increased α-ketoglutarate production, which increases the plasma ammonia concentrations in these patients. These observations also provide a partial explanation in some patients for the clinical syndrome of leucine sensitivity, a syndrome described in the 1950s in which children given a diagnostic load of leucine developed hypoglycemia. Leucine causes increased insulin secretion by activating GDH (**Fig. 20.3**, bottom right panel).

Insulinomas are rare tumors (incidence of 4:1,000,000 patient years) derived from the islet β cell. They may be sporadic or hereditary (multiple endocrine neoplasia type 1, MEN1, or von Hippel–Lindau syndrome, VHL). Like many other neuroendocrine tumors, hereditary insulin-producing tumors occur at a much earlier age (approximately 25 years of age) than do sporadic tumors (average age 50 years). Hereditary tumors tend to be multicentric whereas this is uncommon in the sporadic variety. Although there tend to be multiple tumors present in hereditary disorders, it is uncommon for more than one of these tumors to produce insulin. Malignant islet cell tumors develop in approximately one-third of *MEN1* gene carriers, but are uncommon in sporadic tumors (5–10%).

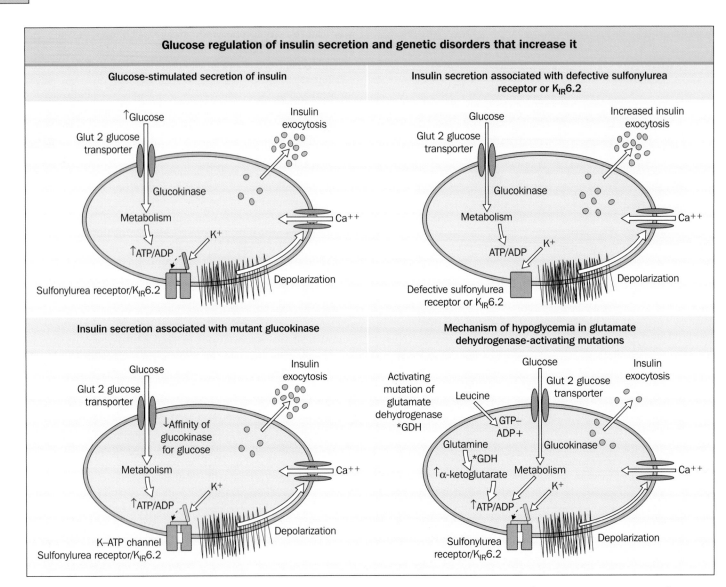

Glucose regulation of insulin secretion and genetic disorders that increase it

Figure 20.3 Glucose regulation of insulin secretion and genetic disorders that increase it. (Top left panel) Glucose-stimulated secretion of insulin. Glucose is phosphorylated by glucokinase and serves as a substrate to increase cellular adenosine triphosphate (ATP), thereby closing the ATP-sensitive K$^+$ channel. This results in depolarization of the cell, calcium entry, and insulin secretion. A reduction in glucose leads to opening of the channel and a reduction of insulin secretion. (Top right panel) Impact of inactivating mutation of *SUR* or $K_{IR}6.2$ on insulin secretion. Permanent closure of the K-ATP channel by inactivating mutations leads to depolarization, calcium entry, and continued secretion of insulin. (Bottom left panel) Insulin secretion associated with heterozygous mutation of glucokinase that increases affinity of the enzyme for glucose. Increased affinity of glucokinase for glucose results in a shift in the set point for glucose-stimulated insulin secretion, resulting in increased cellular ATP levels, closure of the K–ATP channel, and insulin secretion at lower than normal glucose concentrations.(Bottom right panel) Mechanism of hypoglycemia associated with activating mutation of glutamate dehydrogenase (GDH). Leucine normally stimulates insulin release by activating GDH, thereby increasing conversion of glutamate to α-ketoglutarate, resulting in increased cellular ATP, closure of the K–ATP channel, and increased insulin secretion. Activating mutations of GDH bypass this normal regulatory pathway. ADP, adenosine diphosphate.

Multiple endocrine neoplasia type 1 is a distinct genetic tumor syndrome in which gene carriers develop hyperparathyroidism, islet cell tumors (in one-third), including insulinoma (30–35% of all islet tumors in MEN1), pituitary tumors, and adrenocortical tumors (see Chapter 34). Clinical presentation of insulinoma in MEN1 does not differ from that of sporadic insulinoma, although the challenges of identifying and removing the insulin-producing tumor are greater. Multicentricity complicates the localization and removal of the one or two insulin-producing tumors that can exist in a background of multiple tumors.

Von Hippel–Lindau syndrome (VHL) is an autosomal dominant genetic tumor syndrome characterized by renal cell carcinoma (70% by age of 60 years), retinal and cerebellar hemangiomas, pheochromocytomas, islet cell tumors, renal and pancreatic cysts, and endolymphatic tumors. Islet cell tumors occur in approximately 15–20% of gene carriers (see Chapter 34).

During the past 8 years the genes that predispose to the development of islet cell tumors associated with MEN1 and VHL have been identified. Both the *MEN1* and *VHL* genes are examples of tumor suppressors, causing tumor development when both copies of the gene are lost. In autosomal-dominant MEN1 or VHL a mutated allele is inherited; the second allele is lost somatically. The *MEN1* gene, a tumor suppressor located on chromosome 11q, encodes a protein given the name menin. Although its function is unclear at present, recent studies show that it interacts with JunD, a transcription factor involved in regulation of cell division. The *VHL* gene is also a tumor suppressor that interacts with the elongin transcription complex to regulate transcription, ubiquitination, vascular responses to hypoxia, and fibronectin assembly. The precise mechanism by which loss of function of the *VHL* gene causes tumor formation is unclear.

A small percentage of insulinomas metastasize, most commonly to the liver. Management of this group of patients is challenging and will be discussed in a later section. Hypoglycemia may also develop in patients with metastatic islet cell tumors that were not considered to be insulinomas at the time of diagnosis. It is common for islet cell tumors to secrete multiple hormones, including insulin, at a low level. Clinical symptoms may not develop until the total mass of the tumor or hepatic metastasis is substantial.

Clinical features observed in insulinoma patients include neuroglycopenic symptoms (sweating, palpitations, weakness, neurologic symptoms, confusion or coma, and neurologic dysfunction) that tend to worsen with increasing length of the fast. Hypoglycemic symptoms may occur in the immediate postprandial period; it is therefore important to query all patients with postprandial hypoglycemic symptoms not only about the 4–6 hours period following food ingestion, but also about the nocturnal and early morning period. Most commonly, patients with insulinoma will develop symptoms within 8–10 hours following their last meal; in response to these symptoms patients increase caloric intake and frequently gain weight.

The hallmark of an insulinoma is dysregulated insulin secretion that is progressive over time. It is not uncommon for patients to present with a history of symptomatology for several years, but have clear and objective evidence for hypoglycemia only during the preceding several months. Plasma insulin, C-peptide, and proinsulin levels are uniformly elevated or inappropriately normal in the face of a lower than normal serum or plasma glucose. Elevation of all three insulin-related peptides makes it possible to differentiate hyperinsulinemia caused by an insulinoma from exogenous administration of human insulin, in which only plasma insulin levels are elevated.

Hypoglycemia associated with large abdominal tumors, most commonly fibrosarcomas, hemangiopericytomas, or hepatomas, is an uncommon but clearly defined syndrome. An increased concentration of incompletely processed insulin-like growth factor 2 (IGF-2) interacting with the insulin receptor is responsible for the hypoglycemia. A failure of the incompletely processed IGF-2 to interact efficiently with its binding complex (IGF binding protein-3, IGFBP-3, and acid-labile subunit, ALS) results in higher than normal free IGF-2 concentrations. Patients with this clinical syndrome are most likely to develop hypoglycemia during sleeping hours.

Autoimmune hypoglycemia is uncommon in the USA and Europe but occurs with some frequency in Japan. Several mechanisms have been identified. The most straightforward but least common is the production of antibodies that bind to and activate the insulin receptor, a syndrome that is sometimes associated with acanthosis nigricans. A second, less well-defined mechanism is the development of antiinsulin antibodies, resulting in a large storage pool of bound insulin that can be released in response to unclear stimuli, thereby causing hypoglycemia. Finally, antibodies that stimulate insulin release from islet β cells have been identified in a few patients with unexplained hypoglycemia. This type of hypoglycemia should be considered in patients with fasting hypoglycemia for whom no other identifiable cause can be identified.

EVALUATION OF THE PATIENT WITH SUSPECTED HYPOGLYCEMIA

The first step in the evaluation of suspected hypoglycemia is to document the presence of a low plasma glucose concentration combined with symptoms consistent with hypoglycemia, and reversal of symptoms by administration of glucose. This is particularly important in postprandial hypoglycemia, where ingestion of food can produce a variety of symptoms that may not be caused by hypoglycemia. In suspected postprandial hypoglycemia there is nearly universal agreement that a 5-hour glucose tolerance test is unhelpful for diagnostic purposes because it does not mimic a normal meal. In this situation most clinicians provide the patient with a home glucose monitoring device to check the blood glucose when symptoms develop. True postprandial hypoglycemia is relatively uncommon and rarely dangerous. In most cases it can be addressed by smaller, more frequent meals.

In contrast, fasting hypoglycemia is generally indicative of a more serious disorder. Hypoglycemia develops frequently during sleep and may result in neurologic damage or convulsions if not detected and treated. In these patients it is important to initiate an investigation to determine a specific cause or causes.

Diagnostic procedures

Fasting hypoglycemia should be evaluated in a controlled environment where it is possible to reproduce the hypoglycemia and hormonal responses. In most patients with fasting hypoglycemia, symptomatology will develop over a period of months or years. By the time of referral for hypoglycemia most patients have a distinct pattern of hypoglycemic symptoms, making the onset of symptoms predictable. In these cases outpatient fasting with supervision is generally safe. In other patients with unpredictable symptomatology, hospitalization for a supervised 48–72-hour fast with close nursing supervision may be more appropriate.

Recent experience has shown that most but not all patients with an insulinoma will develop hypoglycemia within the first 48 hours after the start of a fast. Adherence to a regimented protocol is important; there are many examples where a fast has been initiated and the important laboratory tests are omitted during the flurry of activity that surrounds a hypoglycemic event. **Figure 20.4** depicts a hypothetical fast, documenting the progressive decline in plasma glucose over a 48-hour period. It is important to obtain measurements of glucose, insulin, proinsulin, and C-peptide at regular intervals during the fast, because hypoglycemia [defined as a blood glucose below 60mg/dL (3.4mmol/L)] may occur without symptoms. It is not necessary to analyze all samples for insulin, C-peptide, or proinsulin, but serum should be available

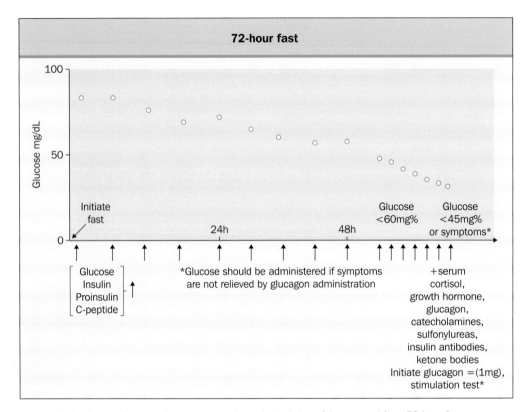

Figure 20.4 72-hour fast. The figure gives a schematic depiction of the protocol for a 72-hour fast to evaluate fasting hypoglycemia. The goals of such a fast are to reproduce the hypoglycemic episode under controlled conditions to assess hormonal dynamics. In the hypothetical fast shown in this figure, the patient is allowed access only to water. The patient is encouraged to be physically active during this period to promote glucose utilization. Measurements of glucose, insulin, C-peptide, and proinsulin are performed at 4–6-hour intervals. When the glucose concentration falls below 60mg/dL (3.4mmol/L) the frequency of sampling increases to 1–2 hours. When the glucose concentration falls below 45mg/dL (2.5mmol/L) or the patient develops symptomatic hypoglycemia, additional measurement of serum or plasma cortisol, growth hormone, glucagon, catecholamines, sulfonylureas, ketones, and insulin antibodies should be performed. Immediately thereafter the patient is given glucagon 1mg subcutaneously or intravenously with measurement of glucose 30 and 60min later to assess the ability of the liver to produce glucose. If neuroglycopenic symptoms become severe, the patient should be given oral or intravenous glucose after sampling for the hormones described above.

for analysis of all samples in which the glucose is below 60mg/dL (3.4mmol/L). Reduction of the glucose concentration below 60mg/dL (3.4mmol/L) should prompt more frequent sampling.

At the time the glucose falls below 45mg/dL (2.5mmol/L)or the patient becomes symptomatic, measurement of plasma or serum cortisol, growth hormone, glucagon, and catecholamines should be performed. Since the response of serum cortisol to hypoglycemia may be delayed by 30–60min, it is also helpful to obtain a sample 1 hour following the period of symptomatic hypoglycemia. At the point of plasma glucose nadir it is useful to administer glucagon (1mg) subcutaneously or intravenously and measure glucose at 30 and 60min thereafter to assess hepatic glucose production. Measurement of sulfonylureas at the glucose nadir will address the question of sulfonylurea use; measurement of ketone bodies (β-hydroxybutyrate) is performed because patients with insulinoma characteristically have low levels (**Fig. 20.5**). A nomogram plotting the plasma glucose on the ordinate and the plasma insulin, C-peptide, or proinsulin on the abscissa makes it possible to compare the patient's results to those obtained in several large insulinoma series (**Fig. 20.5**).

The finding of an inappropriately high serum or plasma insulin, C-peptide, and proinsulin concentration in a hypoglycemic patient is evidence for insulin-mediated hypoglycemia. If there is only an elevated plasma insulin concentration and a suppressed C-peptide or proinsulin, surreptitious use of insulin should be considered. It is also important to assess the levels of serum or plasma growth hormone, cortisol, epinephrine, and glucagon to exclude a deficiency of one of these hormones.

If hypoglycemia does not develop during the fast, it is important to exercise the patient during and at the conclusion of the fast in an attempt to provoke hypoglycemia. Surreptitious users of insulin can be particularly clever and in suspected cases close observation of the patient may be required to document insulin use. Most importantly, the controlled fast provides a decision point; those with insulin-mediated hypoglycemia are further evaluated to identify either a tumor or other process associated with increased insulin production, whereas those with suppressed insulin levels should be evaluated for other non-insulin-related causes of hypoglycemia (**Table 20.3**).

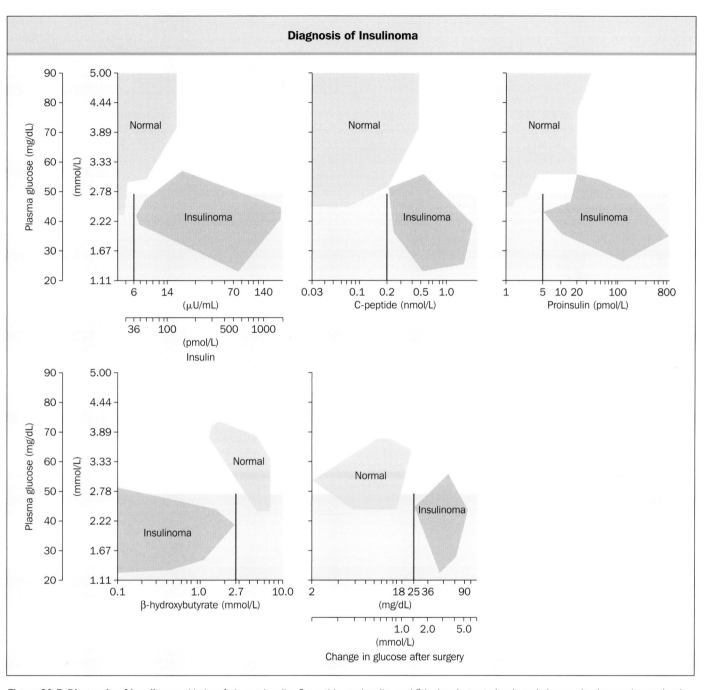

Figure 20.5 Diagnosis of insulinoma. Limits of plasma insulin, C-peptide, proinsulin, and β-hydroxybutyrate levels and changes in plasma glucose levels in response to intravenous glucagon, according to plasma glucose levels at the end of a 72-hour fast in 25 normal persons and when the features of Whipple's triad were noted in 40 patients with histologically confirmed insulinomas. The pale yellow areas represent plasma glucose levels less than or equal to 50mg/dL (2.8mmol/L). The vertical red lines represent the diagnostic criteria for insulinoma: insulin ≥ 6μU/mL (36pmol/L); C-peptide ≥ 0.2nmol/L; proinsulin ≥ 5pmol/L; β-hydroxybutyrate ≤ 2.7mmol/L; and change in glucose level ≥ 25mg/dL (1.4mmol/L). (Reproduced with permission from Service FJ. Hypoglycemic disorders. N Engl J Med. 1995;332:1144–52. © 1995 Massachusetts Medical Society. All rights reserved.)

Diagnostic studies to localize the source of insulin production

In a patient with insulin-mediated hypoglycemia in which there is no suspicion of surreptitious use of insulin and no history to suggest a genetic cause for the hypoglycemia (lifetime history of symptoms), two different approaches have been advocated. One approach is to proceed directly to a surgical exploration, employing intraoperative ultrasound to localize an islet cell tumor. The

success rate for this approach in the hands of experienced surgeons is high. An alternative approach is to perform a more detailed evaluation in an attempt to localize the tumor. The rationale for additional study is to facilitate a decision during a surgical procedure in the event that no pancreatic tumor is identified. The surgeon is confronted with the decision to perform a partial pancreatectomy (most insulinomas occur in the body or tail) or to close and reevaluate the patient. The availability of additional localizing data can be helpful in making this decision. Two types of localization procedures have been used. The first is transhepatic portal venous sampling where a catheter is advanced percutaneously through the liver retrograde into the portal circulation, making it possible to obtain serum insulin measurements from particular pancreatic venous effluents. The second employs a calcium injection to stimulate insulin release. Calcium is injected selectively into arteries that vascularize a particular part of the pancreas (superior mesenteric, splenic, gastroduodenal, and hepatic arteries) with collection of timed hepatic venous effluent for insulin or C-peptide measurement (**Fig. 20.6**). The small size of most insulinomas makes radionuclide scanning with compounds such as radiolabeled octreotide usually unhelpful. Although these tumors frequently express somatostatin receptors, it is difficult to differentiate these tumors from background radioactivity. High-resolution CT scanning, even with early phase examination of contrast enhancement to improve sensitivity, is often not positive in patients with insulinoma, but should be performed to exclude hepatic metastasis or some other unexpected abdominal process.

Another outcome of the 72-hour controlled fast is a suppressed plasma insulin, C-peptide, and proinsulin. This outcome inevitably refocuses the differential diagnosis away from conditions associated with increased insulin production to other conditions. Other laboratory studies obtained during the hypoglycemic period (**Fig. 20.4**) will help the clinician address other causes, including deficiency of counterregulatory hormones (growth hormone, glucagon, epinephrine, and cortisol), autoimmune hypoglycemia, or other pharmacologic agents that rarely cause hypoglycemia. The reader is referred to an extensive list of uncommon causes of non-insulin-mediated hypoglycemia (see Further reading: Service, 1995). In addition, other neoplastic causes of hypoglycemia such as fibrosarcoma, hemangiopericytoma, hepatomas, or other large retroperitoneal tumors should be considered, a diagnosis usually confirmed by abdominal computerized tomography or magnetic resonance imaging.

MANAGEMENT

Clinical management of hypoglycemia should be directed at the underlying cause. Postprandial hypoglycemia is a common referral diagnosis, most commonly based on a borderline plasma glucose obtained during a glucose tolerance test. There is now general agreement that this test is a poor predictor of postprandial hypoglycemia; it should be replaced by home measurement of plasma glucose values during meal-induced symptoms. If hypoglycemia is documented, the disorder will most commonly respond to reassurance and smaller, more frequent meals. A variety of other approaches have been applied to this condition, including reduction of glucose absorption by acarbose, treatment of early type 2 diabetes mellitus, and anticholinergic agents. None are universally successful. Fortunately, the condition is self-limiting in most patients; in patients with persistence of hypoglycemia over time a more detailed evaluation for other causes should be pursued.

In patients with insulin-mediated hypoglycemia, it is important to first exclude drug-induced hypoglycemia (sulfonylureas or insulin self-administration) and to consider the possibility of a genetic disorder (**Table 20.3**). In most cases a genetic disorder will have been present since early childhood, although some genetic forms of β-cell hyperplasia may worsen over time. In the majority of patients with increased insulin production an islet cell tumor will be identified. Surgical exploration should be performed, combined with intraoperative ultrasound, the most sensitive technique for identification of a small tumor. Small tumors should be enucleated and the remainder of the pancreas

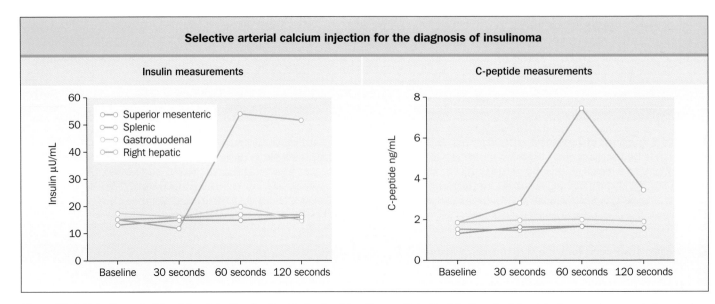

Figure 20.6 Selective arterial calcium injection for the diagnosis of insulinoma. Selective injection of calcium into the superior mesenteric, splenic, and gastroduodenal arteries with measurement of insulin or C-peptide in timed specimens obtained from the hepatic vein. Identification of increased insulin release from a tumor in the normal vascular distribution of the splenic artery made it possible to localize an insulinoma during the surgical procedure.

examined carefully to exclude the rare second tumor. In patients with MEN1-related insulinomas, consideration should be given to excision of all identifiable tumors, performance of a distal pancreatectomy, and exploration of the duodenum for other tumors related to MEN1. A variety of intraoperative techniques such as glucose monitoring or rapid insulin measurement have been employed to verify removal of the tumor; none of these techniques are in widespread use.

An issue that occasionally confronts the surgeon is the absence of an identifiable tumor in a patient with documented insulin-mediated hypoglycemia. It is important in such situations to review the preoperative evaluation to be certain that the evaluation was adequate. If the evidence is compelling for an insulin-mediated process, consideration should be given to performance of a distal pancreatectomy, the site of most insulinomas. It is in this uncommon situation that a preoperative localization procedure permits the surgeon to proceed with a specific surgical procedure with some level of confidence. The diagnosis of diffuse β-cell hyperplasia should also be considered, a disorder that is sometimes resolved or improved by distal pancreatectomy. The necessity for occasional intraoperative decisions that are difficult suggest that patients with potential insulinomas should be evaluated in an experienced referral center.

Management of malignancy-associated hypoglycemia should focus on surgical excision, if possible, or antineoplastic therapy directed toward the tumor. During the initial stages of hypoglycemia, it may be possible to manage the patient by frequent daytime and nocturnal snacks. If therapy directed at the tumor is unsuccessful or caloric intake is inadequate, it may be necessary to institute additional measures. In patients with insulin-producing or large retroperitoneal tumors, several approaches have been used. Glucagon infusion (0.5–2mg/hour using a small pump) stimulates gluconeogenesis and will prevent hypoglycemia in some patients. Response to glucagon should be documented before initiation of therapy by assessing the glucose response 30 and 60min following glucagon (1mg) subcutaneously. Treatment with growth hormone or glucocorticoids may reverse hypoglycemia in patients with large retroperitoneal tumors, possibly by facilitating IGFBP-3/ALS complex formation with reduction of IGF-2 levels. Embolization of hepatic metastasis of insulinoma or fibrosarcomas producing incompletely processed IGF-2 has been used successfully to reduce secretion of these two peptides with improvement of hypoglycemia. In patients with metastatic insulinoma or a benign tumor that has not been found, diazoxide may be effective. Problems with fluid retention may occur but diuretics given concomitantly usually control this side effect. Somatostatin analogs (octreotide or lanreotide) should be tried in patients with metastatic insulinoma, but are rarely effective. Finally, in patients in whom there is complete replacement of the liver by tumor, it is generally necessary to provide parenteral 20% glucose infusion, particularly during the night. Use of the current generation of infusion pumps combined with central line placement make it possible to provide this therapy in the home.

SUMMARY

Diagnosis and treatment of hypoglycemia requires a deliberate thought process and focused evaluation. In most patients a diligent diagnostic approach will lead to the identification of a cause and direct specific therapy.

FURTHER READING

Aguilar-Bryan L, Bryan J. Molecular biology of adenosine triphosphate-sensitive potassium channels. Endocr Rev. 1999;20:101–35.

Amiel S. Reversal of unawareness of hypoglycemia. N Engl J Med. 1993;329:876–7.

Brown CK, Bartlett DL, Doppman JL et al. Intraarterial calcium stimulation and intraoperative ultrasonography in the localization and resection of insulinomas. Surgery 1997;122:1189–93; discussion 1193–4.

De Lonlay P, Fournet JC, Rahier J et al. Somatic deletion of the imprinted 11p15 region in sporadic persistent hyperinsulinemic hypoglycemia of infancy is specific of focal adenomatous hyperplasia and endorses partial pancreatectomy. J Clin Invest. 1997;100:802–7.

De Lonlay-Debeney P, Poggi-Travert F, Fournet JC, et al. Clinical features of 52 neonates with hyperinsulinism. N Engl J Med. 1999;340:1169–75.

Dozio N, Scavini M, Beretta A, et al. Imaging of the buffering effect of insulin antibodies in the autoimmune hypoglycemic syndrome. J Clin Endocrinol Metab. 1998;83:643–8.

Ernst AA, Jones K, Nick TG, et al. Ethanol ingestion and related hypoglycemia in a pediatric and adolescent emergency department population. Acad Emerg Med. 1996;3:46–9.

Glaser B, Kesavan P, Heyman M, et al. Familial hyperinsulinism caused by an activating glucokinase mutation. N Engl J Med. 1998;338:226–30.

Hirshberg B, Livi A, Bartlett DL, et al. Forty-eight-hour fast: the diagnostic test for insulinoma. J Clin Endocrinol Metab. 2000;85:3222–6.

Hoff AO, Vassilopoulou-Sellin R. The role of glucagon administration in the diagnosis and treatment of patients with tumor hypoglycemia. Cancer 1998;82:1585–92.

Le Roith D. Tumor-induced hypoglycemia. N Engl J Med. 1999;341:757–8.

Lengle SJ, Hecht ST, Link DP, et al. Palliative embolization of fibrosarcoma for control of tumor-induced hypoglycemia. Cardiovasc Intervent Radiol. 1995;18:255–8.

Marks V, Teale JD. Drug-induced hypoglycemia. Endocrinol Metab Clin North Am. 1999;28:555–77.

Redmon JB, Nuttall FQ. Autoimmune hypoglycemia. Endocrinol Metab Clin North Am. 1999;28:603–18.

Romijn JA, Godfried MH, Wortel C, et al. Hypoglycemia, hormones and cytokines in fatal meningococcal septicemia. J Endocrinol Invest. 1990;13:743–7.

Service FJ. Hypoglycemic disorders. N Engl J Med. 1995;332:1144–52.

Stanley CA, Baker L. The causes of neonatal hypoglycemia. N Engl J Med. 1999;340:1200–1.

Stanley CA, Lieu YK, Hsu BY, et al. Hyperinsulinism and hyperammonemia in infants with regulatory mutations of the glutamate dehydrogenase gene. N Engl J Med. 1998;338:1352–7.

Thomas PM. Genetic mutations as a cause of hyperinsulinemic hypoglycemia in children. Endocrinol Metab Clin North Am. 1999;28:647–56.

Thomas PM, Cote GJ, Wohllk N, et al. Mutations in the sulfonylurea receptor gene in familial persistent hyperinsulinemic hypoglycemia of infancy. Science 1995;268:426–9.

Thompson GB, Service FJ, Andrews JC, et al. Noninsulinoma pancreatogenous hypoglycemia syndrome: an update in 10 surgically treated patients. Surgery 2000;128:937–44; discussion 944–5.

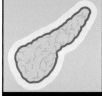

Section 4 Control of Blood Glucose and its Disturbance

Chapter 21 Insulin-Dependent Diabetes Mellitus

Jerry L Nadler, Marcia McDuffie, and Susan E Kirk

INTRODUCTION

The rate of development of type 1 diabetes is increasing and it accounts for nearly 10% of all diagnosed people with diabetes. Type 1 diabetes is a major chronic disease of children and is now being recognized with increasing frequency in adults.

Type 1 diabetes is associated with a reduced life expectancy and significant morbidity because of the damaging effects of acute metabolic complications and chronic vascular complications. These complications can severely impact the patients, their families, and medical and economic resources.

The current chapter reviews the pathogenesis, epidemiology, complications and treatment for type 1 diabetes, and provides updated review and practice information. There continue to be new advances in methods to identify people at risk for diabetes and testing of new methods to prevent or reverse type 1 diabetes. We also have new clearer information about the importance of glycemic and blood pressure control and standards of care that, if followed, could markedly reduce the development of acute and chronic complications.

CAUSES

The pathogenesis of type 1 diabetes mellitus

Type 1 diabetes results from loss of pancreatic β cells. By far the most common mechanism for β-cell destruction appears to be immune-mediated inflammatory damage. Prospective population and family studies strongly support a genetic basis for susceptibility to development of anti-islet immune responses and suggest that the underlying immune abnormalities precede clinical insulin deficiency by many years in most individuals. Potent immunosuppressive agents may be able to slow the destructive process but the known and potential negative effects of the available agents preclude their use. Since the disease process can recur in grafted islet tissue, islet or pancreas transplantation is currently feasible only in individuals with other life-threatening medical conditions requiring life-long immunosuppression, and the functional lifespan of transplanted tissue in these cases may be limited by both disease recurrence and classical rejection mechanisms. Therefore, the only clinical treatment available outside the research setting is carefully monitored insulin replacement.

Studies in the families of affected individuals have provided a great deal of information on methods for diagnosis of the disease in prediabetic stages, but most of the available information is extrapolated from spontaneous rodent models of immune-mediated diabetes. Information from studies in these rodent models is now being used as a basis for intervention trials with disease-specific methods of immunomodulation.

Clinical presentation

A diagnosis of type 1 diabetes mellitus requires evidence of deficient insulin production in an individual with no other disorders known to cause severe pancreatic damage. The majority of cases are recognized before the age of 19 years, and hyperglycemia with ketoacidosis is usually accepted as sufficient evidence for a diagnosis of type 1 diabetes in this age group. Provocative testing is rarely performed except in a research setting. These individuals almost inevitably require insulin for survival and progress to complete loss of insulin production within 2 years of diagnosis. More than 80% of children less than 14 years of age at diagnosis have detectable circulating antibodies directed against islet cells, consistent with immune-mediated islet destruction.

The progression of clinical symptoms in children and adolescents, from polyuria and polydipsia to severe dehydration and ketoacidosis, may appear to be quite abrupt. However, studies in siblings or offspring of affected individuals demonstrate that islet-specific antibodies can be detected in susceptible individuals as early as the first year of life. Since clinical signs of insulin deficiency appear more commonly after the age of 4 years, it is widely accepted that most childhood diabetes results from a relatively slow and progressive destruction of pancreatic β cells caused by an islet-specific immune mechanism.

Although the typical presentation of type 1 diabetes occurs in childhood, diabetes accompanied by islet cell antibodies can become apparent at any age, and up to 10% of elderly diabetic individuals (≥ 65 years) have detectable circulating islet cell autoantibodies similar to those found in children. Ketoacidosis is rare in antibody-positive individuals diagnosed in adulthood but the presence of islet cell antibodies is a good predictor of the eventual need for insulin to maintain adequate control of blood glucose levels in adults. Both body mass index and fasting or stimulated C-peptide levels are lower in this group than in the antibody-negative group, distinguishing them from the majority of adult-onset diabetics with type 2 disease. Thus, although it is recognized as the predominant form of diabetes in middle to late childhood, type 1 diabetes can become clinically apparent from infancy to old age and appears to represent the end stage of a progressive autoimmune process.

Familial risk in type 1 diabetes	
Relationship to proband	Concordance (%)
Monozygotic twin	20–70
Sibling/dizygotic twin	1–8
Child of affected father	2–8
Child of affected mother	0–3
Parent	2–3

Table 21.1 Familial risk in type 1 diabetes.

Epidemiology

Only 10–15% of individuals who carry a diagnosis of type 1 diabetes have an affected relative. However, the risk of disease development in the offspring or siblings of an individual with type 1 diabetes is 20–50 times higher than that of the general population, and the concordance rate in monozygotic twins reaches 70% in certain high-incidence ethnic groups (**Table 21.1**). The high concordance rate in identical twins establishes the importance of genetic factors in susceptibility to the underlying disease process but the lack of complete concordance is strong presumptive evidence that environmental factors also contribute to the development of clinical diabetes. A wide range of possible environmental agents, from foods to common viruses and vaccines, has been suggested but epidemiologic studies provide little support for any specific association, with the exception of wild-type rubella virus exposure during the first trimester of gestation.

The age-specific prevalence of type 1 diabetes varies by region and ethnic group worldwide (**Fig. 21.1**), with incidence rates ranging from less than 1 to more than 40 per 100,000 per year for the population at highest risk (less than 15 years of age in most ethnic groups). The mean age at diagnosis varies inversely with age-specific incidence rates. Although environmental factors have been invoked to explain these population-specific characteristics, studies in ethnic groups with extremely high or low prevalence suggest that genetic differences are the major contributor to this variability.

Immunopathology

Rare autopsy samples from the pancreas of newly diagnosed individuals with type 1 diabetes demonstrate widespread loss of β-cell mass. The few residual islets with insulin-positive β cells contain mononuclear cell infiltrates that are not seen in type 2 diabetes or in nondiabetic individuals. These infiltrates consist of monocyte/macrophages, B lymphocytes, and T lymphocytes of both the CD4 and CD8 subsets. Potent immunosuppressive agents such as azathioprine and cyclosporin A have been shown to delay the onset of insulin dependence in prediabetic individuals in small clinical trials, demonstrating that T lymphocytes

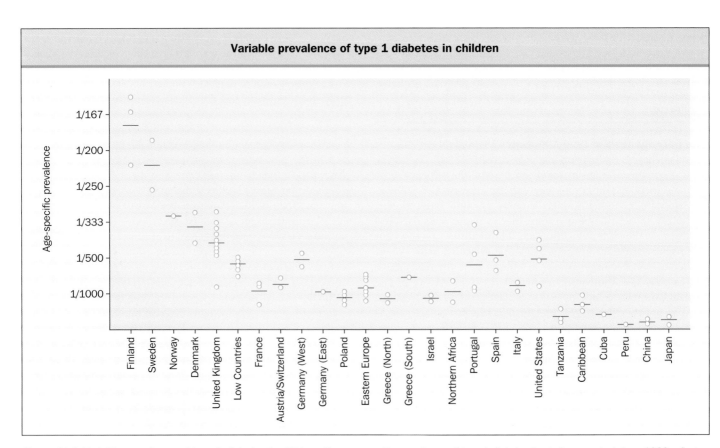

Figure 21.1 Variable prevalence of type 1 diabetes in children. The age-specific prevalence of type 1 diabetes in studies reported since 1980 reflects a wide variation across ethnic groups. Circles indicate the prevalence from a single report in a region; mean values for each region are shown as horizontal bars.

Autoantibodies in type 1 diabetes

Antigen	Prevalence (%)	Preferred assay	β-cell localization	Other cell types
Islet cell antibodies	60–70	Immunofluorescence on pancreatic sections	Cytoplasm, plasma membrane	?
Glutamate decarboxylase	80	RIA: recombinant human GAD65	Secretory granules	Brain, peripheral nerve
IA-2	75	RIA: recombinant human IA2	Secretory granules, plasma membrane	Neuroendocrine cells
Insulin	40–50*	Competitive RIA: recombinant human insulin	Secretory granules	None
Proinsulin	10–15	Competitive RIA	Secretory granules	None
Carboxypeptidase H	10–25	Immunoprecipitation, immunoblotting	Secretory granules	Neuroendocrine cells
GM2-1 ganglioside	65–70	ELISA, thin-layer chromatography	Secretory granule membranes	Brain

* High prevalence only in individuals less than 15 years of age.

Table 21.2 Autoantibodies in type 1 diabetes.

are important mediators of islet damage. However, immuno-suppressive therapy does not appear to be able to control the disease process indefinitely once it is established.

An active islet-specific immune response has also been inferred from circulating IgG antibodies specific for islet cell antigens. These antibodies are found in a high proportion of individuals with insulin-dependent diabetes at the time of diagnosis. Islet cell antibodies do not appear to play a pathogenic role in β-cell destruction but they serve as a useful marker for immunologic autoreactivity. A number of specific targets for these antibodies are proteins associated with insulin secretory granules, such as insulin and glutamic acid decarboxylase (**Table 21.2**). It is clear from prospective studies of first-degree relatives that circulating autoantibodies may be detectable as early as 9–12 months of age in susceptible individuals. Islet autoantibodies are detectable from infancy or early childhood in 3–8% of first-degree relatives. Roughly half of these individuals will develop clinical diabetes, preceded by months to years of diminishing first-phase insulin release on provocative testing, suggesting a similar slow destruction of functional β cells in prediabetic humans. Lifetime risk of type 1 diabetes in these individuals is related to the titer of islet cell autoantibodies detected by indirect immunofluorescence (ICA) or to the number of specific autoantigens recognized by circulating antibodies. Although studies are currently under way to refine the use of testing for anti-islet antibodies as a means of predicting the development of clinical disease, antibody screening is currently used only in research settings to define risk for disease among close relatives of affected individuals.

Genetic basis for disease

The major histocompatibility complex that encodes the 'human leukocyte antigen' or *HLA* genes has been identified as a single major contributor to genetic risk by epidemiologic studies using first-degree relatives of diabetic individuals. In addition to encoding recognition elements for discrimination between self and foreign tissue, genes in this region play a major role in the differentiation and functional activation of T lymphocytes. Association of disease with inheritance of haplotypes carrying specific HLA class II alleles has also been shown in population studies. The specific HLA haplotypes that appear to be associated with disease susceptibility vary from one ethnic group to another, and some specific HLA Class II alleles have been shown

to be negatively associated with disease (e.g. DQβ*0602), suggesting that they are protective. Although the relationship between genes in this region and control of T-cell function is suggestive, the specific mechanism by which they regulate susceptibility to type 1 diabetes is unknown. Observed rates of type 1 diabetes in families best fit a model in which this single locus (*HLA*) confers the major disease risk but is insufficient to support the development of disease in the absence of other susceptibility genes. Modern genetic linkage studies also suggest that susceptibility may be controlled by the *HLA* haplotype and genes from as many as 17 other chromosomal regions.

Environmental factors

Incomplete concordance in identical twins implicates environmental factors in the initiation and/or progression of the disease process in genetically predisposed individuals. Infectious agents, dietary exposures, and environmental toxins have been investigated but only in the case of congenital rubella syndrome is there strong evidence for a specific association. Up to 20% of individuals with congenital rubella develop insulin-dependent diabetes, reflecting the frequency of individuals with susceptible *HLA* haplotypes in this group. The disease process, detectable by the presence of islet cell antibodies and a slow progression to β-cell failure, appears to be identical to that in the general population and is distinguished only by its increased frequency in this group of individuals. There is no evidence of a relationship between postnatal exposure to wild-type or attenuated (vaccine) rubella virus strains and the subsequent development of diabetes. This observation suggests that the timing of infection during a period of active islet development explains the powerful enhancement of susceptibility in individuals infected *in utero* with this virus.

Several other viruses have been implicated in the pathogenesis of type 1 diabetes because of their ability to infect pancreatic tissue. Coxsackie virus of the B4 strain was isolated from the islets of a child who died shortly after the diagnosis of diabetes. Infection with this strain can cause transient hyperglycemia in both mice and nonhuman primates, and nearly half the individuals dying of Coxsackie-related myocarditis in one study had islet-related inflammation. However, subsequent repeated attempts to identify viral genomes in the pancreas of individuals newly diagnosed with type 1 diabetes have failed to detect evidence of active infection and serologic studies have mostly failed to confirm evidence of primary immune responses to Coxsackie viruses. Similar studies have also shown no evidence of acute infection with other pancreatotropic candidate viruses, such as mumps. One recent study from Sweden, which has one of the highest diabetes prevalence rates worldwide, suggested that the risk of diabetes was increased in children exposed to primary Coxsackie infections *in utero* but there is no evidence to date that acute viral infections can induce diabetes in individuals without underlying genetic susceptibility.

Like viruses, foods have been postulated to provide triggers for the development or acceleration of islet autoimmunity. Several groups have reported an association between diabetes and high levels of circulating antibodies against cow milk proteins, and controversial epidemiologic data suggest an increased risk for diabetes in high-risk individuals with early exposure to cow milk proteins or with increased milk consumption in childhood. Although two prospective studies failed to confirm these retrospective analyses, a prospective interventional study is currently underway in a Finnish population and the controversy should be resolved within the next decade. Once again, however, there are no data in any of these studies to suggest that food exposure can induce type 1 diabetes in the absence of genetic susceptibility.

Environmental toxins have also been suggested as possible initiators or accelerators of the diabetogenic process. *N*-3 pyridyl-methyl-*N'* 4 nitrophenyl urea, a rodenticide, can cause hyperglycemia and ketoacidosis within 12 hours of ingestion through acute β-cell necrosis. Although there are reports that anti-islet antibodies have been detected in the sera of long-term survivors, there is no evidence that the persistent diabetes in these individuals is related to autoimmune islet damage. Similarly, autopsy studies in a case of diabetes associated with pentamidine treatment for HIV-related *Pneumocystis carinii* pneumonia found evidence of β-cell loss without inflammation. While it remains possible that environmental toxic exposures can be associated with β-cell damage, no epidemiologic evidence to date supports a specific association.

Predictive testing

Several large population-based screening studies have confirmed the relationship between anti-islet antibodies and type 1 diabetes in individuals without a family history of disease. However, these tests remain restricted to use as research tools because of the cost of assay and their low specificity. Studies are currently underway to test the predictive power of HLA testing for specific disease-associated alleles as part of a newborn screening panel in large populations in both the USA and Europe but the outcome of these studies may not be clear for another decade. Testing for genes with less substantial contributions to disease susceptibility is unlikely to be of use in predicting genetic susceptibility. However, it is hoped that the identification of such genes by positional cloning methods may allow a better understanding of disease pathogenesis and this possibility makes the collection of DNA samples from well-characterized affected individuals and their families of critical importance. As with any form of predictive genetic testing, both ethical and psychologic issues arise in the consideration of the value of performing these tests outside of a research setting. In the case of type 1 diabetes, predictive testing as a component of routine clinical care should not be considered until preventive treatment options are available.

Mechanisms of disease

The pathogenesis of type 1 diabetes in humans has been resistant to study because of its genetic complexity, its variable rate of progression, and the probable influence of unknown environmental factors. However, two rodent models of genetically determined autoimmune β-cell destruction and diabetes are available and provide some insight into the human disease. Both the bio-breeding (BB) rat and the nonobese diabetic (NOD) mouse develop T-lymphocyte-dependent islet-associated mononuclear cell infiltrates that result in β-cell destruction and overt diabetes in 50% of the animals by 4–5 months of age. Environmental factors clearly influence the rate of β-cell damage in these models, and the cumulative incidence of overt diabetes can be either enhanced or decreased by specific rodent viral infections or by defined dietary manipulations. Interestingly, the incidence of diabetes actually increases in NOD mice raised in colonies free of all known mouse viruses. Islet cell antibodies develop in both models, and susceptibility is clearly regulated by genes in the murine equivalent of the HLA complex. As is seen in human disease, genes outside this region are also required for the development of disease. On the basis of these similarities with human type 1 diabetes, the rodent models have been used to study details of pathophysiology and to test possible therapeutic strategies in more tractable experimental systems.

The pancreas in these rodents appears normal at birth (**Fig. 21.2A & B**). A genetically controlled lymphopenia is associated with disease susceptibility in the BB rat that may limit widespread pancreatic infiltration by lymphocytes until the late stages in this model. However, in the NOD mouse, mononuclear cell infiltration begins at about 5–6 weeks of age with an increase in islet macrophages and accumulation of lymphocytes in the perivascular/periductular regions of the pancreas. By 8 weeks of age, infiltrating lymphocytes can be found adjacent to and surrounding islets (**Fig. 21.2C**) and islet-related autoantibodies can be detected in some mice. By 12 weeks, invasive 'insulitis' is well established, and patchy loss of insulin granules is seen in the surviving β cells (**Fig. 21.2D**). It is at this stage that overt diabetes begins to appear in these animals. From 12 weeks of age, the cumulative incidence of diabetes follows progressive loss of β-cell granulation and mass (**Fig. 21.2E & F**), increasing to a plateau by about 30 weeks of age. This slow progression of disease is similar to the evidence in prospective studies of islet-autoantibody-positive first-degree relatives in human type 1 diabetes.

The disease process appears to occur in several discrete steps, each of which may be subject to genetic or pharmacologic control in the future. It is thought to be initiated by abnormal release of antigens from pancreatic islets, particularly β cells. While such release may result spontaneously from genetic defects which increase β-cell turnover, it is also possible that infectious agents or mild β-cell toxins may accelerate this process in humans (**Fig. 21.3**, Step 1). β-cell antigens are then presented to the immune system, resulting in lymphocyte activation (**Fig. 21.3**, Step 2). Normal mice react to excess islet antigen exposure by a self-limited immune response. In diabetes-prone rodents and humans, however, such antigen exposure results in self-perpetuating autoimmune destruction.

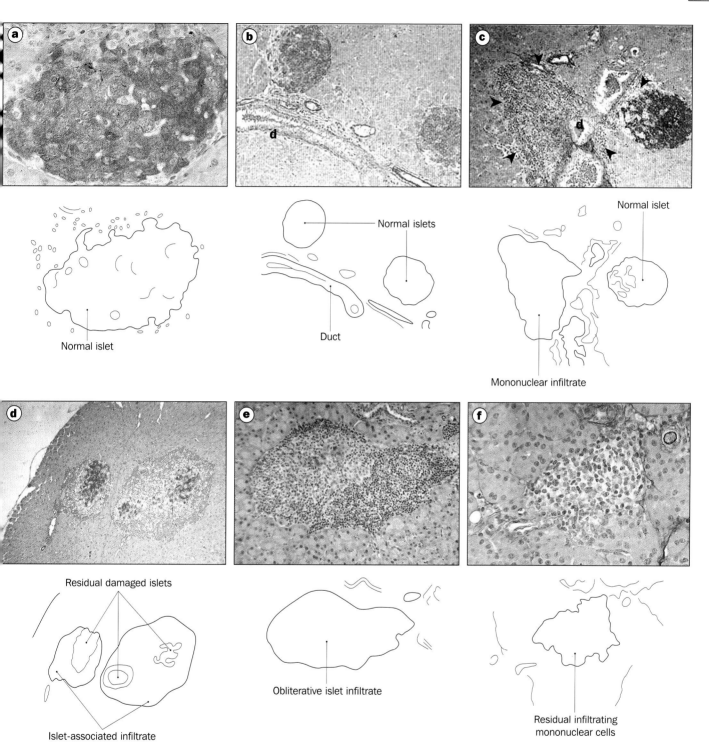

Figure 21.2 Development of destructive insulitis in type 1 diabetes. Histologic sections from the pancreas of female NOD mice show the progression of inflammation with increasing age. (a) Normal islet. (b) Lower-power view of the normal pancreatic architecture in a 4-week-old NOD mouse (d, pancreatic duct). (c). Periductular mononuclear infiltrates (arrows) characteristic of NOD mice at 8 weeks of age. (d) Progressive invasion of islets with loss of insulin storage granules characteristic of 12-week-old NOD mice. (e) Badly infiltrated islet from a newly diabetic NOD mouse with complete loss of β cells. (f) Scant residual infiltrate in long-term diabetes. (a, f 400×; d–e 200×.)

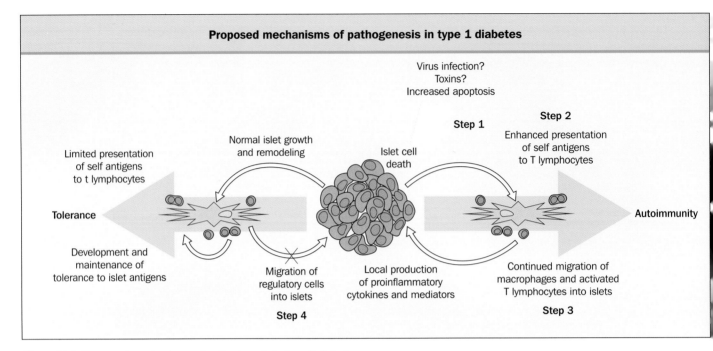

Figure 21.3 Proposed mechanisms of pathogenesis in type 1 diabetes.

Once initiated, destruction from unchecked islet-specific immune responses occurs by multiple mechanisms. Proinflammatory cytokines such as TNF-α, γ-interferon, and interleukin-1 are all upregulated in islets with active inflammation and can cause direct damage to β cells *in vitro* (**Fig. 21.3**, Step 3). Similarly, high-energy oxygen radicals and nitric oxide appear to be produced locally in inflamed islets, and treatment of NOD mice with radical scavengers or enzyme inhibitors dramatically decreases the rate of islet damage and diabetes. Direct cytotoxic activity by antigen-specific CD8 T cells has also been shown to play a role in disease development.

During the early stages, this active, proinflammatory response develops in parallel with expansion of regulatory T cells, which can inhibit β-cell damage, resulting in control of inflammatory damage by this 'balanced' response (**Fig. 21.3**, Step 4). Persistence of a balanced immune response may explain the failure of insulitis to progress to complete β-cell destruction in 50% of NOD mice or BB rats, as well as the lack of complete concordance in human monozygotic twins. The regulatory population can be reduced in NOD mice by certain immunosuppressive drugs, such as cyclophosphamide, precipitating rapid β-cell destruction and diabetes. In humans, decrease in regulatory cell function may result from immune responses to infections. However, should this regulatory population survive in adequate numbers for the life of the individual an active anti-islet immune response can exist without progression to clinical diabetes. In the animal models, administration of either insulin or glutamic acid decarboxylase during the prediabetic phase can expand and activate regulatory cells. This finding forms the basis for an ongoing diabetes prevention trial (DPT-1) sponsored by the National Institutes of Health. In this trial, parenteral and oral human insulin is being used to attempt to delay or inhibit clinical diabetes in prediabetic individuals.

Clinical trials
Methods of risk assessment, prevention, and treatment of established type 1 diabetes are actively being studied in large collaborative clinical trial settings. A listing of sources for information about ongoing trials is provided in **Table 21.3**.

DIAGNOSIS

Clinical
Diagnostic criteria as outlined by the American Diabetes Association (ADA; **Table 21.4**) and the World Health Organization are in place to define the conditions of diabetes mellitus and impaired fasting glucose; however they do not differentiate between the subtypes of diabetes mellitus. If the onset of type 1 diabetes, especially in younger individuals, is abrupt and conspicuous (as described above), a biochemical diagnosis is generally used only to confirm clinical suspicion. Nonetheless, on occasion, especially when the diagnosis of type 1 diabetes is made in a patient outside the typical age range – as occurs with latent autoimmune diabetes of adulthood – or in a patient with atypical symptoms, a biochemical diagnosis may be required. In this section, tests used to confirm the diagnosis of diabetes mellitus are described. In addition, methods that are currently used as research tools to predict a high likelihood of the development of type 1 diabetes are reviewed. Serologic and genetic tests that predict the risk of type I diabetes have been covered in detail above.

Fasting plasma glucose and the oral glucose tolerance test
In 1997, an international working group of the ADA revised the guidelines for the diagnosis of diabetes mellitus previously set by the National Diabetes Data Group and the World Health Organization. The new guidelines had an impact in two major areas. First, the guidelines provide for the diagnosis of diabetes

Contact organizations for information on clinical trials and drug development			
Organization	Contact information	Web site	Notes
US National Institutes of Health	National Institute of Diabetes and Digestive and Kidney Disease (NIDDK) National Institutes of Health Building 31, Room 9A04 Bethesda, MD 20892 USA	clinicaltrials.gov www.niddk.nih.gov/patient/patient.htm#niddk	Searchable database for all clinical trials funded by the US National Institutes of Health
Immune Tolerance Network	5743 South Drexel Avenue Suite 200 Chicago, IL 60637 USA Tel: +1 773 834-4535 Fax: +1 773 834-4640	www.immunetolerance.org/patients/index.html	
Islet Trials Referral Service	Insulin-free World Foundation Islet Trials Registration Service 788 Office Parkway St Louis, MO 63141-7115 USA Tel: +1 888 746-4439 E-mail: Info@InsulinFree.org	www.diabetesportal.org	International index of islet transplantation trials
Veritas Medicine	238 Main Street Suite 501 Cambridge, MA 02142 Tel: +1 617 234-1500 Fax: +1 617 234-1555 E-mail: info@veritasmedicine.com	www.veritasmedicine.com/d_index.cfm	Searchable index on clinical trials for prevention and treatment; overview of new drugs under development

Table 21.3 Contact organizations for information on clinical trials and drug development.

for any random glucose of equal or greater than 200mg/dL (11.1mmol/L) in the presence of symptoms. The vast majority of patients with type 1 diabetes will meet this criterion. In instances for which the diagnosis is less certain, such as a high random plasma glucose value less than 200mg/dL in adults, the new guidelines replace the 75g oral glucose tolerance test (OGTT), the former gold standard in diagnosing diabetes, with measurement of fasting plasma glucose (FPG). This reflected the working group's opinion that the sensitivity and specificity of FPG was nearly equal to the OGTT but that it was far better in terms of ease of administration, convenience to the patient, and expense (note that the guidelines still include the use and interpretation of the OGTT). The working group also lowered the glycemic threshold from 140mg/dL (7.8mmol/L) to 126mg/dL (7mmol/L) for the diagnosis of diabetes. The value of 126mg/dL was chosen because previous research had shown an increased, linear risk of retinopathy above this concentration. It also correlated very well with a value of 200mg/dL (11.1mmol/L) or greater at the 2-hour timepoint in the OGTT.

Glycosylated hemoglobin and hemoglobin A$_{IC}$

Hemoglobin is glycosylated in a nonenzymatic, Schiff-base reaction. Hemoglobin A$_{IC}$, representing hemoglobin molecules with irreversible glycosylation, is the basis for the assay used during the Diabetes Control and Complications Trial (DCCT). Average blood glucose levels can be calculated by extrapolation from total glycosylated hemoglobin or any of its subfractions, providing an accurate and reliable estimate of glycemic control for the preceding 2–3 months because of the long half-life of red blood cells (120 days). Development and widespread use of this assay in the early 1980s revolutionized the monitoring of diabetic

American Diabetes Association diagnostic criteria for diabetes mellitus
Diabetes
Symptoms of diabetes plus random plasma glucose > 200mg/dL (11.1mmol/L)
OR
Fasting plasma glucose > 126mg/dL (7mmol/L), confirmed by repeat testing on a different day
OR
Plasma glucose > 200mg/dL (11.1mmol/L) at 2 hours after a 75g oral glucose challenge, confirmed by repeat testing on a different day. *This method is not recommended for routine clinical use.*
Impaired fasting glucose
Fasting plasma glucose 110–126mg/dL (6.1–7mmol/L)
Normal fasting glucose
Fasting plasma glucose <110mg/dL (6.1mmol/L)
Symptoms of diabetes include such classic symptoms as polyuria, polydipsia, and other acute manifestations of hyperglycemia. Fasting is defined as no caloric intake for at least 8 hours.

Table 21.4 American Diabetes Association diagnostic criteria for diabetes mellitus.

control. (Note: hemoglobin variants such as HbF, HbC, and HbS, undergo stable glycosylation with different kinetics; therefore, values from individuals with sickle-cell disease or sickle trait must be interpreted with caution).

In its 1997 report, the ADA Expert Committee did not allow for the measurement of total glycated hemoglobin or hemoglobin A$_{IC}$ for the diagnosis of diabetes mellitus. At the current time, there is a lack of a standard method, which precludes a single value being chosen as the cutoff between 'normal' and 'diabetic'. However, because this test reflects the average blood glucose concentration over a 2–3 month period, it is not infrequently used in clinical practice to confirm the diagnosis of diabetes mellitus. In 1995, Davidson and colleagues recommended simple guidelines for its use in screening for diabetes. If the value of the glycosylated hemoglobin is more than 1% above the upper limits of normal as reported by the user's reference lab, the specificity of the diagnosis of diabetes is 98%. If the value falls between the upper limits of normal and 1% above normal, there is a high likelihood of developing diabetes, and lifestyle changes as well as followup testing should be encouraged. Until a standard method of measuring and using total glycosylated hemoglobin is established, as suggested as a high priority by the Expert Committee, this represents a reasonable approach.

Fructosamine

Fructosamine represents glycosylated serum protein, 80% of which is albumin. The glycosylation reaction is the same as that described for glucose and hemoglobin. However, because the half-life of serum proteins is significantly shorter than that of red blood cells, fructosamine estimates glycemic control over a 1–3 week period. Fructosamine assays are even less standardized than those for glycosylated hemoglobin, with an even larger overlap between diabetic and normal values. Therefore, the ADA does not approve of the use of fructosamine for routine monitoring. There are two conditions where one might consider measuring fructosamine as an adjunct to usual methods of monitoring. One is in any condition where the half-life of red blood cells is considerably altered and/or glycosylation reactions have different kinetics, such as in sickle-cell disease. The second is pregnancy, where the need to establish near normal control often mandates frequent adjustments to therapy. In this case, the shorter time period reflected by fructosamine is advantageous when compared to the 2–3 months required for the measurement of glycosylated hemoglobin. This assay can also be used to demonstrate deterioration or improvement in short-term control of blood glucose levels during periods of major change in daily care. This is particularly important when questions of compliance with self-monitoring are at issue in adolescence.

C peptide

The connecting peptide (C peptide), a chain of 31 amino acids between the A and B chains of the insulin molecule, is an excellent measure of endogenous insulin secretion in healthy individuals. However, interpretation of C-peptide levels in the setting of diabetes is difficult, as considerable overlap exists between normal individuals, type 1 and type 2 diabetes, depending on the duration of disease and degree of control. Although children with type 1 diabetes who have entered metabolic remission in the 'honeymoon period' may recover β-cell function and the ability to secrete C peptide for a short time, the vast majority can produce no detectable C peptide by 2 years after diagnosis. Adults with type 1 diabetes are more likely to retain the ability to produce detectable C peptide for extended periods. Of note, those subjects in the DCCT with the highest quartile of C-peptide levels had significantly fewer episodes of hypoglycemia as well as a reduced risk for microvascular disease at the completion of the

study. In addition, measurement of C-peptide levels following the diagnosis of type 1 diabetes can be used to prognosticate the course of disease and risk of complications. However, at this time, this indication is reserved for clinical research trials.

Research

The following tests are currently used in research settings to predict the risk of type 1 diabetes or the onset of overt disease:

Autoantibodies

Antibodies to islet cells, insulin, glutamic acid decarboxylase (GAD), and the tyrosine phosphatases IA-2 and IA-2B are present in many patients with newly diagnosed type 1 diabetes. When used in combination, they can be highly sensitive and specific for predicting the risk of disease, particularly in family members of a diabetic patient. However, they are not currently used in clinical practice in the diagnosis of type 1 diabetes.

Human leukocyte antigens

Human leukocyte antigens located on chromosome 6 have been linked with the development of type 1 diabetes. In Caucasians, the prevalence of DR3 and DR4 alleles in patients with type 1 diabetes is disproportionately high when compared to the normal population. Like autoantigens, they can be used to predict the risk of development of type 1 diabetes in individuals known to be at high risk, but they are not useful in clinical practice for diagnosis.

First-phase insulin release

The intravenous glucose tolerance test is not used in the practical diagnosis of type 1 diabetes. However, when used to assess first-phase insulin response it is a sensitive tool to detect early β-cell failure. It is frequently used in clinical trials to predict the onset of overt disease in those subjects deemed at high risk because of autoantigen or HLA status. First-degree relatives of subjects with type 1 diabetes who have a first-phase insulin response below the first percentile (48mU/mL) have a significant risk of progressing to overt diabetes within 1 year. Adult relatives with a normal first-phase insulin response rarely go on to progress to diabetes. Although useful in a research setting or in predicting the need for exogenous insulin in individuals with impaired glucose tolerance, the intravenous glucose tolerance test is not used routinely in the diagnosis of diabetes mellitus.

CLINICAL MANIFESTATIONS

Systemic

Hyperglycemia below the renal threshold for glycemia (typically 180mg/dL (10mmol/L) in older children and young adults) may be tolerated without symptoms. However, when hyperglycemia is sustained above this level, an osmotic diuresis and polyuria lead to dehydration and a hyperosmolar state. In patients with undiagnosed diabetes, mild dehydration often leads to ingestion of large amounts of liquids (polydipsia). If the liquids are carbohydrate-containing (carbonated beverages or juices), hyperglycemia is exacerbated, leading to an ever-worsening cycle of urination and thirst. Weight loss is universally present, because of both fluid loss and catabolism of muscle and fat stores. Weight loss may be quite profound despite increased appetite and caloric intake (polyphagia). Excess breakdown of fatty acids as an alternative energy source produces increased circulating ketoacids, lowering plasma pH. The combination of energy deprivation, dehydration, and sleep deprivation because of significant nocturia leads to malaise and fatigue.

Sensory

Vision is often affected when hyperglycemia is sustained. Patients often complain of blurry vision or an inability to focus. Dry mucous membranes are partly responsible. However, in the setting of hyperglycemia, excess glucose and sorbitol are deposited in the lens. Subsequent osmotic swelling causes a distortion of light. In the first few weeks of treatment and normalization of blood glucose levels, these symptoms may actually worsen but will eventually, with sustained normoglycemia, abate. Infrequently, patients present with diplopia secondary to a palsy of the third or sixth cranial nerve.

Although typically considered a chronic complication, peripheral neuropathy, manifested by numbness or burning in hands and feet, can be present at the time of diagnosis.

Genitourinary

Women and adolescent girls with undiagnosed diabetes often present with recurrent or refractory candidal vaginitis secondary to hyperglycemia-induced overgrowth of yeast. Gynecologists will often suspect the diagnosis of diabetes in the setting of recurrent vaginal infections.

Immune

Wound healing may be poor in the setting of undiagnosed diabetes and hyperglycemia. *In vitro* studies have shown that elevated glucose leads to abnormal phagocytic action of neutrophils and macrophages. Decreased bactericidal activity can lead to altered host defense against pyogenic or mycobacterial infections.

Laboratory

At the time of diagnosis, new patients with type 1 diabetes may exhibit ketoacidosis with resultant acid–base and electrolyte disturbances. More commonly, however, young patients are diagnosed early because of increased public awareness of the symptoms of diabetes. In these cases, blood sugar levels over 400mg/dL (25mmol/L) can be seen without major acid–base disturbance. It is also typical for late-onset patients with type 1 diabetes to present with relatively mild laboratory abnormalities. The most common associated electrolyte abnormality is hyponatremia, which is often present because of the dilutional effect of hyperglycemia. The actual serum sodium can be estimated from the following calculation:

   $1.6 \times$ (actual serum glucose – 100mg/dL)/100
   + measured serum sodium = actual serum sodium.

Serum levels of potassium, phosphate, calcium, and magnesium are generally normal in the absence of acidosis; however, whole-body stores should be considered to be depleted in the presence of clinically apparent dehydration. Volume contraction may also lead to mild elevations in blood urea nitrogen and creatinine, and to a mild erythrocytosis. A leukocytosis may exist in the absence of infection. Triglyceride levels are often elevated. Urine glucose concentration is usually quite elevated.

Diabetic ketoacidosis

Despite an increasing frequency of early diagnosis, newly diagnosed patients with type 1 diabetes may present with acute metabolic decompensation and ketone production, leading to diabetic ketoacidosis (DKA). Although β-cell destruction occurs gradually over months or years before diagnosis, acute physical or emotional stress can create a physiologic demand for increased insulin production by temporarily increasing insulin resistance. In the setting of near-absolute insulin deficiency, alternate metabolic pathways are activated.

The pathophysiology of DKA can be summarized in the following way. Severe insulin deficiency leads to hyperglycemia and, following sufficient osmotic diuresis, hyperosmolarity. Unopposed glucagon action then leads to accelerated glycogenolysis and gluconeogenesis. Lipolysis leads to the production of free fatty acids and glycerol, which serve as the substrate for ketone production. Ketones are negatively charged molecules, and the body eventually depletes its buffering bases, leading to acidosis. The combination of dehydration and acid–base abnormalities leads to severe electrolyte disturbances.

Systemic

Most patients with DKA appear quite ill and weak. They can be hypothermic, and fever should suggest the presence of infection. They may be hypotensive, and poor skin turgor and orthostatic hypotension indicate significant dehydration. If the patient is able to give a history, symptoms of polyuria, polydipsia, and weight loss are invariably present. A classic 'fruity odor' may be present on the breath.

Cardiopulmonary

Tachycardia can be present and breathing can be deep and possibly labored (Kussmaul breathing). There is an increased risk of cardiac arrhythmias because of disordered electrolytes.

Gastrointestinal

Anorexia, nausea, and vomiting may be present. Abdominal pain may be severe; however, unless there are complicating factors present (such as ileus), the physical examination does not generally demonstrate underlying pathology.

Neurologic

Patients in DKA are generally lethargic but abnormalities may range from none to stupor or coma. Severe neurologic abnormalities are a poor prognostic sign.

Laboratory

Laboratory abnormalities in DKA are numerous and severe. In patients with normal renal blood flow, blood glucose ranges between 300 and 500mg/dL (17–28mmol/L). More severe hyperglycemia generally reflects poor renal perfusion and severe dehydration. Serum sodium can be low, as discussed above. However, in the setting of severe fluid losses it may be normal or high. Serum potassium may also be low, normal, or high. Acidemia causes movement of potassium from the intracellular to the extracellular space; therefore, initially in the course of DKA, potassium may be high. Normal or low potassium in severe DKA reflects significant total body losses of potassium and must be managed aggressively. Serum phosphate generally

Laboratory findings in diabetic ketoacidosis and hyperosmolar nonketotic coma		
	Diabetic ketoacidosis	Hyperosmolar nonketotic coma
Serum glucose	200–500mg/dL (11.1–28mmol/l)	500–2000mg/dL (28–110mmol/L)
Urine glucose	Strongly positive	Strongly positive
Serum acetone	Strongly positive	Negative
Urine ketones	Strongly positive	Trace positive
Anion gap	Increased (>30)	Normal/mildly increased
Arterial pH	Decreased (< 7.2)	Normal
Bicarbonate	Significantly decreased	Normal, decreased, increased
Sodium	Usually decreased	Usually increased
Potassium	Normal, decreased or increased	Normal or increased
BUN/creatinine	Usually increased	Increased
White blood cells	Usually increased	Usually increased

Table 21.5 Laboratory findings in diabetic ketoacidosis and hyperosmolar nonketotic coma. BUN, blood urea nitrogen.

follows the same pattern as serum potassium. A high anion gap acidosis is present with a low serum bicarbonate. The degree of acidosis may be mild or severe, with serum pH ranging from just below normal (7.3) to significantly low (6.8). Blood urea nitrogen is generally elevated as a reflection of hypovolemia. However, serum creatinine may be artificially elevated in the setting of acidosis and does not reflect renal pathology. Generally, this corrects quickly with treatment. As discussed above, an erythrocytosis and leukocytosis may be present.

The major ketones produced in DKA are β-hydroxybutyrate, acetoacetate, and acetone. β-hydroxybutyrate is produced in the highest amount and is the first to be cleared with correction of DKA. However, standard urine dipsticks do not detect β-hydroxybutyrate, only acetoacetate and acetone; therefore, at the time of presentation, they may read inappropriately low and actually worsen as ketonemia and ketonuria improve. Most laboratories measure serum acetone, which is generally high and falls with treatment.

Hyperosmolar nonketotic coma

Hyperosmolar nonketotic coma (HNK) is an uncommon presentation for patients with type 1 diabetes and is most often seen in frail, elderly patients with type 2 diabetes. However, in patients with late-onset diabetes or previously diagnosed younger patients with type 1 diabetes, ketone production may be avoided because of small amounts of circulating insulin. In these cases, it is possible to have severe hyperglycemia and hyperosmolarity without acid–base disturbances. The clinical presentation is similar to that described for DKA but the serum glucose concentration is generally much higher, from 500–2000mg/dL (30–110mmol/L). Because many of these patients have comorbid conditions, such as cardiovascular or cerebrovascular disease, they must be carefully evaluated for other causes of hypoperfusion and/or neurologic deficits.

The major laboratory abnormalities for DKA and HNK are summarized in **Table 21.5**.

Late-onset type 1 diabetes

At one time it was considered rare for patients with type 1 diabetes to present over the age of 30. However, with sophisticated testing of serologic markers, we now know that up to 10% of all patients initially classified as having type 2 diabetes will be autoantibody-positive (especially ICA and GAD antibodies). Moreover, these patients generally have a lesser response to insulin secretagogues than those with type 2 diabetes, and have an increased frequency of high-risk *HLA* alleles. This group with late-onset type 1 diabetes has also been termed 'latent autoimmune diabetes of adulthood'. Indeed, we now believe that the age of onset of type 1 diabetes spans the lifetime. Generally, children and younger adults have a more acute presentation, with metabolic decompensation, as described above. However, late-onset patients in general have a much more subtle presentation and are often misdiagnosed with type 2 diabetes.

Many patients with late-onset diabetes initially do well with oral hypoglycemic treatment alone. However, there are several important clinical differences, which predict rapid failure and subsequent requirement of insulin therapy. The most notable feature is that these patients are thin and generally active, compared to their obese, sedentary counterparts with type 2 diabetes. In addition, a family history of insulin-requiring or insulin-dependent diabetes with onset in adulthood is often present. Indeed, in 2000, Vauhkonen and colleagues reported that, as expected, insulin-secretory capacity is diminished in patients with late-onset type 1 diabetes compared to type 2. However, they were also able to demonstrate, with a hyperglycemic clamp technique, that insulin-secretory capacity is diminished in their nondiabetic offspring, leading them to conclude that late-onset type 1 diabetes is a familial disease. Importantly, despite evidence of absolute insulin deficiency, patients with late-onset disease are usually not prone to ketosis.

TREATMENT

Insulin replacement therapy, either by injection or by transplantation of pancreatic tissue or islet cells, is the only available treatment for type 1 diabetes. Although alternative methods of insulin delivery are in the later stages of development, injection of insulin remains the mainstay of therapy. This section will review the various types of insulin and current methods of administration, as well as the more promising therapies under investigation in clinical trials.

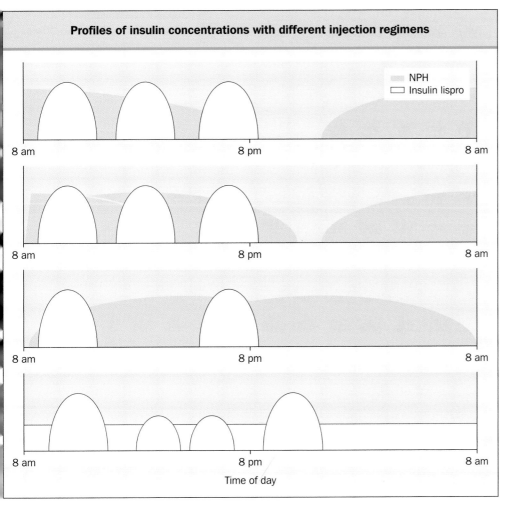

Profiles of insulin concentrations with different injection regimens

NPH
Insulin lispro

8 am 8 pm 8 am

8 am 8 pm 8 am

8 am 8 pm 8 am

8 am 8 pm 8 am

Time of day

Figure 21.4 Profiles of insulin concentrations with varying injection regimens. (Top two panels) Multiple daily injections with either NPH (isophane insulin) at bedtime alone (top panel) or with breakfast (second panel) and insulin lispro with meals. (Third panel) Split-mixed NPH and short-acting insulin twice a day. (Bottom panel) Continuous subcutaneous insulin infusion (insulin pump therapy) with insulin lispro.

Recombinant human insulins

When recombinant human insulin became commercially available in the early 1980s, it virtually replaced the purified pork or beef insulins that had been in use before that time. Recombinant insulin is synthesized in genetically engineered *Escherichia coli* bacteria that have received the insulin gene. By modifying the insulin protein with the addition of protamine or zinc, the half-life can be lengthened, thereby providing insulin with differing peaks and durations of action. In the USA, human insulins currently include one short-acting type – regular (known in the UK as neutral or soluble insulin), two intermediate-acting types – NPH (isophane insulin) and lente, and one long-acting type (ultralente).

The most physiologic regimen of injected insulin is achieved with multiple daily injections, which entails one or two injections of intermediate- or long-acting insulin, and short-acting insulin with meals each day. At least one of the longer-acting insulin injections is at bedtime to counteract the early morning insulin resistance (the dawn phenomenon) that results from higher levels of counterregulatory hormones, specifically cortisol and growth hormone. Examples of insulin levels that result from these regimens are shown in the top two panels of **Figure 21.4**. Although less physiologic, adequate control can occasionally be achieved with two injections per day, with a mixture of short and long or intermediate insulins before breakfast and the evening

meal. This profile is shown in the third panel. As can be seen, the major disadvantage of this regimen is the high levels of intermediate-acting insulin, which peak in the late afternoon and during sleep, leading to an increased incidence of hypoglycemia. There are several premixed, fixed-ratio (biphasic) insulins also available, which are a mixture of NPH (isophane insulin) and regular (soluble) insulin. Because patients with type 1 diabetes often need small adjustments to one type of insulin and not the second, fixed-ration insulins are not recommended for use in this population.

Insulin analogs

The first insulin analog, insulin lispro, is commercially available in the USA and the UK. It is a synthetically modified insulin molecule in which the amino acids at positions 28 and 29 on the B chain are switched (lysine for proline). This change prevents the formation of hexamers and hence a more rapid onset of action, peak, and clearance (**Fig. 21.5**). For patients with type 1 diabetes who must typically inject regular (neutral soluble) insulin 30–45min prior to eating, this leads to a major improvement in compliance and convenience. In addition, insulin lispro levels tend to peak when postprandial glucose levels are highest, leading to a more physiologic control of blood glucose levels. Likewise, levels of insulin lispro are generally lower than regular insulin several hours after injection, leading to less premeal

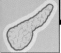

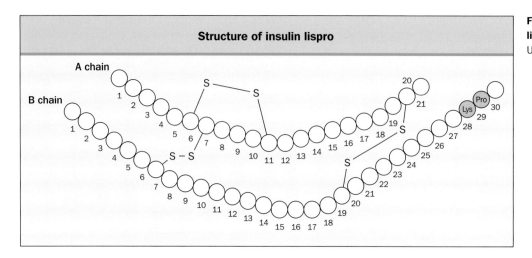

Table 21.6 Recombinant human insulin and insulin analogs.

Recombinant human insulin and insulin analogs

	Onset of action	Peak	Duration	Can be mixed with other insulins
Insulin lispro	5–15min	60min	4 hours	Yes
Insulin aspart	5–15min	60min	4 hours	Yes
Regular (soluble)	30–60min	2 hours	6 hours	Yes
Lente	2–4 hours	6–12 hours	18–24 hours	Yes
NPH (isophane insulin)	2–4 hours	6–12 hours	18–24 hours	Yes
Insulin glargine	4 hours	Peakless	24 hours	No
Ultralente	6–12 hours	18 hours	36 hours	Yes

hypoglycemia. It is an ideal insulin for use in insulin pumps. Currently, insulin lispro is the only rapid-acting insulin analog available; however, a second analog, insulin aspart, is available also in the UK and is expected to be available in the near future in the USA.

An insulin analog with intermediate to long action is also now available for clinical use. Its properties and kinetic profile are similar to insulin lispro. Insulin glargine has been modified by substituting a glycine for aspartic acid at position 21 on the A chain and adding arginine residues to the C-terminal end of the B chain. These changes make the molecule significantly more acidic than human insulin, resulting in crystallization and depot formation when injected into physiologically neutral subcutaneous tissue. After 4 hours, insulin glargine is slowly and consistently released into circulation. Its duration of action is approximately 24 hours, making it an ideal, peakless, once-daily basal insulin. Because of its acidic pH, it may not be mixed with other another insulin in the same syringe. Likewise, its acidity caused an increased incidence of pain at the injection site during clinical trials. Insulin glargine will add considerably to the options of type 1 diabetic patients on mixed insulin regimens.

The profiles of recombinant human insulins and insulin analogs are listed in **Table 21.6**.

Continuous subcutaneous insulin infusion

The most physiologic method of delivering insulin available at this time is by continuous subcutaneous infusion, more commonly referred to as insulin pump therapy. There are several models of pumps available in the USA and Europe; however, they all share the same basic features in insulin delivery. Pumps infuse either insulin lispro or buffered regular (neutral soluble) insulin, which is contained in a cartridge with a capacity of several milliliters. The pumps contain sophisticated programs that allow for the delivery of insulin continuously (basal infusion) at variable rates throughout any 24-hour period (usually between 0.5–1.0u/h). For example, if patients have a tendency to become hypoglycemic during the early morning hours, the basal rate may be set to deliver as little as 0.1u/h. Similarly, at times of higher insulin need (e.g. the dawn phenomenon), insulin delivery can be programmed for a higher rate. All pumps have the capacity to program temporary basal rates, as may be required during times of illness, on certain days of the menstrual cycle, or during times of increased activity. Although these features allow for glycemic control in a very narrow, near-normal range, most patients prefer pump therapy for the convenience of bolus therapy for meals and snacks (**Fig. 21.4**, bottom panel). Insulin need is calculated by determining the amount of carbohydrate in a given meal and using a preset ratio (more insulin for carbohydrates for more obese or insulin-resistant subjects, and less for thinner or more insulin sensitive patients). Patients therefore have the freedom to eat what and when they like. For those who have been on a fixed-carbohydrate diet with set mealtimes, this is a significant advantage.

The pump is connected to the body by thin plastic tubing and a small subcutaneous catheter. The catheter must be changed every 3 days and the insulin in the cartridge or the cartridge itself and tubing every 6 days, to minimize site infections. The major disadvantages of pump therapy are expense and technical difficulties, and pump users must be carefully screened for motivation, sophistication, and financial status prior to selection. There are cases where short-term pump therapy is advised, such as pregnancy (see below).

Pancreas transplantation

Although not widely used as a standard therapy, transplantation of all or part of the pancreas is becoming more frequent. Pancreas transplantation can successfully lead to euglycemia and the elimination of insulin injections, thereby improving the quality of life of patients with type 1 diabetes. Moreover, pancreas transplantation has been shown to stabilize or reverse microvascular complications. Because of the need for immunosuppression, the majority of pancreas transplants are performed in those patients who require a simultaneous kidney transplant or who have previously undergone kidney transplantation. Graft failure may be either secondary to rejection or by recurrence of autoimmune insulitis. Data reported from the International Pancreas Transplant Registry included an overall 1-year patient survival of 91% and a 1-year insulin-independence rate of 74%. The rate of the latter will undoubtedly continue to improve with further advances in immunosuppressive and immunomodulatory therapy.

Islet cell transplantation

The transplantation of islet cells as therapy for type 1 diabetes has been attempted for the past two decades. However, success has been quite limited. Most trials reported a graft survival rate of less than 10% at 1 year. In the spring of 2000, however, Shapiro and colleagues from the University of Alberta, Edmonton, reported a 100% incidence of insulin independence in a small number of subjects who had received cadaveric islet cells. Their protocol differed substantially from others in the avoidance of glucocorticoids, which are toxic to β cells. In addition, after harvesting, the use of nonhuman proteins (specifically fetal calf serum) was avoided, as this may have led to an enhanced host immune response against transplanted cells in previous attempts. Notably, the procedure is minimally invasive and involves a percutaneous catheter placed into the portal vein for dispersal of approximately 10mL of islet cells. The early success of this group has captured the attention of leading diabetes groups and funding agencies on an international level. Attempts are under way at this time to expand this research and verify its results in additional sites (the Immune Tolerance Network). However, even with such promise, the very limited number of human islet cells available for transplantation (two cadaveric donors were required for each subject) and the need for lifelong immunosuppression will preclude its use in a large number of patients until such barriers can be lowered. Future goals will be to develop additional sources of functional β cells (porcine islets, conversion of stem cells, or genetically engineered β cells) and improved methods of immune isolation (microcapsules and inhibitors of cytokine damage).

TREATMENT OF ACUTE DIABETIC COMPLICATIONS

Therapy for diabetic ketoacidosis and hyperosmolar nonketotic coma

Severe DKA and HNK are life-threatening emergencies and should be approached as such. A detailed description of the standard protocols in use at most institutions is beyond the scope of this chapter. However, the mainstay of therapy in both disorders is intravenous fluid replacement and intravenous insulin. Frequent monitoring of vital signs, laboratory abnormalities, and volume status is best accomplished in an intensive care setting. In addition, the practitioner should recognize that these critical states are reached after days, or weeks, of metabolic deterioration; therefore, care should be taken to avoid overly rapid correction, especially of hypernatremia. In the treatment of DKA, measuring the anion gap every 3–4 hours until it normalizes, or 'closes', is an effective way of monitoring therapy of acid–base status. In addition, as this generally lags behind correction of hyperglycemia, when serum glucose concentration falls below 200mg/dL (11.1mmol/L), intravenous insulin should not be stopped. Instead, at that time dextrose can be added to the intravenous solution. In both DKA and HNK, electrolytes must be monitored frequently (no less than every 6 hours) and replaced if needed.

Hypoglycemia

The most effective treatment of hypoglycemia is prevention. However, in intensively controlled patients with type 1 diabetes, two or three mild (not requiring the assistance of a third party and no loss of consciousness) episodes per week can be expected. In addition, the risk of a severe episode (requiring the assistance of a third party or loss of consciousness) is approximately one for every patient-year of treatment. For this reason, both patients and their families must be trained in recognition and treatment. All patients should carry both rapid-acting glucose and identification of their diabetes (such as a MedicAlert bracelet) at all times. In addition, in the event of loss of consciousness, family members should be trained to inject glucagon and provide supportive care until the arrival of emergency medical assistance. For patients with a history of frequent, severe hypoglycemia, or hypoglycemic unawareness, glycemic goals should be adjusted upward.

CLINICAL OUTCOMES

Outcome of intensive control during pregnancy

Before the introduction of home glucose monitoring, intensive control of type 1 diabetes throughout pregnancy was not practical or possible. Despite its expense and impracticality, pregnant women with type 1 diabetes were routinely hospitalized for the latter part of the third trimester. Despite such actions, the prevalence of diabetes-related complications of pregnancy to both the mother and her infant remained extremely high. However, with the advent of home glucose monitoring, normoglycemia became possible and its impact during the preconception period and during each trimester has been examined.

In animal models the negative impact of high glucose levels on organogenesis has been shown. Likewise, in retrospective and prospective human trials, it is known that the higher the glucose level during the first trimester, the greater the likelihood of congenital anomalies. It is thought that glucose is directly toxic to developing tissues. Moreover, no organ system is unaffected by this phenomenon, as all are represented by congenital defects in human infants. Importantly, the risk of congenital anomalies can be lowered to that of nondiabetic pregnant women by keeping serum glucose levels as near normal as possible. In addition, the most crucial time for a woman with type 1 diabetes to establish tight glycemic control is in the preconception period. Unfortunately, whether or not a woman with type 1 diabetes receives preconception counseling is highly dependent on socioeconomic factors such as ethnicity, level of education, and financial status. It has been proven to be cost-effective; the expense of diabetes education and increased obstetric and medical care is far outweighed by the cost of obstetric complications, or corrective therapy and care for an infant with a congenital anomaly.

Hyperglycemia in the second and third trimesters have been associated with medical complications affecting both mother and child. Hyperglycemia in the fetus causes neonatal complications that can be divided roughly into two categories: excessive growth and abnormal metabolism. In the former, maternal glucose freely crosses the placental membrane and resultant fetal hyperglycemia causes hypertrophy and hyperplasia of fetal islet cells. Insulin, along with IGF-2, is a major neonatal growth factor. However, infants of mothers with poor glycemic control are not only large for gestational age but have an abnormal amount and distribution of body fat, causing them to be 'macrosomic'. Excessive body fat in the trunk of the infant of a mother with diabetes results in obstetric complications (fetal–pelvic disproportion leading to cesarean section or maternal trauma) or neonatal complications (shoulder dystocia or brachial plexus injury). Several studies have shown a significant reduction in such complications when maternal glycemia was normalized, although this concept remains somewhat controversial.

Fetal hyperinsulinemia also leads to metabolic disturbances in the neonatal period, most notably hypoglycemia. However, electrolyte disturbances such as neonatal hypokalemia and hypomagnesemia are also associated with maternal hyperglycemia. Other neonatal disorders such as polycythemia, hyperbilirubinemia, and renal vein thrombosis are thought to occur with increased frequency in women with poorly controlled glucose levels because of resultant fetal hypoxia. The most devastating complication during pregnancy in women with type 1 diabetes, sudden intrauterine fetal demise, may occur because of sudden shifts in fetal electrolytes and resultant arrhythmias. For this reason, even with exceptional glycemic control, most women will have labor pharmacologically induced or undergo elective cesarean section at between 36 and 37 weeks gestation.

Because of the risk of multiple complications, the pregnant woman with type 1 diabetes is best served by a multidisciplinary team consisting of a maternal-fetal medicine specialist, endocrinologist, nurse practitioner, dietician, and social worker. In addition, women with type 1 diabetes must be closely monitored for acceleration of microvascular disease during pregnancy. Recommendations include dilated funduscopic examinations in the preconception period and during the second and third trimesters, and 24-hour urine collections for microalbuminuria, total protein, and creatinine clearance in the preconception period and during each trimester. With careful monitoring and a team approach, women with type 1 diabetes can expect to deliver a healthy infant with minimal complications of their own disease.

The standards of care for monitoring type 1 diabetes during pregnancy are outlined in **Table 21.7**.

Monitoring of type 1 diabetes during pregnancy					
Test	**Preconception**	**1st trimester**	**2nd trimester**	**3rd trimester**	**Postpartum**
Hemoglobin A$_{1c}$	X (target normal range)	X (maintain normal range)	X (maintain normal range)	X (maintain normal range)	X
Albumin:creatinine ratio or 24-hour urine*	X	X	X	X	X
Funduscopic exam	X		X	X	X
Electrocardiogram or echocardiogram	If symptoms or multiple risk-factors present				
Thyroid-stimulating hormone	X	X†	X		X
Complete blood count	X				
Fetal surveillance		X	X	X	
Social assessment	X			X	X
Dietary assessment	X	X	X	X	

* Albumin:creatinine ratio for patients with no microalbuminuria; 24-hour urine if preexisting renal disease present or if proteinuria develops.

† Repeat each trimester if preexisting thyroid disease present or if symptoms of hypo- or hyperthyroidism develop.

Table 21.7 Monitoring of type 1 diabetes during pregnancy.

Table 21.8 Major vascular complications.

Major vascular complications of diabetes	
Retinopathy	**Peripheral vascular disease**
Nonproliferative	Claudication
Proliferative	Poor wound healing → amputations
Impaired vision → blindness	Erectile dysfunction
Nephropathy	May involve small or large vessels
Microalbuminuria (30–300mg/dL or 20–200µg/min or above 30mg/g creatinine)	**Cardiovascular disease**
Gross proteinuria (>300mg/day)	Hypertension – in type 1 diabetes usually associated with the onset of nephropathy
Reduced glomerular filtration rate	Myocardial infarction
Hyporeninemic hypoaldosteronism	Stroke
End-stage renal disease	Cardiomyopathy and congestive heart failure
Neuropathy	Cardiovascular disease etiology is multifactorial, involving glucose control, blood pressure levels, presence of hyperlipidemia, genetic factors, and smoking history.
Symmetric distal or proximal	
Asymmetric proximal	
Combined	
Can lead to loss of sensation resulting in ulcers → osteomyelitis amputations and Charcot neuropathic arthropathy or severe pain	
Autonomic insufficiency can result in bladder, gastric, and bowel abnormalities	

CHRONIC COMPLICATIONS

Vascular complications are the major causes of long-term morbidity and mortality in people with type 1 diabetes (**Table 21.8**). The microvascular complications, including retinopathy, neuropathy, and nephropathy, are clearly directly associated with glycemic control. The risk of macrovascular disease, including coronary artery disease, cerebral vascular disease, and peripheral vascular disease, although associated with glycemic control, clearly involves other factors such as smoking, blood pressure, and lipid levels. Macrovascular disease will be covered in detail in Chapter 22.

Microvascular complications
Role of glucose
The clearest example of the role of glycemic control in the development and progression of long-term complications came from the landmark Diabetes Control and Complications Trial. In this prospective trial patients with type 1 diabetes were randomly assigned to receive either conventional insulin therapy or intensive insulin therapy consisting of continuous insulin administration using an insulin pump or multiple daily injections. The mean HbA_{IC} values were 7.2% over 9 years in the intensive group compared to 9.1% in the conventional group.

Intensive insulin treatment in the DCCT study reduced the risk of development and progression of retinopathy by 63%, nephropathy by 54%, and neuropathy by 60%.

Many additional studies have clearly implicated poor glucose control as reflected by elevated HbA_{IC} levels and risk of vascular complications. Very recent evidence indicates that improved glycemic control reduces health-care costs and utilization. It now appears that there is no threshold effect of HgA_{IC} in this relationship. A new study (EPIC-Norfolk) shows that glycated hemoglobin concentrations can explain much of the excess mortality in diabetic men and appears to be a continuous risk factor through the whole population for cardiovascular disease.

It is beyond the scope of this chapter to review the existing knowledge of how elevated glucose leads to vascular complications. However, it is clear that certain pathways – including increased oxidative stress, advanced glycation end-products, inflammatory and lipid oxidation products, altered ion metabolism, and activation of kinases such as protein kinase C – play key roles in the process. Genetics and ethnic background also affect one's risk for development of these complications. In the DCCT study, for example, familial clustering was seen for risk of retinopathy and nephropathy. With the completion of the human genome project in 2000 there is great optimism that we will soon have new ways to predict and treat these devastating complications.

Macrovascular disease
People with type 1 diabetes have an increased risk of macrovascular disease but, as mentioned earlier, the risk is due to several factors in addition to elevated glucose. The DCCT trial found a nonsignificant trend towards less cardiovascular disease in the intensive treatment group. A follow up of the DCCT found no effect of intensive insulin treatment on carotid artery wall thickness, a surrogate for atherosclerotic changes. Ongoing mechanistic studies in animal models and in humans are evaluating the role of insulin resistance, obesity, and interactions with lipids on the risk of cardiovascular disease in type 1 diabetes. By the end of 2001 studies should be available to address this important issue. However, it is clear from studies in a porcine model of accelerated coronary artery disease due to type 1 diabetes that elevated cholesterol clearly interacts with elevated glucose to markedly increase the progression of atherosclerosis through inflammatory lipid pathway mediators such as lipoxygenase enzymes.

Guidelines for diabetes care		
Parameter	Goal	Testing frequency
Glycemic control		
Whole blood glucose		
Preprandial	80–120mg/dL (4.4–6.7mmol/L)	
Average bedtime	100–140 (5.6–7.8mmol/L)	
Hemoglobin A_{1c} (%)	< 7	Every 3 months*
Lipids		
LDL cholesterol	< 100mg/dL (2.6mmol/L)	Annual*
HDL cholesterol	> 45 (1.2mmol/L)	Annual*
Triglycerides	< 200mg/dL (2.2mmol/L)	Annual*
Renal parameters		
Urinary microalbuminuria	< 30mg/g creatinine or <20µg/min	Annual*
Glomerular filtration rate	Can be measured as indicated in specific case	Annual*
Serum creatinine		
Serum BUN and K^+		
Eyes		Annual*
Dilated eye exam		
Blood pressure (mmHg)	< 130/80	Every 6 months
Foot examination		Every 6 months
Smoking cessation		As indicated
Cardiac testing (exercise stress testing, stress perfusion imaging, stress echo, or catherization)	Indicated in people with known disease as appropriate. In addition indicated without prior history of coronary disease indicated if: • Typical or atypical cardiac symptoms. • Resting electrocardiogram showing ischemia or old myocardial infarction • Peripheral or carotid occlusive arterial disease • Sedentary lifestyle, age > 35, or two or more risk factors: total cholesterol > 240mg/dL (6.2mmol/L), LDL > 160mg/dL (4.1mmol/L), or HDL < 35mg/dL (0.91mmol/L); BP > 140/90mm/Hg, smoking, positive family history of premature coronary disease, positive microalbuminuria	

NB: Serum magnesium should be measured in patients at high risk of magnesium deficiency and, if low, should be corrected by diet or supplements.
* The interval for testing varies based on age of diagnosis of diabetes. See Clinical Practice Guidelines. *Diabetes Care* 2001;24(suppl. 1).

Table 21.9 Guidelines for diabetes care. BUN, blood urea nitrogen; HDL, high-density lipoprotein; LDL, low-density lipoprotein.

General recommendations

Specific treatment recommendations will be mentioned in each section on microvascular complications. However, in the January 2001 issue of *Diabetes Care*, the ADA annually presents its 'clinical practice recommendations'. The recommendations for 2001 were published in volume 24, supplement 1. The new changes in these recommendations pertinent to complications in type 1 diabetes are as follows:

• For adult patients with diabetes the blood pressure goal has been lowered to less than 130/80mmHg.
• Aspirin can be useful in prevention of cardiovascular complications even in diabetic patients with hypertension (Hypertension Optimal Treatment Trial).
• Prepubertal duration of diabetes may be an important factor in the development of microvascular complications.

The guidelines for care are shown in **Table 21.9**.

The issue of how tight blood sugar control should be cannot be dictated for every patient. Individual decisions between the patient and health-care professionals involved need to be carefully made in order to maximize the protective benefits without jeopardizing the patient's health by inducing severe or frequent hypoglycemic episodes. The continued improvements in glycemic control described in this chapter will make it easier and safer to achieve these goals. However, until islet transplantation is proved

to be safe and effective, and is more widely available, we, as health care professionals, will need to deal with these important issues.

Retinopathy

Retinopathy is a major cause of morbidity in people with diabetes. The incidence of blindness in patients with diabetes is 25 times higher than people in the general population.

Screening for retinopathy is very important, since symptoms do not usually develop until the very late stages when treatment may be much less effective. Sometimes patients complain of fluctuating vision, blurred vision or 'floaters'. The Wisconsin Epidemiology Study of Diabetic Retinopathy has taught us much of the natural history of this complication:

• Retinopathy begins to occur in patients with type 1 diabetes 3–5 years after diagnosis.
• Prevalence increases with disease duration: proliferative eye disease was seen in 1.2% at 5 years, 56% at 15 years, and 67% at 35 years in younger-onset patients with diabetes.

As described earlier from the DCCT trial, good glycemic control reduces the development and progression of retinopathy. Other factors, such as good control of blood pressure and photocoagulation therapy, can reduce the progression to severe visual loss. These trials have also confirmed the clinical observation that one can see a transient worsening of retinopathy after tight blood sugar control. This can be seen for up to 1 year and may be due to closing off of small retinal vessels or changes in local growth factors. As described earlier in the chapter, retinopathy can also worsen during pregnancy.

Retinopathy is often classified as nonproliferative or proliferative, with grading to indicate severity. There have been major advances over the last several years in understanding the metabolic, molecular, and histologic changes at the various stages of retinopathy. For instance, we now know that retinal pericytes and microvascular endothelial cells drop out at an early stage in the disease. Thickening of the retinal basement membrane is another early change similar to that seen in the kidney. The death of these pericytes and endothelial cells is associated with development of the retinal capillary microaneurysms and increased vascular permeability, in part through generation of potent vasoactive lipids and growth factors such as vascular endothelial growth factor.

Figure 21.6 shows early background retinopathy with microaneurysms and intraretinal infarcts, also known as 'soft' exudates

or 'cotton wool spots', which can occur distal to vascular occlusion. This stage of disease is also associated with flame or blot hemorrhages. More severe ischemia results in proliferation of endothelial cells and vasoproliferation with neovascularization. This is known as proliferative diabetic retinopathy. Severe nonproliferative retinopathy with venous beading and intra-retinal microvascular abnormalities are shown in **Figure 21.7**. **Figure 21.8** shows a more severe case of proliferative diabetic retinopathy. These new vessels are weak and are prone to rupture, resulting in bleeding. As they mature the vessels can have a fibrous network, causing contraction resulting in retinal distortion. Acute glaucoma can also arise if the proliferation blocks the outflow of aqueous humor. **Figure 21.9** shows an even more advanced stage of proliferative retinopathy with preretinal and vitreous hemorrhage.

Diabetic macular edema results from an accumulation of extracellular lipid, fluid, and protein in the macular region of the retina. This does not cause total blindness like vitreous hemorrhage and retinal detachment do, but leads to a loss of central vision, with reading and driving difficulties.

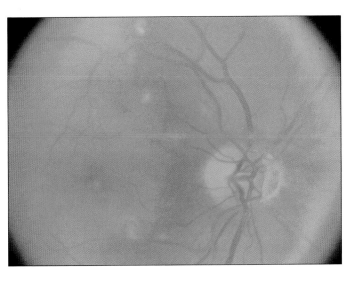

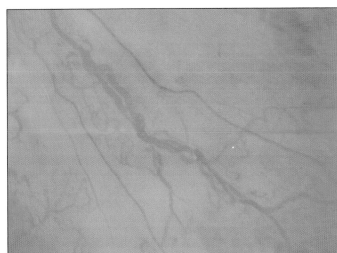

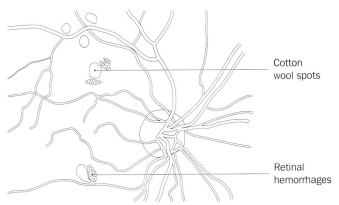

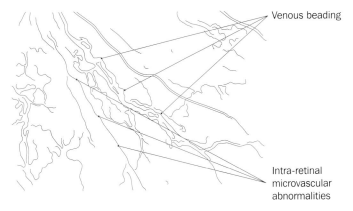

Figure 21.6 Background diabetic retinopathy with cotton-wool spots and retinal hemorrhages. (Courtesy of Dr James Tiedeman.)

Figure 21.7 Severe non-proliferative retinopathy with venous beading and intra-retinal microvascular abnormalities. (Courtesy of Dr James Tiedeman.)

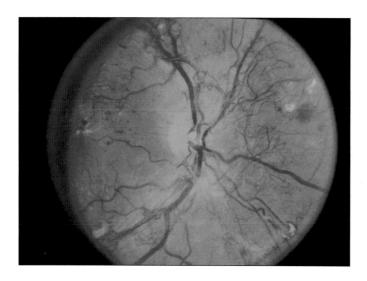

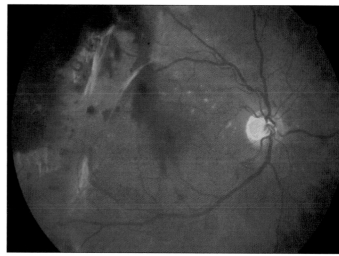

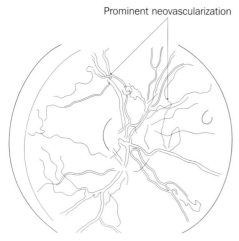

Prominent neovascularization

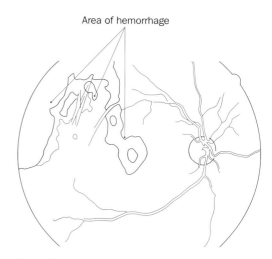

Area of hemorrhage

Figure 21.8 Proliferative diabetic retinopathy with prominent neovascularization arising from disc and adjacent vessels. (Courtesy of Dr James Tiedeman.)

Figure 21.9 Proliferative diabetic retinopathy with preretinal and vitreous hemorrhage. (Courtesy of Dr James Tiedeman.)

There have been advances in diagnosing and managing eye disease. Evidence shows that screening annually for those without retinopathy and every 6 months for those with retinopathy, with appropriate treatment by an experienced ophthalmologist, would result in up to 80,000 more person-years of sight in the USA alone. Fluorescein angiography is sometimes helpful in evaluating areas of vessel nonperfusion. An example of this angiogram is shown in **Figure 21.10**. Control of blood pressure is very important, especially in the reduction of the development and progression of retinopathy. Additional studies will need to be performed to show definitively an advantage of one class of medication over another.

Aspirin use has not been shown to be protective; however, it can be safely used in patients with preexisting retinopathy to reduce the risk of cardiovascular disease. Photocoagulation is the main treatment modality that has been shown in studies to reduce the risk of severe visual loss. Studies have addressed the issue of whether early, extensive, panretinal laser photocoagulation is beneficial. Early photocoagulation may not be indicated in all cases since visual acuity and peripheral vision may be reduced.

Laser treatment may not always halt new vessel formation and if this persists extensive vitreous hemorrhage or retinal detachment could result in blindness. Therefore, carefully timed removal of the opaque vitreous humor followed by photocoagulation to the retina can restore some vision. Timing of this vitreous surgery before extensive retinal detachment has occurred maximizes the benefits.

Therefore, close monitoring by an experienced ophthalmologist is needed in these patients.

Nephropathy

Diabetes is the leading cause of end-stage renal disease in the USA. Almost 45% of patients with type 1 diabetes in the USA will develop dipstick-positive proteinuria during their lifetime. In contrast, the rates of nephropathy have been reduced in Europe because of better glucose and blood pressure control. The peak onset is 10–15 years after diabetes onset. A number of risk factors have been identified in addition to elevated glucose. There are clearly genetic factors that play a role. For instance, the risk of nephropathy is markedly increased when a sibling or parent has diabetic nephropathy. Angiotensin-converting enzyme

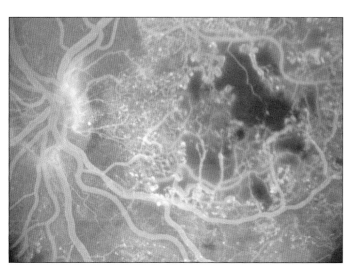

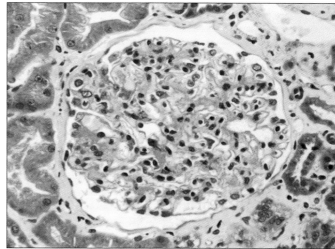

Glomerulus

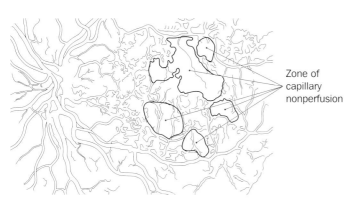

Zone of
capillary
nonperfusion

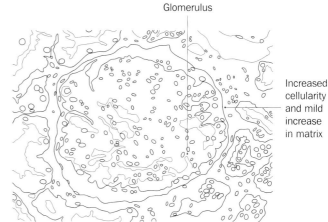

Increased
cellularity
and mild
increase
in matrix

Figure 21.10 Fluorescein angiogram demonstrating nonperfusion of macular capillaries. (Courtesy of Dr James Tiedeman.)

Figure 21.11 Early diabetic glomerulopathy with slight hypercellularity and mild increase in mesangial matrix. Hematoxylin/eosin stain. (Courtesy of Dr Benjamin Sturgill.)

(ACE) genotype may confer an increased risk. Elevated blood pressure, smoking, and elevated glomerular filtration rate also increase the risk of subsequent clinically significant nephropathy in type 1 diabetes.

One should be aware that disorders other than diabetes can lead to proteinuria and renal functional changes. These other etiologies should be considered when overt proteinuria develops less than 5 years after disease onset, in the presence of active urine sediment with red cells and casts, when there is acute onset of disease, or in the absence of other microvascular complications.

A 24-hour urine is the gold standard for evaluating microalbuminuria and this test can also provide information on glomerular filtration rate. One could also use a shorter-timed collection or spot urine albumin to creatinine ratio. The latter test offers the advantages of ease of collection and less interference by volume. An albumin to creatine ratio above 30μg/mg indicates microalbuminuria. One should note that vigorous exercise or fever can produce elevated albumin levels in the absence of diabetic kidney disease. Therefore, confirmation of microalbuminuria should be performed.

Microalbuminuria is the earliest sign of diabetic nephropathy. Approximately 50% of these people with type 1 diabetes are at risk for progression. People with early-onset diabetes and microalbuminuria have the greatest risk of progression. Blood pressure elevations typically do not occur until year 3 or 4 of microalbuminuria unless there is another reason for the rise in blood pressure. The natural history of renal disease in patients receiving intensive glucose control may be different, since a few of these patients studied in followup analysis to the DCCT developed increases in blood pressure before rises in albuminuria.

New evidence suggests that the presence of microalbuminuria is also a risk factor for cardiovascular disease. The mechanism for this relationship is not clear; however, studies suggest that increases in homocysteine, more atherogenic lipid patterns, or changes in vascular permeability could be factors.

The pathologic changes shown in **Figures 21.11–21.16** represent early to later histologic changes in diabetic nephropathy. Thickened basement membrane and increases in mesangial matrix are early findings, with some increase in cellularity. Eventually the nodular glomerulosclerosis described by Kimmelsteil and Wilson develops. With the glomerular changes, tubulointerstitial changes also develop. These include mononuclear cell infiltrates and tubular fibrosis and atrophy. The kidneys typically enlarge, and with end-stage disease they get smaller.

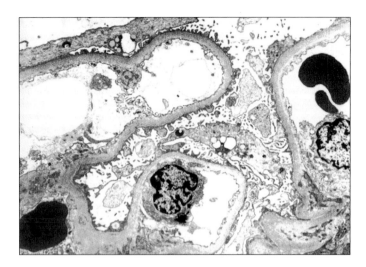

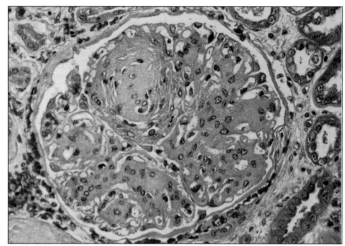

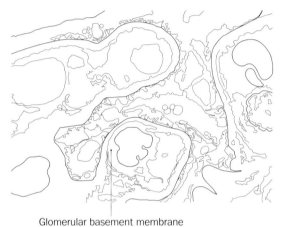

Glomerular basement membrane

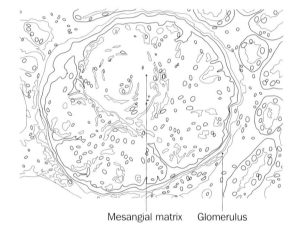

Mesangial matrix   Glomerulus

Figure 21.12 Electron micrograph showing slight thickening of glomerular basement membranes as seen in early diabetic glomerulopathy. (Courtesy of Dr Benjamin Sturgill.)

Figure 21.13 Marked increase in mesangial matrix with a nodule at 11 o'clock. The glomerulus is still somewhat cellular. Hematoxylin/eosin stain. (Courtesy of Dr Benjamin Sturgill.)

Much can be done to reduce the progression of kidney disease if it is treated early. Treatment includes:
- **Glucose control**. The DCCT has clearly demonstrated the primary and secondary benefits of glucose control. Evidence shows that early initiation of glycemic control can often reverse the hyperfiltration seen in early diabetic nephropathy. However, the benefits may be somewhat less if intensive therapy is first started when overt proteinuria has already been established.
- **ACE inhibitors and blood pressure control**. The particular role of the renin–angiotensin system in diabetic kidney disease has been established. ACE inhibitors should be initiated at the onset of microalbuminuria irrespective of blood pressure levels. These recommendations are based on well-conducted multicenter trials showing the benefits of these agents in reducing renal disease. Blood pressure should be tightly controlled, as studies show that blood pressure control, especially with ACE inhibitors, can reduce protein excretion and slow the rate of disease progression. Beta-blockers may reduce proteinuria. Other blood pressure-lowering agents such as thiazides do not affect protein excretion. Calcium-channel blockers have variable effects. Dihydropyridine types may worsen proteinuria while diltiazem and verapamil reduce protein excretion. The newly available angiotensin-II-receptor blockers also seem to reduce proteinuria and may add to the effects of ACE inhibitors. However, there have been no long-term outcome data with angiotensin-II-receptor blockers in terms of renal protection. A recent issue of the New England Journal of Medicine published three articles showing benefit of angiotensin 2-receptor antagonists to reduce proteinuria or progression of renal disease. Therefore, they cannot be recommended as first-line therapy.
- **Protein restriction** (0.6g/kg per day) may also slow the long-term decline in glomerular filtration rate. However, it may not be beneficial or easy to reduce protein intake in the long term. Compliance becomes an issue and it may not be beneficial to reduce L-arginine, the substrate for the vasodilator nitric oxide.

The overall goal is to reduce diastolic blood pressure to below 80mmHg and if possible below 75mmHg in those with microalbuminuria. These recommendations are based on outcome trials using captopril. Hyperkalemia or persistent cough can limit the use

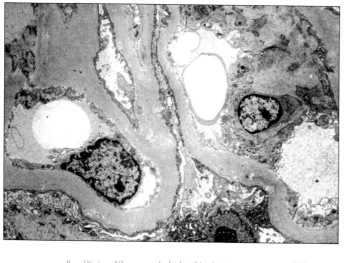

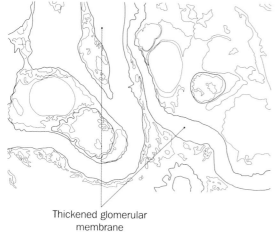

Thickened glomerular
membrane

Figure 21.14 Electron micrograph showing thick, 'moth-eaten' glomerular basement membranes and increased mesangial matrix. (Courtesy of Dr Benjamin Sturgill.)

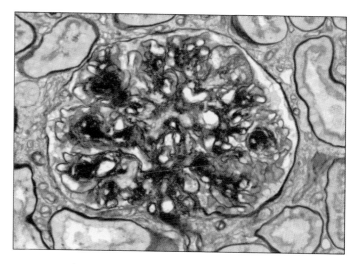

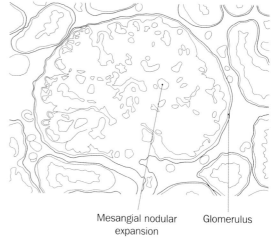

Mesangial nodular   Glomerulus
expansion

Figure 21.15 Glomerulus with nodular expansion of mesangium. Periodic-acid–Schiff stain. (Courtesy of Dr Benjamin Sturgill.)

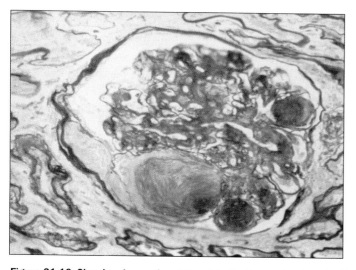

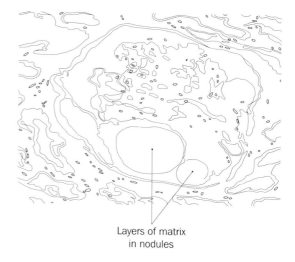

Layers of matrix
in nodules

Figure 21.16 Classic advanced nodular diabetic glomerulosclerosis. Note the concentric layers of matrix. Periodic-acid–Schiff stain. (Courtesy of Dr Benjamin Sturgill.)

or dose of ACE inhibitors. If cough is a problem one can change to the angiotensin-II-receptor blockers and if there is too large a drop in glomerular filtration rate or hyperkalemia, diltiazem or verapamil may be useful. One must watch for these changes in total potassium and glomerular filtration rate, given the risk of the syndrome of hyporeninemic hypoaldosteronism (type 4 renal tubular acidosis) in these patients. Nonsteroidal antiinflammatory agents, by reducing vasodilating prostaglandin, can also worsen glomerular filtration rate and precipitate this syndrome.

There is also evidence that hypercholesterolemia can predispose to glomerulosclerosis, especially in combination with elevated blood pressure. Studies have shown that agents such as simvastatin can help reduce albuminuria in normotensive patients with diabetes with hypercholesterolemia and microalbuminuria.

Neuropathy

Peripheral and autonomic nervous system involvement is commonly seen in people with diabetes. Diabetic polyneuropathy is the most common form seen in industrialized countries. Prevalence is a function of disease duration and the severity of glycemia. Most evidence suggests that approximately 50% of patients will eventually develop neuropathy. Neuropathy can lead to significant morbidity and mortality, causing disorders of the gastrointestinal tract, lower extremity ulceration, infections, and amputations.

There are established classification systems for neuropathy, which are covered in several reviews. In addition to distal symmetric polyneuropathy, individual cranial or peripheral nerve involvement, such as the median nerve or cranial nerve III, may cause focal mononeuropathy. Autonomic neuropathy may affect the circulatory system (postural hypotension) or gastrointestinal system (gastroparesis, enteropathy with diarrhea or constipation). Thoracic and lumbar polyradiculopathy (diabetic amyotrophy) can occur, as well as asymmetric involvement of multiple peripheral nerves (mononeuropathy multiplex).

The earliest signs of disease reflect damage to large and small nerve fibers. Loss of vibration and proprioception are due to large-fiber loss and reduced light touch or temperature sensation result from small-fiber loss. Patients may complain of pain, paresthesias, or dysesthesias. These changes can be progressive and lead to ulceration and joint abnormalities such as Charcot arthropathy or stress fractures.

Close monitoring by the patient and health-care providers is critical to prevent or reduce serious consequences of neuropathic changes. Appropriate education and footwear is very important, along with sensory testing at least every 6 months. Some centers have developed screening scoring systems, such as the Michigan Neuropathy Screening Score. Objective diagnostic testing can be performed to measure nerve conduction or muscle innervation (electromyography). Additional tests for autonomic neuropathy are available, including gastric-emptying nuclear studies or stable isotope breath tests for evaluation of gastroparesis. Referral to a gastroenterologist is often useful to diagnose and evaluate the etiology of other enteropathies seen in diabetic patients.

Pathogenesis and treatment

It is very clear that glycemic control has a major influence in the development and progression of neuropathy. The DCCT showed that neuropathy was reduced by 60% over a 10-year period with tight glucose control. Ongoing studies are addressing the issue of how effective glucose control is in reducing the progression of established neuropathy. However, studies show that glycemic control can reduce the loss of nerve conduction velocity. The treatments for advanced neuropathy are not ideal; they are based primarily on symptom control and do not alter the course of the complication. Ongoing research trials are evaluating various types of medication to minimize the toxicity of glucose or alter the natural history of the disease. These agents include aldose reductase inhibitors and lipid peroxide inhibitors such as α-lipoic acid.

For pain control, one can use local treatment with capsaicin cream (0.075%) applied to the area four times daily. For more severe pain, tricyclic antidepressants such as amitriptyline, desipramine, or fluoxetine may be used. One should start with low doses of these agents and gradually titrate up to reduce side effects. These agents must be used with caution in patients with cardiac disease. The anticonvulsants also offer benefits. Gabapentin (300–600mg three times daily) has been shown to have benefits, with potentially fewer side effects than the tricyclic group. Other therapies have been tried to reduce pain, including tramadol hydrochloride and transcutaneous nerve stimulation.

For gastroparesis, one could recommend dietary changes to more frequent smaller meals or mixed meals – in some cases, enteral feeding is needed. In the USA, metoclopramide is the major drug treatment for improving gastric motility; 10–20mg four times daily, with meals and at bedtime, is often used. The benefits may be reduced over time. Domperidone (20mg four times daily) is a related compound that is also effective. This medication is available in Europe but not in the USA. The antibiotic erythromycin is a motilin-receptor agonist; it increases gastric kinetic action and is effective intravenously or orally. The long-term safety of erythromycin for this purpose is not fully known. Treatment of diabetic enteropathy is based on the diagnostic causes and may include treatments for bacterial overgrowth or antidiarrheal agents. Some evidence shows benefits for clonidine or the somatostatin analog octreotide. However, more studies with these agents are needed.

ACKNOWLEDGEMENTS

The authors want to acknowledge the assistance of Dr James Tiedeman, Professor of Ophthalmology, who provided the photographs of diabetic retinopathy, and Dr Benjamin Sturgill, Professor of Pathology, who kindly provided the histologic and electron micrographs of diabetic kidney disease. They would also like to acknowledge the administrative assistance provided by Terry S. Howell and Nancy L. Diggs in the preparation of the chapter.

FURTHER READING

American Diabetes Association. 2001 clinical practice recommendations. Diabetes Care. 2001;24(suppl. 1).

American Diabetes Association. Medical management of pregnancy complicated by diabetes mellitus, 3rd ed. Alexandria, VA:American Diabetes Association; 2000.

American Diabetes Association. Medical management of type 1 diabetes, 3rd ed. Alexandria, VA:American Diabetes Association; 1998.

American Diabetes Association. Report of the Expert Committee on the diagnosis and classification of diabetes mellitus. Diabetes Care 1997;20:1183–97.

Brenner BM, Cooper ME, de Zeeuw D, et al. Effects of losartan on renal and cardiovascular outcomes in patients with type 2 diabetes and nephropathy. New Engl J Med. 2001;345:861–869.

Eisenbarth GS, Lafferty, KJ, eds. Type 1 diabetes: molecular, cellular, and clinical immunology. http://www.hsc.colorado.edu/misc/diabetes/eisenbook.html (frequent updates).

Groop LC, Botazzo GF, Doniach D. Islet cell antibodies identify latent type I diabetes in patients aged 35–75 years at diagnosis. Diabetes 1986;35:237–42.

International Pancreas Transplant Registry. Newsletter 1995;8:1.

Le RoithD, Taylor S, Olefsky J, eds. Diabetes mellitus: a fundamental and clinical text, 2nd ed. Baltimore, MD:Lippincott, Williams & Wilkins; 2000.

Leahy J, Clark N, Cefalu W, eds. Medical management of diabetes mellitus. New York:Marcel Dekker; 2000.

Lewis EJ, Hunsicker LG, Clarke WR, et al. Renoprotective effect of the angiotensin-receptor antagonist irbesartan in patients with nephropathy due to type 2 diabetes. New Engl J Med. 2001;345:851–860.

Parving HH, Lehnert H, Brochner-Mortensen J, et al. The effect of irbesartan on the development of diabetic nephropathy in patients with type 2 diabetes. New Engl J Med. 2001;345:870–878.

Shapiro AM, Lakey JRT, Ryan EA, et al. Islet transplantation in seven patients with type I diabetes mellitus using a glucocorticoid-free immunosuppressive regimen. N Engl J Med. 2000;343:230–8.

UptoDate® www.uptodate.com. Volume 8.3, 2000.

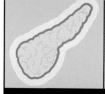

Section 4 Control of Blood Glucose and its Disturbance

Chapter 22 Insulin Resistance

Gerald M Reaven

INTRODUCTION

The focus in this chapter will be on the role played by insulin resistance in the development of hyperglycemia and dyslipidemia in patients with type 2 diabetes. The central hypothesis is that insulin resistance is the necessary, but not sufficient, pathophysiologic abnormality that leads to type 2 diabetes in the overwhelming majority of patients with this syndrome. It is further postulated that the development of hyperglycemia and dyslipidemia is dependent upon the behavior of muscle, pancreatic β cells, adipose tissue, and liver. Consequently, an attempt will be made to develop a coherent view of how changes in these four key tissues interact to bring about the abnormalities of carbohydrate and lipoprotein metabolism that characterize the patient with type 2 diabetes.

Genetic component

Although this chapter will focus on the pathophysiology of type 2 diabetes, there is no doubt that there is a genetic component involved in the development of the full-blown syndrome. For example, there is considerable evidence that individuals with a family history of type 2 diabetes are at increased risk of developing diabetes. Perhaps the most powerful observation in this context is the extremely high concordance for type 2 diabetes in identical twins. In addition, it has been shown that the ability of insulin to stimulate insulin-mediated glucose disposal is decreased in first-degree relatives of patients with type 2 diabetes, and there is also evidence that insulin resistance is at least a familial characteristic. Despite all of this information, there is relatively little understanding of the genetic basis of type 2 diabetes in most patients with this syndrome. A series of candidate genes has been evaluated, with little success to date, and it is certain that type 2 diabetes will be a polygenic disease.

There are two obvious obstacles that have contributed to the lack of understanding of the genetics of type 2 diabetes. In the first place, variations in basic lifestyle variables such as degree of obesity and level of physical activity profoundly affect the phenotypic presentation of patients with type 2 diabetes. Secondly, relatively little is understood of the molecular basis of the syndrome. It is quite clear that insulin resistance is present in the vast majority of patients with type 2 diabetes, and an enormous amount of detail has been published concerning the details of the insulin signal transduction system. On the other hand, this wealth of information has not resulted in a great deal of enlightenment as to the molecular defect, or defects, responsible for insulin resistance. Indeed, given the apparent redundancy of the steps involved in the insulin signal transduction system, it is likely to require several defects in order for insulin resistance to develop, and there may be many possible combinations of defects that can conspire to lead to insulin resistance in a given patient.

If we now consider the likelihood that there will also be genetic factors affecting how the pancreatic β cell responds to insulin resistance, and the complexity of the insulin secretory mechanism, it should not be surprising that we know even less about the genetic/molecular defects responsible for the failure of the β cell to sustain the degree of compensatory hyperinsulinemia to maintain glucose homeostasis. Consequently, in the remainder of this chapter the emphasis will be on the pathophysiology of type 2 diabetes. Furthermore, an effort will be made to rely mainly on information gained from studies performed in human beings.

INSULIN RESISTANCE

Quantitative assessments of insulin action are almost uniformly made by techniques that estimate the ability of insulin to mediate glucose uptake by muscle. As a consequence, the statement that 'insulin resistance' exists usually means that a defined amount of insulin stimulates glucose uptake by muscle to a lesser degree than it does in an 'insulin-sensitive' person. However, there is no accepted definition of who is insulin-resistant and who is insulin-sensitive, and there are a number of questions related to insulin resistance that arise once this simplistic definition has been made.

Differences in tissue sensitivity to insulin

Although insulin receptors are present on many cell types, insulin action is regulated by differences in signal transduction mechanisms that are cell-specific. Perhaps the most relevant example of this involves the difference between insulin action on the kidney and muscle. Both endogenous and exogenous hyperinsulinemia increase sodium retention by the kidney and decrease urinary uric acid clearance in the normal fashion in individuals who have evidence of resistance to insulin action on glucose disposal by muscle. A somewhat more complicated issue involves the liver. Perhaps the most common abnormality associated with muscle insulin resistance is an increase in hepatic very-low-density lipoprotein (VLDL)-triglyceride (TG) secretion and elevated plasma TG concentrations. In order for these two events to exist simultaneously, i.e. a defect in insulin-stimulated glucose uptake by muscle and an increase in hepatic VLDL-TG secretion, the liver must remain normally sensitive to

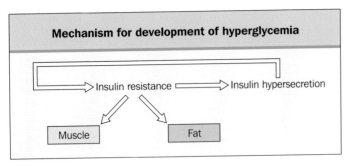

Figure 22.1 Mechanism for the development of hyperglycemia. The figure presents a schematic diagram of the relationship between insulin resistance and insulin secretion in the pathogenesis of hyperglycemia in type 2 diabetes. When insulin hypersecretion is inadequate to counteract insulin resistance, hyperglycemia develops.

the interaction between ambient insulin and free fatty acid (FFA) concentrations in regulation of hepatic VLDL-TG synthesis in the face of muscle insulin resistance.

Differences in tissue dose–response curves

As indicated previously, the phrase 'insulin resistance' usually refers to muscle. However, adipose tissue is as resistant to regulation by insulin as muscle, although the dose–response characteristics of the two tissues are quite different. A plasma insulin concentration of about 20µU/mL will suppress by approximately 50% the release of FFA by adipose tissue; a circulating insulin concentration that has relatively little effect on stimulating glucose disposal by muscle. This is true of both healthy individuals and patients with type 2 diabetes, and the decrease in insulin-stimulated muscle glucose uptake in patients with type 2 diabetes is paralleled by an inability of basal insulin concentrations to maintain fasting plasma FFA concentrations.

HOW DOES HYPERGLYCEMIA DEVELOP IN TYPE 2 DIABETES?

Muscle insulin resistance

The mechanism for the development of hyperglycemia is shown in **Figure 22.1**. Although muscle insulin resistance is a common finding in patients with type 2 diabetes, this defect, by itself, cannot account for the development of hyperglycemia. For example, resistance to insulin-mediated glucose disposal by muscle is not limited to patients with type 2 diabetes and is a common finding in nondiabetic subjects with impaired glucose tolerance, nondiabetic first-degree relatives of patients with type 2 diabetes, and a substantial number of individuals with normal glucose tolerance. The implications of these observations are seen in **Figure 22.2**, which defines the relationship between insulin-stimulated glucose disposal by muscle and fasting plasma glucose concentration in a series of nonobese individuals. It can be seen that there was no simple relationship between insulin resistance and fasting plasma glucose concentration, and that a normal fasting plasma glucose concentration could be maintained by individuals who were essentially as insulin-resistant as many patients with frank type 2 diabetes. In addition, once fasting hyperglycemia supervened, substantial increases in fasting plasma glucose concentration were associated with relatively small decreases in insulin-mediated muscle glucose disposal.

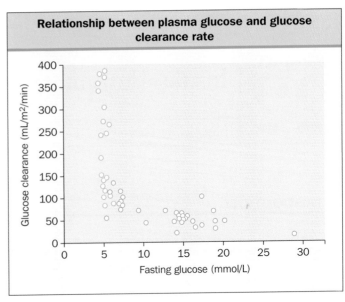

Figure 22.2 Relationship between plasma glucose and glucose clearance rate. The figure shows the relationship between fasting plasma glucose concentration and glucose metabolic clearance rates observed during hyperinsulinemic, glucose clamp studies in 20 nondiabetic subjects (yellow circles) and 30 patients with type 2 diabetes (blue circles). The clamp studies were performed over a 120min period, with a steady-state plasma insulin concentration of approximately 100µU/mL. 10mmol/L glucose is equivalent to 180mg/dL. (Adapted from Reaven GM, Hollenbeck CB, Chen Y-D I. Relationship between glucose tolerance, insulin secretion, and insulin action in non-obese individuals with varying degrees of glucose tolerance. Diabetologia 1989;32:52–5.)

It appears reasonable to conclude that resistance to insulin-mediated muscle glucose uptake by muscle is present in the great majority of individuals with glucose intolerance but that this defect by itself cannot account either for the development of significant hyperglycemia in patients with type 2 diabetes or for the severity of fasting hyperglycemia in these individuals.

Pancreatic β cell

Individuals with muscle insulin resistance can maintain normal glucose tolerance if their pancreatic β cells secrete enough insulin to overcome this defect. Significant hyperglycemia develops when the insulin secretory response is not sufficient to overcome the defect in insulin action on muscle. Evidence for this point of view is shown in **Figure 22.3**, which illustrates day-long plasma glucose and specifically determined insulin concentrations in nonobese, normal volunteers, individuals with impaired glucose tolerance, and patients with type 2 diabetes, measured hourly from 8.00h to 16.00h, before and after meals (breakfast at 8.00h, lunch at 12.00h). Essentially identical relationships were seen in obese individuals. These results show that significant hyperglycemia develops in patients with type 2 diabetes at ambient plasma insulin concentrations lower in absolute terms than in individuals with impaired glucose tolerance, and slightly higher than in normal volunteers. However, despite the relatively small differences in circulating insulin level between the normal subjects and patients with type 2 diabetes, plasma glucose concentrations were approximately three times higher in the patients: dramatic increases in level of

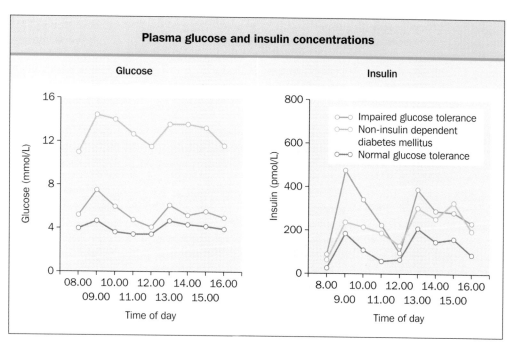

Plasma glucose and insulin concentrations

Glucose

Insulin

○—○ Impaired glucose tolerance
○—○ Non-insulin dependent
  diabetes mellitus
○—○ Normal glucose tolerance

Figure 22.3 Plasma glucose and insulin concentrations. The figure illustrates the plasma glucose concentrations (left panel) and plasma insulin concentrations (right panel) in nonobese subjects with normal glucose tolerance, impaired glucose tolerance, or non-insulin-dependent diabetes, measured hourly from 08.00h to 16.00h. Breakfast was at 08.00h and lunch at 12.00h. 10mmol/L glucose is equivalent to 180mg/dL. (Adapted from Reaven GM, Chen Y-D I, Hollenbeck CB, et al. Plasma insulin, C-peptide, and proinsulin concentrations in obese and nonobese individuals with varying degrees of glucose tolerance. J Clin Endocrinol Metab. 1993;76:44–8.)

glycemia were associated with relatively minor quantitative decreases in day-long circulating insulin concentrations. Thus, although hyperglycemia occurs when β-cell function declines, it is not obvious why such a small change in ambient insulin concentration should lead to the enormous increment in plasma glucose concentration.

Adipose tissue insulin resistance

The realization that adipose tissue is as resistant to insulin as muscle is a relatively recent discovery. It is primarily due to differences in the sensitivity of muscle and adipose tissue to regulation by insulin. It must be remembered that adipose tissue consumes relatively little glucose: its primary physiologic function is to store energy in the form of triglyceride in order to supply the fuel needed to sustain life between meals. Thus, a decrease in whole-body glucose uptake in response to an insulin infusion is primarily a reflection of a defect in muscle glucose disposal. However, as was emphasized previously, adipose tissue is much more insulin-sensitive than muscle, making insulin's regulation of adipose tissue the physiologic characteristic that will change most dramatically when the ability of the β cell to compensate for muscle insulin resistance begins to fail. The development of significant hyperglycemia, associated with the decline in ambient insulin concentration, as seen in **Figure 22.3**, is associated with striking increases in plasma FFA concentration. Furthermore, there are at least three reasons why the elevations in plasma FFA concentration contribute to hyperglycemia (**Fig. 22.4**).

Decreased muscle glucose uptake

The existence of a glucose–fatty-acid cycle was first postulated in 1963, when it was argued that elevations in plasma FFA concentration lead to enhanced muscle FFA uptake and oxidation, which, in turn, inhibits muscle glucose uptake. This notion has received considerable support since its introduction, and there

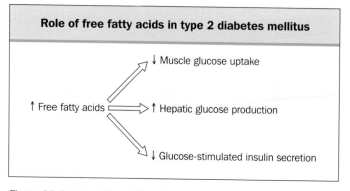

Role of free fatty acids in type 2 diabetes mellitus

↓ Muscle glucose uptake

↑ Free fatty acids → ↑ Hepatic glucose production

↓ Glucose-stimulated insulin secretion

Figure 22.4 Role of free fatty acids in type 2 diabetes mellitus. The proposed relationship is illustrated between increases in plasma free fatty acid concentrations and ensuing changes in muscle glucose uptake, hepatic glucose production, and glucose-stimulated insulin secretion.

is ample evidence that acute elevations in plasma FFA concentration inhibit insulin-stimulated glucose uptake by muscle in normal subjects and patients with type 2 diabetes.

However, evidence that increases in plasma FFA concentration inhibit muscle glucose uptake does not mean that elevated FFA levels are the primary cause of insulin resistance in patients with type 2 diabetes. Substantial increases in plasma FFA concentrations are necessary to decrease insulin-mediated glucose disposal. Furthermore, a significant degree of insulin resistance and hyperglycemia can exist in nondiabetic individuals, at a time when plasma FFA concentrations are only marginally increased. It can also be seen from the results in **Figure 22.2** that there is only a modest increment in insulin resistance as patients with type 2 diabetes progress from a moderate to a severe degree of fasting hyperglycemia. Since this is when the greatest increases in circulating FFA concentrations occur, it seems unlikely that the change in FFA concentration is responsible for the development of fasting hyperglycemia primarily by accentuating muscle insulin resistance. Thus, although increases in plasma FFA concentration probably contribute to the insulin resistance present in patients with type 2 diabetes and fasting hyperglycemia, it does not appear that this change is the primary reason why fasting hyperglycemia develops.

Stimulation of hepatic glucose production

An increase in plasma FFA flux to the liver, due to higher plasma FFA concentrations, will stimulate hepatic glucose production (HGP). The link between increased FFA flux to the liver and HGP is most probably secondary to stimulation of hepatic FFA oxidation as the result of higher plasma FFA concentrations. The biochemical changes that follow an increase in hepatic FFA oxidation indicate that hepatic FFA oxidation and gluconeogenesis are directly related. It is likely that this effect of FFA on hepatic intermediary metabolism plays a crucial role in the development of fasting hyperglycemia in patients with type 2 diabetes. However, the details of the role of the liver in this context is somewhat controversial, and will be discussed in detail subsequently.

Inhibition of glucose-stimulated insulin secretion

Although plasma FFA concentrations are known to increase in patients with type 2 diabetes as β-cell function begins to decline, the view that this increase in plasma FFA concentration may further suppress glucose-stimulated insulin secretion is relatively new. Indeed, there is evidence that FFAs acutely stimulate insulin secretion. However, more recent reports have emphasized that chronic FFA elevations, both *in vitro* and *in vivo*, can suppress glucose-stimulated insulin secretion. These data suggest that elevated FFA levels may act as a positive feedback mechanism in patients with type 2 diabetes by further suppressing glucose-stimulated β-cell function in these individuals.

Based upon the above considerations, it seems obvious that the role of elevated FFA concentrations in regulation of β-cell function is certainly worthy of increased attention. In particular, it is important to distinguish between a primary role of elevated plasma FFA concentrations as a cause of the initial decline in β-cell function that leads to the loss of β-cell compensation in insulin resistant individuals, as differentiated from a secondary effect that acts to further impair β-cell secretory function.

Liver

The liver is both a major producer and consumer of glucose, and the presence of hyperglycemia can be taken to mean that the liver has not succeeded in fulfilling its function. However, the role of the liver in the pathophysiologic changes that lead to hyperglycemia is more complex. For example, there is general agreement that both muscle and adipose tissue are resistant to insulin regulation, whereas it is not so clear that the liver is insulin-resistant. Indeed, there is evidence that insulin regulation of liver glucose production may primarily be exerted by its modulation of peripheral events; particularly by changes in FFA flux to the liver.

The major cause of uncertainty as to the role of the liver in the development of hyperglycemia is the difficulty in quantifying hepatic glucose production. For example, conventional wisdom is that hyperglycemia in patients with type 2 diabetes is directly related to increases in HGP. However, it has more recently been argued that the tracer techniques used in these earlier studies overestimated HGP; a result of the enlarged glucose pool size in patients with fasting hyperglycemia and the consequent inability to reach isotopic steady state. In contrast, when HGP was measured under steady-state isotopic conditions, the values in patients with type 2 diabetes were quite similar in absolute terms to those in nondiabetic individuals. For example, the data shown in Figure 22.5 are the results of measures of HGP made in 51 individuals (18 normal and 33 with type 2 diabetes) using steady-state isotopic conditions. Patients with type 2 diabetes were divided into three groups (on the basis of their fasting glucose concentration (FPG): DM-1 (FPG <10mmol/L): DM-2 (FPG >10 <13mmol/L): and DM-3 (FPG >13mmol/L), and **Figure 22.5** displays the mean FPG and HGP values for these four groups. It

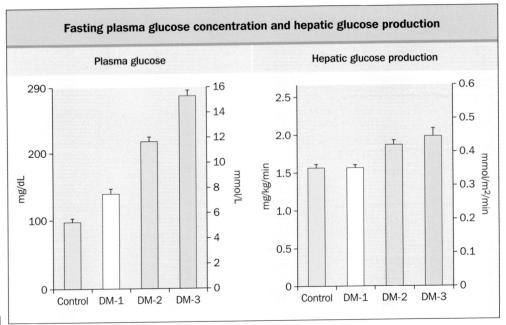

Figure 22.5 Fasting plasma glucose concentration and hepatic glucose production. The measurements were made in control subjects ($n = 11$) and patients with type 2 diabetes. The latter were divided into three groups of 11 each (DM-1, DM-2, and DM-3) on the basis of their fasting plasma glucose concentrations: DM-1 <180mg/dL (<10mmol/L); DM-2 180–250mg/dL (10–13mmol/L); and DM-3 >250mg/dL (>13mmol/L). (Adapted from Jeng C-Y, Sheu WH-H, Fu MM-T, et al. Relationship between hepatic glucose production and fasting plasma glucose concentration in patients with NIDDM. Diabetes 1994;43:1440–4.)

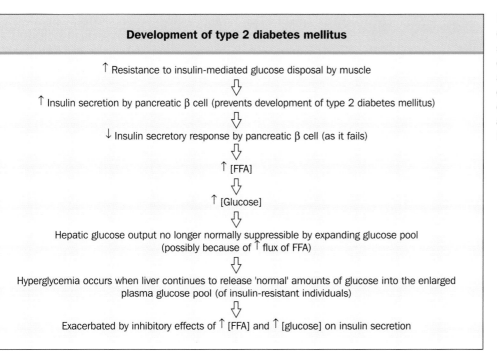

Figure 22.6 Development of type 2
diabetes mellitus. A proposed
summary of the sequence of physiologic
events that leads from muscle and
adipose tissue insulin resistance to the
changes that eventually result in the
decompensation of glucose tolerance
and the development of type 2 diabetes.
FFA, free fatty acids.

can be seen that the FPG values increased progressively from normal subjects to the DM-3 group but that this was not true of the measurements of HGP. Indeed, HGP was not increased above normal in the DM-1 groups (FPG <10mmol/L), and was only increased by approximately 30% in the patients with the highest FPG (>13.0mmol/L). These results differ substantially from the vast majority of previous studies in that the increase in HGP in patients with the most severe degree of fasting hyperglycemia was only 30% higher than normal values, not two to three times higher.

The observation that absolute values for HGP are similar in normal subjects and hyperglycemic patients with type 2 diabetes does not mean that the liver is acting normally in these persons. For example, it could be argued that HGP in patients with type 2 diabetes is not being appropriately suppressed by the hyperglycemia. Of interest in this context was the finding that glycosuria only occurred in the two groups in **Figure 22.5** with the highest fasting glucose concentration, and that the amount of glucose excreted in the urine in these two groups was equal to the magnitude of their increase in HGP above the value in nondiabetic individuals. This observation may be a coincidence, but it permits the speculation that the liver will put out just the amount of glucose needed to maintain a normal rate of tissue glucose utilization; the more the loss of glucose in the urine, the greater will be the HGP needed to compensate for the loss of energy.

Summary

Resistance to insulin-mediated glucose disposal by muscle can be seen in a significant proportion of glucose tolerant individuals. As long as insulin-resistant persons are capable of increasing their insulin secretory response, gross decompensation of glucose homeostasis can be prevented. As the insulin secretory

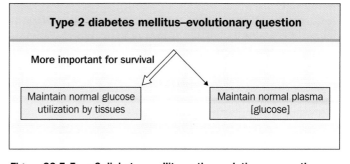

Figure 22.7 Type 2 diabetes mellitus – the evolutionary question.
Schematic diagram of the philosophical argument suggesting that
hyperglycemia, by maintaining tissue glucose utilization at the level needed
for survival, is a more fundamental physiologic need than is a normal
fasting glucose concentration.

response declines, there is a significant increase in FFA and glucose concentrations. As a consequence, HGP is no longer normally suppressible by the expanding glucose pool, possibly, due to the increased flux of FFA. Hyperglycemia occurs in type 2 diabetes when the liver continues to secrete normal amounts of glucose into the enlarged plasma glucose pool of insulin resistant individuals. The degree of hyperglycemia is further accentuated by the inhibitory effects of glucose, and possibly FFA, on insulin secretion (**Fig. 22.6**). The advantage to the patient in this situation is presumably the ability to maintain normal absolute rates of peripheral glucose disposal; the loss is the long-term consequence of chronic hyperglycemia. Teleologically, it seems that the ability to maintain glucose utilization was more crucial in evolutionary terms than the maintenance of normal plasma glucose concentration (**Fig. 22.7**).

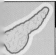

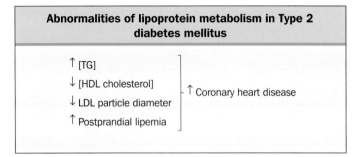

Abnormalities of lipoprotein metabolism in Type 2 diabetes mellitus

↑ [TG]

↓ [HDL cholesterol]

↓ LDL particle diameter — ↑ Coronary heart disease

↑ Postprandial lipemia

Figure 22.8 Abnormalities of lipoprotein metabolism in type 2 diabetes mellitus. Summary of the characteristic lipoprotein phenotype in patients with type 2 diabetes, with emphasis on the fact that all of these changes have been associated with increased risk of coronary heart disease. HDL, high-density lipoprotein; LDL, low-density lipoprotein; TG, triglycerides.

DYSLIPIDEMIA

A high plasma triglyceride and a low high-density lipoprotein (HDL) cholesterol concentration are the most common forms of dyslipidemia in patients with type 2 diabetes (**Fig. 22.8**). These changes are often associated with smaller, denser low-density lipoprotein (LDL) particles and an enhanced degree of post-prandial lipemia. All these abnormalities in lipoprotein metabolism have been identified as risk factors for coronary heart disease, and help explain why coronary heart disease is the major cause of morbidity and mortality in type 2 diabetes. This section will attempt to provide a coherent explanation for the development of dyslipidemia in patients with type 2 diabetes. Particular attention will be directed to the pathophysiology of hypertriglyceridemia in such patients on the premise that the other changes in lipoprotein metabolism tend to be a consequence of this fundamental abnormality.

Triglyceride metabolism

In the most general sense, hepatic VLDL-TG secretion is regulated primarily by two variables—ambient insulin concentration and the FFA flux to the liver (**Fig. 22.9**). The impact of these two variables is complementary. The greater the FFA flux to the liver, the more substrate becomes available for VLDL-TG

synthesis. The higher the ambient insulin concentration, the greater the degree to which FFA entering the liver is used for TG synthesis. Simply put, the higher the day-long ambient insulin level, the more likely it is that FFA will be used for hepatic TG synthesis, and the lower the insulin, the more likely it is that FFA will be diverted to other pathways. At the extreme, hypoinsulinemic individuals use essentially no FFA for TG synthesis.

As outlined previously, patients with type 2 diabetes and fasting hyperglycemia have both muscle and adipose tissue insulin resistance, with elevated plasma glucose and FFA concentrations, and plasma insulin concentrations similar in absolute terms to values in normal volunteers (**Fig. 22.10**). Since these patients have elevated FFA levels and normal ambient insulin concentrations, the FFA–hepatic TG secretion dose–response curve will be 'normal', and the higher FFA levels will increase hepatic VLDL-TG secretion and plasma TG concentration (**Fig. 22.9**).

Muscle and adipose tissue insulin resistance are also present in patients with impaired glucose tolerance. As is apparent in **Figure 22.3**, such individuals are actually hyperinsulinemic in absolute terms throughout the day. The hyperinsulinemia is able to maintain near-normal plasma glucose and FFA concentrations. In this instance, the ambient hyperinsulinemia leads to enhanced hepatic conversion of FFA to TG synthesis, resulting in hypertriglyceridemia (**Fig. 22.9**).

High-density lipoprotein cholesterol

The increase in plasma TG concentration almost certainly plays a major role in the low HDL cholesterol concentrations seen so commonly in patients with type 2 diabetes. The higher the plasma TG concentration, the greater will be the movement, via cholesteryl ester transport protein (CETP), of cholesteryl ester from HDL to VLDL. At the same time that HDL is being depleted of cholesterol, HDL is becoming relatively enriched in TG (**Fig. 22.11**). Evidence has recently been published showing that hyperinsulinemia increases the fractional catabolic rate of HDL apoA-1. This observation helps explain the earlier finding that the fractional catabolic rate of apoA-1 is increased in patients with type 2 diabetes, and the more rapid the fractional catabolic rate, the lower the HDL-cholesterol concentration. Given these data, the finding of a low HDL-cholesterol concentration in patients with type 2 diabetes is easily understood.

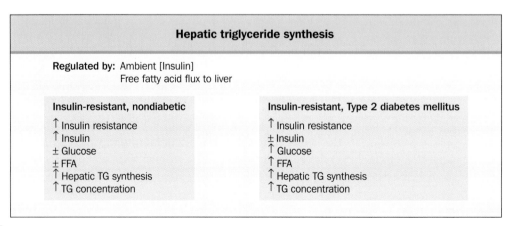

Hepatic triglyceride synthesis

Regulated by: Ambient [Insulin]
Free fatty acid flux to liver

Insulin-resistant, nondiabetic	Insulin-resistant, Type 2 diabetes mellitus
↑ Insulin resistance	↑ Insulin resistance
↑ Insulin	± Insulin
± Glucose	↑ Glucose
± FFA	↑ FFA
↑ Hepatic TG synthesis	↑ Hepatic TG synthesis
↑ TG concentration	↑ TG concentration

Figure 22.9 Hepatic triglyceride synthesis. The changes leading to fasting hypertriglyceridemia in insulin-resistant individuals are summarized – divided into those with hyperinsulinemia and minimal elevations of plasma glucose concentration and those whose plasma insulin concentration has declined to the point where plasma glucose and free fatty acid concentrations have substantially increased. FFA, free fatty acids; TG, triglycerides.

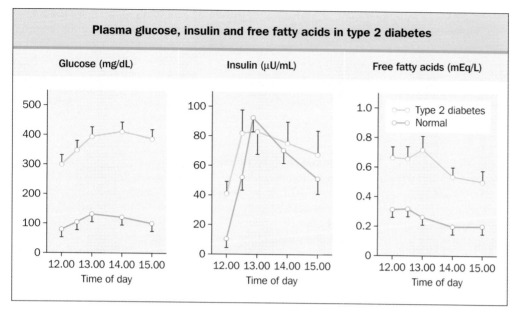

Figure 22.10 Plasma glucose, insulin, and free fatty acids in type 2 diabetes. The figure gives the mean (±SEM) plasma glucose, insulin, and free fatty acid concentrations before and after a meal at 12.00h in normal individuals and patients with type 2 diabetes. 180mg/dL glucose is equivalent to 10mmol/L. (Adapted from Reaven GM, Greenfield MS. Diabetic hypertriglyceridemia: evidence for three clinical syndromes. Diabetes 1981;30(suppl. 2,):66–75.)

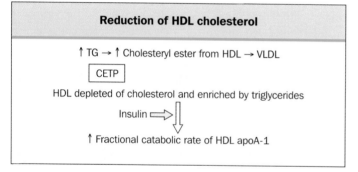

Figure 22.11 Reduction of high-density lipoprotein (HDL) cholesterol. Summary of the changes in lipoprotein metabolism contributing to the decrease in HDL cholesterol concentration characteristic of patients with type 2 diabetes. CETP, cholesteryl ester transport protein; HDL, high-density lipoprotein; TG, triglycerides; VLDL, very-low-density lipoprotein.

Change in LDL particle diameter

+ve related to [TG]
−ve related to [HDL cholesterol]

Unrelated to glycemic control

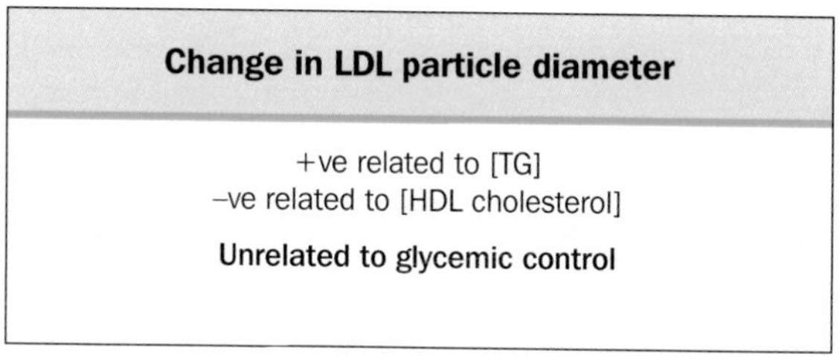

Figure 22.12 Change in low-density lipoprotein (LDL) particle diameter. These factors regulate LDL particle diameter, leading to the smaller and denser LDL particle that is part of the atherogenic lipoprotein profile in patients with type 2 diabetes. HDL, high-density lipoprotein; TG, triglycerides.

Low-density lipoprotein particle diameter

Demonstration that decreases in LDL particle diameter are linked to increased risk of coronary heart disease has focused interest in the impact that changes in LDL subclass, as distinct from LDL cholesterol concentration, have on atherogenesis. Earlier studies emphasized that smaller, denser LDL particles were associated with higher plasma TG and lower HDL cholesterol concentrations in patients with known coronary heart disease, but it is now clear that similar changes in LDL particle diameter can occur in insulin-resistant and hyperinsulinemic volunteers without manifest disease. Given the fact that patients with type 2 diabetes are insulin-resistant, with high plasma TG and low HDL cholesterol concentrations, it should not be surprising that LDL particles were also found to be smaller and denser in patients with this syndrome. Note that the change in LDL particle diameter seen in patients with type 2 diabetes appeared to be independent of the degree of glycemic control, but significantly related to both plasma TG (positive) and HDL-cholesterol (negative) concentrations (**Fig. 22.12**).

Postprandial lipemia

It has been apparent for some time that the postprandial accumulation of TG-rich lipoproteins is enhanced in patients with hypertriglyceridemia. Given the fact that plasma TG concentrations are characteristically increased in patients with type 2 diabetes, it is not surprising that postprandial lipemia is accentuated in these patients. However, it appears that postprandial lipemia is greater in patients with type 2 diabetes than in healthy volunteers, even when matched for fasting TG concentrations. Thus, the enhanced postprandial lipemia in patients with type 2 diabetes is not a simple function of an increase in VLDL pool size and competition between VLDL and chylomicron remnants for removal. The demonstration that magnitude of postprandial lipemia was increased in nondiabetic individuals in proportion to their degree of insulin resistance is of interest. Thus, insulin resistance contributes indirectly to enhanced postprandial lipemia in patients with type 2 diabetes, by virtue of its ability to enhance VLDL-TG secretion and increase the fasting VLDL pool size, and directly by decreasing the removal rate of TG-rich lipoproteins from plasma (**Fig. 22.13**).

Postprandial lipemia	
Related to insulin resistance by:	↑ VLDL-TG secretion
	↑ VLDL pool size
	↓ Rate of TG-rich lipoprotein removal from plasma

Figure 22.13 Postprandial lipemia. The figure summarizes the link between insulin resistance and the changes in lipoprotein metabolism that lead to an accentuated degree of postprandial lipemia in patients with type 2 diabetes. TG, triglycerides; VLDL, very-low-density lipoprotein.

Summary

Hypertriglyceridemia is the most prominent abnormality of lipoprotein metabolism in patients with type 2 diabetes. Insulin resistance appears to play a fundamental role in the development of hypertriglyceridemia in these individuals, with the increases in circulating insulin and FFA concentrations resulting from the defect in insulin regulation of muscle and adipose tissue interacting to stimulate hepatic VLDL-TG secretion. The relative roles of insulin and FFA in stimulating VLDL-TG secretion vary as a function of the degree of hyperglycemia. In patients with substantial elevations of plasma glucose concentration (who have 'normal' insulin concentrations in absolute terms), FFA concentrations are quite high, and it is the increased flux of substrate to the liver that is mainly responsible for the increase in hepatic VLDL-TG secretion. In patients with lesser degrees of hyperglycemia (associated with elevated plasma insulin levels), it is the hyperinsulinemia that is most responsible for the hypertriglyceridemia by enhancing the conversion of FFA to hepatic TG synthesis and secretion.

Once plasma TG concentration increases, HDL cholesterol concentrations begin to fall, postprandial accumulation of TG-rich lipoproteins is accentuated, and LDL particles get smaller and denser. These latter changes are at least partly explained by the effects of hypertriglyceridemia, but it appears that insulin resistance in itself plays a direct role in bringing about these additional abnormalities of lipoprotein metabolism common to type 2 diabetes.

TREATMENT

Goals

Treatment of type 2 diabetes must focus on an effort to restore the metabolic abnormalities towards normal in order to prevent the associated vascular complications. In the case of microangiopathy, i.e. retinopathy, nephropathy, neuropathy, the situation is straightforward: the better the glycemic control, the lower risk of these complications appearing. The situation is more complicated in the case of macrovascular disease, the major cause of morbidity and mortality in patients with type 2 diabetes. The link between glycemia and coronary heart disease is not nearly as tight as that between level of glucose control and microangiopathy, and it is almost certain that additional abnormalities present in type 2 diabetes, e.g. dyslipidemia and hypertension, play a more important role in increasing the risk of coronary heart disease than does glycemic control. Consequently, achieving good glycemic control is a necessary, but not sufficient, goal in the treatment of type 2 diabetes. In order to prevent the macrovascular complications it is essential that all coronary heart disease risk factors be addressed.

Lifestyle interventions

The ability of insulin to stimulate glucose disposal varies approximately 10-fold in the population at large. Approximately 50% of this variability is most likely related to genetic differences, with the remaining 50% related to lifestyle. The two major lifestyle variables are weight and level of physical activity – the heavier, the more insulin-resistant; the more physically inactive, the more insulin-resistant. Since insulin resistance is present in the vast majority of patients with type 2 diabetes, the inclusion of diet and exercise in the treatment program of patients with type 2 diabetes is essential.

Diet

In order to discuss the role of diet in the treatment patients with type 2 diabetes it is necessary to distinguish between the effects of the amount and kind of calories ingested.

Weight loss

Hyperglycemia will improve substantially in overweight patients with type 2 diabetes in association with weight loss of as little as 5–7kg. However, it is important to realize that not all patients with type 2 diabetes are overweight, and in these individuals weight loss offers no therapeutic gain. There is no magic that results in successful weight loss in overweight/obese individuals with type 2 diabetes, nor does it appear that any particular distribution of macronutrients in calorie-restricted diets guarantees compliance with the diet prescription.

Macronutrient composition

As indicated above, weight loss will significantly improve glycemic control in overweight/obese patients with type 2 diabetes. However, not all of these patients are able to lose weight, nor are they all overweight. In both of these situations, changes in macronutrient composition can be of substantial benefit.

Dietary recommendations for patients with type 2 diabetes have until quite recently been based upon the principle that hypercholesterolemia, more specifically an elevated LDL cholesterol level, is the only clinical endpoint that needs to be addressed. The result has been almost total emphasis on the use of low-fat, high-carbohydrate diets. Advice to replace saturated fat with carbohydrate in order to lower LDL cholesterol concentrations continues to be given, regardless of the metabolic characteristics of the patient. Unfortunately, this dietary approach has the capacity to make all the clinical manifestations of type 2 diabetes worse. The greater the carbohydrate content in an isocaloric diet, the more insulin must be secreted in order to maintain glucose homeostasis. This poses no danger to insulin-sensitive, nondiabetic individuals but the same cannot be said of patients with type 2 diabetes. The more relatively insulin-deficient patients are, the less able they are to secrete enough additional insulin to maintain glycemic control. The more insulin they are able to secrete, the less will be the increase in day-long plasma glucose concentration but the greater the degree of compensatory hyperinsulinemia.

The relative increases in day-long plasma glucose and insulin concentrations elicited by low saturated fat, high carbohydrate diets will vary from patient to patient, but in all subjects fasting plasma TG concentrations will increase, as will the day-long post-prandial accumulations of remnant lipoproteins. In addition, HDL cholesterol concentrations will tend to further decrease, as will LDL particle diameter. These abnormalities of lipoprotein metabolism are precisely the ones that are most frequently found in patients with type 2 diabetes, and represent a highly atherogenic lipoprotein profile. In order to avoid this problem, saturated fat should be replaced with monounsaturated and polyunsaturated fat. This maneuver results in a fall in LDL cholesterol concentration as great as is seen with low-saturated-fat, high-carbohydrate diets, without the untoward effects on lipoprotein metabolism described above. Given this information, weight maintenance diets containing (as a percentage of total calories) approximately 15% protein, 40% fat (<10% saturated fat, ~20% monounsaturated fat, and the rest as polyunsaturated fat), and 45% carbohydrate will decrease LDL cholesterol concentrations without accentuating the abnormalities of glucose, insulin, and lipoprotein metabolism that characterize patients with type 2 diabetes.

Physical activity

An improvement in physical fitness will also improve glycemic control, and aerobic exercise for about 30 min three or four times per week is approximately as powerful as 5–7kg of weight loss in improving insulin action in insulin-resistant individuals. As a consequence, exercise training programs can be useful in patients with type 2 diabetes. In contrast to weight loss, the benefits of exercise programs disappear quite quickly if they are discontinued. It is also important to stress the potential dangers if inappropriate exercise programs are initiated. For all of these reasons, weight loss is probably a more beneficial approach to improving long-term glycemic control than is a program of intensive physical activity. However, even if it is difficult to maintain the level of exercise necessary to significantly affect glycemic control, any increase in physical activity will potentiate the ability to lose weight and keep it off.

Antihyperglycemic agents

Once specific pharmacologic treatment is initiated, the aim should be to return glycemic control as close to normal as possible. Perhaps the most practical goal is a fasting plasma glucose concentration between 100 and 120mg/dL (5.5–6.5mmol/L). Although useful information can occasionally be gained by assessing plasma glucose concentrations at other times during the day, there is a strong correlation between fasting plasma glucose concentration and plasma glucose concentration measured through the day. The only antihyperglycemic agent that can always achieve adequate glycemic control as monotherapy is insulin. No matter how high the plasma glucose concentration, if insulin is administered in the appropriate amount at the right

time, glycemic control can be achieved in every patient with type 2 diabetes. In contrast, all the oral antihyperglycemic agents have a finite ability to decrease plasma glucose concentration (about 60mg/dL – 3.3mmol/L). Thus, it is most unlikely that any oral antihyperglycemic agent can achieve adequate glycemic control when used as monotherapy once fasting plasma glucose concentration exceeds 200mg/dL (11mmol/L). However, most healthcare providers appear reluctant to initiate pharmacologic treatment with insulin in patients with type 2 diabetes. Thus, discussion of insulin will be limited to its use as combined therapy.

Monotherapy

Although it is possible to provide theoretical arguments as to which oral agent should be used to initiate pharmacologic treatment, there is no compelling medical reason to choose one over the other. In this section some of the salient features of the drugs now available will be summarized.

Insulin secretagogues

For many years sulfonylurea compounds were the only insulin secretagogues available, but nonsulfonylurea secretagogues are also now available. By definition, these compounds lower plasma glucose concentration by stimulating insulin secretion. Although the various insulin secretagogues vary in many respects – effective dose, plasma half-life, etc. – there is no evidence that any of these differences significantly affect their ability to achieve glycemic control. The obvious advantage of this form of therapy is the long history of the use of many of the compounds in this class, both in terms of safety and efficacy. Many of them are now generic, offering obvious economic advantage. The major drawback to their use is the potential for hypoglycemia, and the lower the pretreatment degree of hyperglycemia, the more likely this is to occur. Finally, although these drugs primarily lower plasma glucose concentrations by increasing circulating plasma insulin concentrations, lowering plasma glucose concentration by any means will secondarily lead to an improvement in insulin action.

Metformin

Clinical experience with metformin is also quite extensive, and its record of both efficacy and safety is comparable to that of the sulfonylurea compounds. However, despite the long history of its use, the mechanism by which metformin lowers plasma glucose concentration is still debated. Evidence has been presented that it acts by enhancing insulin sensitivity, decreasing hepatic glucose output, and inhibiting lipolysis. The one unequivocal fact is that it does not act by stimulating insulin secretion, and the decrease in plasma glucose concentration following metformin treatment is associated with plasma insulin concentrations that are either the same or lower than baseline values. The most obvious clinical advantage of metformin is that metformin-treated patients tend to gain less weight than do individuals treated with insulin or other oral antihyperglycemic agents. The reason for this is not clear, but is likely related to the gastrointestinal side effects that can occur in association with metformin treatment. Hypoglycemia is not a risk when metformin is used as monotherapy, but it can occur if it is used in combination with insulin or an insulin secretagogue. Although lactic acidosis has been reported to occur in association with metformin treatment, its causal role in many of these reports is not clear. However, use of metformin should be avoided in individuals with hepatic and/or renal failure.

Thiazolidenedione compounds
The last few years have seen the introduction of three drugs that enhance insulin-mediated glucose disposal in patients with type 2 diabetes. Two of these, rosiglitazone and pioglitazone, currently have US Food and Drug Administration approval as antihyperglycemic agents and it is likely that additional compounds of this class will be introduced. The thiazolidenedione (TZD) compounds appear to be approximately as efficacious as insulin secretagogues and metformin as antihyperglycemic agents. Since the TZD compounds are the only currently available antihyperglycemic drugs that address the fundamental abnormality predisposing individuals to develop type 2 diabetes, a strong theoretical argument could be made that pharmacologic intervention should be initiated with this therapeutic class. On the other hand, at the present time there is little experimental support suggesting that it matters how glycemic control is achieved.

The first TZD compound to be introduced (troglitazone) was withdrawn from the market because of severe, and apparently idiosyncratic, liver function abnormalities. The two drugs still available appear to have avoided this problem, but liver monitoring is strongly recommended when either drug is used. As with metformin, hypoglycemia is not a problem when TZD compounds are used as monotherapy, but this problem can certainly occur when TZDs are used in combination with either insulin or insulin secretagogues. Finally, the most common side effect associated with TZD treatment is an increase in plasma volume, and the report of significant instances of salt and water retention has led to the warning that this class of drugs should be avoided in patients with evidence of this problem.

Disaccharidase inhibitors
These antihyperglycemic agents act by inhibiting the conversion of dietary carbohydrate in the small intestine to monosaccharides, thereby limiting carbohydrate absorption. As a consequence, these agents are more effective at lowering postprandial than fasting hyperglycemia. These compounds appear to lower HbAIc concentrations to a lesser degree than the other pharmacologic agents, and their therapeutic utility is most apparent in those with little, or no, elevation in fasting plasma glucose concentrations.

The carbohydrate that has escaped absorption in the small bowel is metabolized by bacteria in the colon, leading to the generation of FFAs that can be absorbed. It is this process that is responsible for the flatulence that is the most dramatic side effect of treatment with this class of compounds.

Combination therapy
As emphasized previously, adequate glycemic control is rarely achieved with one drug in patients with significant fasting hyperglycemia (180–200 mg/dL). Thus it is often necessary to use more than one antihyperglycemic agent in order to lower plasma glucose concentrations to the desired level. In this case,

the addition of predinner, or bedtime, intermediate-acting insulin can provide a simple and effective solution. The availability of multiple oral antihyperglycemic agents has led to a decrease in the use of this approach, effective as it may be. However, if the use of multiple oral antihyperglycemic agents is not successful in achieving glycemic control, it must again be emphasized that insulin remains the only treatment modality that is not limited in its efficacy.

If the decision is made to use several oral antihyperglycemic agents, there is at least some published information demonstrating that every theoretical combination seems to work. The use of an insulin secretagogue with metformin has the best documented evidence of success, but it is not likely that this is any more effective than metformin and a TZD, or an insulin secretagogue and a TZD. It is much more important to understand the need to achieve good glycemic control, than to debate the therapeutic advantages of any particular combination.

Treatment of dyslipidemia
The characteristic abnormality of lipoprotein metabolism in patients with type 2 diabetes is hypertriglyceridemia, usually associated with a low HDL cholesterol concentration, increased postprandial lipemia, and small, dense LDL particles. These changes comprise a highly atherogenic lipoprotein profile, and almost certainly play a major role, if not the predominant one, in the pathogenesis of coronary heart disease in this clinical syndrome. Although the appropriate diet and improved glycemic control can attenuate the changes described above, these interventions are far from being universally successful. If lipid abnormalities continue to persist, the use of fibric acid derivatives in patients with type 2 diabetes will significantly lower plasma TG concentrations, as well as improving the other lipoprotein abnormalities associated with hypertriglyceridemia. In addition, there is now evidence that the use of this class of drugs will decrease coronary heart disease risk in patients with this type of dyslipidemia.

A solitary elevation of LDL cholesterol concentration is rarely seen as the only lipoprotein abnormality in patients with type 2 diabetes, and when present is usually associated with the more characteristic lipoprotein phenotype. In either case, an increase in LDL cholesterol concentration must be addressed. Indeed, the only therapeutic intervention to date shown to decrease coronary heart disease in patients with type 2 diabetes was treatment with HMG-CoA reductase inhibitors (statins). As a consequence, the American Diabetes Association recommends that LDL cholesterol concentrations should be <100 mg/dL in patients with diabetes. Although decreasing saturated fat intake can help in this effort, reaching this goal usually also requires initiation of statin treatment.

Treatment of hypertension
The prevalence of hypertension is increased in type 2 diabetes, approaching 50%, and the results of the United Kingdom Prospective Diabetes Study have shown that attempts at aggressive treatment of high blood pressure were successful in significantly decreasing the development of microangiopathy. As in the case with LDL cholesterol concentrations, the therapeutic goals are more stringent in patients with type 2 diabetes,

with recommendations to lower the blood pressure to ≤ 130/80mmHg. Based upon the results of the UKPDS, achieving this goal will usually require the use of more than one antihypertensive agent. It is not possible within the context of this chapter to discuss extensively details of the pharmacologic approach to the treatment of this patient population. On the other hand, some generalization may be useful. Initiation of treatment with an angiotensin-converting enzyme (ACE) inhibitor has considerable experimental support. The combination of an ACE inhibitor and hydrochlorothiazide has been shown to be highly effective when a second drug is required. However, it should be emphasized that a relatively low dose of hydrochlorothiazide, 12.5mg, provides the antihypertensive benefit of this class of drugs, without any of the untoward

side effects. It should also be noted that a third drug may be necessary to attain the desired therapeutic goal. Finally, the use of a β-receptor antagonist is certainly warranted in individuals with a history of previous myocardial infarction.

Summary

We now have available the potential to use both lifestyle and pharmacologic interventions to effectively address all of the metabolic abnormalities in patients with type 2 diabetes. The crucial point is that it will be necessary to pay attention to all of the multiple metabolic abnormalities that contribute to the vascular complications of type 2 diabetes, and to aggressively use these tools to achieve the therapeutic goals outlined in this chapter.

FURTHER READING

Carpentier A, Mittelman SD, Lamarche B, Bergman RN, Giacca A, Lewis GF. Acute enhancement of insulin secretion by FFA in humans is lost with prolonged FFA elevation. American Physiological Society; 1999, E1055-E1066.

Chen Y-DI, Swami S, Skowronski R, Coulston A, Reaven GM. Differences in postprandial lipemia between patients with normal glucose tolerance and noninsulin-dependent diabetes mellitus. J Clin Endocrinol Metab. 1993;76:172–7.

Feingold KR, Grunfeld C, Pang M, Doerrler W, Drauss RM. LDL subclass phenotypes and triglyceride metabolism in non-insulin dependent diabetes. Arteriosclerosis Thrombosis 1992;12;1496–502.

Ferrannini E, Barret EJ, Bevilacqua S, DeFronzo RA. Effect of fatty acids on glucose production and utilization in man. J Clin Invest. 1983;72:1737–47.

Fontbonne A, Eschwege E, Cambien F, et al. Hypertriglyceridemia as a risk factor of coronary heart disease mortality in subjects with impaired glucose tolerance or diabetes. Diabetologia 1989;32;300–4.

Fraze E, Donner CC, Swislocki ALM, Chiou Y-AM, Chen Y-DI, Reaven GM. Ambient plasma free fatty acid concentrations in noninsulin-dependent diabetes mellitus: evidence for insulin resistance. J Clin Endocrinol Metab. 1985;61:807–11.

Golay A, Zech L, Shi M- Z, Chiou Y-AM, Reaven GM, Chen Y-DI. High density lipoprotein (HDL) metabolism in noninsulin-dependent diabetes mellitus: measurement of HDL turnover using tritiated HDL. J Clin Endocrinol Metab. 1987;65:512–8.

Greenfield MS, Doberne L, Kraemer FB, Tobey TA, Reaven GM. Assessment of insulin resistance with the insulin suppression test and the euglycemic clamp. Diabetes 1981;30:387–92.

Jeng CY, Sheu WH-H, Fu MM-T, et al. Relationship between hepatic glucose production and fasting plasma glucose concentration in patients with NIDDM. Diabetes 1994;43:1440–4.

Lehto S, Ronnemaa T, Pyorala K, Laakso M. Cardiovascular risk factors clustering with endogenous hyperinsulinemia predict death from coronary heart disease in patients with type II diabetes. Diabetologia 2000;43:148–55.

Reaven GM, Greenfield MS. Diabetic hypertriglyceridemia: evidence for three clinical syndromes. Diabetes 1981;30(suppl. 2):66–75.

Reaven GM. Insulin resistance in noninsulin-dependent diabetes mellitus: does it exist and can it be measured? Am J Med. 1983;74(suppl. 1A):3–17.

Reaven GM. Role of insulin resistance in human disease. Diabetes 1988;37:1595–607.

Reaven GM. The Fourth Musketeer–from Alexandre Dumas to Claude Benard. Diabetologia 1995;38:3–18.

Reaven GM. The pathophysiological consequences of adipose tissue insulin resistance. In: Reaven GM, Laws A, eds. Insulin resistance: The metabolic syndrome X. Toyota, NJ: Humana Press; 1999:233–46.

Reaven GM. Insulin resistance and its consequences: Type 2 diabetes mellitus and coronary heart disease. In: LeRoith D, Taylor SI, Olefsky JM, eds. Diabetes mellitus, 2nd edn. Philadelphia, PA:Lippincott-Raven; 2000:604–15.

Reaven GM, Hollenbeck CB, Chen Y-DI. Relationship between glucose tolerance, insulin secretion, and insulin action in non-obese individuals with varying degrees of glucose tolerance. Diabetologia 1989;32:52–5.

Reaven GM, Chen Y-DI, Hollenbeck CB, Sheu WHH, Ostrega D, Polonsky KS. Plasma insulin, C-peptide, and pro-insulin concentrations in obese and nonobese individuals with varying degrees of glucose tolerance. J Clin Endocrinol Metab. 1993;76:44–8.

Skowronski R, Hollenbeck CB, Varasteh BB, Chen Y-DI, Reaven GM. Regulations of non-esterified fatty acid and glycerol concentration by insulin in normal individuals and patients with Type 2 diabetes. Diabetic Medicine 1991;8:330–3.

Swislocki ALM, Chen Y-DI, Golay A, Chang M-O, Reaven GM. Insulin suppression of plasma-free fatty acid concentration in normal individuals and patients with Type 2 (non-insulin-dependent) (diabetes. Diabetologia 1987;30:622–6.

Wu MS, Ho LT, Chen JJ, Chen Y-DI, Reaven GM. Somatostatin potentiation of insulin-induced glucose uptake in normal individuals. Am J Physiol. 1986;13:E674–9.

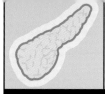

Chapter 23

Non-Insulin-Dependent Diabetes Mellitus

Eugene J Barrett and Jerry L Nadler

DIAGNOSIS OF DIABETES

The current diagnostic criteria for diabetes include a fasting plasma glucose above 7mmol/L (126mg/dL) on two occasions, or a plasma glucose above 11mmol/L, 2 hours after an oral challenge with 75g of glucose (**Table 23.1 & 23.2**). These cut points were selected based upon extended epidemiologic data that examined the impact of variation in plasma glucose on the prevalence of retinal microvascular abnormalities characteristic of diabetic microangiopathy. **Figure 23.1** illustrates this relationship from one such study. Far from arbitrary, these diagnostic criteria are selected to designate risks for the development of tissue pathology and adverse clinical consequences, particularly the specific eye and renal microangiopathic complications of diabetes.

Abnormalities in either the fasting plasma glucose or the oral glucose tolerance test (OGTT) can provide a diagnosis of diabetes or an abnormality in glucose metabolism referred to as impaired fasting glucose or impaired glucose tolerance, respectively. These levels of glycemia do not imply any immediate risk for microvascular disease. They do index persons at risk for the subsequent development of diabetes; i.e. persons with impaired glucose tolerance carry an approximate 50% risk of developing diabetes over a 10-year period. As such, these early changes in glucose homeostasis can serve as a guidepost to stimulate lifestyle modifications that may delay or prevent subsequent development of frank diabetes. Moreover, and of at least equal concern, there is a mounting volume of information that even these more subtle abnormalities of glucose regulation identify individuals with an increased risk of accelerated large-vessel atherosclerotic disease and premature coronary and cerebrovascular events (**Fig. 23.2**).

Although formally these diagnostic criteria pertain to both types 1 and 2 diabetes, practically they are much more used with type 2, as the onset of type 1 is more commonly abrupt, with loss of regulation of glucose metabolism that is not subtle. In contrast, the transition from impaired glucose tolerance or impaired fasting glucose to frank diabetes can be quite insidious with type 2 diabetes mellitus. This is highlighted by the unfortunate observation that approximately one in three individuals with type 2 diabetes is undiagnosed. When necessary, the formal categorization of patients as having either type 1 or 2 diabetes can be done with measurements of antibodies to insulin, islet cells, or several different islet cells proteins, as well as measurements of insulin secretion using C- peptide as a marker. It is uncommon that this testing is needed in routine clinical settings.

Diagnosis of gestational diabetes with a 100-g or 75-g glucose load		
	mg/dL	mmol/L
100-g Glucose load		
Fasting	95	5.3
1-h	180	10.0
2-h	155	8.6
3-h	140	7.8
75-g Glucose load		
Fasting	95	5.3
1-h	180	10.0
2-h	155	8.6

Table 23.2 Diagnosis of gestational diabetes with a 100-g or 75-g glucose load. Two or more of the venous plasma concentrations must be met or exceeded for a positive diagnosis. The test should be done in the morning after an overnight fast of between 8 and 14h and after at least 3 days of unrestricted diet (≥ 150g carbohydrate per day) and unlimited physical activity. The subject should remain seated and should note smoke throughout the test.

Diagnosis of diabetes: plasma glucose cutoff points				
	FPG		2-hour PG on OGTT	
Category	mg/dL	mmol/L	mg/dL	mmol/L
Normal	<110	<6.1	<140	<7.8
IFG	≥ 110 and <126	≥ 6.1 and <6.9	–	–
IGT	–	–	≥ 140 and <200	≥ 7.8 and <11.1
Diabetes	≥ 126	≥ 7.0	≥ 200	≥ 11.1

FPG, fasting plasma glucose; IFG, impaired fasting glucose; IGT, impaired glucose tolerance; OGTT, oral glucose tolerance test, PG, plasma glucose.

Table 23.1 Diagnosis of diabetes: plasma glucose cutoff points. (Data from The Expert Committee on the Diagnosis and Classification of Diabetes Mellitus. Diabetes Care 1997;20:1183–97.)

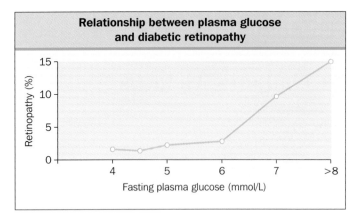

Figure 23.1 Relationship between plasma glucose and diabetic retinopathy. The prevalence of microvascular lesions seen on retinal fundus photographs is seen to vary with the fasting plasma glucose concentration. The prevalence is negligible until fasting plasma glucose concentrations reach approximately 7mmol/L (126mg/dL). With further increases in fasting plasma glucose concentration, the prevalence of retinal microvascular abnormalities increases progressively.

The hemoglobin A_{1c} test, although routinely and effectively used to follow the course of glycemic treatment of diabetes, is not yet recommended for diagnosis. The cost, the variability between laboratories in the methodology used and precision of the testing, and the concern that it will be insensitive in detecting diabetes early in the disease are issues that have discouraged adapting this as a screening test. However, in an individual where such testing is done and findings are abnormal, diabetes is confirmed. The value of hemoglobin A_{1c} measurements in nondiabetic individuals may be re-evaluated in the future on the basis of the results of the EPIC study (**Fig. 23.2**).

Although either the fasting or postchallenge plasma glucose can be used for diagnosis, both cost and convenience have increasingly led to the use of the fasting glucose. An exception is in the diagnosis of diabetes during gestation. The OGTT remains the preferred test and the criteria for diagnosis and treatment differ in this special setting (**Table 23.1**). In part, that is because fetal and

maternal health, not microangiopathy, are the major concerns and treatment focuses on preventing either early (morphogenetic) or later (macrosomic) complications to the pregnancy that are associated with even mild abnormalities in glucose metabolism.

EPIDEMIOLOGY OF DIABETES

The second half of the 20th century witnessed a veritable explosion in the incidence and prevalence of type 2 diabetes that appears even to be gaining further momentum in the new millennium (**Fig. 23.3**). Throughout the last century the increasing prevalence of type 2 was most notable in the developed world. In part this is due to increased longevity, with type 2 diabetes being more prevalent as the population ages. Of concern, in the past decade however, has been the increasing incidence of type 2 in the second, third, and fourth decades of life in highly developed nations. Within the last decade it has become apparent that the prevalence of diabetes in developing nations is all too rapidly overtaking that of more affluent nations. In part at least, this relates to changing economic and cultural factors. These include migration of populations from the countryside to cities and differences in physical activity between agrarian and industrial employment, as well as changes in the types and abundance of foods available and, to a yet unclear extent, differences in intrinsic risks for the development of diabetes among ethnic and racial groups.

The differences in diabetes prevalence across racial groups are striking (**Fig. 23.4**) and, at least in those settings where it has been studied, there can be differences in the frequency of development of specific types of complications among diabetic patients in different racial groups. Cultural, economic and genetic factors each appear to play a role in this outcome as well.

Within racial groups the epidemiology of diabetes and its complications has been particularly well studied in several specific populations, including the Pimas, a native American tribe in the southwestern US and Mexico, the Naurians in the Pacific islands, the Japanese and the populations of several Scandinavian countries. Among racial groups in the USA, it is apparent that the prevalence of type 2 diabetes is greatest among Native Americans,

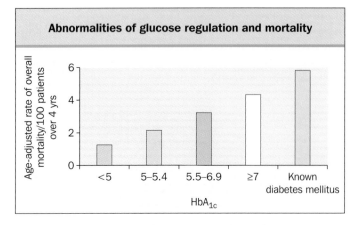

Figure 23.2 Abnormalities of glucose regulation and heart mortality. Data are shown from the recent EPIC study (Br Med J. 2001;322:1–6). The prevalence of overall mortality predominantly due to cardiovascular disease in a European population is plotted as a function of the hemoglobin A1 C.

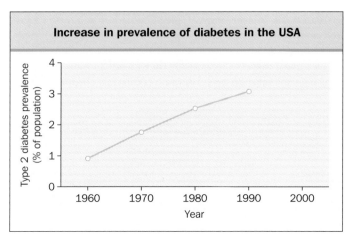

Figure 23.3 Increase in prevalence of diabetes in the USA. The estimated number of cases of diabetes in the USA between the 1950s and the 1990s.

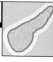

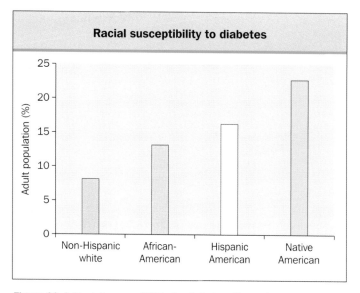

Figure 23.4 Racial susceptibility to diabetes. The estimated percentage of Caucasian American, African-American, Hispanic American and Native American adults affected by diabetes in the USA.

reaching rates of over 50% in some tribes such as the Pimas. Hispanic Americans are similarly affected at rates at least twice those seen among Caucasians, while African-Americans experience prevalence rates about 50% higher than Caucasians. In each of these populations there is a strong relationship between the prevalence of diabetes and the prevalence of obesity in the population. An alarming consequence of increasing obesity, particularly in developed nations, is the increasing incidence of type 2 diabetes in children. Almost unheard of a generation ago, in some minority communities, e.g. Hispanic Americans, type 2 diabetes is becoming nearly as common in children as type 1.

PATHOGENESIS OF TYPE 2 DIABETES MELLITUS

The pathogenesis of the common form of type 2 diabetes remains incompletely understood. However, intensive clinical and basic studies of insulin secretion and action in animal models and humans, as well as genetic studies principally in mice, have moved us far along towards that understanding. It is clear that there are a number of potential pathogenetic lesions that can result in the diabetic phenotype.

In humans, this has been most clearly illustrated by what has been learned in the last 10 years from studies of uncommon monogenic forms of diabetes. Among these uncommon forms of type 2 diabetes the MODY phenotype (maturity-onset diabetes in the young) was early recognized as an autosomal dominant disorder with onset of abnormalities of glucose metabolism at a young age (first to fourth decades). Ketosis was rare in these subjects. Subsequent detailed genetic mapping studies have identified at least four variants of MODY. The one most readily understood appears to be due to a deficient expression of the enzyme glucokinase. This enzyme is the dominant hexokinase found in the liver and in pancreatic β cells. In the heterozygote state, islets of affected individuals will contain only half the usual complement of active enzyme. As a result, higher glucose concentrations are required to sustain normal glycolytic flux in the β cell, which is required for insulin secretion (**Fig. 23.5**). Because of this, insulin secretion is diminished at normal plasma glucose concentrations, but rises with hyperglycemia.

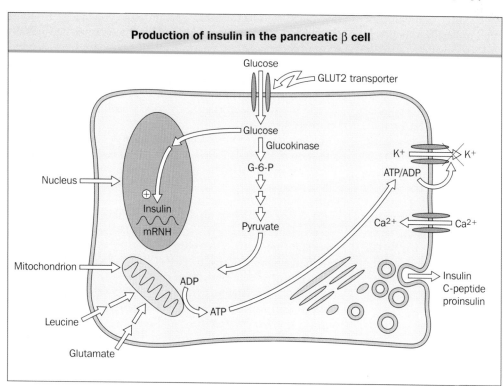

Figure 23.5 Production of insulin in the pancreatic β cell. Glucose enters the β cell of the pancreatic islet via the GLUT2 transporter. Once inside the β cell glucose is converted by the enzyme glucokinase into glucose 6-phosphate. Subsequently the glucose 6-phosphate is metabolized via glycolysis to pyruvate which is subsequently oxidized within the mitochondria. Other substrates that can provoke insulin secretion (amino acids, oxaloacetate) also enter the tricarboxylic (Krebs) cycle. Oxidation of these substrates increases the ratio of adenosine triphosphate (ATP) to adenosine diphosphate (ADP). This ratio regulates the activity of a plasma membrane potassium channel. An increased ratio diminishes potassium leakage through the K–ATP channel. As a result, the plasma membrane potential falls to less negative values. This activates voltage-dependent calcium channels, allowing calcium to flow down an electrochemical gradient. The rise in cell calcium concentration triggers a migration and fusion of insulin containing secretory granules with the plasma membrane allowing insulin secretion to proceed.

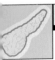

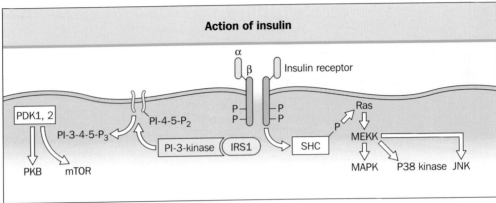

Figure 23.6 Action of insulin. Insulin initiates its cellular actions by first binding to a specific heterodimeric plasma membrane receptor. Insulin is recognized by binding sites on the α subunits. The binding triggers a conformational change, which results in the activation of an intrinsic tyrosine kinase activity on the intracellular domain of the β subunit. This activity phosphorylates tyrosines on the β subunit. This autophosphorylation sets in motion a sequence of reactions whereby adapter molecules within the cell associate with the phosphorylated insulin receptor. One family of these, the insulin receptor substrate (IRS) proteins, are phosphorylated on tyrosine residues by the insulin receptor kinase. This allows the subsequent binding of the enzyme phosphotidylinositol-3-kinase (PI-3-kinase). This binding activates the kinase ,with subsequent increased production of phosphatidyl-inositol 3,4,5 triphosphate (PI-3-4-5-P_3). This can activate two downstream serine-threonine kinases, which in turn can activate the enzyme AKT (also referred to as PKB), as well as other kinases. Further downstream of this pathway the GLUT4 (insulin-regulated) glucose transporter in skeletal muscle and adipose tissue is recruited to the plasma membrane, thereby enhancing glucose entry. Also downstream of this pathway are two other important biologic actions of insulin, glycogen synthesis and protein synthesis. An entirely separate action of insulin involves the stimulation of mitogenesis and gene regulation. This appears to proceed through a distinct pathway that is again triggered by phosphorylation of the β subunit of the insulin receptor. However, it proceeds through a different kinase cascade, which involves first the activation of Ras, then Raf, followed by phosphorylation of MEKK, then MEK. Increasingly, there is evidence that at several levels there may be crossover between these two major activation pathways initiated by insulin.

A variety of specific mutations in the enzyme glucokinase have been described in MODY subjects. In addition, mutations in the genes that code for hepatic nuclear factor-1 (HNF-1) and HNF-4 also produce a MODY phenotype. However, the pathogenetic sequence by which each of these defects alter body glucose metabolism and insulin secretion is not clear. Finally, there are a number of families in which early onset type 2 diabetes appears to be transmitted in an autosomal dominant pattern, in whom no molecular defect has yet been ascertained. One of the most informative aspects of these studies is in their clear demonstration that type 2 diabetes can begin as a defect in insulin secretion.

Complementing MODY, there are a number of uncommon forms of type 2 diabetes that are clearly attributable to genetic defects in the pathway(s) of insulin action. Among the use are leprechaunism and lipoatrophic diabetes, as well as individuals with specific defects in the insulin receptor or the PPARγ transcription factor. It is apparent from the diversity of molecular defects capable of causing human type 2 diabetes that abnormalities in either insulin secretion or action can initiate the development of diabetes. These observations have led to the recognition that there are multiple forms of diabetes and that the common form (which itself probably represents multiple genetic etiologies) involves combined impairments in insulin action and insulin secretion.

Using modern, high-throughput genetic screening methods and sophisticated statistical analyses, a number of the genome-wide searchers are in progress to define the specific genetic bases for the common forms of type 2 diabetes. At present, these efforts have not yielded an accepted candidate gene or family of genes. However, as the organization of the human genome is better understood and patterns of gene expression are further

clarified, there is the expectation that more significant progress will be made with this approach.

As these efforts towards the discovery of the genetic bases of a number of forms of human diabetes have progressed, genetic manipulation using transgenic and knockout technology in animal models has yielded interesting and at times surprising findings. Most of these targeted genetic manipulations have been directed at components of the insulin-signaling pathway. This pathway has been increasingly characterized over the past 15 years. **Figure 23.6** gives a simplified diagram of insulin signaling as it occurs in muscle and adipose, tissues that express insulin-sensitive glucose transport systems.

Insulin binding to its receptor at the cell surface triggers the activation of a tyrosine kinase activity that is resident in the S-subunit. This kinase phosphorylates the receptor at multiple sites. These phosphorylations facilitate the association of a number of proteins with the intracellular domain of the receptor and some of these proteins are themselves tyrosine phosphorylated by the receptor kinase. Among these the first described were the IRS (insulin receptor substrate) proteins. These constitute a family of multidomain proteins that includes IRS 1,2,3, and 4, which when phosphorylated will bind to other proteins with Src homology domains or PTB binding domains. The P85 subunit of the PI-3 kinase is a primary example of a protein that binds to and is activated by phosphorylated IRS-1 and 2. Activated PI-3 kinase catalyzes the production of phosphatidyl inositol 3,4,5-phosphate. This subsequently activates at least two serine or threonine kinases, PDK-1 and 2. Further along is a series of threonine/serine kinases, which are responsible for transmitting the biologic effects of insulin to the glucose transport mechanism, glycogen synthesis, and protein synthesis. Yet another pathway that begins at the

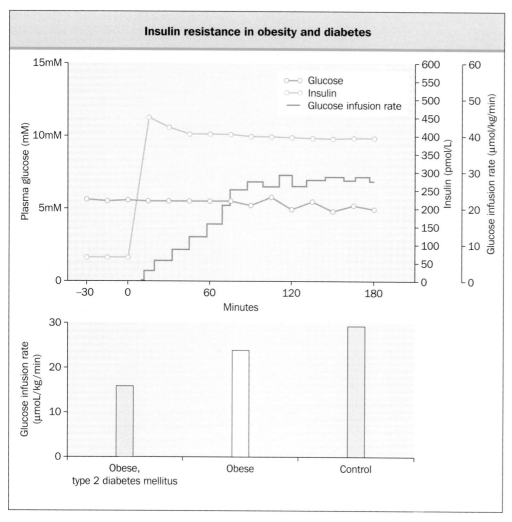

Figure 23.7 Insulin resistance in obesity and diabetes. (Top panel) The experimental procedure followed in an insulin-clamp. The plasma glucose concentration is measured after an overnight fast (Blue circle); samples are also obtained for plasma insulin (Orange circle). After obtaining several basal samples, insulin is infused to raise the plasma insulin concentration to a preselected value based upon known kinetics of insulin clearance. Ordinarily, this would cause a decline in plasma glucose. However, by measuring plasma glucose frequently and infusing a concentrated glucose solution, plasma glucose is held constant at its basal concentration. As a result, at steady state the effect of a given concentration of insulin on the glucose infusion rate required can be estimated. Since the plasma glucose concentration remains constant, all the infused glucose is being used by body tissues. The sensitivity of tissue glucose disposal to a given concentration of insulin can thereby be measured. (Lower panel) The glucose infusion rate, at steady state, is compared in three groups of individuals: healthy lean control subjects, obese nondiabetic subjects, and obese type 2 diabetic patients. This was done during a 1mU/kg/min insulin infusion. Compared to the control subjects, both the obese and the diabetic subjects received lower glucose infusion rates, because their tissues used less glucose despite identical plasma glucose and insulin concentrations, indicating insulin-resistance in the latter two groups.

insulin receptor but signals via the Ras/Raf, MEKK, MEK pathway appears more involved in the mitogenic activities of insulin that have been reported in a number of tissues. Crosstalk between these branched signaling cascades also occurs, emphasizing both the complexity and redundancy that has evolved.

A number of mouse models have been created in which a targeted deletion was made in one of these intermediates in insulin signaling or in the insulin receptor or glucose transporter. Some, for example the IRS-2 knockout mouse, have a diabetic phenotype. Surprisingly, however, this seems to be related to an effect more on islet development than on insulin-mediated glucose disposal. Perhaps even more surprisingly, when the insulin receptor was deleted selectively in skeletal muscle, the phenotype had no major abnormality in glucose metabolism. These models have been particularly instructive in indicating how closely linked changes of the insulin-signaling cascade in the peripheral insulin target tissues are to those in the β cell. They have not yet, however, provided us with a strong indication of the likely candidate genes responsible for aberrant metabolism in type 2 diabetes.

Insulin resistance – the islet, the liver, muscle and fat, vascular tissue

Beginning with the demonstration by Berson and Yalow that plasma insulin was measurable or even increased in type 2 diabetic patients, clinical investigations have demonstrated that insulin resistance is widespread in type 2 diabetes. Using a variety of radioisotopic turnover methods, organ-balance techniques and *in vivo* magnetic resonance spectroscopic methods during strictly controlled euglycemic insulin infusions (euglycemic clamp), investigators have convincingly demonstrated that insulin-mediated glucose disposal is impaired in skeletal muscle of type 2 diabetics (**Fig. 23.7**). In addition, hepatic glucose production and adipose tissue lipolysis are likewise resistant to the normal action of insulin to restrain glucose and fatty acid production. The changes in fatty acid concentration worsen glucose metabolism indirectly as the free fatty acids impair insulin-mediated glucose uptake by muscle and promote hepatic glucose production. This rise in free fatty acids can further worsen muscle and liver insulin sensitivity.

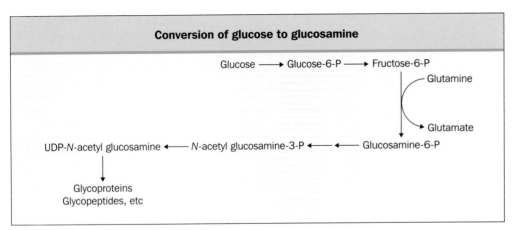

Figure 23.8 Conversion of glucose to glucosamine. The diagram indicates the pathway by which glucose is converted through glutamine-fructose amino-transferase to glucosamine and how this compound might be involved in producing glucose toxicity.

The insulin resistance of type 2 diabetes is qualitatively similar to the insulin resistance seen in association with hypertension, obesity, and specific forms of dyslipidemia discussed elsewhere (Chapter 22). Quantitatively, the insulin resistance of diabetes is more severe in most reports, but this may be in part attributable to the 'glucose toxicity' typically seen with established diabetes. The term 'glucose toxicity' refers to the further impairment in glucose disposal that accrues simply as a result of an individual being hyperglycemic for some time. This form of insulin resistance is reversible and improvement in glucose control by anyone of a variety of measures (insulin treatment, dietary changes, weight reduction, etc.) will over several weeks improve insulin-mediated glucose disposal. Perhaps equally important, prolonged elevations of plasma glucose can impair glucose-stimulated insulin secretion in type 2 diabetes. This islet 'glucose toxicity' is likewise reversible, particularly early in the course of type 2 diabetes. The biochemical basis for glucose toxicity in either insulin target tissues (muscle, liver, adipose) or the β cells has not been fully defined. A significant contributor to this process appears to be increased concentrations of glucosamine, formed intracellularly with the transfer of an amino group from glutamine to fructose by the action of the enzyme glutamine-fructose aminotransferase (GFAT; **Fig. 23.8**). The increase in cellular glucosamine content can be used in a variety of the glucosylation reactions involving UDP-glucosamine.

There is evidence for impairment in insulin action early in the course of stimulation of the insulin-signaling cascade. Even the tyrosine phosphorylation of the insulin receptor itself, as well as tyr-phosphorylation of the IRS proteins, appears diminished in type 2 diabetes. This occurs despite ample evidence that these proteins are themselves products of normal genes, raising the possibility that post-translational modification of these proteins, particularly serine phosphorylation, has resulted in diminished signal transduction. However, at this time the exact mechanism for this altered signaling is not known.

The hypothesis that altered insulin action is a fundamental defect in type 2 diabetes has gained attractiveness with the recognition that this signaling system exists in the β cell as well, where a defect might alter development and function of the islet, thereby giving the combination of defects in insulin secretion and action seen in type 2.

As discussed in Chapter 22, insulin resistance is seen in a number of disorders in which regulation of glucose metabolism

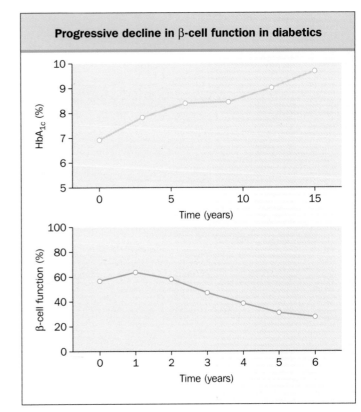

Figure 23.9 Progressive decline in β cell function in diabetics. In the United Kingdom Prospective Diabetes Study a progressive increase in hemoglobin A_{1c} and a time-dependent decline in insulin secretory function were observed.

remains normal. Many patients with obesity or essential hypertension or polycystic ovarian disease are insulin-resistant and these disorders are themselves very common. As a result, there is a large population of insulin-resistant nondiabetic people. Some of these people will experience a progressive loss of β-cell function, and they will develop diabetes. What has become increasingly apparent in recent years is the continuing decline of β-cell function that proceeds even after diabetes has developed (**Fig. 23.9**). This was well illustrated in the UKPDS study results and underlies the long-standing clinical observation that many patients with type 2 eventually become insulin-dependent and that the

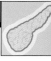

insulin doses are increased over time. Clearly, genetic and nutritional factors such as altered free fatty acid or mineral metabolism play a role in impaired glucose-induced insulin secretion seen in type 2 diabetes. There is evidence for a role of islet cell lipotoxicity in this process.

In addition to the common form of type 2 diabetes associated with obesity and insulin resistance, there are a number of secondary forms of type 2 diabetes. These include those secondary to a variety of drugs, especially glucocorticoids, those secondary to other endocrine disorders (e.g. acromegaly, Cushing's disease, pheochromocytoma), or caused by other systemic illness, and some rare forms of uncertain cause, such as the acquired lipodystrophies.

COMPLICATIONS OF DIABETES

Introduction

Before considering the treatment of the glycemic abnormalities that identify diabetes, we will discuss the varied complications that arise from the disease. This is done principally to emphasize that, because the consequences of diabetes are protean, the treatment approach must be flexible and multifaceted and include attention to issues of blood pressure, lipids, antithrombotic treatment, nutrition, mineral replacement, and other factors that interact with glycemia to accelerate or retard the development or progression of many of the tissue injuries that constitute the major complications of diabetes.

Microvascular

As indicated previously, chronic hyperglycemia has a specific damaging effect on the microvasculature that is most evident in the retina and the renal glomerulus but is present more generally in body tissues. Although microvascular lesions affect many organs in diabetic patients, it is in the eye and kidney that these effects produce their most direct, devastating clinical consequences. Indeed, diabetes is a leading cause of blindness and end-stage renal disease throughout the developed world.

Because of the prevalence of diabetes and the prevalence of microvascular pathology in the diabetic population, treatment options that might forestall or slow the development of eye and renal complications of diabetes have been studied extensively. To assess the effects of treatment and evaluate the progression or delay of progression, quantitative assessment measures have been adopted. In the case of eye disease this has involved repeated evaluation of fundus photographs and measures of retinal capillary leakage. In the case of the kidney it has been measurements of capillary leakage (as indicated by microalbuminuria or proteinuria) and eventual loss of glomerular capillary function, as evidenced by diminished filtration rates, that have been measures of disease progress. With these tools it has been possible to demonstrate that systemic therapies directed at controlling blood sugar and blood pressure are each capable of slowing the development and progression of diabetic eye and renal disease.

In the eye, early changes from diabetes include capillary rarefaction and leakage, microaneurysms, and blot hemorrhages. **Figure 23.10** illustrates some of the various stages of diabetic eye disease. Such changes are frequently referred to as 'background diabetic retinopathy'. Of themselves these changes do not affect vision. However, they serve to mark that some tissue injury is

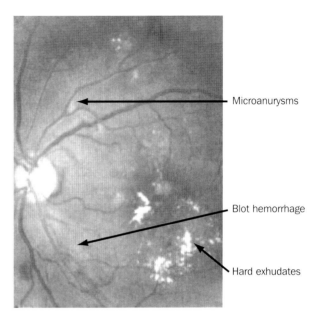

Figure 23.10 Diabetic retinopathy. Early changes in the retina seen with diabetes including microaneurysms, blot hemorrhages, and hard exudates.

occurring and may presage more serious changes, including the development of macular edema and neovascularization that can seriously impair vision. As such, the earlier stages of retinopathy serve to warn of the need for vigilant followup examinations. When more serious preproliferative or proliferative retinopathy is seen, treatment with laser photocoagulation can preserve vision in many patients. In advanced stages, if major vitreous hemorrhages have occurred, some improvement in vision can frequently be achieved by vitrectomy procedures. As good glycemic control can avoid many of these retinal complications, a priority must be given to preventive measures as the most effective treatment.

Though the retinopathy of diabetes is fairly specific and distinct from that seen with hypertension, elevated blood pressures clearly accelerate the development and progression of diabetic retinopathy. The impact of blood glucose control on the development and progression of diabetic eye disease in the cohort followed in the United Kingdom Prospective Diabetes Study (UKPDS) is shown in **Figure 23.11**. This study also demonstrated a particularly dramatic effect of blood pressure control on the development and progression of eye disease. A significant effect of glucose control on both eye and kidney disease had been demonstrated earlier in the prospective Diabetes Control and Complications Trial (DCCT) and an effect of blood pressure control had been suggested in earlier, shorter-duration, and smaller cohort studies.

To effectively assess the presence and progression of eye disease in the clinical setting requires examination of the dilated eye, generally by an eye specialist. Numerous studies have shown that the simple use of the office indirect ophthalmoscope can miss significant pathology, particularly in older patients, where pupil size, lens opacity, and the simultaneous presence of other eye pathology can complicate the examination. These limitations have led to practice recommendations suggesting annual or biennial eye examinations by eye physicians. This is not to discourage the generalist physician from doing an indirect ophthalmoscopic

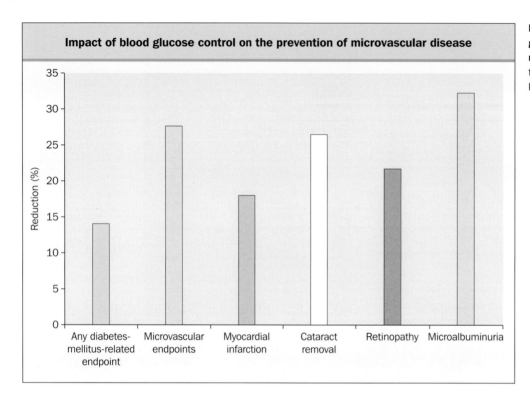

Figure 23.11 Impact of blood glucose control on the prevention of microvascular disease. These data are from the results of the UK Prospective Diabetes Study.

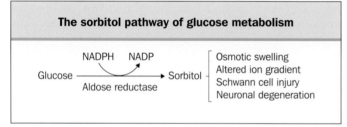

Figure 23.12 The sorbitol pathway of glucose metabolism. This pathway appears involved in cataract formation and potentially peripheral neuropathy.

examination, as this can often allow visualization of interim changes and precipitate timely referral and early intervention, when treatments are most effective.

In addition to retinal damage, patients with diabetes are at higher risk for the development of cataracts than nondiabetic patients and again this appears to be related to the effects of glycemia itself. The lens of the eye is also susceptible to acute changes in volume as a result of glucose entering and being metabolized within the lens. The lens has provided a useful model system for studying the aldose reductase pathway, which converts fructose (derived from glucose) into sorbitol (**Fig. 23.12**). Sorbitol is less permeable than glucose, tending to remain within the lens and cause an osmotic swelling. This process appears to account for some of the changes in visual acuity noted at the time of the initial diagnosis of diabetes. Beyond that, the buildup of these sugar alcohols may accelerate cataract development and in other tissues, particularly peripheral nerve, may contribute to the development of other diabetic complications. As the rate of sorbitol generation is proportional to the extent of glycemia, excellent glycemic control can minimize the development of these complications.

In the kidney, the glomerulus is the major target for glycemia-related tissue injury (**Fig. 23.13**). Early responses include a thickening and altered permselectivity of the glomerular capillary basement membrane. Clinically this may be manifest as increased excretion of larger proteins, such as albumin, in urine. Indeed, albumin excretion rate is a well-established marker for early renal disease and is widely used to screen patients with both type 1 and type 2 diabetes. Over time, if glycemia is not successfully managed, more glomeruli are affected and glomerular involvement becomes more diffuse, with mesangial proliferation and a more exuberant deposition of extracellular matrix materials. This is accompanied by a decline in filtration rates and typically a further rise in protein excretion. As filtration is impaired in some glomeruli others may be hyperfiltering, exposing them to risk of further injury. The declining renal function can also lead to a rise in blood pressure in normotensive patients and in those with pre-existing hypertension. This will only accelerate progressive renal injury.

The progression of renal disease in patients with type 2 diabetes differs from that seen in type 1 diabetes. Type 1 patients have been observed to experience a nearly inexorable decline in renal function once frank proteinuria has developed. This can be slowed or prevented by pharmacologic intervention, particularly with angiotensin converting enzyme (ACE) inhibitors. Type 2 individuals may develop proteinuria but the subsequent decline in renal function is less predictable than with type 1 patients. Some patients are observed to have proteinuria for a number of years without declining renal function. Yet, because type 2 diabetes is so much more prevalent than type 1, in a number of developed countries type 2 diabetes accounts for a greater fraction of end-stage renal disease from diabetes. Because the course of renal disease progression has been less predictable in type 2 diabetes, the use of ACE inhibitors and other agents early in the course of renal disease has been less well supported by clinical

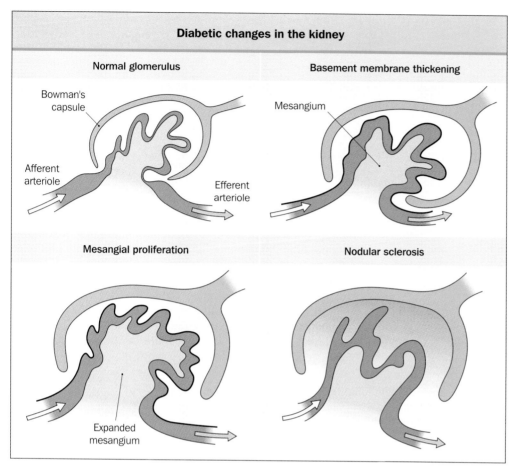

Figure 23.13 Diabetic changes in the kidney. Illustrated here are the progressive changes in the renal glomerular architecture that occur in the diabetic kidney.

trial results. However, following data from several recent trials (most notably the UKPDS and HOPE trials), ACE inhibitors are now widely used in type 2 patients showing even the earliest signs of renal disease (microalbuminuria), even in the absence of hypertension. The success of ACE inhibitors in reducing overall mortality in the HOPE trial underscores the association of microalbuminuria with an increased risk of cardiovascular disease (CVD) in type 2 diabetes. Newer trials also suggest angiotensin 2 receptor agonists may also have therapeutic benefit to reduce the decline in renal function in type 2 diabetes.

As mentioned previously, hypertension frequently accompanies type 2 diabetes as part of the insulin-resistance syndrome. With regard to renal disease, while hypertension *per se* does not produce anatomic renal lesions similar to those of diabetes, it can clearly accelerate the development and progression of renal injury from diabetes. As a result, recommendations for control of blood pressure are more stringent in patients with diabetes, and achieving blood-pressure control targets typically requires multiple agents. As a result of trials such as the UKPDS and HOPE trials, the use of ACE inhibitors and beta-blockers is well supported in this patient population. In some populations, such as African-Americans, whose blood-pressure may not be well controlled with ACE inhibitors, other agents, such as diuretics, may be needed early in the course of treatment.

Unfortunately, despite the availability of measures, such as glucose and blood-pressure treatment, that have been demonstrated to slow the progression of renal disease in type 2 diabetes, many patients progress to end-stage renal failure. Both peritoneal and hemodialysis can be used to manage the renal failure successfully in these patients. However, the clinical outcomes of patients with type 2 diabetes are generally much poorer than for most other causes of dialysis-dependent renal disease. In part this may be due to the acceleration of the atherosclerotic process, which occurs with endstage renal disease and is particularly aggressive in diabetes. Transplantation affords another option that can be more successful, although it brings along its own constellation of adverse consequences. Clearly, early, aggressive, persistent management of blood pressure and glucose affords patients the best prospect for a good clinical outcome.

Diabetic neuropathies

There are multiple manifestations of diabetes in the peripheral nervous system. Most common is the symmetric peripheral combined motor–sensory polyneuropathy that is characteristically seen distally in the toes and feet. With time it proceeds proximally to involve more of the lower then distal upper extremity. It is characteristically symmetric and affects the longest nerves first. It originates as a Schwann cell lesion with loss of myelination at discrete sites on many fibers throughout the peripheral nervous system. However, as the longest nerves are most susceptible to having their action potential disrupted by multiple small areas of injury, these are clinically affected earliest. A number of theories have been advanced to explain how hyperglycemia produces this common polyneuropathy.

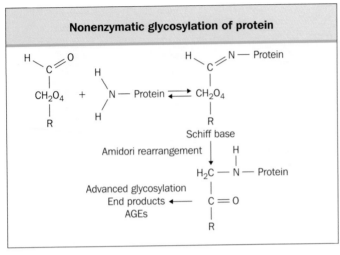

Figure 23.14 Nonenzymatic glycosylation of proteins. Illustrated here is an important pathway for nonenzymatic glycosylation of proteins by glucose and the formation of advanced glycosylation end-products.

Both the sorbitol hypothesis (described above for the generation of cataracts) and nonenzymatic glycosylation (**Fig. 23.14**) probably play a role. In addition, at least in experimental models, there is a considerable body of data suggesting that depletion of an inositol sugar, myoinositol, is involved. Probably, multiple factors contribute. Efforts at directing therapies towards each of these pathogenetic pathways has met with limited success to date. Trials of aldose-reductase inhibitors have been ongoing for more than a dozen years but have as yet not proved to be clinically useful. Efforts at myoinositol supplementation have not produced useful improvement in human trials and use of inhibitors of nonenzymatic glycosylation, while still early in evaluation, has not yet provided a clinically useful product. As a result, glucose control remains the mainstay for preventing and treating the development and progression of neuropathy.

Established sensory neuropathy can present as either a progressive loss of sensation alone, loss of sensation combined with minor dysesthesias or with varying degrees of pain, which in some cases can be debilitating. There are important symptomatic therapies that are useful in patients symptomatic from painful peripheral neuropathy. These include topical therapy with capsaicin-containing creams, which act to deplete substance P from small-diameter pain fibers. If these fail, systemic treatment with antidepressants such as amitriptyline or analgesics such as

gabapentin are frequently helpful. Occasional patients require multiple drugs, infrequently in combination with strong analgesics. As the symptoms of painful neuropathy can last many months or years, efforts should be made to avoid the use of narcotic analgesics or chronic use of cyclooxygenase inhibitors.

Control of hyperglycemia can ameliorate symptoms and slow progression of sensory loss. Sensory losses expose the patient to an increased risk for tissue injury unawareness. This risk is increased by the motor neuropathy, which alters the carriage of the foot, with frequent development of claw-toe deformities that alter weightbearing and increase callus development, particularly over the metatarsal heads (**Fig. 23.15**). Fastidious foot care is of vital importance both to prevent the acute infections and to avoid the worsening bony deformities that can accompany diabetic peripheral neuropathy. In advanced stages, patients with diabetic neuropathy can develop an essentially anesthetic foot with Charcot deformities of the ankle joint. All these patients require skilled podiatric care to avoid the sequence of infection and amputation seen all too frequently.

The autonomic nervous system is also regularly affected by diabetes. This may present with a variety of manifestations, including impotence, urinary retention, retrograde ejaculation, constipation (or diarrhea), gastroparesis, dysautonomia with sweating or flushing, resting tachycardia, and orthostatic hypotension. There is no specific treatment to reverse the neuropathy responsible for these problems. However, as with the peripheral neuropathy, a number of symptomatic treatments can be gratifyingly effective. Thus, sildenafil or intraurethral or intracavernous administration of a prostaglandin can improve impotence in 50% or more of patients. Constipation and gastroparesis can be treated with promotility agents like erythromycin or metaclopramide. The cardiac autonomic neuropathy can be particularly symptomatic, with resting tachycardia and orthostatic hypotension. The latter can be treated with volume repletion and occasional by pressors such as amphetamines.

Less common than either the sensorimotor polyneuropathy or autonomic neuropathies are nerve injuries that result from single or multiple vaso-occlusive injuries. Thus mononeuritis, most frequently seen as a palsy of one or more extraocular muscles, or, less commonly, mononeuritis multiplex are recognized complications of vascular infarction of nervous tissue. These appear to occur more frequently in diabetic patients secondary to more advanced atherosclerosis, particularly in small vascular beds.

Another uncommon form of diabetic neuropathy is referred to as either diabetic neuropathic cachexia or diabetic amyotrophy.

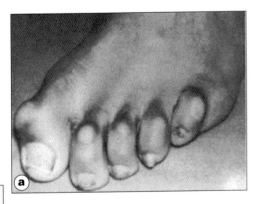

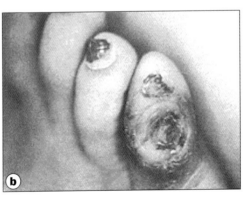

Figure 23.15 Effects of diabetes on the foot. Note the hammer toes (a), ulcer over the 5th metatarsal heads (b).

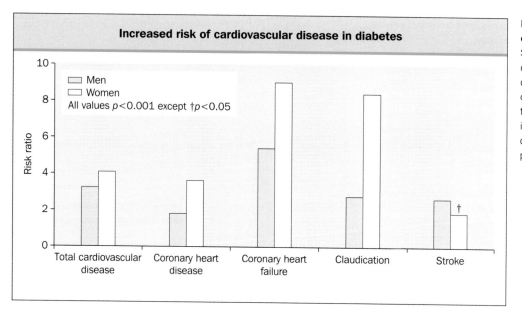

Figure 23.16 Increased risk of cardiovascular disease in diabetes. Shown here are prospectively gathered data from the Framingham study demonstrating the increased overall cardiovascular mortality as well as the frequency of stroke, and myocardial infarction in the men and women with diabetes compared to the nondiabetic population.

This is a poorly understood disorder that is most frequently encountered in patients with long-standing diabetes and is characterized by severe proximal muscle weakness. This may be unilateral or symmetric and is generally associated with deep pain and frequently with profound weight loss. Perhaps the most peculiar aspect of this disorder is that it typically remits spontaneously over 3–12 months, with restoration of muscle strength and remission of pain. The proximal muscles of the lower extremity are most frequently involved, although the upper extremities can be affected. Muscle wasting is very marked and the principal differential involves evaluation for spinal cord or nerve root disease.

Macrovascular disease in diabetes

It has been repeatedly demonstrated that diabetic patients have a two- to threefold increased risk of CVD compared to age-matched nondiabetic controls (**Figs 23.16 & 23.17**). Beyond that, they are less likely to survive cardiovascular events and respond less well to interventional procedures directed at remediation of their atherosclerotic disease. Macrovascular disease in the diabetic patient population is so prevalent that it is estimated to account for more than 75% of the morbidity, mortality, and costs of diabetes in the USA.

In this context, the steadily increasing prevalence of type 2 diabetes in the population and its appearance at younger ages is particularly alarming. With type 2 diabetes now frequently being seen in the fourth, third, and even second decades of life, we will soon be dealing with a population of younger patients with diabetes and heart disease. Inasmuch as the majority of patients with type 2 diabetes are cared for by their primary care physicians, there will be an increasing need for skilled, knowledgeable interventions on their part to optimize the prevention, diagnosis, and treatment of CVD.

As noted previously, in a number of studies the increased prevalence of CVD has been seen even when glucose homeostasis is only very modestly affected. As the majority of type 2 diabetic patients are affected by additional components of the insulin-resistance syndrome (e.g. hypertension, low high-density-

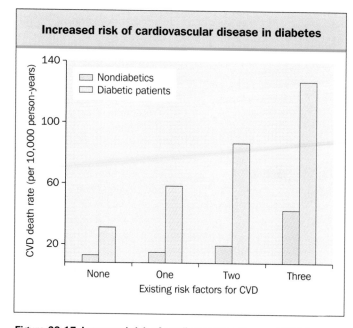

Figure 23.17 Increased risk of cardiovascular disease (CVD) in diabetes. The Mr Fit study demonstrated that for patients without diabetes, there is an increased risk of coronary disease as the number of coronary risk factors increased (cigarette smoking, hypertension, and hypercholesterolemia). For each risk factor or combination, diabetes had an additive effect on overall risk.

lipoprotein cholesterol, increased visceral fat) this constellation of the insulin-resistance syndrome may in part account for the high prevalence of CVD. Hyperglycemia *per se* adds to the risk somewhat and may have a particular impact on postevent complications, including repeat infarction, sudden death, and congestive heart failure.

The accelerated atherosclerosis affects the coronary, cerebral, and peripheral vasculature, accounting for the increased incidence of myocardial infarction, stroke, and peripheral vascular disease seen with diabetes. Within each of these circulatory beds, the atherosclerotic process tends to be more diffuse and extend further distally than in nondiabetic patients. The plaque formation frequently includes calcium deposits and it is not uncommon to encounter extensive calcification of vessel walls even distally in the lower legs and feet. The extensiveness of the disease can sometimes frustrate use of conventional vascular dilation or bypass procedures to aid tissue perfusion. Emerging reports support the role of inflammatory changes in the vasculature as an important factor in accelerated cardiovascular disease in type 2 diabetes.

As the morbidity and mortality from macrovascular disease is such a problem in the diabetic population, it is of vital importance to focus CVD prevention efforts on the diabetic population. This includes addressing all modifiable CVD risk factors, including smoking cessation, blood pressure control, correction of lipid abnormalities, prophylactic use of aspirin or other antiplatelet agents, and consideration of the use of ACE inhibitors and β-adrenergic blocking drugs in subjects with known or suspected CVD even in the absence of classical indication (elevated blood pressure, proteinuria or microalbuminuria). Because of the high risk for CVD in type 2 diabetes, recommended treatment goals for blood pressure and lipid management are more aggressive than in the non-diabetic population (**Table 23.3**).

As the risk for CVD events in the diabetic population without known CVD appears comparable to that of the nondiabetic population with known ischemic heart disease, a strong argument can be made for more vigilant CVD screening of type 2 diabetic patients. This is particularly applicable when patients have additional traditional CVD risk factors or have microalbuminuria or proteinuria, peripheral or carotid vascular disease, or extensive retinopathy. Generally, a stress electrocardiogram (ECG) is a good initial screening test. The outcome of such testing may serve either to trigger additional diagnostic evaluation or to provide a rationale to intensify prevention measures or institute anti-ischemic therapy. Subsequent testing in patients with abnormal stress tests might include stress perfusion imaging, echocardiography, or cardiac catheterization. Additional testing is also appropriate for patients who cannot complete an exercise protocol or in whom baseline ECG abnormalities prevent use of exercise testing.

For patients in whom significant coronary artery disease is identified, intensive medical therapy is clearly indicated. Beyond this, there is need for patient evaluation by a cardiovascular specialist team familiar with the complexities of managing patients with diabetes undergoing revascularization procedures involving either percutaneous or bypass techniques. Early studies with percutaneous balloon angioplasty in type 2 diabetic patients suggested that this group of patients fare considerably less well than nondiabetic patients undergoing the same procedure. This situation may be improving, with the use of coronary stents and platelet glycoprotein 2b3a inhibitors, although it may be too early to consider this a general finding. More encouraging than the response to percutaneous dilation and stenting procedures are the apparently good outcomes seen for diabetic patients with severe coronary disease undergoing bypass using the internal mammary artery to revascularize the anterior myocardium.

Risk category for patients with type 2 diabetes mellitus based on plasma lipid measurenents			
Risk	**LDL cholesterol**	**HDL cholesterol**	**Triglyceride**
High	>130	<35*	>400
Borderline	100–129	35–45	200–399
Low	<100	>45	<200

Data are given in mg/dL. For women HDL cholesterol values should be increased by 10mg/dL.
Goal for blood pressure control is <130/85 based on Joint National Commission 6 recommendations.

Table 23.3 Risk category for patients with type 2 diabetes mellitus based on plasma lipid measurements. HDL, high-density lipoproteins; LDL, low-density lipoproteins.

TREATMENTS DIRECTED AT IMPROVING HYPERGLYCEMIA

The recently completed UKPDS has provided a wealth of information relating to the effect of diabetes management on clinical outcome in patients with type 2 diabetes. It has provided definitive evidence that in this population sustained improvement in levels of hemoglobin A_{1c} could be achieved. Furthermore, the seemingly modest changes in hemoglobin A_{1c} levels (average approximately 0.9% reduction over 10–12 years) brought about by insulin, metformin, or sulfonylurea treatment (or combinations thereof) reduced microvascular complications in the eye, kidney, and peripheral nerve by approximately 25%. These quantitative changes in microvascular outcomes parallel remarkably those seen in the earlier Diabetes Control Complications Study, where a 2% lowering of hemoglobin A_{1c}, sustained over 7 years, reduced microvascular disease development/progression in the eye, kidney, and nerve by approximately 50–60% in patients with type 1 diabetes. Combined, these two large population trials, supported by earlier, smaller trials, show a strong relationship between glycemia, its control, and improved clinical microvascular outcomes.

Among the agents used to treat glycemia in UKPDS (metformin, sulfonylurea and insulin), all provided benefits. In a subset of obese type 2 patients selected to receive metformin as first-line therapy, there was an improvement in mortality as well. In addition, weight gain was less in subjects treated with metformin compared to those treated with insulin or sulfonylurea. These factors have led to metformin being considered as a first choice for oral therapy in patients with type 2 diabetes.

Diet and nutritional management

Dietary management remains the mainstay of the treatment of type 2 diabetes. Early in the course of the disease, dietary management alone can be sufficient to control glycemia. As approximately 80% of patients with type 2 are obese or overweight, weight reduction is usually an added goal. The basic dietary recommendations include a low-fat (<30% of calories), particularly low-saturated-fat (<10% of calories) diet that includes 50–55% carbohydrate and 15–20% protein. The carbohydrate should include a significant fraction of complex carbohydrate.

Oral hypoglycemic agents		
Medication class	Mechanism of action	Comments
Biguanides – metformin and phenformin	Major action is to suppress hepatic glucose production probably by interfering with gluconeogenesis – though the step(s) of this pathway where biguanides act is not known	Renal excretion of active compound. Gastrointestinal intolerance is major side effect. Hypoglycemia is rare and weight gain uncommon. Long record of relatively safe use for metformin. Rarely, can cause lactic acidosis in susceptible patients
Sulfonylurea	Bind to and inhibit the K-ATP channel in pancreatic β cells and other tissues.	Available for more than 50 years. Good safety profile (hypoglycemia is the most frequent serious side effect). Weight gain is common. The least expensive oral hypoglycemic agents
Meglitinides	Bind to and inhibits the K-ATP channel in pancreatic β cells and other tissues. Binding site differs from that of the sulfonylureas	Short half-life in plasma as well as biologically short half-life. Taken before meals to enhance prandial insulin secretion
Thiazolidinediones	Bind to and regulate the activity of PPARγ receptors, principally in adipose tissue	Relatively new agents that work by a unique mechanism of gene induction or repression. Ability to enhance insulin sensitivity is an attractive feature. Weight gain is common and is, in part, secondary to edema formation
α-glucosidase inhibitors	Inhibit activity of the α-glucosidase present on the mucosal surface of the intestinal epithelial cell	Taken with meals, have moderate efficacy in lowering postprandial hyperglycemia. With higher doses, flatus limits use

Table 23.4 Oral hypoglycemic agents. ATP, adenosine triphosphate; PPARγ, peroxisome proliferation activating receptor-γ.

Ongoing studies are addressing the concept that a diet lower in carbohydrate but somewhat higher in monounsaturated fat and protein may be advantageous in this population. The total caloric recommendation would typically target 200–400kcal/day less than estimated caloric need in the overweight or obese patient. An individual patient's perseverance with any prescribed dietary intervention will be dependent upon their ability to successfully implement food purchase, meal planning, and preparation strategies that may vary from those to which they have become accustomed over a lifetime. This in turn is dependent upon economic resources and cultural and lifestyle preferences. This complexity in general requires that the patient obtain consultation with a trained nutritionist and avail themselves of community resources and those available from the diabetes associations. There may be a role for increased magnesium in the diet, since higher magnesium intake has been associated with reduced rates of development of diabetes and improved insulin action.

Beyond these very basic aspects of a heart-healthy diet, patients receiving insulin can benefit from instruction in carbohydrate counting in an effort to match insulin dose to food intake and thereby limit postprandial glycemic excursions. Again, this regimen requires the assistance of a skilled nutritionist and patient participation, with mealtime glucose measurements.

Exercise

Exercise, like diet, has long been recognized as an appropriate part of diabetes management. It serves both to facilitate specifically the disposal of glucose by skeletal muscle and, more generally, weight reduction and improved cardiovascular fitness. Only recently have the cellular mechanisms by which exercise facilitates glucose disposal been recognized. A key pathway in muscle appears to be the activation of AMP-kinase with subsequent phosphorylation of the serine threonine kinase AKT, which then appears to activate the GLUT4 glucose transporter (**Fig. 23.18**). In addition, exercise has a well-established ability to enhance blood flow to muscle and increase perfusion by recruit-

Effect of exercise on glucose disposal
Muscle contraction ↑ AMP, ↓ ATP
↑ AMP activates AMP-dependent protein kinase
Phosphorylation of AKT
Downstream recruitment of GLUT4 transporter

Figure 23.18 Effect of exercise on glucose disposal. Illustrated here is the pathway by which exercise activates adenosine monophosphate (AMP)-activated protein kinase and the subsequent stimulation of glucose transport in skeletal muscle.

ing additional capillaries. This probably facilitates both insulin and glucose delivery to muscle. Finally, the caloric expenditure can be a valued component of most successful weight-reduction programs.

Typical prescriptions for exercise would include 30–40 minutes of dedicated activity at least 4 days each week. The type of exercise selected would depend upon individual patient preferences and available resources available. For patients with known retinopathy, significant resistance exercise and high impact aerobics would be discouraged. Likewise, for patients with neuropathic disease, impact aerobics and jogging would be discouraged and swimming or stationary bicycle exercise might be substituted.

Oral hypoglycemic agents

Within the past decade there has been a burgeoning interest in the development of drugs that influence body glucose metabolism. Because these agents act by diverse mechanisms, they can be used in combination with one another as well as with insulin. This has increased both the complexity and flexibility of pharmacologic interventions available (**Table 23.4**). In all cases

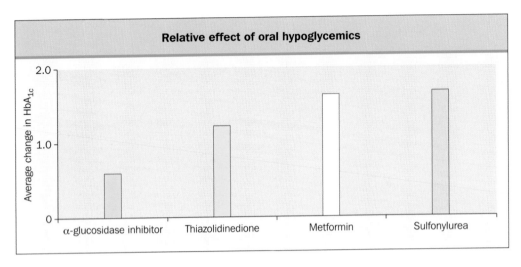

Figure 23.19 Relative effect of oral hypoglycemics. Shown here are the representative changes in hemoglobin A1c that result from the use of the four classes of oral hypoglycemic agent as monotherapy.

the goal is to reduce the plasma glucose to a level where the probability of microvascular complications is minimized, while avoiding unwanted side-effects of treatment, particularly hypoglycemia.

Agents that stimulate insulin secretion

As discussed earlier, in established type 2 diabetes, insulin secretion has failed to keep up with the insulin requirements needed to cope with insulin resistance, and hyperglycemia results. Agents of the sulfonylurea class have been available for more than 50 years. At least eight different pharmaceuticals are available; all act by stimulating β-cell insulin secretion. Within the past 10 years it has been recognized that agents of this class bind to a subunit of the adenosine triphosphate (ATP)-inhibitable potassium channel in β cells and facilitate channel closing. This leads to β-cell depolarization and calcium entry via voltage-dependent calcium channels. The rise in cytosol calcium appears to be critical to the subsequent exocytosis of insulin-containing secretory granules. These agents can cause hypoglycemia, which is particularly a problem with the longer-acting agents in this class (e.g. glyburide and chlorpropamide). The sulfonylureas have a moderately good potency when used as single agents in previously drug-naïve patients with type 2 diabetes, and can lower hemoglobin A_{1c} by 1–2% (**Fig. 23.19**). Their principal side effect is hypoglycemia, and this requires patient education to enhance awareness and guide appropriate treatment. As these agents were used extensively in the UKPDS study we have reasonable outcome data that suggest that long-term improvement in glycemia obtained using these agents can reduce the microvascular complications of diabetes.

A new class of agents, the meglitinides, which differ structurally from the sulfonylureas, have a similar effect on the K–ATP channel, although they appear to act at a different site on the channel complex. Like the sulfonylureas, these agents lower plasma glucose by stimulating insulin secretion. The two agents currently available are short-acting and may be particularly effective in correcting postprandial hyperglycemia. Their short duration of action would lead to the expectation that they will be less likely to cause severe hypoglycemia than longer-acting agents, although convincing clinical data regarding this are not yet available. No long-term clinical outcome data are yet available with the meglitinides.

Biguanides

Two agents in this class are available, metformin and phenformin, although the latter agent was withdrawn from the US market after being implicated in multiple reports of life-threatening lactic acidosis. Our discussion will focus chiefly on metformin, which is more widely used and for which more clinical data are available. Metformin is a highly effective agent for the treatment of type 2 diabetes. The liver is the principal target organ for its therapeutic actions. Metformin diminishes hepatic glucose production in both the fasting and postprandial state. However, despite its long-standing clinical use, its molecular mechanism of action within the liver has not been defined. Indeed, there is still discussion as to whether it acts to regulate gluconeogenesis or glycogen breakdown. Whatever its cellular actions, its clinical efficacy is clear and the findings of the UKPDS study support its use as a first-line agent in the treatment of obese type 2 diabetic patients. Particularly striking was the improvement in overall mortality and cardiovascular mortality in obese subjects treated with metformin (**Fig. 23.20**), an effect not seen in the larger group of subjects treated with insulin or sulfonylureas.

Metformin, unlike the sulfonylureas, thiazolidinediones, or insulin, does not lead to weight gain. In most studies, metformin used as a single agent in drug-naive patients or when added to a sulfonylurea or other agent in patients not meeting therapeutic goals results in a 1–2% lowering of hemoglobin A_{1c}. Metformin's glucose-lowering action begins promptly and requires several weeks to be fully established. Because it works by different mechanisms from other oral hypoglycemic agents it can be used as part of oral-hypoglycemic combination regimens. Furthermore, when used together with insulin, thiazolidinediones, or sulfonylureas it ameliorates the weight gain otherwise seen with treatment using these agents.

Figure 23.21 illustrates the dose–response relationship between metformin and hemoglobin A_{1c} levels in subjects on metformin monotherapy. In some, but not all studies, metformin is also seen to have a beneficial effect in lowering plasma triglycerides. In as much as metformin improves glucose regulation without increasing insulin secretion, it is considered to be an insulin-sensitizing agent. This is perhaps most clearly seen when it is given to type 2 patients already receiving insulin therapy. Not uncommonly, it will enable reductions of 50% or more in insulin dosage.

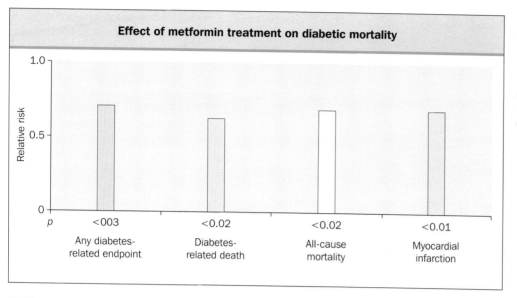

Figure 23.20 Effect of metformin treatment on diabetic mortality. Illustrated here are the results of the obese substudy of the UK Prospective Diabetes Study indicating that glucose control with metformin decreased microvascular complications and decreased mortality.

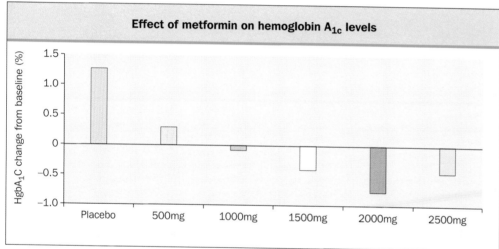

Figure 23.21 Effect of metformin on hemoglobin A$_{1c}$ levels. The figure illustrates the dose–response relationship between metformin and hemoglobin A1c.

The gastrointestinal side effects of metformin limit its use in some patients. In addition, like phenformin, it can cause severe lactic acidosis. This latter toxicity is much less common with metformin than with phenformin and can generally be avoided by avoiding its use in patients with renal, hepatic, or cardiac disease.

Alpha-glucosidase inhibitors

The α-glucosidase inhibitors act to lower blood glucose by inhibiting the cleavage of disaccharides to monosaccharides on the brush border membrane of the intestinal epithelial absorptive cell, the terminal step of carbohydrate digestion in the gastrointestinal tract. This slows the rate of absorption of carbohydrate and diminishes postprandial hyperglycemia. As a result, these agents are particularly suited to control diet-induced glycemic excursions. As single agents they are somewhat less potent that either metformin or the sulfonylureas. At recommended doses in drug-naive patients, these agents will lower hemoglobin A$_{1c}$ by 0.5–1.0%. There have been no long-term trials that have examined the effect of using these agents on clinical endpoints like eye, renal, or cardiovascular disease.

Because the α-glucosidase inhibitors act to delay or block carbohydrate absorption, their principal untoward side effects result from subsequent gas formation from undigested carbohydrate metabolized by intestinal flora. Again, as these agents act by a different biologic mechanism from other oral hypoglycemic agents, they can be used as part of a multidrug combination together with insulin, sulfonylureas, metformin, or a thiazolidinedione.

Thiazolidinediones

The thiazolidinediones are a newer class of drugs whose role in the management of type 2 diabetes is only now emerging. Two agents are available in most parts of the world, pioglitazone and rosiglitazone, and others are in development. These agents bind to transcription factors called peroxisome-proliferation-activating receptors (PPARs), particularly the γ subtype (PPARγ). As a result, they increase or decrease the transcription of multiple genes in insulin target tissues (and other tissues as well). This leads, by a not well-characterized path, to an increase in insulin sensitivity in classical insulin target tissues (**Fig. 23.22**). As insulin resistance is a major contributor to the development of

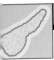

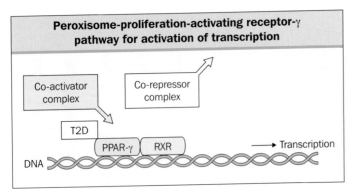

Figure 23.22 Peroxisome proliferation activating receptor-γ (PPARγ) pathway for activation of transcription. One consequence of the activation of PPARγ is a transcription of new genes or suppression of previously transcribed genes.

type 2 diabetes mellitus, agents such as these have tremendous appeal as a potentially important therapeutic breakthrough. Currently, clinical outcome data regarding the prevention of development or progression of the micro- or macrovascular complications of diabetes is not available for these agents. Available data suggest that they, like insulin and the sulfonylureas, cause weight gain. Fortunately, severe hepatic toxicity, seen with an earlier agent in this class (troglitazone) does not appear to be shared by the two newer agents.

The onset of therapeutic action is somewhat slower for the thiazolidinediones than for metformin, the sulfonylureas, or the α-glucosidase inhibitors. Some glucose lowering is seen in 2–4 weeks but maximum effects require 12 weeks or longer. These drugs can be used as monotherapy or in combination with any of the other three classes of oral agent. These agents lower hemoglobin A_{1c} 1–1.5% and show good additive effects with other oral agents. Ongoing trials with the thiazolidinediones are assessing whether they have cardiovascular protective actions. Such effects, if observed, could strongly advance their utility.

FURTHER READING

Anonymous. Cost effectiveness analysis of improved blood pressure control in hypertensive patients with type 2 diabetes: UKPDS 40. UK Prospective Diabetes Study Group [see comments]. BMJ. 1998;317:720-6.

Anonymous. Effect of intensive blood-glucose control with metformin on complications in overweight patients with type 2 diabetes (UKPDS 34). UK Prospective Diabetes Study (UKPDS) Group [see comments] [published erratum appears in Lancet 1998 Nov 7;352(9139):1557]. Lancet 1998;352:854-65.

Anonymous. Effects of ramipril on cardiovascular and microvascular outcomes in people with diabetes mellitus: results of the HOPE study and MICRO-HOPE substudy. Heart Outcomes Prevention Evaluation Study Investigators [see comments]. Lancet 2000;355:253-9.

Anonymous. Tight blood pressure control and risk of macrovascular and microvascular complications in type 2 diabetes: UKPDS 38. UK Prospective Diabetes Study Group [see comments]. BMJ. 1998;317:703-13.

Boden G. Free fatty acids, insulin resistance, and type 2 diabetes mellitus. Proc Assoc Am Phys. 1999;111:241-8.

Brownlee M. Biochemistry and molecular cell biology of diabetic complications. Nature 2001;414:813-820.

DeFronzo RA. Pharmacologic therapy for type 2 diabetes mellitus. Ann Int Med. 1999;131:281-303.

Effect of intensive blood-glucose control with metformin on complications in overweight patients with type 2 diabetes (UKPDS 34). UK Prospective Diabetes Study (UKPDS) Group. Lancet 1998;352:854-65.

Ginsberg HN. Insulin resistance and cardiovascular disease. J Clin Invest. 2000;106:453-8.

Goodyear LJ, Kahn BB. Exercise, glucose transport, and insulin sensitivity. Ann Rev Med. 1998;49:235-61.

Inzucchi SE, Maggs DG, Spollett GR, Page SL, Rife FS, Walton V, et al. Efficacy and metabolic effects of metformin and troglitazone in type II diabetes mellitus. NEJM. 1998;338:867-72.

Khaw KT, Wareham N, Luben R, et al. Glycated haemoglobin, diabetes, and mortality in men in Norfolk cohort of european prospective investigation of cancer and nutrition (EPIC- Norfolk). BMJ. 2001;322:15-18.

Lifetime benefits and costs of intensive therapy as practiced in the diabetes control and complications trial. The Diabetes Control and Complications Trial Research Group. JAMA. 1996;276:1409-15.

Mokdad AH, Bowman BA, Ford ES, Vinicor F, Marks JS, Koplan JP. The continuing epidemics of obesity and diabetes in the United States. JAMA. 2001;286:1195-2000.

Mueckler M. Insulin resistance and the disruption of Glut4 trafficking in skeletal muscle. J Clin Invest. 2001;107:1211-13.

Olefsky JM, Saltiel AR. PPARgamma and the Treatment of Insulin Resistance. Trends Endocrinol Metab. 2000;11:362-368.

Pessin JE, Saltiel AR. Signaling pathways in insulin action: molecular targets of insulin resistance. J Clin Invest. 2000;106:165-9.

Polonsky KS, Sturis J, Bell GI. Seminars in Medicine of the Beth Israel Hospital, Boston. Non-insulin-dependent diabetes mellitus - a genetically programmed failure of the beta cell to compensate for insulin resistance. NEJM. 1996;334:777-83.

Standards of medical care for patients with diabetes mellitus. American Diabetes Association. Diabetes Care 2001;24(supplement 1):S33-S43.

Saltiel AR, Kahn CR. Insulin signalling and the regulation of glucose and lipid metabolism. Nature 2001;414:799-806.

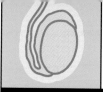

Section 5 Gonad and Growth

Chapter 24A

Normal and Abnormal Puberty

Joanne C Blair and Martin O Savage

INTRODUCTION

The onset of puberty heralds the start of the physical, hormonal, and psychologic changes that result in the immature child attaining physical maturity, independence, and reproductive ability.

The mechanisms by which puberty is initiated remain unclear. Adequate nutrition is essential and the secular trend towards an earlier puberty reflects improving socioeconomic environments. In Western countries, however, despite apparent socioeconomic stability, a similar trend continues. In 1999 a study from North America of more than 17,000 girls reported a significant reduction in the age of onset of puberty, leading the Lawson Wilkins Pediatric Endocrine Society to review its guidelines for the age at which puberty should be considered to be precocious. This trend is observed in the presence of increasing childhood obesity and may reflect a permissive role for leptin, the concentration of which is directly related to total body fat. Other factors thought to contribute to the timing of puberty are age and central nervous system (CNS) maturation, environmental factors, inheritance, and ethnic origin.

During puberty the interaction between the central nervous system and peripheral endocrine organs generates a consistent series of endocrine changes. This is reflected in the acquisition of secondary sexual characteristics in an ordered pattern of development and an accompanying acceleration in height velocity. A clear understanding of normal puberty is essential, as deviation away from this pattern of development should alert the physician to the possibility of underlying pathology.

ENDOCRINOLOGY OF PUBERTY

Fetal development

During fetal and perinatal life, activity of the hypothalamo–pituitary–gonadal axis plays an important role in sexual differentiation. From about 8 weeks gestation testosterone production from the testicular Leydig cells and antimüllerian inhibitory factor (MIF) from Sertoli cells is stimulated primarily by placental human chorionic gonadotropin (hCG). Maximal concentrations of testosterone are achieved by about 12–13 weeks gestation and this period is critical for normal male sexual differentiation. By midgestation, secretion of testosterone is under the influence of the hypothalamo–pituitary–gonadal axis. Gonadotropin-releasing hormone (GnRH) from the hypothalamus stimulates release of luteinizing hormone (LH) and follicle-stimulating hormone (FSH) from the pituitary (**Fig. 24.1**). In the male, LH drives production of testosterone and the importance of the integrity of this pathway for normal male genital development is

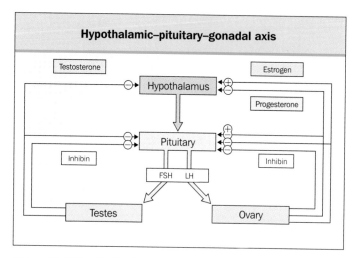

Figure 24.1 Hypothalamic–pituitary–gonadal axis. The figure demonstrates the feedback effect of peripheral hormones. FSH, follicle-stimulating hormone; LH, luteinizing hormone.

seen in boys with congenital hypopituitarism born with microphallus. In female fetuses, where such testosterone production does not occur, masculinization of the internal genitalia does not occur.

Neonatal development

By midgestation the fetal pituitary is sensitive to the negative-feedback effect of sex hormones on gonadotropin production. Disruption of the feto-placental unit at birth results in elevation of gonadotropins to pubertal levels in response to falling maternal and placental estrogens. There is a surge in testosterone production in male infants, which continues for the first 3 months, declining thereafter to very low levels until the onset of puberty. In female infants there is minimal gonadal steroidogenesis during this period, and estradiol levels fall rapidly after birth. GnRH, LH, and FSH are present in higher concentrations in female than male infants during the first few months of life. This picture persists until centers in the central nervous system responsible for inhibition of the hypothalamus mature. By 6 months of age in boys, and late infancy in girls, LH and FSH levels start to fall, reaching a nadir in mid-childhood when response to GnRH is minimal.

Development at puberty

The endocrine changes of puberty may be considered to be active in three systems, resulting in the maturation of the

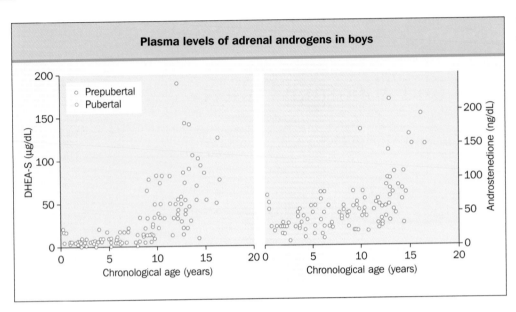

Figure 24.2 Plasma levels of adrenal androgens in boys. Left panel: Increase in levels of dihydroepiandrosterone sulfate (DHEA-S) with chronological age. Right panel: Increase in levels of androstenedione with chronological age. (Modified from Ilondo MM, Vandershueren-Lodeweyck X, Vlietinck R, et al. Plasma androgens in children and adolescents. Horm Res. 1982;16:61–72.)

adrenal gland (adrenarche), gonad (gonadarche), and changes in the growth-hormone–insulin-like-growth-factor (IGF) axis, resulting in the pubertal growth spurt. The interaction between the systems is complex; for example, increasing sex steroid production primes the pituitary to increase growth hormone production and an optimal pubertal growth spurt is also dependent on the direct effect of sex steroids on bone growth and maturation. Adrenarche, however, appears to be independent of the hypothalamo–pituitary–gonadal axis but is probably dependent on production of adrenocorticotropic hormone (ACTH). Adrenarche may proceed in the absence of gonadarche, as observed in girls with Turner's syndrome, or may fail to occur in children with Addison's disease, while gonadarche progresses normally. In healthy children, however, the onset of adrenarche and gonadarche are temporally related.

Adrenarche

Adrenarche is the first endocrine event of puberty. Increased production of the adrenal androgens dihydroepiandrosterone (DHEA), the sulfated form DHEA-S, and androstenedione has been documented from 5 years of age and the secretion of these androgens increases from this time on (**Fig. 24.2**).

The clinical manifestations of adrenarche generally lag behind those of gonadarche, however. Patients with ACTH resistance have impaired adrenarche, implicating ACTH as an important influence in the onset of adrenarche. It has been suggested that corticotropin-releasing factor (CRF) is also a major regulator of adrenarche.

During adrenarche the relative production of adrenal androgens to cortisol and aldosterone increases. There is speculation that during adrenarche the activity of the enzymes 17,20-lyase and 17-hydroxylase increases, favoring increased production of DHEA, DHEA-S, and 17-hydroxyprogesterone while cortisol and aldosterone production are unchanged.

More recently, molecular studies of the 3β-hydroxysteroid dehydrogenase type II gene have demonstrated reduced gene expression as an effect of age in the adrenal glands of prepubertal and early pubertal children. Such changes in gene expression would favor dehydroepiandrosterone production.

The physiologic significance of adrenarche is unclear. Adrenal androgens are observed to stimulate the differentiation of pilosebaeous units. In pubic and axillary regions the growth of terminal hair is stimulated. In acne prone areas and in the scalp the growth of the sebaceous glands is promoted, resulting in greasy hair and skin and body odor.

Gonadarche

The endocrine changes of true puberty are initiated when GnRH secretion by the hypothalamus is released from the tonic inhibition of the CNS centers and the pulsatile secretion of GnRH gonadotropin increases.

Gonadotropin secretion in boys

Luteinizing hormone is secreted in a pulsatile pattern during childhood with a clear circadian pattern, pulses of greatest amplitude and frequency being secreted during the sleep hours. With the onset of puberty in boys nocturnal LH pulses show increased amplitude and frequency. As puberty progresses the marked circadian pattern of LH secretion is lost as daytime pulses increase in amplitude and duration (**Fig. 24.3**).

In boys, LH secretion stimulates the production of testosterone from Leydig cells in the testes. Reflecting the pattern of LH secretion, testosterone release is initially maximal at night but remains lower by day; as puberty progresses the adult pattern of testosterone secretion is achieved. Simultaneously, and as a result of increased androgen secretion, the production of sex-hormone-binding globulin (SHBG) by the liver reduces. This results in increased unbound, and therefore active, sex steroid.

In the male, increases in the secretion of FSH are predominantly basal secretion rather than changes in either pulse frequency or amplitude. Increased FSH secretion acts synergistically with intratesticular testosterone to stimulate the proliferation and maturation of the seminiferous tubules, resulting in secretion of inhibin B.

In its biologically active form, inhibin circulates as a dimer, with an α subunit bound to either a $β_A$ subunit (inhibin A) or $β_B$ subunit (inhibin B). Inhibin B is thought to be a product of Sertoli cells, and cross-sectional studies of prepubertal and pubertal boys

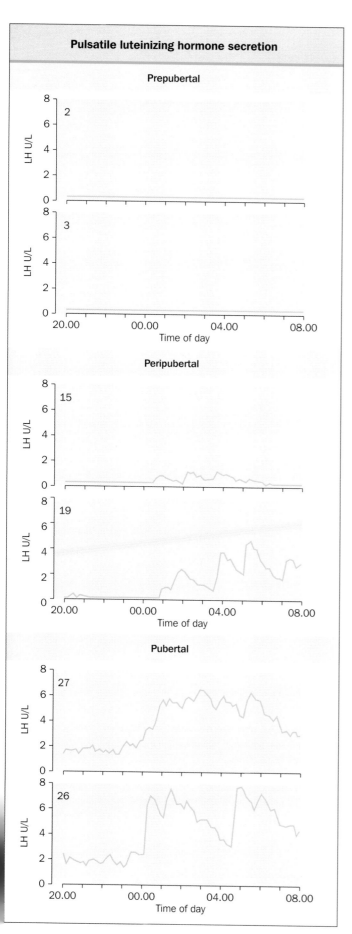

Figure 24.3 Pulsatile luteinizing hormone (LH) secretion. The diagram shows LH secretion in young prepubertal boys (top panel), peripubertal boys (middle panel) and pubertal boys (bottom panel). (Modified from Wu FCW, Butler GE, Kelnar CJH, Sellar RE. Patterns of pulsatile luteinising hormone secretion before and during the onset of puberty in boys: a study using an immunoradiometric assay. J Clin Endocrinol Metab. 1990; 629–735 © The Endocrine Society.)

have documented increasing production of inhibin during the immediate prepubertal period, initially directly correlated with testosterone, FSH, and LH levels. By midpuberty this correlation has reversed, such that inhibin B appears to acquire its negative feedback effect during puberty in boys. Levels of inhibin A are undetectable in males.

Gonadotropin secretion in girls

In girls, the earliest and most marked changes in gonadotropin secretion occur in FSH rather than LH. Throughout puberty concentrations of FSH in girls exceed those in boys. Increased secretion of FSH is achieved in early puberty by increases in pulse amplitude rather than frequency. By midpuberty, levels of FSH have leveled off. LH secretion increases steadily throughout puberty, with frequency and magnitude of pulses increasing. In the premenarchal phase, secretion of both inhibin A and B increase steadily until a cyclic pattern of inhibin A and B secretion is established.

Gonadal development and activity

The number of primordial ovarian follicles reaches its maximum around 20 weeks of gestational age, then decreases logarithmically until complete depletion occurs at the menopause. The early rise in FSH at the onset of puberty stimulates ovarian follicular growth of the ovary. As puberty progresses, cohorts of follicles enlarge, some continuing to develop, others regressing until, late in puberty, menstrual cycles are achieved by maturation of the positive feedback loop. Sustained FSH stimulation induces activity of ovarian aromatase, an enzyme essential for conversion of androgens to estrogens. Progesterone production increases and mitosis is induced, enabling follicular development to progress. As a result of increased mitosis the oocyte becomes enveloped in layers of granulosa cells, which cause fluid rich in inhibin B and FSH to collect between the cells. With cell proliferation, LH receptor numbers increase and the ovary becomes increasingly sensitive to LH stimulation. LH further stimulates the production of progesterone and androgens, which act as estrogen precursors.

Estrogen levels steadily rise and act on the hypothalamus to increase GnRH pulse amplitude. The pituitary responds by progressively increasing gonadotropin secretion, with LH secretion becoming dominant over FSH. The effect of this positive-feedback loop is to generate a gonadotropin surge, with the magnitude of the LH surge considerably greater than that of the FSH surge. Ovulation occurs approximately 24–36 hours later.

Following ovulation, the granulosa cells of the follicle undergo luteinization and increase progesterone production under the influence of LH. Production of inhibin by the granulosa cells changes to increase secretion of inhibin A. The follicle is described as a corpus luteum. Progesterone secretion transforms the endometrial lining from the proliferative to the secretory phase. If the oocyte is not fertilized, the corpus luteum regresses, progesterone production wanes, and the endometrial lining is shed. The first menstrual bleed (menarche) does not necessarily imply that ovulation has occurred, as early cycles are frequently anovulatory, occurring as a result of estrogen withdrawal.

Growth hormone and insulin-like growth factor

Growth hormone secretion increases concomitantly with increased gonadotropin secretion at the onset of puberty. This is thought to be an estrogen-mediated event, in boys dependent on aromatization of testosterone to estradiol, and reflecting increasing sex steroid production. Evidence that androgens exert their influence on growth hormone secretion via estrogen receptors came from studies of the effect of estrogen blockade on growth hormone production in pubertal boys. This resulted in significantly reduced rates of secretion. This was further supported by the observation that nonaromatizable androgens fail to increase growth hormone secretion, in contrast to the effect of testosterone.

Case reports of two male patients, one with a point mutation in the estrogen receptor and the other with aromatase deficiency, document continued growth past the adolescent period and diminished bone density, despite normal androgen production but reduced estrogen action or production respectively. This would suggest that estrogens, rather than androgens, have a pivotal role in epiphyseal fusion and the development and maintenance of bone density.

Growth hormone is a highly pulsatile hormone, showing marked circadian variation in rates of secretion, with pulses of greatest amplitude and frequency occurring at night (**Fig. 24.4**). This pattern persists throughout puberty and the effect of sex steroids is to increase pulse amplitude, rather than modify pulse frequency or timing.

Gender differences in growth hormone secretion

Gender differences are observed in growth hormone secretion during puberty. Maximal production of growth hormone occurs at an earlier stage in puberty in girls compared to boys, being at stage 3–4 in girls compared to stage 4 in boys. In both sexes the period of maximal growth hormone secretion coincides with the period of maximal height velocity. Girls also demonstrate higher basal concentrations of growth hormone throughout puberty, reaching maximal levels at stage 4, and declining thereafter. In contrast, basal concentrations of growth hormone are constant throughout puberty in boys.

Growth hormone stimulates IGF-I production from all tissues, but that which circulates spills over from the liver. During puberty it would appear that the negative feedback effect of IGF-I on growth hormone secretion is dampened as both GH and IGF-I levels are high. Growth hormone, IGF-I, and testosterone are powerful anabolic hormones; growth hormone and IGF-I primarily increasing protein production while testosterone also increases proteolysis. Failure of estrogen to affect protein metabolism suggests that the anabolic effects of androgens are mediated directly through androgen rather than estrogen receptors. This may account for the gender differences in adult body composition.

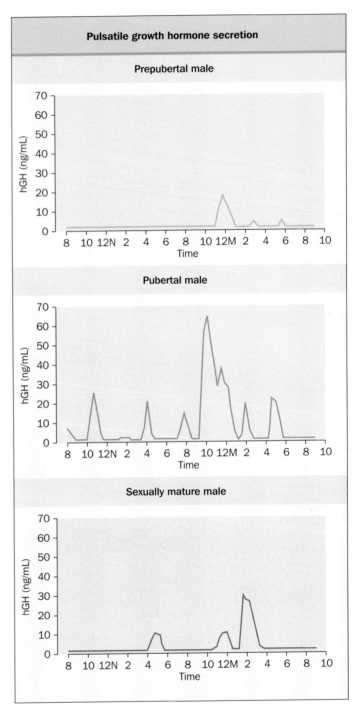

Figure 24.4 Pulsatile growth hormone secretion. The diagram shows growth hormone secretion in a prepubertal (top panel), pubertal (middle panel), and sexually mature male (bottom panel). (Modified from Finkelstein JW, Roffwarg HP, Boyar RM, Kream J, Hellman L. Age related change in the twenty four hour spontaneous secretion of growth hormone. J Clin Endocrinol Metab. 1972;35:665–70 © The Endocrine Society.)

By the final stages of puberty in both males and females, growth hormone production starts to diminish, returning to prepubertal levels in adult life, despite continued exposure to high concentrations of sex steroids.

Leptin and puberty

The role of leptin in the initiation and maintenance of puberty is unclear. It has long been observed that the onset of puberty and the maintenance of fertility is associated with a critical body mass. As leptin is a product of adipocytes, it is an attractive candidate as an initiating factor for the onset of puberty. Moreover, in the infertile leptin-deficient mouse, leptin therapy can induce sexual maturation and maintain fertility. Observations of two patients with leptin receptor mutations who failed to enter puberty suggest that leptin has a similar role in humans.

Longitudinal studies of leptin secretion have reported temporal relationships between increased leptin secretion and the onset of puberty. Sexual dimorphism in leptin concentration is also reported, with a sustained rise throughout puberty in girls but not in boys. Opinions differ as to whether these temporal relationships and gender differences simply reflect the increase in body fat and sexual dimorphism in body composition acquired during puberty or are a primary effect. A direct effect of testosterone inhibiting leptin secretion is also reported, and may account for some of these gender differences. Despite intensive research the relationship between leptin and the initiation and maintenance of puberty has yet to be clarified.

PHYSICAL CHANGES THROUGH PUBERTY

Boys

The earliest sign of male sexual development is testicular enlargement. Using the Prader orchidometer (see **Fig. 25.14**), a series of ovoids of known volumes, a testicular volume of 4mL is closely correlated with the onset of puberty. The increase in testicular volume is primarily due to proliferation of seminiferous tubules under the influence of testosterone and FSH, although Leydig cell proliferation, stimulated by LH, also contributes. The scrotal skin becomes lax and may darken in color. As puberty progresses there is continued testicular enlargement and increased testosterone production. Penile growth results from androgen exposure and occurs primarily in length in early puberty, but then in breadth also. Towards the end of puberty the glans develops and the genitalia reach adult size and shape.

The presence of pubic (pubarche) and axillary hair reflects androgen production. Pubic hair generally precedes axillary hair growth by 1 year and is usually noted after testicular development has started. Initially fine, straight, and sparsely distributed at the base of the penis, pubic hair growth develops first by changing in quality to darker, coarse, curly hair and second by changing in distribution. Hair growth extends first over the junction of the pubes, then to the inner aspect of the thighs, achieving an inverted triangle distribution by late puberty. These stages of pubertal development have been classified by Tanner (**Fig. 24.5**).

Girls

The earliest sign of female secondary sexual development is the development of a palpable breast bud (thelarche), occurring in response to estrogen secretion from the ovaries. Estrogen stimulates the proliferation of the duct system of the breast and the accumulation of fat. Characteristic changes in the contour of the breast occur during puberty, and these appearances have been described and staged by Tanner (**Fig. 24.6(a)**).

Pubic and axillary hair growth usually becomes evident after breast budding. Like boys, early pubic hair is sparse, fine, and straight and changes in character to acquire the adult form as puberty progresses. Distribution of hair extends from the labia to the inner thigh (**Fig. 24.6(b)**).

The pubertal growth spurt

The growth of boys and girls is similar until the onset of puberty and body proportions are not significantly different between sexes. It is the pubertal growth spurt and associated changes in body proportions and composition that result in the differences in height and physique between the sexes.

The pubertal growth spurt is dependent on exposure of the pituitary to sex steroids and as such is closely related to the acquisition of secondary sexual characteristics.

The pubertal growth spurt lasts approximately 6 years in both sexes. Girls experience their maximal height velocity early in puberty, approximately 1 year after the appearance of breast development. In boys it is not until midpuberty, testicular volume 10–12mL, that the maximal height velocity is achieved (**Fig. 24.7**). As a result, by 12.5 years of age girls are on average 2.5cm taller than boys. It is the combination of a longer childhood growth period, together with a greater maximal height velocity during puberty (9.8cm/year in boys compared to 8.1cm/year in girls) that enables males to attain a final height that is, on average, 13cm greater than that of females.

Body proportions

During early puberty maximal growth occurs in the limbs, resulting in an increase in the ratio of leg length to sitting height. Following the most rapid phase of pubertal growth, growth of the trunk predominates and the body proportions once again change. These changes are most marked in boys.

Growth in the width of the trunk also displays sexual dimorphism, with boys exhibiting maximal growth across the shoulders (biacromial diameter), while maximal growth in trunk width in girls occurs in the pelvis (bi-iliac diameter).

Growth is decelerating by menarche, with girls growing on average a further 5cm. The near-completion of growth in boys is associated with the appearance of facial hair and shaving.

Body composition

Significant changes in body composition also occur during puberty. Testosterone is a potent anabolic steroid and mean body mass index increases from 16kg/m^2 at the age of 10 years to 21kg/m^2 by the completion of puberty. This dramatic increase in body mass index represents the acquisition of lean body mass rather than fat. Estrogen also effects body composition, increasing total body fat in a characteristic distribution at the thighs, buttocks, and abdomen. In girls the increase in mean body mass index from approximately 16kg/m^2 to 20kg/m^2 results from a mean increase in body fat of 11kg.

PRECOCIOUS PUBERTY

Introduction

Puberty may be considered to be precocious when it occurs in a child who is aged more than 2SD below the population mean for age at onset of puberty. It results not only in premature

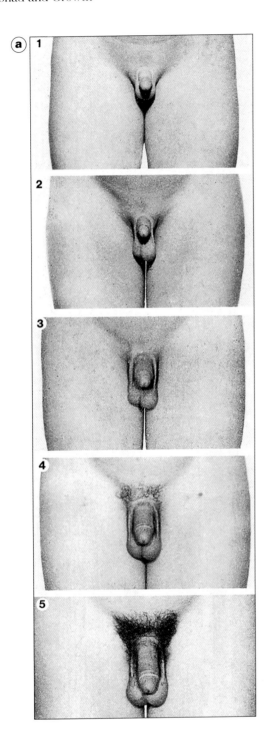

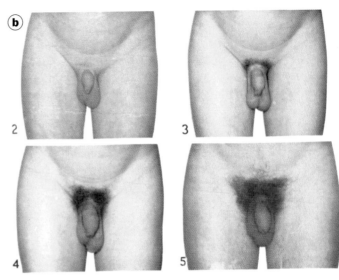

Figure 24.5 Standards for rating of pubertal changes in boys.
(a) Genital changes. (b) Pubic hair. (Reproduced from Marshal WA, Tanner JM. Variations in pattern of pubertal changes in boys. Arch Dis Child. 1970;45:13–24.)

and observation, as concerns regarding impaired final adult height in children experiencing idiopathic precocious puberty appear to be misplaced.

Classification

Precocious puberty may be classified as gonadotropin-dependent (true precocious puberty), which results from premature but normal activation of the hypothalamo–pituitary–gonad axis, or gonadotropin-independent precocious puberty (pseudoprecocious puberty), which results from autonomous sex steroid production or exposure to exogenous sex steroid. Exposure of the CNS to sex steroids in children with pseudoprecocious puberty can prematurely activate the hypothalamic– pituitary– gonadal axis and result in gonadotropin-dependent precocious puberty. This is not uncommon in children with poorly controlled congenital adrenal hyperplasia. Precocious puberty may be further classified as isosexual, when there is gender-appropriate secondary sexual development, or contrasexual, when there is virilization of females, e.g. in a girl with congenital adrenal hyperplasia, or feminization of boys, e.g. in a boy with an estrogen-secreting testicular or adrenal tumor.

If precocious puberty is classified in this way, careful clinical examination should direct the physician towards the probable anatomic source of sex steroid production. The finding of a normally progressing but premature puberty should prompt consideration of a central lesion. The findings of contrasexual development or disordered puberty, on the other hand, should suggest investigation for autonomous hormone production or exposure to exogenous sex steroids.

The differential diagnosis of precocious puberty will be considered using this anatomic classification of gonadotropin-dependent puberty and pseudoprecocious puberty, resulting from exposure to non-gonadotropin-dependent steroids (**Table 24.1**).

acquisition of secondary sexual characteristics, with acceleration in linear growth, but is accompanied by bone maturation, which may compromise final adult height. The mean age at the onset of puberty varies between ethnic groups and with time. At the present time, puberty is considered to be precocious in girls less than 8 years and in boys less than 9 years in the UK. Precocious puberty is 20 times commoner in girls than in boys. In 90% of girls precocious puberty is said to be idiopathic, i.e. with no definable structural cause. In boys the equivalent figure is thought to be approximately 10%.

Knowledge of the etiology and prognosis of precocious puberty is essential. Many cases simply require sympathetic counseling

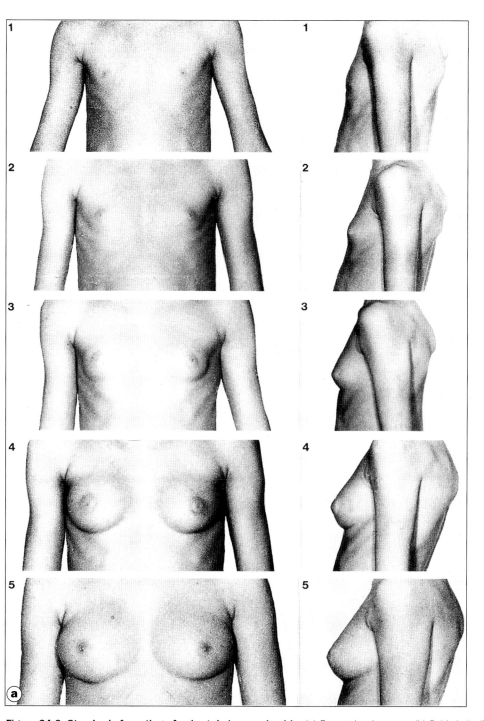

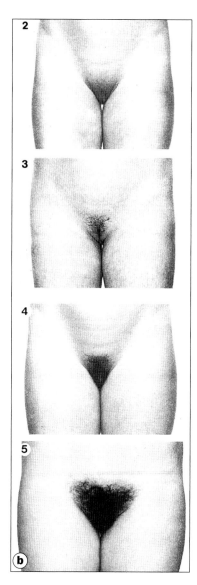

Figure 24.6 Standards for rating of pubertal changes in girls. (a) Breast development. (b) Pubic hair. (Reproduced from Marshal WA, Tanner JM. Variations in pattern of pubertal changes in girls. Arch Dis Child. 1969; 44: 291–301.)

Gonadotropin-dependent precocious puberty

Clinical features

Children with gonadotropin-dependent precocious puberty present with a normally progressing or consonant early puberty. Boys will have testes of 4mL volume or greater before penile growth and pubic hair growth are observed. In girls, breast development precedes pubic or axillary hair growth and menarche. Parents may also report recent rapid growth as evidence of the pubertal growth spurt. There are also likely to be behavioral changes related to pubertal levels of sex steroids.

Children with longstanding hypothyroidism may present with testicular enlargement or breast development. In contrast to precocious puberty of other etiologies, the remarkable clinical sign of precocious puberty as a consequence of hypothyroidism is slow growth and delayed skeletal maturity.

Gonadotropin-dependent precocious puberty may result from any condition that disrupts the CNS control of hypothalamic GnRH production. Such underlying pathology is highly likely in boys, who should be aggressively investigated (**Fig. 24.8**). True precocious puberty is most commonly observed in girls, however, where 90% of cases are idiopathic in nature.

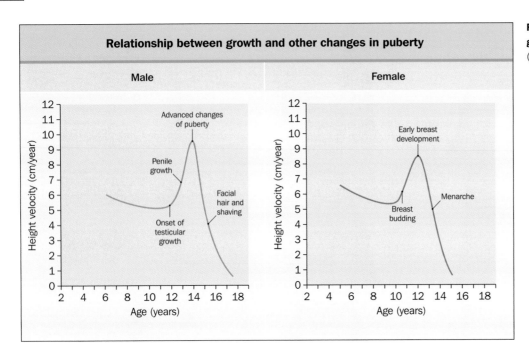

Figure 24.7 Relationship between growth and other changes in puberty. (Courtesy of Pharmacia Corporation.)

Idiopathic precocious puberty

Girls with idiopathic precocious puberty form a highly hetero-geneous group of patients (**Fig. 24.9**). Many girls have a slowly progressive puberty and height prognosis is not impaired despite moderate bone age advance and accelerated height velocity. In contrast, a minority of girls with idiopathic precocious puberty develop rapidly and their height prognosis may be significantly compromised. These girls may benefit from early therapy.

The principal long-term complication of idiopathic precocious puberty is impaired adult height. Given the heterogeneous nature of the condition, identifying girls in whom treatment is indicated can be difficult. The effect of precocious puberty on final adult height may be minimal and the benefit of treatment is also

difficult to predict. Medical intervention with the primary objec-tive of improving final height may not be indicated; parental attitudes and social and psychologic difficulties experienced by the child may be more important.

It has been reported that girls in whom treatment is unlikely to be beneficial in terms of growth differ at presentation from those in whom puberty is likely to progress rapidly. Bone age advance is less marked, pelvic ultrasound demonstrates smaller ovarian volumes and response to GnRH as a provocative test for gonadotropin secretion is less marked. Unfortunately, these obser-vations are relative and no absolute values that identify this group are available. Such girls have previously been described as having 'thelarche variant'.

Pseudoprecocious puberty

Pseudoprecocious puberty most commonly results from autonomous sex steroid secretion from the gonad, adrenal gland, or ectopic sources (**Fig. 24.10**). It may also result from exposure to exogenous sex steroids, e.g. placental products in shampoo and cosmetic products.

Isolated premature thelarche

Isolated premature thelarche is most commonly observed in young girls aged less than 5 years. It is generally transient, but may persist and progress to early puberty in a minority of girls. Although estrogen levels may be increased, gonadotropin response in a GnRH test is prepubertal. Bone age is not signifi-cantly advanced, height velocity is normal, and final height is not compromised. No intervention is indicated other than observation of pubertal status and height velocity to ensure that the diagnosis is correct.

Premature pubarche

Premature pubarche is defined as the early appearance of pubic hair before 8 years in girls and 9 years in boys. In most children this is idiopathic premature adrenarche. It is associated with

Causes of sexual precocity	
Gonadotropin-dependent precocious puberty	**Pseudoprecocious puberty**
Idiopathic	Congenital adrenal hyperplasia
Defined CNS disruption	Sex-hormone-secreting tumor
Tumor	Ovarian tumor/cysts
Ex premature infant	McCune–Albright syndrome
Post head injury	Testotoxicosis
Post infection, e.g. meningitis	hCG-secreting tumors
Neurofibromatosis	Cushing's syndrome
Williams syndrome	Hypothyroidism
Cerebral palsy	Exposure to exogenous steroids
Hydrocephalus	
Post cranial surgery or radiotherapy	

Table 24.1 Causes of sexual precocity. hCG, human chorionic gonadotropin.

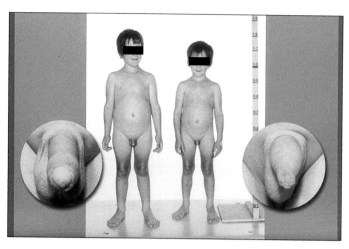

Figure 24.8 Seven-year-old boy with central precocious puberty secondary to neurofibromatosis with unaffected twin. (Courtesy of Pharmacia Corporation.)

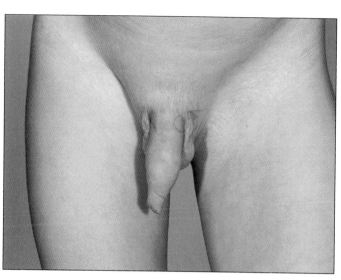

Figure 24.10 Genitalia of a 2-year-old boy with pseudoprecocious puberty secondary to congenital adrenal hyperplasia. Note penile enlargement and pubic hair growth in the presence of prepubertal testes.

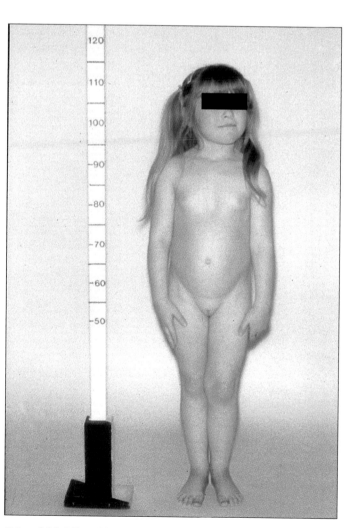

Figure 24.9 Idiopathic central precocious puberty in a 5-year-old girl. (Courtesy of Pharmacia Corporation.)

modest elevation of DHEA-S and androstenedione levels similar to those found in early pubertal children. Modest acceleration in height velocity and bone maturation are observed, but final height is not compromised and gonadarche proceeds as normal. It was thought to be a benign condition. However, there is now evidence that a minority of girls with idiopathic premature adrenarche, particularly obese girls of African, South American and Mediterranean origin, may be at risk of developing hyperinsulinemia and ovarian hyperandrogenemia. A link with low birthweight has also been reported.

Long-term consequences
The observation that some girls with premature adrenarche are at risk of developing polycystic ovarian disease has prompted detailed biochemical assessment of this group of patients. It has been documented that, although mean androgen levels are within the normal range, a significant minority demonstrate an exaggerated androgen response to ACTH stimulation. Moreover, the magnitude of this response is inversely related to insulin sensitivity. These girls also have elevated testosterone levels associated with suppressed SHBG, an effect augmented by hyperinsulinemia.

These findings suggest that premature adrenarche may be the first presentation of insulin insensitivity or polycystic ovary disease in some patients. Treatment of coexisting obesity and long-term followup are indicated to address these potential complications.

It is important to distinguish idiopathic premature adrenarche from other causes of virilization. Pubic hair growth may also be a presenting feature of congenital adrenal hyperplasia or adrenal, ovarian, or testicular neoplasia. In the early stages of virilization pubic hair may be the only clinical sign, but persistent exposure to elevated androgen levels causes skeletal maturity to be advanced and growth is rapid. Growth of the penis occurs in the absence of testicular growth and girls may develop clitoromegaly. Greasy hair and skin and acne may also result. If exposure of the CNS to elevated androgens is prolonged, activation of the hypothalamic–pituitary axis may then result in true precocious puberty.

hCG-producing tumors

hCG-secreting tumors occur most commonly in boys and may be associated with the 47,XXY karyotype. They are generally located in the brain, mediastinum, liver, or gonads. hCG can induce an apparently normal but precocious puberty in boys by activating LH receptors. In girls, however, exposure to FSH is required to induce LH-receptor expression by ovarian granulosa cells. For this reason, girls with hCG-secreting tumors do not experience precocious puberty.

Ovarian cysts

Girls with precocious puberty may present with vaginal bleeding and early breast development. Most of these girls have sexual precocity secondary to autonomous ovarian function, with elevated estradiol levels in the presence of a prepubertal gonadotropin response to GnRH. Pelvic ultrasound examination reveals unilateral large ovarian cysts, in contrast to the multiple small ovarian cysts that result from gonadotropin stimulation. The unaffected ovary is usually of prepubertal dimensions, while uterine appearances reflect estrogen stimulation. Pubic hair may or may not be present but bone age is seldom advanced.

The trigger for ovarian cyst formation is unclear but spontaneous resolution is the norm and intervention is seldom indicated. The persistence of cyclic vaginal bleeding in the presence of ovarian cysts should prompt further investigation for the features of McCune–Albright syndrome.

McCune–Albright syndrome

McCune–Albright syndrome was first described in 1937 as a triad of osteitis fibrosa, pigmented skin lesions, and endocrine dysfunction associated with precocious puberty. The syndrome most commonly occurs in girls but may also affect boys. The occurrence of McCune–Albright syndrome is sporadic. The skin lesions are irregular café-au-lait skin patches and may occur anywhere on the body, but seldom cross the midline. The location of café-au-lait macules may correspond to the location of bone lesions (**Fig. 24.11**).

Precocious puberty usually results from autonomous gonadal steroidogenesis, although it may occasionally be centrally driven. The endocrine abnormalities of McCune–Albright syndrome are not restricted to the hypothalamic–pituitary–gonadal axis. Hyperthyroidism occurs in up to 40% of patients. Growth hormone and prolactin excess is reported and nodular hyperplasia of the adrenal gland resulting in Cushing's syndrome has been described. McCune–Albright syndrome results from the autonomous function of tissues where productivity is regulated by cyclic adenosine monophosphate (cAMP) accumulation. Increased cell activity secondary to accumulation of cAMP results from an activating mutation of guanine-nucleotide-stimulating protein, which increases adenylate cyclase activity.

The diagnosis of McCune–Albright syndrome remains clinical, however, as molecular studies may not identify a mutation of the gene coding for guanine-nucleotide-stimulating protein. The demonstration of characteristic bone X-ray appearances in the presence of precocious puberty and café-au-lait patches is sufficient to make the diagnosis.

Testotoxicosis

Testotoxicosis or familial male precocious puberty may be inherited in an autosomal dominant manner or occur sporadically. Affected females pass the condition on to male offspring, but do not show any of the clinical manifestations of the condition themselves. The typical presentation is in boys of preschool age with moderate testicular enlargement, penile growth, pubic and axillary hair growth, advanced skeletal maturity, and increased height velocity. The underlying abnormality in this condition is an activating mutation of the LH receptor causing autonomous production of testosterone by Leydig cells. Females exhibiting this mutation do not enter puberty precociously because FSH stimulation is required for the expression of LH receptors before ovarian steroidogenesis is initiated.

Investigation of precocious puberty

The investigation of precocious puberty consists of establishing gonadotropin or nongonadotropin dependency, circulating sex steroid, and gonadotropin concentrations and defining etiology by radiologic or molecular investigations. A protocol is given in **Table 24.2**.

Treatment of precocious puberty

Gonadotropin-dependent precocious puberty

The aim of treating patients with true precocious puberty is to lower sex steroid levels to arrest progression of puberty and particularly menstruation, and diminish behavioral abnormalities and to maximize linear growth.

Treatment of gonadotropin-dependent precocious puberty aims to suppress the activity of the hypothalamic–pituitary–gonadal axis by the administration of a GnRH analog. Secretion of FSH and LH is subsequently reduced. These drugs are optimally administered in the form of subcutaneous depot GnRH injections, which may be administered on a monthly or 3-monthly basis. Successful treatment with a GnRH analog results in some slowing of the height velocity and regression of most of the sex-steroid-dependent secondary sexual characteristics. Treatment is discontinued at approximately 10–11 years of age and normal puberty progresses from that time on.

Gonadotropin-independent puberty

The treatment of children with autonomous sex steroid production, i.e. with McCune–Albright syndrome or familial male precocious puberty, is much more difficult. Cyproterone acetate (50–100mg daily) has been used with variable success but causes weight gain, tiredness, and suppression of the pituitary–adrenal axis. Aromatase inhibitors such as testolactone have been used with some success.

The management of children with gonadotropin-independent precocious puberty is otherwise based on treatment of the underlying pathology.

DELAYED PUBERTY

Introduction

Puberty is said to be delayed when there are no secondary sexual characteristics at an age more than 2SD above the population mean for the onset of puberty. In the UK this relates to an

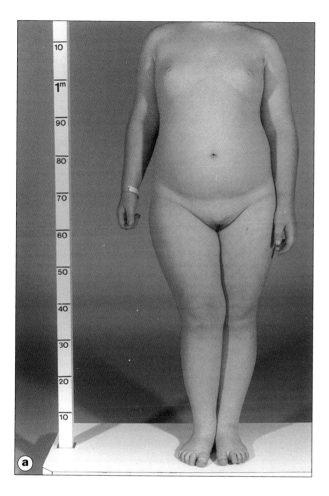

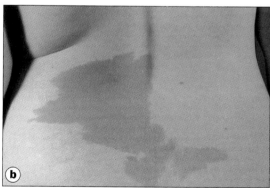

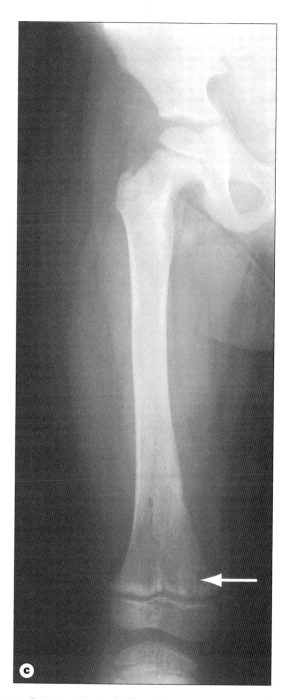

Figure 24.11 McCune–Albright syndrome. (a) Five-year-old -girl with pseudoprecocious puberty secondary to McCune–Albright syndrome, (b) café-au-lait macules affecting the lumbosacral region, and (c) early osteolytic lesion affecting the distal femur.

age of 14 years in boys and 13.3 years in girls. In contrast to precocious puberty, pubertal delay is much commoner in boys.

Puberty may be delayed in a child suffering from any chronic disease, such as celiac disease, Crohn's disease, sickle cell anemia, and cystic fibrosis. The assessment of a child presenting with pubertal delay must therefore include careful consideration of general wellbeing and chronic illness of non-endocrine nature should be actively excluded (**Table 24.3**).

Pubertal delay is most commonly idiopathic in nature and is generally associated with poor growth because of the delay of the pubertal growth spurt. This clinical picture is described as

constitutional delay of growth and puberty (CDGP). Pubertal delay may also result from disorders of the hypothalamic–pituitary axis when gonadotropin levels are low (hypogonadotropic hypogonadism) or from disorders of the gonad when gonadotropin levels are elevated (hypergonadotropic hypogonadism).

Constitutional delay of growth and puberty

Children who experience CDGP are frequently exhibiting a familial trait. By definition, children with CDGP are basically healthy with no evidence of chronic illness or genetic disorder but their delay of puberty can cause great anxiety. In a normal

Protocol for investigation of precocious puberty

History, family history	
Exposure to environmental sex steroids	
Physical examination	Cutaneous lesions, e.g. neurofibromatosis, McCune–Albright syndrome
	CNS examination
Auxology	Pubertal staging (Tanner)
	Height, weight, height velocity
	Bone age
Hormone measurements	Testosterone/estradiol
	Luteinizing hormone/follicle-stimulating hormone
	Adrenal androgens (DHEA-S, androstenedione)
	17-hydroxyprogesterone ± ACTH stimulation test
	hCG-β
	Gonadotropin-releasing hormone test
Radiology	Pelvic ultrasound
	Magnetic resonance imaging of the hypothalamic–pituitary region
DNA analysis for known genetic disorders (testotoxicosis, McCune–Albright syndrome)	

Table 24.2 Protocol for investigation of precocious puberty. DHEA-S, dihydroepiandrosterone sulfate; hCG, human chorionic gonadotropin.

Causes of delayed puberty

Hypogonadotropic hypogonadism	Hypergonadotropic hypogonadism
Constitutional delay of growth and puberty	Turner's syndrome
Chronic illness	Klinefelter's syndrome
Malnutrition	Autoimmune ovarian failure
Hyperprolactinemia	Bilateral anorchia
Hypopituitarism	Gonadal failure following chemotherapy or radiotherapy
Congenital	Inactivating mutations of gonadotropin-releasing hormone or gonadotropin receptor
Acquired	
Radiotherapy	
CNS malignancy	
CNS infection	
CNS trauma	
Isolated gonadotropin deficiency	
Congenital – Kallman's syndrome	
Acquired	
Hypothyroidism	

Table 24.3 Causes of delayed puberty.

population 2–3% of normal children will be classified as having pubertal delay, which may be considered as a variant of normal physiology (**Fig. 24.12**).

The distinction of CDGP from hypogonadotropic hypogonadism may be difficult and laboratory investigation is relatively unhelpful. CDGP is essentially a diagnosis of exclusion. Incomplete puberty is more likely to be due to true gonadotropin deficiency, as is delay in association with a previous history of undescended testes or micropenis. The presence of anosmia suggests hypogonadotropic hypogonadism secondary to Kallmann's syndrome. Children with true gonadotropin deficiency tend to be tall or eunuchoid, whereas children with CDGP generally display poor growth.

Although it may theoretically be preferable to induce puberty by the use of gonadotropins and hCG in patients with known gonadotropin deficiency, puberty can be induced in both conditions by the use of sex steroids. Continued observation until the completion of puberty (regular menses in girls and full sexual development in boys) will exclude the rare cases of gonadotropin deficiency.

Constitutional delay of growth and puberty is a self-limiting condition and with time all patients will experience a normal puberty. It has previously been considered to be a benign condition. Awareness of the psychosocial difficulties experienced by some of these children and the implications of delayed puberty for the acquisition of bone mineral density has led to

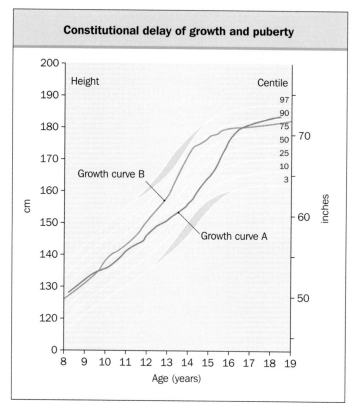

Figure 24.12 Constitutional delay of growth and puberty. Growth curves of two brothers demonstrating the effect of constitutional delay of growth and puberty (growth curve A) in contrast to an unaffected brother (growth cure B). (Courtesy of Pharmacia Corporation.)

re-evaluation of the indications for active management of this condition.

Although many children show good adaptation to the incumbent psychosocial stress of delayed puberty there are others who display poor self-esteem, impaired school performance, depression, reduced peer contact, aggression, and general social immaturity. It is uncertain whether these social difficulties result from the isolation of children with pubertal delay from their peers or whether sex steroids have a direct effect on the maturation of the CNS. Whatever the cause, it is clear that some of these children experience a significant social handicap. The long-term consequences of constitutional pubertal delay appear to be confined to a reduction in peak bone mineral density. Final adult height may be less than predicted from genetic potential but this is an inconsistent finding. Final adult height is related to the adequacy of catchup growth during puberty. Longitudinal studies suggest that the current treatment regimes do not unduly accelerate skeletal maturity or compromise final adult height.

Treatment
The rationale for treatment is to induce secondary sexual development and accelerate growth in order to alleviate psychosocial stress. Theoretically, exposure of the hypothalamus to sex steroids should also accelerate the activation of the hypothalamo–pituitary–gonadal axis.

The benefits of treatment are not well documented and there is little evidence to support the idea that treatment improves psychologic function. Until there is long-term data on the benefits of treatment on bone mineral density, the decision to treat should be based on the patient's perception of the need for physical maturity.

There is considerable experience in the use of androgens to induce puberty in boys. Such treatment is safe and current treatment regimes do not compromise adult height. At the present time the preferred treatment in boys over 14 years is testosterone enanthate 125mg given as an intramuscular depot injection once a month for 3–4 months. This is sufficient to initiate secondary sexual development, increase lean body mass, and accelerate height velocity. The patient should be advised that this treatment will not significantly increase testicular volume.

In girls with constitutional pubertal delay ethinylestradiol, in a dose of 0.05–0.1μg/kg/day for 3–4 months, has been used with beneficial effect.

Hypogonadotropic hypogonadism
Gonadotropin deficiency may be congenital or acquired, isolated, or a feature of hypopituitarism with multiple endocrine deficiencies. Any lesion of the hypothalamus or pituitary may result in impaired hormone production, e.g. infection, trauma, radiotherapy, or tumor. More commonly the deficiency relevant to pubertal development is congenital, e.g. septo-optic dysplasia.

Congenital hypogonadotropic hypogonadism may be diagnosed at birth in boys in association with micropenis and cryptorchidism. Short courses of intramuscular testosterone during childhood may increase penile size to the normal range. In less severe cases and in girls, presentation is usually during the adolescent years with delayed, slowly progressing, or incomplete pubertal development.

Congenital hypogonadotropic hypogonadism can usually be anticipated in children with other pituitary deficiencies, although definitive diagnosis is not possible until puberty.

Kallmann's syndrome
Kallmann's syndrome is the commonest form of isolated congenital gonadotropin deficiency due to primary GnRH deficiency and occurs with a frequency of 1 in 10,000 males and 1 in 50,000 females. Affected individuals have hypogonadism and anosmia. Associated abnormalities include cerebellar ataxia, sensorineural deafness, mental retardation, color blindness, and somatic defects (cleft palate, congenital heart disease, renal agenesis). Inheritance may be autosomal dominant or autosomal or X-linked recessive. Cases also occur sporadically.

Anosmia results from hypoplasia or aplasia of the olfactory tracts and bulbs, although in some patients the anatomy is normal. Hypogonadism is secondary to impaired GnRH secretion from the hypothalamus. The link between impaired olfaction and hypogonadism lies in the origin of the GnRH-secreting neurons, which develop in the nasal epithelium, then migrate along the olfactory placode to the preoptic and hypothalamic regions. Studies of males with X-linked Kallmann's syndrome have identified heterogeneous mutations of a gene coding for the KAL protein. This protein has features of the serine protease inhibitors that modulate axonal outgrowth, path finding, and target recognition of cell-adhesion molecules important in cell migration.

It is thought to be important in GnRH cell migration and olfactory axonal targeting. The molecular basis of the condition is heterogeneous, however, and more than 50% of patients do not have a mutation of the KAL protein gene.

Induction of puberty in hypogonadotropic hypogonadism

Puberty may be induced in children with gonadotropin deficiency by the use of depot testosterone enanthate 125mg given as an intramuscular depot injection monthly in boys and ethinylestradiol in a dose of 0.05–0.1µg/kg/day for girls.

The use of recombinant FSH alone, or in combination with human chorionic gonadotropin, has been advocated as a method of inducing puberty in gonadotropin-deficient males. This treatment has the benefit of increasing testicular volume and possibly improving spermatogenesis.

Hypergonadotropic hypogonadism

Elevated gonadotropin levels in the presence of pubertal delay are indicative of primary gonadal pathology.

Turner's syndrome

Turner's syndrome is a common chromosomal disorder with an incidence of approximately 1 in 2000 live female births. It is defined as a loss or abnormality of the second X chromosome in a major cell line. Some 50% of cases are reported to have the 45,XO karyotype but this statistic is likely to change as more sophisticated prenatal diagnosis identifies girls with less common karyotypes and milder phenotypes that might previously have gone undiagnosed. A minority of girls with Turner's syndrome will carry Y chromosome material, in which case consideration should be given to gonadectomy to avoid possible malignant change.

The phenotype of Turner's syndrome is highly variable. Some girls are severely affected while others present with slow growth in the absence of any dysmorphic features. For this reason it is important to document the karyotype of all girls presenting with short stature. The two most constant features of Turner's syndrome are short stature and impaired ovarian function.

In most cases there are 'streak' gonads comprised of fibrous tissue. Although primordial follicles may have been present in early gestation, they are usually reduced in number. While as many as 30–50% of girls with Turner's syndrome will enter puberty spontaneously, not all will progress to menarche and most who do so will experience premature ovarian failure in early adult life. There is absence of the pubertal growth spurt and final height is approximately 142–146cm (**Fig. 24.13**). FSH levels are elevated in girls with Turner's syndrome and impaired ovarian function. FSH levels peak in early childhood, and then fall, rising again from the age of approximately 8 years. (**Fig. 24.14**).

Treatment of delayed puberty in Turner's syndrome

The optimal treatment regimen to maximize height and induce puberty is under evaluation. It should be borne in mind that, although treatment with growth hormone is reported to increase final adult height by up to 10cm, the individual response to treatment is highly variable. Growth may be further augmented with the use of oxandrolone, an anabolic steroid, from mid-childhood. The additional gain in final height from this combination therapy is uncertain but, when used in a dose of 0.0625mg/kg/day, there appear to be no virilization effects or adverse effects on bone maturity.

Optimal pubertal induction will produce a normally progressive puberty concurrent with the puberty of the patient's peer group, and optimize bone mineral density without compromising final adult height. Induction with ethinylestradiol 5µg/day with gradual incremental increases to physiologic levels and addition of a progesterone should achieve this. The age at which estrogen should be commenced is controversial. Inducing puberty late prolongs the period available for growth but may be detrimental to bone mineral density and psychosocial function.

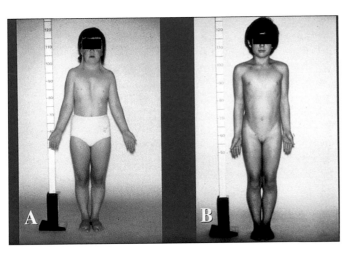

Figure 24.13 Two patients with Turner's syndrome. Patient A has the characteristic dysmorphic features of Turner's syndrome; patient B has minimal dysmorphic features. In some patients the only clinical features are short stature and pubertal delay. (Courtesy of Pharmacia Corporation.)

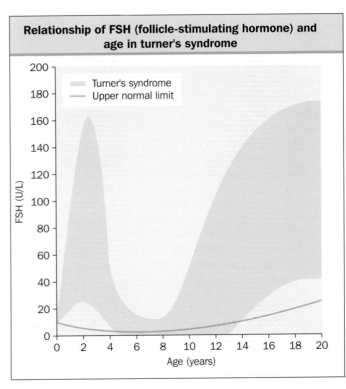

Figure 24.14 Relationship of FSH (follicle-stimulating hormone) and age in Turner's syndrome. (Courtesy of Pharmacia Corporation.)

Guidelines should become clearer with the completion of the longitudinal studies that are currently in progress.

Autoimmune ovarian failure

Autoimmune ovarian failure is a rare cause of pubertal failure or primary amenorrhea. It may occur in isolation but is commonly associated with autoimmune polyendocrinopathy, i.e. adrenal and thyroid failure and hypoparathyroidism.

Autoantibodies to steroid-secreting cells may be detected, in which case ovarian failure is likely to be permanent. Rarely, autoantibodies inhibit granulosa cell growth without cell damage. In these unusual cases ovarian function may recover spontaneously.

Klinefelter's syndrome

Klinefelter's syndrome is a chromosomal disorder with a frequency of approximately 1 in 600 to 1 in 800 male births. Affected males have an additional X chromosome. The characteristic phenotype is of tall stature, variable learning difficulties, and seminiferous tubule dysgenesis resulting in testicular hypoplasia with small, firm testes (**Fig. 24.15**). Expression of the phenotype is highly variable. Boys characteristically enter puberty at an appropriate age, but pubertal progress is slow and incomplete. Testosterone therapy is required by mid-adolescence to ensure adequate virilization and to protect against osteoporosis. Testosterone therapy also promotes epiphyseal fusion, limiting the extremely tall stature and disproportionately long legs that result from delayed epiphyseal fusion. Approximately one third of boys with Klinefelter's syndrome develop gynecomastia during puberty.

Psychologic studies highlight the difficulties experienced by these boys during adolescence, with low self-esteem often combined with learning difficulties.

Bilateral anorchia

Boys with bilateral anorchia, or rudimentary testes, present with a phenotype that reflects the stage of embryogenesis at which the testes were exposed to an intrauterine insult. There is speculation that testicular regression may result from bilateral torsion, exposure to a teratogen, or genetic mutation. Most infants are normally virilized. Pubertal induction and maintenance with testosterone is required.

Investigation of delayed puberty

The assessment of a child presenting with delayed or slowly progressing puberty is aimed at identifying possible lesions of the hypothalamic–pituitary region or gonads, excluding chronic illness, and distinguishing between structural and constitutional delay. A protocol is shown in **Table 24.4**.

OTHER DISORDERS OF PUBERTY

Cancer treatment

As long-term survival from childhood malignancy improves, the late effects of cancer treatment become increasingly important. Some chemotherapeutic agents, in particular alkylating agents and busulfan, have adverse effects on spermatogenesis. The prepubertal gonad is less vulnerable to the effects of chemotherapy than the adult and there may be potential benefit for gonadal

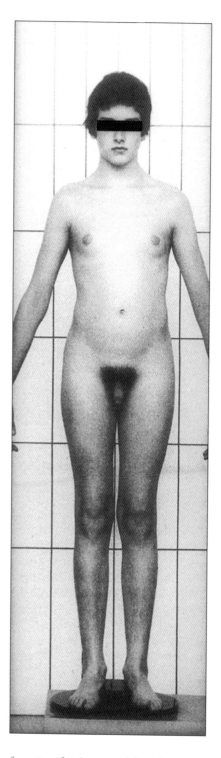

Figure 24.15 Adolescent boy with Klinefelter's syndrome exhibiting eunuchoid habitus and gynecomastia. (Courtesy of Gower Medical Publishing Ltd.)

function if puberty is delayed with GnRH analogs in peripubertal children receiving cyclophosphamide but there is, as yet, no clear conclusion to this effect.

Radiotherapy to the brain, face, and orbit may impair the hypothalamic–pituitary axis, while radiotherapy to the trunk may impair spinal growth and directly affect gonadal function.

Endocrine assessment should be routine 1 year after completion of a course of radiotherapy in childhood. Children exposed to therapeutic agents known to be associated with impaired gonadal function should also be referred on completion of treatment. Early diagnosis of hypogonadism, which may be

Protocol for the investigation of delayed puberty	
History	Family history
	Chronic illness, malignancy
	Anosmia
	Physical examination, test of smell
Auxology	Height, weight, height velocity
	Bone age
	Puberty staging (Tanner)
Baseline general investigations	Full blood count, ESR
	Electrolytes, creatinine, liver function tests
	Immunoglobulins, endomysial and gliadin antibodies
	Karyotype
Baseline hormone tests	Thyroxine, thyroid-stimulating hormone
	Prolactin
	Cortisol (09.00h)
	Testosterone, estradiol
	Luteinizing hormone, follicle-stimulating hormone
	Insulin-like growth factor-I
Dynamic hormone tests	Gonadotropin-releasing hormone test
	Clomiphene test
Radiology	Pelvic ultrasound
	Magnetic resonance imaging hypothalamus, pituitary, olfactory bulbs

Table 24.4 Protocol for the investigation of delayed puberty.

associated with gonadotropin deficiency, gonadal failure, or a combination of the two, should then be possible.

Gynecomastia

Gynecomastia in the pubertal period is generally benign and resolves spontaneously. It may be unilateral or bilateral. The etiology of the condition is unclear but it occurs at a time when the estrogen:testosterone ratio is high and may reflect locally increased sensitivity of breast tissue to estrogens. Boys with idiopathic pubertal gynecomastia tend to be tall, with a greater body mass than other boys their age. If it persists a 5-month course of tamoxifen (10 or 20mg/day) may help, or cosmetic surgery may be needed.

Up to 10% of cases of pubertal gynecomastia are due to underlying pathology, e.g. Klinefelter's syndrome, primary testicular failure, or partial androgen insensitivity.

Complete androgen insensitivity syndrome

Androgen insensitivity syndrome exists in a broad spectrum of clinical phenotype (see Chapter 25). Complete androgen insensitivity syndrome is rarely diagnosed before puberty except when inguinal testes are identified.

There is a wide variety of molecular defects underlying the spectrum of clinical features of androgen insensitivity syndrome. All defects interrupt the regulation of expression of androgen target genes. There is poor correlation between molecular abnormality and phenotype, and the same genetic defect may result in different phenotypes within the same family.

The prenatal testes produce testosterone and antimüllerian hormone, resulting in regression of the müllerian structures. The resulting phenotype is that of a female infant with a blind-ended vagina and absent uterus. Presentation in adolescence is characterized by failure of pubic and axillary hair growth and primary amenorrhea. Breast development is normal and the body habitus becomes feminine during puberty, resulting from estrogen production from aromatization of testosterone secreted from the testes. Gonadectomy is indicated to avoid malignant transformation of the testis, which has a high incidence in XY patients who have a female phenotype. Pubertal induction with estrogen therapy is then indicated.

FURTHER READING

Albanese A, Stanhope R. Predictive factors in the determination of final height in boys with constitutional delay in growth and puberty. J Pediatr. 1995;126:545–50.

Albertsson-Wikland K, Rosberg S, Karlberg J, Groth T. Analysis of 24-hour growth hormone profiles in healthy boys and girls of normal stature: relation to puberty. J Clin Endocrinol Metab. 1994;78:1195–201.

Albertsson-Wikland K, Rosberg S, Lannering B, Dunkel L, Selstam G, Norjavaara E. Twenty-four hour profiles of luteinizing hormone, follicle stimulating hormone, testosterone and estradiol levels: a semilongitudinal study throughout puberty in healthy boys. J Clin Endocrinol Metab. 1997;82:541–9.

Andersson AM, Juul A, Peterson JH, Muller J, Groome NP, Skakkebaek NE. Serum inhibin B in healthy prepubertal and adolescent boys: relation of age, stage of puberty, and follicle stimulating hormone, luteinizing hormone, testosterone and estradiol levels. J Clin Endocrinol Metab. 1997;82:3976–81.

Finkelstein JS, Neer RM, Biller BMK, Crawford JD, Kilbanski A. Osteopenia in men with a history of delayed puberty. N Engl J Med. 1992;326:600–4.

Herman-Giddens ME, Slora EJ, Wasserman RC et al. Secondary sexual characteristics and menses in young girls seen in office practice: a study from the pediatric research in office settings network. Pediatrics 1997;99:505–12.

Ibanez L, Potau N, Vardis R. Postpubertal outcome in girls diagnosed of premature pubarche during childhood. Increased frequency of functional hyperandrogenism. J Clin Endocrinol Metab. 1993;76:1599–603.

Kaplowitz PB, Oberfield SE. Reexamination of the age limit for defining when puberty is precocious in girls in the United States: implications for evaluation and treatment. Pediatrics 1999;104:936–41.

Kulin HE. Extensive personal experience: delayed puberty. J Clin Endocrinol Metab. 1996;81:3460–4.

Oerter KE, Uriate M, Rose SR, Barnes KM, Cutler GB. Gonadotropin secretory dynamics during puberty in normal girls and boys. J Clin Endocrinol Metab. 1990;71:1251–7.

Palmert MR, Malin HV, Boepple PA. Unsustained or slowly progressive puberty in young girls: initial presentation and long term follow up of twenty untreated patients. J Clin Endocrinol Metab. 1999;84:415–23.

Rugarli EI, Ballabio A. Kallmann syndrome: from genetics to neurobiology. JAMA. 1993;270:2713–6.

Shenker A, Weinstein LS, Moran A. Severe endocrine and nonendocrine manifestations of the McCune–Albright syndrome associated with activating mutations of stimulatory protein G. J Pediatr. 1999;123:509–18.

Smith EP, Boyd J, Frank GR, et al. Estrogen resistance caused by a mutation in the estrogen receptor gene in a man. N Engl J Med. 1994;331:1056–61.

Veldhus JD, Metzger DL, Martha PM, et al. Estrogen and testosterone but not a non aromatizable androgen, direct network integration of the hypothalamo-somatotrope (growth hormone)-insulin like growth factor I axis in the human: evidence from pubertal physiology and sex steroid hormone replacement. J Clin Endocrinol Metab. 1990;82:3414–20.

Vuguin P, Linder B, Rosenfeld, RG, Seanger P, DiMartino-Nardi J. The roles of insulin sensitivity, insulin like growth factor I (IGF-I) and IGF-binding protein-1 and 3 in the hyperandrogenism of African-American and Caribbean Hispanic girls with premature adrenarche. J Clin Endocrinol Metab. 1990;84:2037–42.

Zachmann M, Prader Kind HP, Haflinger H, Bubliger H. Testicular volume during adolescence. Helv Paediatr Acta. 1974;29:61–72.

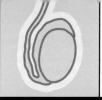

Chapter 24B Growth Disorders

Peter E Clayton and Charles G D Brook

INTRODUCTION

Normal growth in height and size results from the complex interplay of many intrinsic and extrinsic factors on the innate, genetically determined capacity for growth of an individual. The ultimate height of a person is a function not only of the rate of linear growth of the bones but also of its duration.

The growth of an individual from birth to adulthood may be pictorially represented in a height distance chart (**Fig. 24B.1**). All normal children follow such a growth curve.

To determine the rate of growth of an individual child, a number of height measurements should be made at regular intervals: for instance, twice in one year. A height velocity curve (**Fig. 24B.2**) is obtained by plotting the height gained during each year and yields important information about the growth pattern of a child. The three phases of growth in childhood are easily recognized: initially, there is a period of rapid but rapidly decelerating growth in infancy, with a subsequent period of steady and slowly decelerating growth in middle childhood, followed by a rapid rise and fall of growth at adolescence. These phases of growth are primarily dependent on nutrition, growth hormone (GH), and sex steroids, respectively.

The adolescent growth spurt, which is associated with puberty in both sexes, occurs earlier in girls than in boys, by an average of 2 years (**Fig. 24B.3**). The absence of the 2 years of decelerating prepubertal growth and the difference in the peak height velocity at puberty account for the adult height difference between men and women, which is 12.6cm on average.

Height is usually plotted on a standard centile chart for distance (**Fig. 24B.4**). This chart is no more than a description of the height in the population (in this case, the population of the UK). At 4 years, 50% of girls have a height above 100cm while the

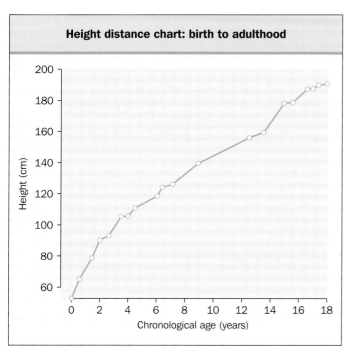

Figure 24B.1 Height distance chart: birth to adulthood. The chart shows the growth of an individual boy. All normal children follow a growth curve resembling this distance chart.

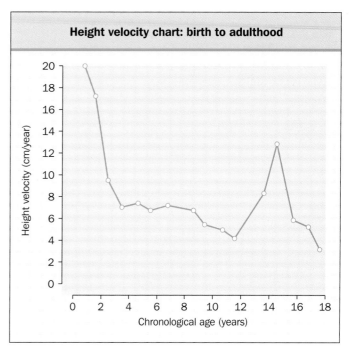

Figure 24B.2 Height velocity chart: birth to adulthood. This is the chart for the same boy as in Figure 24B.1. To produce such a chart, the annual gain in height is plotted against chronological age. Three distinct growth phases – rapid deceleration in infancy, slow deceleration in middle childhood, and rapid acceleration at adolescence – may be identified.

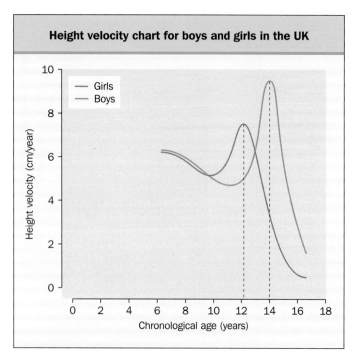

Figure 24B.3 Height velocity chart for boys and girls in the UK. The earlier onset of the adolescent growth spurt of girls is shown, together with the greater peak height velocity in boys.

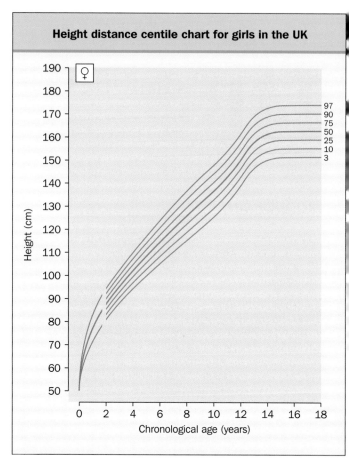

Figure 24B.4 Height distance centile chart for girls in the UK. This chart is no more than a description of the height of the female population. The 50th percentile is the median, so that 50% of individuals are taller and 50% shorter than this height.

remaining 50% have a height below 100cm. Some 3% of all girls aged 4 years measure less than 92cm and the growth of the majority of these is not abnormal. The position of the height of a child on the centile chart at any time depends upon genetic and environmental factors, most of which are beyond the control of physicians.

Although in most children growth and developmental events follow the same orderly pattern, the pace of maturation varies widely. Thus, the growth performance of individual children is better viewed in relationship to their stage of physical maturity than in relationship to their chronological age. Using skeletal age, it is possible to predict, with some degree of reliability, the final adult stature and to distinguish between children who will mature early and those in whom sexual development will be delayed. A number of systems for estimating bone age are available but all use comparisons of the maturity of a number of epiphysial centers with standard radiographs and, from these, derive an average maturity score. Since a number of centers are conveniently available in the hand and wrist, radiographs from these areas are usually used to make such an assessment. The hand of a girl with precocious puberty is shown in **Figure 24B.5**; she has the maturity of a girl of 10 years of age, which means that 83% of her growth has already taken place. She now measures 128cm, which is tall for her chronological age but short for her bone age. Her final height will be short and is estimated to be approximately 154cm.

A typical problem is shown in **Figure 24B.6**. A boy aged 14 years is referred for evaluation of his short stature, since his present height is only 140cm, which is below the third percentile. His skeletal maturity corresponds to that of a boy of 11 years of age, so his growth prognosis (170cm) is well within normal limits for the centile position of his parental heights (shown on the right of

the chart). Whether he will achieve this potential depends upon whether he is growing at a normal rate and on how long he continues to grow, which is defined by his bone age. To establish the growth rate of a child, height should be measured on two different occasions that are separated by a period of time. The length of time needed to establish a normal growth velocity depends upon the increment that might be expected and the accuracy of the equipment used. Instruments of the type shown in **Figure 24B.7** would require approximately 3 years to establish normality because of the high error margin when using them.

MEASURING TECHNIQUE

Before measuring the standing height of children, they should remove their shoes and should stand with their heels and back in contact with an upright wall. The head should be held so that the child looks straight ahead, with the outer canthus of the eye socket in the same horizontal plane as the external auditory meatuses, and not with the nose tipped upwards. A right-angled block is then slid down the wall until the bottom surface touches the child's head, and a scale fixed to the wall is read. During measurement, the child should be told to stretch the neck to be as tall as possible, although care must be taken to prevent the heels from coming off the ground. Gentle but firm

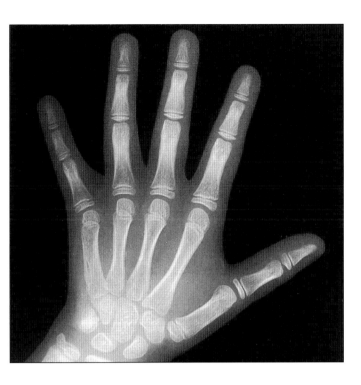

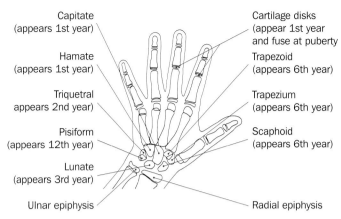

Figure 24B.5 Radiograph of a hand, used to assess skeletal maturity (bone age). The hand of a 6-year-old girl with precocious puberty is shown. Although the girl is tall for her chronological age, her bone age is advanced to that of a 10-year-old, which means that 83% of her growth has already taken place. Assessment of her bone age is important since it is used to predict her final height, which in this case will be short. The normal ages at which the bone ossification centers develop are shown in brackets.

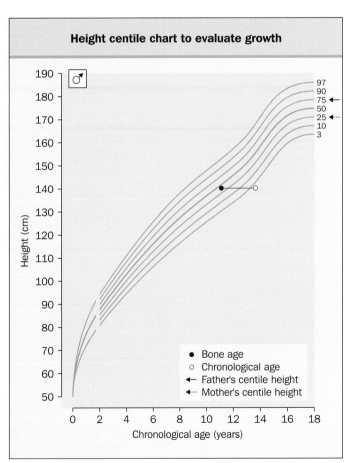

Figure 24B.6 Height centile chart to evaluate growth. This chart is being used to evaluate the growth of a short boy. Although the boy's chronological age is 14 years, his bone age is only that of an 11-year-old, suggesting that he has potential for catch-up growth.

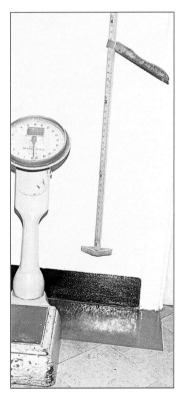

Figure 24B.7 A stadiometer not to be recommended. This instrument should be avoided since it would take several years to produce a reliable growth curve because of the error margin involved.

traction should be applied by the measurer under the mastoid processes to keep the child stretched. In this way, the reduction in height from morning to evening is minimized.

A stadiometer, as shown in **Figure 24B.8**, allows the height to be measured on successive occasions to within 1mm when the measurements are made with care by the same observer using the

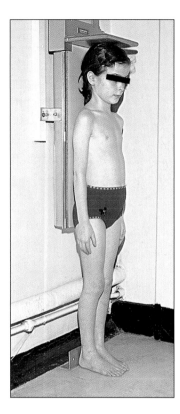

Figure 24B.8 A recommended stadiometer in use. During measurement, the child should be told to stretch the neck while the measurer applies gentle traction under the mastoids to keep the child stretched. The outer canthus of the eye sockets of the child should be in the same horizontal plane as the external auditory meatuses, and the heels should be touching the ground.

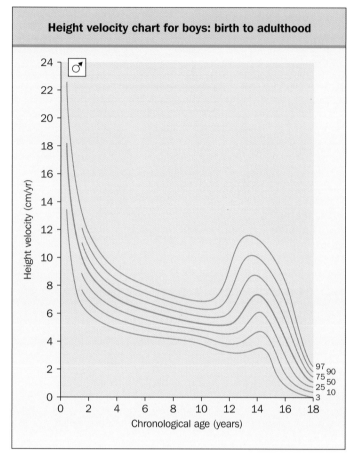

Figure 24B.9 Height velocity chart for boys: birth to adulthood. Height velocity is the change in height over an interval of time. The length of time needed to establish a normal growth velocity depends upon the increment that might be expected and the accuracy of the equipment used. The child must maintain a height velocity at around the 50th percentile to maintain growth along the centile line on a distance chart.

same technique. In a measurement of more than 1m, the accuracy of this instrument compares favorably with any other measurement made clinically or in the laboratory. Nevertheless, measurement made over less than 3–6 months may produce considerable errors, and reliance should not be placed upon single estimates of height velocity made over a short period of time.

Height velocity measurements (**Fig. 24B.9**) are converted into annual rates of growth by dividing the increment by the lapse of time. Such measurements are compared with centiles as before but, whereas a third-percentile position on a height distance chart may be, and probably is, normal, a velocity that is persistently on the third percentile leads to progressive loss of height compared with children of the same age. The growth velocity of a given child must oscillate about the 50th percentile to maintain growth along a centile chart or a distance chart. Visual inspection on a distance chart is not a substitute for calculating the height velocity and plotting it on a centile chart.

SHORT STATURE AND GROWTH FAILURE

Short stature is a common cause of concern among children and adolescents, and their parents. The definition of short stature is dependent on the growth performance of a given population and thus will vary from country to country. In addition, different criteria are applied between countries, although all definitions of shortness are based on the extent of height deviation from the population mean (e.g. height below the 3rd percentile or height standard deviation score less than –2). Currently in the UK, children whose height falls below the 0.4th percentile (based on the 1990 growth standards) should be evaluated, while those with heights below the 2nd percentile should have their growth velocity carefully monitored. It is also important to

recognize that growth failure can occur in a child whose height is within the normal range.

Among those children whose height falls below the cut-off, only a minority will have a primary endocrine disorder. In order to detect such children, careful clinical assessment and measurements of the height velocity are needed to separate those who are small but growing normally from those who are failing to grow. For the latter, a diagnosis is needed in order for the appropriate treatment to be instituted without delay. The state of nutrition may help to point the diagnostic pathway, but any child who is growing slowly should have a diagnostic investigation to determine the cause.

In assessing all short patients, a detailed history, physical examination, and urine analysis are required, together with a radiograph of the nondominant hand and wrist, allowing the bone age to be assessed and hence also the growth potential. The midparental height (the mean of the parental centile heights) can be calculated in order to estimate height expectation. An abnormal height in one or both parents could indicate a dominantly inherited condition. Additionally, stature that is out of keeping with the family background is likely to be significant (e.g. a child whose

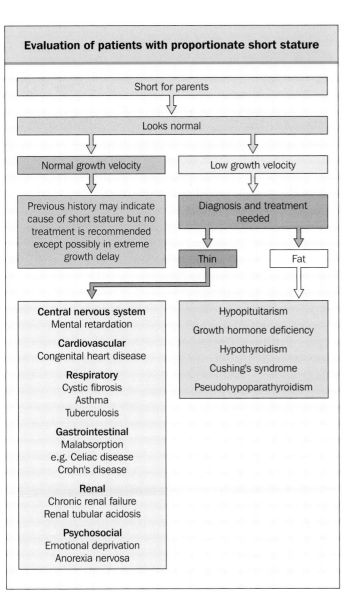

Figure 24B.10 Evaluation of patients with proportionate short stature. The figure shows a flow diagram for the evaluation of short stature of patients with proportionate short stature. Examples of possible diagnoses are shown.

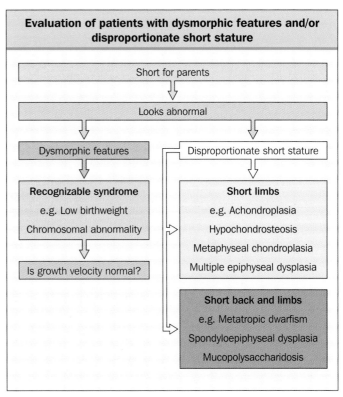

Figure 24B.11 Evaluation of patients with dysmorphic features and/or disproportionate short stature. The figure shows a flow diagram for the evaluation of short stature in patients who have an abnormal phenotype.

Disproportionate short stature

Children who are short because they have short limbs will have plots that lie towards the upper left side of a chart of sitting height versus stature, and those with short backs will have the opposite (**Fig. 24B.12**): the method of measurement of sitting height is shown in **Figure 24B.13**. Shortness may be caused by skeletal dysplasia: for example, hypochondroplasia, in which there is proportionate shortening in the back and limbs that is only identifiable by clinical inspection. Where a skeletal dysplasia is suspected, a full skeletal radiographic survey is needed and an experienced radiologist should be consulted. Since few radiologists are practiced in this field, only a very few know how to interpret the very subtle radiographic changes; it is a field for the superspecialist.

Dysmorphic features

Children with dysmorphic features may have a recognizable syndrome, such as one that is associated with a chromosomal abnormality (e.g. Turner's syndrome), or they may have dysmorphic features associated with low birthweight (e.g. Russell–Silver syndrome) or a nonchromosomal genetic disorder (e.g. Noonan's syndrome).

height is on the 2nd percentile, but whose midparental height falls on the 75th percentile). Information should also be obtained about the growth pattern in the parents, especially concerning the time of onset of the pubertal growth spurt. Physical examination may reveal a child with dysmorphic features suggestive of a syndrome diagnosis, which may be associated with disproportionate short stature (short limbs or short back and limbs). The major causes of short stature in children with proportionate and disproportionate short stature are illustrated in **Figures 24B.10** and **24B.11** respectively.

341

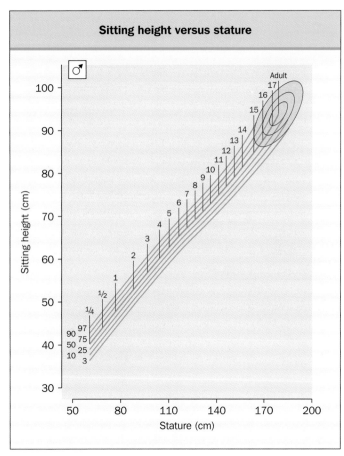

Sitting height versus stature

Sitting height (cm) vs Stature (cm)

Figure 24B.12 **Sitting height versus stature.** The measurement of body proportion is greatly facilitated in measuring sitting height and plotting the relationship of sitting height to stature.

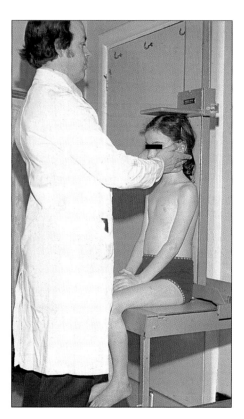

Figure 24B.13 The correct method of measurement of sitting height.

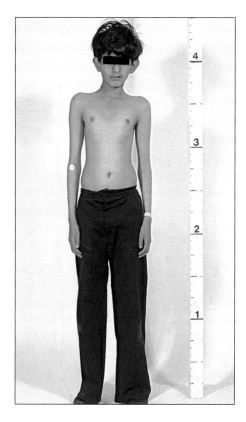

Figure 24B.14 A boy showing dysmorphic features (facial asymmetry) and body thinness associated with low birth weight.

The dysmorphic features associated with relatively low birth-weight are shown in **Figure 24B.14**: note the facial features, the body asymmetry, and the appearance of thinness. An early history of being difficult to feed is extremely characteristic of this very common problem.

Absolute low birthweight is not a prerequisite for the diagnosis. A low birthweight for the family is frequently found. If a normal growth velocity exists, it is unlikely that there is further pathology. Where a low growth velocity exists, however, further investigation would be warranted.

Systemic causes of short stature

Short and thin children usually have a systemic cause for their short stature, whereas endocrinopathies that cause short stature usually result in obesity. In systemic disease, there is often delayed skeletal maturation but the potential for catch-up growth may be present if the underlying systemic disorder can be successfully treated. A child with celiac disease, for example, will continue to have stunted growth until gluten is removed from the diet, after which time rapid growth and development

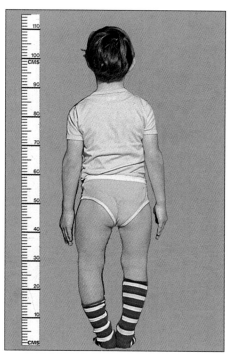

Figure 24B.15 A child with rickets. Note the bowing of the boy's legs, which is only part of the reason for poor growth in children with rickets.

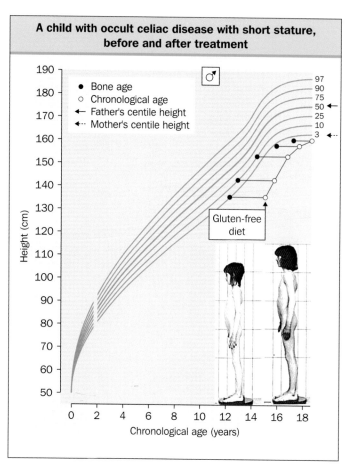

Figure 24B.16 A child with occult celiac disease with short stature, before and after treatment. The effect on growth of introducing a gluten-free diet is shown. Note the delayed bone age at the start of treatment.

may occur. Other chronic disorders that may also retard growth are Crohn's disease, respiratory disease (e.g. asthma, cystic fibrosis), renal disease including hypophosphatemic rickets, hematologic disorders (e.g. Fanconi anemia), infections such as human immunodeficiency virus (HIV) or chronic giardiasis, cardiovascular causes, and nutritional causes (e.g. rickets; **Fig. 24B.15**).

Occult celiac disease may be found among children who grow slowly for no obvious reason. It is therefore important to include antigliadin and antiendomysial antibody measurement in preliminary investigations. This may lead to jejunal biopsy to exclude villous atrophy. The effect of a gluten-free diet in a late-diagnosed asymptomatic celiac patient whose only complaint was short stature is shown in **Figure 24B.16**.

Psychosocial and emotional deprivation

Psychosocial and emotional deprivation are commonly recognized in infancy and childhood. Infants suffering from maternal deprivation display behavioral abnormalities such as apathy, watchfulness, and autoerotic activity, as well as delayed developmental behavior. There is often a history of maternal rejection or neglect, nonaccidental injury, or lack of physical handling. Emotional deprivation in childhood may lead to small stature (**Figs. 24B.17 & 24B.18**), retarded skeletal maturation, and, in older children, delayed sexual maturation. Endocrine function may also be abnormal in affected patients, who may have high levels of fasting GH and also cortisol nonresponsiveness with the insulin tolerance test. GH deficiency that is reversible when the caring environment is improved has also been described.

Endocrine causes of short stature

The important hormones that are concerned with growth are thyroxine (T$_4$), GH, and sex steroids. Deficiency of any of these hormones may result in short stature.

Children may have deficiency of GH secretion from birth or may acquire it later, e.g. as a result (rarely) of a tumor in the area of the hypothalamus or pituitary, or (more commonly) secondary to cranial irradiation. Causes of GH deficiency are listed in **Table 24B.1**.

A congenital deficiency may arise through deletion of the *GH* gene, in which case no GH molecule can be produced, or by mutations within the gene, often at exon–intron splice sites, that result in an abnormal dysfunctional GH molecule. The difference between complete absence of the GH gene and relative deficiency is important, since children with the former have no immunologic tolerance to the GH molecule and thus develop antibodies when exposed to therapy.

Isolated GH deficiency presenting in early childhood without any family history, which is the commonly encountered condition, is usually associated with pituitary hypoplasia secondary to a deficiency of the secretion of GH-releasing hormone from the hypothalamus. Thin-slice magnetic resonance imaging (MRI) images through the hypothalamic region may also reveal an absent or attenuated pituitary stalk and/or an ectopically positioned posterior pituitary bright spot. These latter features can indicate that the isolated GH deficiency may evolve with the development of other anterior pituitary hormone deficits. MRI scans can, however, be normal.

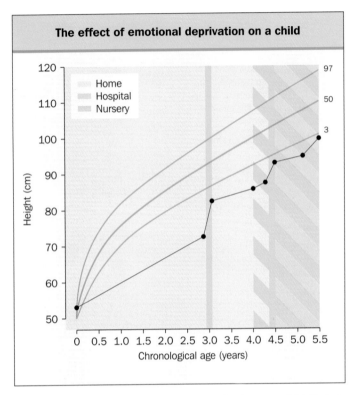

Figure 24B.17 The effect of emotional deprivation on a child. During hospitalization, the growth rate of the child increased, but it 'steadied off' during periods of emotional deprivation at home.

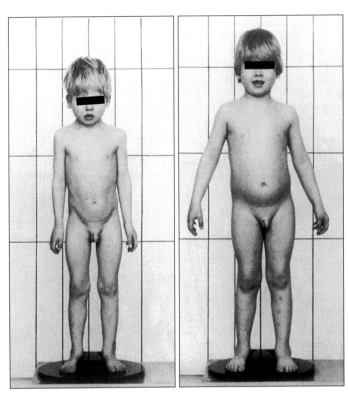

Figure 24B.18 An emotionally deprived 7-year-old child before and after treatment (1 year later). Note the marked short stature (a) and the rapid growth following treatment (b).

Causes of growth hormone deficiency (± hypopituitarism)		
Congenital	GH deficiency resulting from congenital malformations of the hypothalamic–pituitary region	Septo-optic dysplasia/optic nerve hypoplasia
		Other midline abnormalities (e.g. holoprosencephaly)
	Gene deletion or mutations within the *GH* gene	
	Mutations within the *GHRH* receptor gene	
	Mutations of transcription factors necessary to pituitary development	Prop1
		POUF1 (Pit-1)
		Hesx1
		Lhx3
Acquired	GH deficiency resulting from irradiation of the hypothalamic–pituitary region	
	GH deficiency of undefined etiology (idiopathic), including those with abnormal pituitary morphology on magnetic resonance imaging – pituitary hypoplasia, interrupted or hypoplastic stalk, ectopically placed posterior pituitary lobe	
	Trauma, infiltration or infection in the hypothalamic–pituitary region	

Table 24B.1 Causes of growth-hormone (GH) deficiency (± hypopituitarism). These can have a hypothalamic or pituitary basis.

The etiology of this form of GH deficiency is unclear. Some may have a history of birth trauma or prematurity. Presently, there is considerable interest in the role of pituitary development genes. Abnormalities in these genes may contribute. GH deficiency may be associated with midline congenital abnormalities such as optic nerve/septo-optic dysplasia. GH deficiency may be the only deficiency or associated with hypopituitarism. Despite the congenital nature of this disorder, GH deficiency may not present until later childhood.

If GH insufficiency is an isolated pituitary hormonal problem, birthweight is characteristically normal and the early postnatal course is uneventful. A diminished growth velocity becomes obvious towards the end of the first year of life as the hormone-dependent childhood phase of growth fails to take over from the nutrition-dependent infant phase. The lack of sufficient GH causes a characteristic appearance (**Fig. 24B.19**), with truncal obesity, a face appearing younger than the chronological age, and a tendency for crowding of the facial features to the center of the

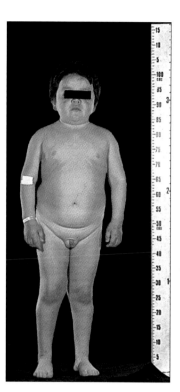

Figure 24B.19 A boy with classic growth-hormone insufficiency. Such children are very small, tend to be obese, and have underdeveloped genitalia. They have a low growth velocity and usually a retarded bone age.

Agents used in formal assessment of growth hormone reserve
Insulin tolerance test
Arginine infusion
l-dopa
Glucagon
Clonidine

Table 24B.2 Agents used in formal assessment of growth hormone reserve. The insulin tolerance test remains the most frequently used investigation in specialized units.

face, suggesting maxillary hypoplasia. In boys, the genitalia may be small; however, a very small penis is suggestive of an associated gonadotropin deficiency. Body proportions are normal before puberty, although these patients tend to have poorly developed musculature. Puberty, if it occurs spontaneously, is usually slightly, but not significantly, delayed.

When there are multiple pituitary hormone deficiencies, there are likely to be problems in the newborn period with hypoglycemia or conjugated hyperbilirubinemia (secondary to adrenocorticotropic hormone deficiency), and micropenis may draw attention to a concomitant deficiency of luteinizing hormone.

Methods of testing the hypothalamic–pituitary GH axis are legion (**Table 24B.2**) and the interpretation of the results of GH tests requires consideration of the circumstances, particularly in the patient with delayed puberty whose GH response can be amplified by the administration of 100mg testosterone (to a boy), given intramuscularly 3 days before the test, or of 30mg ethinylestradiol (to a girl) for 3 days. There are also many different commercial assays for GH, using both polyclonal and monoclonal antibodies. The reported values for GH can vary widely between assays done on identical samples. It is therefore important for each unit to be acquainted with the performance of their GH assay. It is also suggested that a measurement of the GH-dependent peptide insulin-like growth factor-I (IGF-I) be undertaken in conjunction with the GH test. A serum IGF-I level below an age- and sex-matched normal range, in association with a low peak GH level during a provocation test, would confirm the diagnosis of GH deficiency.

Because of the recognized fallibility of GH tests (indicating GH deficiency when it is not present), the diagnosis of moderate GH deficiency is difficult. This should be based on a multi-faceted process that takes into consideration clinical and auxologic assessment, combined with biochemical tests of the GH–IGF axis and MRI evaluation of the hypothalamic–pituitary axis. In addition, it is most important for those with a diagnosis of GH deficiency through childhood and adolescence to have pituitary function, in particular GH reserve, retested at the completion of growth to determine whether they should continue GH replacement throughout life (see Chapter 4). Some patients who have isolated GH deficiency in childhood are able to generate normal levels of GH when retested in adolescence and do not seem to require GH replacement in adulthood.

When investigations are required to assess a low growth velocity, these should comprise testing of the whole hypothalamic–pituitary axis and should be undertaken in a center that is properly staffed and equipped for the safe investigation of children with endocrine problems.

Treatment of insufficient GH secretion is by daily injections of recombinant GH. The dose can be calculated on a bodyweight or body-surface-area basis – 25–50µg/kg/day or 0.7–1.4mg/m^2/day. In the USA, growth-hormone-releasing hormone (GHRH) is available to treat GH deficiency associated with impaired secretion of endogenous GHRH, although it is not widely used. In addition, depot GH preparations, whereby a single injection is given every 2 weeks, have been used in GH deficiency. The response to treatment with daily subcutaneous GH injections is predictable from the pretreatment growth rate and from the dose of GH administered (**Fig. 24B.20**).

Growth-hormone-insensitive states

The phenotype of GH insensitivity is very similar to GH deficiency with short stature, truncal adiposity, and midfacial hypoplasia, but the biochemical hallmark is raised basal and stimulated GH levels coupled with low IGF-I and IGF-binding protein-3 (IGFBP-3) levels. GH insensitivity may be congenital or acquired. The latter occurs with fasting, poor nutrition and catabolic states. Congenital GH insensitivity (Laron's syndrome; **Fig. 24B.21**) is very rare. In the majority it is a recessive condition caused by mutations in the GH receptor gene, most commonly in the extracellular domain of the receptor. The mutations result in a highly truncated nonsense protein, and therefore circulating GH-binding protein (GHBP), produced normally by cleavage of the extracellular domain from the cell surface, is absent. However GH insensitivity with a normal or raised GHBP has been described, caused by mutations within the transmembrane or intracellular domains of the GH receptor. The latter can be inherited as a dominant trait, thus demonstrating, in a similar way to autosomal-dominant GH deficiency, that genetic short stature may have an endocrine origin.

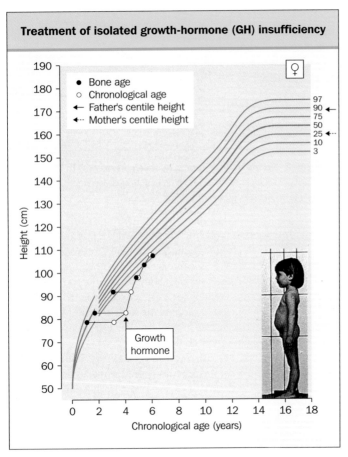

Treatment of isolated growth-hormone (GH) insufficiency

- ● Bone age
- ○ Chronological age
- ← Father's centile height
- ◄-- Mother's centile height

Figure 24B.20 Treatment of isolated growth-hormone (GH) insufficiency. The figure shows the response of a girl with isolated GH insufficiency to treatment with injections of human GH. The heights are shown as open circles and continuous lines, and height plots are connected to the corresponding bone ages by solid lines.

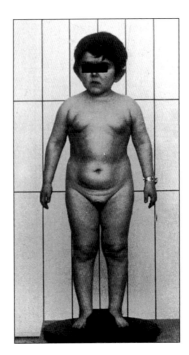

Figure 24B.21 Growth-hormone (GH) insensitivity, with a phenotype very similar to GH deficiency. The child has Laron's syndrome and lacks GH receptors.

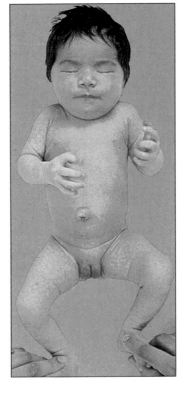

Figure 24B.22 A child suffering from congenital hypothyroidism. Coarse features, a large tongue, and an apathetic appearance are characteristic of congenital hypothyroidism.

Hypothyroidism

Hypothyroidism in children is traditionally divided into congenital (**Fig. 24B.22 & Table 24B.3**) and acquired hypothyroidism. Causes of congenital hypothyroidism include thyroid dysgenesis (aplasia, hypoplasia ± ectopic position), inborn errors of thyroid hormonogenesis, and secondary/tertiary hypothyroidism. The latter is usually associated with other features of hypopituitarism.

Basal thyroid function tests will reveal low levels of T_4, together with a raised level of thyroid-stimulating hormone (TSH) in those with congenital primary hypothyroidism. Bone-age radiographs, particularly of the knees, are valuable. The distal femoral epiphyses are calcified in nearly all normal-term individuals but not in those with congenital hypothyroidism.

Screening programs have allowed this condition to be detected in the first weeks of life and thyroxine treatment is instituted early. Linear growth, skeletal maturity, and intellectual development should then proceed normally. There is, however, a persistent difference in IQ between those with severe versus moderate congenital hypothyroidism, reflecting the importance of intrauterine thyroxine to development of the central nervous system.

It is unusual for congenital hypothyroidism not to be detected on a screening program, although some inborn errors, such as abnormalities in the Pendrin gene, may present later in life. Thus the presentation of hypothyroidism outside infancy is usually truly acquired (**Figs 24B.23 & 24B.24**), and is caused by Hashimoto's thyroiditis or iodine deficiency; with symptoms and signs being similar to adult hypothyroidism. Short stature is very common, the bone age tends to be very retarded, and children tend to maintain infantile proportions because of poor linear bone growth.

Clinical features of congenital hypothyroidism
Prolonged neonatal jaundice
Lethargy
Feeding problems
Failure to gain weight
Constipation
Dry skin
Thick tongue
Umbilical hernia
Respiratory problems
Goiter
Mental retardation

Table 24B.3 Clinical features of congenital hypothyroidism.

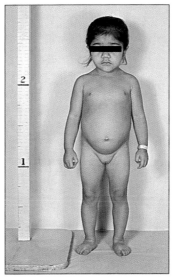

Figure 24B.23 A hypothyroid girl.

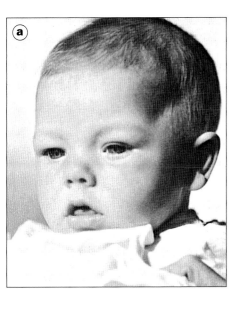

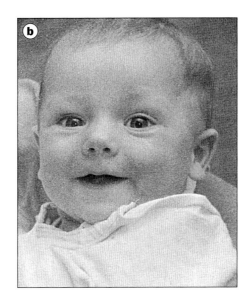

Figure 24B.24 A hypothyroid baby (a) before and (b) after treatment.

Pseudohypoparathyroidism

Pseudohypoparathyroidism Type 1a (**Fig. 24B.25**) is characterized by peripheral resistance to the actions of parathyroid hormone (PTH) and often TSH, and is inherited as an autosomal dominant trait. The typical phenotypic features include short stature, a round face, obesity, a short thick neck, decreased intelligence in at least 50%, and subcutaneous and intracranial calcification. Shortening of the metacarpals is frequent. The diagnosis may be confirmed by the presence of low or normal levels of serum calcium, elevated phosphate levels, and the presence of a raised PTH level. Following PTH infusion, urinary cyclic adenosine monophosphate (cAMP) fails to rise. The condition is treated by administering high doses of vitamin D.

Cushing's syndrome

Cushing's syndrome associated with steroid administration for atopy, inflammatory disorders, or immune suppression (i.e. iatrogenic) is the most common presentation. Otherwise Cushing's syndrome (**Fig. 24B.26**) is unusual in infancy and childhood. Short stature results from decreased linear growth (corticosteroid-suppressed GH secretion and direct inhibitory effects of corticosteroids on the growth plate). Rarely, where a preponderance of androgen secretion occurs, there may be an acceleration of growth and signs of virilization. The etiology in early childhood is more likely to be an adrenal adenoma, while in later childhood an adrenocorticotropic-hormone (ACTH)-secreting pituitary adenoma may occur. Ectopic ACTH syndrome is very unusual in children.

Nonendocrine causes of short stature
Constitutional growth delay

One of the most common causes of short stature is constitutional growth delay with delayed puberty: the bone age is retarded but the growth velocity is normal. A normal growth spurt in puberty can be predicted, and eventual height will be normal (**Fig. 24B.27**).

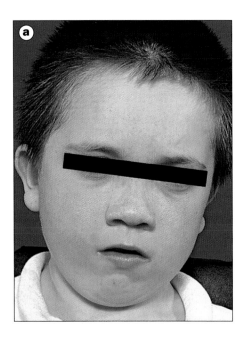

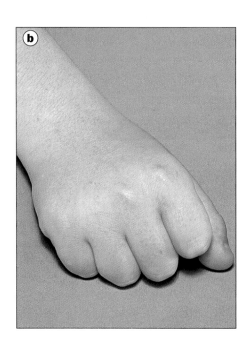

Figure 24B.25 A boy with pseudohypoparathyroidism. Note his round face and shortened neck (a) and his shortened metacarpals (b).

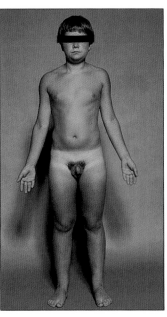

Figure 24B.26 A patient with Cushing's syndrome. This is uncommon in childhood. Short stature is a consequence of the suppression of growth hormone secretion by corticosteroids. In addition to short stature, note the plethoric 'moon' face.

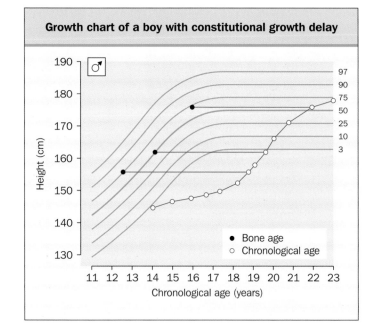

Figure 24B.27 Growth chart of a boy with constitutional growth delay. The boy's short height during childhood would have been accompanied by a delayed bone age. When the average boys of his age started to grow rapidly in puberty, this boy was left behind. Thus, he was referred for short stature and delayed puberty. His pubertal stages were appropriate for his bone age and, because of his previously normal growth velocity, a normal growth spurt in puberty was predicted and occurred as shown.

Although treatment is not essential, these patients are seriously disadvantaged by their condition, which is easily improved with small doses of sex steroids.

Turner's syndrome

Chromosome analysis should be performed on any girl unexpectedly short for her family; signs of puberty should not inhibit this investigation, since 20% of girls with Turner's syndrome have signs of spontaneous sexual development, although very few progress beyond the earliest stages of breast development. The only constant feature is short stature. The majority of this short stature may be attributable to the haplo-insufficiency of the SHOX gene in Turner's syndrome. This gene is located on the pseudoautosomal region of the short arm of the X chromosome.

The management of Turner's syndrome requires a growth-promoting regimen in childhood (GH with or without oxandrolone) and phased introduction of estrogen from an appropriate peripubertal age, for instance the 12th year of life. The gain in final height over that achieved in the untreated state is variable and appears to depend on the time spent on treatment, the use of oxandrolone, and the age at which estrogen is introduced.

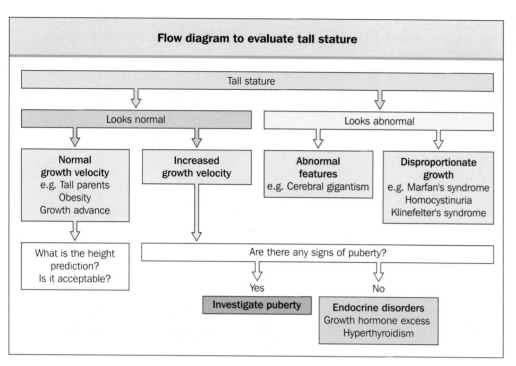

Figure 24B.28 Flow diagram to evaluate tall stature.

Flow diagram to evaluate tall stature

Skeletal dysplasias

Patients who are short for their family in childhood, have a reduced height prediction, and are growing normally should be suspected of having a skeletal dysplasia. In hypochondroplasia, for example, the disproportionate short stature may not become manifest until adult life. Treatment with GH has been tried experimentally for these patients and for patients with familial short stature. The results in terms of final height have not been fully evaluated but do not appear to be impressive.

TALL STATURE

There are relatively few pathologic cases of tall stature, with most children representing the upper end of the normal distribution of height. Most often there is a family history of tallness in one or both parents. Ultimate height can be predicted by assessment of bone age. A diagram showing the method of evaluation of tall stature is shown in **Figure 24B.28**.

Tall stature associated with normal growth velocity

If a child looks normal and has a normal growth velocity, constitutional tall stature is usually present (**Fig. 24B.29**). Obese children are often taller than average for their age and, if maturity is also advanced, then puberty may occasionally occur earlier. Tall stature may represent a considerable handicap and, if necessary, treatment to limit growth should be considered.

The most commonly used strategy is to induce puberty early with replacement doses of sex steroids. This achieves a reduction in height in relation to the age at which puberty is induced.

Tall stature associated with increased growth velocity

With increased growth velocity, pubertal status should be assessed. If signs of puberty are present, together with accelerated skeletal maturation, this should be investigated. Precocious sexual development (**Fig. 24B.30**) should be differentiated

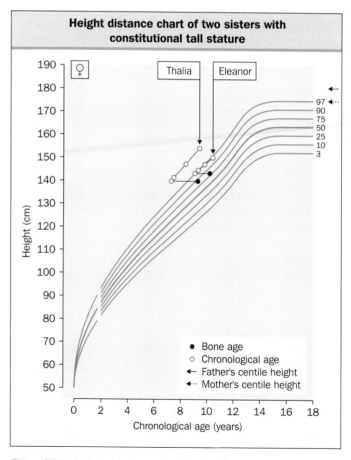

Figure 24B.29 Height distance chart of two sisters with constitutional tall stature, who were brought for assessment by their tall mother.
Since Eleanor's bone age is less advanced than Thalia's, her eventual height will probably be greater. Provided their growth velocity is normal (thus excluding other diagnoses), the decision to commence medical treatment to reduce their final height is not so much a medical one as a social one.

349

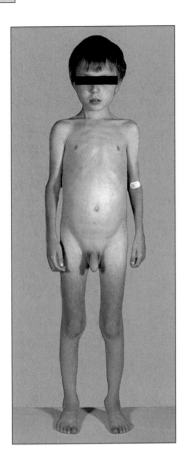

Figure 24B.30 An 8-year-old child with precocious puberty and tall stature, which are associated with a cerebral tumor.

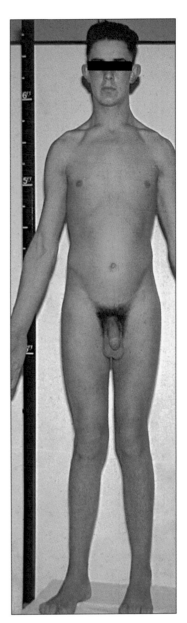

Figure 24B.31 A 16-year-old patient suffering from **gigantism.** GH is raised and bone age is not advanced, indicating that the boy's eventual stature will be abnormally tall.

from pseudoprecocious puberty, where excessive androgen and estrogen production results from a tumor in the ovary, testis, or adrenals, or from congenital adrenal hyperplasia. In precocious puberty, the linear growth and bone maturation are advanced and height is often above average, although the final height is likely to be reduced.

Growth hormone excess

An excess of GH in childhood or adolescence causes gigantism (**Fig. 24B.31**) but bone age is not advanced. A GH-secreting tumor may be present and can be diagnosed using MRI. Levels of GH are raised, contrasting with levels in constitutional tall stature. Clinically, the disease is characterized by extremely rapid linear growth, overgrowth of soft tissues, and metabolic changes that are similar to those observed in older acromegalic patients. Treatment is aimed at reducing the excessive GH secretion. Possible treatment modalities to be considered, as for acromegaly (see Chapter 3), include transsphenoidal removal of the tumor, medical therapy with somatostatin analogs, and/or radiotherapy. Pegvisomant (a GH antagonist), when introduced on to the market, is likely to be the most effective medical therapy for this condition.

Hyperthyroidism

An increase in growth rate associated with advanced bone age is seen in hyperthyroid children and also in hypothyroidism overtreated with T4. The diagnosis is made by measuring the T4, triiodothyronine, and TSH levels, and a thyroid-releasing hormone test should be carried out where doubt still exists.

A hyperthyroid girl is shown in **Figure 24B.32**, with her hypothyroid twin sister.

Tall stature associated with an abnormal appearance

Some examples of tall stature syndromes are presented.

Sotos syndrome

Children with Sotos syndrome have a large elongated head, prominent forehead, large ears and jaws, elongated jaw, and coarse facial features. They also have normal GH secretion and no evidence of thyroid, adrenal, or gonadal dysfunction. Most have subnormal intelligence.

Marfan's syndrome

Patients with Marfan's syndrome (**Fig. 24B.33**) are usually well above average in height but within the normal range. They have long limbs with narrow hands and long slender fingers. Their arm span is greater than their height and the lower segment is

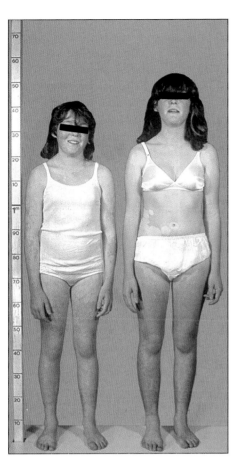

Figure 24B.32 A girl (right) whose tall stature is caused by excessive thyroid activity. Her twin sister (left) suffers from hypothyroidism and is consequently short for her age.

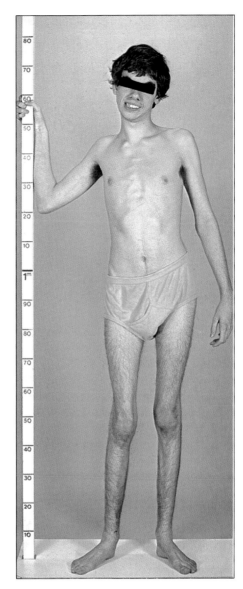

Figure 24B.33 A boy with Marfan's syndrome. Arm span is greater than height, and the limbs are long with slender hands and fingers. The cause of death in these patients is usually a dissecting aneurysm in early adult life.

much greater than the upper segment. Hyperextensible joints, kyphoscoliosis, deformities of the rib cage, and dislocation of the lens are also present. Aortic root dilatation is an important feature. Death from a dissecting aneurysm may occur in early adult life. Echocardiographic and ophthalmic assessment should be undertaken in a child with marfanoid features.

Homocystinuria

Homocystinuria is caused by an absence of the enzyme cystathionine synthetase. Phenotypically, patients resemble those with Marfan's syndrome but they usually have mental retardation and there is a tendency for them to die from thrombotic disorders. Lenticular dislocation also occurs, usually in a downward direction.

Klinefelter's syndrome

Patients with Klinefelter's syndrome (see **Fig. 24A.15**) have an XXY karyotype and a tendency to be tall; they also display eunuchoid features. Seminiferous tubule dysgenesis, gynecomastia, and small, pea-sized testes are present. Behavioral and learning difficulties are common.

GENERAL CONSIDERATIONS

Abnormalities of growth represent a frequent cause of referral to the endocrine clinic. The approach to the management of

these patients is summarized in **Figure 24B.34**. The importance of accurate anthropometry cannot be overemphasized and, in the early assessment, it is mandatory to establish the parental pattern of growth and also the age at which puberty was entered. The midparental height, adjusted for the sex of the patient, enables the clinician to gain an estimate of the expected final height of the individual and, by using a height distance chart, to determine whether the child is on course to achieve this. The estimation of skeletal maturity, usually by radiography of the child's wrist, is essential in the assessment of growth prognosis of the likely final height.

Follow-up measurements should also be carried out at a minimum of 6-monthly intervals, allowing the growth velocity to be calculated. The growth velocity is a very important clue to the pattern of growth taking place. Abnormality of growth velocity requires systematic investigations directed at the diagnosis of systemic or endocrine pathology.

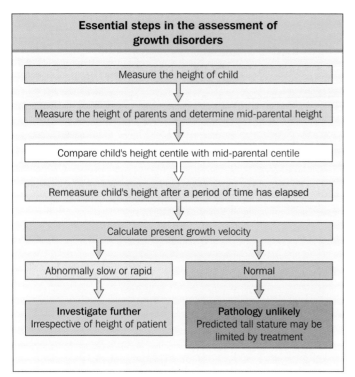

Figure 24B.34 Essential steps in the assessment of growth disorders.

FURTHER READING

Brook CGD, Hindmarsh PC, ed. Clinical paediatric endocrinology. Oxford: Blackwell Science, 2001: chapters on 'Normal growth and its endocrine control', 'Growth assessment – purpose and interpretation' and 'Management of disorders of size'.

Buckler JHM. Growth disorders in children. London: BMJ Publishing, 1994.

Duquesnoy P, Roy A, Dastot F, et al. Human Prop-1: cloning, mapping, genomic structure. Mutations in familial combined pituitary hormone deficiency. FEBS Lett. 1998;437:216–20.

GH Research Society. Consensus guidelines for the diagnosis and treatment of growth hormone (GH) deficiency in childhood and adolescence: summary statement of the GH Research Society. J Clin Endocrinol Metab. 2000;85;3990–3.

Jones KL. Smith's recognizable patterns of human malformation. Philadelphia, PA: WB Saunders, 1998.

Krude H, Biebermann H, Schnabel D, et al. Molecular pathogenesis of neonatal hypothyroidism. Hormone Res. 2000;53(Suppl):112–8.

Lipscomb KJ, Clayton-Smith J, Harris R. Evolving phenotype of Marfan's syndrome. Arch Dis Child. 1997;76:41–6.

Pfaffle RW, Blankenstein O, Wuller S, Kentrup H. Combined pituitary hormone deficiency: role of Pit-1 and Prop-1. Acta Paediatr Suppl. 1999;88:33–41.

Rosenfeld RG, Rosenbloom AL, Guevara-Aguirre J. Growth hormone insensitivity due to primary GH receptor deficiency. Endo Rev. 1994;15:369–90.

Ross JL, Scott C Jr, Marttila P, et al. Phenotypes associated with SHOX deficiency. J Clin Endocrinol Metab. 2001;86:5674–80.

Saenger P, Wikland KA, Conway GS, et al. Recommendations for the diagnosis and management of Turner syndrome. J Clin Endocrinol Metab. 2001;86:3061–9.

Sizonenko PC, Clayton PE, Cohen P, et al. Diagnosis and management of growth hormone deficiency in childhood and adolescence. Part 1: Diagnosis of growth hormone deficiency. GH IGF Res. 2001;11:137–65.

Wales JKH, Rogol AD, Wit JM. Color atlas of pediatric endocrinology and growth. London: Mosby-Wolfe, 1996.

Section 5 Gonad and Growth

Chapter 25 The Testis

James E Griffin and Jean D Wilson

INTRODUCTION

The testes produce sperm and the hormones that regulate male sexual function. During fetal life the testes produce three hormones – the peptide antimüllerian hormone, a product of the Sertoli cells that causes regression of the müllerian ducts, and the steroid testosterone, which, along with its 5α-reduced metabolite dihydrotestosterone, virilizes the male urogenital tract. In adulthood the testes continue to produce testosterone and in addition produce the peptide hormones inhibin and activin, which control the secretion of follicle-stimulating hormone (FSH). These various hormones are responsible for the induction of male phenotype during embryogenesis, for sexual maturation at puberty, and for adult male sexual function. As a consequence, abnormalities of testicular function cause different clinical effects during different periods of life.

GENES THAT CONTROL TESTIS DIFFERENTIATION

Differentiation of the indifferent gonad into a testis is initiated by the *SRY* (sex-determining region, Y chromosome) gene on the short arm of the Y chromosome (**Fig. 25.1**). At least four additional genes are necessary for normal testicular development: Wilms-tumor-related (*WT1*) gene, steroidogenic factor-1 (*SF-1*), SRY-related HMG-box 9 (*SOX9*), and dosage-sensitive sex reversal–adrenal hypoplasia congenita critical region of the X chromosome gene 1 (*DAX-1*; **Fig. 25.1**). *WT1* is important in urogenital tract development and is expressed in fetal renal mesenchyme, the primordial gonad, and adult Sertoli cells. *SF-1* is expressed in the genital ridge, steroidogenic cells in the gonads and adrenals, the hypothalamus, and pituitary gonadotropes. *SOX9* is expressed in the developing testis, and

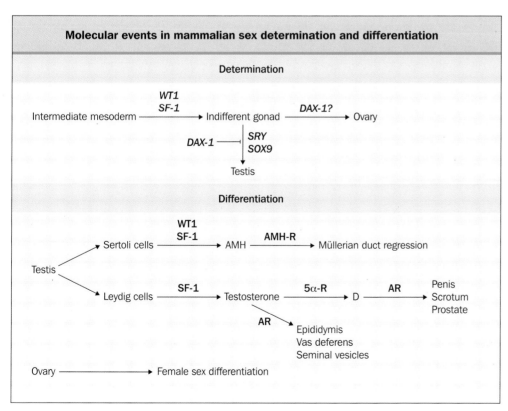

Figure 25.1 Molecular events in mammalian sex determination and differentiation. The role of the genes believed to mediate key events is indicated as described in the text. AMH, antimüllerian hormone; AMH-R, AMH receptor; AR, androgen receptor; D, dihydrotestosterone; DAX-1, dosage sensitive sex reversal-adrenal hypoplasia congenita critical region of the X chromosonme gene; 5α-R, 5α-reductase. (Modified from Parker KL. Sexual differentiation. In: Griffin JE, Ojeda SR, eds. Textbook of endocrine physiology, 4th edn. Oxford; Oxford University Press: 2000.)

DAX-1 may act to antagonize *SRY* in testis differentiation. Loss of function mutations in *SRY* or any of the four downstream genes can impair testicular development. (See Dysgenetic testes syndrome, below.)

STRUCTURE OF THE TESTES AND MALE REPRODUCTIVE TRACT

The testes contain two functional units: interstitial or Leydig cells, which contain the enzymatic machinery for androgen synthesis, and a network of spermatogenic tubules for the production and transport of sperm (**Fig. 25.2**).

The lipid droplets in Leydig cells contain esterified cholesterol that is derived from circulating lipoproteins and locally synthesized cholesterol. Following hydrolysis, free cholesterol moves to mitochondria, where the side chain is cleaved to form pregnenolone, which, in turn, is converted to testosterone in the endoplasmic reticulum. The amount of Leydig cell testosterone is small, since newly synthesized hormone diffuses promptly into the plasma.

Spermatogenic tubules are composed of germ cells and Sertoli cells (**Fig. 25.3**). Tight junctions between the Sertoli cells form a diffusion barrier that divides the testis into two functional compartments. The basal compartment consists of Leydig cells and the outer portion of the tubules that contain the spermatogonia. The adluminal compartment is composed of the inner two thirds of the tubules and includes primary and secondary spermatocytes and spermatids. Sertoli cells line the spermatogenic tubule, and the inner portion of the Sertoli cell consists of an arborized cytoplasm that engulfs the spermatogonia so that spermatogenesis actually takes place within a network of Sertoli cell cytoplasm.

The seminiferous tubules empty into the rete testes, a network of ducts that anastomose into the coiled epididymis, which is 5–6m in length. The vas deferens is a 30–35cm tube that connects the epididymis to the ejaculatory duct (which terminates in the prostatic urethra). The paired seminal vesicles (4–5cm in length) empty into the ejaculatory ducts. The adult prostate, weighing about 20g, surrounds the urethra and contains a network of ductules that also terminate in the urethra.

HYPOTHALAMO–PITUITARY–TESTICULAR AXIS

The hypothalamus communicates with the pituitary by neural pathways and by a portal vascular system that delivers regulatory hormones from the brain to the pituitary (**Fig. 25.4**). The preoptic and medial basal regions of the hypothalamus (particularly the arcuate nucleus) control gonadotrophin secretion. Peptidergic neurons in these regions act as a pulse generator to secrete the decapeptide gonadotrophin-releasing hormone (GnRH), also known as luteinizing-hormone-releasing hormone (LHRH), in a pulsatile fashion. Neurons from other regions of the brain terminate in this area and influence GnRH synthesis and release via catecholaminergic, dopaminergic, and β-endorphin-related mechanisms. GnRH is widely distributed in the central nervous system and in other tissues but a physiologic role has not been established for it outside the pituitary.

The major hormones under GnRH control are luteinizing hormone (LH) and FSH (**Fig. 25.4**). GnRH acts on cell-surface receptors on pituitary gonadotropes to stimulate the release of LH

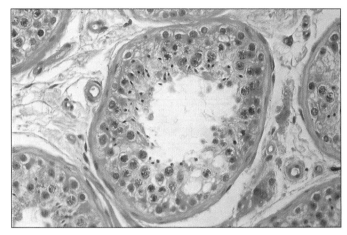

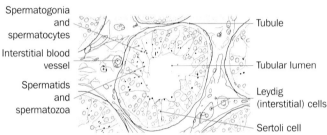

Figure 25.2 A histologic section of a normal testis. Spermatogenesis takes place between the Sertoli cells in the seminiferous tubules. Different stages of spermatogenesis may be seen in the same cross-section, a feature particular to man and different from most other mammals. In the normal mature testis, the Leydig cells appear in clumps between the seminiferous tubules. Hematoxylin–eosin stain. (Courtesy of Professor I Doniach.)

and FSH by a calcium-dependent, cAMP-independent mechanism. Diacylglycerols may amplify the calcium-mediated signal. In addition, GnRH probably enhances the synthesis of LH and FSH long-term. The episodic secretion of GnRH into the hypophysial portal system results, in turn, in episodic secretion of LH. In adult men, LH is secreted at a frequency of eight to 14 pulses per 24 hours. Coincidental pulsatile secretion of FSH also occurs but with a lower amplitude.

Luteinizing hormone interacts with cell-surface receptors on Leydig cells to stimulate a membrane-bound adenylate cyclase. Cyclic adenosine monophosphate (cAMP) is subsequently released into the cytoplasm, where it binds to a protein kinase. Activation of the protein kinase, operating through unidentified intermediate steps, stimulates the delivery of cholesterol to the inner mitochondrial membrane. LH secretion is controlled primarily by negative feedback and both testosterone and estradiol can inhibit LH secretion. Testosterone can be converted to estradiol in the brain and the two hormones are believed to act independently on LH secretion. Testosterone slows the hypothalamic pulse generator in the hypothalamus and thus decreases the frequency of pulsatile LH release and also exerts a direct negative-feedback effect on LH secretion by the pituitary.

The Sertoli cell is the primary site of action of FSH. The biochemical events that follow the binding of FSH to its receptor on the cell surface are similar to those for LH. The elevation of

A Sertoli cell

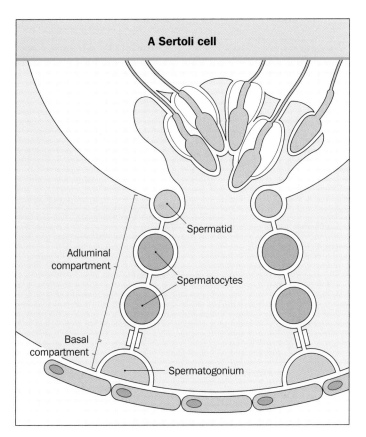

Figure 25.3 A Sertoli cell. The relationship between Sertoli cell cytoplasm and developing spermatocytes is shown. (Modified from Griffin JE, Wilson JD. Disorders of the testes and male reproductive tract. In: Wilson JD, Foster DW, eds. Williams textbook of endocrinology, 7th edn. Philadelphia, PA;WB Saunders: 1985.)

Hypothalamic regulation of gonadotrophin secretion

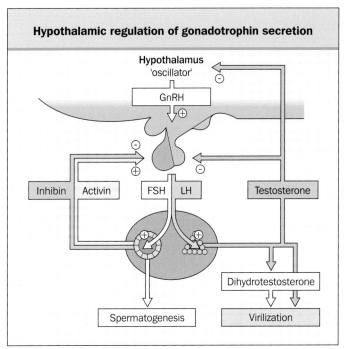

Figure 25.4 Hypothalamic regulation of gonadotrophin secretion. Episodic release of gonadotrophin-releasing hormone (GnRH) stimulates the gonadotropes, causing pulsatile release of luteinizing hormone (LH) and, to a lesser extent, follicle-stimulating hormone (FSH). LH acts on Leydig cells, causing the production of testosterone, which is responsible for virilization (in some tissues through the production of dihydrotestosterone). LH release is suppressed by the negative feedback mechanism of the testosterone action on the hypothalamus and pituitary. FSH acts on Sertoli cells and this results in spermatogenesis. Inhibin has a negative feedback effect and activin has a positive effect on FSH production in the anterior pituitary.

Sertoli cell cAMP activates cAMP-dependent protein kinase and stimulates synthesis of mRNAs and proteins, including androgen-binding protein (ABP) and aromatase. Serum FSH levels increase as germinal elements in the testis are lost, whereas there is a minimal change in LH levels. The control of FSH secretion involves peptide and steroid hormones. Inhibin, an inhibitor of pituitary FSH secretion formed in Sertoli cells, is a glycoprotein that consists of two disulfide-linked subunits – α, combined with β_A or β_B. Both FSH and androgen enhance inhibin production. Activins, composed of the heterodimers or homodimers of the β-subunits of inhibin, stimulate FSH. The relation between serum inhibin and serum FSH levels became apparent with the development of an immunoassay for inhibin B. Using this assay, serum inhibin levels correlate positively with spermatogenesis and negatively with serum FSH levels. Inhibin is thought to be the most important hormone for feedback inhibition of FSH secretion. Although inhibin B is stimulated by FSH, there is also evidence for a gonadotrophin-independent component of its regulation in men. Inhibin B may prove to be a useful marker of Sertoli cell function but its utility as a diagnostic tool has not yet been established.

ANDROGEN PHYSIOLOGY

In the Leydig cell, cholesterol is transported into the mitochondrion by the carrier protein StAR (steroidogenic acute regulatory protein) and is transformed to testosterone by a series of enzymatic reactions (**Fig. 25.5**): cholesterol side-chain cleavage (CYP11A1, also termed P450$_{scc}$), 3β-hydroxysteroid dehydrogenase/isomerase 2 (3β-HSD2), 17α-hydroxylase (CYP17, also termed P450$_{17\alpha}$), 17,20-lyase (CYP17), and 17β-hydroxysteroid dehydrogenase 3 (17β-HSD3). The initial and rate-limiting step in testosterone synthesis involves the delivery of cholesterol by StAR to the inner mitochondrial membrane under the control of LH. 3β-HSD2 oxidizes the steroid A ring to the Δ^4-3-keto configuration. Both the 17α-hydroxylation and 17,20-lyase activities are controlled by a single enzyme, CYP17, and the final reaction involves the reduction of the 17-ketone to a hydroxyl by 17β-HSD3. Testosterone is the principal steroid formed, but small amounts of its precursors in the pathway are secreted, as are small amounts of dihydrotestosterone and estradiol. The main sites of formation of dihydrotestosterone and estradiol in men are androgen-target tissues and adipose tissue, respectively (see below).

Normal testes contain approximately 25µg of testosterone so that the testicular hormone turns over 200 times or more to provide the average 5–10mg secreted daily. In normal men, approximately 2% of plasma testosterone is free (unbound), 44% is bound to sex-hormone-binding globulin (SHBG, also known as

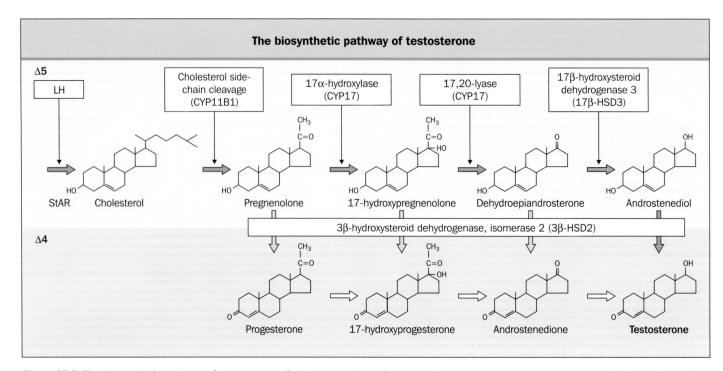

The biosynthetic pathway of testosterone

Figure 25.5 The biosynthetic pathway of testosterone. Partial or complete deficiencies of steroidogenic acute regulatory protein (StAR) or of any of the enzymes involved causes inadequate testosterone synthesis and may lead to inadequate virilization, resulting in male pseudohermaphroditism. A deficiency of StAR or of the enzymes CYP17 or 3β-HSD2 is also associated with adrenal hyperplasia.

testosterone-binding globulin or TeBG), and the remainder is bound to albumin and other proteins. Since albumin-bound testosterone is available for tissue uptake, bioavailable testosterone (the free component plus the albumin-bound component) is equal to some 50% of the total amount.

Testosterone serves as a circulating precursor or prohormone for two types of metabolites, which in turn mediate many androgen actions (**Fig. 25.6**). It can be 5α-reduced to dihydrotestosterone, which mediates many differentiative, growth-promoting, and functional actions. Alternatively, androgens can be aromatized in the extraglandular tissues to estrogens that act independently or in concert with androgens to influence physiologic processes. Thus, the actions of testosterone are the result of the combined effects of testosterone, dihydrotestosterone, and estradiol. Dihydrotestosterone is formed by two 5α-reductase enzymes, principally in androgen-target tissues. Aromatization occurs in many tissues, perhaps the most important being the adipocyte.

In normal men, the production rates of testosterone and the adrenal androgen, androstenedione, average some 5mg/day and 3mg/day respectively, and the production rates of estrone and estradiol average approximately 66g/day and 45μg/day, respectively (**Fig. 25.7**). All the estrone is formed from circulating precursors: 35% of estradiol is derived from circulating testosterone, 50% is formed from circulating estrone, and 15% is secreted by the testes. When gonadotrophin levels are elevated, estradiol secretion by the testis increases.

Current concepts of androgen action are summarized in **Figure 25.8**. Inside the cell, testosterone and dihydrotestosterone bind to the same intracellular androgen receptor, which is located primarily in the nucleus in the unbound state. The hormone–receptor complexes are believed to attach to specific DNA

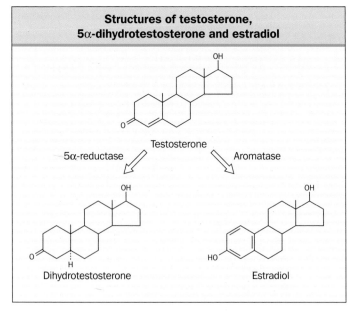

Structures of testosterone, 5α-dihydrotestosterone and estradiol

Figure 25.6 Structure of testosterone, 5α-dihydrotestosterone and estradiol.

sequences in the promoters of genes to control gene transcription and mRNA synthesis. The androgen receptor contains DNA-binding and hormone-binding regions that share a high degree of homology with other members of the steroid/thyroid/retinoid family of receptors and an N-terminal region that has little homology with other receptors.

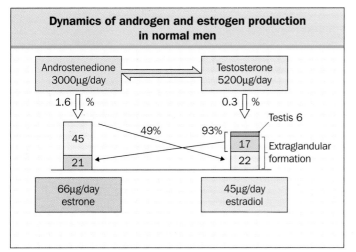

Figure 25.7 Dynamics of androgen and estrogen production in normal men. Average production rates of androgen are indicated in the upper boxes, those of estrogen in the lower boxes. The extent of conversion (%) of plasma testosterone and androstenedione to estradiol and estrone is shown by vertical arrows, and interconversions of estradiol and estrone, and of testosterone and androstenedione, are indicated by horizontal arrows. Sources of estradiol and estrone are indicated by vertical bars. Thus, estradiol arises from plasma testosterone, from estrone, and from direct secretion by the testis; and estrone arises from plasma androstenedione and from estradiol. (Modified from MacDonald PC, Madden JD, Brenner PF, et al. Origin of estrogen in normal men and women with testicular feminization. J Clin Endocrinol Metab. 1979;49:905–16 © The Endocrine Society.)

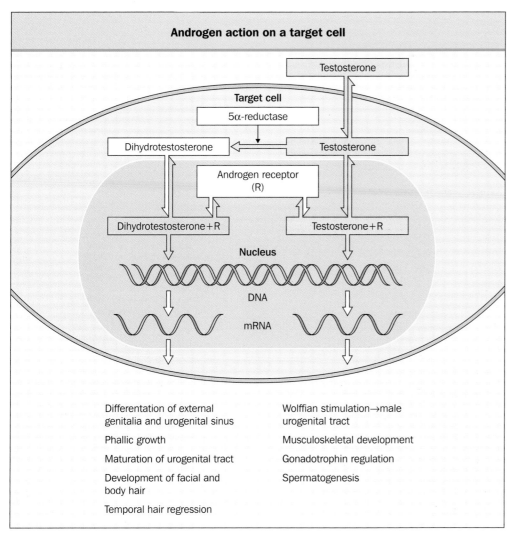

Figure 25.8 Androgen action on a target cell. Testosterone exerts its effect on target tissues by binding to a specific androgen receptor. The testosterone–receptor complex leads to the synthesis of specific mRNA, and hence the translation of androgen-dependent proteins. In certain tissues, the active androgen is the 5α-reduced metabolite of testosterone – dihydrotestosterone – which is generated largely *in situ* and which acts by the same androgen receptor.

The testosterone–receptor complex is responsible for gonadotrophin regulation, spermatogenesis, and virilization of the wolffian ducts during embryogenesis, whereas the dihydrotestosterone–receptor complex mediates external development during embryogenesis and most aspects of virilization at puberty (**Fig. 25.8**). Analysis of single-gene mutations in man and animals indicates that a single-receptor protein mediates the action of both testosterone and dihydrotestosterone. Dihydrotestosterone formation may amplify androgen action because it binds to the receptor more tightly.

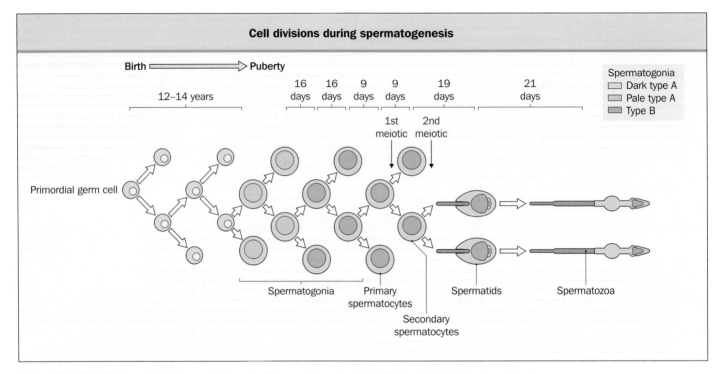

Figure 25.9 Cell divisions during spermatogenesis. The overall number of cell divisions is higher than in oogenesis.

SPERMATOGENESIS AND FERTILIZATION

Testes contain three principal cell types – germ cells that migrate from the yolk sac to the genital ridge, Sertoli cells derived from the epithelium of the genital ridge, and stromal or interstitial cells derived from the genital ridge mesenchyme. Approximately 3×10^5 germ cells migrate to each ridge during embryogenesis, and this number increases up to the time of puberty. After puberty, each spermatogonium that undergoes differentiation gives rise to 16 primary spermatocytes, each of which then enters meiosis and gives rise to four spermatids and ultimately four sperm (**Fig. 25.9**). Transformation of the spermatid into the mature sperm involves reorganization of the nucleus and cytoplasm, and development of the flagellum (**Fig. 25.10**). In adult men, approximately 10^8 sperm are formed each day. Formation of mature sperm takes approximately 70 days, and transport through the epididymis to the ejaculatory duct requires an additional 12–21 days. Upon leaving the testes, sperm have a poor capacity to fertilize. During passage through the epididymis, the sperm mature, as evidenced by development of the capacity for sustained motility, modification of the nuclear chromatin and tail organelles, and loss of the cytoplasmic remnant.

The ejaculate is derived from three sources. Seminal fluid from the epididymis accounts for approximately 20%, the seminal vesicles contribute fructose and prostaglandins and some 60% of the volume, and the remainder of the ejaculate is derived from the prostate, which contributes spermine, citric acid, zinc, and acid phosphatase. Acquisition of the capacity of sperm to fertilize is poorly understood and may be completed in the female genital tract.

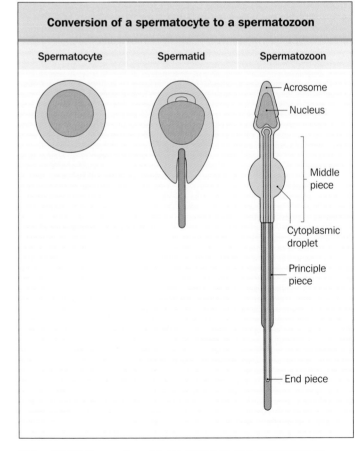

Figure 25.10 Conversion of a spermatocyte to a spermatozoon.

Spermatogenesis is controlled by both LH and FSH: FSH acts directly on the Sertoli cell, whereas LH influences spermatogenesis indirectly by its enhancement of testosterone synthesis. Testosterone interacts with androgen receptors in Sertoli cells to activate genes that are required for spermatogenesis.

PHASES OF NORMAL TESTICULAR FUNCTION

The phases of testicular function can be defined in terms of the levels of plasma testosterone (**Fig. 25.11**). In men, testosterone production by the testis commences at approximately 7 weeks of gestation (**Fig. 25.12**). Shortly thereafter, plasma testosterone reaches a high value; this level is maintained until late gestation, when it falls, so that the level is only slightly higher in male newborns than in female newborns. Shortly after birth, plasma testosterone in the male newborn again rises and remains high for several months, falling to low levels by the age of 6 months to 1 year. Plasma testosterone then remains low (but slightly higher in boys than in girls) until the onset of puberty, when it begins to increase in boys, reaching adult levels by the age of 17 (see Chapter 23). During the adult phase, sperm production matures to allow reproduction to take place. The total testosterone level declines gradually as men age. Beginning about age 40 levels of bioavailable (or non-SHBG-bound) testosterone start to decline at a rate of about 1.2% per year. Since this decrease is accompanied by a 1.2% per year increase in the level of SHBG, the decline

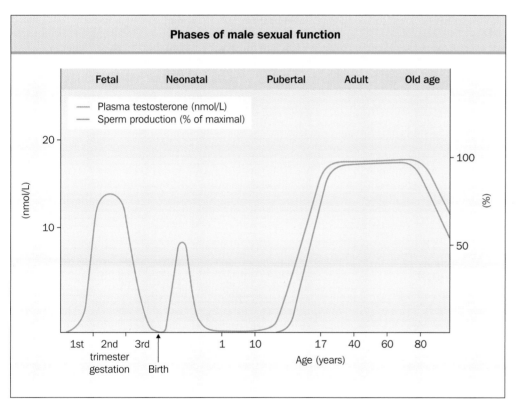

Figure 25.11 Phases of male sexual function. The phases are distinguished by mean plasma testosterone level and sperm production at different periods of life. (Modified from Griffin JE, Wilson JD. The testes. In: Bondy PK, Rosenberg LE, eds. Metabolic control and disease, 8th edn. Philadelphia, PA;WB Saunders: 1980.)

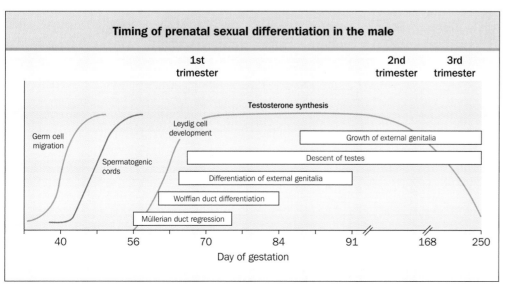

Figure 25.12 Timing of prenatal sexual differentiation in the male. (Modified from Wilson JD, George FW, Griffin JE. The hormonal control of sexual development. Science 1981;211:1278–84.)

of serum testosterone with age may be less apparent if only total testosterone is measured. As many as 40% of unselected healthy men over age 65 have a serum bioavailable testosterone below the lower limit of normal for young men. The significance of the decline in bioavailable testosterone in older men is unclear. Sperm production also gradually declines in older men.

ASSESSMENT OF TESTICULAR FUNCTION

Assessment of testicular function begins with the history and physical examination. Inadequate testosterone production or action during embryogenesis can cause hypospadias, cryptorchidism, or microphallus. Leydig cell failure prior to puberty prevents sexual maturation and causes features, termed eunuchoidism, that include an infantile amount and distribution of body hair; poor development of skeletal muscles; and failure of closure of the epiphyses so that the arm span is more than 5cm greater than height, and the lower body segment (heel to pubis) is more than 5cm longer than the upper body segment (pubis to crown). Therefore, the assessment of androgen status should include an inquiry about developmental abnormalities at birth (e.g. hypospadias, microphallus, and/or cryptorchidism); sexual maturation and growth at puberty; rate of beard growth; and current libido, sexual function, strength, and energy. Nonspecific symptoms associated with testosterone deficiency include depression and irritability. Longstanding hypogonadism of all causes can result in characteristic fine facial wrinkling (**Fig. 25.13**).

The prepubertal testis measures some 2cm in length and increases to 4.1–5.5cm in the normal adult. Testicular size can be assessed by comparison with an orchidometer, which comprises a set of ellipsoids that can be related to testicular size (**Fig. 25.14**). When the seminiferous tubules are damaged before puberty, the testes are small and firm. Postpubertal damage characteristically causes small, soft testes. Considerable testicular damage may occur before the overall size is below the lower limits of normal. Breast enlargement is a common feature of feminizing states in men and may be an early sign of androgen deficiency.

Because of the pulsatile secretion of LH and testosterone (**Fig. 25.15**), and because of the effects of each on the synthesis of the other, gonadotrophins and testosterone may be measured in a pool that is formed by combining three or four samples of equal amounts of blood obtained at 15–20-minute intervals. In this way, a single sample of serum is submitted to the laboratory, and the 'averaging' of values is accomplished prior to assay. In men, the normal range of plasma LH, determined by immunoassay, is 1–15 IU/L. Bioactive LH may be detected when immunoreactive LH is immeasurable. Normal FSH levels in adult men also range from 1 to 15 IU/L. Pulsatile secretion is less pronounced for FSH. The normal range for plasma testosterone in adult men, determined by immunoassay, is 10–35nmol/L (300–1000ng/dL). Bioavailable testosterone can be estimated by precipitation of SHBG and calculating the percentage of the total amount of testosterone that is non-SHBG-bound. This combination of the free and albumin-bound testosterone is thought to best represent

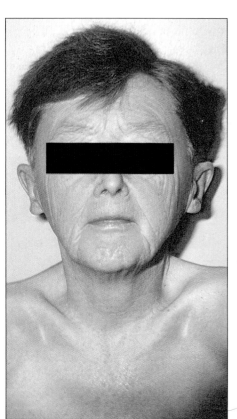

Figure 25.13
The facial appearance in postpubertal hypogonadism.
The very characteristic perioral wrinkling of the skin can be seen.

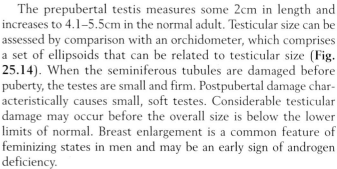
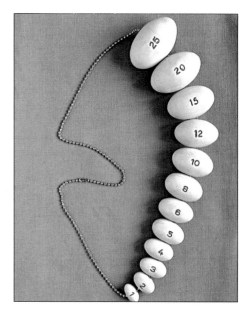

Figure 25.14
A Prader's orchidometer.
Testicular volume (in milliliters) may be estimated by direct comparison with the ellipsoids. During the assessment of testicular volume, the epididymis should not be included.

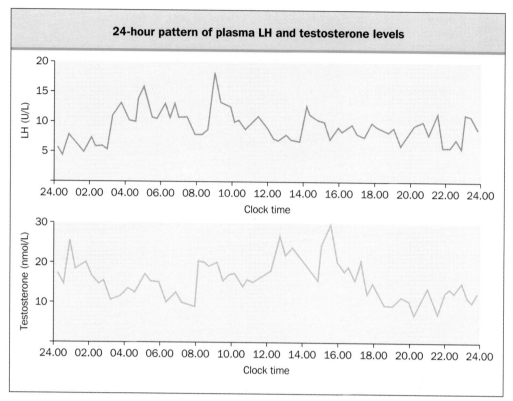

Figure 25.15 The 24-hour pattern of plasma luteinizing hormone (LH) and testosterone levels. The levels in a 21-year-old normal man were sampled every 20min. Variations as great as threefold were demonstrated in individual values of both LH and testosterone, depending on the time of sampling. (Modified from Griffin JE, Wilson JD. The testes. In: Bondy PK, Rosenberg LE, eds. Metabolic control and disease, 8th edn. Philadelphia, PA;WB Saunders: 1980.)

the component of total testosterone that is able to enter target cells. It is particularly useful to measure bioavailable testosterone in men in whom SHBG is likely to be abnormal, i.e. in older men, obese men, or men with HIV or liver disease. Dihydro-testosterone, as measured by immunoassay, averages approximately 10% of the testosterone value.

Prior to puberty, Leydig cell function is assessed by measuring the response of plasma testosterone after 3–5 days of treatment with 1000–2000IU/day of human chorionic gonadotrophin (hCG), which has intrinsic LH-like activity; in prepubertal boys, plasma testosterone should increase to about 7nmol/L (200ng/dL). The response increases with the initiation of puberty and peaks in early puberty. In certain circumstances, the response of plasma LH to GnRH administration is utilized to assess the functional integrity of the hypothalamic–pituitary–Leydig-cell axis. In general, the peak LH that follows a single GnRH injection correlates with the basal levels. A subnormal response indicates that an abnormality exists but does not identify the site.

For routine evaluation of the seminal fluid, ejaculate should be analyzed within 1 hour after masturbation into a clean glass or plastic container (**Table 25.1**). The normal volume is 2–6mL. Sperm motility is assessed microscopically in a drop of undiluted seminal fluid and should include estimation of the percentage of motile forms. Sperm with grade 3 motility move rapidly across the field, those with grade 2 motility move aimlessly, and those with grade 1 motility beat aimlessly but do not move. Normally, 60% or more of sperm have an average motility grade of 2.5 or more.

Sperm density is determined in seminal fluid diluted with an appropriate solution by counting the number of sperm in a hemocytometer or with an electronic particle counter. The

Parameters of normal semen analysis	
Ejaculate volume	2–6mL
Sperm density	> 20 million/mL
Total sperm per ejaculate	> 60 million
Motility	> 60%
Average motility grade	2.5 or more

Table 25.1 Parameters of normal semen analysis.

normal count is greater than 20 million per milliliter and more than 60 million per ejaculate. At least 60% of the spermatozoa should have a normal morphology. Random sampling of sperm density is complicated by variable extragonadal sperm reserves in the excretory ducts and by factors that can influence sperm count, such as hot baths, acute febrile illness, and medication. Consequently, it is difficult to define the minimally adequate ejaculate. At least three ejaculates should be assessed to evaluate adequacy of sperm number or cytology, and six or more estimates may be necessary if initial findings are equivocal. Electron microscopy can be used to identify specific abnormalities in immotile sperm such as abnormalities in the dynein arms. Testicular biopsy is useful in some men with oligospermia or azoospermia, both as an aid in diagnosis and as a guide to treatment, particularly in infertile men in whom the possibility of ductal obstruction is suggested by the finding of azoospermia and normal plasma FSH.

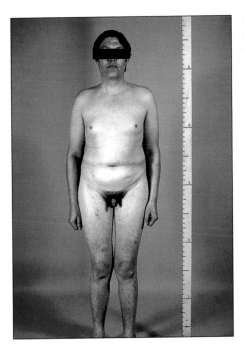

Figure 25.16 The classical appearance of a patient with Klinefelter's syndrome. The patient is hypogonadal, has a female habitus, is poorly virilized with gynecomastia and eunuchoidism, and has a small phallus. Body hair is sparse.

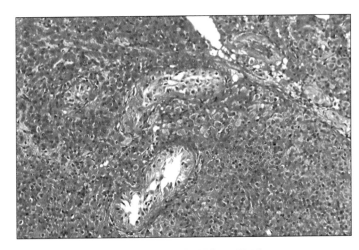

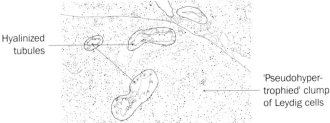

Hyalinized tubules

'Pseudohyper-trophied' clump of Leydig cells

Figure 25.17 A histologic section of a testis of a patient with Klinefelter's syndrome. The dysgenetic seminiferous tubules are evident, and the clumps of Leydig cells give an illusory impression of hyperplasia. Hematoxylin–eosin stain. (Courtesy of Professor I Doniach.)

ABNORMALITIES OF TESTICULAR FUNCTION

Abnormalities of testicular function can be divided into disorders of fetal development, puberty, adult life, and old age, depending on the phase of sexual life in which they first become manifest.

Disorders of fetal development

Klinefelter's syndrome and its variant

Klinefelter's syndrome (see also Chapter 43) is characterized by small, firm testes, azoospermia, gynecomastia, and elevated plasma gonadotrophin levels in men with two or more X chromosomes. The common karyotype is either 47,XXY (the classic form) or 46,XY/47,XXY mosaicism. The incidence is approximately 1 in 500 men. Prepubertally, the testes are small but otherwise appear normal. After puberty, the disorder is characterized by infertility, gynecomastia, and underandrogenization (**Fig. 25.16**). Hyalinization of the seminiferous tubules (**Fig. 25.17**) and azoospermia are consistent features of the 47,XXY variety. The small, firm testes are usually less than 2cm and always less than 3.5cm in length (corresponding to a volume of 2mL and 12mL, respectively). Mean body height is increased because of a larger lower body segment. Prepubertal boys are often identified as being affected on the basis of developmental delay and/or learning disabilities. Gynecomastia ordinarily appears during adolescence and may progress to become disfiguring. The mosaic variant accounts for about 10% of cases, as estimated by peripheral blood chromosomal karyotypes. In this variant the testes may be normal in size, endocrine abnormalities are usually less severe, and gynecomastia and azoospermia are less common. Plasma FSH and LH levels are usually high; FSH shows the best discrimination, and little overlap occurs with normals because of the consistent damage

to the seminiferous tubules. The plasma testosterone level averages 50% of the normal value but the range overlaps the normal. Treatment primarily consists of testosterone replacement. Assisted reproductive techniques make it possible to achieve fertility in men who produce some sperm or have spermatids present in testicular biopsy. Gynecomastia is treated surgically.

A 46,XX karyotype in phenotypic males occurs in 1 in 20,000–24,000 male births. Such men have male psychosexual identities and an absence of all female urogenital structures. The phenotype and the hormonal profile resemble those in Klinefelter's syndrome: the testes are small and firm (generally less than 2cm in length), gynecomastia is common, the penis is male in character, and azoospermia and hyalinization of the seminiferous tubules are usual. Such men differ from Klinefelter men in that average height is less than normal, the incidence of cognitive dysfunction is not increased, and hypospadias is common. The fact that most XX males have a *SRY* gene indicates that interchange of a fragment of a Y-chromosome with another chromosome is the usual cause. The management is similar to that of Klinefelter's syndrome.

Dysgenetic testes syndromes

Dysgenetic testes is a term that has been applied to a heterogeneous group of disorders in 46,XY males with variable defects in testicular development ranging from streak gonads to less severe defects. Three autosomal genes and one X-linked gene have been linked to specific clinical syndromes. Mutations in the *WT1* gene lead to the Denys–Drash or Frazier syndromes, in which variable gonadal defects are associated with Wilms tumor and mesangial sclerosis of the kidneys or only focal sclerosis of the kidney without Wilms tumor, respectively. One man with a heterozygous *SF-1* mutation had adrenal insufficiency and gonadal dysgenesis with streak gonads. Heterozygous mutations in *SOX9* can cause 'campomelic dysplasia', an autosomal dominant form of dysgenetic testes associated with skeletal, renal, and cardiac abnormalities. Finally, duplication of the region of the short arm of the X-chromosome that contains the *DAX-1* gene causes variable testicular defects in 46,XY males.

Embryonic testicular regression

A spectrum of disorders occurs in 46,XY males with absent testes but in whom endocrine function of the testis must have been present transiently during embryonic life (e.g. müllerian duct regression and variable testosterone synthesis). The phenotypes vary from complete failure of virilization to partial virilization of the external genitalia, to otherwise normal men with bilateral anorchia. In the purest form of the vanishing testis syndrome, 46,XY phenotypic females have absent testes, sexual infantilism, and absence of müllerian duct and wolffian duct derivatives. (By contrast, women with 46,XY pure gonadal dysgenesis have streak gonads and a uterus.) Testicular failure in the vanishing testis syndrome must have occurred after the onset of formation of antimüllerian hormone and before the initiation of testosterone synthesis. i.e. after Sertoli cell development and before the onset of Leydig cell function. In others, testicular failure occurs later in gestation, and these individuals may constitute problems in gender assignment. Some have incomplete müllerian regression but none has normal müllerian development. At the final extreme is the syndrome of bilateral anorchia, in which testicular failure occurs after male differentiation is complete; these phenotypic men have an absence of müllerian structures and gonads but a male wolffian system and male external genitalia. The pathogenesis is not understood. Management depends on the phenotype.

Male pseudohermaphroditism due to defective testosterone formation

Defective virilization of the 46,XY embryo (male pseudohermaphroditism) can result from defects in androgen synthesis, androgen action, or müllerian duct regression and from uncertain causes.

Rarely, the defect in androgen synthesis is due to Leydig cell hypoplasia or agenesis as a result of homozygous loss of function mutations in the LH receptor or the production of a biologically inactive LH molecule. Most defects in androgen biosynthesis are due to developmental defects of the testis (as in the dysgenetic testes syndromes described above) or to single-gene defects that impair androgen synthesis. Defects in StAR or any of the last four enzymatic reactions in the pathway from cholesterol to testosterone can impair virilization of the male embryo (see **Fig. 25.5**). Defects in StAR, CYP17, and 3β-HSD2 also result in congenital adrenal hyperplasia. Defects in CYP11A1 have not been described and may be lethal, as a result of impairment of placental function. In all the enzymatic defects, müllerian regression is usually normal but masculinization of the wolffian ducts, urogenital sinus, and urogenital tubercle and virilization at puberty vary from absent to almost normal; therefore, the phenotype varies from phenotypic women to men with mild hypospadias. This variability is due to varying severity of the enzymatic defects and varying effects of the steroids that accumulate proximal to the metabolic blocks. In subjects with partial defects, diagnosis may require measurement of the steroids that accumulate proximal to the metabolic block.

Each of these disorders is the result of rare autosomal recessive mutations. StAR deficiency is frequently lethal through profound adrenal insufficiency. 3β-HSD2 deficiency usually results in salt wasting, but variable deficiency of enzyme activity in the adrenal and liver may complicate diagnosis. 17α-hydroxylase and 17,20-lyase reactions are mediated by a single CYP17 and it is thought that some mutations impair cofactor binding and selectively impair lyase function. Severe CYP17 deficiency causes hypokalemic alkalosis and hypertension (as a result of compensatory overproduction of deoxycorticosterone), in addition to deficiency of gonadal steroids. 17β-HSD3 deficiency is probably the most common of the defects. The external phenotype is usually that of a female with inguinal or abdominal testes and virilized wolffian duct structures. At the time of expected puberty, both virilization (phallic enlargement and facial hair growth) and some feminization (appearance of gynecomastia) take place.

In those disorders with adrenal hyperplasia, treatment with glucocorticoids and sometimes mineralocorticoids is required. Management of genital abnormalities must be individualized. Newborn males with ambiguous genitalia who are severely affected are often raised as females after gonadectomy and corrective surgery of the genitalia.. Estrogen therapy is then provided at the appropriate age. Less severely affected newborn males should have correction of the hypospadias and receive androgen supplementation at the time of expected puberty.

Male pseudohermaphroditism due to androgen resistance

Impairment of androgen action causes several forms of male pseudohermaphroditism in which testosterone formation and müllerian regression are normal and in which impairment of male development is a result of resistance to androgen action in the target cells. The defect can be in the formation of the active metabolite of testosterone, dihydrotestosterone, or in the androgen receptor that binds both hormones.

5α-reductase deficiency is an autosomal recessive disorder in 46,XY males characterized by severe perineoscrotal hypospadias, a blind vaginal pouch that opens into the urogenital sinus or the urethra, testes, epididymides, vasa deferentia, seminal vesicles, and ejaculatory ducts that terminate in the blind-ended vagina, a female habitus with normal axillary and pubic hair but absence of female urogenital structures, failure of female breast development at adolescence, normal male plasma testosterone, and variable masculinization during adolescence. A failure of dihydrotestosterone formation in a male embryo is responsible for the phenotype (**Fig. 25.18**). Since testosterone itself regulates LH secretion, plasma LH levels are usually normal or minimally elevated. As a result, testosterone and estrogen production rates are those of normal men, and gynecomastia does not develop. Affected individuals have defects in the steroid 5α-reductase 2 gene, resulting in loss of function, and the virilization later in life is caused by dihydrotestosterone formed by the unaffected isoenzyme (5α-reductase 1)

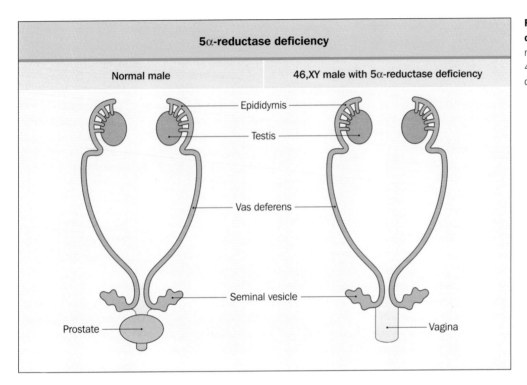

5α-reductase deficiency

Normal male	46,XY male with 5α-reductase deficiency

Epididymis
Testis
Vas deferens
Seminal vesicle
Prostate
Vagina

Figure 25.18 5α-reductase deficiency. The urogenital tract in a normal man is compared with that in a 46,XY male with 5α-reductase deficiency.

Mutations in the androgen receptor gene are the most common cause of male pseudohermaphroditism resulting in resistance to the biologic actions of androgens. These mutations are inherited as X-linked defects and cause several syndromes that have similar pathophysiology and hormone profiles. Complete testicular feminization, the most common phenotype, is associated with a female phenotype, including feminization of the breasts after puberty and a female habitus and distribution of body fat (**Fig. 25.19(a)**) due to the increased estrogen production by the testes. The disorder is identified either because of inguinal hernia (prepubertal) or primary amenorrhea (postpubertal). Axillary and pubic hair are absent or scanty but some vulval hair is usually present. Scalp hair is normal, and facial hair is absent. The external genitalia are unambiguously female, and the clitoris is normal. The vagina is short and blind-ended and may be absent or rudimentary. All internal genitalia are absent except for undescended testes that contain normal Leydig cells and seminiferous tubules without spermatogenesis.

Incomplete testicular feminization is some 10 times less common than the complete form. In this variant, there is a minor virilization of the external genitalia (partial fusion of the labioscrotal folds and some degree of clitoromegaly), normal pubic hair (**Fig. 25.19(b)**), and a mixed pattern of virilization and feminization at the time of expected puberty. The vagina is short and blind-ended, and the wolffian duct derivatives are partially virilized.

Reifenstein's syndrome is the term now applied to forms of incomplete male pseudohermaphroditism – Reifenstein's syndrome, Gilbert–Dreyfus syndrome, Lubs syndrome, Rosewater syndrome – that were originally assumed to be distinct entities. These syndromes constitute variable manifestations of mutations that cause partial loss of function of the androgen receptor. The most common phenotype is an undervirilized man with gynecomastia (**Fig. 25.19(c)**) and perineoscrotal hypospadias, but the spectrum of defective virilization ranges from men with azoospermia to phenotypic women with pseudovaginas. Axillary and pubic hair are normal but chest and facial hair are minimal. Cryptorchidism is common, the testes are small, azoospermia is usual, and the vas deferens may be absent or hyperplastic.

The undervirilized or infertile male syndrome is the least severe form of an androgen receptor disorder. Some cases are minimally affected men in families with Reifenstein's syndrome, who have azoospermia as the major manifestation of receptor abnormality. Other men with uninformative family histories are ascertained because of infertility (**Fig. 25.19(d)**). Some undervirilized males are fertile.

Hormone dynamics are similar in all disorders of the androgen receptor. Plasma testosterone levels, and rates of testosterone production by the testes, are normal or high. The elevated testosterone production is caused by the high plasma level of LH, which in turn is due to defective feedback regulation caused by resistance to androgen action at the hypothalamic–pituitary level. Elevated LH levels cause increased estrogen production by the testes, and increased estrogen production combined with variable androgen resistance leads to feminization. Each of these syndromes is the result of an abnormality of the androgen receptor. The most common cause is missense mutations leading to single amino-acid substitutions that either interfere with hormone binding or DNA binding, selectively, or lead to premature termination codons that truncate the receptor. Small insertions or partial deletions and (rarely) complete deletions of the coding sequence of the receptor gene account for the remaining mutations.

The therapy of androgen resistance depends on the phenotype and whether the cause is 5α-reductase deficiency or a receptor defect. Since many individuals with 5α-reductase deficiency undergo a change in social sex from female to male at the time of expected puberty, care must be taken in gender assignment. Individuals who are raised as females but elect to change social

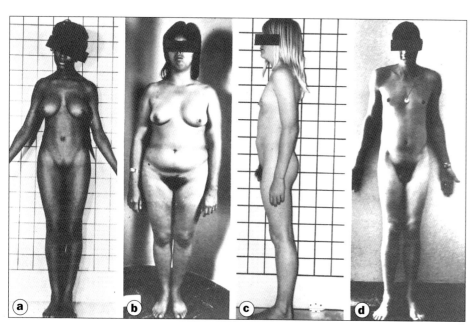

Figure 25.19 Four subjects with androgen receptor disorders. (a) Complete testicular feminization. (b) Incomplete testicular feminization. (c) Reifenstein's syndrome. (d) Undervirilized or infertile male. (Reproduced from Griffin JE, Wilson JD. Disorders of sexual differentiation. In: Walsh PC, Retik AB, Stamey TA, Vaughan ED, eds. Campbell's textbook of urology, 6th edn. Philadelphia, PA;WB Saunders: 1992.)

sex should be monitored carefully and given supplemental androgens if virilization is incomplete. Individuals with 5α-reductase deficiency who continue to function as females should be gonadectomized, given estrogen, and have surgical reconstruction of the external genitalia as needed. Women with testicular feminization should be gonadectomized after completion of the pubertal growth spurt to prevent formation of malignant tumors in the testes – a risk in all intra-abdominal testes. Following gonadectomy, estrogen replacement is necessary. Men with Reifenstein's syndrome should have correction of the hypospadias and may require surgical repair of the gynecomastia.

Male pseudohermaphroditism due to defective müllerian regression

Men with the persistent müllerian duct syndrome have a normal male phenotype, testes, bilateral fallopian tubes, a uterus and upper vagina, and variable development of the vas deferens. Such men may have inguinal hernias that contain the uterus, and cryptorchidism is common. The condition is usually inherited as an autosomal recessive trait, but rare families suggest X-linked recessive inheritance. Since the external genitalia are well developed and the patients usually masculinize at puberty, it is assumed that, during the critical stage of embryonic development, the fetal testes produce a normal amount of androgen. Müllerian regression, however, does not occur, because of mutations that impair the formation of either normal antimüllerian hormone or its receptor.

Pubertal disorders

Pubertal disorders of testicular function are discussed in Chapter 24. Isolated gonadotrophin deficiency may not be recognized until adulthood and is discussed below.

Adult disorders

The hypothalamo–pituitary–testicular axis is subject to a variety of influences. Spermatogenesis is sensitive to alterations in temperature, and brief increases in either systemic or testicular temperature can cause temporary decreases in sperm count. Drugs, alcohol, environmental agents, and psychologic stress may also impair sperm production.

Persistent abnormalities of testicular function after puberty can be due to hypothalamo–pituitary abnormalities, testicular defects, or abnormalities of sperm transport. Some of these conditions affect Leydig cell function or spermatogenesis selectively but most cause both underandrogenization and infertility (**Table 25.2**). Even partial decreases in testosterone production can cause infertility. Other disorders (hyperprolactinemia, radiation, cyclophosphamide therapy, autoimmunity, paraplegia, androgen resistance) can cause isolated infertility or combined defects in different subjects.

Hypothalamic–pituitary disorders

Impairment of gonadotrophin secretion may be the consequence of generalized diseases that affect the hypothalamus and pituitary (e.g. craniopharyngioma, see also Chapter 3) or an isolated deficiency in which secretion of LH and FSH is impaired; idiopathic hypogonadotrophic hypogonadism can be either congenital or, less commonly, acquired. Manifestations of isolated gonadotrophin deficiency vary from infants with microphallus, through boys with eunuchoidal features and testes of prepubertal size, to men with partial LH and FSH deficiency and incomplete testicular enlargement and pubertal development. Cryptorchidism and anosmia or hyposmia are common, the latter due to associated impaired development of the olfactory tracts and bulbs. Histologic examination of the testis reveals immature Leydig cells and immature germinal epithelium. The disorder is inherited as an X-linked recessive or autosomal recessive trait with variable expressivity. About two thirds of cases are sporadic. Serum FSH and LH levels are low or low–normal, and plasma testosterone levels are low for the age. The levels of other pituitary hormones are normal. The defect in most appears to be in the synthesis or release of GnRH and has a severity varying from the complete absence of pulsatile LH secretion (usually the X-linked families), to impairment in

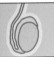

Adult abnormalities of testicular function		
Type of defect	**Infertility with underandrogenization**	**Infertility with normal virilization**
Hypothalamo–pituitary	Panhypopituitarism Isolated gonadotropin deficiency Cushing's syndrome Adrenal hypoplasia congenita Hyperprolactinemia Hemochromatosis	Isolated FSH deficiency Congenital adrenal hyperplasia Hyperprolactinemia Androgen administration

Testicular	Developmental and structural defects
	  Klinefelter's syndrome
	  XX male syndrome
	
	Acquired defects
	  Viral orchitis
	  Trauma
	  Radiation
	  Drugs
	    (e.g. spironolactone, alcohol,
	    ketoconazole, cyclophosphamide)
	  Enviromental toxins
	  Autoimmunity
	  Granulomatous disease
	Systemic disease
	  Liver disease
	  Renal failure
	  Sickle cell disease
	  Immune disease (AIDS, rheumatoid arthritis)
	  Neurological disease (mytonic dystrophy,
	    paraplegia)
	Androgen resistance
		Developmental and structural defects
		  AZF mutations of the Y chromosome
		  Germinal cell aplasia
		  Cryptorchidism
		  Varicocele
		  Immotile cilia syndrome
		  Other structural defects
		Acquired defects
		  Mycoplasma infection
		
		  Radiation
		  Drugs
		    (e.g. cyclophosphamide,
		    sulfasalazine)
		  Enviromental toxins
		  Autoimmunity
		
		Systemic diseases
		  Febrile illness
		  Celiac disease
		
		  Neurological disease (paraplegia)
		
		Androgen resistance

Sperm transport		Obstruction of epididymis or of vas
		  deferens (cystic fibrosis,
		  diethylstilbestrol exposure, congenital
		  absence)

Table 25.2 Adult abnormalities of testicular function. (Modified from Griffin JE, Wilson JD. Disorders of sexual differentiation. In: Walsh PC, Retik AB, Stamey TA, Vaughan ED, eds. Campbell's textbook of urology, 6th edn. Philadelphia, PA;WB Saunders: 1992.)

amplitude and frequency of LH secretion. In some individuals with an X-linked form of the disorder, mutations in a neural cell adhesion molecule have been identified, and a mutation in *DAX-1* is the cause in boys with adrenal hypoplasia congenita. The latter represent only about 1% of patients with isolated gonadotrophin deficiency. Some families with autosomal recessive defects have mutations in the GnRH receptor. Distinction between gonadotrophin deficiency and delayed puberty is difficult in boys of early or midpubertal age; the presence of microphallus, anosmia, or a positive family history may help in diagnosis. Sometimes, differentiation of the two states may require prolonged observation.

Mutations in the *FSHβ* gene can lead to delayed puberty and male hypogonadism, and one male with an inactivating mutation of the *LHβ* gene had delayed puberty with increased serum LH levels.

Gonadotrophin secretion can be altered secondarily. Elevation of plasma cortisol levels in Cushing's syndrome depresses GnRH and LH secretion independently of a space-occupying lesion of the pituitary. Some patients with congenital adrenal hyperplasia have suppressed gonadotrophin secretion and infertility. Hyperprolactinemia (as the consequence of either pituitary adenomas or drugs such as phenothiazines) can impair function of both Leydig cells and seminiferous tubules, because of inhibition of GnRH, LH, and FSH secretion. Hemochromatosis impairs testicular function as the result of effects on the pituitary and occasionally affects the testes directly. The use of androgens for

purposes other than replacement therapy is often associated with low plasma gonadotrophin levels and impaired sperm production (see below). Men with morbid obesity have low SHBG levels suppressed by the accompanying hyperinsulinemia and may have decreased levels of total and bioavailable testosterone that return to normal after weight loss. Temporal lobe epilepsy can also cause hypogonadotropic hypogonadism.

Testicular defects

Abnormalities of testicular function in the adult can be grouped into several categories: developmental and structural defects of the testes, acquired testicular defects, disorders secondary to systemic and/or neurologic disease, and androgen resistance.

Developmental abnormalities

Klinefelter's syndrome (both the classic and mosaic forms) and the XX male may not be diagnosed until after the time of expected puberty (see above). Testicular defects that cause infertility in the presence of normal androgen production include varicocele, which occurs in 10–15% of the general population and may be a contributory factor in one third of cases of male infertility. It is caused by increased testicular temperature due to retrograde flow of blood into the internal spermatic vein, which leads to progressive, often palpable dilatation of the peritesticular plexus of veins.

Some men with azoospermia and germinal cell aplasia (the Sertoli-cell-only syndrome) have a positive family history and may

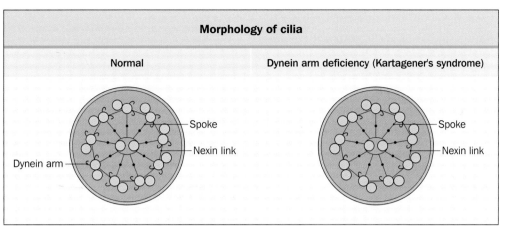

Figure 25.20 Morphology of cilia. Transverse sections of the morphology of (left panel) normal spermatozoa and (right panel) spermatozoa from patients with Kartagener's syndrome are shown.

constitute a specific entity; plasma testosterone and LH levels are normal, and the plasma FSH level is high. Other men with similar histologic and clinical findings have androgen resistance or a history of viral orchitis or cryptorchidism so that diverse conditions may be grouped in this category. As many as 15% of men with unexplained azoospermia have microdeletions in the *AZF* (azoospermia factor) genes on the short arm of the Y chromosome.

Unilateral cryptorchidism, even when corrected prior to puberty, may be associated with abnormal semen, suggesting that the testicular abnormality is usually bilateral.

The immotile cilia syndrome is an autosomal recessive defect characterized by immotility or poor motility of the cilia of the respiratory epithelium and of sperm. Kartagener's syndrome is a subgroup of the immotile cilia syndrome associated with situs inversus, chronic sinusitis, and bronchiectasis. The specific defects of the cilia can usually be defined by the electron-microscopic appearance and include abnormalities in the cilial dynein arms, spokes, or microtubule doublets (**Fig. 25.20**). Cilia from epithelia, and sperm from the same individual, usually exhibit the same defects but the pulmonary manifestations may be minor. Less well understood structural defects of sperm can lead to immotile sperm without involvement of cilia in the lung.

Acquired testicular defects

One cause of acquired primary testicular failure is viral orchitis. Responsible viruses include mumps, echovirus, lymphocytic choriomeningitis, and group B arboviruses. Orchitis is due to viral invasion of the tissue, occurs in as many as 25% of adult men with mumps, and is unilateral in over 65% of the cases. The testis may return to normal size and function or undergo atrophy. Bilateral atrophy, which occurs in approximately 10% of subjects with bilateral orchitis, can result in oligospermia and also impair testosterone production.

The exposed position in the scrotum renders the testis susceptible to both thermal and physical trauma. The seminiferous tubules and the Leydig cells are also sensitive to radiation damage; decreased secretion of testosterone is the result of diminished testicular blood flow. Fractionated delivery may have a more profound effect than single-dose radiation. Recovery of sperm density depends on radiation dosage, and complete recovery of sperm density may take as long as 5 years. Permanent infertility can occur after radiation therapy of a malignant lymphoma, despite the fact that the testes are shielded. Permanent androgen deficiency

is uncommon after radiation in adults, but boys who receive direct testicular radiation for acute lymphoblastic leukemia may have persistent testosterone deficiency.

Spironolactone and ketoconazole block the synthesis of androgen, and spironolactone and cimetidine interfere with androgen action by competing with androgen for binding to the androgen receptor. Abuse of marijuana, heroin, or methadone may be associated with low plasma testosterone and high plasma estradiol levels, although the exact reasons are unclear. Alcohol can cause plasma testosterone levels to decrease, independent of liver disease or malnutrition.

Antineoplastic and chemotherapeutic agents can impair spermatogenesis. Cyclophosphamide causes azoospermia or oligospermia within a few weeks after the initiation of therapy. Combination chemotherapy for acute leukemia, Hodgkin's disease, and other malignancies may also impair testosterone formation. Environmental hazards for the testis include microwaves, ultrasound, and chemicals such as cadmium, lead, or the nematocide dibromochloropropane. In some populations sperm density has declined significantly in recent decades, a phenomenon that is postulated to be due to environmental chemicals that act as estrogens or antiandrogens.

Testicular failure due to circulating antibodies to the testis can be part of a generalized disorder of autoimmunity in which multiple primary endocrine deficiencies coexist (Schmidt's syndrome). Alternatively, sperm antibodies can be a cause of isolated male infertility. In some instances, such antibodies develop secondary to duct obstruction or vasectomy. Granulomatous diseases such as leprosy can also destroy the testes.

Testicular abnormalities associated with systemic disease

In cirrhosis of the liver, a combined testicular and pituitary abnormality causes decreased testosterone production, independent of the direct toxic effects of ethanol. Testicular atrophy and gynecomastia are present in some 50% of men with cirrhosis, and many are impotent. Although plasma LH is elevated, the level may be inappropriate for the degree of androgen deficiency, probably because of inhibition of LH secretion by estrogen in patients with chronic liver disease. Increased estrogen production results from impaired hepatic extraction and consequent increased extraglandular aromatization of the adrenal androgen androstenedione. In effect, estrogen precursors are shunted from normal degradation in the liver to sites of extraglandular aromatization.

In chronic renal failure, decreased androgen synthesis and impairment of sperm production are associated with elevated plasma gonadotrophins. The elevated LH level is due to increased production and reduced clearance but does not result in normal testosterone production. Approximately 25% of men with chronic renal failure also have hyperprolactinemia.

Men with sickle cell disease usually have incomplete secondary sexual development, and testicular atrophy is present in one third. The defect may be either at the testicular level or at the hypothalamic–pituitary level. Decreased Leydig cell function, with or without decreased sperm density, occurs in a variety of chronic systemic diseases; the lowered plasma testosterone level is usually coupled with a minimal increase in the plasma LH level, suggesting combined hypothalamic–pituitary and testicular defects.

Men with HIV infection commonly have impaired testosterone production. Initially partial impairment causes increased gonadotrophin levels, which keep testosterone in the normal range, but 35–50% of men with overt AIDS have low plasma testosterone levels. It is unclear whether the low testosterone is the cause of the 10% weight loss characteristic of AIDS wasting, but physiologic testosterone replacement may increase lean body mass.

Infertility in men with celiac disease is associated with elevated testosterone and LH levels. In myotonic dystrophy, small testes may be associated with abnormalities of both spermatogenesis and Leydig cell function. Spinobulbar muscular atrophy is due to an expansion of the CAG repeat in the aminoterminal region of the androgen receptor, leading to a late development of androgen resistance with neurologic manifestations. Spinal cord lesions associated with paraplegia lead to persistent defects in spermatogenesis and to temporary decreases in testosterone levels that tend to return to normal; some patients retain the capacity to obtain an erection and to ejaculate.

Impairment of sperm transport

Disorders of sperm transport cause about 6% of the cases of infertility with normal virilization. Ductal obstruction may be unilateral or bilateral and may also be congenital or acquired. Congenital defects of the vas deferens can occur as an isolated abnormality that is associated with an absence of the seminal vesicles, in patients with cystic fibrosis, or in men whose mothers received diethylstilbestrol during pregnancy. Mutations of the cystic fibrosis gene can cause congenital bilateral absence of the vas deferens without the usual pulmonary and gastrointestinal manifestations of cystic fibrosis.

In at least 36% of infertile men (**Table 25.3**), the cause is unknown. Biopsy of the testis in these individuals and in men with a suspected cause may show a variety of nonspecific findings. Therapy in male infertility, except surgically correctable varicocele, vas deferens obstruction, or treatable endocrinopathy, is unsatisfactory. The only empirical therapy for male infertility that is successful is *in vitro* fertilization. Men with sperm densities lower than 5 million/mL or poor motility or a high frequency of abnormal forms may require intracytoplasmic sperm injection with *in vitro* fertilization. This technique may be successful in men with azoospermia using sperm obtained from testicular biopsies.

Causes and associated conditions in infertile men	
Cause or condition	Approximate %
Hypogonadotrophic hypogonadism	0.8
Klinefelter's syndrome	2.0
Cryptorchidism	6.0
Varicocele	39.0
Immotile sperm	0.6
Viral orchitis	2.0
Radiation or chemotherapy	0.2
Obstruction of epididymis or vas deferens	5.0
Coital disorders	2.0
Y-chromosome deletions	6.0
Idiopathic disorders	36.0

Table 25.3 Causes and associated conditions in infertile men.

Disorders of old age

The major androgen-dependent disorder in the elderly is benign prostatic hyperplasia. During puberty the prostate undergoes androgen-mediated growth to reach the adult size of about 20 g and remains constant in size until the fifth decade of life, when prostate growth resumes in most men, commencing in the periurethral region with proliferation of glandular and stromal elements and eventually involving the entire gland. By the eighth decade 90% of men have prostatic hyperplasia. Although many men remain asymptomatic, prostatic hyperplasia is the most common cause of obstruction to urinary flow in men. Symptomatic disease occurs in all populations but may be less common in Asian men. The average age for development of symptoms is about 65 years for whites and 60 for blacks. The secondary growth spurt that eventuates in prostatic hyperplasia requires a functioning testis and is thought to be mediated by dihydrotestosterone synthesized within the gland. In elderly men, prostate dihydrotestosterone content remains high, and inhibition of dihydrotestosterone formation in animals causes involution of the prostate, despite an elevated concentration of testosterone in the tissue. In men, plasma estradiol levels increase slightly with age.

There is no straightforward relationship between prostate size and urethral obstruction or urethral obstruction and symptoms. Obstructive symptoms include decrease in caliber and force of stream, hesitancy on starting voiding, and the feeling of incomplete emptying. Nonspecific irritative symptoms may also be present, such as dysuria, increased frequency, and urgency. The natural history of the disorder is not well understood but many men have lower urinary tract syndrome without prostatic hyperplasia and most men with prostatic enlargement do not have significant symptoms. The American Urological Association Symptom Index can be used to classify the severity of symptoms, and prostate size, consistency, and shape can be assessed by digital rectal examination. The measurement of prostate-specific antigen (PSA) may be helpful in excluding advanced prostate cancer, but PSA levels are increased in benign prostatic hyperplasia.

Treatment is not required for asymptomatic individuals with prostate enlargement. Clear indications for treatment include inability to urinate, renal failure, and bladder stones. In the remainder of patients the severity of symptoms determines the need for therapy. Medical therapy involves either finasteride, a competitive inhibitor of the steroid 5α-reductase enzyme, to block the conversion of testosterone to dihydrotestosterone, or an alpha-adrenergic blocking drug to relax the smooth muscle in the bladder neck and cause an increase in urinary flow rate. Men who are most likely to benefit from finasteride are those patients with larger prostates. Finasteride is given in a dose of 5mg per day, and it causes an average decrease in prostate size of about 24%, an increase in urine flow rates, and in some men improvement in symptoms. Alpha-adrenergic blockade can be accomplished with terazosin 5–10mg per day or doxazosin 4–8mg per day. There is no evidence to suggest that alpha-adrenergic blockade prevents further prostate growth. Prostate surgery offers the best chance for improvement in symptoms for those who are severely affected and in men who fail to respond to medical therapy, but it has significant complications. Transurethral resection is the most common surgical procedure.

HORMONAL THERAPY

Androgens

Effective androgen therapy requires either the administration of testosterone in a slowly absorbed form (transdermal preparations or micronized oral preparation) or the oral or parenteral administration of chemically modified analogs. Such chemical modifications either retard the rate of absorption or catabolism so as to sustain effective blood levels, or enhance the androgenic potency of each molecule so that physiologic effects can be achieved at a lower blood level. Three types of modification have proved useful (**Fig. 25.21**): esterification of the 17β-hydroxyl group, alkylation at the 17α position, and modification of the ring structure, particularly substitutions at the 2, 9, and 11 positions. Most drugs contain combinations of ring-structure alterations and either 17α-alkylation or esterification of the 17β-hydroxyl group.

The oral effectiveness of 17α-alkylated androgens (such as methyltestosterone and methandrostenolone) is due to slower hepatic catabolism so that the alkylated derivatives escape degradation by the liver and reach the systemic circulation. All 17α-alkylated steroids may cause abnormal liver function.

Testosterone undecanoate, an orally active ester available in some countries, is absorbed via the lymphatic system into the systemic circulation. Physiologic blood levels of testosterone can be achieved at doses of 120mg per day but because of rapid turnover the agent must be administered three times a day. Partial conversion of testosterone to dihydrotestosterone by steroid 5α-reductase in the intestine results in increased plasma dihydrotestosterone levels.

Four transdermal therapeutic preparations of testosterone are available. Each provides physiologic serum levels throughout the day. This therapy avoids the wide swings in serum testosterone values that occur between injections of testosterone esters. The first transdermal preparation released was the Testoderm scrotal patch, delivering 4 or 6mg of testosterone via a thin patch without permeation enhancers. Use of this patch requires shaving of

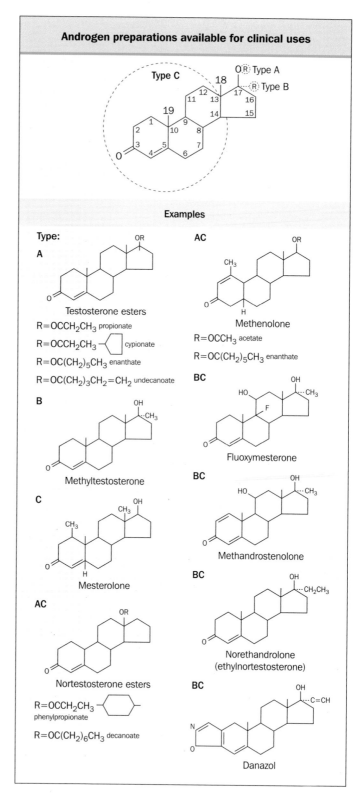

Figure 25.21 Some of the androgen preparations available for clinical use, classified into three types. Type A derivatives are esterified in the 17β-position; type B steroids have alkyl groups in a 17α-position; and type C derivatives include a variety of additional alterations of ring structure that enhance activity or impede catabolism, or influence both functions. Most androgen preparations involve combinations of type AC or type BC changes. (Modified from Griffin JE, Wilson JD. Disorders of the testes and male reproductive tract. In: Wilson JD, Foster DW, eds. Williams textbook of endocrinology, 8th edn. Philadelphia, PA; WB Saunders: 1991.)

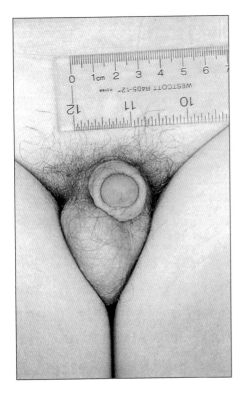

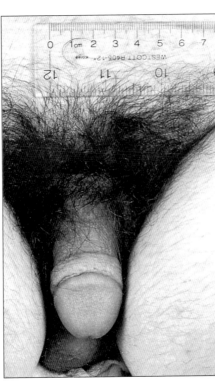

Figure 25.22 The effect of testosterone cypionate therapy for 11 months in a 22-year-old man with hypogonadotropic hypogonadism.

the scrotal hairs once or twice a week and usually the wearing of jockey-style underwear. It is applied in the morning with peak levels achieved a few hours later. Because of the presence of 5α-reductase in the scrotal skin, serum dihydrotestosterone levels are increased in men using this patch. There are two nonscrotal patches, Androderm and Testoderm TTS. Each delivers 5mg of testosterone via a central liquid reservoir with ethanol as a permeation enhancer and has a peripheral rim of adhesive. The Androderm patch is applied at bedtime (with peak serum levels the next morning) to the trunk, arms, or thighs but must be rotated to a different site each day to minimize skin irritation. The Testoderm TTS patch is larger but causes less skin irritation. It is applied in the morning (with peak levels a few hours later) to the upper buttocks, back, or upper arm, and the application site does not need to be rotated. AndroGel is a 1% hydroalcoholic gel, the usual dose being 5g containing 50mg of testosterone applied to the dry skin of the upper chest, arms, and shoulders. After a few days a reservoir is believed to form in the skin that provides a near constant serum testosterone level somewhat higher than the patches. Care must be taken to avoid skin to skin transmission of the hormone to the sexual partner or others.

Esters such as testosterone cypionate and testosterone enanthate can be injected every 1–3 weeks. Since the esters are hydrolyzed before the hormones act, the effectiveness of therapy can be monitored by measuring the plasma testosterone level following administration. At physiologic replacement doses, testosterone esters have few side effects in mature men (see below). At supraphysiologic doses, however, gonadotrophin secretion is inhibited, the testes decrease in volume, and the sperm count falls (indeed, low sperm counts may persist for as long as 9 months after supraphysiologic doses are discontinued). The administration of testosterone esters results in an increase in plasma estrogen levels and may, on occasion, cause gynecomastia.

Androgen therapy in testosterone deficiency

The aim of therapy in hypogonadal men is to restore, or bring to normal, male secondary sexual characteristics (beard, body hair, external genitalia; **Fig. 25.22**) and male sexual behavior and to mimic the hormonal effects on somatic development (hemoglobin, muscle mass, nitrogen balance, and epiphyseal closure). Since an assay for plasma testosterone is available for monitoring therapy, the treatment of androgen deficiency is almost universally successful. The parenteral administration of a long-acting testosterone ester, such as 100–200mg testosterone cypionate or enanthate at 1–2-week intervals, results in a sustained increase in plasma testosterone levels to the normal male range. The standard regimen is 200mg of either of these preparations intramuscularly every 2 weeks. This regimen results in serum testosterone levels above the physiologic in the two days following the injection followed by a gradual decline to baseline levels by day 12–14. Many men notice fluctuations in mood, energy, and libido corresponding to the change in serum levels of testosterone. The fluctuations in serum testosterone levels can be decreased by giving the injections every week (e.g. 100mg once a week instead of 200mg every 2 weeks). The transdermal testosterone preparations, in contrast, provide physiologic levels of testosterone throughout the day. The efficacy of testosterone replacement therapy can be monitored by measuring serum hormone levels and by assessment of adequacy of virilization in individuals not previously exposed to testosterone and of the relief of symptoms of hypogonadism in men with acquired hypogonadism. The optimal time to measure serum testosterone in men receiving injections is either midway between injections to assess median levels or just before the next injection to be certain that the trough level is within the normal range. For men using transdermal testosterone preparations, a midmorning sample should be in the midnormal range.

In young men there is little concern for adverse effects of testosterone replacement therapy. However, in elderly men some concern must be given to the possibility of testosterone exacerbating a preexisting condition. Prostate cancer is multifactorial in etiology and can occur in men with testosterone deficiency. Consequently, it is important in older men to assess for the presence of prostate cancer prior to beginning testosterone replacement by performing a digital rectal exam and measuring serum prostate-specific antigen. The presence of prostate cancer (or breast cancer) is a contraindication to the administration of testosterone. Because a small prostate cancer may not be associated with an increased PSA level in the setting of a low testosterone level, it is also necessary to repeat the digital rectal examination and the PSA measurement 2–3 months after starting an older man on testosterone replacement. Thereafter monitoring may be performed every 6–12 months. Benign prostatic hyperplasia is usually not worsened by physiologic testosterone replacement, and no clear relation exists between the serum testosterone level and prostate size when the testosterone is in the normal range. In men with benign prostatic hyperplasia the severity of obstructive symptoms should be monitored. Older men, particularly former smokers, may be at risk for polycythemia when given testosterone replacement, and the hematocrit should be measured regularly. Finally, testosterone therapy may initiate or worsen obstructive sleep apnea, and obese men who may be particularly at risk should be monitored for symptoms such as daytime somnolence and excessive snoring. The mechanism for the testosterone effect on breathing is thought to be a central action on neuromuscular control of the upper airway muscles allowing a closure of the airway during sleep.

Androgen use in conditions other than testosterone deficiency

The most common uses of androgens other than to correct testosterone deficiency has been to treat wasting disorders with the hope of improving lean body mass, to improve muscle mass and/or athletic performance, to attempt to increase erythropoiesis in severe anemias, and to treat angioedema. Supraphysiologic doses of testosterone (600mg of testosterone enanthate intramuscularly each week) increase muscle size and strength in normal men. This dose is six times the replacement dose and poses significant risk of adverse effects such as decreased high-density lipoprotein cholesterol, fluid retention, polycythemia, reduction of spermatogenesis, and possibly exacerbation of prostatic hyperplasia or cancer. The only established uses of androgen therapy in men who do not have testosterone deficiency are to treat selected patients with bone marrow failure or angioedema. Studies are in progress to evaluate the benefit of testosterone therapy in men with osteoporosis including older men and men receiving glucocorticoids. Studies of combinations of testosterone and a gonadotrophin-suppressing agent for male contraception are also under way.

Gonadotrophins

Gonadotrophin therapy is used to establish or restore fertility in men with gonadotrophin deficiency of all causes. Two gonadotrophin preparations are commonly used: human menopausal gonadotrophins (hMG) and hCG: hMG contains 75IU FSH and 75IU LH per vial, while hCG has little FSH

activity and resembles LH in its ability to stimulate testosterone production by Leydig cells. Because of the expense of hMG, treatment is usually initiated with hCG alone, and hMG is added later to stimulate the FSH-dependent stages of spermatid development. A high ratio of LH to FSH activity, and a long duration of treatment (3–6 months), are necessary to bring about the maturation of the prepubertal testis. Once spermatogenesis is restored in hypophysectomized patients or initiated in hypogonadotropic hypogonadal men by combined therapy, it can usually be maintained with hCG alone. Recombinant FSH appears to be comparable to the urinary preparation.

Gonadotrophin-releasing hormone

Gonadotrophin-releasing hormone (gonadorelin) is available for endocrine testing and has been tried for chronic therapy of hypogonadotrophic hypogonadism. It is necessary to administer GnRH in frequent boluses (25–200ng/kg of body weight every 2 hours); however, it is unclear whether this regimen has any advantages over gonadotrophin therapy.

Antiandrogens

Pharmacologic compounds that interfere with the synthesis of testosterone or block its action have potential use in adult men with prostatic hyperplasia, prostatic carcinoma, male pattern baldness, or pedophilia and in boys with precocious puberty (**Fig. 25.23**).

Inhibitors of testosterone synthesis

The continuous administration of large doses of GnRH down-regulates gonadotrophin secretion and results in a pharmacologic castration. A number of GnRH analogs have been developed to treat precocious puberty or as an alternative to orchiectomy or estrogen administration in men with disseminated prostate cancer. Most of these analogs are agonists rather than antagonist, and testosterone production is transiently stimulated before gonadotrophin secretion is inhibited and testosterone levels decrease. Nafarelin acetate and histrelin are primarily used for central idiopathic precocious puberty. Leuprolide acetate, which is used for both precocious puberty and prostate cancer, is available in preparations for daily subcutaneous administration and as a depot preparations that lasts 1, 3, or 4 months. For advanced prostate cancer the subcutaneous dose is 1mg/day and the intramuscular dose of the depot suspensions is 7.5mg monthly. Goserelin acetate is used in advanced prostate cancer or precocious puberty (in Europe) and is administered as a 1-month or 3-month implant of 3.6mg per month in the upper abdominal wall. The adverse side effects of all of these GnRH analogs in men are similar and include gynecomastia, hot flashes, sexual dysfunction, and loss of libido.

5α-reductase inhibitors

The azasteroid finasteride is a competitive inhibitor of steroid 5α-reductase 2, the principle isoenzyme in the prostate, and also has some inhibitory activity on the type 1 enzyme. As discussed above, it is useful in treating obstructive symptoms of benign prostatic hyperplasia, especially in men with large prostates. The usual dose of finasteride for prostatic hyperplasia (5mg orally each day) lowers intraprostatic dihydrotestosterone levels without affecting serum testosterone or gonadotrophin

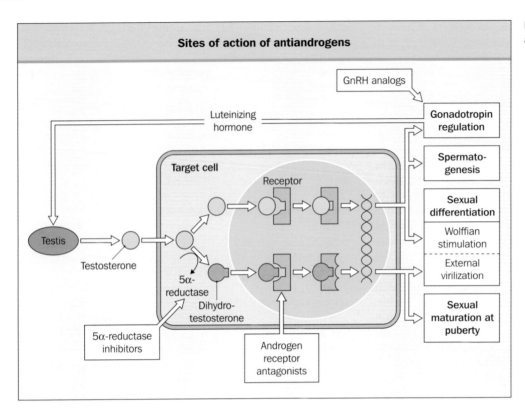

Figure 25.23 Sites of action of antiandrogens.

levels. A small percentage of men experience a decline in libido that usually resolves with time and does not necessitate discontinuing the medication. Because the type 2 enzyme is also expressed in the scalp hair follicles, finasteride is also useful in men with male pattern baldness. At a dose of 1mg daily it can decrease the rate of loss of hair from the forehead and partially restore occipital hair growth in men with early male pattern baldness.

Androgen receptor antagonists

The androgen receptor antagonist most commonly used in men is the nonsteroidal antiandrogen flutamide. It is converted *in vivo* to 2-hydroxyflutamide, which is a competitive inhibitor of androgen, binding to the androgen receptor. Since it blocks testosterone feedback inhibition of gonadotrophin secretion at the hypothalamic–pituitary axis, flutamide administration results in increased plasma LH and increased serum testosterone levels. The increased testosterone levels may overcome the antiandrogen effects. Thus, flutamide is primarily useful as an antiandrogen only in men who have either been castrated or

are receiving GnRH analog therapy to lower testosterone production as part of therapy for advanced prostate cancer. It has been postulated that the combination of a GnRH analog and flutamide might provide a 'total androgen blockade', since flutamide would be able to block the effects of any adrenal androgens.

The dose of flutamide is 250mg orally three times daily. Its major limitation is hepatotoxicity (liver failure has been reported). Diarrhea may be a troubling side effect, and gynecomastia develops in as many as half of men treated with flutamide or the other androgen-receptor antagonists. Two other similar anilide-derived androgen-receptor antagonists are nilutamide and bicalutimide, which differ from flutamide by having a longer half-life and different pharmacokinetics. Nilutamide is given at a dose of 300mg daily, and bicalutimide has been used at 150mg per day when used without a GnRH analog and 50mg per day in regimens that include GnRH analogs. Bicalutamide, which appears to have a good safety profile, is the only one of the group that has been used for treatment of prostate cancer as monotherapy. Nilutamide therapy has been associated with alcohol intolerance and visual disturbances.

FURTHER READING

Belville C, Josso N, Picard JY. Persistence of Mullerian derivatives in males. Am J Med Genet. 1999;89:218–23.

Bhasin S, Storer TW, Berman N, et al. The effects of supraphysiologic doses of testosterone on muscle size and strength in normal men. N Engl J Med. 1996;335:1–7.

Denis LJ, Griffiths K. Endocrine treatment of prostate cancer. Semin Surg Oncol. 2000;18:52–74.

Donohoue PA, Parker K, Migeon CJ. Congenital adrenal hyperplasia. In: Scriver CR, Beaudet AL, Sly WS, Valle D, eds. The metabolic and molecular basis of inherited disease, 8th edn. New York:McGraw-Hill, 2001:4077–116.

Griffin JE, Wilson JD. Disorders of the testes and male reproductive tract. In: Wilson JD, Foster DW, Kronenberg HM, Larsen PR, eds. Williams textbook of endocrinology, 9th edn. Philadelphia, PA:WB Saunders; 1998:819–75.

Griffin JE, McPhaul MJ, Russell DW, Wilson JD. The androgen resistance syndromes: Steroid 5α-reductase 2 deficiency, testicular feminization, and related disorders. In: Scriver CR, Beaudet AL, Sly WS, Valle D, eds. The metabolic and molecular basis of inherited disease, 8th edn. New York:McGraw-Hill; 2001:4117–46.

Grinspoon S, Corcoran C, Anderson E, et al. Sustained anabolic effects of long-term androgen administration in men with AIDS wasting. Clin Infect Dis. 1999;28:634–6.

Grumbach MM, Conte FA. Disorders of sex differentiation. In: Wilson JD, Foster DW, Kronenberg HM, Larsen PR, eds. Williams textbook of endocrinology, 9th edn. Philadelphia, PA:WB Saunders; 1998:1303–425.

Najmabadi H, Huang V, Yen P, et al. Substantial prevalence of microdeletions of the Y-chromosome in infertile men with idiopathic azoospermia and oligozoospermia detected using a sequence-tagged site-based mapping strategy. J Clin Endocrinol Metab. 1996;81:1347–52.

Parker KL, Schedl A, Schimmer BP. Gene interactions in gonadal development. Annu Rev Physiol. 1999;61:417–33.

Snyder PJ, Peachey H, Berlin JA, et al. Effects of testosterone replacement in hypogonadal men. J Clin Endocrinol Metab. 2000;85:2670–7.

Wang C, Swerdloff RS, Iranmanesh A, Dobs A, et al. Transdermal testosterone gel improves sexual function, mood, muscle strength, and body composition parameters in hypogonadal men. J Clin Endocrinol Metab. 2000;85:2839–53.

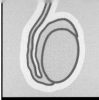

Section 5 Gonad and Growth

Chapter 26

Ovary

Carole Gilling-Smith and Stephen Franks

INTRODUCTION

The principal function of the ovary is to produce, each month, a mature oocyte capable of fertilization and subsequent implantation. The associated endocrine activity is responsible for the development of secondary sexual characteristics and preparation of the genital tract for pregnancy. Both depend on the cyclic development of healthy graafian follicles. Clinical manifestations of ovarian dysfunction are largely caused, directly or indirectly, by absent or abnormal folliculogenesis.

EMBRYOLOGY

Differentiation of the ovary

During the fifth week of embryonic life, indifferent gonads first appear as a thickening of celomic epithelium medial to each mesonephros. As celomic epithelial and underlying mesenchymal cells proliferate, a bulge called the gonadal ridge develops. Finger-like epithelial cords, the primary sex cords, grow into the underlying mesenchyme and the gonad develops an outer cortex and inner medulla. At this point, the genetic sex of the embryo determines subsequent differentiation. In the presence of the Y chromosome, the primary sex cords differentiate into seminiferous tubules, and testes develop. In the absence of the Y chromosome, the medulla and primary sex cords gradually regress and the cortex of the indifferent gonad develops into an ovary. Both X chromosomes are required for normal ovarian differentiation. Absence of one X chromosome (XO or Turner's syndrome) is associated with ovarian dysgenesis.

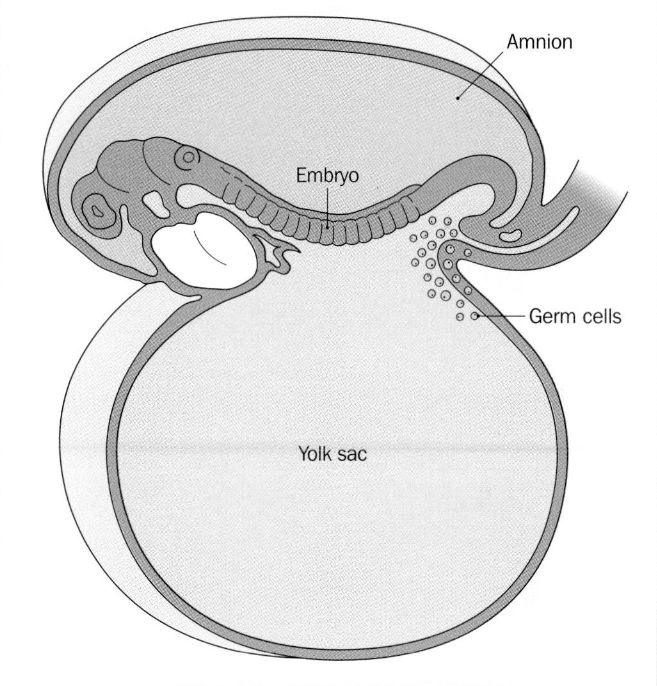

Oocyte formation

From the fourth week of life, primordial germ cells migrate by ameboid movement from the wall of the yolk sac to the gonadal ridges (**Fig. 26.1**). During migration, the germ cells start to undergo mitotic division and, by the time they reach the primitive ovary, are referred to as oogonia. They continue to proliferate within the ovary to reach a peak of 6–7 million by the 20th week of fetal development. Thereafter they begin to undergo germ cell loss, atresia, a process that continues throughout reproductive life until the menopause (**Fig. 26.2**). A female is born with 1–2 million germ cells. By puberty her ovarian germ cell reserve has reduced to 400,000 and by the time the menopause is reached no oocytes are left within the ovary. A declining ovarian reserve is usually evident, both clinically and endocrinologically, several years before the menopause.

Figure 26.1 Origin of primordial germ cells. Primordial germ cells migrate from the wall of the yolk sac to the developing gonad.

Between 3 and 7 months of intrauterine life, oogonia enter the prophase of the first meiotic division to become primary oocytes. Meiosis only resumes at the time of ovulation, which may be up to 45 years later. During ovarian development, secondary sex cords grow inwards from the surface epithelium into the underlying mesenchyme to incorporate the primordial germ cells. By the 16th week, these cortical cords start to break up to form isolated cell clusters called primordial follicles (**Fig. 26.3**) which consist of a primary oocyte surrounded by a single layer of spindle-shaped granulosa cells.

Only 400–500 oocytes are destined for ovulation and potential fertilization. The remaining 99% will undergo atresia. Folliculogenesis can be viewed as an attempt to rescue oocytes from programmed cell death.

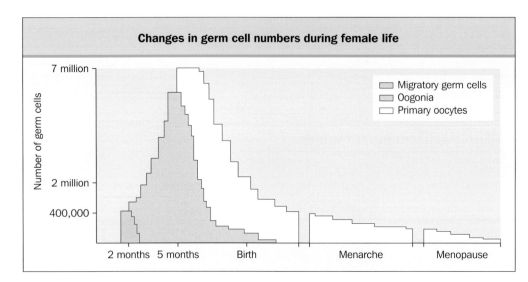

Figure 26.2 Changes in germ cell numbers during female life.

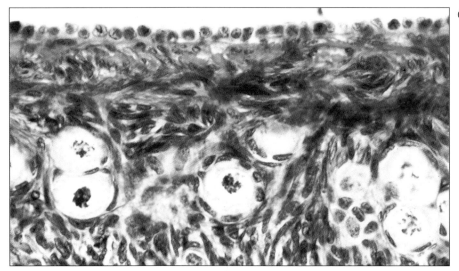

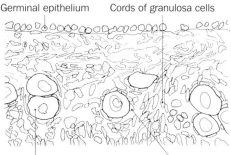

Figure 26.3 Section of ovarian cortex showing developing primordial follicles. The primordial follicle consists of an oocyte surrounded by a single layer of spindle-shaped granulosa cells.

OVARIAN PHYSIOLOGY

Folliculogenesis

No oogonia are formed postnatally and primordial follicles cease to develop once the infant has reached 6 months. The ovary will contain at any one time many follicles at different stages of development.

Folliculogenesis describes the transformation of a primordial follicle to a graafian follicle and takes approximately 6 months (**Fig. 26.4**). Primordial follicles lie in the outer cortex of the ovary and, as folliculogenesis proceeds, migrate towards the medulla (**Fig. 26.5**). The initial change takes place when the spindle-shaped cells surrounding the oocyte differentiate into a single layer of cuboidal granulosa cells and a primary follicle forms. Granulosa cells then proliferate and form multiple layers around the oocyte, giving rise to the secondary (preantral) follicle. As the follicle enlarges, the surrounding stroma is compressed and spindle-shaped theca cells appear around the granulosa layer. Cell proliferation leads to the formation of a distinct, well-vascularized theca layer, separated from an avascular granulosa layer by a basement membrane. As the granulosa cells proliferate to form several layers, spaces form between these and coalesce to form the antrum. Follicles at this stage of development are referred to as early tertiary (antral) follicles and, if selected to become the dominant or graafian follicle, will enter a final exponential growth phase during the first half of the ovarian cycle. The majority of secondary and tertiary follicles however never develop into graafian follicles but undergo atresia. Following atresia, both granulosa cells and oocyte die. Theca cells undergo hypertrophy and are incorporated into the stroma, where they continue to produce androgens in response to luteinizing hormone (LH).

Follicular development is not thought to be dependent on gonadotropin stimulation until antrum formation. Thereafter, folliculogenesis depends on fine endocrine interplay between hypothalamus, pituitary, and ovaries.

Ovarian hormone production
Enzyme control

The ovary produces androgens, estrogen and progesterone. The pathways and enzymes involved are shown in **Figure 26.6**. The initial step, conversion of cholesterol to pregnenolone, takes place in the theca cell and is catalyzed by cholesterol side-chain

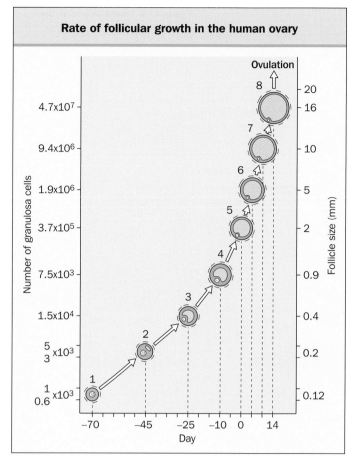

Figure 26.4 Rate of follicular growth in the human ovary. Classes 1–8 are defined by the number of granulosa cells and the corresponding estimated follicular diameter (mm). (Redrawn from Gougeon A. Dynamics of follicular growth in the human: a model from preliminary results. Human Reprod. 1986;1:81–7.)

cleavage cytochrome P450 (P450$_{scc}$). The recently described steroid acute regulatory protein (StAR) is now known to be important in facilitating transport of cholesterol from the outer to the inner membrane of the mitochondria where P450$_{scc}$ is located. It is a significant rate-limiting factor in steroidogenesis.

Both uptake of cholesterol substrate and subsequent conversion to pregnenolone depend on gonadotropin stimulation. Subsequent conversion of pregnenolone to androstenedione proceeds by one of two parallel pathways called Δ_4 and Δ_5. In the Δ_4 pathway, pregnenolone is converted to 17α-hydroxypregnenolone and then to dehydroepiandrosterone (DHEA) while in the Δ_5 pathway androstenedione is formed via progesterone and 17α-hydroxyprogesterone. The conversion of pregnenolone to progesterone is a two-step reaction involving 3β-hydroxysteroid dehydrogenase (3β-HSD) and Δ_{4-5} isomerase enzymes. The two rate limiting steps in ovarian androgen biosynthesis are the conversion of pregnenolone and progesterone to their respective 17α-hydroxylated steroids and then their subsequent conversion to C_{19} androgens. This two step reaction is catalyzed by 17α-hydroxylase cytochrome P450 (P450$_{c17\alpha}$), a single enzyme with two activities, 17α-hydroxylase and 17,20 lyase. The final step, aromatization of androstenedione to estradiol takes place in the granulosa cell layer and is catalyzed by aromatase cytochrome P450 (P450$_{arom}$).

Gonadotropin control

Steroid production by the ovary is primarily controlled by the pituitary gonadotropins, LH and follicle-stimulating hormone (FSH) and, in pregnancy, human chorionic gonadotropin (hCG) produced by the trophoblast. All three are glycoprotein hormones composed of α and β subunits. The α subunit is identical in all three. The β subunit is specific to each hormone, differing in both amino acid and carbohydrate composition. Nevertheless, the β subunits have considerable amino-acid sequence homology, particularly those of LH and hCG. Both bind to a common LH/hCG transmembrane receptor in theca and luteinized theca and activate similar postreceptor effects, a feature that allows the two hormones to be used interchangeably in clinical practice.

The cellular effects of FSH, LH, and hCG are triggered when they bind to G-protein-linked receptors in target cell membranes (**Fig. 26.7**). This binding stimulates adenylate cyclase and an increase in intracellular cyclic AMP (cAMP). Cyclic AMP binds specifically to a cytoplasmic protein, which in turn activates protein kinase A, resulting in the phosphorylation of specific proteins. These induce the genes encoding the enzymes involved in ovarian steroid biosynthesis. This amplification system means that only a small percentage of receptors need be occupied in order to trigger a significant steroid response.

Theca granulosa interaction

During follicular growth, the granulosa and theca cell layers work in synchrony to produce estradiol, a phenomenon referred to as the two-cell, two-gonadotropin theory (**Fig. 26.8**). In the early follicular phase, LH receptors are found exclusively on theca cells and FSH receptors exclusively on granulosa cells. Theca cells have virtually no P450$_{arom}$ while granulosa cells have no P450$_{c17\alpha}$. The granulosa layer is avascular, separated from the vascular theca layer by the lamina basalis. As LH levels rise in the early follicular phase, cholesterol is converted to androstenedione in the theca layer. Androstenedione then diffuses across the basement membrane to the granulosa layer where FSH stimulates its aromatization to estradiol.

The ovarian cycle

The follicular phase

Failed fertilization leads to corpus luteum regression and heralds the start of the next ovarian cycle and graafian follicle development. The first signal for recruitment is a rise in pituitary FSH, which occurs as negative feedback inhibition by progesterone, estradiol, and inhibin produced by the corpus luteum is withdrawn. This intercycle rise in FSH in the first few days after the start of menstruation (**Fig. 26.9**), stimulates a pool of secondary antral follicles 2–5mm in diameter to enter the final stages of follicular development. FSH stimulates granulosa cells to proliferate and differentiate and develop aromatase-linked LH receptors. Each follicle has a different threshold requirement for FSH and only one is capable of responding maximally to

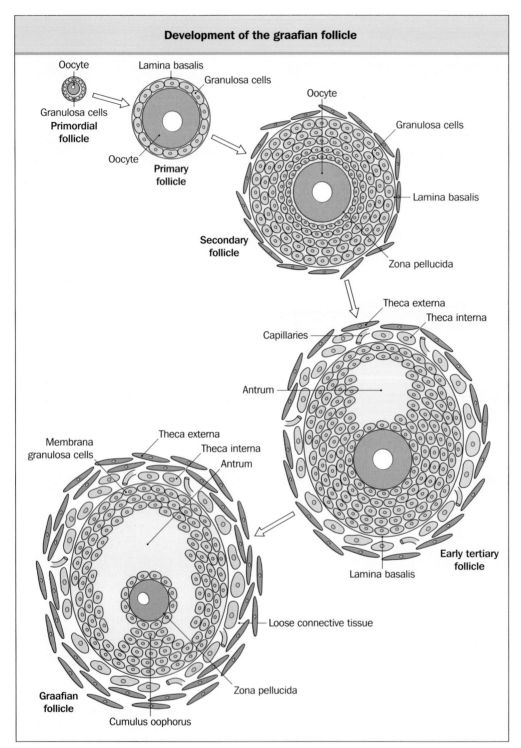

Figure 26.5 Development of the graafian follicle.

Development of the graafian follicle

Oocyte
Granulosa cells
Primordial follicle

Lamina basalis
Granulosa cells
Oocyte
Primary follicle

Oocyte
Granulosa cells
Lamina basalis
Zona pellucida
Secondary follicle

Theca externa
Theca interna
Capillaries
Antrum
Lamina basalis
Early tertiary follicle

Membrana granulosa cells
Theca externa
Theca interna
Antrum
Loose connective tissue
Zona pellucida
Cumulus oophorus
Graafian follicle

become the dominant follicle. Follicle selection is usually apparent by day 7 of the cycle, when the dominant follicle has reached 10mm in diameter. As this follicle grows and produces increasing amounts of estradiol, FSH secretion is inhibited and the other follicles undergo atresia.

As the follicle enlarges, FSH induces further LH receptors on granulosa cells and, in response to LH stimulation, the dominant follicle secretes increasing amounts of androstenedione and estradiol into the ovarian vein. During the follicular phase, more than 95% of the circulating estradiol is secreted by the dominant follicle. The ovarian contribution to circulating androstenedione levels rises from 30% in the early follicular phase to 60% by midcycle. The adrenal accounts for the rest.

Ovulation
Rising estradiol levels exert a positive feedback effect on pituitary LH release, which in turn enhances estradiol production (**Fig. 26.10**). This leads to the midcycle surge of LH (and to a

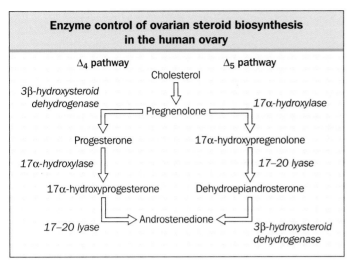

Figure 26.6 Enzyme control of androgen biosynthesis in the human ovary.

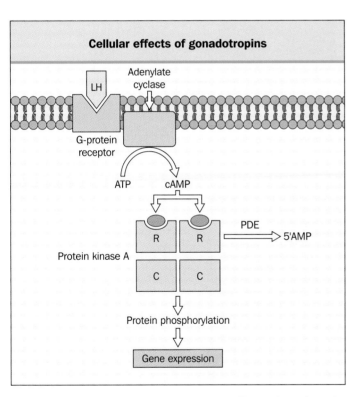

Figure 26.7 Cellular actions of gonadotropins. The cellular actions of follicle stimulating hormone, luteinizing hormone (LH) and human chorionic gonadotropin are triggered when they bind to G-protein linked receptors in target cell membranes. AMP, adenosine monophosphate; ATP, adenosine triphosphate; cAMP, cyclic adenosine monophosphate; PDE, phosphodiesterase.

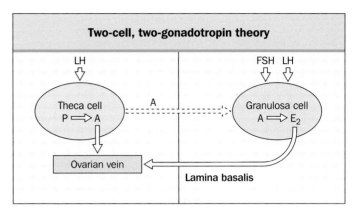

Figure 26.8 Two-cell, two-gonadotropin theory. The figure illustrates two-cell, two-gonadotropin control of estradiol synthesis in the human ovary. A, androstenedione; E$_2$, estradiol; FSH, follicle-stimulating hormone; LH, luteinizing hormone; P, pregnenolone.

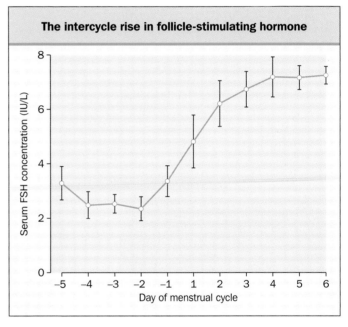

Figure 26.9 The intercycle rise in follicle-stimulating hormone (FSH).

lesser extent of FSH), which triggers follicular rupture and ovulation, which occurs 36 hours later (**Fig. 26.11**). Exogenous hCG can also be used to trigger ovulation, because of its structural similarity to LH. About 12 hours after the LH surge there is a fall in serum levels of estradiol, thought to be caused by LH receptor desensitization. This estrogen fall occasionally produces a small midcycle withdrawal bleed (midcycle spotting).

The LH surge stimulates a proteolytic cascade that leads to protrusion of the follicle on to the ovarian surface, followed by rupture. The oocyte surrounded by its cumulus and antral fluid are gently picked up by the fimbriae of the fallopian tube.

The luteal phase
Following ovulation, capillaries and fibroblasts from the surrounding stroma proliferate and invade the basal lamina, leading to vascularization of the granulosa layer. The luteinized granulosa cells, supplied directly with precursor low density lipoprotein (LDL), start to produce large amounts of estradiol and progesterone in response to LH. Progesterone production increases progressively to peak 7 days postovulation, to coincide with the time of blastocyst implantation. If fertilization and implantation take place, the exponential rise in hCG produced by the developing trophoblast ensures that copious amounts of

379

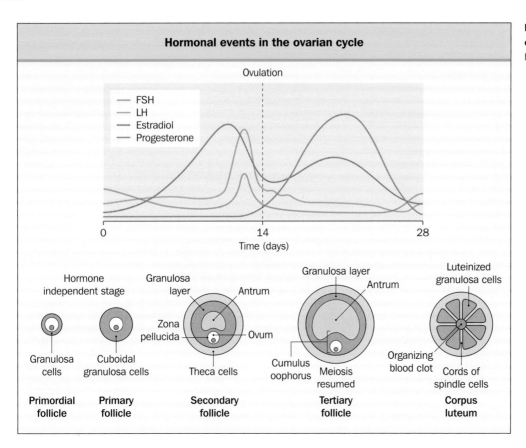

Figure 26.10 Hormonal events in the ovarian cycle. FSH, follicle-stimulating hormone; LH, luteinizing hormone.

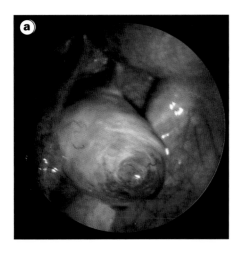

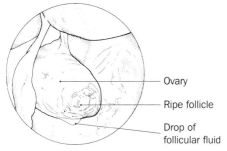

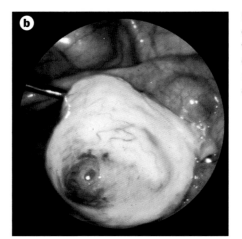

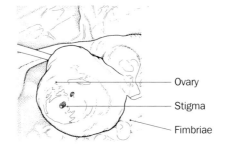

Figure 26.11 Ovulation of the cumulus–oocyte complex. Endoscopic view of the ovary immediately prior to ovulation (a) and following ovulation (b). (Courtesy of Professor H Frangenheim and Dr MR Darling.)

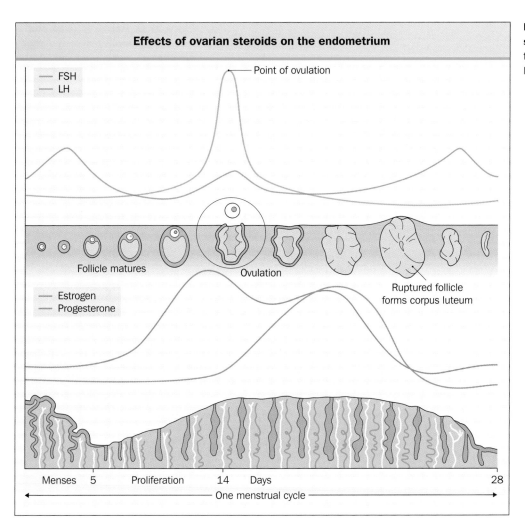

Figure 26.12 Effect of ovarian steroids on the endometrium. FSH, follicle-stimulating hormone; LH, luteinizing hormone.

Effects of ovarian steroids on the endometrium

- FSH
- LH

Point of ovulation

Follicle matures

Ovulation

Ruptured follicle forms corpus luteum

- Estrogen
- Progesterone

Menses 5 Proliferation 14 Days 28

One menstrual cycle

---

progesterone are produced until the placenta is fully formed at around 12 weeks gestation. If fertilization does not occur, progesterone and estradiol levels start to fall in the midluteal phase and luteal regression begins. A scar is left on the ovary, which gradually becomes avascular several cycles later (corpus albicans). As an endocrine gland, the corpus luteum has one of the highest blood flows per unit mass of all the glands in the body.

Ovarian proteins – inhibin and activin

These are proteins isolated from ovarian follicular fluid. The two proteins have opposing actions on FSH secretion by the pituitary: inhibin suppresses while activin stimulates FSH secretion. Within the follicle, however, inhibin augments LH-stimulated theca androgen synthesis, in contrast to activin, which inhibits androgen production. Studies of activin mRNA in nonhuman primates suggests that activin synthesis is induced as the follicle reaches the antral stage. Inhibin production then increases as the follicle matures, which provides a mechanism for selectively enhancing androgen production prior to ovulation.

Effect of ovarian steroids on the endometrium

The response of the endometrium to the cyclical changes in estrogen and progesterone involves complex interplay between many autocrine and paracrine factors. The endometrium itself is divided functionally into three thirds. The upper two thirds is the decidua functionalis layer, which is shed and regenerates each cycle to prepare for blastocyst implantation. The lower third is the basalis layer, which provides the regenerating endometrium. During the first half of the cycle, estrogen production by the developing follicle leads to endometrial proliferation of both glands and stroma and thickness increases from 0.5mm to 5mm. Following ovulation, the exposure of the endometrium to progesterone limits further growth in height. The stroma becomes more edematous, the glands become increasingly tortuous, and spiral endometrial arteries become prominent. In the event of failed fertilization and corpus luteum regression, falling estrogen and progesterone levels provoke myometrial contractions and rhythmic vasoconstriction of the spiral arterioles. These events are mediated by prostaglandins and in turn lead to endometrial ischemia and finally shedding of the basalis functionalis (**Fig. 26.12**). In women with anovulatory cycles, prolonged exposure of the endometrium to estrogen alone produces excessive proliferation. Clinically, this is manifest as irregular, heavy, prolonged bleeding which can only be controlled by the exogenous administration of cyclic progestagens. Prolonged exposure of the endometrium to unopposed estrogen increases the risk of developing endometrial hyperplasia or carcinoma.

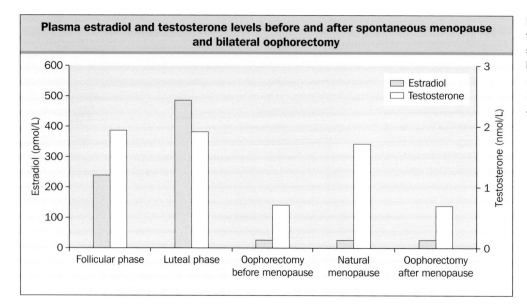

Plasma estradiol and testosterone levels before and after spontaneous menopause and bilateral oophorectomy

Figure 26.13 Plasma estradiol and testosterone levels before and after spontaneous menopause and bilateral oophorectomy. Estradiol 100pmol/L = 30pg/mL; testosterone 1nmol/L = 0.29ng/mL. (Courtesy of J. Studd.)

The menopausal ovary

The first indication of a declining ovarian reserve is a rise in the level of FSH (> 10IU/L) in the early follicular phase as the number of follicles available for recruitment falls. More and more cycles become anovulatory and cycle length increases. The menopause is defined as the time in a woman's life when menstruation stops completely because of depletion of her oocyte stock. The climacteric is the run up to this, when folliculogenesis becomes disrupted and estrogen levels start to wax and wane. During this time, FSH levels may fluctuate from cycle to cycle but gradually become persistently elevated. The rise in LH is later than that of FSH but is certainly apparent once menstruation stops. Absent folliculogenesis is accompanied by a fall in estradiol and inhibin levels. Although androgen levels also decline, the postmenopausal ovary may continue to produce significant amounts of androgen and testosterone that can be aromatized to estrogen in peripheral fat cells. This is why surgical oophorectomy, as opposed to a natural menopause, usually produces a more profound fall in estrogen levels (**Fig. 26.13**).

Low estrogen levels produce a series of clinical symptoms and metabolic abnormalities that prompt many women to seek medical advice, primarily to discuss and start hormone replacement therapy (HRT).

The ovary in a postmenopausal woman is small, pale yellow, and atrophic. Microscopically, the cortex is thin, with no evidence of follicles. In a few women, the menopausal ovary becomes full of hyperplastic stromal nodules whose cells behave functionally like theca interna cells and produce appreciable amounts of androgens. Stromal hyperplasia should be considered in any postmenopausal woman presenting with hirsutism or virilization.

CLINICAL ASPECTS OF OVARIAN DYSFUNCTION

Any disruption to the process of normal ovarian development *in utero*, or in the cycle of oocyte recruitment, maturation, and release during reproductive life, can lead to profound disturbances in ovarian hormone production and clinical symptoms. Patients present to either endocrinologist or gynecologist, depending on the predominant symptoms. Only those conditions endocrinologists are most likely to encounter in clinical practice are discussed in this chapter.

Polycystic ovary syndrome

Polycystic ovary syndrome (PCOS) is the commonest disorder of ovarian function during reproductive life and one of the commonest endocrinopathies to affect women. First described by Stein and Leventhal in 1935 as a triad of amenorrhea, hyperandrogenism, and obesity, associated with bilaterally enlarged cystic ovaries, PCOS is now recognized to have a heterogeneous clinical and biochemical spectrum. With the aid of high-resolution pelvic ultrasound as a means of identifying the characteristic ovarian morphology, it has become apparent that the spectrum of clinical presentation includes both women with anovulation but no evidence of hirsutism and those with severe hirsutism or male pattern alopecia and regular cycles. Hyperinsulinemia due to insulin resistance is a common feature, as is obesity, and both exacerbate the expression of clinical symptoms. This clinical heterogeneity has fueled debate over whether the syndrome is a single disease entity or a group of related disorders. However, what is clear is that women with polycystic ovarian morphology on ultrasound are characterized by a significant elevation of serum androgens, irrespective of symptomatology.

Diagnosis

It is generally, although not universally, accepted that pelvic ultrasound provides the primary means of diagnosing the characteristic ovarian morphology (**Fig. 26.14**). A polycystic ovary defined on ultrasound criteria should have at least 10 follicles, 2–8mm in diameter, in any one plane. These are typically distributed peripherally and central stroma is increased. Ovarian volume is usually enlarged, although in some cases it may be normal (**Fig. 26.15**). The appearance can be confused with multifollicular ovaries, which are associated with hypothalamic

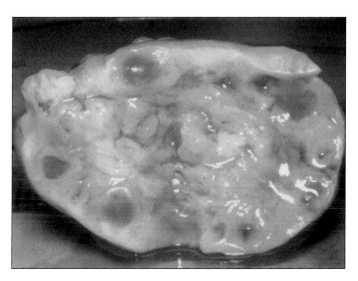

Figure 26.14 Section through a polycystic ovary. The ovary is enlarged and pearly white. The ovarian capsule is thickened.

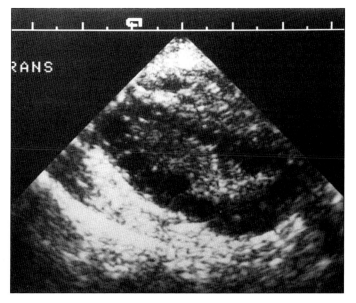

Figure 26.15 Transvaginal ultrasound picture of a polycystic ovary.

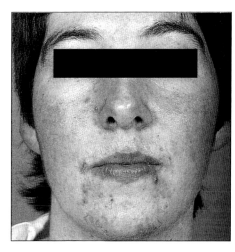

Figure 26.16
Clinical evidence of hyperandrogenemia in PCOS – acne, oily skin and hirsutism.

The heterogeneous clinical and biochemical spectrum of polycystic ovary syndrome	
Clinical	**Biochemical**
Cycle irregularity (oligomenorrhea, amenorrhea)	Hyperandrogenemia
Anovulatory infertility	Hyperinsulinemia
Menorrhagia	Elevated LH:FSH ratio
Acne	
Hirsutism	
Male pattern alopecia	
Acanthosis nigricans (rare)	
Obesity	

Table 26.1 The heterogeneous clinical and biochemical spectrum of polycystic ovary syndrome. Patients commonly present with only one or two of the characteristic symptoms or biochemical changes. Diagnosis rests on ultrasound evidence of polycystic ovaries. FSH, follicle-stimulating hormone; LH, luteinizing hormone.

In many women, the history of menstrual disturbance dates back to the menarche, which may be delayed. Primary amenorrhea is an uncommon but well-described presentation. Anovulation, and lack of progesterone secretion in the luteal phase, produces a persistently proliferative and thickened endometrium, which, in some women, leads to irregular and heavy bleeding. In the long term, if regular shedding of the endometrium is not achieved therapeutically, these women are at high risk of developing endometrial hyperplasia or cancer. Menorrhagia is more common in obese subjects because serum estradiol levels may be augmented by peripheral aromatization of androgens in adipose tissue.

Hyperandrogenemia and hyperinsulinemia produce symptoms of hirsutism, acne, and male pattern baldness. About 30% of women with PCOS have acne, 60–70% develop hirsutism and about 8% will present with male pattern balding or androgenic alopecia (**Table 26.1**).

Acanthosis nigricans is a mucocutaneous eruption found in up to 5% of women with polycystic ovaries. It is characterized by areas of hyperpigmented papillomas in the axillas, the nape of the

amenorrhea and hyperprolactinemia. Although these ovaries also have an increased number of follicles. they are scattered throughout the stroma, which is not increased, and within an ovary of normal volume.

Clinical presentation

In clinical practice it is important to differentiate between the incidental finding of polycystic ovaries on ultrasound, which have been reported in over 20% of women of reproductive age, and polycystic ovary syndrome, in which polycystic ovaries are identified in association with symptoms. Numerous ultrasound-based prevalence studies have confirmed polycystic ovaries to be the commonest cause of anovulatory infertility, acne, and hirsutism (**Fig. 26.16**).

neck, under the breasts and in the groin area. The combination of acanthosis nigricans, hyperandrogenemia, and insulin resistance is sometimes referred to as the HAIR-AN syndrome.

The severity of clinical symptoms is undoubtedly modified by genetic factors but increasing body mass is a key trigger and many women first present following a period of weight gain.

Endocrine and metabolic abnormalities

Hyperandrogenemia is a common feature in women with polycystic ovaries, irrespective of symptomatology. Hypersecretion of LH, hyperinsulinemia, and insulin resistance, on the other hand, are more characteristic of women with anovulation and menstrual disturbance. The link between hyperandrogenemia and hyperinsulinemia in PCOS has been extensively investigated. Elevated serum androgens are unlikely to cause hyperinsulinemia, since drugs that lower serum androgen levels do not reverse the insulin resistance. Conversely, insulin amplifies the action of LH on theca cell androgen production and drugs that reduce serum insulin concentrations, such as metformin, thiazolidinediones, and diazoxide, lower androgen levels and improve symptoms of anovulation and hirsutism. Recent evidence supports the existence of a subgroup of women with PCOS and anovulation who have a genetic susceptibility to hyperinsulinemia. A raised body mass index further increases serum insulin and testosterone levels and reduces sex-hormone-binding globulin levels, and thus exacerbates symptoms. For this reason, weight loss is a very important therapeutic measure in hyperinsulinemic obese women as it promotes a fall in circulating insulin and testosterone levels, leading to an improvement in symptoms.

Etiology – a genetic disorder of ovarian androgen secretion

The etiology of PCOS is a hotly debated and highly controversial issue. Most agree that the ovary, rather than the adrenal, is the principal source of excess androgen production. Theca cells from polycystic ovaries have been shown to produce more androgen per cell than theca cells from normal ovaries. Furthermore, women with polycystic ovaries demonstrate an exaggerated ovarian androgen response to either gonadotropin-releasing hormone (GnRH) or hCG. These observations have led to the hypothesis that the condition is a genetically determined disorder of androgen biosynthesis, with much interest focused on $P450_{c17}$, which encodes for the enzymes 17-hydroxylase, 17/20-lyase. The heterogeneous clinical and biochemical spectrum is probably the result of interaction with other genes, such as those affecting insulin resistance and environmental factors such as obesity. Recent data from our group has identified $CYP11\alpha$, the gene encoding side-chain cleavage, rather than $P450_{c17}$, as a major genetic susceptibility locus. While the precise mode of inheritance is still uncertain, a familial basis for the syndrome is well established and it is not uncommon to find a mother or sister with one or more symptoms of PCOS.

Investigations

All women presenting with menstrual irregularity, infertility or symptoms of hyperandrogenemia should have a pelvic ultrasound. A transabdominal scan should be done first to exclude any ovarian or uterine masses, followed by a transvaginal scan (except in women who are virgo intacta) to get a better view of the internal structure and stroma of the ovary. The latter is particularly important when trying to differentiate between polycystic and multifollicular ovaries, as management and long-term health risks are quite different. In women with regular cycles, the scan should be done in the early follicular phase, since this is the best time to evaluate ovarian morphology.

Endocrine evaluation of cycle irregularity should include serum FSH, LH, thyroid function, prolactin, and testosterone. It is important to note that, while serum concentrations of testosterone and LH are often raised in women with PCOS, this is not invariably the case. Thus, some hirsute women have normal serum testosterone (although androgen production rates are usually increased). However, it should be emphasized that the main clinical rationale for measurement of testosterone in hirsute subjects is as a screening test for more serious causes of hyperandrogenism than PCOS. As many as 50% of women with anovulatory PCOS will have normal serum levels of LH and so, while a high LH (with a normal FSH) is specific in the diagnosis of PCOS, a normal LH measurement dose not exclude the diagnosis. In obese subjects, fasting glucose and lipids are advisable. Hirsutism should be assessed clinically by the Ferriman–Gallwey score, which is a semiquantitative method of recording the severity and distribution of unwanted body and facial hair (**Table 26.2**).

Differential diagnosis

Pituitary disorders, thyroid disorders, and adrenal diseases may also present with menstrual disturbance, infertility, or hirsutism, e.g. hyperprolactinemia, late-onset (nonclassic) congenital adrenal hyperplasia. A serum testosterone of more than 5nmol/L (1.4ng/mL) and /or signs of severe virilization such as clitoromegaly or deepening of the voice are rarely caused by PCOS alone and further tests of adrenal function and imaging of the ovary or adrenal must be done to exclude an androgen secreting tumor. Other conditions presenting with hirsutism or virilization are listed in **Table 26.3**.

Management of hirsutism, acne, male pattern balding

Since in PCOS most of the excess androgens are of ovarian, rather than adrenal origin, effective therapy in these conditions should target the ovary. It is important to advise patients that, although medical therapy will bring about a rapid fall in serum androgens, an improvement in hair growth is unlikely to be visible for 6–12 months. Acne responds more quickly. For this reason, cosmetic measures should be encouraged from the outset and continued throughout treatment.

If symptoms are mild, the combined oral contraceptive pill is a useful first-line approach for both acne and hirsutism. By suppressing pituitary FSH and LH, ovarian androgen production is reduced. The estrogen component also has the benefit of stimulating sex-hormone-binding globulin production by the liver and reducing testosterone bioavailability. Contraceptive pills that contain nonandrogenic progestagens such as desogestrel are the most effective, while those that contain levonorgestrel and norethisterone are better avoided, since these are androgenic progestagens, which could exacerbate symptoms.

For moderate to severe hirsutism, acne, or male pattern alopecia, cyproterone acetate is advisable. This is an antiandrogen that acts by blocking the androgen receptor. It also has appreciable progestogenic activity, which suppresses gonadotropin secretion

The Ferriman–Gallwey scoring system for the assessment of hirsutism

Site	Grade	Definition
Upper lip	1	A few hairs at outer margin
	2	Small moustache at outer margin
	3	Moustache extending halfway from outer margin
	4	Moustache extending to midline
Chin	1	A few scattered hairs
	2	Small concentrations of scattered hairs
	3	Light complete cover
	4	Heavy complete cover
Chest	1	Circumareolar hairs
	2	Additional midline hairs
	3	Fusion of these areas with three quarter cover
	4	Complete cover
Upper back	1	A few scattered hairs
	2	Rather more, still scattered
	3	Light complete cover
	4	Heavy complete cover
Lower back	1	A sacral tuft of hair
	2	With some lateral extension
	3	Three-quarter cover
	4	Complete cover
Upper abdomen	1	A few midline hairs
	2	Rather more, still midline
	3	Half cover
	4	Full cover
Lower abdomen	1	A few midline hairs
	2	A midline streak of hair
	3	A midline band of hair
	4	An inverted V-shaped growth
Upper arm	1	Sparse growth affecting no more than a quarter of limb surfaces
	2	More than this, cover still incomplete
	3	Light complete cover
	4	Heavy complete cover
Forearm	1–4	Complete cover of dorsal surface: light (1) to heavy (4) growth
Thigh	1–4	As for arm
Leg	1–4	As for arm

Table 26.2 The Ferriman–Gallwey scoring system for the assessment of hirsutism.

Differential diagnosis of hirsutism

Polycystic ovary syndrome	
Idiopathic	
Hyperthecosis	
Late-onset congenital adrenal hyperplasia	
Cushing's syndrome	Cushing's disease (ACTH-secreting pituitary tumor)
	Ectopic ACTH secretion by nonpituitary tumor e.g. bronchus, thymus
	Autonomous cortisol secretion by adrenal or ovarian tumor
Androgen-secreting tumors of the ovary	Sex-cord stromal cell tumors
	Adrenal-like tumors of the ovary
Androgen-secreting tumors of the adrenal	Adenomas
	Adrenocortical carcinomas
Acromegaly	
Iatrogenic	Testosterone
	Danazol
	Glucocorticoids

Table 26.3 Differential diagnosis of hirsutism. Most women with hirsutism of gradual onset, with or without menstrual cycle irregularity, have polycystic ovaries. More serious pathology is usually obvious on clinical history and examination alone and tends to be associated with a gross elevation of circulating testosterone (> 5nmol/L [>1.4ng/mL]).

and hence ovarian androgen production. Since the progestogenic effect is long-lasting, cyproterone acetate is usually prescribed in a reverse sequential regimen for the first 10 days of a 21-day treatment combined with either the low-dose contraceptive pill or ethinyl estradiol 30μg daily. The dose of cyproterone acetate can be varied from 2mg (prescribed in combination with 35μg ethinyl estradiol), which is effective in over 50% of cases, to 25–100mg in more severe cases. Side-effects include weight gain, breast tenderness, depression, mood changes, loss of libido, and fatigue and limit the dose and duration of treatment. In practice, a 6–12-month course of treatment at high dose should followed by a low-dose maintenance therapy such as the oral contraceptive pill, with or without 2mg cyproterone acetate. Contraception is advised, as cyproterone acetate crosses the placenta and may produce feminization of a male fetus.

Spironolactone is an aldosterone antagonist with powerful androgen-receptor activity and is first-line treatment for hirsutism in the USA. Compared to cyproterone acetate, it is equally effective in reducing hair growth but concerns over its long-term safety have limited its use in the UK. The starting dose is 25–50mg daily and this can be increased to a maximum of 200mg daily. It should not be used in women with renal impairment.

Flutamide is a nonsteroidal antiandrogen with no glucocorticoid or progestogenic properties. Although it was initially used for the treatment of prostatic cancer, it has been found to be effective in the treatment of hirsutism and acne, although reports of serious hepatotoxicity have limited its use in clinical practice. Side effects include dry skin, menstrual disturbance, and fatigue. A daily dose of 125mg appears to be effective and a regular check on liver function is advisable.

More recently, insulin-sensitizing agents have been used in obese, hyperinsulinemic women with PCOS to treat either anovulation or hirsutism. Metformin prescribed at a dose of 850mg twice daily or 500mg three times daily reduces serum insulin and testosterone levels and has been shown to improve symptoms. Weight loss is an equally important therapeutic measure in these women.

Gonadotropin-releasing hormone analogs, by inhibiting FSH and LH secretion, produce a more complete suppression of ovarian androgen production. Although they have been evaluated in the treatment of hirsutism, they appear to be no more effective than antiandrogens. As they are costly and need to be administered parentally, there is little justification for their use in clinical management.

Management of anovulation

Anovulatory women who are not trying to conceive should be encouraged to take cyclic progestagens in an effort to minimize the risk of developing endometrial hyperplasia. For many women, the combined oral contraceptive is an ideal choice, as it provides effective contraception, promotes regular shedding of the endometrium, and also suppresses ovarian androgen production, thereby minimizing any coexisting symptoms of hyperandrogenemia. If estrogenic side-effects such as nausea or weight gain are undesirable, cyclic progestagens alone, such as norethisterone or medroxyprogesterone acetate, can be prescribed for 2 weeks out of every 4. Attention to body weight is of paramount importance and referral to a dietitian may be helpful.

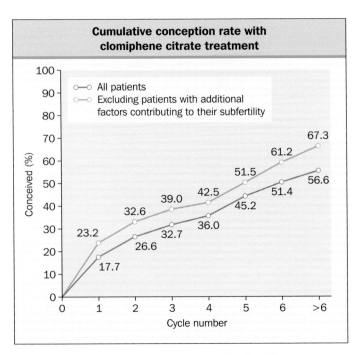

Figure 26.17 Cumulative conception rate with clomiphene treatment. (Redrawn from Kousta A, White DM, Franks S. Modern use of clomiphene citrate in induction of ovulation. Human Reprod Update. 1997;3:359–65.)

An in-depth discussion of fertility management in PCOS is beyond the scope of this chapter, but endocrinologists should be familiar with basic ovulation induction therapy. If a woman is diagnosed as having anovulatory cycles associated with polycystic ovaries, a detailed semen analysis should first be done to exclude a treatable male factor before ovulation induction is considered. This is particularly important in the light of recent evidence suggesting a link between ovulation induction therapy and long-term risk of developing ovarian cancer. For the same reason, features in the history suggestive of tubal damage, such as previous pelvic infection, should prompt further assessment of tubal patency before treatment is started.

For the majority of women with PCOS, an antiestrogen such as clomiphene citrate is a highly effective first-line treatment and successful in inducing ovulation in over 70–85% of patients. The cumulative conception rate after six cycles of therapy is 67% and continues to rise for up to 12 cycles, provided there are no other fertility factors (**Fig. 26.17**). The usual starting dose of clomiphene is 50mg, taken on days 2–6 of the cycle. In oligomenorrheic women, a 5-day course of progesterone is usually given to promote a withdrawal bleed. Therapy should initially be combined with serial ultrasound follicle tracking (**Fig. 26.18**) to define the minimum threshold dose of clomiphene needed to achieve unifollicular growth. Evidence of successful ovulation should be confirmed with a midluteal progesterone measurement and ultrasound evaluation of endometrial thickness done 7 days after the lead follicle has reached 17mm or greater. It is rarely necessary to induce ovulation with hCG, which should only be given if there is evidence of an unruptured follicle on ultrasound scan. Luteal support with progesterone is not required. Side effects of clomiphene include bloating, mood changes, and depression.

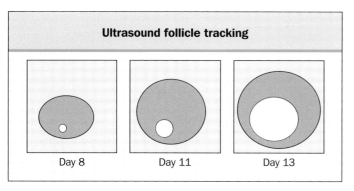

Figure 26.18 Ultrasound follicle tracking. Serial scans are done from day 8 of the cycle to monitor follicular growth.

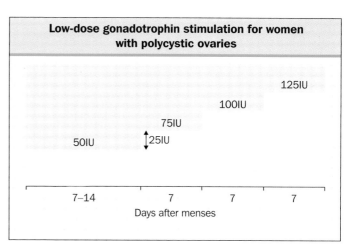

Figure 26.19 Low-dose gonadotropin stimulation for women with polycystic ovaries.

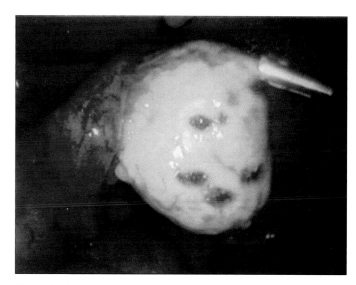

Figure 26.20 Laparoscopic ovarian diathermy.

Since the polycystic ovary contains multiple antral follicles, which are extremely sensitive to stimulation, the principal risks of ovulation induction treatment in PCOS are those of ovarian hyperstimulation syndrome (OHSS) and multiple pregnancy. Protected intercourse should therefore be advised if three or more follicles greater than 15mm in diameter are seen on ultrasound monitoring. A dose of 150mg or more has not been shown to be effective if a patient fails to respond to 100mg and at this stage gonadotropin therapy should be considered. In some women clomiphene has marked antiestrogenic effects on endometrial thickness and cervical mucus and these are other reasons for considering alternative therapy.

In the UK, clomiphene is currently only licensed for 6 months of treatment because of a putative link between its long-term use and the development of ovarian cancer. This relates to a publication in which clomiphene taken for more than 12 months was associated with a higher incidence of ovarian cancer. Since data are limited, and by no means conclusive, and cumulative conception rates continue to rise beyond 6 month's use, we suggest that patients receive full counseling about possible risks if treatment is to be for longer than six cycles. Alternative treatments such as injectable gonadotropins or ovarian diathermy should also be discussed at this stage, although neither are themselves without risks.

Gonadotropin therapy is indicated if a woman fails to ovulate in response to clomiphene, or she ovulates but has a poor endometrial response because of the antiestrogenic effects of the drug. A low-dose stimulation regimen should be used to reduce the risk of ovarian hyperstimulation and multiple pregnancy. We advise a starting dose of 50IU, increased to 75IU if there is no response after 14 days. Thereafter, gonadotropin dose is increased by increments of 25IU every 7 days (**Fig. 26.19**). Human chorionic gonadotropin is given once the lead follicle reaches 17mm. As with clomiphene, ultrasound should be used to monitor follicular growth and hCG should be withheld and protected intercourse advised if three or more follicles of 15mm or greater develop.

Laparoscopic ovarian diathermy (**Fig. 26.20**) is a useful alternative to gonadotropin therapy in women resistant to clomiphene and has been shown to be equally effective. It can be usefully combined with laparoscopic assessment of the pelvis and tubal insufflation. It is unclear why destroying ovarian tissue, even just unilaterally, can restore ovulatory cycles in these women. When spontaneous ovulation is not restored, the sensitivity of the ovary to exogenous gonadotropins appears to be increased.

Metformin has recently been evaluated as an ovulation induction agent and compared to clomiphene. It reduces insulin secretion and hyperandrogenemia and can restore ovulation in some women. The results of a large prospective randomized controlled trial are awaited to determine its true benefit over clomiphene or gonadotropins in an ovulation-induction program.

Long-term health risks

As previously discussed, it is important to ensure that regular shedding of the endometrium takes place in oligomenorrheic women to minimize the risk of developing endometrial carcinoma. PCOS appears to be a significant risk factor for development of type 2 diabetes (and possibly cardiovascular disease) in later life. Obese women with PCOS are at particularly high risk compared with obese normal subjects and lean women with or without PCOS. Diet and exercise and careful counseling about these health risks are an essential part of treatment, whatever the presenting symptoms.

Endocrine causes of anovulation/cycle disturbance	
Hypothalamic	Hypothalamic hypogonadism
Pituitary	Hyperprolactinemia
	Hypopituitarism, e.g. Sheehan's syndrome
Ovarian	Polycystic ovary syndrome
	Primary ovarian failure
Thyroid	Hypothyroidism
	Thyrotoxicosis
Adrenal	Cushing's syndrome
	Congenital adrenal hyperplasia

Table 26.4 Endocrine causes of anovulation/cycle irregularity.

Other endocrine causes of anovulation

Although PCOS is the commonest endocrine cause of anovulation, a number of other causes should be considered (**Table 26.4**). For this reason, evaluation of any woman presenting with anovulation/secondary amenorrhea should include measurement of FSH, LH, prolactin, and an assessment of estradiol production (serum estradiol or a progestogen withdrawal test). Thyroid function tests are also helpful because thyroid dysfunction is commonly found in women with amenorrhea associated with hyperprolactinemia and primary ovarian failure. A pelvic ultrasound scan is useful in defining ovarian morphology.

Hypothalamic disturbances

The pulsatile release of gonadotropin-releasing hormone is essential in maintaining the ovarian cycle. Disruption of GnRH secretion by organic causes of hypothalamic dysfunction (such as tumors or isolated deficiency of GnRH – Kallmann's syndrome) is rare but functional causes are common. Weight loss, excess exercise, and other psychogenic stress factors can have a profound effect on the hypothalamic GnRH pulse generator and lead to a fall in FSH and LH secretion and abolition of ovulatory cycles. These women present with various forms of cycle irregularity but most commonly with amenorrhea. On biochemical evaluation they have low circulating levels of FSH, LH, and estradiol. On scan the ovaries may be small, with very few antral follicles, or may appear multifollicular. Cycle disturbance may persist, even when weight is regained or stressful lifestyle factors are removed. Some women who present with 'hypothalamic amenorrhea' do not have a clearcut history of vigorous exercise, anorexia, or bulimia and often have a normal body mass index at the time of presentation. These are often high achievers, who put little time aside for relaxing and socializing. Before any medical therapy is considered, it is important to address the psychologic issues that may be behind the hypothalamic disturbance.

Management rests on correcting the underlying behavioral risk factors and, provided fertility is not an issue, replacing estrogen to prevent any long-term damage to bone and provide protection from cardiovascular disease. A baseline bone mineral density scan may be warranted in severely underweight, estrogen-deprived women. Some women, particularly if weight is an issue, are reluctant to comply with hormone replacement therapy. Contraception should be discussed as resumption of ovulation may occur during hormone replacement and the combined oral contraceptive may be a better choice if pregnancy is to be avoided. Ovulation induction should only be performed once body mass index is within the normal range ($19–25\text{kg/m}^2$). Clomiphene is rarely successful in the face of hypothalamic amenorrhea with estrogen deficiency. The most physiologic method of ovulation induction is the pulsatile delivery of GnRH by a suitably programmed, small, portable infusion pump. Although somewhat cumbersome, it is associated with normal cumulative conception rates and a lower risk of multiple follicle development than the alternative, i.e. gonadotropin treatment.

Pituitary disorders

Hyperprolactinemia (often due to an autonomous prolactin-secreting tumor) may present as either primary or secondary amenorrhea. Raised prolactin disrupts the normal hypothalamic control of gonadotropin secretion and consequently ovarian production of estrogen and progesterone. Anovulation results and endocrine evaluation confirms a raised prolactin, low FSH, and low estrogen levels. Management of hyperprolactinemia is fully discussed elsewhere (see Chapter 6) but, as a general rule, as long as prolactin levels are normalized by either medical or surgical treatment, regular ovulation and fertility are usually fully restored, provided there are no other coexisting conditions, such as PCOS.

Amenorrhea due to primary pituitary deficiency of gonadotropins is rare and is most commonly associated with more widespread hypopituitarism following pituitary ablative therapy. Other causes include Sheehan's syndrome (postpartum pituitary deficiency) and large pituitary adenomas. Isolated pituitary deficiency of gonadotropins may be found as a complication of multiple blood transfusion for conditions such as thalassemia major. Iron overload appears to affect the gonadotrope selectively within the pituitary.

Ovary

Primary ovarian failure (POF) is common. It accounts for about 50% of cases of primary amenorrhea and 15% of cases of secondary amenorrhea. POF is discussed in detail below.

Thyroid

Hypothyroidism is often accompanied by anovulation, irrespective of whether prolactin levels are raised or not. Menorrhagia is reported in up to 45% of women and is caused by the development of a persistently proliferative endometrium. Amenorrhea is less common.

Menstrual dysfunction is also seen in thyrotoxicosis, with many patients complaining of cycle irregularity and reduced menstrual loss. The precise action of elevated thyroxine levels on the hypothalamo–pituitary–ovarian axis is unknown. What is important is that, despite changes in menstrual pattern, ovulation is often preserved and patients receiving radioiodine treatment must be advised to use contraception.

Adrenal

Elevation of serum testosterone > 5nmol/L in association with cycle disturbance should prompt further testing of adrenal function to exclude Cushing's syndrome or late onset congenital adrenal hyperplasia.

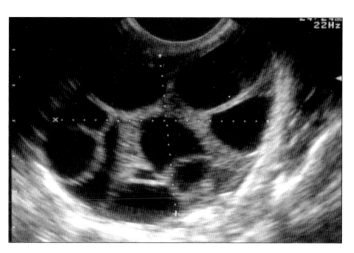

Figure 26.21 Ultrasound picture of an enlarged hyperstimulated ovary.

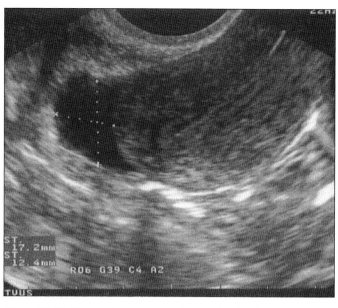

Figure 26.22 Transvaginal ultrasound scan showing free fluid in the pouch of Douglas in a patient with ovarian hyperstimulation.

Ovarian hyperstimulation syndrome

Ovarian hyperstimulation syndrome (OHSS) is a iatrogenic complication of ovulation therapy. It is rare following clomiphene treatment but may complicate gonadotropin ovulation induction regimens or, more commonly, superovulation treatment in *in vitro* fertilization (IVF) cycles. Because of the high proportion of fertility treatments taking place in private units, it is not unusual for patients with OHSS to end up in their local hospital and for endocrinologists and/or gynecologists to be called to advise on management.

Etiology

Although the precise pathogenesis of OHSS is unknown, it is precipitated by luteinization of stimulated follicles by either LH or hCG. There is increasing evidence that cytokines and vasoactive peptides are important mediators. Characteristically the ovaries are enlarged (**Fig. 26.21**) and vascular permeability is increased, resulting in a shift of protein-rich fluid into serous cavities (**Fig. 26.22**).

Clinical presentation

The fluid shift produces ascites and, in more severe cases, pleural and rarely pericardial effusions. There is usually evidence of hemoconcentration (a rising hematocrit) and a fall in intravascular volume, which increases the risk of thrombosis and promotes a fall in blood pressure, central venous pressure, and renal perfusion. Severe OHSS may lead to acute respiratory distress and hepatorenal failure if not treated promptly.

Ovarian hyperstimulation syndrome is classified as mild to severe depending on the size of the ovaries, presence of ascites and pleural effusions, and extent of hemoconcentration (**Table 26.5**). Mild to moderate OHSS has been reported in 4% of ovulation induction cycles and up to 14% of IVF cycles. Severe OHSS is seen in about 1% of all IVF cycles.

Classification of ovarian hyperstimulation syndrome	
Mild	Abdominal bloating, weight gain, mild pain, mild nausea
	On examination, no evidence of ascites or dehydration
	On ultrasound, ovarian volume < 8cm*. No ascites
Moderate	Increasing abdominal discomfort and pain, nausea and vomiting and/or diarrhea
	On examination, abdomen distended but not tense. Ovaries may be tender
	On ultrasound, ovarian volume 8–12cm.* Moderate amount of free fluid
Severe	Marked abdominal distention, shortness of breath
	Clinical ascites ± hydrothorax
	Hemoconcentration (packed cell volume > 50%, white blood count > 15,000/mL)
	Hypovolemia, electrolyte imbalance, oliguria with normal creatinine ± liver dysfunction
	On ultrasound, ovarian volume > 12cm,* marked ascites ± pleural effusions
Critical (rare)	Gross abdominal ascites, hepatorenal failure, pericardial effusions
	Acute respiratory distress
	Thromboembolic phenomena

* Ovarian volume may not correlate with severity of ovarian hyperstimulation syndrome in *in vitro* fertilization cycles because of the effect of follicular aspiration.

Table 26.5 Classification of ovarian hyperstimulation syndrome.
Symptoms vary from mild to severe. This classification is adapted from the 1995 Royal College of Obstetricians and Gynaecologists guidelines.

Risk factors for the development of OHSS include PCOS, low body mass index, previous history of over response to ovarian stimulation, and, most importantly, pregnancy and rising levels of hCG.

Management

This should be essentially supportive, allowing time for spontaneous resolution. However, severe OHSS is potentially life-threatening and is best managed in a high-dependency unit. Clinical examination should include an evaluation of the respiratory system, looking for effusions, and an assessment of the degree of abdominal distention and pain. A pelvic scan should be done of the pelvis and abdomen, to measure the size of the ovaries and extent of ascites and blood taken for hematocrit, urea and electrolytes, and liver function. Daily weight and abdominal girth measurements should be done and fluid balance monitored carefully. In cases of severe OHSS, a central venous pressure line should be put in place.

Analgesia, including opiates, and antiemetics are often required but nonsteroidal anti-inflammatory drugs must not be used as these may precipitate renal failure. Subcutaneous heparin prophylaxis is sensible during hospital admission to minimize the risk of thromboembolism. Intravenous colloid should be administered if urine output falls to below 600mL in 24 hours. Loop diuretics are absolutely contraindicated but, if there is severe oliguria that is not responsive to colloid, dopamine may be used. Ultrasound-guided drainage of ascitic fluid, either transabdominally or transvaginally, may provide symptomatic relief in patients with severe pain from a tense ascites or marked respiratory symptoms.

Premenstrual syndrome

Premenstrual syndrome (PMS) is defined as the cyclic recurrence of physical and psychologic symptoms during the luteal phase of the menstrual cycle. Symptoms may appear up to 14 days before menstruation and disappear as bleeding starts. A wide range of symptoms are reported (**Table 26.6**) and can even vary in an individual woman from cycle to cycle. Tiredness and stress exacerbate symptoms.

Although premenstrual symptoms are experienced by about 90% of menstruating women, 5–10% are severely affected and seek medical help. It is commoner in women over 30 and in those with young children. Stopping the oral contraceptive, sterilization, or recent postnatal illness can precipitate symptoms.

Etiology

The wide variation in symptoms between individuals and even between cycles suggests that a number of different etiologic factors are likely to be involved. The cyclicity of symptoms, restricted to the luteal phase of the cycle, suggests that ovarian steroids have a role to play in etiology. This is further supported by the observation that PMS resolves during pregnancy, after the menopause, and following hysterectomy, provided the ovaries are also removed. However, despite an abundance of theories as to how estrogen or progesterone could be involved, hard evidence is lacking. Recent research suggest that some PMS sufferers have a deficiency in the neurotransmitter serotonin, which makes them more sensitive to cyclic changes in their own hormones.

Physical and psychologic symptoms in premenstrual syndrome	
Physical	**Psychologic**
Weight gain	Mood swings
Abdominal bloating, water retention	Depression
Breast tenderness	Food cravings
Headaches	Irritability
Acne	Clumsiness, poor coordination
Constipation or diarrhea	Insomnia
Backache	Poor concentration
Muscle pain, joint stiffness	Exacerbation of migraine, epilepsy, or asthma

Table 26.6 Physical and psychologic symptoms in premenstrual syndrome.

Management

Lack of a clearcut etiology complicates management. Often, patients need to try several therapies before finding symptomatic relief. Pyridoxine (vitamin B_6), a cofactor for many enzyme reactions, including the biosynthesis of serotonin, has been found to help some PMS sufferers. More recently, selective serotonin reuptake inhibitors (SSRIs) such as fluoxetine or sertraline have been shown to be of therapeutic benefit, particularly where psychologic symptoms such as anxiety are prominent. Some women note an improvement in symptoms if ovulation is suppressed with the combined oral contraceptive but others, possibly because of their increased sensitivity to the progesterone in the pill, find that symptoms worsen. Some women find natural progesterone taken as vaginal or rectal pessaries in the second half of the cycle helpful. Bromocriptine, by inhibiting prolactin, can been used to treat cyclic mastalgia. Attention to diet is also important in PMS and patients should avoid excess alcohol and caffeine and a diet rich in saturated fats or cholesterol.

THE MENOPAUSE

The rapid fall in circulating estrogen levels after the menopause has important short-term and long-term sequelae. Early symptoms include hot flushes and night sweats. These are due to the effect of falling estrogen levels on the thermoregulatory center in the hypothalamus. The body is perceived to have a higher than normal temperature and responds accordingly. Fatigue, poor concentration, depression, and loss of libido are also attributable to the drop in estrogen levels. Many women present at this stage and seek advice on estrogen replacement. While helping to alleviate these symptoms, estrogen replacement confers long-term protection against osteoporosis, cardiovascular disease, urogenital atrophy, and possibly even Alzheimer's disease and colorectal cancer. More studies are, however, required to establish the place of estrogen treatment for these disorders.

Benefits of estrogen and progesterone replacement

Postmenopausal estrogen replacement can reduce cardiovascular morbidity and mortality by up to 50%. This benefit is greatest in women with risk factors such as hypertension, smoking or preexisting heart disease. Estrogen induces several beneficial lipid changes, which are influenced by type of estrogen and route of administration. These include a reduction in LDL cholesterol, which is greater with oral than with transdermal administration, and a rise in high density lipoprotein (HDL) cholesterol, seen only with oral treatment. Triglyceride levels are increased by oral conjugated equine estrogens, unchanged by oral estradiol, and reduced by transdermal estrogens. Progestagens tend to oppose the beneficial effects of estrogens on HDL and triglycerides but this is not significant provided either micronized natural progesterone or medroxyprogesterone acetate are used. With respect to effects on vascular tone, estrogen stimulates nitric oxide production, a potent vasodilator, particularly in atherosclerotic arteries, but inhibits endothelin production, an important vasoconstrictor. Estrogens increase blood flow and women on HRT have a higher cardiac output. Estrogen also has a direct antiatherosclerotic effect and has been shown to reduce the size of atherosclerotic plaques in postmenopausal women. HRT does not have a significant effect on blood pressure in normotensive women. Hypertensive women should have their blood pressure treated before receiving HRT.

Lack of estrogen in postmenopausal women leads an accelerated loss of bone mass, which is effectively reversed by estrogen replacement. Fractures in women over 70 can be life-threatening because of the increased risk of thromboembolism with immobility. A family history of osteoporosis and an early menopause are important risk factors for osteoporosis, which should be considered when weighing up the pros and cons of estrogen replacement.

Management

In a woman with an intact uterus, estrogen should always be prescribed with a progestogen to prevent the development of endometrial hyperplasia. In the first few years after the menopause it is usually necessary to prescribe progestagens in a cyclic manner, 10–12 days in every cycle, to promote regular shedding. As women get older, continuous combined regimens can be successfully introduced. These avoid the need for monthly bleeds and further reduce the risk of developing endometrial cancer.

Controversy remains as to the best route of administration and type of estrogen and progesterone to use. Although a small increase in estrogen-dependent cancers has been noted with HRT, the benefits far outweigh the risks and this needs to be spelled out carefully to patients thinking of starting treatment.

PREMATURE OVARIAN FAILURE

Premature ovarian failure (POF) is defined as menopause occurring at or before the age of 40 and affects 1% of women. Some 10% of patients presenting with secondary amenorrhea will be diagnosed as having POF. Definition with respect to duration of amenorrhea and FSH level is controversial but most series use a cutoff FSH of more than 40IU/L following at least 6 months of amenorrhea. In practical terms, women with primary ovarian failure who present with primary amenorrhea, raised FSH, and pubertal delay should also be included in the definition, as management strategies are similar.

Causes of premature ovarian failure	
Idiopathic	
Iatrogenic	Radiotherapy
	Chemotherapy
	Extensive ovarian surgery
Chromosomal	Turner's syndrome (XO)
	Gene mutations of the X chromosome
	46XY gonadal dysgenesis
Autoimmune	
Viral infection (rare)	

Table 26.7 Causes of premature ovarian failure.

Causes

An identifiable cause for premature ovarian failure can only be identified in about a third of cases (**Table 26.7**).

The improved treatment of cancer, both in children and adults, has led to an increase in the number of women presenting with ovarian failure due to radiotherapy or chemotherapy. In a recent series, radiotherapy accounted for 2% and chemotherapy for 6% of cases of POF. Extensive or repeated ovarian surgery can also lead to a significant reduction in functional ovarian tissue and POF.

Between 2.5% and 13% of women with POF are found to have an abnormal karyotype. Absence of a second X chromosome – XO or Turner's syndrome – leads to premature depletion of oocytes during the first decade of life and typically presents as primary ovarian failure. However some patients have a mosaic karyotype (45XX, 45XO) and present later with POF. Other karyotypic abnormalities associated with POF include small deletions of the short or long arm of the X chromosome and gene mutations on the X chromosome. Although most women with XXX have normal ovarian function, a few will develop POF. A genetic mutation in the FSH receptor has also been identified as a rare cause of POF presenting with primary amenorrhea.

Autoantibodies to the ovary are identified in 1% of cases of POF. The antibodies are targeted against the enzymes involved in ovarian steroid production and ovarian biopsy (which should not be performed routinely) shows plasma cell infiltration around developing follicles. Autoimmune POF is typically seen in association with Addison's disease.

Viral infection in adult life, including mumps, is a rare cause of POF.

Management

The psychologic impact of a diagnosis of POF in a young female cannot be overstated. A diagnosis at, or shortly after, the expected time of puberty can lead to a great deal of confusion over sexuality and may precipitate severe depression. Referral to a clinical psychologist or counselor trained to deal with some of the difficult issues, such as childbearing, is mandatory. Patients should be strongly encouraged to start hormone replacement therapy and continue with it at least until the normal age of menopause to prevent some of the long-term sequelae of

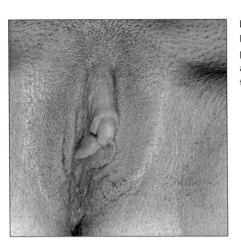

Figure 26.23 Enlarged clitoris in a patient with an androgen-secreting tumor.

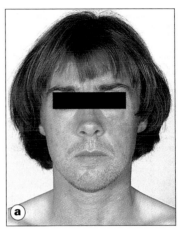

Figure 26.24 A patient with an arrhenoblastoma with associated polycystic ovaries before and after treatment. Before treatment (a), the patient had marked facial hirsutism. In (b) the patient is shown successfully treated. The tumor was resected and ovulation ensued with clomiphene and human chorionic gonadotropin therapy.

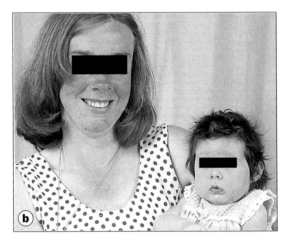

estrogen deprivation. A baseline bone mineral density scan is advisable, particularly in young, thin women, to identify those patients who may need higher-dose estrogen supplementation or additional treatment to prevent bone loss. The issue of whether women with POF on HRT should have regular mammograms is controversial, as most data on possible increased risk of breast cancer refer to older women on HRT.

For the vast majority of these women, their only hope of having children rests with oocyte donation as part of an IVF program. Recent work on maturation of primordial follicles *in vitro* may provide a therapeutic avenue in the future for women with a family history of POF or those about to undergo chemotherapy or radiotherapy. Although rare, spontaneous pregnancy can occur. In a review of all publications relating to pregnancy in women diagnosed as having POF, 6.3% conceived either spontaneously or following ovulation induction. The balance of opinion is that there is no justification for inducing ovulation in hypergonadotropic women with POF.

ENDOCRINE TUMORS OF THE OVARY

These are very rare but must be considered in any woman who presents with rapid onset of hirsutism or virilization (**Fig. 26.23**) or evidence of hyperestrogenism. Fewer than 1% of ovarian tumors are endocrine-secreting ovarian tumors. They are classified in two groups:

Sex-cord stromal cell tumors

These include Sertoli–Leydig cell and Leydig cell tumors, granulosa cell tumors, and thecomas. The Sertoli–Leydig and Leydig cell tumors are the most common androgen-secreting tumors of the ovary. The majority of Sertoli-Leydig tumors arise in women

aged between 20 and 40. They are usually large enough to be palpable, unilateral, and benign in 90% of cases. Leydig cell tumors tend to occur in peri- or postmenopausal women. They are usually small, unilateral, and benign. Clinically, symptoms of hirsutism and virilization develop over months rather than years and serum testosterone is usually greater than 5nmol/L. Granulosa cell tumors are much rarer. They produce excess estrogen and may present with abnormal bleeding or endometrial hyperplasia.

Adrenal-like tumors of the ovary

These are very rare and include luteomas, virilizing lipoid cell tumors, hypernephromas, and adrenal rest tumors. Over 50% are associated with cushingoid features.

With all functional tumors of the ovary, surgical removal leads to a rapid improvement in symptoms (**Fig. 26.24**).

FURTHER READING

Adams J, Polson DW, Franks S. Prevalence of polycystic ovaries in women with anovulation and idiopathic hirsutism. Br Med J. 1986;293:355–9.

Anast JN. Premature ovarian failure: an update. Fertil Steril. 1998:70:1–5.

Armar NA, McGarrigle HH, Honour J, Holownia P, Jacobs HS, Lachelin GC. Laparoscopic ovarian diathermy in the management of anovulatory infertility in women with polycystic ovaries: endocrine changes and clinical outcome. Fertil Steril. 1990;53:45–9.

Balen AH. Anovulatory infertility and ovulation induction – recommendations for good clinical practice. J Br Fertil Soc. 1997;2:83–7.

Balen AH, Jacobs HS. A prospective study comparing unilateral and bilateral laparoscopic ovarian diathermy in women with the polycystic ovary syndrome. Fertil Steril. 1994;62:921–5.

Balen AH, Conway GS, Kaltas G, et al. Polycystic ovary syndrome: the spectrum of the disorder in 1741 patients. Human Reprod. 1995;10:2107–11.

Barth JH, Cherry CA, Wojnarowska F and Dawber RPR. Cyproterone acetate for severe hirsutism: results of a double-blind dose-ranging study. Clin Endocrinol. 1991;35:5–10.

Bunker CB, Newton JA, Kilborn J, Patel A, Conway GS. Most women with acne have polycystic ovaries. Br J Dermatol. 1989;121:675–80.

Conway GS, Honour JW, Jacobs HS. Heterogeneity of the polycystic ovary syndrome: clinical, endocrine and ultrasound features in 556 patients. Clin Endocrinol. 1989;30:459–70.

Conway GS. Premature ovarian failure. Curr Opin Obstet Gynecol. 1997;9:202–8.

Crook D. Postmenopausal hormone replacement therapy, lipoprotein metabolism and coronary heart disease. J Cardiovasc Pharmacol. 1996;28(suppl. 5):S40–5.

Franks S, Gharani N, Waterworth D, et al. The genetic basis of polycystic ovary syndrome. Human Reprod. 1997;12:2641–8.

Kousta A, White DM, Franks S. Modern use of clomiphene citrate in induction of ovulation. Human Reprod Update 1997;3:359–65.

Nugent D, Salha O, Balen AH, Rutherford AJ. Ovarian neoplasia and subfertility treatments. Br J Obstet Gynaecol. 1998;105:584–91.

O'Driscoll JB, Mamtora H, Higginson J, Pollock A, Kane J and Anderson DC. A prospective study of the prevalence of clear-cut endocrine disorders and polycystic ovaries in 350 patients presenting with hirsutism or androgenic alopecia. Clin Endocrinol. 1994;41:231–36.

Van Kasteren YM, Schoemaker J. Premature ovarian failure: a systematic review on therapeutic interventions to restore ovarian function and achieve pregnancy. Hum Reprod. 1999;5:483–92.

Chapter 27 Hormone Assay Techniques

Raymond Edwards

INTRODUCTION

Hormones have been measured by many different types of method. From an analytic perspective, they are a disparate group of molecular species with differing structures and chemical properties. Any review of prominent developments in hormone assays would reveal a wide spectrum of methods, reflecting, in part, the diverse nature of the substances to be assayed but also the change in emphasis from methods measuring function (bioassays) to those based more on chemical structure. **Table 27.1** illustrates an example for a small-molecular-size hormone, progesterone, with a known chemical structure. **Table 27.2** shows an example for a larger molecule, thyroid-stimulating hormone (TSH), principally defined by biologic function. These two categories, those that measure biologic function and those that respond to an aspect of molecular structure, provide the basis for simple classification (**Fig. 27.1**).

Bioassays

In principle, a bioassay is the estimation of the nature (constitution) or potency of a substance by means of the reaction that follows its application to living material. Bioassays performed *in vivo* are not used for routine clinical analyses. Bioassays *in vitro*, which use either tissue, organ slices, dissociated target cells or cell fragments, can be more practical in terms of routine work, provided suitable cell lines are available and long-term culture is possible. In some cases the isolated cell may lose some of its function in either a discrete or gradual manner.

In general, the final detection or end points for bioassays are based on gravimetric, histologic, or biochemical measurements.

Measurement of progesterone: historical perspective	
1929	Growth of glandular components in uterine epithelium of rabbits	Bioassay *in vivo*; could detect 1mg
1942	UV absorption at 240nm to measure 3-keto-4-ene structure	Physicochemical test
1947	Hypertrophy of stromal nuclei in endometrium of ovariectomized mice	Bioassay *in vivo*
1957	Increase in carbonic anhydrase activity in endometrium of immature rabbits	Bioassay *in vivo*
1960	Specific fluorescence of enzyme-converted derivatives	Physicochemical test
1963	Radioisotope derivatives using either ^{35}S or ^{3}H	Physicochemical test
1964	Competitive protein binding assay using radioisotope ^{3}H	Binding protein assay
1965	Dual isotope derivatives using ^{3}H and ^{14}C or ^{35}S and ^{14}C	Physicochemical test
1979	Direct radioimmunoassay	Immunoassay; could detect 5pg

Table 27.1 Measurement of progesterone: historical perspective.

Measurement of thyroid-stimulating hormone: historical perspective	
1932	Starved guinea pigs; histologic changes in excised thyroids	Bioassay *in vivo*; could detect 12mU
1942	Weight changes in starved tadpoles	Bioassay *in vivo*
1953	Iodine-131 uptake by thyroids from iodocasein-treated mice	Bioassay *in vivo*
1958	Release of ^{131}I-labeled protein-bound iodine from guinea pig thyroid slices	Bioassay *in vitro*
1965	Radioimmunoassay; sensitivity capable of measuring thyroid-stimulating hormone in 50% of euthyroids	Immunoassay
1974	Penetration of lysosomal membranes, from thyroid slices, by dye using microdensitometry	Bioassay *in vitro*
1984	Immunoradiometric assay	Immunoassay; could detect 4nU

Table 27.2 Measurement of thyroid-stimulating hormone: historical perspective.

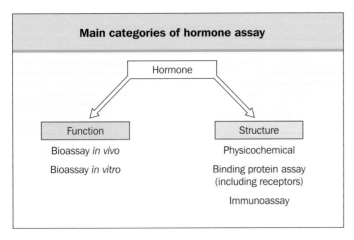

Figure 27.1 Main categories of hormone assay.

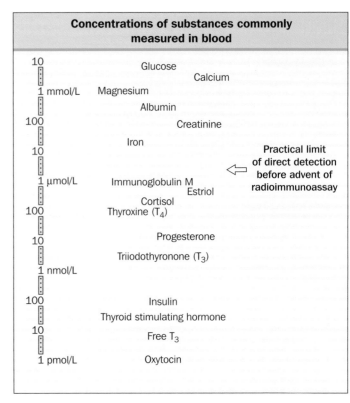

Figure 27.2 Concentrations of substances commonly measured in blood. These are plotted in sequence depending on normal circulating concentrations. The lower limit of direct detection before radio-immunoassay was between 1 and 10µmol/L.

The advantage of a bioassay is that it only responds to biologically active substances and not to inactive but structurally similar material. The main disadvantage is inconsistency. The assumption that living material behaves in a consistent way is, in many circumstances, not true. Variability in bioassays arises from a number of general factors but in particular:

- hereditary variability in both individuals and species;
- route of administration;
- frequency of administration;
- distribution between bodily compartments;
- metabolism;
- rate of excretion.

In addition, more specific factors can contribute, such as:

- age;
- weight;
- sex;
- associated pathologies.

Hereditary variation is minimized by using purebred strains or specified cell lines. Individual variation is reduced by combining data from a group. Bioassays still play an important role in establishing primary calibration. They are used to assign a definitive value for reference purposes.

Physicochemical methods

Greater conformity of results is found in physicochemical assays. However they are more insensitive in general. Specificity is usually enhanced by extraction, in some cases by organic solvents, and then purification, commonly by some form of chromatography. These steps allow for a degree of concentration of the analyte and thus can compensate for a lack of sensitivity. The final step would be measurement of a key physicochemical parameter, e.g. fluorescence of the D4 steroid structure in progesterone.

IMMUNOASSAYS

The development of immunoassay was a milestone for the quantitative analysis of hormones. The potential seen by endocrinologists in this novel technique was undoubtedly considerable and application led to an exponential growth in understanding of the principles underlying clinical endocrinology. Its advantages were completely expedient in terms of the

requirements for measuring physiologic levels of hormones in blood, which before that time was impractical. They can be summarized as follows:

- sensitivity;
- specificity;
- simplicity;
- comprehensive application.

The increase in sensitivity was considerable, possibly in the order of 10^5 in molar terms. Up to this time, direct detection of hormones in blood was well below the sensitivity of methods then available. Immunoassay appeared to extend this range from millimoles per liter to picomoles per liter, thus opening a window for direct observation and quantification (**Fig. 27.2**). The superior specificity of immunoassays is a consequence of the uniqueness of the chemical sequence of the binding site of the antibody (the epitope), the principal reagent. An antibody, by virtue of its exclusive antigen-binding site, can discriminate very effectively between two closely related chemical structures (**Fig. 27.3**). The simplicity of immunoassays, in terms of handling large numbers of samples, is a direct consequence of both enhanced sensitivity and improved specificity. It became possible to measure almost any hormone directly in small samples of blood or tissue fluids. Because the complex work of extracting and purifying samples was no longer necessary, it was possible to process many samples at a time. This increase in throughput was obviously necessary to effectively study changing levels of hormones in both normal physiology and pathology.

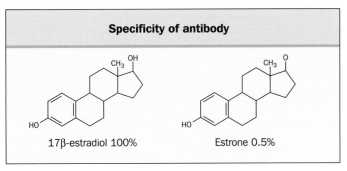

Figure 27.3 Specificity of antibody. An antiserum raised against 17β-estradiol crossreacted with estrone, a closely related structure, with a potency of 0.5%.

Details of the radioimmunoassay method (RIA) were published in 1960. Although earlier immunoassays, e.g. using red blood cells and subsequent hemagglutination, were similar in principle, the use of a radioisotope proved a major advance. Development of radioimmunoassays was initiated in the mid-1950s. At this time, work was proceeding in two centers, one in London and the other in New York.

In New York, Solomon Berson and Rosalyn Yalow were investigating the metabolic fate of intravenously administered ^{131}I-labeled insulin at the Veterans Administration Hospital. Their studies showed that, although the insulin disappeared rapidly from the blood of normal subjects, it persisted for a longer period in the bloodstream of patients who had received insulin therapy for more than a few weeks. This proved to be because of the presence of antibodies to insulin in those patients receiving therapy. Their initial studies demonstrated that the binding of the ^{131}I-insulin to antibody was inhibited in a quantitative manner by the presence of unlabeled insulin. These simple findings were to be the basis of their method, now familiar as RIA.

At the other center, the radioisotope unit of the Middlesex Hospital Medical School, Roger Ekins was working on a new theory for the measurement of endogenous hormones at levels consistent with those found in blood. Monitoring the radioactivity in serum from a patient with metastatic thyroid carcinoma, he found that some of the iodine-131 administered to the patient had been incorporated into thyroxine *in vivo*. Using this radiolabeled thyroxine and thyroxine-binding globulin as a high-affinity binding reagent, he demonstrated the measurement of thyroxine. The technique, which he called saturation analysis, was a general procedure utilizing a specific binding protein and thus included all immunoassays. Attempting to optimize sensitivity and precision in radiolabeled immunoassays led Miles and Hales in 1968 to formulate the principles of assays using radiolabeled antibodies, referred to as 'immunoradiometric' assays (IRMA). The use of highly purified antibodies coupled to a radioactive tracer increased sensitivity and improved precision. Subsequent developments, in 1970, incorporating an additional antibody coupled to a particle or other solid-phase, and referred to as the 'two-site' IRMA or 'sandwich' assay, further improved precision and hence sensitivity. The exponential growth in application of radiolabeled-immunoassays established radiolabeled-immunoassays as the dominant analytic method in endocrinology.

Principles of immunoassays

The historical development of immunoassays began at the end of the last century (**Table 27.3**). In 1917 Landsteiner published work which was to have a most significant application in the subsequent development of immunoassays. Essentially he described the techniques which enabled the production of antibodies to nonimmunogenic molecules. Small molecules could be coupled to weakly immunogenic proteins such as albumin and then injected into animals such as rabbits leading to the production of antibodies. These had binding attributes with specificity for the non-immunogenic part of the conjugate. This

Table 27.3 Historical development of immunoassays.

Historical development of immunoassays

Date	Authors	Subject
1890s	Krause	Reaction of soluble antigen and antiserum
1903	Uhlenhuth	Improved sensitivity of precipitin reaction
1905	Bechold	Analysis of individual antigen–antiserum reactions in complex mixtures by applying diffusion in gel techniques
1917	Landsteiner	'Artificial Conjugated Antigen', later to be described as hapten
1929	Heidelberger and Kendall	Quantitative immunochemical method using precipitin reaction
1941	Coons	Labeling antibody with fluorophore
1946	Oudin	Immunologic analysis by tube diffusion method in agar gel using simple and double diffusion
1947	Ouchterlony	Formation of immune precipitate in gel plates using simple diffusion in two dimensions and double diffusion in one and two dimensions
1954	Stavitsky and Arquila	Quantitative immunoassay using hemagglutination
1960	Ekins; Berson and Yalow	Radioimmunoassay (RIA)
1967	Wide; Miles and Hales	Radiolabeled antibody technique, i.e. immunoradiometric assay (IRMA)
1968	Haberman; Wide; Addison and Hales	Two-site IRMA. Use of two different antibodies to enhance specificity
1976	Kohler and Milstein	Monoclonal antibody; production of antibodies with monospecificity and potentially inexhaustible supply *in vitro*

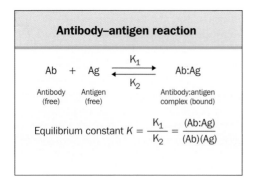

Figure 27.4 Antibody–antigen reaction. The reaction between antibody (AB) and antigen (Ag) is reversible. At equilibrium the proportion of free (unbound) and bound complex is a reflection of the affinity constant, K. The higher the value of K, the more the amount of complex. Antibodies have very high K values.

'artificial conjugated antigen' was an important demonstration of the key 'hapten' principle, later to prove invaluable in raising antibodies to an extensive range of small molecules used in many immunodiagnostic tests.

The need for purified antibodies with monospecific binding sites was fulfilled by the advances in monoclonal antibody production following the publication of Kohler and Milstein in 1976. In recent years the main developments have been in the proliferation of different types of label or detection system. All immunoassays are based on the reaction between antibody and antigen (**Fig. 27.4**). A fixed concentration of antibody reacts with varying concentrations of antigen to form antibody–antigen complexes ('bound' antigen). The reaction is reversible and eventually reaches equilibrium. The proportion of concentrations at equilibrium is described by a constant, K. There is an optimal K value for the measurement of any given concentration of antigen. It is generally recognized that, as the target analyte concentration decreases, so the optimal K value needs to increase.

There are two main types of immunoassay:
- Antibody in limiting concentration (i.e. less than comparative concentrations of antigen), often referred to as competitive, e.g. RIA. General term is immunoassay.
- Antibody concentration in excess, e.g. IRMA. General term is immunometric assay.

Immunoassay or competitive binding test

When a fixed but limited concentration of antibody reacts with increasing concentrations of antigen, there is an increasing amount of antigen in the free fraction (not bound to antibody) and a correspondingly lower percentage bound (**Fig. 27.5**). The distribution between bound and free fractions is monitored by the addition of a trace amount of labeled antigen. This is measured after separating one fraction from the other, e.g. by precipitation of the antibody protein (**Fig. 27.6**). Values for samples

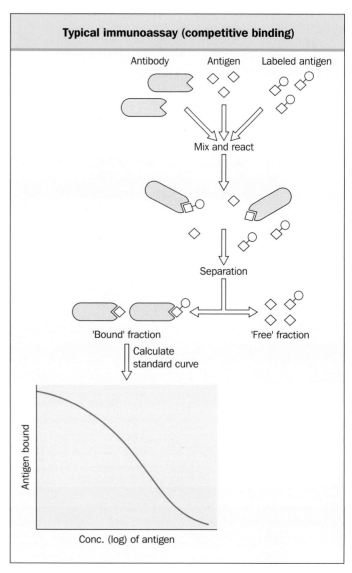

Figure 27.6 Typical immunoassay (competitive binding). The critical components and steps are shown. The decreasing proportion of bound labeled antigen with increasing concentrations of analyte is plotted as a typical standard curve.

Figure 27.5 Principle of immunoassay. A fixed and limited concentration of antibody reacts with varying concentrations of antigen (analyte) giving rise to saturation of the antibody binding site and decreasing proportions of bound analyte, i.e. (i) 50%, (ii) 25%, and (iii) 12.5%.

are read off from a standard curve, derived from the responses of a range of calibrants with known concentrations. Most small molecules, such as the thyronine hormones (T_4 and T_3) or steroid hormones (cortisol, progesterone, etc.), are measured in this way.

Immunometric assay or labeled antibody test

This type of immunoassay follows more conventional analytic procedures in which the specific reagent is used in relative excess to the concentration of analyte. When a fixed but essentially unlimited concentration of antibody reacts with increasing amounts of antigen, a progressively greater proportion of the antibody is bound (**Fig. 27.7**). The proportion of antibody bound is monitored through the attached label, following separation from the unreacted or free fraction. Values for samples are read off from a standard curve, derived from the responses of a range of calibrants with known concentrations.

There are two basic procedures for separating bound antibody from the free fraction. The addition of exogenous antigen linked to a solid phase serves to bind the unreacted antibody. This can be separated by removing the solid-phase reagent from the reaction (**Fig. 27.8**). Because antibodies are often bivalent, this method requires careful optimization.

A second type, usually referred to as a 'two-site' or 'sandwich' assay, uses an additional antibody with a binding site directed to a second epitope on the antigen not already occupied by the first antibody. In this method, one antibody is linked to a solid phase to provide effective separation and the other carries the label for measurement (**Fig. 27.9**). The two-site immunometric assays can only be used to measure molecules with at least two epitopes and large enough for binding of two antibodies, to avoid interaction of the two bound antibodies (steric hindrance). In practice, this means a minimum molecular size of approximately 2500Da. Many current immunometric assays used in clinical endocrinology are based on the two-site design. Sensitivity is improved as a function of the combined effects of two affinity constants. Also they have enhanced specificity because two separate and specific epitopes are required before a response is

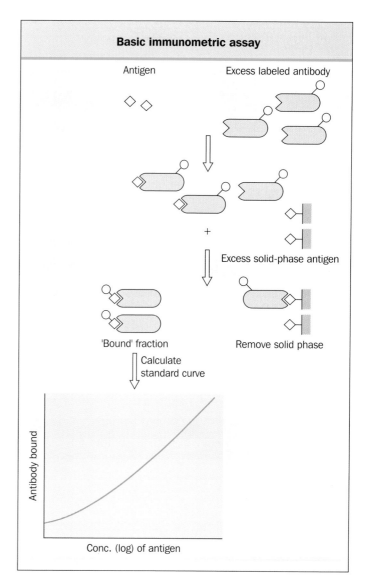

Figure 27.8 Basic immunometric assay. The figure shows the separation of unreacted labeled antibody from the bound fraction by solid-phase antigen. This type of assay gives a conventional dose–response relationship (standard curve).

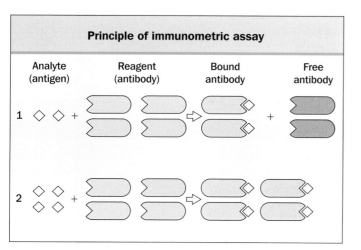

Figure 27.7 Principle of immunometric assay. A fixed concentration in excess of antibody reacts with increasing amounts of antigen, giving rise to increasing proportions of bound antibody.

generated. The successful routine measurement of many peptide hormones (e.g. adrenocorticotropic hormone, ACTH and parathyroid hormone, PTH) depended critically on the development of the two-site assay. It was particularly decisive in elucidating the role of PTH and in deriving unequivocal diagnostic reference ranges. PTH, a peptide with a sequence of 98 amino acids, is cleaved into two fragments following its secretion into the blood and both or either may react with an antibody. However the whole molecular sequence is important for full biologic activity and corresponding diagnostic significance. Because the metabolic clearance rates for the fragments differ from that of the whole molecule, concentrations of all immunoreactive material do not necessarily reflect the concentration of the whole molecule. In these cases inaccurate values are likely when using only one antibody and early RIAs for PTH gave equivocal results. This situation was resolved with the introduction of a two-site IRMA based

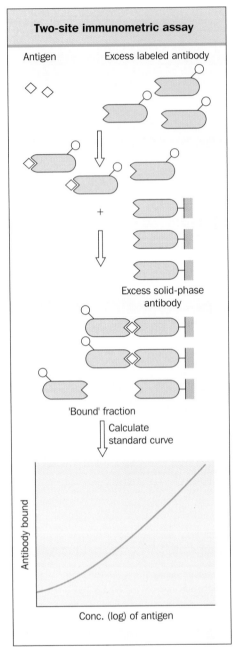

Two-site immunometric assay

Antigen   Excess labeled antibody

+

Excess solid-phase antibody

'Bound' fraction

Calculate standard curve

Antibody bound

Conc. (log) of antigen

Figure 27.9 Two-site immunometric assay. Two antibodies directed against different epitopes are used; one is attached to a solid phase for separation and the other carries the label for detection. The combination of two binding sites increases discrimination, leading to assays with better specificity and precision.

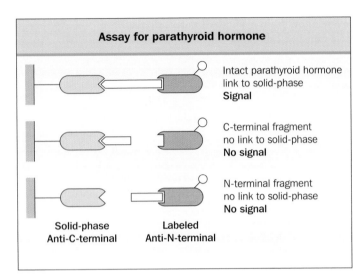

Assay for parathyroid hormone

Intact parathyroid hormone link to solid-phase **Signal**

C-terminal fragment no link to solid-phase **No signal**

N-terminal fragment no link to solid-phase **No signal**

Solid-phase   Labeled
Anti-C-terminal   Anti-N-terminal

Figure 27.10 Assay for parathyroid hormone. The principle of two-site immunometric assay is applied to the measurement of a peptide hormone in the presence of biologically inactive fragments, e.g. parathyroid hormone. The biologically active whole molecule generates a signal, whereas the inactive N- and C-terminal fragments do not.

contains specified antibodies, is referred to as antiserum. All antibodies have the same basic structure of four polypeptide chains: two identical 'light' chains and two identical 'heavy' chains, linked together by disulfide bonds in a distinctive Y conformation (**Fig. 27.11**). Essentially they are bivalent, with two identical binding sites.

Techniques for production of antibodies are:

- immunization for polyclonal antisera;
- culture of monoclonal antibodies;
- genetic engineering.

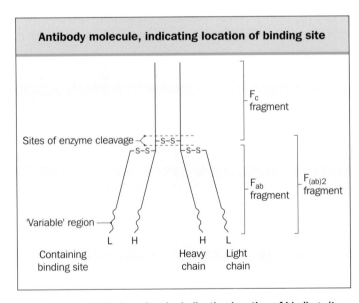

Antibody molecule, indicating location of binding site

F_c fragment

Sites of enzyme cleavage — S–S

F_{ab} fragment

$F_{(ab)2}$ fragment

'Variable' region

Containing binding site

L   H   H   L

Heavy chain   Light chain

Figure 27.11 Antibody molecule, indicating location of binding site. The f_{ab}, f_{ab2} and f_c fragments are made by enzyme hydrolysis at the cleavage sites.

on two antibodies, one specific for the C-terminal portion of the full peptide and the other for the N-terminal sequence (**Fig. 27.10**).

Components

There are three critical components in all immunoassays:

- antibody;
- labeled reagent (either antigen or antibody);
- assay standard.

Antibody

Antibodies or immunoglobulins, a heterogeneous group of glyco-proteins present in the serum and tissues, are produced as part of the immune response by B-cell lymphocytes. Serum, when it

Sera taken from animals immunized with specific immunogens contain antibodies derived from a number of different stimulated lymphocyte clones. They are referred to as polyclonal antisera and contain different antibodies with a variety of specificities. Antibodies produced by hyperimmunization are predominantly IgG, occasionally with IgM. IgM antibodies are often less stable.

Monospecific antibodies can be produced by monoclonal antibody production. The method of Kohler and Milstein was to fuse hyperimmunized lymphocyte cell homogenates with β-cell myelomas. The fused hybridomas were cloned and cultured in selective media to remove unfused cells of either type. Cultures from a single clone produce monospecific antibodies of one type called monoclonal. Monoclonal antibodies are easy to purify from culture medium. Purified antibodies are necessary for a number of purposes, especially labeling.

Labeled reagent

The use of an appropriately sensitive labeled reagent is important in realizing the full potential of the antibody as an analytic tool. The labels used in current endocrine tests are:

- radioisotopes, especially iodine-125, tritium, or cobalt-57;
- enzymes with colorimetric detection, typically peroxidase or phosphatase;
- enzymes with chemiluminescent detection;
- fluorophores with time-resolved emission;
- enzymes with amplification substance cycling, i.e. amplified enzyme detection.

Time-resolved fluorescence and amplified enzyme detection are inherently more sensitive. However antibody affinity is the main constraint on analytic sensitivity. The choice of a particular label is unlikely to confer any advantage in terms of sensitivity when used with most commonly used antibodies. Selection of a label is frequently an aspect of automation and associated technology. All of the listed labels can be used to measure concentrations as low as fmol/L (femtomoles per liter, 10^{-12}mol/L).

Assay standard

An assay or working standard should behave in an identical manner to the sample. In the first place this means that the added exogenous analyte should be in a form which is identical to that found in the sample. Secondly the matrix should be similar in composition. These criteria are met for most assays.

Reference calibrant or standard

The use of a common material to calibrate an analytic response is fundamental to pooling of data, common interpretation of results, and sharing of clinical experience. These in turn have been important in establishing common reference ranges, particularly in cases of rare or infrequent pathologies. Unfortunately the crucial role of the standard material can often be overlooked.

Ehrlich first introduced the concept of standardization for biologic materials in the late 19th century. Working with diphtheria antitoxin, he defined the potency of each batch in terms of standard units. The issue was first addressed internationally in

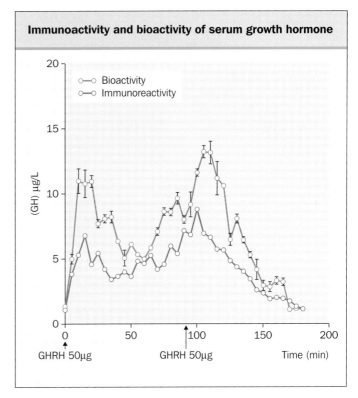

Figure 27.12 Immunoactivity and bioactivity of serum growth hormone. Growth hormone (GH) was measured by immunoassay and bioassay in blood samples taken every 5min from a patient given injections of growth-hormone-releasing hormone (GHRH). These results indicate the varying proportions of different isoforms that have different potencies in the two types of analysis.

1921 by the health committee of the League of Nations, the forerunner of the United Nations.

Potency was originally defined in terms of biologic response. For example, digitalis preparations were assessed by frog units, defined as the lethal dose corrected for weight, i.e. the amount required to kill 1g of frog. Results were highly variable, because of the susceptibility of frogs not the potency of the material. A key change was to define potency by comparison with a standard material, which was either pure or selected as representative. For effective use, a standard needs to be prepared in a dry state and protected from damaging effects of light, moisture, and oxygen.

Many standards are recognized internationally under the auspices of the World Health Organization. These international standards (IS, formerly referred to as IRP) have been prepared by organizations like the UK National Institute of Biological Standards and Controls and are used as primary standards to calibrate the batches of working standards used in various methods.

Occasionally a change of IS can affect calibration because of a bias to the previous standard, e.g. the introduction of IS 80/505 for growth hormone increased results by approximately 20%. Fortunately, this is very rare.

OTHER METHODS – HIGH-PRESSURE LIQUID CHROMATOGRAPHY AND GAS CHROMATOGRAPHY/MASS SPECTROMETRY

Immunoassay technology is the dominant, and in many centers exclusive, analytic procedure for clinical diagnosis in endocrinology. However there are a few cases where other techniques are necessary. These are usually limited to specialist or referral centers. The main reasons for the use of alternative techniques are:

- the lack of specificity in available antibodies;
- the need to generate an analytic profile of a number of chemically related hormones and their metabolites;
- the need to identify small quantities of a unique molecular variant in the presence of relatively large concentrations of the dominant molecule.

The catecholamines – dopamine, epinephrine and norepinephrine – are best measured by HPLC (high-pressure liquid chromatography), using reverse phase and electron detection. Attempts to raise appropriate antibodies have been unsuccessful and the clinically significant concentrations of catecholamines are high enough for chemical detection for samples of urine. Serum samples require concentration by a factor of about 10 following extraction.

Analysis of steroids in neonates and young children presents particular problems and immunoassays are generally not suitable. A steroid profile will give definitive results in certain cases, especially involving adrenal pathology in neonates. Samples, usually urine, are initially extracted on to a solid phase. This is followed by a number of steps, including enzyme hydrolysis of conjugates, formation of derivatives, separation of steroids by gas chromatography using capillary columns and detection by mass spectrometry. Mass spectrometry gives additional information helping to confirm identity.

HETEROGENEITY OF HORMONES

Heterogeneity in biologically active molecules is a challenge to accurate analysis and diagnostic interpretation. Molecular structure and biologic activity are intimately linked but can vary disproportionately. A small change in molecular structure can have a large effect on biologic activity without a significant change in analytic result.

Many protein hormones are intrinsically heterogeneous, circulating in a number of biologically active forms. Forms that share common epitopes and thus can be potentially detected in immunoassays are:

- **precursors or prohormones**, e.g. pro-opio-melanocorticotropin as precursor for ACTH;
- **isoforms**, e.g. glycosylation variants, especially variations in sialic acid residues;
- **fragments**, e.g. degradation by enzyme hydrolysis including N-terminal and C-terminal peptide fragments;
- **subunits**, e.g. α and β subunits of thyroid-stimulating hormone (TSH), luteinizing hormone (LH), follicle-stimulating hormone (FSH) and human chorionic gonadotropin (hCG);
- **genetic variants** from point mutations;
- **complexes**, including aggregation and dimerization.

Glycosylation of proteins usually increases their effective potency as hormones by prolonging their presence in the circulation by reducing their metabolic clearance rate. Antibodies generally bind whether or not the hormone is glycosylated. Variable glycosylation, therefore, has little effect on immunoassays but may affect biologic activities considerably and this may lead to misinterpretation of the biologic significance of an immunoassayed hormone. Because the glycoprotein hormones, TSH, LH, FSH and TSH, share a common α subunit, some degree of crossreactivity is a potential problem. There is greater homology between LH and hCG. Many early immunoassays for LH showed significant crossreaction with hCG. However, in practice this did not cause difficulties with interpretation; on the contrary, it served to monitor for high levels of hCG from tumors at the same time as measuring LH. Using monospecific monoclonal antibodies, two-site immunometric assays can be optimized to eliminate any significant crossreaction with hCG.

Heterogeneity in growth hormone has been well studied. The dominant form of growth hormone circulating in blood is 22kDa, but the proportion can change significantly, particularly following stimulation. Biologic activity, as assessed by bioassay using cells, varies differently from immunoreactivity, which reflects structure (**Fig. 27.12**). Different immunoassays also respond differently, presumably because the antibodies react with different epitopes.

PROBLEMS FOR CLINICAL INTERPRETATION

The use of monospecific antibodies has had some unforeseen consequences. A few immunometric assays have failed to measure a particular genetic variant of LH, which nevertheless is biologically active. This variant arises from a point mutation, allowing for a new site of glycosylation. It seems that the glycosidic residue blocks a critical epitope. For homozygotes, LH is undetectable and is reduced by 30–50% in heterozygotes. The possibility of enhanced specificity compromising detection, particularly of hormones where a degree of heterogeneity exists, remains to be resolved.

There are inherent difficulties in assaying steroid hormones. Many closely related crossreacting compounds circulate with the bioactive molecule. In addition, plasma binding proteins would prevent the antigen reacting with the antibody. Originally, samples were extracted with organic solvents, removing the binding proteins, and if necessary chromatographed to purify from significant amounts of crossreacting material. Recently, many steroids have been measured by direct assays, i.e. samples are measured directly without any pretreatment such as extraction. Specific chemicals are added to the assay medium to block the binding sites on plasma proteins. However in many assays these blocking agents will not totally remove the interference. For example, variations in sex-hormone-binding globulin concentrations are known to affect the results of some direct assays for testosterone. The presence of unusual binding proteins or large changes in binding protein concentration may require a more cautious approach to interpretation. This also applies to the measurement of free hormones, i.e. the fraction of hormone not bound by specific proteins and considered to be more relevant to bioactivity. Thyroid activity is often assessed by free thyroxine (T_4) and free triiodothyronine (T_3) assays. Depending on assay design, results can be influenced by binding proteins, particularly the aberrant albumin found in familial dysalbuminemia. This form of albumin has a very high binding affinity for T_4.

Where results for a particular analyte differ widely between laboratories, comparison of clinical practice is more difficult. Cortisol immunoassays still show considerable variation between different assays. Comparison with mass spectrometry suggests that most immunoassays for cortisol overestimate results. For urinary cortisol, this can be twofold.

There are a number of substances in plasma that can interfere with antibody binding. If they are present at high concentrations, results might be misleading. The following present potential problems in immunometric assays:

- rheumatoid factors, i.e. immunoglobulins that react with other immunoglobulins;
- heterophilic antibodies – antibodies that crossreact with animal immunoglobulins, e.g. those used in the assay;
- specific antimouse antibodies, which often arise in patients injected with monoclonal antibodies, either for imaging or treatment.

AUTOMATION AND POINT-OF-CARE TESTING

Cost-effective clinical practice demands efficient analytic techniques, in terms not just of accuracy but also of high throughput and rapid response time. The advent of high precision automation has done much to improve these aspects. However the production by one manufacturer of both equipment and reagents has reduced flexibility. Most automated immunoassay analyzers have fully integrated reagent systems, where all reagents are supplied by one manufacturer. Frequently they are not all of a common high standard and, in these systems, an assay with poor performance cannot be substituted with another. There is a need for greater flexibility.

Fully optimized and sophisticated analyzers, in which all variables are strictly controlled, can generate results without the need for a high level of technical expertise or experience. This means that samples can be analyzed outside laboratories; nearer the patient or, more importantly, nearer the person responsible for care (point-of-care testing). Laboratories have responsibility for quality of results, response time, and cost, and these are usually well defined and controlled. However the major effect of a poor analytic service is on clinical management, where the costs, particularly the full financial consequences, are very difficult to assess. As these factors are clarified, there will be a greater incentive for more of the responsibility to become part of clinical management. Point-of-care systems should generally be restricted to analysis of a single analyte, in order to maximize control of variables. There are a few examples of point-of care testing in diabetic clinics, e.g. automated analyzers for HbA_{1c} and glucose monitors. Home-use devices for pregnancy testing and ovulation monitoring are well known. The concept is expected to expand into other areas of clinical endocrinology.

FURTHER READING

Edwards R. Immunoassay: an introduction. London:Heinemann Medical; 1985.

Edwards R, ed. Immunoassays: essential data. Chichester, West Sussex:John Wiley; 1996.

Edwards R, ed. Immunodiagnostics. Oxford:Oxford University Press; 1999.

Ekins RP. The estimation of thyroxine in human plasma by an electrophoretic technique. Clin Chim Acta. 1960;5:453.

Ekins RP. General principles of hormone assay. In: Loraine JH, Bell ET, eds. Hormone assays and their clinical application. Edinburgh:Churchill Livingstone; 1976:1–72.

Holman RB, Cross AJ, Joseph MH, eds. HPLC in neuroscience research. Chichester, West Sussex:John Wiley; 1993.

Honour J. Steroid profiling. Ann Clin Biochem. 1997;34:32–44.

Honour J, Brook CGD. Clinical indications for the use of urinary steroid profiles in neonates and children. Ann Clin Biochem. 1997;34:45–54.

Hunter WM, Corrie JET, eds. Immunoassays for clinical chemistry proceedings workshop, Edinburgh 1982. Edinburgh:Churchill Livingstone; 1983.

Jackson TM, Ekins RP. Theoretical limitations on immunoassay sensitivity. J Immunol Methods. 1986;87:13–20.

Price CP, Newman DJ, eds. Principles and practice of immunoassays, 2nd ed. London:Macmillan; 1997.

Yalow RS, Berson SA. Immunoassay of endogenous plasma insulin in man. J Clin Invest. 1960;39:1157.

Chapter 28

Cell Signaling and the Control of Gene Expression

Adrian J L Clark

INTRODUCTION

Hormonal signals act via receptors. The interaction of a hormone with its receptor is critical for determining the specificity of the response in the target tissue. Activation of a receptor is followed by further transmission of the signal into the cell, resulting in diverse but specifically targeted responses.

The interaction of a hormone with its specific receptor and the consequent activation of 'secondary' messages is a unique process for each hormone and each cell type. However the complex wealth of information on these effects can be simplified greatly by recognizing that there are a limited number of major classes of hormone receptor, which are each closely associated with one particular mode of intracellular signaling. In reality, many of these receptors are also associated with additional signaling processes and can modulate signaling processes activated by other hormone–receptor interactions.

Each of these receptor-signaling classes will be described in the following sections. The essential features of this generally applicable classification are shown in **Table 28.1**. Inevitably, this type of classification is not absolute, and some receptors do not fit easily within one particular grouping. However, such classifications

are essential in order to understand the vast array of receptor functions and signaling systems.

Since receptors provide the majority of the specificity of hormonal regulation, it is no surprise that many hormones or 'ligands' have multiple receptors. In most cases these 'sibling' receptors have evolved from a common precursor and structural and signaling characteristics are relatively well conserved. However there are a few instances of ligands that have acquired receptors in two distinct classes. A particular example of this is the evidence for the existence of cell surface steroid receptors that clearly have different, nongenomic actions from the well-recognized nuclear steroid receptors.

With such diversity, it is of little surprise that pathologic defects occur in receptor action and signal transduction. Often, these are inherited germline defects, although acquired defects are also found with increasing frequency. Inevitably, in some situations such defects are incompatible with survival *in utero*. However, when fetal life is not compromised, the consequences often appear in the form of endocrine disease. Some examples of this type of defect will be highlighted in the following sections.

The consequences of the various signal transduction processes are multiple. They include the activation of membrane ion

Classification of the receptors			
Receptor class	**Type of hormone/ligand**	**Structural characteristics**	**Primary mode of signal transduction**
Kinase cascade receptors			
Cytokine receptors	Interleukins, growth hormone, prolactin, erythropoietin	Single transmembrane domain. Homo or heterodimers	JAK/STAT signaling cascades
Growth factor receptors	Insulin, growth factors	Single transmembrane domain. Dimerize after ligand binding	Receptor tyrosine kinases – adapters, PI3 kinase, Grb2/Sos
TGF-β class receptors	Activin, TGF-β, BMPs	Single transmembrane domain heterodimers	Receptor serine kinases → SMADs
G-protein-coupled receptors			
G-protein-coupled receptors	Light, ions, amines, lipids, peptides, enzymes	Seven transmembrane domains	Activation of G protein cycle → activation of specific effectors
Nuclear receptors			
Nuclear receptors	Smaller lipophilic molecules. Steroids, triiodothyronine	Intracellular molecules with conserved zinc finger DNA binding function	Direct modulation of gene expression. Co-activators and co-repressors

Table 28.1 Classification of the receptors. Major classes are shown in bold.

Generalized mechanisms by which receptor activation can influence cellular processes

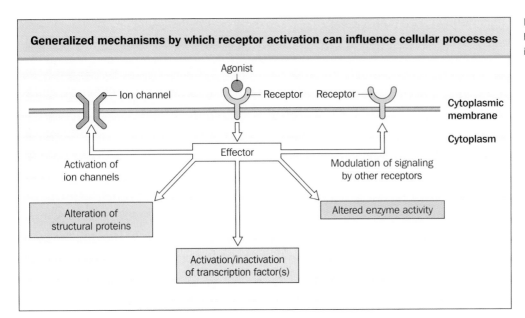

Fig. 28.1 Generalized mechanisms by which receptor activation can influence cellular processes.

channels leading to depolarization of cells, activation (or inactivation) of specific target proteins by phosphorylation, and alterations in gene expression. These consequences of intracellular signal activation are illustrated in **Figure 28.1**. Discussion of the details of each of these processes is impossible. However, many of the more profound and persistent effects of receptor activation result from changes in gene expression, and in the last section of this chapter some of the mechanisms by which this is achieved will be discussed.

KINASE CASCADE RECEPTORS

This general term is used here to denote receptor/signal transduction pathways of several distinct classes that have a number of features in common, and in particular the dependence on modification of proteins by the addition of one or more phosphate molecules to a tyrosine, serine, or threonine residue.

The ligands for each of these types of receptor are larger peptides such as growth hormone, insulin, epidermal growth factor, or transforming growth factor-β (TGF-β). Their cell surface receptors often function as homo- or heterodimers. Receptor dimerization and ligand binding is followed by receptor activation. Activation takes the form of phosphorylation of the receptor either by itself or by specific cytoplasmic kinases, resulting in docking of the receptor to second messenger proteins. These in turn are often activated by phosphorylation. The activated second messenger may have diverse actions such as translocation to the nucleus to affect gene transcription or phosphorylation of other cytoplasmic effectors.

The individual components of these apparently similar pathways are, however, distinct and have evolved independently of each other. Specific aspects of each of these classes – the cytokine receptors, the growth factor receptors, and the TGF-β class of receptors are described below.

Cytokine receptors

This class of receptors is relatively heterogeneous in structural terms, yet they have in common several general functional features, including the type of intracellular signal they generate. The ligands for this class of receptor are listed in **Table 28.2** and, of particular significance to clinical endocrinology, include growth hormone (GH) and prolactin (PRL).

As outlined above, all these receptors act as homo- or heterodimers, each dimer binding a single molecule of ligand. Thus each ligand must contain two separate receptor-binding surfaces, and each member of a receptor dimer must contain two distinct ligand-binding surfaces. The identity of the dimerization partner in each of these receptors is summarized in **Table 28.2**. The receptors for GH, PRL, erythropoietin, and thrombopoietin act as homodimers, whereas those for the cytokines function as heterodimers with a specific member of one of three dimerization partners – gp 130, βC or γC.

Each of the specific receptor monomers in this family contains a single transmembrane domain. The N-terminal extracellular domain contains several N- and O-linked glycosylation sites and a number of cysteine residues, which form intramolecular disulfide bonds. In particular, the extracellular domain of these receptors is characterized by the presence of a WSXWS (tryptophan–serine–X–tryptophan–serine) box, which is absent only in the GH receptor. The cytoplasmic domains of these receptors are not highly conserved other than the presence of two motifs known as Box 1 and Box 2. Box 1 is located close to the transmembrane domain and is involved in binding of JAK/Tyk proteins (see below). In the case of many of these receptors a proteolytic or a splicing event results in the release of the extracellular ligand-binding domain from the cell. These free binding domains can bind ligand and may function as carrier proteins or as natural antagonists to the receptor (**Fig. 28.2**).

In contrast to the other receptor classes that signal by generation of a phosphorylation cascade (see below), the cytokine family receptors lack any endogenous kinase activity. This led to some difficulty in identifying their signal transduction mechanisms for many years. This situation was clarified by the recognition of the role of the Janus-associated kinase family members, or JAK kinases, with this class of receptor.

Ligands acting through cytokine receptors

Cytokine/ligand	Dimerization partner
Growth hormone	Homodimers
Prolactin	Homodimers
Erythropoietin	Homodimers
Thrombopoietin	Homodimers
Leptin	
Interleukin 6	gp 130
Interleukin 11	
Leukemia inhibitory factor	
Oncostatin M	
Interleukin 3	βC
Interleukin5	
GM-CSF	
Interleukin 2	γψ
Interleukin 4	
Interleukin 7	
Interleukin 9	
Interleukin 15	
Interferon-α	IFNA-R + IFNB-R
Interferon-β	IFNA-R + IFNB-R
Interferon-γ	IFNG-Rα + β
Interleukin 10	

Table 28.2 Ligands acting through cytokine receptors. The table lists ligands known to act through the cytokine family of receptors and their receptor dimerization partner. GM-CSF, granulocyte–macrophage colony stimulating factor.

There are four JAK kinase family members, JAK1, JAK2, JAK3 and Tyk2. They have a characteristic modular structure containing an N-terminal receptor binding domain and two C-terminal kinase domains (**Fig. 28.2**). The most C-terminal of these is the true kinase domain, whereas the more N-terminal is a 'pseudokinase' domain with regulatory functions. Certain JAKs are associated with certain receptors and these associations are summarized in **Table 28.2**.

The likely initial series of events in activation of a cytokine receptor is that ligand binds to its specific receptor monomer. This is followed by binding to the dimerization partner, resulting in receptor dimerization. On the cytoplasmic side of the membrane, the dimerized receptor is bound in the Box 1 region by a member of the JAK family. This process activates the JAK kinase, which then phosphorylates itself on tyrosine residues and other targets, which include the receptor to which it is bound. Tyrosine phosphorylation of the receptor creates two types of specific docking site recognized by either the phosphotyrosine binding domain or the Src-homology 2 (SH2) domain.

These newly created docking sites are then bound by several molecules. These include the adapter molecule, Shc, which after

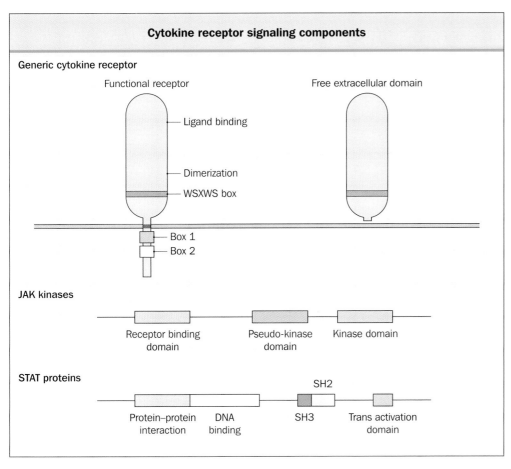

Fig. 28.2 Cytokine receptor signaling components. The modular structure of (top panel) a generic cytokine receptor, (center panel) the Janus-associated (JAK) kinases and (bottom panel) the STAT proteins is illustrated.

phosphorylation by JAK will be capable of activating the MAP kinase pathway, and in the case of some receptors, members of the insulin receptor substrate docking proteins. Activation of these by phosphorylation will stimulate several further signaling pathways (see below). However, the most significant of the secondary signals generated is that of the 'signal transducers and activators of transcription', or STATs, which appears to be relatively unique to the cytokine receptor family.

Seven distinct STATs have been identified. A conserved modular domain can be identified for this class of molecule (**Fig. 28.2**). This includes a central DNA-binding domain and a C-terminal SH2 domain. The STAT binds to the tyrosine phosphorylated receptor via their SH2 domain and themselves are phosphorylated on tyrosine by the receptor-associated JAK. This phosphorylation creates an SH2-binding domain on the STAT, which results in their dimerization. Both homo- and hetero-dimerization of STATs take place. Dimerized STATs migrate across the nuclear membrane and this enables them to bind to specific DNA response elements and modulate gene expression. Each receptor can usually signal through more than one STAT, although certain receptor:STAT pairings are notable and are summarized in **Table 28.2**. This model of cytokine receptor signaling via the JAK/STAT pathways is summarized in **Figure 28.3**.

An interesting twist to the cytokine receptor signal transduction mechanism came with the identification of a class of molecules that were induced by the JAK/STAT signal and that inhibited further signal transduction. At least eight proteins that function as 'suppressors of cytokine signaling' or SOCS have now been identified. All contain a C-terminal SOCS box that is essential for their function. Their mode of action appears to be via binding to the JAK kinase to inhibit further kinase activity, although there is evidence in the case of some SOCS proteins that they can interfere with the STAT:DNA interaction.

Only a few defects in the cytokine receptors and their signaling mechanisms have been found to be associated with disease. This probably reflects the important functional role of these pathways, making defects incompatible with life. Many of the knockout mouse models of these components support this notion. Two defects are important to mention. Of particular relevance to clinical endocrinology are a variety of inherited defects in the GH receptor that result in GH insensitivity or Laron syndrome. Many homozygous defects that interfere with synthesis of a normal GH receptor (e.g. premature stop codons, frameshift mutations, splicing defects, and gene deletions) have been described. In addition, certain missense mutations and splicing defects illuminate our understanding of GH receptor function. Many missense mutations appear to interfere with normal ligand binding. As a consequence, in a homozygous form, receptor activation fails and the secreted GH-binding protein cannot be detected by the usual assay of its ability to bind GH.

Other disease states that have been recognized include mutations of the leptin receptor associated with severe childhood obesity, missense mutations of the interleukin 4 receptor giving rise to atopy, and missense mutations of the erythropoietin receptor, which result in persistent activation of JAK2 and the condition of benign erythrocytosis. Heterozygous intracellular domain deletion mutations of the granulocyte-colony-stimulating factor receptor act in a dominant negative manner in that their dimerization with the wild-type receptor results in a receptor incapable of signaling,

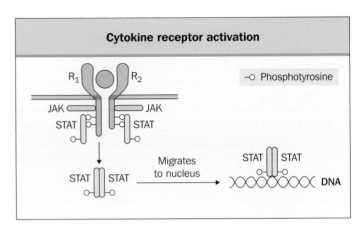

Fig. 28.3 Cytokine receptor activation. One molecule of ligand binds to two receptor molecules either as a homodimer or a heterodimer. Janus-associated (JAK) kinases associate with the dimerized receptor and phosphorylate it and other molecules including members of the STAT family. Phosphorylated STATs dimerize, migrate to the nucleus and bind to cognate response elements in DNA to regulate transcription.

resulting in congenital neutropenia. The most severe of the cytokine receptor diseases is X-linked severe combined immunodeficiency (SCID). This is caused by mutations in the γC common subunit required for interleukin 2, 4, 7, 9, and 15 receptors. A related, autosomal recessive syndrome results from mutations in the interleukin 7 receptor α-chain.

Defects in the cytoplasmic cytokine receptor signal transduction components are much less prominent, probably reflecting their essential functional role in a multitude of signaling pathways. The notable but rare exception is the finding of inactivating mutations of JAK3 in autosomal recessive SCID. There is considerable interest in the possibility of mutations in the JAK/STAT pathways in neoplasia, and some chromosomal translocations in malignant disease have been identified that activate these signals.

Growth factor receptors

Members of this family of receptors were the first of the cellular receptors to be identified and characterized, and there is probably more variability in this family than in any other class of receptor. Although the receptors for epidermal growth factor (EGF) and platelet-derived growth factor were the first to be cloned, research in this area has, for obvious reasons, been extensively driven by the insulin receptor. **Table 28.3** lists some of the growth factor and related molecules that act as ligands for these receptors. All are relatively large polypeptides with significant secondary structure. Much of the following discussion is based on the insulin and EGF receptors. Other members of this family use variations on these themes.

All members of this receptor family are large molecules that span the cytoplasmic membrane with a single hydrophobic transmembrane domain. The extracellular domains contain significant posttranslational modifications in the form of disulfide bridges and glycosylation that serves to define a specific ligand-binding pocket. Despite this, there is some degree of flexibility in that the insulin receptor, for example, can bind insulin-like growth factor 1 (IGF-I) with reduced affinity, and several EGF-like ligands exist for the EGF receptor and its related receptors. In the case

Ligands for some growth factor receptor family members
Insulin
Insulin-like growth factor I
Insulin-like growth factor II
Epidermal growth factor (five EGF-like molecules)
Platelet derived growth factor A and B
Vascular endothelial growth factor
Placental growth factor
Fibroblast growth factor (multiple FGF-like molecules)
Hepatocyte growth factor
Colony-stimulating factor

Table 28.3 Ligands for some growth factor receptor family members.

of most of these family members the receptor appears to exist as a monomer on the cell surface. Insulin and the IGF-I receptor exist as homodimers, and one molecule of ligand will bind to the preformed dimer. In the case of monomeric receptors, ligand binding is followed by receptor dimerization. This is often a homodimerization process but clearly, in the case of EGF receptors, heterodimerization with other members of the EGF-R family (HER-2, HER-3 and HER-4) is a frequent and normal event.

Conformational changes consequent on ligand binding and dimerization lead to activation of the receptor tyrosine kinase(s) located in the cytoplasmic domain. These domains are relatively well conserved between different growth factor receptor family members, and include an adenosine triphosphate (ATP) binding domain and a catalytic domain. The kinase domain on one receptor molecule initially phosphorylates the dimerization partner on tyrosine residues and *vice versa* – the process of

autophosphorylation. This results in enhanced kinase activity of the receptor by removal of an inhibitory component of the receptor by a conformational change.

The consequences of this autophosphorylation and enhanced kinase activity are twofold. The autophosphorylated receptor becomes a target for binding of specific adapter molecules to phosphotyrosine sites. Many of these sites are targets for binding by proteins containing a SH2 domain (see above). Signaling molecules containing SH2 sites that have relevance to growth factor receptor signaling include molecules such as GRB-2, phosphotidyl inositol 3-kinase and phospholipase Cγ.

The second major consequence of receptor activation and autophosphorylation is that the enhanced intrinsic tyrosine kinase phosphorylates several downstream targets such as the insulin receptor substrate (IRS) molecules – IRS-1, IRS-2, IRS-3 and IRS-4, and Shc. These tyrosine-rich molecules in turn become SH2 binding targets after tyrosine phosphorylation, and in this way serve to amplify the initial signal.

A diagrammatic summary of these pathways and mechanisms is shown in **Figure 28.4**. A complete description of the various pathways stimulated by this family of receptors is clearly not appropriate here.

One major pathway stimulated by all members of this receptor family to a greater or lesser extent is the *ras*–MAP kinase pathway. GRB-2 contains two copies of another relatively widespread *src* homology domain known as an SH3 domain. This type of domain is in general capable of binding to proline-rich sequences on growth factor receptors and other signaling molecules. The guanine nucleotide exchange factor, SOS, contains such a proline-rich region, which binds tightly to the SH3 domains of GRB-2. The consequence is the activation of SOS, which stimulates the exchange of guanosine 5′ triphosphate (GTP) for guanosine 5′ diphosphate (GDP) on *ras*. Ras is thereby activated, which in turn activates *raf*. This serine/threonine kinase phosphorylates and activates MEK (MAP kinase kinase), a serine/threonine kinase that phosphorylates MAP kinases (ERK).

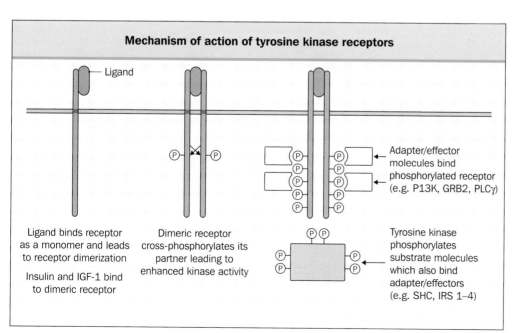

Fig. 28.4 Mechanism of action of tyrosine kinase receptors. Receptor monomers dimerize after ligand binding (except in the case of insulin and insulin-like growth factor I (IGF-I) receptors). The dimeric receptor cross-phosphorylates its partner, leading to enhanced tyrosine kinase activity phosphorylating the receptor and other substrates. Several adapter/effector molecules bind to the phosphorylated receptor and to some substrate molecules.

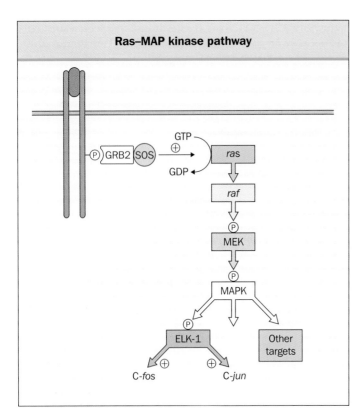

Fig. 28.5 Ras–MAP kinase pathway. The diagram shows the essential components of the Ras–MAP kinase pathway stimulated by activation of a growth factor receptor.

MAP kinase activation in this way results in phosphorylation of transcription factors such as ELK-1, which activate several of the early immediate genes, including c-*fos* and c-*jun* family members. This cascade is illustrated in **Figure 28.5**.

The other major pathway activated by growth factor and insulin receptor family members is the phosphotidyl inositol-3 kinase (PI3K) pathway. This pathway is particularly crucial in

stimulating the metabolic actions of insulin, and attempts to understand why a number of growth factor receptors that activate PI3K do not exhibit insulin's metabolic action reveal the much greater complexity of these pathways.

PI3K, a heterodimer consisting of a p85 regulatory subunit and a p110 catalytic subunit, binds to receptors or to IRS adapter proteins through its SH2 domain on the p85 subunit. As a consequence, the p110 catalytic subunit is activated and stimulates the synthesis of phosphotidyl inositol 3,4,5 triphosphate (PIP3) and other inositol phosphates. Production of PIP3 in the membrane results in recruitment of Akt to the cytoplasmic membrane. Akt is a serine/threonine kinase that has a crucial role in insulin signaling. In the cell membrane it is phosphorylated and activated by phosphoinositide-dependent kinases (PDK-1 and PDK-2), which are also activated by PIP3. Thus activation of PI3K results in kinase activation in the microenvironment of the cell membrane. Akt plays a crucial role in the translocation of the glucose transporter, GLUT4, to the cell membrane. It is clearly not the only factor that can achieve this end result, but is undoubtedly one of the major ones. Although Akt can be activated by several growth factor receptors, it is only insulin activation that results in efficient glucose uptake. The precise reasons for this are still unclear, but it seems that IRS-activated PI3K/Akt pathways are crucial, and this may relate to the cytoplasmic compartments in which this activation takes place. These pathways are illustrated in **Figure 28.6**.

The fundamental role played by many growth factors and their receptors in differentiation and development is probably the reason that germline defects in the genes encoding these receptors are not a frequent cause of disease. Nevertheless, achondroplasia is the result of heterozygous defects in the fibroblast growth factor type 3 (FGFR3) receptor, and a number of point mutations and deletions in the insulin receptor giving rise to syndromes of severe insulin resistance have been described.

Of greater clinical significance are the acquired mutations or overexpression of growth factor receptors associated with various tumors. The earliest of these to be described were the amplification of the EGF-receptor gene found in many squamous cell

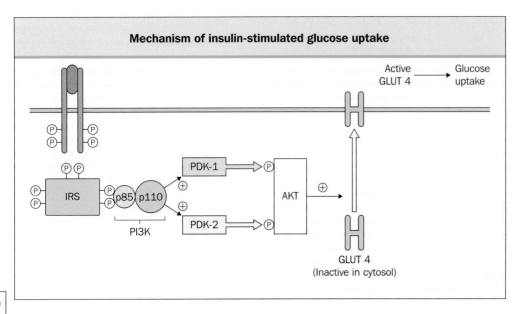

Fig. 28.6 Mechanism of insulin-stimulated glucose uptake. Akt has an important although not a unique role in GLUT 4 activation and hence stimulation of glucose uptake.

carcinomas, malignant gliomas, and breast and other carcinomas. Breast carcinoma is more often associated with amplification of the EGFR-related receptor, ErbB2 or HER2. Defects in the *ret* protooncogene, which has been shown to be the receptor for brain-derived neurotropic factor, have been described in thyroid carcinomas (gene rearrangements), in multiple endocrine neoplasia 2A (point mutations of specific cysteine residues on the extracellular side of the transmembrane domain) and in MEN2B (cytoplasmic domain mutations). Many other growth factor receptors and the signal transduction components described above have been found to play a role as oncogenes in various types of tumor, or were originally identified as viral oncogenes. In these cases tumor viruses have 'captured' all or part of a mammalian growth factor receptor or signal transduction molecule, and use this inappropriately to transform their host cell.

Transforming growth factor-beta class receptors

Although only a small family, this unique group of signaling molecules appears to exert a major influence on cell growth and differentiation. The first receptor in this class to be recognized was the activin receptor in 1991. Currently recognized mammalian ligands that signal directly through these receptors are listed in **Table 28.4**.

Cloning of the activin receptor revealed it to be a single transmembrane domain molecule containing a unique cytoplasmic serine/threonine kinase domain. Other family members retained this general structure, thereby defining a new receptor class. This class has now become known as the type II receptor serine kinases (RSKs).

It was apparent however that another cell surface binding component was required, and this led to the identification of the partially homologous group of receptors known as the activin-receptor-like kinases (ALKs) or type I RSKs. These receptors also contain a serine/threonine kinase and a characteristic glycine–serine motif (GS motif) in the intracellular domain. Thus a functional TGF-β class receptor is a heterodimer of a molecule from each class. Some of these functional pairings are listed in **Table 28.4**.

Following ligand binding and receptor activation, the type II receptor phosphorylates the type I receptor on the conserved GS motif. This activates the Type I ALK receptor kinase, which phosphorylates specific target molecules. Most significant amongst these are a unique group of signal transduction molecules known as SMADs, a composite name derived from the names for two members of this protein family found in *Drosophila* in one case and in *Caenorhabtidis elegans* in the other case.

Multiple SMADs from both vertebrate and invertebrate organisms have now been identified and their general structural features have been defined. SMADs have conserved N- and C-terminal domains, the latter containing a specific serine–serine–X–serine (SSXS) motif. This motif is phosphorylated by the activated type I receptor, and this results in heterodimerization of the phosphorylated SMAD with a member of a second class of co-SMAD molecules. Co-SMADs lack the SSXS sequence and are consequently not phosphorylated. A certain amount of specificity in this system is maintained in that a given ALK receptor phosphorylates only certain SMADs, which dimerize with only certain co-SMADs (see **Table 28.4**).

In a similar mechanism to the STAT signaling pathways, the SMAD/co-SMAD heterodimer then migrates to the nucleus where, often in association with additional co-factors, it can modulate transcription of specific target genes. The DNA-binding elements of the SMAD lie in its C-terminal domain, whereas the N-terminal domain is involved in interactions with other transcriptional activators/repressors. Amongst a number of co-effectors of SMAD transcriptional function is the c-*fos*/c-*jun* heterodimer (AP1), the vitamin D receptor and CREB-binding protein/p300, which has intrinsic histone acetyltransferase activity (see below). These pathways are illustrated in **Figure 28.7**. Clearly, research in these receptor signaling pathways is in its early days and it seems highly probable that these pathways will be shown to exert a profound influence on cellular function and human disease in the coming years.

G-protein-coupled receptors

This, the largest single class of receptors, demonstrates a remarkable conservation of structural features in the form of the seven transmembrane domains characteristic of all members of this superfamily, and conservation of signal transduction mechanisms, in the form of the heterotrimeric G proteins. The remarkable evolutionary success of this class of receptors is reflected not only in the diversity and extent of the ligands that interact with them (**Table 28.5**), but also in the observation that distinct evolutionary processes appear to have converged on this structural format. As a consequence three major classes of G-protein-coupled receptor (GPCR) can be recognized (**Table 28.5**).

Structure

The structural nature of this class of receptors has posed a considerable problem for many years in view of the difficulty in obtaining crystals of these highly hydrophobic molecules for which membrane integrity is essential for function. Our present

Serine kinase receptor ligands and receptor dimerization partners		
Ligand	Type II receptor	Type I receptor (ALK)
Activin	ActR II	ALK4
Activin	ActR IIB	
TGF-β	TGF-βR II	ALK5
Bone morphogenetic protein 2/4	BMPR II	ALK3
	ActR II	ALK6

Table 28.4 Serine kinase receptor ligands and receptor dimerization partners. TGF, transforming growth factor.

411

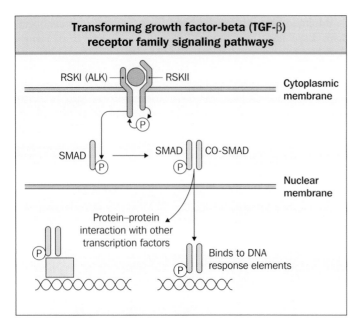

Fig. 28.7 Transforming growth factor-beta (TGF-β)-receptor family signaling pathways. See text for details.

G-protein-coupled receptors

Class A (rhodopsin-like)

Biogenic amines (catecholamines, dopamine, serotonin, histamine)

Acetylcholine (muscarinic)

Adenosine

Nucleotides

Odorants

Leukotrienes

Small peptides (angiotensin II, bradykinin, melanocortins adrenocorticotropic hormone, thyrotropin-releasing hormone Tachykinins, vasopressin, oxytocin, gonadotropin-releasing hormone, others)

Chemokines

Larger peptides (thyroid-stimulating hormone, luteinizing hormone, follicle-stimulating hormone)

Proteases

Class B (secretin/glucagon-receptor-like)

Glucagon

Secretin

Vasoactive intestinal polypeptide/PACAP

Gastric inhibitory polypeptide

Growth-hormone-releasing hormone

Parathyroid hormone/PTHrP

Calcitonin/calcitonin-gene-related peptide/adrenomedullin/amylin

Corticopepsin releasing hormone receptor

Class C (metabotropic-receptor-like)

Metabotropic glutamate receptor

Metabotropic gamma-amino butyric acid receptor

Calcium-sensing receptor

Taste receptors

Table 28.5 G-protein-coupled receptors. The range of ligands that act through G-protein-coupled receptors (GPCRs) are listed below in groups that reflect the three major classes of GPCR as defined by structural variation and evidence for distinct evolutionary origins. The list of ligands is not exhaustive, but is to provide examples of the type and diversity of ligand. PACAP, pituitary adenylate cyclase activating peptide; PTHrP parathyroid hormone related peptide

understanding is based on evidence from a variety of distinct sources, including electron cryomicroscopy projection images of bovine rhodopsin, theoretical modeling, site-directed mutagenesis and crosslinking studies, and, recently, a crystal structure for rhodopsin.

The conclusions from these lines of evidence is that the seven transmembrane domains cluster around each other in an irregular oval pattern when viewed from above. These general structures are illustrated in **Figure 28.8**. As a consequence, the N-terminus of the receptor and three 'loops' lie outside the cell, and the C-terminus and the remaining three loops lie inside the cell. GPCRs are also extensively modified posttranslationally. Disulfide bridges, usually located in highly conserved extracellular positions, assist in holding the receptor in its clustered conformation, and extracellular N- and O-linked glycosylation is characteristic. On the intracellular surface of the receptor, several serine and/or threonine residues are often present, located in target sites for phosphorylation by specific kinases that can modify receptor function. In some GPCRs a cysteine residue in the C-terminal tail may be palmitoylated, probably resulting in tethering of this part of the tail to the cell membrane.

Hormone interaction

The manner in which the hormone or other ligand interacts with the GPCR has also become clearer in recent years. As a general rule, small ligands, such as the biologic amines (epinephrine, norepinephrine, dopamine, serotonin) enter the central pocket of the receptor, interacting with specific amino acid residues in the transmembrane domains. Slightly larger ligands such as the smaller peptides (e.g. angiotensin II, vasopressin) interact with both the extracellular loops and the central pocket. Larger peptides (e.g. luteinizing hormone, follicle-stimulating hormone, thyroid-stimulating hormone) interact primarily with the large N-terminal domain found in these receptors, and only after this does interaction with the transmembrane domain region take

place. There are many exceptions to these rules. For example, the calcium-sensing receptor, which recognizes one of the smallest GPCR ligands, interacts with calcium ions in its large N-terminal domain. A subgroup of 'protease-activated receptors', which includes the thrombin receptor, require the N-terminus to be cleaved by the protease, following which the newly revealed N-terminal end of the receptor interacts directly with the central pore region to activate signal transduction.

There has been growing evidence in recent years that some GPCRs may need to form homo- or heterodimers in order to function effectively. For example, the GABA B1 receptor will only function efficiently when heterodimerized with the closely related but equally inefficient GABA B2 receptor. Heterodimerization in this example takes place through their C-terminal tails. A number of other interesting examples of a similar dimerization phenomenon have recently been described.

Structure of the G-protein-coupled receptors

Two-dimensional view

View from above

Probable three-dimensional arrangement

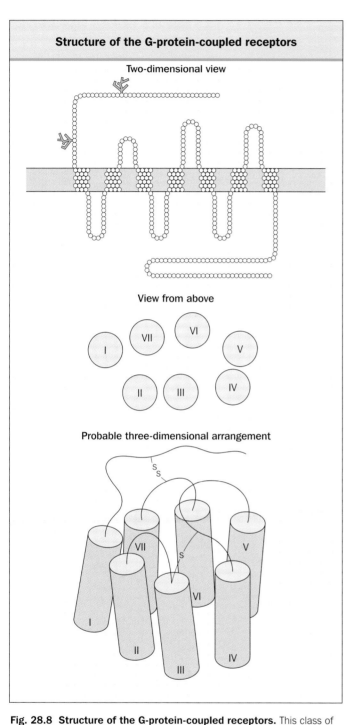

Fig. 28.8 Structure of the G-protein-coupled receptors. This class of receptor is often depicted in a two-dimensional form as seen in the top panel, demonstrating the seven transmembrane domains and the three extracellular and three cytoplasmic loops. Glycosylation moieties may be present on the extracellular regions of the receptor. (Center panel) The structural arrangement of the transmembrane helices is more complex and molecular modeling and electron microscopic evidence suggests that they are arranged around a central pocket when viewed from above. The probable three-dimensional arrangement will therefore resemble that seen in the bottom panel.

Constitutive activity and disease

The consequence of binding ligand is that the GPCR appears to undergo a small conformational change. The nature of this change is poorly understood but the general consensus is that the unliganded receptor is held in a constrained position and that binding of ligand interferes with this constraint. The 'relaxed' receptor can then activate the heterotrimeric G protein with which it is associated. Support for this model comes from both artificially generated receptor mutations and a growing list of 'experiments of nature'. Thus, in each of the examples listed in **Table 28.6**, an inherited or an acquired point mutation in a specific receptor renders it constitutively active in the absence of ligand. First described in an inherited form in male pseudoprecocious puberty, and in an acquired form in toxic thyroid adenomas in the luteinizing hormone and thyroid-stimulating hormone receptors respectively, these mutations causing endocrine disease have provided vital insight into the biologic mechanisms of receptor function.

The G protein cycle

The GTPase proteins activated by GPCRs are distinct from the small G proteins (e.g. Ras) activated by growth factor signaling pathways. GPCRs activate a heterotrimeric G protein composed of one α, one β and one γ subunit. The $\beta\gamma$ subunits remain tightly associated and effectively function as a single entity. The α subunit contains the GTPase catalytic activity and determines the mode of signal transduction (**Table 28.7**). Under unstimulated conditions the α subunit is bound to GDP and is complexed with the $\beta\gamma$ subunits. Activation of the G protein following receptor stimulation results in exchange of GDP by GTP. In the GTP bound state, the α subunit has only weak affinity for the $\beta\gamma$-subunits and it dissociates. It is this GTP bound α subunit that is the essential effector of GPCRs. However, since the α subunit possesses intrinsic GTPase activity, this GTP-bound state is only short-lived. Hydrolysis of GTP to GDP inactivates the α subunit, which then regains affinity for the $\beta\gamma$ subunit, thereby completing the G protein cycle, as shown in **Figure 28.9**.

The rate of GTP hydrolysis determines, in part, the strength of the stimulus. A family of cytoplasmic proteins known as 'regulators of G protein signaling' (RGS) proteins or $G\alpha_I$ proteins (GAIPs) have been identified that enhance the catalytic rate of the α subunit. Cholera toxin inhibits the GTPase activity of the α_s subunit, while pertussis toxin inhibits GTP binding by α_I or α_o subunits. These actions are also shown in **Figure 28.9**.

It has become apparent that the $\beta\gamma$ subunits are not simply inert partner proteins of the α subunit but that they may activate certain processes by themselves. Such activities include a role in activating receptor desensitization processes, in mitogenic signaling by GPCRs and in ion channel activation.

Defects in the function of the α_s subunit are a well-recognized cause of endocrine disease. Heterozygous inactivating mutations of the α_s gene result in pseudohypoparathyroidism. This illustrates the dependence of endocrine signaling on this component, in that the presence of the protein product from the single

Disorders associated with G-protein-coupled receptors

Receptor	Clinical disorder	Genetic origin
Luteinizing hormone receptor	Male pseudoprecocious puberty	Germ line – inherited
Thyroid-stimulating hormone receptor	Toxic thyroid adenoma	Spontaneous mutation
Severe neonatal thyrotoxicosis		Germ line – inherited
Parathyroid hormone receptor/ parathyroid hormone-related protein receptor	Jansen-type metaphyseal chondrodysplasia	Germ line – inherited
Calcium sensing receptor	Congenital hypoparathyroidism	Germ line – inherited
α-melanocyte-stimulating hormone (MC1) receptor	Mouse and other species coat-color mutants	Germ line – inherited
Rhodopsin	Congenital night blindness	Germ line – inherited

Table 28.6 Disorders associated with G-protein-coupled receptors. Constitutive activation of GPCRs has been demonstrated to result in the following conditions.

Major subtypes of G protein α subunit

Subunits	Target effector	Intracellular signal
α_s	Adenylate cyclase stimulated	cAMP increased
$\alpha_{i1}, \alpha_{i2}, \alpha_{i3}$	Adenylate cyclase inhibited	cAMP reduced
α_o	Calcium channel inhibited	Ca^{2+} influx reduced
$\alpha_{q/11}$	Phospholipase C_β activated	Protein kinase C activated and inositol triphosphate released

Table 28.7 Major subtypes of G protein α subunit. Principal effectors and signal transduction pathways are shown. cAMP, cyclic adenosine monophosphate.

remaining normal allele is insufficient to rescue certain signaling processes. Homozygous defects are very uncommon and are likely to impair fetal survival.

Genetic defects that impair the GTPase activity of the α_s subunit would be predicted to result in overstimulation of adenylate cyclase. In the McCune–Albright syndrome such a mutation exists as a genetic mosaic, presumably as a consequence of the acquisition of a point mutation after fertilization in the early blastocyst stage. Germline mutations are likely to be incompatible with life. The pattern of disease in McCune–Albright syndrome depends partly on the extent and distribution of cells bearing the mutant gene, thereby providing an explanation for its heterogeneity. The same GTPase-inactivating mutations occurring in endocrine tissue are commonly found in somatotroph adenomas and occasionally in functioning thyroid adenomas. The evidence for disease-causing mutations in the other α subunits or in the βγ subunits is more limited. An association with a mutation in the β_3 subunit has been described in essential hypertension.

G protein-coupled receptor effectors

Adenylate cyclase

Cyclic adenosine monophosphate (cAMP) was the first intracellular second messenger signaling molecule to be identified. cAMP is synthesized by the hydrolysis and cyclization of ATP by the enzyme adenylate (or adenylyl) cyclase. At least nine distinct adenylate cyclases have now been identified, each having slightly differing characteristics of activation and cellular distribution.

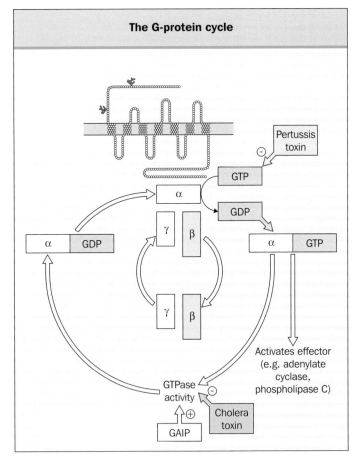

The G-protein cycle

Fig. 28.9 The G protein cycle. The crucial activator is the guanosine 5′ triphosphate (GTP)-bound α subunit, which possesses intrinsic GTPase activity that limits the extent of the signal. The sites of action of cholera and pertussis toxins are shown. GAIP, Gα$_i$ protein; GDP, guanosine 5′ diphosphate.

All are tightly associated with the cell membrane and have a characteristic multiple transmembrane domain structure. Adenylate cyclases can be activated by GTP-bound α$_s$ subunit and inhibited by α$_i$ subunit. cAMP is inactivated by the phosphodiesterases, of which four types exist, each having a distinct profile of activation and distribution. Thus the precise concentration of cAMP in the cell at any moment is usually the product of the combined activities of several adenylate cyclases and phosphodiesterases.

Cyclic AMP activates a specific protein kinase – protein kinase A (PKA). PKA is a tetramer composed of a homodimer of the regulatory subunit and a homodimer of the catalytic subunit. The regulatory subunit retains the catalytic subunit in an inactive form until it is released by binding cAMP. Once released, the catalytic subunit is able to phosphorylate a variety of protein targets. Many of these targets have not been clearly identified but one of the most significant is the cAMP response element binding protein (CREB).

Phosphorylation of CREB on a specific serine residue activates this transcription factor, resulting in its binding to a specific target DNA response element. This element is present in many cAMP-regulated genes activated by cAMP, and provides the means by which cAMP can stimulate gene expression. Other kinases can also phosphorylate CREB on this same residue, and thus the specificity of this transcription factor for cAMP pathway activation is poor. This pathway is summarized in **Figure 28.10**.

It has recently been shown that one of the genes responsible for the Carney complex (primary pigmented nodular adrenal hyperplasia) is the PKA regulatory subunit. Inactivating germline mutations result in impaired inhibition of PKA activity that mimics the effect of a continuous cAMP stimulus to the cell. It is not clear at present whether similar acquired mutations of this gene might account for any spontaneous endocrine tumors.

Phospholipase C

Activation of phospholipase C by $G\alpha_{q/11}$ results in the lipolysis of membrane phospholipids into diacylglycerol (DAG) and inositol trisphosphate (IP_3). DAG interacts with calcium-dependent protein kinase (protein kinase C/PKC), causing it to relocate from the cytosol to the cell membrane. Membrane-associated DAG-bound PKC is activated and results in phosphorylation of a number of specific protein targets at specific serine or threonine residues.

Inositol triphosphate diffuses into the cell, where it may bind to a specific IP_3 receptor. This large molecule is located on the microsomal membrane, where one of the consequences of binding IP_3 is to cause release of calcium ions from intracellular calcium stores. This is a rapid process that is followed by reuptake of free intracellular calcium.

Intracellular calcium release may have a number of effects, including the activation of calcium channels in the cell membrane, leading to an influx of extracellular calcium. A further important consequence is the binding of free calcium to calmodulin, which in turn may activate calmodulin kinase. This is a further protein kinase that can phosphorylate specific, although poorly defined target proteins on serine or threonine residues. These pathways are summarized in **Figure 28.11**.

Nuclear receptors

This, the third of the major classes of receptor defined in **Table 28.1**, is also a large class of molecules that have the obvious distinction of not being located in the cell membrane. These receptors act in the nucleus to control the rate of transcription of target genes. As a consequence their ligands have to be able to cross the cytoplasmic membrane, and in some cases the nuclear membrane, without difficulty. This group of lipophilic molecules includes all the steroid hormones, including vitamin D, thyroid hormone, and retinoic acid. In view of their conserved structure (see below) a large number of nuclear receptors for which an endogenous ligand has not been identified are recognized. It is clear that some of these orphan nuclear receptors, such as steroidogenic factor 1 and NFκB, have important roles in development and physiology. Some of the members of this class of receptor and their endogenous ligands are listed in **Table 28.8**.

As implied above, this class of receptor has a well conserved, modular structure, which is illustrated in **Figure 28.12**. In contrast to other receptor classes, the ligand-binding domain is located at the C-terminal end of the molecule. This is a large domain that consists of 11–13 α helices folded in such a way as

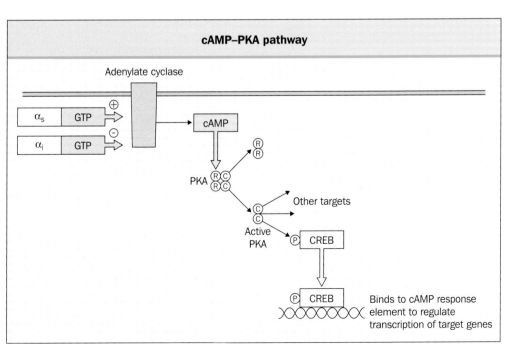

Fig. 28.10 cAMP–PKA pathway.
Adenylate cyclase activation leads to production of cyclic adenosine monophosphate (cAMP) and activation of protein kinase A (PKA). PKA has several targets, including activation of the transcription factor CREB.

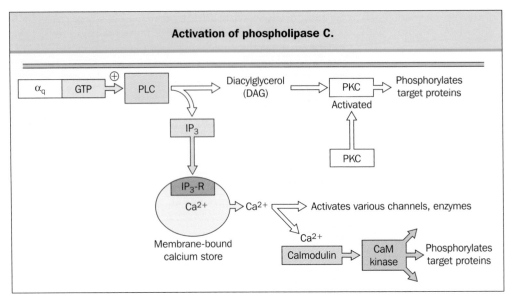

Fig. 28.11 Activation of phospholipase C. Phospholipase C (PLC) activation leads to a bimodal signal. Diacylglycerol release activates protein kinase C (PKC), whereas inositol triphosphate (IP_3) synthesis releases intracellular calcium to activate several processes, including calmodulin kinase. GDP, guanosine 5′ diphosphate.

Important nuclear receptor family members

Receptor	Subtypes	Preferred endogenous ligand
Glucocorticoid receptor	α, β	Cortisol, corticosterone
Progesterone receptor		Progesterone
Androgen receptor		Dihydrotestosterone
Mineralocorticoid receptor		Aldosterone, cortisol, corticosterone
Estrogen receptor	α, β	Estradiol
Thyroid hormone receptor	α, β	Triiodothyronine
Vitamin D receptor		1,25 dihydroxycholecalciferol
Peroxisomal proliferator receptor	α, β, γ	Leukotriene B_4 (α), prostaglandin J_2 (γ)
Retinoic acid receptor	α, β, γ	Retinoic acid
Retinoid X receptor	α, β, γ	9-*cis* retinoic acid
Steroidogenic factor 1	Orphan receptor	

Table 28.8 Important nuclear receptor family members. Some nuclear receptor family members of particular relevance to endocrinology and their preferred endogenous ligand (where known) are listed.

to create a precise 'pocket' into which the steroid molecule or other ligand can fit directly. Ligand-dependent activation of the receptor is dependent on a highly conserved activation function (AF-2) motif located at the C-terminus of this domain. The generally accepted model is one in which binding of ligand results in the AF-2 motif swinging across the binding pocket to create a surface that is recognized and bound by nuclear coactivators (see below). Receptor antagonists may bind in the binding pocket but the AF-2 region fails to be positioned correctly for coactivator binding and consequently the receptor fails to activate a response. A third important role of the ligand binding domain is that of receptor dimerization. Most members of this family act as homodimers or as heterodimers, usually with one of the RXRs. Part of this domain also acts as a dimerization interface.

N-terminal to the ligand-binding domain is a fairly variable hinge region that permits a large degree of flexibility between the DNA-binding and ligand-binding domains. The DNA-binding domain is a highly conserved region in all members of this class of receptors and is characterized by the presence of two zinc fingers. These structures are loops of amino acids tied into a finger-like conformation by the presence of a zinc atom, which is held in place by highly conserved cysteine residues (in the nuclear receptors). The structural features of this important region are shown in **Figure 28.12** and include the P box, which is critical in recognition of the DNA response element, and the D box, which is required for determining the dimerization partner.

The DNA response element to which the receptor binds usually consists of a repeated half-site. The repeat may be either an inverted (palindromic) or a direct repeat, the latter being recognized by receptor dimers that contain the RXR. The DNA sequence in each half site is well conserved. The steroid receptors generally recognize the consensus sequence AGAACA, whereas other nuclear receptors recognize an AGGTCA consensus.

The final major domain found in this class of receptors is the so-called modulator domain. This is highly variable in size and poorly conserved in sequence between receptors, although it contains the other major transcription activation function motif (AF-1). Receptor activation in some nuclear receptors can be influenced by serine and/or threonine residue phosphorylation by various kinases in this domain. There is also evidence for direct interaction between this domain and some coactivators.

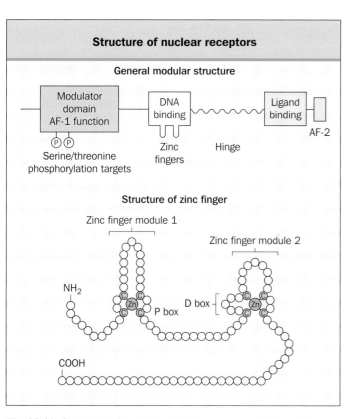

Structure of nuclear receptors

General modular structure

Fig. 28.12 Structure of nuclear receptors. (Top panel) All members conform to this general modular structure. The critical DNA-binding ability is mediated by the two zinc fingers (bottom panel), which are highly conserved between members of this family.

Nuclear receptors fall into two distinct groups in terms of both their preferred dimerization partners and their cellular location. The steroid receptors other than the estrogen receptor (also known as type I receptors) in a ligand-free state exist in the cytosol bound to a heat shock protein complex. Binding ligand releases them from this complex, whereupon they homodimerize and migrate to the nucleus. The mechanism of translocation across the nuclear membrane is not entirely clear but once inside the nucleus they seek out their DNA response elements found in the promoters of many genes. After binding to these specific sites, gene expression is stimulated or repressed by mechanisms described in the next section.

Other nuclear receptors such as those for thyroid hormone, vitamin D, and retinoic acid (known as type II receptors) exist only in the nucleus occasionally as homodimers, but usually as heterodimers with one of the retinoid X receptors, and are often bound to their consensus DNA response elements even in the absence of ligand. In this unliganded state they often repress transcription of the gene to which they are bound. In these cases, ligand binding will relieve this repression, allowing gene expression to occur.

Inherited defects of many of the nuclear steroid receptors and the thyroid hormone receptor have been described and cause syndromes such as glucocorticoid resistance, androgen insensitivity (testicular feminization syndrome) and thyroid hormone resistance syndrome. Many of these defects and in particular those in the thyroid hormone receptors have provided valuable

insights into the molecular mechanisms of nuclear receptor action and into the physiology of the hormones involved.

TRANSCRIPTIONAL REGULATION

Hormone action on a cell may result in changes in metabolism, structure, growth, or gene expression. The nature and extent of these changes is dependent on the hormone involved, the number and type of its receptors expressed by that cell, the signal transduction components available and the influences of other factors on that cell. While metabolic and structural changes may be relatively short-lived, changes in gene expression can have longlasting and sometimes permanent changes on cellular behavior. Almost all the receptor signaling processes described above may influence gene expression by a large number of different mechanisms.

In the case of all the signaling pathways outlined, one of the end points described has been the activation of a particular transcription factor. A description of all the transcription factors that can be activated by these pathways is clearly impossible, and so the following discussion will deal in generalizations, with a few examples as appropriate. In general, transcription factors recognize and bind to specific target DNA sequences that are usually located upstream (or 5′) to the coding region of the genes that they control. This 5′ region responsible for regulating and carrying out transcription is the *promoter*.

Types of transcription factor

As with the receptors, transcription factors can be roughly classified according to their structural features. Three major classes can be defined according to the presence of zinc fingers, leucine zippers, and homeobox domains. A number of examples of relevance to endocrinology are listed in **Table 28.9** according to this classification. Some transcription factors contain more than a single type of structural element.

Classification of transcription factors

Structural feature	Examples
Zinc fingers	Steroid hormone receptors
	Triiodothyronine receptor
	Retinoid X receptor
	Steroidogenic factor 1
	GATA transcription factors
Leucine zippers	CAAT box-binding protein
	CREB
	c-Fos
	c-Jun
Helix–loop–helix	Pit 1
	Oct 1
	HNF1
	PROP1
	Hsx1

Table 28.9 Classification of transcription factors. The table supplies a simple classification of transcription factors of particular relevance to endocrinology based on structural features.

Zinc fingers are one such element that have been discussed in the context of nuclear receptors. Multiple zinc fingers may be found in some molecules. The leucine zipper is a structure required for two such transcription factors to dimerize. An α-helical amino-acid structure consists of a helix of approximately 3.5 amino acids per turn. In a leucine zipper a leucine residue (typically) lies every 7 amino acids so that at a particular point on the helix this amino acid will occur every two turns. Two such helices can then interact by interdigitating with each other at these hydrophobic leucine residues, exactly like a zip. This type of dimerization (as homodimers or heterodimers) acts to hold the double-stranded DNA helix as if in a cleft stick. DNA-binding specificity is usually conferred by a separate basic region.

Homeo domain proteins make use of a so-called helix–turn–helix or helix–loop–helix (HLH) structural motif. In this structure each of two consecutive helices of the transcription factor lies in opposite grooves of the DNA helix. Certain members of this family, which typically have a role in cellular differentiation, are named after the three HLH factors they resemble (Pit1, Oct1, Unc 87) as POU domain proteins.

The structures of the leucine zipper and the HLH motif are shown in **Figure 28.13**.

The transcription complex

Transcription factors act by influencing the rate of transcription of their target gene by RNA polymerase II. This polymerase exists as a large complex of proteins that are responsible for recognizing the point at which gene transcription is to start. In many genes this process is assisted by the presence of a TATA box (so-named because of its consensus nucleotide sequence) located 20–30 base pairs upstream of the site of transcription initiation. The TATA box-binding protein is part of a complex of factors that comprise transcription factor IID, which acts as a recognition signal for the polymerase complex. In certain genes the mechanisms for locating the start of transcription are less well defined, and in some cases a so-called initiator element is found. In other cases, no very precise start signal for the polymerase complex exists, and consequently transcription may commence from several clustered points on the gene.

Correct positioning of the polymerase complex on the gene will usually result in weak transcriptional activity. The rate of transcription is determined by a variety of other regulatory elements and enhancers. Of particular significance is the 'upstream regulatory element', a sequence usually located about 60bp upstream of the transcription start site, and often taking the form of a CAAT box. This DNA element binds to the CAAT box-binding protein, which acts in concert with the RNA polymerase complex to bring about an enhanced rate of transcription.

A variety of other enhancer elements are found in the promoter region and these serve to define whether the gene will be transcribed in the particular cell type in question, whether this is an appropriate stage of development for transcription to occur, and whether the extracellular signals mediated ultimately through transcription factors favor this. Transcription factors binding to their response elements in the promoter may either stimulate or repress transcription. In certain instances, competition between a stimulatory and a repressive transcription factor may determine the rate of transcription.

The precise mechanism by which these effects are mediated remained obscure until relatively recently. However the discovery of crucial additional factors known as coactivators and corepressors has greatly enhanced understanding of transcription. These molecules interact with both transcription factors and the polymerase complex by protein–protein contacts, and in part they serve to relay the signal to the polymerase complex. More significantly, they influence the chromatin structure of the gene in question and its accessibility to transcription factors. The term chromatin refers to the complex of DNA and histones assembled into a nucleosomal structure.

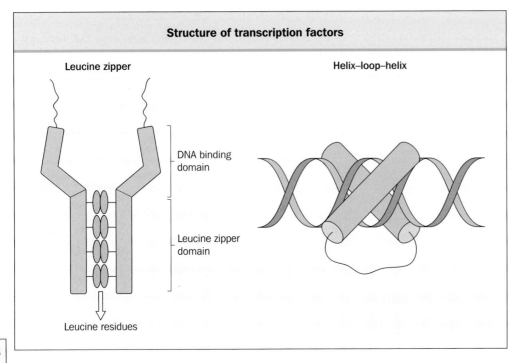

Structure of transcription factors

Leucine zipper

Helix–loop–helix

DNA binding domain

Leucine zipper domain

Leucine residues

Fig. 28.13 Structure of transcription factors. Generalized structure of (left panel) leucine zipper transcription factors and (right panel) helix–loop–helix transcription factors.

Histones are highly basic proteins that are intrinsically associated with DNA in a form in which the DNA helix is wound around core histones to form a nucleosome. Each nucleosome consists of about 180bp of double-stranded DNA wound around two core histones and a linker histone molecule. The N-terminus of the histone faces the outer surface of the nucleosome, and it is this region that is liable to acetylation on specific lysine residues. When acetylated, the nucleosome loses its tightly packed structure and the DNA strands become more readily accessible to extrinsic proteins either in the form of general and specific transcription factors in the promoter region or in permitting the RNA polymerase complex to process down the gene. Thus histone acetylation favors active transcription and, conversely, deacetylation inhibits transcription (**Fig. 28.14**). Interestingly, certain transcription factors, including some of the steroid receptors and the thyroid hormone receptor, are able to bind to DNA even in a closed chromatin conformation.

Understanding of the role of coactivators and corepressors is complicated by the multiple names applied to essentially the same factor. **Table 28.10** summarizes these protein families and their nomenclature. Coactivators bind to multiple transcription factors usually by a highly conserved LXXLL motif and in many cases have intrinsic histone acetyltransferase (HAT) activity. In addition they also form synergistic complexes with other HAT-containing coactivators. Corepressors work in essentially the opposite direction, forming complexes often with unliganded nuclear receptors and with histone deacetylase, thereby maintaining the closed chromatin conformation.

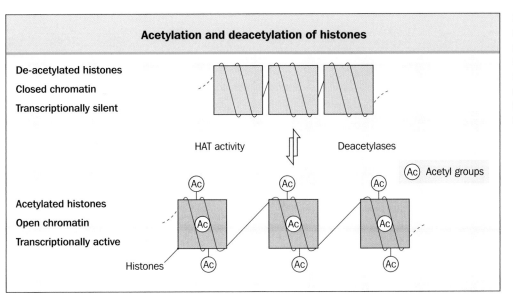

Fig. 28.14 Acetylation and deacetylation of histones. Acetylation of histones by transcription co-activators with acetyltransferase activity leads to a relaxation of the histone assembly and an open chromatin formation that favors transcription. HAT, Histamine acetyl transferases.

Table 28.10 Summary of transcription coactivators and corepressors.

Summary of transcription coactivators and corepressors

Prototype	Family members	Function
Coactivators		
SW1/SNF family (yeast)	BRG1 (mammalian)	Bind nuclear receptors/ remodel chromatin
SRC-1α family	SRC-1α/NcoA-1	Histone acetyltransferases (HATs) – bind transcription factors and other HATs including p300/CBP to form complex
	TIF-2/GRIP1/ NcoA-2	
	P/CIP/ACTR/ RAC3/ AIBI/TRAM-1	
P300/CBP	PCAF	HAT activity – bind transcription factors; complex and synergize with other HATs
DRIP/TRAP		Bind transcription factors; reorganize chromatin by unknown mechanism – no HAT activity
Corepressors		
NcoR	SMRT	Bind transcription factors; recruit histone deacetylase and SIN3 to form repressor complex
TIF1α	TIF1β	Bind transcription factors and HP1; recruit histone deacetylase

Inevitably in any single differentiated cell only a tiny proportion of the entire genetic information will ever be needed, and other mechanisms are also available to enforce this long-term repression of unrequired genes. These mechanisms primarily take the form of DNA methylation. Cytosine residues that precede guanosine residues in DNA are potential targets for methylation. When methylated these methylcytosine residues are bound by members of the methyl-CpG-binding protein family. These proteins not only inhibit transcription by blocking access to DNA but also recruit histone deacetylases and thus maintain a closed chromatin structure. This mechanism is essential for phenomena such as parental imprinting and X chromosome inactivation, in addition to cell-specific genomic silencing as occurs in cellular differentiation. There has been much interest in recent years in the tendency for neoplastic change to be associated with both DNA methylation and demethylation events.

CONCLUSIONS

In summary, this chapter has attempted to review the main molecular characteristics by which hormone signals are recognized by cells, an intracellular second messenger is generated, and exerts its effects. In particular, the mechanism of the influence of these second messengers on gene expression has been considered. Inevitably there are both omissions and generalizations in the limited space available. It is hoped that a satisfactory general picture has been portrayed that can serve as an introduction to a more detailed understanding of this area.

FURTHER READING

Chen E, Gadina M, Chen M, O'Shea JJ. Advances in cytokine signalling: the role of JAKs and STATs. Transplant Proc. 1999;31:1482–7.

Finidori J, Kelly PA. Cytokine receptor signalling through two novel families of transducer molecules: Janus kinases and signal transducers and activators of transcription. J Endocrinol. 1995;147:11–23.

Gether U. Uncovering molecular mechanisms involved in activation of G protein-coupled receptors. Endocrinol Rev. 2000;21:90–113.

Giguere V. Orphan nuclear receptors: from gene to function. Endocrinol Rev. 1999;20:689–725.

Leo C, Chen JD. The SRC family of nuclear receptor coactivators. Gene 2000;245:1–11.

Newell-Price J, Clark AJL, King P. DNA methylation and silencing of gene expression. Trends Endocrinol Metab. 2000;11:142–8.

Nystrom FH, Quon MJ. Insulin signalling: metabolic pathways and mechanisms for specificity. Cell Signal. 1999;11:563–74.

Robertson KD, Wolffe AP. DNA methylation in health and disease. Nat Rev Genet. 2000;1:11–9.

Spiegel AM. G proteins, receptors and disease. Totowa, NJ:Humana Press; 1998.

Touw IP, De Koning JP, Ward AC, Hermans MHA. Signalling mechanisms of cytokine receptors and their perturbances in disease. Mol Cell Endocrinol. 2000;160:1–9.

Whitehead JP, Clark SF, Urso B, James DE. Signalling through the insulin receptor. Curr Opin Cell Biol. 2000;12:222–8.

Zimmerman CM, Padgett RW. Transforming growth factor β signalling mediators and modulators. Gene 2000;249:17–30.

Chapter 29

Pathogenesis of Hormone Secreting Pituitary Tumors

Toni R Prezant and Shlomo Melmed

CLINICAL BACKGROUND

Pituitary tumors are generally benign adenomas, which cause significant morbidity because of their size and/or inappropriate expression of pituitary hormones. Symptomatic anterior pituitary tumors represent about 10% of intracranial neoplasms, although autopsy studies reveal pituitary tumors in as many as 10–20% of adults. Specific hormone-producing cells may be amplified in these tumors, causing unique clinical syndromes. Somatotropinomas overexpress growth hormone, causing acromegaly. Prolactinomas overexpress prolactin, and are the most common of all pituitary adenomas, occurring more frequently in females, with a 3:1 preponderance. Tumors expressing both prolactin and growth hormone are derived from earlier mammosomatotroph precursors. Corticotropinomas, responsible for Cushing's disease, produce increased levels of adrenocorticotropic hormone (ACTH), resulting in excess adrenal gland cortisol, androgens, and 11-deoxycorticosterone secretion. Gonadotropinomas cause sexual dysfunction and hypogonadism, while thyrotropinomas are very rare and cause a mild increase in T_4 levels.

ETIOLOGY OF ANTERIOR PITUITARY TUMORS

Pituitary adenomas are primarily derived from clonal expansion of mutated somatic cells, rather than from hyperplasia in response to hypothalamic hormones. Two lines of evidence support this 'intrinsic defect' hypothesis, X-inactivation studies and loss of heterozygosity (LOH) analysis. In females, the inactivated and methylated X chromosome is sometimes distinguishable by restriction fragment length polymorphism (RFLP) analysis with methylation-sensitive restriction enzymes. The non-random methylation pattern observed in most pituitary tumors indicates that the tumor initiates from the expansion of a single cell. LOH, indicative of hemizygous chromosomal DNA deletions, is observed in all pituitary tumor subtypes. Likewise, these DNA alterations would not be detectable unless the tumor is genetically homogeneous.

However, polyclonal pituitary tumors have been associated with hyperprolactinemia, resulting from extrinsic changes in hypothalamic factors, from multifocal small tumors, or possibly from causes other than prolactinoma, such as pituitary stalk compression, which blocks dopamine inhibition. Furthermore, pituitary hyperplasia and eventual adenoma formation occur in animal models that overexpress hypothalamic growth factors

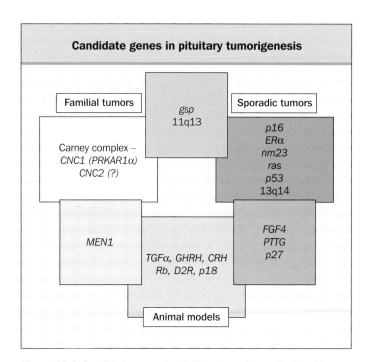

Figure 29.1 Candidate genes in pituitary tumorigenesis. Candidate genes and loci are categorized by their method of identification. The 'primary colors' include familial pituitary tumors (yellow), animal models (blue), and sporadic tumors (red). Genes or loci that are implicated in more than one category are placed in the following boxes: orange, both familial and sporadic tumors; purple, both sporadic tumors and animal models; green, both familial tumors and animal models.

corticotropin-releasing hormone (CRH) or growth-hormone-releasing hormone (GHRH), or that are deprived of dopamine inhibition, as observed in mice with a disrupted D2 receptor transgene (**Fig. 29.1**). In humans, pituitary hyperplasia may develop in response to ectopic GHRH-producing tumors but frank pituitary adenomas are very rare in this situation.

FAMILIAL PITUITARY TUMORS

Pituitary tumors are usually sporadic, but can also occur as a component of a familial cancer syndrome (multiple endocrine neoplasia type I – MEN1, Carney complex), in the mosaic McCune–Albright syndrome, or in isolated familial pituitary tumors. These are listed in Table 29.1 and detailed in Chapter 30.

Genes in familial pituitary tumors			
Gene	Locus (disease)	Function	Evidence in sporadic tumorigenesis?
GNAS1, gsp	20q13.2 (McCune–Albright syndrome)	G-protein α subunit, transduces signal from GHRH to adenylate cyclase, activating mutation results in increased cAMP levels	30–40% of sporadic GH tumors have gsp-activating mutations, rare in other pituitary tumor subtypes, clinical correlation with octreotide sensitivity
MEN1	11q13 (MEN 1)	Menin tumor suppressor protein, interacts with JunD, represses transcription	Mutations are infrequent and MEN 1 mRNA levels are normal in most sporadic pituitary tumors
CNC1, PRKAR1α	17q24 (Carney complex)	Regulates protein kinase A activity, transduces cAMP signal from GHRH to GH activation	
CNC2 (?)	2p16 (Carney complex)		
?	11q13 and second locus (familial acromegaly)	?	LOH in up to 30% of sporadic pituitary tumors
?	? (familial prolactinoma)	?	?

Table 29.1 Genes in familial pituitary tumors.

MEN1

Multiple endocrine neoplasia type 1, or MEN1 (see also Chapter 34), is a familial tumor syndrome most often affecting the parathyroid gland and endocrine pancreas, and less frequently the anterior pituitary. For as yet unknown reasons, most MEN1 pituitary tumors are prolactinomas. MEN1 is inherited as an autosomal dominant disorder or can arise *de novo*. However, it has reduced penetrance because an additional somatic mutation in the *MEN1* tumor suppressor gene is required for phenotypic expression. MEN1 is similar to other familial cancer syndromes that conform to the Knudson two-hit model of tumorigenesis. A germline mutation in one chromosome becomes unmasked by a 'second hit,' generally a deletion of the normal gene in the second chromosome, visualized as a loss of heterozygosity, or LOH, for polymorphic DNA markers spanning the *MEN1* gene (this is considered in Chapter 34). Multiple tumors excised from the same MEN1 patient arise clonally but independently, with different deletions presumably uncovering the germline *MEN1* mutation in each tumor.

MEN1 was localized to chromosomal region 11q13 by linkage and LOH analyses. The *MEN1* gene encodes a 610-amino-acid nuclear protein, menin, which interacts with the transcription factor JunD, to repress transactivation of other genes. The majority of MEN1 families (75–85%) harbor detectable *MEN1* mutations. Most *MEN1* mutations are truncating, while several missense mutations disrupt the interaction of menin with JunD.

MEN1 *variants*

The direct involvement of *MEN1* mutations in pituitary tumor formation in MEN1 families has been called into question. Not all pituitary tumor subtypes occur with equal frequencies in MEN1 families. This is discussed in detail in Chapter 34.

Infrequent MEN1 *mutations in sporadic pituitary tumors*

Tumor-suppressor genes identified in familial cancer syndromes are usually involved in the corresponding sporadic tumors. The *MEN1* gene meets this criterion for parathyroid and pancreatic tumors, but its role in sporadic pituitary adenomas is less clear. The frequency of LOH for 11q13 is considerably lower in sporadic pituitary tumors than for parathyroid and pancreatic tumors, ranging from 0–30%. The highest frequencies for LOH

at 11q13 were seen in invasive pituitary tumors (14/45), suggesting a possible role for *MEN1* in the progression but not the initiation of sporadic pituitary tumors.

Sequence analysis showed that MEN1 mutations occur rarely in sporadic pituitary adenomas. The majority of sporadic pituitary tumors have approximately equal expression of both *MEN1* alleles, excluding genomic imprinting as a general mechanism to silence this chromosomal region. By comparative reverse transcription–polymerase chain reaction (RT–PCR) experiments, normal *MEN1* mRNA levels are apparent in pituitary adenomas, except for those tumors with LOH, in which *MEN1* mRNA levels were decreased. Taken together, the evidence from studies of sporadic pituitary tumors predicts that a second tumor suppressor gene should be found in 11q13.

McCune–Albright syndrome

Activating '*gsp*' mutations in the *GNAS1* gene, on chromosome 20q13.2, account for asymmetric defects in the bony skeleton, skin, and endocrine system in McCune–Albright syndrome. Endocrine abnormalities include precocious puberty, thyrotoxicosis, acromegaly, gigantism, or Cushing's syndrome. While there are few familial occurrences, the defect is inherited as a somatic mosaic, with high variability in symptoms depending on the proportions of mutant cells and specific tissues involved in the mosaicism. The disorder is presumably caused by an autosomal dominant lethal gene that allows embryonic survival only when the mutation arises in somatic cells.

G-protein mutations

G-protein mutations are common in sporadic somatotropinomas. Pituitary cell growth and function is regulated by G-protein-signaling pathways, which respond to stimulatory and inhibitory hypothalamic growth factors. Dominant mutations of the *gsp* gene, identified in 30–40% of somatotropinomas, reduce GTPase activity and stabilize the active form of the $G_s\alpha$-protein, leading to increased adenylyl cyclase activity, increased levels of cyclic adenosine monophosphate (cAMP), and increased growth hormone secretion, independent of hypothalamic GHRH. These mutations occur less frequently in nonfunctioning pituitary adenomas (0–13%), and, rarely, in gonadotropinomas or corticotropinomas. Other G-proteins might be involved in pituitary tumorigenesis, as mutations were described in *gip-2*, which encodes a G_i subunit. Although the *gip-2* mutation should have the opposite effect of *gsp* mutations, causing constitutive inhibition of adenylyl cyclase, the mutation is postulated to affect other signaling pathways.

Clinical outcome of *gsp* mutation
Since stimulation of somatostatin receptors by somatostatin analogs inhibits adenyl cyclase these *gsp+* tumors may be more sensitive to somatostatin analogs, e.g. octreotide, even when a tumor remnant is present after surgery.

Carney complex
Carney complex (CNC), is characterized by a constellation of cardiac myxomas, spotty skin pigmentation, and tumors of the adrenal gland and anterior pituitary, most often somatotropinomas. CNC pituitary specimens are hyperplastic with multifocal microadenomas, in accord with the clinically elevated growth hormone (GH) levels commonly found even when tumors are undetectable by standard imaging techniques. CNC exhibits genetic heterogeneity, mapping to two chromosomal regions, 2p16 and 17q24. The gene encoding the protein kinase A type Iα regulatory subunit, *PRKAR1A*, was reported to be the chromosome 17 CNC gene. Mutations have been found in seven of 11 families with Carney complex definitively linked to 17q24.

Since the predicted truncated proteins were not detectable by Western blot, the *PRKAR1A* defects may act through haploinsufficiency. The altered ratio of the protein kinase A (PKA) regulatory α and β subunits results in lower basal activity of protein kinase A. However, *in vitro* experiments showed that CNC tumor extracts have increased PKA responses to cAMP stimulation compared to non-CNC tumors. Hyperstimulation of this pathway is likely to be tumorigenic. Recently, CNC mutations have been identified in some families that only exhibit cardiac myxomas. Specific alleles of these genes may similarly lead to pituitary tumorigenesis with no other endocrine organ neoplasia.

Figure 29.2 depicts the GHRH signaling pathway implicated in pituitary tumorigenesis. GH-producing tumors arise in transgenic mice overexpressing GHRH. Human somatotropinomas have been identified with activating mutations in the G-protein α subunit, or inactivating mutations in the *PRKAR1A* gene.

Familial prolactinoma
Four pedigrees with isolated prolactinoma in two family members have been reported. The patients and their families had normal parathyroid and pancreatic function, suggesting that MEN1 was not the cause of the pituitary tumors. Linkage analysis and *MEN1* mutation screening have recently shown that familial hyperprolactinemia is genetically distinct from MEN1.

Familial acromegaly
Isolated familial somatotropinoma is linked to at least two chromosomal regions, 11q13 and a distinct locus. We and others excluded *MEN1* mutations as a common cause of familial acromegaly. Interestingly, a family described by Gadelha et al. (2000), with early onset acromegaly, shows evidence of linkage to both chromosomal regions 11q13 and 2p16, one of the loci for CNC.

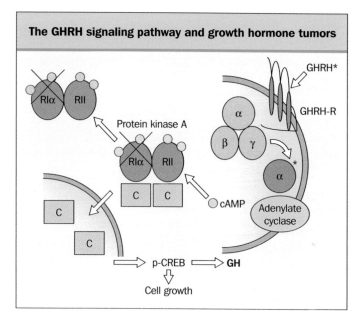

Figure 29.2 The growth-hormone-releasing hormone (GHRH) signaling pathway and growth hormone (GH) tumors. Hypothalamic GHRH stimulates the GHRH receptor (GHRH-R) in the plasma membrane of the anterior pituitary. The signal is transmitted through the heterotrimeric G-protein, to adenylate cyclase. As cyclic adenosine monophosphate (cAMP) is increased, the regulatory subunit dimer of protein kinase A binds cooperatively and dissociates from the catalytic domain. Catalytic subunits of protein kinase A then localize to the nucleus, activate transcription of cAMP-responsive genes, inducing expression of growth hormone and other growth stimulating genes. *, X, lesion identified in pituitary tumors.

MODELS OF PITUITARY TUMORIGENESIS

Candidate genes from animal models for pituitary tumorigenesis are listed in **Table 29.2**.

TGFα
The mitogenic protein transforming growth factor-α, TGFα, is found in conditioned medium derived from retrovirally transformed cells, and is expressed in fetal development and in several adult tissues, including lactotrophs. Estrogen-treated ovariectomized adult rats have increased TGFα mRNA levels before initiation of lactotroph hyperplasia. Female mice expressing the *TGFα* transgene under transcriptional control of the rat prolactin promoter developed lactotroph hyperplasia by 6 months, and prolactinomas by 12 months, with no evidence of pituitary disease in transgenic males. TGFα did not induce tumors of other pituitary cell subtypes, indicating a specific role in prolactinoma tumorigenesis.

DRD2
Dopamine and its agonists inhibit prolactin secretion and lactotroph growth through the dopamine D2 receptor. Pituitary stalk compression, neovascularization, or gene disruption block dopamine inhibition and result in lactotroph hyperplasia, hyperprolactinemia and prolactinoma formation. The prolonged lactotroph hyperplasia (17–18 months) that preceded adenoma

Candidate genes from animal models			
Gene	Function	Evidence for involvement	Evidence against involvement
Transgene			
TGFα	Transforming growth factor-α, mitogenic protein	Expressed in lactotrophs, induced early by estrogen, prolactinomas in female transgenic mice	
GHRH	Induces growth hormone expression	Old transgenic mice develop adenomas	
CRH	Induces adrenocorticotropic hormone expression	Transgenic mice develop hypercortisolism	
NGF	Nerve growth factor	Ectopic NGF induces lactotroph hyperplasia in transgenic mice	Reduces tumorigenicity of primary prolactinoma cultures (after 90 days in vitro)
Overexpressed gene			
PTTG1	Pituitary tumor transforming gene-1, securin	Overexpression is tumorigenic, induces bFGF, induced early by estrogen, increased in pituitary tumors and regulates chromosome segregation	
hst	Heparin binding secretory transforming gene, fibroblast growth factor, FGF-4	Transfected GH4 cells are more tumorigenic, expressed in invasive prolactinomas	Transforming changes unknown, normal in Southern blot of human prolactinomas
Excess hormone			
ERα, ERβ	Estrogen receptor	Estrogen induces prolactinomas in rats, human prolactinomas express ER and constitutively active ER splice variants	
Disrupted gene			
Rb	Retinoblastoma protein, tumor suppressor gene, controls cell cycle progression	Rb-knockout mice develop tumors of intermediate lobe, 13q14 LOH in invasive or malignant pituitary tumors	No mutations, hypophosphorylated Rb (active form) is immunodetected
p27^{Kip1}	Cyclin-dependent kinase inhibitor protein, p27, blocks phosphorylation of Rb protein to keep it in active form	p27-knockout mice develop tumors of intermediate lobe, decreased or absent protein in most human pituitary tumors	
DRD2	Dopamine receptor subtype 2, inhibits prolactin secretion and lactotroph growth	DRD2 –/– mice develop prolactinomas, dopamine agonists shrink prolactinomas, decreased expression in nonresponders	No DRD2 mutations in human prolactinomas

Table 29.2 Candidate genes from animal models.

development in female DRD2–/– mice, dopamine D_2-receptor knockout animals, suggested that preventing dopamine inhibition allowed an increased pool of lactotrophs to acquire initiating tumorigenic changes. However, similarly aged male DRD2-knockout mice developed multifocal microprolactinomas without an increase in pituitary size, suggesting that loss of DRD2 signaling activates gender-specific tumorigenic pathways. Alternatively, hyperplasia might not be a prerequisite for tumorigenesis.

DRD2 and human prolactinomas
No DRD2 coding sequence mutations were detected in 46 human prolactinomas and 19 mixed GH/prolactin adenomas. However, reduced dopamine receptor expression correlates clinically with bromocriptine resistance in prolactinomas.

ADDITIONAL CANDIDATE GENES IN PITUITARY TUMORIGENESIS

Several studies have excluded the involvement of well-known oncogenes (ras, c-myc, c-myb, c-fos), tumor suppressor genes (p53, Rb, nm23), and pituitary transcription factors in the majority of pituitary tumors, although alterations are sometimes associated with invasiveness. However, expression of two cell-cycle regulatory proteins (p16, p27) is significantly decreased in most pituitary adenomas, implicating DNA methylation and ubiquitin-mediated proteolysis pathways in tumorigenesis. These are summarized in **Table 29.3**.

Oncogenes
Oncogenes are dominantly acting genes that promote cell growth through a gain of function or altered regulation.

ras
Ras proteins transduce signals from plasma membrane tyrosine kinase receptors to the nucleus through a protein kinase cascade. The ras gene family is frequently involved in early stages of human cancers. Oncogenic mutations were identified in the H-ras gene in two highly invasive pituitary tumors, one of which arose de novo in the metastatic tumor. However, two large studies excluded activating mutations in codons 12, 13 and 61 in the N-, H-, and K-ras genes, suggesting that ras activation is limited to pituitary tumor progression.

c-myc, c-myb, c-fos
Mutations or altered expression of the nuclear oncogenes c-myc, c-myb, and c-fos do not appear to be a common mechanism for pituitary tumorigenesis. Although c-myc mRNA was

Additional candidate genes in pituitary tumorigenesis			
Gene	Function	Evidence for involvement	Evidence against involvement
H-, K-, N-*ras*	Ras protein family, transduces signals from tyrosine kinase receptors	Activating mutations rarely found in highly invasive prolactinomas	No mutations in most benign or invasive prolactinomas
p53	Checkpoint protein, senses DNA damage and blocks cell cycle progression	Immunodetectable in pituitary carcinomas and some invasive adenomas	No mutations, conflicting reports of immunodetectable p53 in less invasive adenomas
p16^{INK4a}	Cyclin dependent kinase inhibitor protein, p16, blocks phosphorylation of Rb protein to keep it in active form	Protein undetectable in pituitary tumors, mRNA usually decreased	
nm23	Purine-binding factor, tumor suppressor in rodent models, decreased expression in metastatic cell	Decreased expression of H2 isoform protein and mRNA in invasive pituitary tumors	

Table 29.3 Additional candidate genes in pituitary tumorigenesis.

overexpressed in nine of 30 pituitary tumors, two invasive prolactinomas had normal levels. Thus, c-*myc* expression does not correlate with proliferative state.

Tumor suppressor genes

Tumor suppressor genes restrain cell division. Their loss by homozygous inactivation or failed expression results in progression through the cell cycle. Several of the tumor-suppressor genes depicted in **Figure 29.3** have been implicated or tested for roles in pituitary tumorigenesis.

p53

p53 encodes a checkpoint protein that prevents cell-cycle progression when DNA is damaged. *p53* is the most commonly mutated gene found in human tumors, with missense mutations usually occurring in exons 5 through 8. Mutations in this region were not detected in a large series of pituitary adenomas or carcinomas, except for a single *p53* mutation in a prolactin-secreting carcinoma. Mutant p53 forms accumulate in the nucleus, with a longer half-life than wild-type p53, although the correlation is not absolute. While some investigators reported p53 immunopositive non-invasive adenomas, others found a clear correlation between p53 nuclear immunopositivity and tumor aggressiveness.

Rb

The retinoblastoma protein, Rb, participates in cell-cycle control through its differential phosphorylation by cell-cycle-dependent kinases and cyclins. Hypophosphorylated (active) Rb binds E2F transcription factors, blocking entry into the cell cycle; phosphorylated Rb releases E2Fs (**Figure 29.3**). Transgenic mice with *Rb* disruptions develop pituitary tumors of the intermediate lobe, in ACTH-producing cells. This observation made *Rb* a prime candidate for involvement in human pituitary tumors. However, intragenic LOH for the *Rb* locus was not found in more than 50 benign adenomas, or in two invasive prolactinomas. Aggressive pituitary tumors may have a higher frequency of LOH, but Rb protein is present in these tumors. Another gene on 13q14 seems to be implicated in the progression, but not the initiation, of aggressive human pituitary tumors.

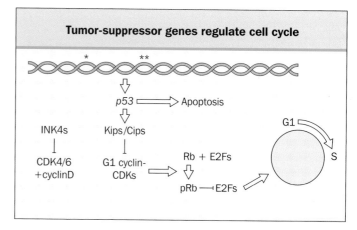

Figure 29.3 The regulation of the G1-to-S transition by tumor-suppressor gene products. Cyclin-dependent kinases (CDKs) phosphorylate and inactivate Rb, releasing the inhibition of E2F transcription factors. INK4s block CDK binding to cyclin and Kips block cyclin kinase activity, indirectly inhibiting Rb phosphorylation. p53 activates one of the Kip proteins in response to DNA damage.

p27

The eukaryotic cell cycle is tightly controlled by cyclin-dependent kinases (CDKs) that promote progression through G1 to S phase. The CDK inhibitors block cell-cycle progression and act as tumor suppressors, and constitute two classes (**Fig. 29.3**). Ink4 proteins (p16^{Ink4a}, p15^{Ink4b}, p18^{Ink4c}, p19^{Ink4d}) block the interaction of CDK4 and CDK6 kinases with cyclin D. Cip/Kip proteins (p21^{Cip1}, p27^{Kip1}, p57^{Kip2}) bind to cyclin–CDK complexes and inhibit their activation or kinase activity. Mice disrupted for *p27* develop multiorgan hyperplasia and frequent tumors of pro-opiomelanocortin-positive cells of the pituitary intermediate lobe. Disruption of *p27* leads to increased cell divisions in organs that express it.

p27 behaves as a tumor suppressor gene both in an animal model and in human sporadic pituitary tumors. p27 protein is underexpressed or absent in the majority of human pituitary tumors of all subtypes, and absent in pituitary carcinomas. Decreased p27 immunostaining occurs in all pituitary tumors compared to respective normal pituitary cell types and was especially reduced in carcinomas. Mutations were excluded by SSCP analysis. Decreased p27 expression is regulated instead by posttranscriptional and posttranslational mechanisms, including ubiquitin-dependent protein degradation.

p18

Mice disrupted for the cyclin inhibitor $p18^{Ink4c}$ display a phenotype similar to $p27$-disrupted mice, including widespread organomegaly, pituitary hyperplasia, and development of intermediate lobe tumors at an advanced age. The normal GH levels and only slightly elevated IGF-1 levels suggest that other affected organs are enlarged because of an intrinsic defect in p18, rather than from endocrine effects of pituitary hyperplasia. Mice that are doubly disrupted for $p18$ and $p27$ have greatly accelerated pituitary tumorigenesis, and die by 3 months. This synergistic effect indicates that the genes functionally collaborate, acting on distinct pathways to regulate Rb.

p16

$p16^{Ink4a}$, the product of the *CDKN2A* gene on chromosome 9p21, is inactivated in several human tumor cell lines and in primary tumors. *p16* product prevents the phosphorylation/inactivation of Rb by inhibiting CDK4. Loss of p16 function allows phosphorylation of Rb, and hence cell-cycle transcription factors become active (**Fig. 29.3**). p16 is undetectable by Western blot analysis but mutations were not detected in 25 pituitary tumors. Loss of p16 protein correlated with decreased or undetectable mRNA in 93% of tumors but, in contrast to other tumor types in which *p16* is silenced through LOH or homozygous deletions, pituitary adenomas more frequently inactivate this gene by methylation.

nm23

The purine-binding factor nm23 is a tumor suppressor in rodent tumor models that has decreased expression in highly metastatic melanoma cell lines. The *nm23* gene encodes two isoforms, H1 and H2. Invasive tumors had decreased expression of the H2 isoform compared to benign adenomas.

Transcription factors

Pit-1

The pituitary-specific transcriptional activator Pit-1 regulates expression of *GH*, *PRL*, and *TSHβ* genes, and is required for proliferation of the cells that express these hormones. *Pit-1* mRNA was increased 2.5- to 5-fold in pituitary adenomas compared to normal pituitary. However, the cell-type distribution, size and sequence of the *Pit-1* mRNA appears identical in normal and adenomatous pituitaries. Although alternative splicing of the *Pit-1* mRNA results in isoforms with different DNA-binding and transactivation properties, similar ratios of the *Pit-1* and *Pit-1β* isoforms were observed in pure GH- or prolactin-secreting tumors, suggesting that pituitary tumorigenesis is not associated with altered Pit-1 expression.

PROP-1

The 'prophet of Pit-1' gene (*PROP-1*) is expressed in early pituitary development and activates *Pit-1* transcription. In humans, *PROP-1* mutations result in combined pituitary hormone deficiency (deficits of GH, prolactin, TSH, and gonadotropins), but altered expression is not associated with pituitary tumorigenesis.

Estrogen receptor

Estrogen is a mitogen for normal and transformed lactotrophs and gonadotrophs. The female preponderance of prolactinomas and their increased size during pregnancy may be due to high estradiol levels. In addition, pharmacologic doses of estrogen cause rat lactotroph hyperplasia and adenomas. Estrogen stimulates the prolactin promoter and activates the expression of *PTTG* and *TGFα*, genes implicated in tumorigenesis. Estrogen is a ligand for the estrogen receptor (ER), a transcriptional factor in the steroid receptor superfamily. Prolactinomas are the pituitary tumor subtype that most strongly express estrogen receptors, as demonstrated by immunohistochemistry, binding assays, and ribonuclease protection assays. ER is encoded by two genes, *ERα*, expressed in 70–100% of prolactinomas, and *ERβ*, detectable in 60%. Binding of estradiol *in vitro* leads to ER dimerization and activation of estrogen-responsive genes, with a stronger estrogen response due to *ERα* (14-fold induction) than *ERβ* (fourfold induction). Alternatively spliced *ERα* mRNAs can produce isoforms with altered responsiveness to estrogens and antiestrogens, suggesting an attractive mechanism for tumorigenesis. In particular, deletion of exon 2 results in a stimulatory isoform, and deletion of exon 5 (*ERα–Δ5*) produces a ligand-independent constitutively active isoform. In contrast, exon 3 or exon 7 deletions produce dominant negative isoforms of *ERα* lacking DNA binding or transactivation functions, respectively. Exon-2- and exon-5-deleted transcripts were detected in nearly all prolactinomas while exon 7 deletions were much less common, although the relative proportions of mutant and full-length *ERα* cDNAs were not determined. *ERβ* is not strongly activating by itself and is not expressed in all prolactinomas, but can nonetheless interact with *ERα–Δ5* to increase expression of an estrogen response element (ERE)-controlled luciferase reporter gene.

TRH-R

Hypothalamic thyrotropin-releasing hormone (TRH) stimulates both TSH release from thyrotrophs and prolactin release from lactotrophs. The pituitary G-protein-coupled TRH receptor mediates these effects. Although the *TRH-R* gene was screened for activating mutations, none were detected in 15 prolactinomas.

Growth factors

hst

The heparin-binding secretory transforming gene (*hst*), also known as fibroblast growth factor 4 (*FGF-4*), was identified in DNA derived from human prolactinomas. Strong FGF-4 immunoreactivity was detected specifically in human prolactinomas (36%), and not in other pituitary tumor subtypes or normal anterior pituitary. The FGF-4 expression correlated with invasiveness, assessed by the Ki-67 index, a proliferation-related nuclear antigen. Taken together, these studies implicate *hst* in prolactinoma formation, by an as yet unknown mechanism.

bFGF

Basic fibroblast growth factor, or bFGF, is a potent mitogen for neuroectoderm cells *in vitro* and stimulates angiogenesis *in vivo*, and its expression is highest in the pituitary and brain. Although it lacks a classical amino-terminal signal sequence, bFGF is secreted, but normally undetectable in human serum. However, in some MEN 1 patients with prolactinomas, immunoreactive bFGF was detectable before surgery or dopamine agonist treatment, and decreased after surgery or bromocriptine. Elevated plasma bFGF was not detectable in three patients with sporadic macroprolactinomas but intratumoral bFGF expression positively correlated with expression of the *PTTG* oncogene in seven sporadic prolactinomas. **Figure 29.4** shows that transcription of both *PTTG* and bFGF is increased in a time- and dose-dependent manner in rats treated with estrogen, prior to development of prolactinomas.

NGF

The role of nerve growth factor, NGF, in prolactinoma tumorigenesis is controversial. NGF is involved in growth, differentiation, and survival of neurons, through binding to cell-surface tyrosine kinase receptors. The anterior pituitary, specifically the mammosomatotroph lineage, expresses NGF and its receptors. Primary cultures of human prolactinomas that were nonresponsive to dopamine did not express NGF and its receptor, but both genes could be induced by NGF treatment. The dopamine responders, which express NGF, had lower tumorigenic potential than nonresponders. These phenotypes were reversed in cultured prolactinoma cells, by inducing NGF and its receptor or inhibiting their expression.

PTTG

A novel proto-oncogene, *PTTG* (pituitary-tumor-transforming gene), was isolated from rat pituitary tumor cells. The homologous human counterpart, human *PTTG*, behaves as an oncogene, since NIH 3T3 cells transfected with *PTTG* cDNA are transformed *in vitro* and form tumors in athymic mice. *PTTG* expression correlates with size of secreting pituitary tumors (**Fig. 29.5**), and with lymph node invasion in colorectal tumors, and therefore may potentially be useful as a molecular diagnostic marker for tumor invasiveness.

CONCLUSIONS

Early changes leading to pituitary tumorigenesis are becoming better understood (**Fig. 29.6**). Three genes that predispose to pituitary tumorigenesis have been identified from studies of familial pituitary tumors, and their protein products have elucidated important regulatory pathways. The *MEN1* gene encodes menin, a transcriptional co-repressor interacting with JunD. Presumably, the altered expression of target genes in the absence of functional menin is tumorigenic. Although *MEN1* defects are not common in sporadic pituitary tumors, the *gsp* mutation identified in McCune–Albright syndrome occurs in a significant

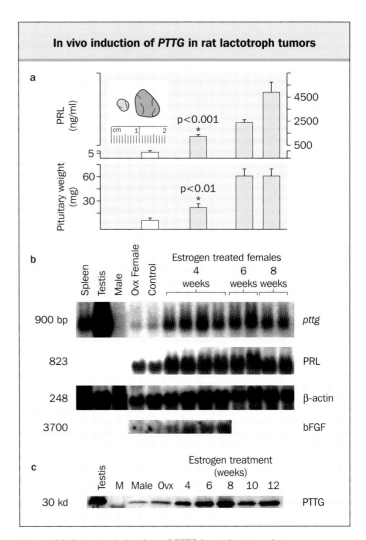

Figure 29.4 In vivo induction of *PTTG* in rat lactotroph tumors. (a) Representative normal rat pituitary and tumor, serum prolactin, and pituitary wet weight, (b) Northern blot, and (c) Western blot of pituitary tissue extracts derived from estrogen-treated rats, intact male pituitary ($n = 2$) and ovariectomized controls (Ovx, $n = 2$), during prolonged estrogen treatment. M, molecular weight standard. (Adapted with permission from Heaney AP, et al. Early involvement of estrogen-induced pituitary tumor transforming gene and fibroblast growth factor expression in prolactinoma pathogenesis. Nat Med. 1999;5:1317–21.)

proportion of sporadic GH-secreting tumors. This constitutively activated G-protein leads to chronic stimulation of adenylate cyclase. Tumors with *gsp* mutations are generally more responsive to somatostatin analog treatment. The cAMP-mediated GHRH signal transduction pathway is also involved in Carney complex. One of the two CNC genes was recently identified. The functional inactivation of its encoded protein kinase A regulatory subunit I-α results in greater sensitivity to cAMP. Pituitary adenomas in both McCune–Albright syndrome and Carney complex tend to be multifocal, and to be preceded by hyperplasia, as occurs in an animal model with excess GHRH secretion.

Animal models have implicated growth-restraining tumor suppressor genes in pituitary tumors. Initially, the *Rb* gene appeared to be a promising candidate, because *Rb*-disrupted mice develop pituitary adenomas. However, active hypophosphorylated Rb

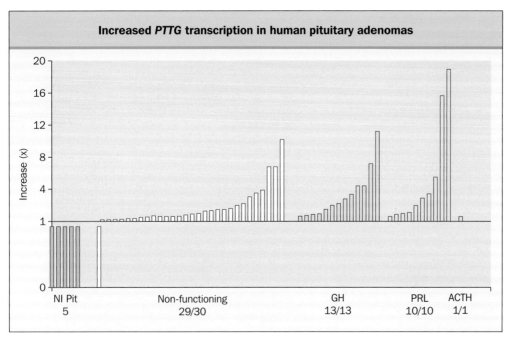

Figure 29.5 Increased *PTTG* transcription in human pituitary adenomas. Densitometric ratios of *PTTG*:cyclophilin A mRNA, determined by comparative RT-PCR, in human pituitary adenomas ($n = 54$) and normal pituitary ($n = 5$). ACTH, adrenocorticotropic hormone; GH, growth hormone; PRL, prolactin. (Adapted with permission from Zhang X, Horwitz GA, Heaney AP, et al. Pituitary tumor transforming gene (PTTG) expression in pituitary adenomas. J Clin Endocrinol Metab. 1999;84:761–7 © The Endocrine Society.)

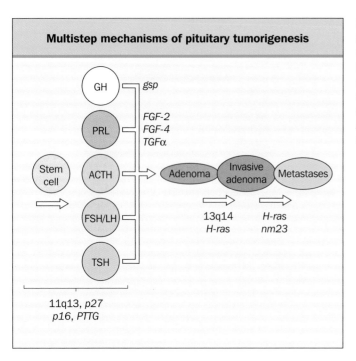

Figure 29.6 Multistep mechanisms of pituitary tumorigenesis. Several genes or chromosomal loci are implicated in all pituitary tumor subtypes (11q13, *p27*, *p16*, *PTTG*). Some genes appear to have subtype-specific involvement in tumorigenesis (growth-hormone (GH)-secreting tumors: *gsp*; prolactin (PRL)-secreting tumors: *FGF-2*, *FGF-4*, *TGFα*). Alterations of additional candidate genes or loci (13q14, H-*ras*, and *nm23*) have been observed in a few instances of invasive or metastatic pituitary adenomas. ACTH, adrenocorticotropic hormone; FSH, follicle-stimulating hormone; LH, luteinizing hormone; TSH, thyroid-stimulating hormone.

protein is expressed in human pituitary tumors. Several proteins that regulate the cell-cycle-dependent phosphorylation of Rb have been implicated, either by their decreased expression in human pituitary tumors or by their effects in gene-disrupted mice. The decreased expression of *p16* and *p27* is a universal finding in human pituitary tumors, invoking gene methylation and proteolytic pathways, respectively, in pituitary tumorigenesis. Mice deficient in *p27* or *p18* develop late-onset pituitary adenomas. The genes act in synergy, since doubly deficient mice develop giant pituitary tumors by 3 months. Mice deficient in the D2 receptor gene lack dopamine inhibition and develop lactotroph hyperplasia and eventual adenomas. While the *DRD2* gene is not mutated in human pituitary tumors, around 20% of prolactinomas are insensitive to dopamine inhibition. Estrogen induces expression of growth factors bFGF and TGFα and the oncogene *PTTG*, which further induces bFGF, promoting angiogenesis even before lactotroph hyperplasia is evident. In humans, *PTTG* expression is elevated in all pituitary adenoma subtypes, suggesting that its dysregulation is an initiating event in pituitary tumorigenesis. Dysregulated *PTTG* expression may lead to aberrant chromosome segregation and additional changes in the multistep progression of pituitary tumors.

FURTHER READING

Farrell WE, Clayton RN. Molecular pathogenesis of pituitary tumors. Front Neuroendocrinol. 2000;21:174–98.

Gadelha MR, Une KN, Rohde K, et al. Isolated familial somatotropinomas: establishment of linkage to chromosome 11q13.1–11q13.3 and evidence for a potential second locus at chromosome 2p16–12. J Clin Endocrinol Metab. 2000;85:707–14.

Heaney AP, Horwitz GA, Wang Z, et al. Early involvement of estrogen-induced pituitary tumor transforming gene and fibroblast growth factor expression in prolactinoma pathogenesis. Nat Med. 1999;5:1317–21.

Herman V, Fagin J, Gonsky R, et al. Clonal origin of pituitary adenomas. J Clin Endocrinol Metab. 1990;71:1427–33.

Kirschner LS, Carney JA, Pack SD, et al. Mutations of the gene encoding the protein kinase A type I-α regulatory subunit in patients with the Carney complex. Nat Genet. 2000;26:89–92.

Prezant TR, Kadioglu P, Melmed S. An intronless homolog of human proto-oncogene hPTTG is expressed in pituitary tumors: evidence for hPTTG family. J Clin Endocrinol Metab. 1999;84:1149–52.

Shimon I, Melmed S. Genetic basis of endocrine disease: pituitary tumor pathogenesis. J Clin Endocrinol Metab. 1997;82:1675–81.

Stratakis CA. Genetics of Carney complex and related familial lentiginoses, and other multiple tumor syndromes. Front Biosci. 2000;5:D353–66.

Thakker RV, Pook MA, Wooding C, et al. Association of somatotrophinomas with loss of alleles on chromosome 11 and with gsp mutations. J Clin Invest. 1993;91:2815–21.

Vallar L, Spada A, Giannattasio G. Altered Gs and adenylate cyclase activity in human GH-secreting pituitary adenomas. Nature 1987;330:566–8.

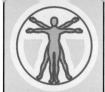

Chapter 30 Familial Endocrine Syndromes

Rajesh V Thakker

INTRODUCTION

Endocrine cancers are uncommon when compared to the incidence of lung, breast, colorectal, and prostate cancers (Table 30.1). For example, only ovarian cancer features in the estimates of the worldwide incidence of the 18 major cancers, where it ranks as the sixth most frequent cancer in women. However, it is important to note that parathyroid tumors giving rise to primary hyperparathyroidism are more common but, as these tumors are rarely malignant, they are often not considered in the cancer registries. Familial endocrine cancer syndromes, which are generally inherited as autosomal dominant traits (Table 30.2) with a high penetrance, are rare, but their recognition is important for two main reasons. First, the affected patients may be at risk from multiple tumors that may arise in different glands, and regular screening for these together with earlier treatment is likely to improve the prognosis. Second, the relatives of an affected patient are at a 50% risk of having inherited the mutation and thus developing tumors. Identification of these individuals, together with screening for the early development of tumors, is also likely to improve the prognosis. This chapter will review the molecular genetics of neoplasia together with the clinical and genetic features of some familial endocrine cancer syndromes. These syndromes include:

- multiple endocrine neoplasia type 1 (MEN1);
- multiple endocrine neoplasia type 2 (MEN2);
- familial isolated primary hyperparathyroidism (FIHP);
- the hyperparathyroidism–jaw-tumor syndrome (HPT–JT);
- familial benign hypocalciuric hypercalcemia (FBH or FHH) and neonatal primary hyperparathyroidism (NHPT);
- Von Hippel–Lindau disease (VHL);
- neurofibromatosis type 1 (NF1);
- Carney complex;
- Cowden's syndrome; and
- the familial breast–ovarian cancer syndrome.

Incidence of some common cancers and endocrine cancers		
Cancer		Incidence (per 100,000 population per year)
Nonendocrine	Lung	72 (M), 19 (F)*
	Breast	54 (F)
	Colorectal	40
	Prostate	20–30 (M)
Endocrine	Ovary	11 (F)
	Testis	3.3 (M)
	Thyroid	1.5
	Parathyroid	28
Neuroendocrine		0.7 (to 8.4)

Table 30.1 Incidence of some common cancers and endocrine cancers. * M, males; F. females; if not stated, both sexes.

Familial endocrine cancer syndromes and their chromosomal locations	
Disorder	Chromosomal location (gene or protein)
Multiple endocrine neoplasia type 1	11q13 (MENIN)
Multiple endocrine neoplasia type 2	10q11.2 (RET)
Familial isolated primary hyperparathyroidism	11q13 (MENIN), 1p32-pter, 1q25-q31
Hyperparathyroidism–jaw-tumor syndrome	1q25-q31
Familial benign hypocalciuric hypercalcemia, neonatal primary hyperparathyroidism	3q13-q21 (CaSR)
Von Hippel–Lindau disease	3p26-p25 (pVHL, ELONGIN)
Neurofibromatosis type 1	17q11.2 (NEUROFIBROMIN)
Pheochromocytoma	1p, 17p, 22q
Carney complex	2p16, 17q22-q23 (PPKARIA)
Cowden's syndrome	10q23.3 (PTEN)
Breast–ovarian cancer	17q21 (BRCA1)

Table 30.2 Familial endocrine cancer syndromes and their chromosomal locations.

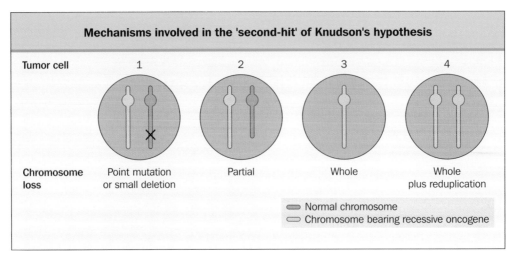

Figure 30.1 Mechanisms involved in the 'second hit' of Knudson's hypothesis. A pair of chromosomes, one normal and the other bearing the recessive oncogene, are schematically represented in each of four tumor cells ((1)–(4)). Four main forms of the 'second hit' involving the normal chromosome, i.e. the normal dominant allele, are shown. In tumor cell (1) there has been a point mutation or a small deletion, whereas in tumor cells (2) and (3) partial and complete loss of the normal chromosomes, respectively, have occurred. A complete loss of a chromosome, resulting in autosomal monosomy, may be disadvantageous to cell growth, and reduplication of the chromosome bearing the recessive oncogene may occur, as shown in tumor cell (4). These 'second hits' involving the normal dominant allele would lead to an unmasking of the recessive oncogenic mutation and thus result in tumor development. (Redrawn from Thakker RV. The molecular genetics of the multiple endocrine neoplasia syndromes. Clin Endocrinol. 1993;38:1–14.)

MOLECULAR GENETICS OF NEOPLASIA

Genetic models of tumor development

The development of tumors may be associated with mutations or inappropriate expression of specific normal cellular genes, which are referred to as oncogenes. Two types of oncogene referred to as dominant and recessive oncogenes have been described. An activation of dominant oncogenes leads to malignant transformation of the cells containing them, and the genetic changes that cause this activation have been elucidated. For example, chromosomal translocations affecting such dominant oncogenes are associated with the occurrence of chronic myeloid leukemia and Burkitt's lymphoma. In these conditions, the mutations that lead to activation of the oncogene are dominant at the cellular level, and therefore only one copy of the mutated gene is required for the phenotypic effect. Such dominantly acting oncogenes may be assayed in cell culture by first transferring them into recipient cells and then scoring the numbers of transformed colonies; this is referred to as the 'transfection assay'.

However, in some inherited neoplasms that may also arise sporadically, such as retinoblastoma, tumor development is associated with two recessive mutations that inactivate oncogenes, and these are referred to as recessive oncogenes. In the inherited tumors, the first of the two recessive mutations is inherited via the germ-cell line and is present in all the cells. This recessive mutation is not expressed until a second mutation, within a somatic cell, causes loss of the normal dominant allele (**Fig. 30.1**).

The mutations causing the inherited and sporadic tumors are similar but the cell types in which they occur are different. In the inherited tumors the first mutation occurs in the germ cell, whereas in the sporadic tumors both mutations occur in the somatic cell. Thus, the risk of tumor development in an individual who has not inherited the first germline mutation is much smaller, as both mutational events must coincide in the same somatic cell. In addition, the apparent paradox that the inherited cancer syndromes are caused by recessive mutations but are dominantly inherited at the level of the family is explained because, in individuals who have inherited the first recessive mutation, the loss of a single remaining wild-type allele is almost certain to occur in at least one of the large number of cells in the target tissue. This cell will be detected because it forms a tumor, and almost all individuals who have inherited the germline mutation will express the disease, even though they only inherited a single copy of the recessive gene.

This model involving two (or more) mutations in the development of tumors is known as the 'two-hit' or Knudson hypothesis. The normal function of these recessive oncogenes appears to be in regulating cell growth and differentiation, and these genes have also been referred to as anti-oncogenes or tumor-suppressor genes. An important feature that has facilitated the investigation of the genetic abnormalities associated with such tumor development is that the loss of the remaining allele (i.e. the 'second hit'), which occurs in the somatic cell and gives rise to the tumor, often involves a large-scale loss of chromosomal material (**Fig. 30.1**). This 'second hit' may be detected by a comparison of the variations of the structure of the DNA sequences, called DNA polymorphisms, e.g. restriction fragment length polymorphisms (RFLPs; **Fig. 30.2**) or microsatellite polymorphisms (**Fig. 30.3**), in the leukocytes and tumor cells obtained from the patient, and observing a loss of heterozygosity (LOH) in the tumors (**Fig. 30.4**). In addition to these studies of tumors, the locations of cancer susceptibility genes may be identified by grouping or

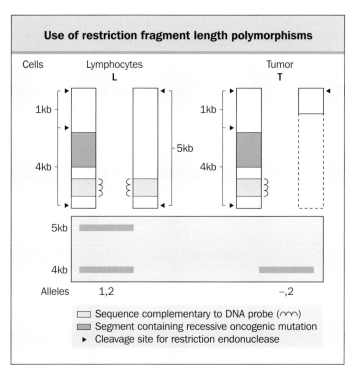

Figure 30.2 Use of restriction fragment length polymorphisms.
Schematic representation of the use of restriction fragment length polymorphisms (RFLPs) to investigate the chromosomal mechanisms involved in the 'second hit'. RFLPs result from variations in the primary DNA sequence of individuals and may result from single base changes, deletions, additions, or translocations. These changes in DNA sequence occur frequently (approximately once every 250bp) in the noncoding regions, do not usually affect gene function, and are often some distance from the disease gene. Such polymorphisms may, however, lead to the presence or absence of a cleavage site for a restriction enzyme, which cleaves DNA in a sequence-specific manner. RFLPs can be used to detect loss of heterozygosity in tumors. The example illustrated is that of a partial loss of the normal chromosome in the tumor, i.e. tumor cell (2) in Figure 30.1. RFLPs obtained from the leukocyte (L) and tumor (T) DNA of a patient are compared to detect deletions in the tumor tissue. The leukocytes are heterozygous (alleles 1,2) and one of the pair of chromosomes in the leukocytes contains the segment containing the recessive oncogenic mutation, whereas the other chromosome contains the normal dominant allele. In the example illustrated, the partial loss of the normal chromosome is detected by a loss of one of the RFLPs, which have been designated alleles. An example of such losses in a parathyroid tumor from an MEN1 patient is illustrated in Figure 30.4. (Redrawn from Thakker RV. The molecular genetics of the multiple endocrine neoplasia syndromes. Clin Endocrinol. 1993;38:1–14.)

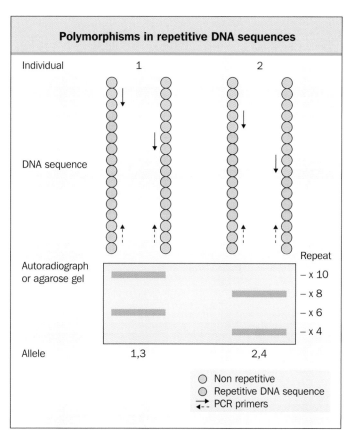

Figure 30.3 Polymorphisms in repetitive DNA sequences. These may consist of, for example, two (CA), three (ATT), four (ATTT), or six nucleotides (TATATG). Oligonucleotide primers (arrows) corresponding to the nonrepetitive sequences (empty circles) on either side of the repetitive DNA sequence (filled circles) are synthesized and the polymerase chain reaction (PCR) is used to amplify the repeat in genomic DNA obtained from different individuals. The resulting PCR products are separated either by polyacrylamide gel or agarose gel electrophoresis, and the polymorphisms are revealed by autoradiography or by viewing ethidium-bromide-stained agarose gel under ultraviolet light. Thus, of the pair of chromosomes from individual 1, one has 10 repeats and the other has six repeats, whereas of the pair of chromosomes from individual 2, one has eight repeats and the other has four. Following PCR amplification and separation by gel electrophoresis, the variations in the length of the repeats will be revealed by the differences in the size of the bands, which have been designated alleles. For example, the larger band consisting of 10 repeats is designated allele 1 and those consisting of eight, six, and four repeats are designated alleles 2, 3, and 4 respectively. These microsatellite tandem repetitive sequences, which are highly polymorphic, show mendelian inheritance (see Fig. 30.5) and can be used as genetic markers in MEN1 families. (Redrawn from Thakker RV. The molecular genetics of the multiple endocrine neoplasia syndromes. Clin Endocrinol. 1993;38:1–14.)

'linkage' studies in which the cosegregation of DNA sequence polymorphisms with the disease is investigated in affected families (**Fig. 30.5**). These two approaches will be further discussed.

Tumor studies

A comparison of the RFLPs obtained from leukocyte DNA and tumor DNA can facilitate the detection of the chromosomal abnormalities associated with the 'second hit' in tumor DNA, and this is illustrated in **Figure 30.2**. A restriction enzyme is used to cleave leukocyte and tumor DNA, and the resulting

DNA fragments are separated according to size by agarose gel electrophoresis and transferred by Southern blotting to a nylon membrane, which is hybridized with a single-stranded radioactively labeled DNA probe. The labeled DNA probe will attach to any fragments that have a complementary sequence, and these restricted fragments of varying lengths (RFLPs) are revealed by autoradiography. The exact number and size of RFLPs will vary in relation to the number of recognition sites for

Loss of heterozygosity in MEN1

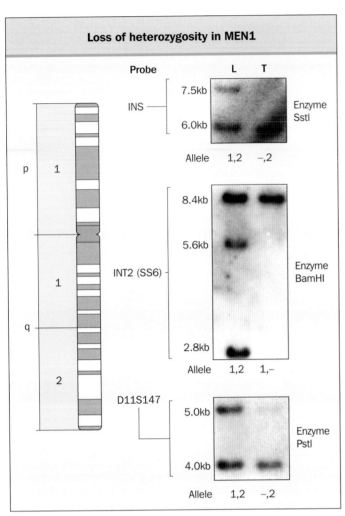

Figure 30.4 Loss of heterozygosity in familial multiple endocrine neoplasia type 1 (MEN1). The figure shows loss of heterozygosity involving polymorphic loci from chromosome 11 in a parathyroid tumor from a patient (individual III.1 in Fig. 30.6) with this condition. The restriction fragment length polymorphisms (RFLPs) obtained from the patient's leukocyte (L) and parathyroid tumor (T) DNA using the probes for the genes *INS* (insulin), *INT2*(SS6) and *D11S147* are shown. These probes are cloned human DNA sequences from chromosome 11 and are shown juxtaposed with their region of origin on the short (p) and long (q) arms of chromosome 11. The RFLPs are assigned alleles (Fig. 30.2). For example, two PstI-derived RFLPs were revealed by *D11S147*: the 5.0kb fragment is assigned allele 1 and the 4.0kb fragment is assigned allele 2. The leukocytes are heterozygous (alleles 1,2) but the tumor cells have lost the 5.0kb fragments (allele 1) and are hemizygous (alleles –,2). Similar losses of alleles are detected by the use of the DNA probes *INS* and *INT2*(SS6) and an extensive loss of alleles involving the whole of chromosome 11 is observed in the parathyroid tumor of this patient. In addition, the complete absence of bands suggests that this abnormality has occurred within all the tumor cells studied, and indicates a monoclonal origin for this MEN1 parathyroid tumor. (Reproduced from Thakker RV, Bouloux P, Wooding C, et al. The molecular basis of parathyroid tumours in multiple endocrine neoplasia type 1. Calcium Reg Bone Metab. 1990;10:118–24.)

bearing the recessive oncogenic mutation has three cleavage sites and, although two fragments of 4 kilobases (kb) and 1kb will result from the enzymatic cleavage, only the 4kb fragment will be visualized at autoradiography, as only it contains the complementary sequence to the radiolabeled DNA probe. However, the normal chromosome, i.e. the one not containing the recessive oncogenic mutation, has a loss of one restriction enzyme cleavage site, because of a change in the DNA sequence, and following digestion only one restriction fragment of 5kb is observed at autoradiography.

Alleles can be designated to these RFLPs; for example, the larger, 5kb RFLP is designated allele 1 and the smaller, 4kb RFLP is designated allele 2. Thus, the leukocytes in this example are heterozygous (alleles 1,2) and the chromosome bearing the recessive oncogenic mutation has allele 2 while the normal chromosome with the dominant allele has allele 1. A partial loss of the normal chromosome, i.e. the 'second hit' (**Fig. 30.1**) associated with the development of the tumor, would be detected by the loss of the 5kb RFLP (allele 1). Thus, the tumor cells would be hemizygous (allele –,2), as illustrated in **Figure 30.2**, or they might be homozygous (allele 2,2) if a reduplication of the chromosome bearing the recessive oncogenic mutation had occurred (**Fig. 30.1**). This type of analysis, involving paired leukocyte and tumor DNA – which has been referred to as the detection of a loss of alleles, or allelic deletions, or a loss of heterozygosity in tumors – has been very useful in localizing tumor-suppressor genes, e.g. those associated with retinoblastoma, colorectal carcinomas, Wilms' tumor, and MEN1.

Linkage analysis

DNA sequence polymorphisms (**Figs 30.2 & 30.3**) are inherited in a Mendelian manner and their inheritance can be followed together with the occurrence of disease in an affected family. The consistent inheritance of an allele with the disease (**Fig. 30.5**) indicates that the two genetic loci are close together, i.e. linked. Genes that are located close together on a chromosome will remain together during meiosis (cosegregate) but those that are far apart will cross-over during meiosis (recombine). By studying recombination events in family studies, the distance between two genes and the probability that they are linked can be ascertained. The distance between two genes is expressed as the recombination fraction (θ), which is equal to the number of recombinants divided by the total number of offspring resulting from informative meioses within a family. The value of the recombination fraction can range from zero to 0.5. A value of zero indicates that the genes are very closely linked while a value of 0.5 indicates that the genes are far apart and not linked. The probability that the two loci are linked at these distances is expressed as a 'LOD score', which is $\log_{10}$ of the odds ratio favoring linkage. The odds ratio favoring linkage is defined as the likelihood that two loci are linked at a specified recombination (θ) versus the likelihood that the two loci are not linked. A LOD score of +3, which indicates a probability in favor of linkage of 1000:1, establishes linkage between two loci, and a LOD score of –2, indicating a probability against linkage of 100:1, is taken to exclude linkage between two loci. LOD scores are usually evaluated over a range of recombination fractions, thereby enabling the genetic distance and the maximum (or peak) probability favoring linkage between two loci to be ascertained.

the restriction enzyme, as shown in **Figure 30.2**. In this example, the two chromosomes from the leukocytes differ in the number of restriction enzyme cleavage sites. The chromosome

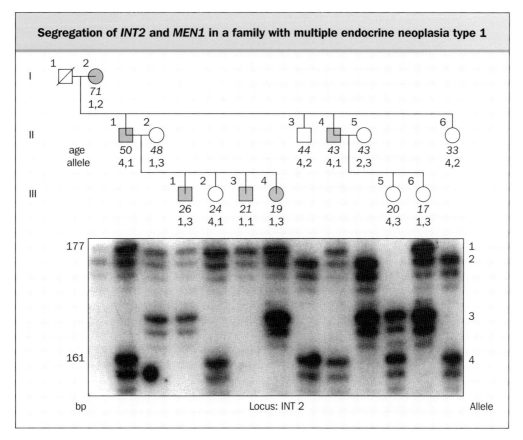

Figure 30.5 Segregation of *INT2* and *MEN1* in a family with multiple endocrine neoplasia type 1 (MEN1). *INT2* is a polymorphic locus from chromosome 11q13. Genomic DNA from the family members (upper panel) was used with $\gamma^{32}P$ adenosine triphosphate (ATP) for PCR amplification of the polymorphic repetitive element $(TG)_n$ at this locus. The PCR amplification products were detected by autoradiography on a polyacrylamide gel (lower panel). PCR products were detected from the DNA of each individual; these ranged in size from 161 to 177bp.

Alleles were designated for each PCR product and are indicated on the right. For example, individuals II.1 and II.4 revealed two pairs of bands on autoradiography. The upper pair of bands is designated allele 1 and the lower pair is designated allele 4; these two individuals are therefore heterozygous (alleles 1,4). A pair of bands for each allele is frequently observed in the PCR detection of microsatellite repeats. The upper band in the pair is the 'true' allele and the lower one is its associated 'shadow', which results from slipped-strand mispairing during the PCR. The segregation of these bands and their respective alleles, together with the disease, can be studied in the family members whose alleles and ages are shown. In some individuals, the inheritance of paternal and maternal alleles can be ascertained; the paternal allele is shown on the left.

Yellow square, unaffected male; blue square, affected male; Yellow circle, unaffected female; blue circle, affected female. Individual II.1 is affected and heterozygous (alleles 4,1) and an examination of his affected children (III.1, III.3, and III.4), his mother (I.2), and his brother (II.4) reveals inheritance of allele 1 with the disease. The unaffected individuals II.3, II.6, III.2, and III.5 have not inherited this allele 1. However, one of the daughters (III.6) of individual II.4 has inherited allele 1, but remains unaffected at the age of 17 years; this may either be a representation of age-related penetrance or a recombination between the disease and *INT2* loci. Thus, in this family, the disease and *INT2* loci are co-segregating in nine out of the 10 children but in one individual (III.6), assuming a 100% penetrance in early childhood, recombination is observed.

Thus, MEN1 and INT2 are co-segregating in 9/10 of the meioses and not segregating in 1/10 meioses, and the likelihood that the two loci are linked at $\theta = 0.10$, i.e. 10% recombination, is $(9/10)^9 \times (1/10)^1$. If the disease and the *INT2* loci were not linked, then the disease would be associated with allele 1 in one half (1/2) of the children and with allele 2 in the remaining half (1/2) of the children, and the likelihood that the two loci are not linked is $(1/2)^{10}$. Thus, the odds ratio in favor of linkage between the *MEN1* and *INT2* loci at $\theta = 0.10$, i.e. 10% recombination in this family, is $(9/10)^9 \times (1/10)^1 \div (1/2)^{10} = 39.67:1$, and the LOD score (i.e. $\log_{10}$ of the odds ratio favoring linkage) is 1.60 (i.e. $\log_{10} 39.67$). A LOD score of +3, which indicates a probability in favor of linkage of 1000:1, establishes linkage.

LOD scores from individual families can also be summated, and such studies revealed that the peak LOD score between *MEN1* and the *INT2* locus was >+3, thereby establishing linkage between *MEN1* and *INT2* loci. (Adapted from Thakker RV. The role of molecular genetics in screening for multiple endocrine neoplasia type 1. Endocrinol Metab Clin North Am. 1994;23:117–35.)

The multiple endocrine neoplasia syndromes			
Type	**Tumors**		**Biochemical features**
MEN1	Parathyroids (often multiglandular)		Hypercalcemia and ↑ PTH
	Pancreatic islets	Gastrinoma	↑ gastrin and ↑ basal gastric acid output
		Insulinoma	Hypoglycemia and ↑ insulin
		Glucagonoma	Glucose intolerance and ↑ glucagon
		VIPoma	↑ VIP and WDHA
		PPoma	↑ PP
	Pituitary (anterior)	Prolactinoma	Hyperprolactinemia
		GH-secreting	↑ GH
		ACTH-secreting	Hypercortisolemia and ↑ ACTH
		Nonfunctioning	Nil or α subunit
	Associated tumors	Adrenocortical	Hypercortisolemia or primary hyperaldosteronism
		Carcinoid	↑ 5-HIAA
		Lipoma	None
MEN2A	Medullary thyroid carcinoma		Hypercalcitoninemia*
	Pheochromocytoma		↑ Catecholamines
	Parathyroid		Hypercalcemia and ↑ PTH
MEN2B	Medullary thyroid carcinoma		Hypercalcitoninemia
	Pheochromocytoma		↑ Catecholamines
	Associated abnormalities	Mucosal neuromas	
		Marfanoid habitus	
		Medullated corneal nerve fibers	
		Megacolon	

Table 30.3 The multiple endocrine neoplasia (MEN) syndromes. Characteristic tumors and associated biochemical abnormalities are shown. Autosomal dominant inheritance of the MEN syndromes has been established.

*In some patients, basal serum calcitonin concentrations may be normal but show an abnormal rise at 1min and 5min after stimulation with pentagastrin 0.5 μg/kg. ↑, increased; 5-HIAA, 5-hydroxyindoleacetic acid; ACTH, adrenocorticotropic hormone; GH, growth hormone; PP, pancreatic polypeptide; PTH, parathyroid hormone; VIP, vasoactive intestinal peptide; WDHA, watery diarrhea, hypokalemia, and achlorhydria.

MULTIPLE ENDOCRINE NEOPLASIA

Multiple endocrine neoplasia is characterized by the occurrence of tumors involving two or more endocrine glands within a single patient. The disorder has been referred to previously as multiple endocrine adenomatosis (MEA) or the pluriglandular syndrome. However, glandular hyperplasia and malignancy also may occur in some patients and the term multiple endocrine neoplasia is now preferred.

There are two major forms of MEN, type 1 and type 2, and each form is characterized by the development of tumors within specific endocrine glands (**Table 30.3**). Thus the combined occurrence of tumors of the parathyroid glands, the pancreatic islet cells, and the anterior pituitary is characteristic of MEN1, which is also referred to as Wermer's syndrome. In addition to these tumors, adrenocortical tumors, carcinoid tumors, facial angiofibromas, collagenomas, and lipomatous tumors have also been described in patients with MEN1.

However, in MEN2, also called Sipple's syndrome, medullary thyroid carcinoma (MTC) occurs in association with pheochromocytoma, and three clinical variants referred to as MEN2A, MEN2B, and MTC-only are recognized. In MEN2A, which is the most common variant, the development of MTC is associated with pheochromocytoma and parathyroid tumors. In MEN2B, parathyroid involvement is rare and MTC and pheochromocytoma are found in association with a marfanoid habitus, mucosal neuromas, medullated corneal fibers, and intestinal autonomic ganglion dysfunction leading to a megacolon. In the variant MTC-only, medullary thyroid carcinoma appears to be the sole manifestation of the syndrome.

Although MEN1 and MEN2 usually occur as distinct and separate syndromes, some patients occasionally may develop tumors that are associated with both MEN1 and MEN2. For example, patients suffering from islet cell tumors of the pancreas and pheochromocytomas or from acromegaly and pheochromocytomas have been described, and MEN in these patients may represent an 'overlap' syndrome. All these forms of MEN may either be inherited as autosomal dominant syndromes or may occur sporadically, i.e. without a family history. However, this distinction between sporadic and familial cases may sometimes be difficult, since in some sporadic cases the family history may be absent because the parent with the disease died before developing symptoms.

MULTIPLE ENDOCRINE NEOPLASIA TYPE I

Clinical features
Parathyroid, pancreatic, and pituitary tumors constitute the major components of MEN1 (**Fig. 30.6**). In addition to these tumors, adrenocortical tumors, carcinoid tumors, facial angiofibromas, collagenomas, and lipomatous tumors may also occur in some patients.

Parathyroid tumors
Primary hyperparathyroidism is the most common feature of MEN1 and occurs in more than 95% of all MEN1 patients. Patients may present with asymptomatic hypercalcemia, nephrolithiasis, osteitis fibrosa cystica, or vague symptoms associated with hypercalcemia – e.g. polyuria, polydipsia, constipation, malaise – or occasionally with peptic ulcers. Biochemical investigations reveal hypercalcemia, usually in association with

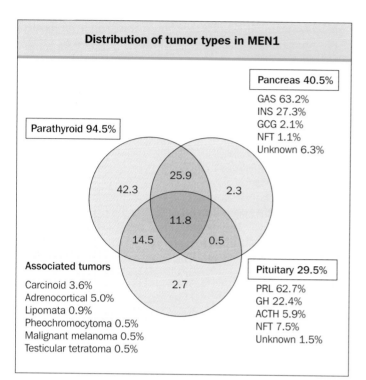

Distribution of tumor types in MEN1

Pancreas 40.5%

GAS 63.2%
INS 27.3%
GCG 2.1%
NFT 1.1%
Unknown 6.3%

Parathyroid 94.5%

42.3   25.9   2.3

11.8

14.5   0.5

Associated tumors

2.7

Carcinoid 3.6%
Adrenocortical 5.0%
Lipomata 0.9%
Pheochromocytoma 0.5%
Malignant melanoma 0.5%
Testicular tetratoma 0.5%

Pituitary 29.5%

PRL 62.7%
GH 22.4%
ACTH 5.9%
NFT 7.5%
Unknown 1.5%

Figure 30.6 Distribution of tumor types in multiple endocrine neoplasia type 1 (MEN1). The figure illustrates the distribution of 384 MEN1 tumors in 220 MEN1 patients. The proportion of patients in whom parathyroid, pancreatic, or pituitary tumors occurred is shown in the respective box. For example, 94.5% of patients had a parathyroid tumor. The Venn diagram indicates the proportion of patients with each combination of tumors. For example, 37.7% (25.9% + 11.8%) of patients had both a parathyroid and pancreatic tumor, whereas 2.3% of patients had a pancreatic tumor only. In addition to these tumors observed in one series, multiple facial angiofibromas have been observed in 88% of 32 patients and collagenomas in 72% of patients. The hormones secreted by each of these tumors are indicated (ACTH, adrenocorticotropic hormone; GAS, gastrin; GCG, glucagon; GH, growth hormone; INS, insulin; NFT, nonfunctioning tumors; PRL, prolactin). Parathyroid tumors represent the most common form of MEN1 tumors and occur in about 95% of patients, with pancreatic islet cell tumors occurring in about 40%, and anterior pituitary tumors occurring in about 30%. (Reproduced from Trump D, Farren B, Wooding C, et al. Clinical studies of multiple endocrine neoplasia type 1 (MEN1). QJM. 1996;89:653–69.)

raised circulating parathyroid hormone (PTH) concentrations. The hypercalcemia is usually mild; severe hypercalcemia resulting in crisis or parathyroid carcinoma are rare occurrences. Additional differences in the primary hyperparathyroidism of MEN1 patients from that in non-MEN1 patients include an earlier age of onset (20–25 years versus 55 years) and an equal male:female ratio (1:1 versus 1:3). Primary hyperparathyroidism in MEN1 patients is unusual before the age of 15 years and the age of conversion from being unaffected to affected has been observed to be between 20 and 21 years in some individuals.

No effective medical treatment for primary hyperparathyroidism is generally available and surgical removal of the abnormally overactive parathyroid glands is the definitive treatment. All four parathyroid glands are usually affected with multiple adenomas or hyperplasia, although this histologic distinction may be

difficult, and either partial or total parathyroidectomy has been proposed as treatment for primary hyperparathyroidism in MEN1. If a total parathyroidectomy is undertaken, then the resultant lifelong hypocalcemia is treated with oral calcitriol (1,25 dihydroxyvitamin D_3). It has been suggested that parathyroidectomy should be reserved for the symptomatic hypercalcemic patient with MEN1, and that the asymptomatic patient should not have parathyroid surgery but have regular assessments to look for the onset of symptoms and complications, at which time total parathyroidectomy should be undertaken. Persistent or recurrent hypercalcemia often occurs in patients treated with subtotal parathyroidectomy.

Pancreatic tumors

The incidence of pancreatic islet cell tumors in MEN1 patients varies from 30–80% in different series. The majority of these tumors produce excessive amounts of hormone, e.g. gastrin, insulin, glucagon, or vasoactive intestinal polypeptide (VIP), and are associated with distinct clinical syndromes (see Chapter 31).

Gastrinomas

These gastrin-secreting tumors represent over 50% of all pancreatic islet cell tumors in MEN1 and approximately 20% of patients with gastrinomas have MEN1. Gastrinomas are the major cause of morbidity and mortality in MEN1 patients. This is because of the recurrent severe multiple peptic ulcers, which may perforate. This association of recurrent peptic ulceration, marked gastric acid production, and non-β-islet-cell tumors of the pancreas is called the Zollinger–Ellison syndrome. Additional prominent clinical features of this syndrome include diarrhea and steatorrhea. The clinical and investigational features are described in Chapter 31. The ideal treatment for a non-metastatic gastrinoma is surgical excision of the gastrinoma. However, in patients with MEN1 the gastrinomas are frequently multiple or extrapancreatic and the role of surgery has been controversial. For example, in one study, only 16% of MEN1 patients were free of disease immediately after surgery, and at 5 years this had declined to 6%; the respective outcomes in non-MEN1 patients were better at 45% and 40%. The treatment of disseminated gastrinomas is difficult and hormonal therapy with octreotide, which is a long-acting somatostatin analog, chemotherapy with streptozotocin and 5-fluorouracil, hepatic artery embolization, and removal of all resectable tumor have all occasionally been successful.

Insulinoma

These β-islet-cell tumors secreting insulin represent one-third of all pancreatic tumors in MEN1 patients. Insulinomas also occur in association with gastrinomas in 10% of MEN1 patients, and the two tumors may arise at different times. Insulinomas occur more often in MEN1 patients who are below the age of 40 years, and many of these arise in individuals before the age of 20 years, whereas in non-MEN1 patients insulinomas generally occur in those over 40. Insulinomas may be the first manifestation of MEN1 in 10% of patients and approximately 4% of patients presenting with insulinoma will have MEN1. Patients with an insulinoma present with hypoglycemic symptoms that develop after a fast or exertion and improve after glucose intake. For details of clinical features and investigations see Chapter 20.

Glucagonoma

These α-islet-cell, glucagon-secreting pancreatic tumors occur in less than 3% of MEN1 patients. The characteristic clinical manifestations of a skin rash (necrolytic migratory erythema), weight loss, anemia, and stomatitis may be absent and the presence of the tumor is indicated only by glucose intolerance and hyperglucagonemia (for details see Chapter 31). The tail of the pancreas is the most frequent site for glucagonomas and surgical removal of these is the treatment of choice. However, treatment may be difficult as 50% of patients have metastases at the time of diagnosis. Medical treatment of these with octreotide or streptozotocin has been successful in some patients.

VIPoma

Patients with VIPomas, which are vasoactive-intestinal-peptide (VIP)-secreting pancreatic tumors, develop watery diarrhea, hypokalemia, and achlorhydria, referred to as the WDHA syndrome. This clinical syndrome has also been called Verner–Morrison syndrome or the VIPoma syndrome (see Chapter 31). VIPomas have been reported in only a few MEN1 patients and the diagnosis is established by documenting a markedly raised plasma VIP concentration.

PPoma

These tumors, which secrete pancreatic polypeptide (PP), are found in a large number of patients with MEN1. No pathologic sequelae of excessive PP secretion are apparent and the clinical significance of PP is unknown, although the use of serum PP measurements has been suggested for the detection of pancreatic tumors in MEN1 patients.

Pituitary tumors

The incidence of pituitary tumors in MEN1 patients varies from 15–90% in different series. Approximately 60% of MEN1 associated pituitary tumors secrete prolactin, nearly 25% secrete growth hormone (GH), 5% secrete adrenocorticotropic hormone (ACTH) and the remainder appear to be nonfunctioning. Prolactinomas may be the first manifestation of MEN1 in up to 10% of patients and somatotropinomas occur more often in patients over the age of 40 years. Less than 3% of patients with anterior pituitary tumors will have MEN1. The clinical manifestations depend upon the size of the pituitary tumor and its product of secretion (see Chapter 3).

Treatment of pituitary tumors in MEN1 patients is similar to that in non-MEN1 patients and consists of medical therapy or selective hypophysectomy by the trans-sphenoidal approach if feasible, with radiotherapy being reserved for residual unresectable tumor.

Associated tumors

Patients with MEN1 may have tumors involving glands other than the parathyroids, pancreas and pituitary. Thus carcinoid tumors, adrenocortical tumors, facial angiofibromas, collagenomas, thyroid tumors and lipomatous tumors have been described in association with MEN1.

Carcinoid tumors

Carcinoid tumors, which occur in more than 3% of patients with MEN1, may be inherited as an autosomal dominant trait in association with MEN1. The carcinoid tumor may be located in the bronchi, the gastrointestinal tract, the pancreas, or the thymus. Bronchial carcinoids in MEN1 patients predominantly occur in women (M:F = 1:4) whereas thymic carcinoids predominantly occur in men, with cigarette smokers having a higher risk of developing them. Most patients are asymptomatic and do not suffer from the flushing attacks and dyspnea associated with the carcinoid syndrome, which usually develops after the tumor has metastasized to the liver.

Adrenocortical tumors

The incidence of asymptomatic adrenocortical tumors in MEN1 patients has been reported to be as high as 40%. The majority of these tumors are nonfunctioning. However, functioning adrenocortical tumors in MEN1 patients have been documented to cause hypercortisolemia and Cushing's syndrome, and primary hyperaldosteronism, as in Conn's syndrome.

Lipomas

Lipomas may occur in more than a third of patients, and frequently they are multiple. In addition, pleural or retroperitoneal lipomas may also occur in patients with MEN1.

Thyroid tumors

Thyroid tumors, consisting of adenomas, colloid goiters, and carcinomas, have been reported to occur in over 25% of MEN1 patients. However, the prevalence of thyroid disorders in the general population is high and it has been suggested that the association of thyroid abnormalities in MEN1 patients may be incidental and not significant.

Facial angiofibroma

Multiple facial angiofibromas, which are similar to those observed in patients with tuberous sclerosis, have been observed in 88% of MEN1 patients and collagenomas have been reported in more than 70%.

Genetics

The gene causing MEN1 was localized to chromosome 11q13 by genetic mapping studies that investigated MEN1 associated tumors for LOH (**Fig. 30.4**) and by segregation studies in MEN1 families (**Fig. 30.5**). The results of these studies (**Fig. 30.7**), which were consistent with Knudson's model for tumor development, indicated that the *MEN1* gene represented a putative tumor-suppressor gene. Further studies defined a region of less than 300kb as the minimal critical segment that contained the *MEN1* gene. Characterization of genes from this region led to the identification of the gene, which consists of 10 exons with a 1830bp coding region (**Fig. 30.8**) that encodes a novel 610 amino acid protein, referred to as MENIN. Mutations of *MEN1* (**Figs 30.8 & 30.9**) have been identified and the total number of germline mutations of *MEN1* that were identified in MEN1 patients between 1997 and 1999 is 262 (**Fig. 30.8**). Approximately 22% are nonsense mutations, about 48% are frameshift deletions or insertions, 8% are in-frame deletions or insertions, 5% are donor-splice site mutations, and about 17% are missense mutations. More than 10% of the MEN1 mutations arise *de novo* and may be transmitted to subsequent generations. It is also important to note that between 5% and 10% of

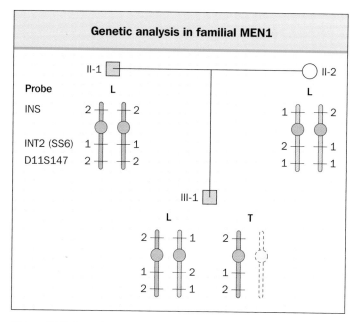

Genetic analysis in familial MEN1

Figure 30.7 Genetic analysis in familial multiple endocrine neoplasia type 1 (MEN1). The figure shows combined pedigree and tumor LOH analysis in a family with MEN1. The alleles obtained with probes from the short arm (*INS*) and the long arm (*INT2*(SS6) and *D11S147*) of chromosome 11 in individual III.1 and his parents, II.1 and II.2, are shown. These alleles were obtained by restriction fragment length polymorphism (RFLP) analysis of leukocytes (L) and parathyroid tumor (T) DNA, as illustrated in Figure 30.4. The father (II.1) was affected, and his leukocyte genotypes, which were homozygous at these three loci, are represented on the chromosomes as dark areas; the mother (II.2) was unaffected, and her leukocyte genotypes, which were heterozygous at the *INS* and *INT2*(SS6) loci and homozygous at *D11S147*, are represented on the chromosomes as yellow areas. The centromere is shown as a solid circle. The leukocyte genotypes of the affected son, III.1, which were heterozygous at all three loci, are represented on the chromosomes inherited from the father and the mother. An examination of the parathyroid tumor genotypes indicated hemizygosity with a loss of the maternal chromosome (dotted lines). Thus, a loss of the chromosome carrying the normal *MEN1* allele from the mother occurred in the tumor cells of this patient, and this is consistent with the 'two-hit' recessive oncogene model described (Fig. 30.1, cell (3)) for the development of MEN1 tumors. (Reproduced from Thakker RV, Bouloux P, Wooding C, et al. Association of parathyroid tumors in multiple endocrine neoplasia type 1 with loss of alleles on chromosome 11. N Engl J Med. 1989;321:218–24.)

MEN1 patients may not harbor mutations in the coding region of *MEN1* and that these individuals may have mutations in the promoter or untranslated regions (UTRs), which remain to be investigated.

The majority (75%) of *MEN1* mutations are inactivating and are consistent with those expected in a tumor-suppressor gene. The mutations are not only diverse in their types but are also scattered throughout the 1830bp coding region of *MEN1* (**Fig. 30.9**) with no evidence for clustering as observed in MEN2 (see below). However, some of the mutations have been observed to occur several times in unrelated families (**Fig. 30.8**), and four deletional and insertional mutations involving codons 83 and 84 (nt359 del 4), 119(K119 del), 209–211 (nt738 del 4), and

514–516 (nt1656–7 del or ins C), account for approximately 19% of all the germline *MEN1* mutations, and thus may represent potential 'hot' spots.

Such deletional and insertional hot spots may be associated with DNA sequence repeats, which may consist of long tracts of either single nucleotides or shorter elements, ranging from dinucleotides to octanucleotides. Indeed, the DNA sequence in the vicinity of codons 83 and 84 in exon 2 (**Fig. 30.8**) and codons 209–211 in exon 3 contains CT and CA dinucleotide repeats, respectively, flanking the 4bp deletions; these would be consistent with a replication–slippage model, in which there is misalignment of the dinucleotide repeat during replication, followed by excision of the 4bp single-stranded loop. A similar replication–slippage model may also be involved at codons 119–120, both of which consist of AAG nucleotides encoding a lysine (K) residue. The deletions and insertions of codon 516 involve a poly(C)$_7$ tract, and a slipped-strand mispairing model is also the most likely mechanism to be associated with this mutational hot spot. Thus, the *MEN1* gene appears to contain DNA sequences that may render it susceptible to deletional and insertional mutations.

Correlations between the *MEN1* mutations and the clinical manifestations of the disorder appear to be absent (genotype–phenotype dissociation). For example a detailed study of five unrelated families with the same 4bp deletion in codons 209 and 211 (**Table 30.4**) revealed a wide range of MEN1-associated tumors; all the affected family members had parathyroid tumors, but members of families 1, 3, 4, and 5 had gastrinomas whereas members of family 2 had insulinomas. In addition, prolactinomas occurred in members of families 2, 3, 4, and 5 but not in family 1, which was affected with carcinoid tumors. The apparent lack of genotype–phenotype correlation, which contrasts with the situation in MEN2 (see below), together with the wide diversity of mutations in the 1830bp coding region of the *MEN1* gene has made mutational analysis in MEN1 for diagnostic purposes time-consuming and expensive, such that it is generally not available. Tumors from MEN1 and non-MEN1 patients have been observed to harbor the germline mutation together with a somatic LOH involving chromosome 11q13, as expected from Knudson's model and the proposed role of *MEN1* as a tumor suppressor.

Function of *MEN1* protein (MENIN)

Initial analysis of the predicted amino acid sequence encoded by the *MEN1* gene did not reveal homologies to any other proteins, sequence motifs, signal peptides, or consensus nuclear localization signals, and thus the putative function of the protein (MENIN) could not be deduced. However, studies based on immunofluorescence, Western blotting of subcellular fractions, and epitope tagging with enhanced green fluorescent protein revealed that MENIN was located primarily in the nucleus. Furthermore, enhanced green fluorescent protein-tagged MENIN deletional constructs identified at least two independent nuclear localization signals that were located in the C-terminal quarter of the protein (**Fig. 30.8**). Interestingly, only one of the 94 *MEN1* missense mutations and in-frame deletions results in an alteration of either of these putative nuclear localization signals (**Fig. 30.8**); this missense mutation (Lys502Met), which involves an evolutionary conserved residue, was detected in a nonfunctioning sporadic pituitary tumor. However, all of the truncated MEN1 proteins that would result from the

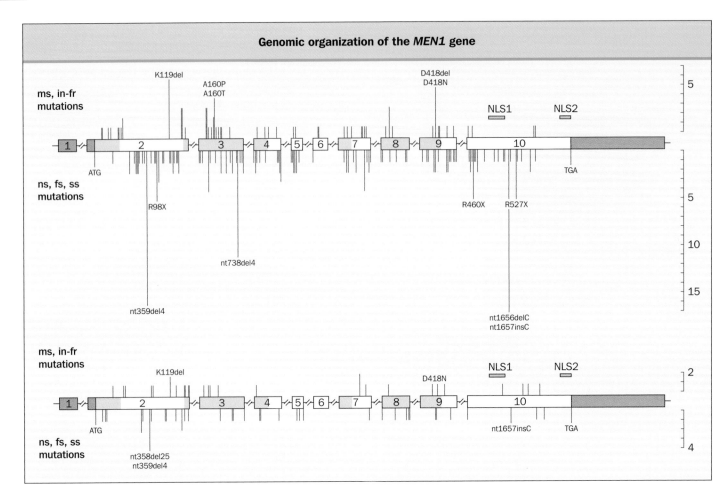

Figure 30.8 Genomic organization of the *MEN1* gene. Germline (top panel) and somatic (bottom panel) mutations are illustrated. The human *MEN1* gene consists of 10 exons that span more than 9kb of genomic DNA and encode a 610-amino-acid protein. The 1.83kb coding region is organized into 9 exons (exons 2–10) and 8 introns (indicated by a line but not to scale). The sizes of the exons (boxes) range from 88bp to 1312bp and those of the introns from 41bp to 1564bp. The start (ATG) and stop (TGA) sites, in exons 2 and 10 respectively, are indicated. Exon 1, the 5' part of exon 2, and the 3' part of exon 10 are untranslated (red boxes). The locations of the two nuclear localization sites (NLS), which are at codons 479–497 and 588–608 at the C-terminus, are represented by the thick horizontal lines, and the locations of the three domains formed by codons 1–40 (exon 2), 139–242 (exons 2, 3, and 4), and 323–428 (exons 7, 8, and 9) that interact with the transcription factor JunD are indicated by the gray boxes. The sites of the 262 germline mutations (top panel) and 67 somatic mutations (bottom panel) are indicated by the vertical lines; the missense (ms) and in-frame (in-fr) mutations are represented above the gene, and the nonsense (ns), frameshift (fs), and splice site (ss) mutations are represented below the gene. Mutations that have occurred more than four times (scale shown on the right) are indicated and a total of 329 MEN1 mutations are represented. (Reproduced from Pannett AAJ, Thakker RV. Multiple endocrine neoplasia type 1. Endocrine-Rel Cancer. 1999;6:449–73.)

219 nonsense and frameshift mutations, if expressed, would lack at least one of these nuclear localization signals (**Fig. 30.8**). The nuclear localization of MENIN suggested that it may act in the regulation of transcription, DNA replication, and/or the cell cycle. In order to investigate this further and to identify proteins that may interact with MENIN, the yeast-two hybrid system was utilized. This revealed that MENIN directly interacts with the N-terminus of the AP-1 transcriptional factor JunD to repress JunD-activated transcription. Analysis of several *MEN1* missense and deletional mutations indicated that the N-terminus and central domains of MENIN (**Fig. 30.8**) have a critical role in MENIN–JunD interaction.

However, JunD inhibits cell growth, an action that differs from that of other activated (AP-1) proteins, and thus the repressive effect of MENIN on JunD-mediated transcriptional activation would predict enhanced growth rather than the observed

suppression in growth. This seeming paradox may be due to the involvement of other target genes and proteins in cell proliferation, which may have interactions with the MENIN–JunD complex. These suggestions are further supported by the observation that disease-associated mutations that occur outside the domains interacting with JunD (**Fig. 30.8**) are associated with normal MENIN–JunD binding; this suggests that MENIN may interact with other proteins that may influence JunD-mediated transcription. Further investigations are needed to elucidate the role of MENIN– JunD interactions in the control of endocrine cell proliferation.

MEN1 mutations in hereditary endocrine disorders
The role of the *MEN1* gene in the etiology of other inherited endocrine disorders in which either parathyroid or pituitary tumors occur as an isolated endocrinopathy has been investigated

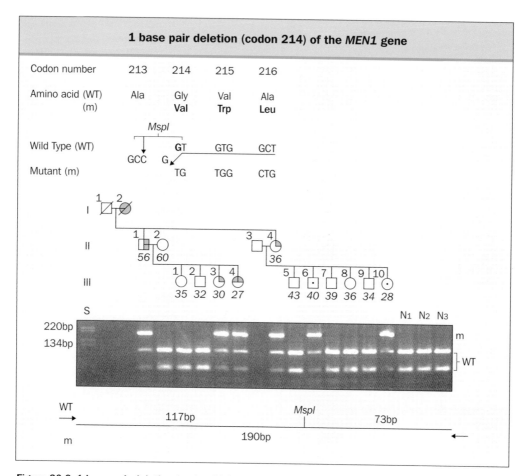

Figure 30.9 1 base pair deletion (codon 214) of the *MEN1* gene. The figure illustrates the detection of a mutation in exon 3 in a multiple endocrine neoplasia type 1 (MEN1) family by restriction enzyme analysis. DNA sequence analysis of individual II.1 revealed a 1bp deletion at the second position (G**G**T) of codon 214 (top panel). The deletion has caused a frameshift, which continues to codon 223 before a stop codon (TGA) is encountered in the new frame. The 1bp deletion results in the loss of an *MspI* restriction enzyme site (C/CGG) from the normal (wild-type, WT) sequence (top panel) and this has facilitated the detection of this mutation in the other affected members (II.4, III.3, and III.4) of this family (middle panel). The mutant (m) PCR product is 190bp whereas the wild-type products are 117 and 73bp (bottom panel). The affected individuals were heterozygous and the unaffected members were homozygous for the wild-type sequence. Individuals III.6 and III.10, who are 40 and 28 years old respectively, are mutant gene carriers who are clinically and biochemically normal; this is due to the age-related penetrance of this disorder. These individuals would still require screening by clinical, biochemical, and radiological assessments, as they still have residual risks (i.e. 100%–age-related penetrance), respectively of 2% and more than 13%, of developing tumors by the age of 60 years. Individuals are represented as: male (square); female (circle); unaffected (yellow); affected with parathyroid tumors (blue-filled upper right quadrant), affected with gastrinoma (blue-filled lower right quadrant), affected with prolactinoma (blue-filled upper left quadrant), and unaffected mutant gene carrier (dot). Individual I.2, who is dead but was known to be affected (tumor details not known) is shown as a filled symbol. The age is indicated below for each individual at diagnosis or at the time of the last biochemical screening. The standard size marker (S) in the form of the 1kb ladder is indicated. Co-segregation of this mutation with *MEN1* in this family and its absence in 110 alleles from 55 unrelated normal individuals (N1–3 are shown) indicates that it is not a common DNA sequence polymorphism. (Adapted from Bassett JH, Forbes SA, Pannett AA, et al. Characterization of mutations in patients with multiple endocrine neoplasia type 1. Am J Hum Genet. 1998;62:232–44).

by mutational analysis. *MEN1* mutations in familial isolated hyperparathyroidism have been reported, and these consist of one nonsense mutation (Tyr353Stop), one deletion (Leu414del 3bp), and three missense mutations (Val184Glu, Glu255Lys, and Leu267Pro). The sole occurrence of parathyroid tumors in these five families, which harbor *MEN1* mutations similar to those found in MEN1 families, is remarkable, and the mechanisms that

determine the altered phenotypic expressions of these mutations remain to be elucidated. Mutational analysis studies in another inherited isolated endocrine tumor syndrome, that of familial isolated acromegaly, have not detected abnormalities of the *MEN1* gene, even although segregation analysis in one family indicated that the gene was likely to be located on chromosome 11q13. However, nonsense mutations (Tyr312Stop and

Tumors associated with multiple endocrine neoplasia type 1					
	Family				
	1	2	3	4	5
Tumors					
Parathyroid	+	+	+	+	+
Gastrinoma	+	–	+	+	+
Insulinoma	–	+	–	–	–
Glucagonoma	–	–	–	–	+
Prolactinoma	–	+	+	+	+
Carcinoid	+	–	–	–	–

Table 30.4 Tumors associated with multiple endocrine neoplasia type 1 (MEN1). The table lists MEN1-associated tumors found in five unrelated families with a 4bp deletion at codons 209 and 211. +, presence of tumors; –, absence of tumors. (Adapted from Thakker RV. Multiple endocrine neoplasia – syndromes of the twentieth century. J Clin Endocrinol Metab. 1998;83:2617–20.)

Arg460Stop) have been detected in MEN1 families with the Burin or prolactinoma variant, in which there is a high occurrence of prolactinomas and a low occurrence of gastrinomas.

Screening in multiple endocrine neoplasia type 1

Multiple endocrine neoplasia type 1 is inherited as an autosomal dominant disorder in the majority of patients. Occasionally, MEN1 may arise sporadically (i.e. without a family history), although it may be difficult to make the distinction between sporadic and familial forms; in some cases the family history may be absent because the parent with MEN1 is not available and may already have died before developing any manifestations, and other cases may be due to *de novo* mutations, which will be transmitted in an autosomal dominant manner in future generations. MEN1 is an uncommon disorder but, because of its autosomal dominant inheritance, the finding of MEN1 in a patient has important implications for other family members; first-degree relatives have about a 50% risk of developing the disease. Screening for MEN1 in patients involves the detection of tumors and the ascertainment of the germline genetic state, i.e. normal or mutant gene carrier. The detection of tumors entails clinical, biochemical, and radiological investigations. The recent cloning of the *MEN1* gene has facilitated the identification of individuals who have mutations and hence are at a high risk of developing the disease (**Figs 30.8 & 30.9**).

Genetic analysis

Molecular genetic analysis for MEN1, either by detecting mutations (**Fig. 30.9**) or by performing segregation studies using linked markers, could now be introduced to identify those individuals who are mutant carriers and thus at a high risk of developing tumors. The advantages of DNA analysis are that it requires a single blood sample and does not need, in theory, to be repeated. This is because the analysis is independent of the age of the individual and provides an objective result. Such mutational analysis could be undertaken in children around the first decade, as some children have developed tumors by the age of 5 years; appropriate intervention in the form of biochemical

testing and/or treatment has been considered. However, the great diversity, together with the widely scattered locations, of the *MEN1* mutations (**Fig. 30.8**), and a lack of genotype-phenotype correlation (**Table 30.4**), will make such mutational screening time-consuming, arduous, and expensive, and as yet this is not widely available. Nevertheless, an integrated program of both mutational analysis, to identify mutant gene carriers, and biochemical screening, to detect the development of tumors, would be of advantage. Thus, a DNA test identifying an individual as a mutant gene carrier is likely to lead not to immediate medical or surgical treatment but to earlier and more frequent biochemical and radiologic screening, whereas a DNA result that indicates that an individual is not at risk will lead to a decision to carry out no further clinical investigations (**Fig. 30.10**). Thus, the identification of *MEN1* mutations may be of help in the clinical management of patients with this disorder and their families.

Detection of tumors

Biochemical screening for the development of MEN1 tumors in asymptomatic members (**Figs 30.9 & 30.10**) of families with MEN1 is of great importance, as earlier diagnosis and treatment of these tumors may help to reduce morbidity and mortality. The age-related penetrance (i.e. the proportion of gene carriers manifesting symptoms or signs of the disease by a given age) has been ascertained and the mutation appears to be nonpenetrant below the age of 5 years. Thereafter the mutant *MEN1* gene has a high penetrance, being more than 50% penetrant by 20 years of age and more than 95% penetrant by 40 years.

Screening for MEN1 tumors is difficult because the clinical and biochemical manifestations in members of any one family are not uniformly similar (**Fig. 30.9**). The attempts to screen for the development of MEN1 tumors in the asymptomatic relatives of an affected individual have depended largely on measuring the serum concentrations of calcium, gastrointestinal hormones, e.g. gastrin, and prolactin, and also on ultrasound and radiological imaging of the abdomen and pituitary. Parathyroid overactivity causing hypercalcemia is almost invariably the first manifestation of the disorder and this has become a useful and easy biochemical screening investigation. In addition, hyperprolactinemia, which may be asymptomatic, may represent the first manifestation in up to 10% of patients, and this may also be a useful and easy biochemical screening investigation.

Pancreatic involvement in asymptomatic individuals has been detected by estimating the fasting plasma concentrations of gastrin, PP and glucagon, and by abdominal imaging. However, one study has shown that a stimulatory meal test is a better method for detecting pancreatic disease in individuals who have no demonstrable pancreatic tumors by computerized tomography. An exaggerated increase in serum gastrin and/or PP proved to be a reliable early indicator for the development of pancreatic tumors in these individuals.

At present it is suggested that individuals at high risk of developing MEN1 (i.e. mutant gene carriers) should undergo biochemical screening (**Fig. 30.10**) at least once per annum, and also have baseline pituitary and abdominal imaging, which should then be repeated at 5–10-year intervals. Screening should commence in early childhood, as the disease has developed in some individuals by the age of 5 years, and should continue for life, as

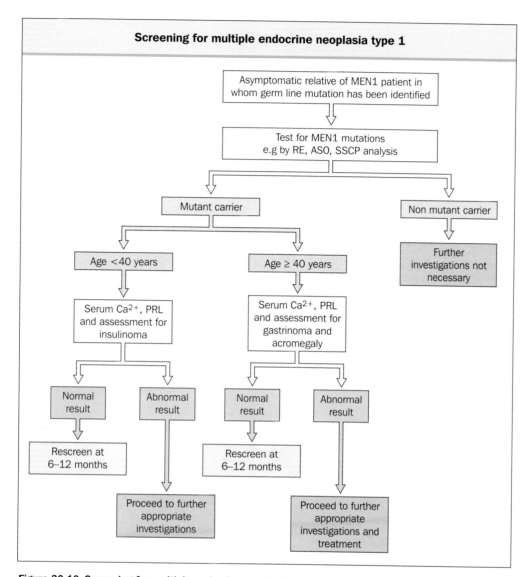

Figure 30.10 Screening for multiple endocrine neoplasia type 1 (MEN1). The figure illustrates an approach to screening in an asymptomatic relative of a patient with MEN1. The relative should first have undergone a clinical evaluation for MEN1-associated tumors to establish that s/he is asymptomatic. Relatives who are symptomatic, who could also have a test for *MEN1* mutations, should proceed to appropriate investigations and management. Mutational analysis for *MEN1* is not routinely available at present, and this protocol could instead be adapted for first-degree relatives. The *MEN1* mutation may be identified directly by DNA sequence analysis or by restriction enzyme (RE; Fig. 30.9), allele-specific oligonucleotide (ASO) hybridization, or another method such as single-stranded conformational polymorphism (SSCP) analysis. The use of mutational analysis and such screening methods in children is controversial and varies in different countries. It has been suggested that nonessential genetic testing in a child who is not old enough to make important long-term decisions should be deferred. However, the finding that a child from a family with MEN1 does not have any *MEN1* mutations removes the burden of repeated clinical, biochemical, and radiologic investigations and enables health resources to be more effectively directed towards those children who are *MEN1* mutant gene carriers. The approaches to genetic testing and screening in MEN1 vary in different countries. (Redrawn from Thakker RV. Multiple endocrine neoplasia type 1. In: DeGroot LJ, Jameson JL, eds. Endocrinology, 4th edn. Philadelphia, PA:WB Saunders;2001:2503–17.)

some individuals have not developed the disease until the eighth decade. Screening history and physical examination should be directed towards eliciting the symptoms and signs of hypercalcemia, nephrolithiasis, peptic ulcer disease, neuroglycopenia, hypopituitarism, galactorrhea and amenorrhea in women, acromegaly, Cushing's disease, visual field loss and the presence of subcutaneous lipomas, angiofibromas, and collagenomas. Biochemical screening should include serum calcium and prolactin estimations in all individuals, and measurement of gastrointestinal hormones, e.g. gastrin. More specific endocrine function tests should perhaps be reserved for individuals who have symptoms or signs suggestive of a clinical syndrome.

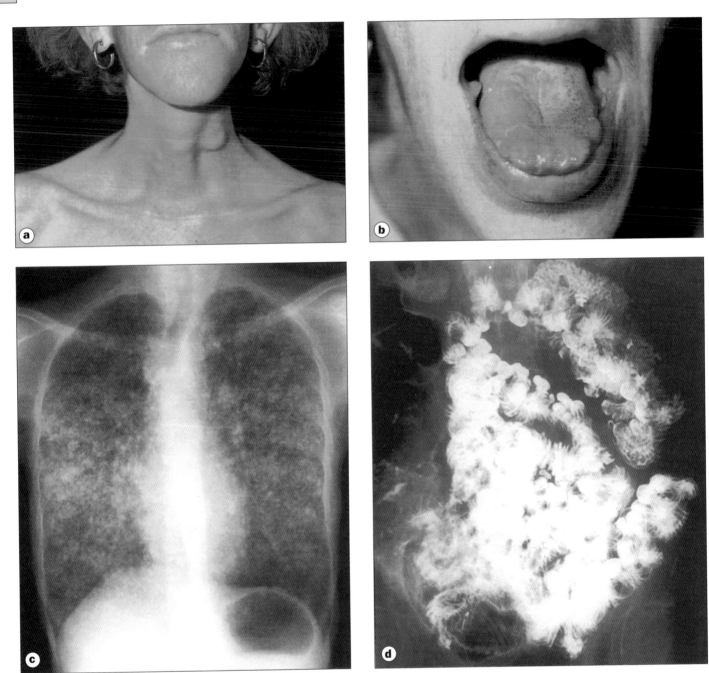

Figure 30.11 Clinical features in a patient with MEN2B. (a) Note thyroidectomy scar and nodule on left side of neck representing metastases of medullary thyroid carcinoma (MTC). (b) Mucosal neuromas on tongue and lips. (c) Bilateral lung metastases of MTC. (d) Radiograph of barium meal and follow-through, illustrating the presence of multiple intestinal diverticulae, which are secondary to autonomic ganglion dysfunction. (Reproduced from Thakker RV. Multiple endocrine neoplasia. In: Thakker RV, Wass JAH, ed. Endocrine disorders. Medicine. 1997;25:86–8.)

MULTIPLE ENDOCRINE NEOPLASIA TYPE 2

Multiple endocrine neoplasia type 2 describes the association of medullary thyroid carcinoma (MTC), pheochromocytomas, and parathyroid tumors (**Table 30.3**). Three clinical variants of MEN2 are recognized – MEN2A, MEN2B, and MTC only. MEN2A is the most common variant: the development of MTC is associated with pheochromocytomas (50% of patients), which may be bilateral, and parathyroid tumors (20% of patients).

MEN2B, which represents 5% of all MEN2 cases, is characterized by the occurrence of MTC and pheochromocytoma in association with a marfanoid habitus, mucosal neuromas, medullated corneal fibers, and intestinal autonomic ganglion dysfunction leading to multiple diverticulae and megacolon (**Fig. 30.11**). Parathyroid tumors do not usually occur in MEN2B. MTC-only is a variant in which medullary thyroid carcinoma is the sole manifestation of the syndrome. The clinical features of MTC, pheochromocytoma, and parathyroid tumors in MEN2 will be reviewed.

Clinical features

Medullary thyroid carcinoma

Medullary thyroid carcinoma (see also Chapter 12) is the most common feature of MEN2A and occurs in almost all affected individuals. MTC represents 10% of all thyroid gland carcinomas, and 20% of MTC patients have a family history of the disorder. Patients with MTC may be asymptomatic and the presence of MTC may have been detected by the demonstration of hypercalcitoninemia at family screening. However, MTC may also present as a palpable mass in the neck, which may be asymptomatic or associated with symptoms of pressure or dysphagia in 16% of patients. Diarrhea may occur in 30% of patients and is associated either with elevated circulating concentrations of calcitonin or tumor-related secretion of serotonin and prostaglandins. Some patients may also suffer from flushing. In addition, ectopic ACTH production by MTC may cause Cushing's syndrome. Radionucleotide thyroid scans reveal MTC tumors as 'cold' nodules.

The diagnosis of MTC relies on the demonstration of hypercalcitoninemia either in the basal state (>90pg/ml) or following stimulation with intravenous pentagastrin (0.5μg/kg) and/or calcium infusion (2mg/kg). Fine needle aspiration and cytology of lesions may also be useful. In the early stages of metastasis, MTC usually metastasizes to the cervical lymph nodes and in later stages to the mediastinal nodes, lung, liver, trachea, adrenal glands, esophagus, and bone. Radiography may reveal dense irregular calcification within the involved portions of the thyroid gland and the lymph nodes involved with the metastases. However, the presence of metastases does not necessarily lead to a poor prognosis, and in 80% of patients the tumor(s) pursues a relatively indolent course. MTC does follow an aggressive course with early metastases and death in up to 10% of patients and there may be a family history of such aggressive MTC or MEN2B (**Fig. 30.11**).

Treatment for MTC is total thyroidectomy, with central lymph node resection, followed by replacement thyroxine therapy.

Pheochromocytoma

These norepinephrine (noradrenaline)- and epinephrine (adrenaline)-secreting tumors (see also Chapter 18) occur in more than 50% of patients with MEN2A and are a major cause of morbidity and mortality. Patients may have symptoms and signs of catecholamine secretion, (e.g. headaches, palpitations, sweating, and poorly controlled hypertension), or they may be asymptomatic and have been detected through biochemical screening because of a familial history of either MEN2A or MTC. The biochemical and radiologic investigation of pheochromocytoma in MEN2A patients is similar to that in non-MEN2 patients and includes the estimation of urinary free epinephrine and norepinephrine, computerized tomography (or magnetic resonance imaging) scanning and radionuclide scanning with meta-iodo-(^{123}I or ^{131}I)-benzyl guanidine (MIBG). An early biochemical abnormality in MEN2 patients with pheochromocytoma and medullary hyperplasia is an increase in the urinary epinephrine:norepinephrine ratio to more than 0.15. Bilateral adrenomedullary hyperplasia is the precursor to pheochromocytoma in patients with MEN2. This is associated with the expansion of the medullary tissue into the body and tail of the gland, with a decrease in corticomedullary ratio and nodular hyperplasia. Nodules exceeding 1mm in diameter are designated pheochromocytomas. The incidence of bilateral adrenal medullary tumors in MEN2A patients is 70%, in contrast to the 10% incidence observed in non-MEN2 patients. In addition, pheochromocytomas in patients with MEN2A differ significantly in distribution when compared to those in non-MEN2 patients. Thus, extra-adrenal pheochromocytomas, which occur in 10% of non-MEN2 patients, are rarely observed in MEN2A patients, and similarly malignancy is much less common in MEN2A pheochromocytomas. Thus, a recommended treatment for pheochromocytoma in patients with MEN2A is bilateral adrenalectomy, even in those MEN2A patients in whom only a unilateral tumor has been demonstrated by radiology.

Parathyroid tumors

The incidence of parathyroid tumors in MEN2A patients varies from 40% to 80% in different series. However, more than 50% of these patients do not have hypercalcemia, and the presence of abnormally enlarged parathyroids, which are unusually hyperplastic, is revealed in the normocalcemic patient undergoing thyroidectomy for MTC. The biochemical investigation and management of hypercalcemic MEN2A patients is similar to that of MEN1 patients.

Genetics

The gene causing all three MEN2 variants was mapped to chromosome 10cen-10q11.2, a region containing the c-*ret* proto-oncogene, which encodes a tyrosine kinase receptor with cadherin-like and cysteine-rich extracellular domains and a tyrosine kinase intracellular domain. Specific mutations of c-*ret* have been identified for each of the three MEN2 variants (**Fig. 30.12**). Thus, in 95% of patients, MEN2A is associated with mutations of the cysteine-rich extracellular domain, and mutations in codon 634 (Cys→Arg) account for 85% of MEN2A mutations. MTC-only is also associated with missense mutations in the cysteine-rich extracellular domain, and most mutations are in codon 618. However, MEN2B is associated with mutations in codon 918 (Met→Thr) of the intracellular tyrosine kinase domain in 95% of patients. Interestingly, the c-*ret* proto-oncogene is also involved in the etiology of papillary thyroid carcinomas and in Hirschsprung's disease.

Mutational analysis of c-*ret* to detect mutations in codons 609, 611, 618, 620, 634, 768, and 804 in MEN2A and MTC-only, and codon 918 in MEN2B, has been used in the diagnosis and management of patients and families with these disorders. Such testing quickly and reliably identifies the 50% of family members who do not have the mutation and who therefore do not have to undergo further screening.

For those family members who have inherited the mutation and are at high risk of developing tumors, there are two clinical approaches. In one approach, repeated testing of calcitonin release following pentagastrin stimulation is recommended, with total thyroidectomy being reserved until an abnormal pentagastrin test is observed. This usually delays total thyroidectomy until 10–13 years of age. In the alternative approach, a total thyroidectomy is recommended, on the sole basis of the abnormal genetic test, at the age of 5 years; this is the earliest age at which metastasis in MEN2A has been identified. In MEN2B, metastasis at 2 years

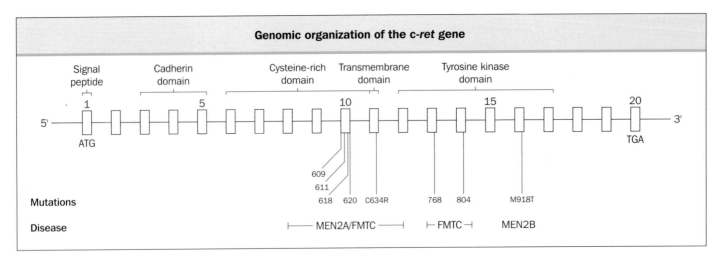

Genomic organization of the c-ret gene

Figure 30.12 Genomic organization of the c-ret gene. This schematic representation illustrates germline mutations that cause MEN2. The human c-ret (*MEN2*) gene, which is located on chromosome 10q11.2, consists of 20 (or 21) exons that span about 30kb of genomic DNA and encodes a 1114-amino-acid membrane-associated tyrosine kinase receptor. The 3342bp coding region is organized into 20 exons and 19 introns (indicated by a line but not to scale). The sizes of the exons (boxes) range from 70bp to 292bp and those of the introns range from 333bp to 2456bp. The start (ATG) and stop (TGA) sites in exons 1 and 20 respectively are indicated. The receptor consists of a signal peptide region, a cadherin-like domain, a region containing several conserved cysteine residues (cysteine-rich domain), a transmembrane domain, and two tyrosine kinase domains. The occurrence of MEN2A and MTC-only involves codons 609, 611, 618, 620, 634, 768, and 804, whereas that of MEN2B involves only codon 918. C634R indicates Cys634Arg and M918T indicates Met918Thr. (Redrawn from Thakker RV. Multiple endocrine neoplasia. In: Williams. Metabolic genetic basis of common diseases. Philadelphia, PA:WB Saunders; 2002 [in press].)

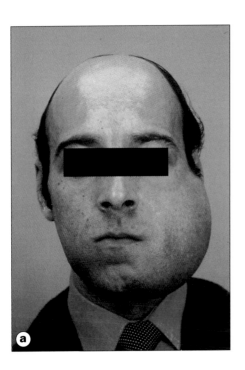

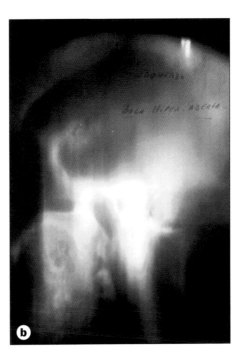

Figure 30.13 Hyperparathyroidism–jaw tumor (HPT–JT) syndrome. (a) An HPT–JT patient with a jaw tumor. (b) Skull X-ray of this patient showing a mandibular tumor with bone destruction. Histology revealed this jaw tumor to be an ossifying fibroma similar to that illustrated in Figure 30.14, which was obtained from the patient's daughter. (Reproduced from Cavaco BM, Barros L, Pannett AA, et al. The hyperparathyroidism–jaw tumor syndrome in a Portuguese kindred. QJM. 2001;94:213–22)

of age has been reported, and total thyroidectomy at an earlier age has been recommended. The advantages of this approach are that pentagastrin testing is avoided and it is more likely that a cure will be achieved before micrometastases develop. The management of affected families is complicated, and requires careful coordination between the medical team (endocrinologists, geneticists, surgeons, and family physicians) and the family.

HYPERPARATHYROIDISM–JAW-TUMOR SYNDROME

The hyperparathyroidism–jaw tumor (HPT–JT) syndrome is an autosomal dominant disorder characterized by the development of parathyroid tumors and fibro-osseous jaw tumors (**Figs 30.13 & 30.14**). In addition, some patients may also develop Wilms'

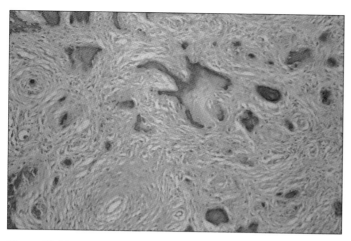

Figure 30.14 Hyperparathyroidism–jaw tumor (HPT–JT) syndrome. Histology of a typical ossifying fibroma from a patient with HPT–JT, the daughter of the patient shown in Figure 30.13. The tumor consists of irregular, focally branching islands of immature bone in an abundant fibrous stroma. (Reproduced from Cavaco BM, Barros L, Pannett AA, et al. The hyperparathyroidism-jaw tumor syndrome in a Portuguese kindred. QJM. 2001;94:213–22)

tumors, renal cysts, renal hamartomas, renal cortical adenomas, papillary renal cell carcinomas, pancreatic adenocarcinomas, testicular mixed germ cell tumors with a major seminoma component, and Hurthle cell thyroid adenomas.

It is important to note that the parathyroid tumors may occur in isolation and without any evidence of jaw tumors, and this may cause confusion with other hereditary hypercalcemic disorders such as MEN1, familial benign hypercalcemia (familial hypocalciuric hypercalcemia), and familial isolated primary hyperparathyroidism (see below). HPT–JT can be distinguished from FBH, as in FBH serum calcium levels are elevated from the early neonatal or infantile period whereas in HPT–JT such elevations are uncommon in the first decade. In addition, HPT–JT patients, unlike FBH patients, will have associated hypercalciuria (24-hour urine excretion over 6mmol/24h, 270mg/24h).

The distinction between HPT–JT patients and MEN1 patients who have only developed the usual first manifestation of hypercalcemia (>90% of patients) is more difficult and is likely to be influenced by the operative and histologic findings and the occurrence of other characteristic lesions in each disorder. It is important to note that HPT–JT patients usually have single adenomas or a carcinoma, while MEN1 patients often have multiglandular and hyperplastic parathyroid disease. The distinction between FIHP and HPT–JT in the absence of jaw tumors is difficult but important as HPT–JT patients may be at a higher risk of developing parathyroid carcinomas. These distinctions may be helped by the identification of additional features, and a search for jaw tumors, renal, pancreatic, thyroid, and testicular abnormalities may help to identify HPT–JT patients.

The jaw tumors in HPT–JT are different from the brown tumors observed in some patients with primary hyperparathyroidism with bone disease, and do not resolve after parathyroidectomy. Indeed, ossifying fibromas of the jaw are an important feature distinguishing of HPT–JT from FIHP, and the occurrence of these may occasionally precede the development of hypercalcemia in HPT–JT patients by several decades.

The gene causing HPT–JT has been mapped to chromosome 1q25–q31, and the use of polymorphic genetic markers from this region for the detection of LOH in parathyroid and renal tumors, and for segregation studies, may help to clarify the differences between HPT–JT and other hyperparathyroid disorders.

FAMILIAL ISOLATED PRIMARY HYPERPARATHYROIDISM

Primary hyperparathyroidism, which may result from parathyroid adenomas, hyperplasia, or carcinoma, affects 1:1000 of adults and is most frequently encountered as a nonfamilial disorder. However, approximately 10% of patients with primary hyperparathyroidism will have a hereditary form, which may either be part of the MEN1 or MEN2 syndromes or part of the HPT–JT syndrome (see above). In addition, hereditary primary hyperparathyroidism may develop as a solitary endocrinopathy, and this has also been referred to as familial isolated hyperparathyroidism. Investigations of these hereditary and sporadic forms of primary hyperparathyroidism have helped to identify some of the genes and chromosomal regions that are involved in the etiology of parathyroid tumors (**Table 30.2**). FIHP has been reported in several kindreds, and some have been shown to harbor mutations of the *MEN1* gene (see above), while in other families linkage to polymorphic loci from chromosome 1q21–q31, the region of the HPT–JT syndrome, has been shown. In addition, analysis of parathyroid tumors from FIHP patients has revealed LOH involving chromosome 1q21–q31 loci. FIHP located on chromosome 1q21–q31 has been reported to be associated with a high incidence of early-onset parathyroid carcinomas.

FAMILIAL BENIGN HYPERCALCEMIA AND NEONATAL PRIMARY HYPERPARATHYROIDISM

Familial benign hypercalcemia, also referred to as familial hypocalciuric hypercalcemia, is an autosomal dominant disorder with a high degree of penetrance characterized by lifelong asymptomatic hypercalcemia in association with an inappropriately low urinary calcium excretion (calcium clearance to creatinine clearance ratio < 0.01). A normal circulating PTH concentration and mild hypermagnesemia are also typically present. Although most patients with FBH are asymptomatic, chondrocalcinosis and acute pancreatitis have occasionally been observed to occur in some patients.

In addition, children of consanguineous marriages within FBH kindreds have been observed to have life-threatening hypercalcemia due to neonatal primary hyperparathyroidism (NHPT). NHPT is defined as symptomatic hypercalcemia with skeletal manifestations of hyperparathyroidism (**Fig. 30.15**) in the first 6 months of life. NHPT children often present in the first few days or weeks of life with failure to thrive, dehydration, hypotonia, constipation, rib cage deformities, and multiple fractures due to bony undermineralization. Children with NHPT often require urgent parathyroidectomy, which corrects the PTH-dependent hypercalcemia and bone demineralization (**Fig. 30.15**).

FBH is caused by heterozygous inactivating mutations of the calcium-sensing receptor (CaSR) and NHPT is often associated with inactivating homozygous CaSR mutations. However, NHPT

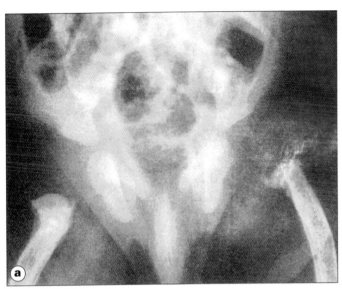
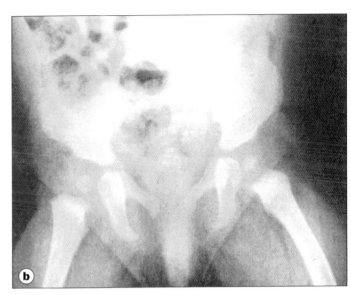

Figure 30.15 Neonatal primary hyperparathyroidism (NHPT). Radiology findings in the pelvis and femora of a child with NHPT. (a) Generalized osteopenia, metaphyseal fractures of the proximal femora, and periosteal calcifications were noted at 3 weeks of age, when the serum calcium was 3.33mmol/L. At 6 weeks of age a parathyroidectomy was performed, and an improvement in the bone disease was observed by 18 weeks of age (b). (Reproduced from Bai M, Pearce SH, Kifor O, et al. In vivo and in vitro characterization of neonatal hyperparathyroidism resulting from a *de novo*, heterozygous mutation in the Ca^{2+}-sensing receptor gene. J Clin Invest. 1997;99:88–96.)

has also been observed in children where only one parent had clinically apparent FBH, and many other NHPT patients appear to be sporadic, i.e. both parents are normocalcemic. In such NHPT patients with heterozygous CaSR mutations, the mutant CaSR may exert a dominant negative action on the normal CaSR. The human CaSR is a 1078-amino-acid cell-surface protein that is expressed in parathyroids, thyroid cells, and kidney and is a member of the family of G-protein-coupled receptors (**Fig. 30.16**). The *CaSR* gene is located on chromosome 3q21–q24. In addition to the loss-of-function *CaSR* mutations that result in FBH and NHPT, gain-of-function *CaSR* mutations resulting in autosomal dominant hypocalcemia with hypercalciuria have also been reported. The clinical importance of FBH lies in its differentiation from forms of primary hyperparathyroidism (see above), and it has been reported that 10% of patients in whom hypercalcemia failed to respond to parathyroid surgery had FBH. The diagnosis of FBH relies on the interpretation of urinary calcium clearance to creatinine clearance ratios (< 0.01), together with a family history of hypercalcemia, and often parathyroid surgery that failed to correct the hypercalcemia, and identification of a *CaSR* mutation. However, it is important to note that up to one third of FBH patients may not harbor mutations of the CaSR coding region.

Von Hippel–Lindau disease

Von Hippel–Lindau disease is an autosomal-dominant disorder characterized by: hemangioblastomas of the retina and central nervous system (CNS); cysts involving the kidneys, pancreas, and epididymis; renal cell carcinomas; and pheochromocytomas. The retinal and CNS hemangioblastomas are benign vascular tumors that may be multiple and those in the CNS may cause symptoms by compression of adjacent structures and/or raised intracranial pressure. In the CNS, the cerebellum and spinal cord are the most frequently involved sites. The renal

abnormalities consist of cysts and carcinomas, and it is important to note that the lifetime risk of a renal cell carcinoma in von Hippel–Lindau disease is 70%.

The endocrine tumors in von Hippel–Lindau disease consist of pheochromocytomas and pancreatic islet cell tumors. The clinical presentation of pheochromocytoma is similar to that in sporadic cases, except that there is a higher frequency of bilateral or multiple tumors, which may involve extra-adrenal sites, in von Hippel–Lindau disease . The most frequent pancreatic lesions are multiple cyst-adenomas, which rarely cause clinical disease. However, nonsecreting pancreatic islet cell tumors occur in under 10% of von Hippel–Lindau patients. They are usually asymptomatic and the presence of the pancreatic tumor in these patients is often detected by regular screening using abdominal imaging. The pancreatic islet cell tumors frequently become malignant, and early surgery has therefore been recommended.

The *VHL* gene, which is located on chromosome 3p26–p25, is widely expressed in human tissues and encodes a 213-amino-acid protein (pVHL). A wide variety of germline *VHL* mutations have been identified and an analysis of the tumors indicates that *VHL* acts as a tumor-suppressor gene. There appears to be a correlation between the type of mutation and the phenotype, in that large deletions and protein-truncating mutations are associated with a low incidence of pheochromocytomas, whereas some missense mutations in VHL patients are associated with pheochromocytoma (referred to as von Hippel–Lindau disease type 2C). However, other missense mutations may be associated with hemangioblastomas and renal cell carcinoma but not pheochromocytoma (referred to as von Hippel–Lindau disease type 1), while other missense mutations are associated with hemangioblastomas, renal cell carcinoma and pheochromocytoma (von Hippel–Lindau disease type 2B). Type 2A, which refers to the occurrence of hemangioblastomas and pheochromocytoma without renal cell carcinoma, is associated with some rare missense mutations.

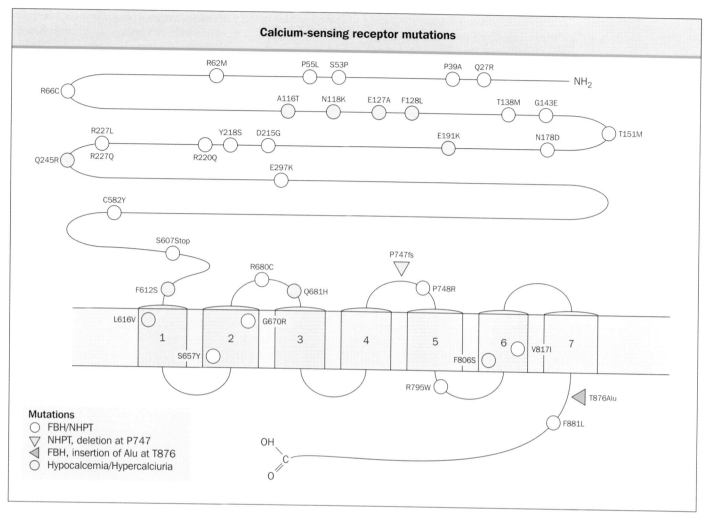

Figure 30.16 Calcium-sensing receptor mutations. The figure shows the location of calcium sensing receptor (CaSR) mutations found in familial benign hypocalciuric hypercalcemia, neonatal primary hyperparathyroidism, and hypocalcemic hypercalciuric kindreds. *CaSR*, which consists of a large extracellular domain, seven transmembrane domains and an intracellular carboxy-terminal domain, is shown schematically, together with 36 different mutations. Each missense mutation is shown in the single-letter amino-acid code: A, alanine; C, cysteine; D, aspartate; E, glutamate; F, phenylalanine; G, glycine; H, histidine; I, isoleucine; M, methionine; N, asparagine; P, proline; Q, glutamine; R, arginine; S, serine; T, threonine; V, valine; W, tryptophan; Y, tyrosine. (Adapted from Thakker RV. Disorders of the calcium-sensing receptor. Biochimica et Biophysica Acta. 1998;1448:166–70.)

The basis for these complex genotype–phenotype relationships remains to be elucidated. The functions of pVHL, which is also referred to as elongin, are being investigated, and one major function is to downregulate the expression of vascular endothelial growth factor and other hypoxia-inducible mRNAs. Thus, pVHL, in complex with other proteins, regulates the expression of hypoxia-inducible factors (HIF-1 and HIF-2) such that loss of functional pVHL leads to a stabilization of the HIF protein complexes, which results in overexpression of vascular endothelial growth factor and tumor angiogenesis.

NEUROFIBROMATOSIS

Neurofibromatosis type 1, also referred to as von Recklinghausen's disease, is an autosomal dominant disorder characterized by many associated manifestations: neurologic (e.g. peripheral and spinal neurofibromas), ophthalmologic (e.g. optic gliomas and iris hamartomas – Lisch nodules) dermatologic (e.g. café-au-lait patches), skeletal (e.g. scoliosis,

macrocephaly, short stature and pseudoarthorosis), vascular (e.g. stenoses of renal and intracranial arteries), and endocrine (e.g. pheochromocytoma, carcinoid tumors, and precocious puberty). Neurofibromatosis type 2 (NF2) is also an autosomal-dominant disorder but is characterized by the development of bilateral vestibular schwannomas (acoustic neuromas), which lead to deafness, tinnitus, or vertigo. Some NF2 patients also develop meningiomas, spinal schwannomas, peripheral nerve neurofibromas, and café-au-lait patches. Endocrine abnormalities are not found in NF2 and are associated solely with NF1. Thus, pheochromocytomas, carcinoid tumors, and precocious puberty occur in about 1% of NF1 patients, and growth hormone deficiency has also been occasionally reported.

The features of pheochromocytomas in NF1 are similar to those in non-NF1 patients, with 90% of tumors being located within the adrenal medulla and the remaining 10% at an extraadrenal location, which often involves the para-aortic region. Primary carcinoid tumors are often periampullary and may also occur in the ileum but rarely in the pancreas, thyroid, or lungs.

Hepatic metastases are associated with symptoms of the carcinoid syndrome, which include flushing, diarrhea, bronchoconstriction, and tricuspid and pulmonary valve disease. Precocious puberty is usually associated with the extension of an optic glioma into the hypothalamus with resultant elevations in gonadotrophins, but may also rarely arise in the absence of a chiasmal or hypothalamic involvement. Growth hormone deficiency has also been observed in some NF1 patients, who may or may not have optic chiasmal gliomas, but it is important to note that short stature in the absence of growth hormone deficiency is frequent in NF1 patients.

The *NF1* gene, which is located on chromosome 17q11.2 and acts as a tumor suppressor, consists of 60 exons that span over 350Kb of genomic DNA. *NF1* mutations are of diverse types and are scattered throughout the exons, making it difficult to implement mutational analysis in the clinical setting. The *NF1* gene product is the protein NEUROFIBROMIN, which has homologies to the p120^{GAP} (GTPase activating protein), and it acts on p21^{ras} by converting the active guanosine-triphosphate-bound form to its inactive guanosine diphosphate form. This downregulates the p21^{ras} signaling pathways, which in turn results in abnormal cell proliferation.

FAMILIAL PHEOCHROMOCYTOMAS

Pheochromocytomas occur as a part of several autosomal dominant syndromes, which include MEN2, von Hippel–Lindau disease, and NF1 (see above). In the familial setting, these pheochromocytomas may often occur bilaterally, and in some syndromes the pheochromocytomas or related paragangliomas may also arise in extra-adrenal sites. Carotid body tumors, often bilateral, may also occur. In addition to the mutations in the genes causing MEN2, von Hippel–Lindau disease and NF1, other genetic abnormalities involving LOH in tumors have also been identified. The regions involved include chromosomes 1p, 17p, and 22q, and the underlying tumor suppressors remain to be elucidated.

CARNEY COMPLEX

Carney complex is an autosomal-dominant disorder characterized by spotty skin pigmentation (usually of the face, labia, and conjunctiva), myxomas (usually of the eyelids and heart, but also tongue, palate, breast, and skin), psammomatous melanotic schwannomas (usually of the sympathetic nerve chain and upper gastrointestinal tract), and endocrine tumors involving the adrenals, Sertoli cells, somatotrophs, thyroid, and ovary. Cushing's syndrome, caused by primary pigmented nodular adrenal disease, is the most common endocrine manifestation of Carney complex and may occur in one third of patients.

Carney complex patients with Cushing's syndrome often have an atypical appearance in being thin (as opposed to having truncal obesity). In addition, they may have short stature, muscle and skin wasting, and osteoporosis. It is important to note that these patients may not have markedly elevated urinary free cortisols, but that this may be normal or only marginally elevated.

However, this pattern of normal cortisol production may be periodically replaced by days or weeks of hypercortisolism; this variant is referred to as 'periodic Cushing's syndrome'. Carney complex patients with Cushing's syndrome usually have loss of the circadian rhythm of cortisol production.

Acromegaly, caused by a macro-somatotrophinoma, affects about 10% of Carney complex patients and this may be detected earlier by observing elevations in 24-hour growth hormone secretion. Testicular tumors may also occur in one third of Carney complex patients. These may either be large-cell calcifying Sertoli cell tumors, or adrenocortical rests, or Leydig cell tumors. The large-cell calcifying Sertoli cell tumors may occasionally be estrogen-secreting and lead to precocious puberty or gynecomastia. Some Carney complex patients have been reported to develop thyroid follicular tumors, ovarian cysts, and breast duct adenomas.

Carney complex may be caused by one of two genes that have been mapped to chromosomes 2p16 and 17q22–q23. The Carney complex gene located on chromosome 17q22–q23, which is a tumor suppressor, has been identified as encoding the protein kinase A (PKA) regulatory subunit 1α, and is referred to as PPKARIA. Germline mutations that would result in premature terminations, and hence truncated PPKARIA, have been identified in Carney complex kindreds, and an analysis of PKA activity in tumors has demonstrated a decreased basal activity. The Carney complex gene on chromosome 2p16 has not yet been identified, but it is interesting to note that some tumors do not demonstrate LOH of 2p16 but instead show genomic instability, suggesting that this Carney complex gene may perhaps not be a tumor suppressor.

COWDEN'S SYNDROME

Multiple hamartomatous lesions, especially of the skin, mucous membranes (e.g. buccal, intestinal, and colonic), breast, and thyroid are characteristic of Cowden's syndrome, which is an autosomal-dominant disorder. Thyroid abnormalities occur in two thirds of Cowden's syndrome patients and these usually consist of multinodular goiters or benign adenomas, although up to 10% of patients may have a follicular thyroid carcinoma. Breast abnormalities occur in over 75% of patients and consist of either fibrocystic disease or adenocarcinomas.

The gene causing Cowden's syndrome is located on chromosome 10q23.3 and consists of 9 exons that encode a 403-amino-acid protein referred to as PTEN (phosphate and tensin homologue deleted on chromosome 10). PTEN contains a tyrosine phosphatase domain, which acts as a dual-specificity phosphatase and, more specifically, as a lipid phosphatase. PTEN may have roles in the apoptosis pathway, and in cell migration and focal adhesion. Mutations that would lead to truncated, and hence inactive, forms of PTEN have been identified in kindreds with Cowden's syndrome, and LOH suggesting a role of PTEN as a tumor suppressor has been detected in tumors. A recent study indicates that the occurrences of malignant breast disease or multiorgan disease appear to correlate with two different mutations, but these preliminary observations need to be confirmed in a larger series.

OVARIAN CANCERS AND FAMILIAL BREAST–OVARIAN CANCER SYNDROME

Ovarian cancer affects more than 5% of women and inherited mutations of the breast cancer genes, *BRAC1* and *BRAC2*, and of the mismatch-repair genes, *hMSH2* and *hMLH1*, are known to confer predisposition to ovarian cancer. All these genes have roles as tumor suppressors.

BRAC1 is considered to be involved in the majority of families with the breast–ovarian syndrome and in site-specific ovarian cancers. Approximately 5% of ovarian cancers occurring before the age of 70 years are caused by germline mutations of *BRAC1*, which is located on chromosome 17q21. *BRAC1* encodes a 220kDa protein, which contains two zinc-finger DNA domains and which localizes to the nucleus, suggesting that it acts as a transcription factor. *BRAC2*, which has only distant homology to *BRAC1*, is located on chromosome 13q13 and its function remains to be elucidated. *hMSH2* and *hMLH1*, which are human homologues of the bacterial *mutS* and *mutL* genes respectively, are located on chromosomes 2p22–p21 and 3p23–p22. These genes are involved in DNA repair mechanisms.

A recent study examining for germline mutations of *BRAC1*, *BRAC2*, *hMSH2*, and *hMLH1*, in epithelial ovarian cancers in women below the age of 30 years found that only 2% of these cancers harbored a mutation in *hMLH1* and none of the cancers had mutations of *BRAC1*, *BRAC2*, or *hMSH2*. Thus, although *BRAC1* mutations confer a high risk of breast and ovarian cancer in kindreds with familial breast–ovarian cancer syndrome, the roles of *BRAC1* together with that of *BRAC2*, *hMSH2*, and *hMLH1* and other genes in the etiology of other forms of ovarian cancers remain to be defined.

FURTHER READING

Cavaco B, Barros L, Pannett AAJ, et al. The hyperparathyroidism–jaw tumor (HPT–JT) Syndrome in a kindred from Portugal. Q J Med. 2001;94:213–22.

Eng C. The RET proto-oncogene in multiple endocrine neoplasia type 2 and Hirschsprung disease. N Engl J Med. 1996;335:943–51.

Ford D, Easton DF. The genetics of breast and ovarian cancer. Br J Cancer 1995;72:805–12.

Gagel RF. Multiple Endocrine Neoplasia Type 2. In: DeGroot LJ, Jameson JL, eds. Endocrinology, 4th edn. Philadelphia, PA:WB Saunders; 2001:2518–32.

Huson SM. Neurofibromatosis 1: a clinical and genetic overview. In: Huson SM, Hughes RAC, eds. The neurofibromatoses. A pathogenetic and clinical overview. London:Chapman & Hall; 1994:160–203.

Kirscher LS, Carney IA, Pack SD, et al. Mutations of the gene encoding the protein kinase A type 1, a regulatory subunit in patients with the Carney Complex. Nature Genet. 2000;26:89–92.

Liaw D, Marsh DJ, Li J, et al. Germline mutations of the PTEN gene in Cowden disease, an inherited breast and thyroid cancer syndrome. Nature Genet. 1997;16:64–7.

Maher ER, Kaelin NG. Von Hippel–Lindau disease. Medicine 1997;76:381–91.

Pannett AAJ, Thakker RV. Multiple endocrine neoplasia type 1. Endocrine Rel Cancer 1999;6:449–73.

Thakker RV. Disorders of the calcium sensing receptor. Biochim Biophys Acta 1998;1448:166–70.

Thakker RV. Multiple Endocrine Neoplasia Type 1. In: DeGroot LJ, Jameson JL, eds. Endocrinology, 4th edn. Philadelphia, PA:WB Saunders; 2001:2503–17.

Trump D, Farren B, Wooding C, et al. Clinical studies of multiple endocrine neoplasia type 1 (MEN1). Q J Med. 1996;89:653–69.

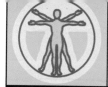

Section 7 General Conditions – Clinical

Chapter 31 Endocrinology of the Gastrointestinal Tract

Shahrad Taheri, Mohammad A Ghatei, and Stephen R Bloom

INTRODUCTION

The first evidence for the existence of hormonal communication between tissues was observed in the gastrointestinal tract when the peptide hormone secretin was discovered in 1902. Since then, the complex gastrointestinal endocrine system has contributed greatly to our understanding of peptide hormones. In contrast to most endocrine tissues, in which hormone-producing cells are grouped together into anatomically distinct glands, the endocrine cells of the gastrointestinal tract are scattered throughout its length. These enteroendocrine cells synthesize and secrete peptides that regulate gastrointestinal motility, the chemical and enzymatic processes of digestion, post absorptive processes, and growth and development of the gut. The majority of these peptides display a regional distribution in the gut (**Fig. 31.1**) and may act in an autocrine, paracrine, or endocrine fashion, or as neurotransmitters and neuromodulators. Gut peptides and their receptors (G-protein-coupled receptors) belong to various families determined by amino-acid sequence and gene homology. Peptides belonging to the same family may be produced from processing of the same precursor (e.g. the proglucagon-derived peptides, **Fig. 31.2**) or through differential splicing of the same gene.

Most gastrointestinal peptides have short circulating half-lives in plasma (**Table 31.1**). A variety of gastrointestinal pathologies are associated with alterations in circulating concentrations of gut peptides, which are likely to represent adaptation of the gut, for example, in response to loss of absorptive or secretory surface by altering secretion and motility in unaffected regions. Despite the large number of peptides found in the gastrointestinal tract, only a few are secreted in excess by rare gastroenteropancreatic neuroendocrine tumors resulting in well-defined clinical syndromes.

GASTRIN–CHOLECYSTOKININ FAMILY

Gastrin

Gastrin (**Fig. 31.3**) is synthesized in the upper small intestine and in G cells in the gastric antrum. The major circulating forms of gastrin, varying in the length of their amino terminals, are G34, G17, and G14. Full biologic activity of gastrin resides in the carboxy-terminal peptide and requires α-amidation of the carboxy-terminal phenylalanine. Both gastrin and cholecystokinin (CCK) end in the peptide gly-trp-met-asp-phe-NH$_2$ but differ in that the tyrosine in position 7 from the carboxy-terminal phenylalanine is sulfated in CCK (**Fig. 31.4**). G17, the major form in the circulation after a meal, has a shorter circulating half-life than G34 (**Table 31.1**); the two forms, however, are almost equipotent. Gastrin secretion is under luminal, humoral,

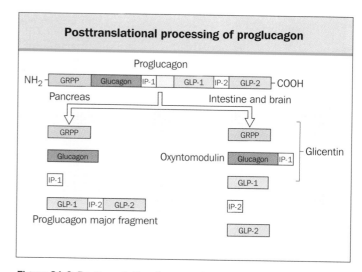

Figure 31.1 Gut hormones. The figure illustrates hormone production in the gastrointestinal tract.

Gut hormones

Gut hormones
- Gastrin
- Secretin
  Cholecystokinin
  Motilin
  Glucose-dependent insulinotrophic peptide
  Peptide-tyrosine-tyrosine
  Proglucagon-derived peptides
  Neurotensin
- Pancreatic polypeptide
  Somatostatin
- Peptide-tyrosine-tyrosine
  Enteroglucagon

Figure 31.2 Posttranslational processing of proglucagon. GLP, glucagon-like peptide; GRPP, glicentin-related pancreatic polypeptide; IP, intervening peptide.

Posttranslational processing of proglucagon

453

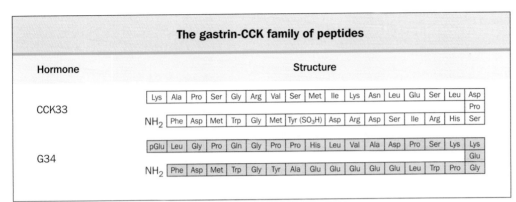

Figure 31.3 The gastrin–cholecystokinin (CCK) family of peptides.

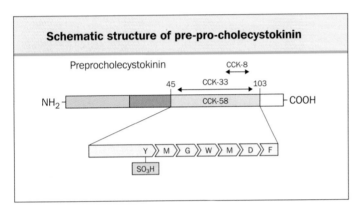

Figure 31.4 Schematic structure of pre-pro-cholecystokinin. The figure shows the relative locations of CCK (cholecystokinin)-58, CCK-33, and CCK-8. The carboxy-terminal heptapeptide important in conferring biologic specificity is also shown.

Plasma half-lives of gut peptides	
Peptide	**Plasma half-life (min)**
Gastrin–CCK family	
Gastrin 17/34	5/42
Cholecystokinin (CCK) 8/33	2/5
Secretin–glucagon family	
Secretin	3
Glucagon	2.5
Glucose-dependent insulinotropic polypeptide (GIP)	20
Glucagon-like peptide-1 (GLP-1)	4.5
Glucagon-like peptide-2 (GLP-2)	2.5
Vasoactive intestinal peptide (VIP)	< 1
Pancreatic polypeptide family	
Pancreatic polypeptide (PP)	2.5
Peptide tyrosine–tyrosine (PYY)	9
Other	
Somatostatin	3
Motilin	4.5
Neurotensin	1.5

Table 31.1 Plasma half-lives of gut peptides.

and autonomic nervous system control. The presence of amino acids and proteins in the lumen of the stomach, and gastric distention, stimulate gastrin secretion. Gastrin secretion also occurs in response to vagal stimulation. Calcium, administered orally or intravenously, and intravenous infusions of epinephrine also stimulate gastrin release. A gastric pH of less than 3 inhibits gastrin secretion indirectly, by stimulating the release of somatostatin by antral D cells. Somatostatin, acting in a paracrine fashion, inhibits gastrin secretion and is the final pathway for the inhibition of gastric acid secretion by several peptides, including the enterogastrones (hormones released in response to fat or its digestive products in the intestine that inhibit gastric acid secretion; **Fig. 31.5**). CCK inhibits gastric acid secretion through activation of CCK-A receptors on D cells, but stimulates acid secretion via CCK-B (also called gastrin receptors) receptors. Gastrin, acting via CCK-B receptors, stimulates the secretion of gastric acid from parietal cells and promotes growth of the gastric mucosa. The control of gastric acid secretion is complex, involving endocrine, paracrine, and neural mechanisms (**Fig. 31.6**).

Cholecystokinin

Cholecystokinin (CCK; **Fig. 31.4** & **Table 31.1**) is secreted by I cells in the duodenum and upper jejunum. CCK is also abundant in the CNS and posterior pituitary. CCK occurs in several molecular forms of varying amino-acid length, all derived from pre-pro-cholecystokinin (**Fig. 31.4**). CCK-8, CCK-58, CCK-33,

and CCK-39 have all been identified in significant amounts in plasma. The main stimulus to CCK release is the presence of breakdown products of fat and protein in the upper small intestine. Bile salts may be inhibitory to CCK release, since severe obstructive cholestasis or ingestion of cholestyramine results in elevated CCK levels. Somatostatin reduces CCK peptide secretion. Two receptor types for CCK have been described: CCK-A and CCK-B.

The major hormonal action of CCK is stimulation of gallbladder contraction via activation of CCK-A receptors. Other actions, such as pancreatic enzyme secretion, may be purely neural or a combination of neural and endocrine actions. CCK potentiates the actions of secretin in pancreatic bicarbonate release. CCK has been implicated in gastric emptying, control of gastric acid secretion and the promotion of pancreatic growth. CCK antagonists have been proposed for use as gastrointestinal prokinetic and antireflux agents and in the treatment of acute and chronic pancreatitis.

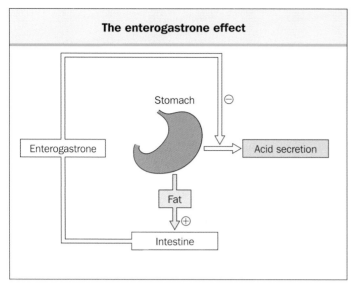

Figure 31.5 The enterogastrone effect.

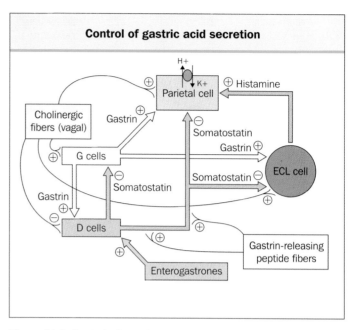

Figure 31.6 Control of gastric acid secretion. D, somatostatin cells; ECL, enterochromaffin-like cell; G, gastrin cells.

Figure 31.7 The secretin family of peptides.

The secretin family of peptides

Hormone	Structure													
Secretin	His	Ser	Asp	Gly	Thr	Phe	Thr	Ser	Glu	Leu	Ser	Arg	Leu	Arg
														Glu
	NH₂	Val	Leu	Gly	Gln	Leu	Leu	Arg	Gln	Leu	Arg	Ala	Gly
Glucagon	His	Ser	Gln	Gly	Thr	Phe	Tyr	Ser	Asp	Tyr	Ser	Lys	Tyr	Leu
														Asp
	Thr	Asn	Met	Leu	Trp	Gln	Val	Phe	Asp	Gln	Ala	Arg	Arg	Ser
Glucose-dependent insulinotropic peptide (GIP)	Tyr	Ala	Gln	Gly	Thr	Phe	Ile	Ser	Asp	Tyr	Ser	Ile	Ala	Met
														Asp
	Gln	Ala	Leu	Leu	Trp	Asn	Val	Phe	Asp	Gln	Gln	His	Ile	Lys
	Lys													
	Gly	Lys	Lys	Asn	Asp	Trp	Lys	His	Asn	Ile	Thr	Gln	
Vasoactive intestinal polypeptide (VIP)	His	Ser	Asp	Ala	Val	Phe	Thr	Asp	Asn	Tyr	Thr	Arg	Leu	Arg
														Lys
	NH₂	Asn	Leu	Ile	Ser	Asn	Leu	Tyr	Lys	Lys	Val	Ala	Met	Gln
Peptide histidine methionine (PHM)	His	Ala	Asp	Gly	Val	Phe	Thr	Ser	Asp	Phe	Ser	Lys	Leu	Leu
														Gly
	NH₂	Met	Leu	Ser	Glu	Leu	Tyr	Lys	Lys	Ala	Ser	Leu	Gln

SECRETIN–GLUCAGON FAMILY

The secretin–glucagon superfamily of peptides (**Fig. 31.7**) includes secretin, the proglucagon-derived peptides (PGDPs), glucose-dependent insulinotropic polypeptide (GIP), vasoactive intestinal peptide (VIP), pituitary adenylate-cyclase-activating peptide (PACAP), peptide-histidine-methionine (PHM) and growth-hormone-releasing factor (GRF).

Secretin

Secretin is secreted by the S cells of the upper duodenum and jejunum and is a 27-amino-acid linear peptide with a helical configuration. The major stimulus to secretion of secretin is the presence of acid in the duodenum: secretin is released when the pH of duodenal contents falls below 4.5. Fatty acids, bile salts, and alcohol also stimulate secretin secretion, while its release is inhibited by somatostatin. Secretin is the principal hormonal stimulant of pancreatic and biliary water and bicarbonate secretion. It may also contribute to pancreatic enzyme secretion.

Glucose-dependent insulinotropic peptide

Glucose-dependent insulinotropic polypeptide, also called gastric inhibitory polypeptide, is secreted by mucosal K cells, predominantly found in the duodenum and jejunum. GIP, a 42-amino-acid peptide, is released into the circulation following a mixed meal and also following ingestion of glucose, fat, or amino acids. Fat ingestion is a more potent stimulus to GIP secretion than carbohydrate in man. Peak plasma concentrations are achieved after 30–60min, but can be delayed up to 2 hours after fat ingestion. GIP was originally believed to be an enterogastrone (**Fig. 31.5**), although supraphysiologic doses are required to observe this effect in man. The observation that orally administered glucose results in a greater increase in plasma insulin than when the same quantity of glucose is administered intravenously suggested that a factor(s) is released from the intestine in response to oral glucose that stimulates insulin secretion from the pancreatic islets. This effect is called the incretin effect and GIP has been shown to be an incretin (**Fig. 31.8**). GIP is likely to act in concert with glucagon-like peptide-1 (GLP-1), and perhaps other peptides, to stimulate insulin secretion. GIP has been implicated in the disordered insulin secretion of several diseases, including chronic pancreatitis, cirrhosis, and Turner's syndrome. Secretion of GIP is enhanced in type 2 diabetes mellitus but, unlike GLP-1, there is little response to exogenous GIP in this condition. GIP may have an important role in lipid metabolism. Several case reports of food-dependent but adrenocorticotropic hormone (ACTH)-independent Cushing's syndrome have suggested that GIP may stimulate adrenal corticosteroid secretion through ectopic GIP receptors on cells of the adrenal cortex.

Glucagon and other proglucagon-derived peptides

Pre-pro-glucagon mRNA is expressed in the pancreatic islets (α-cells), intestine (L cells), and brain. Cleavage of a signal peptide from pre-pro-glucagon yields pro-glucagon. Pro-glucagon is differentially processed in tissues such that it gives rise to glucagon, glicentin-related pancreatic peptide (GRPP), and a large major fragment in the pancreas, while in intestinal L cells and in the brain it gives rise to GLP-1, GLP-2 and glicentin/enteroglucagon (**Fig. 31.2**). Glicentin/enteroglucagon, in turn, gives rise to GRPP and oxyntomodulin, while GLP-1 is further processed to glucagon-like peptide-1 (7–36) amide, glucagon-like peptide-1 (9–36) amide (a GLP-1 antagonist), and glucagon-like peptide-1 (7–37). Glucagon is a 29-amino-acid-residue peptide secreted by α cells of pancreatic islets. PGDPs are secreted by L cells in the ileal and colonic mucosa. A subpopulation of these cells also synthesizes peptide-tyrosine-tyrosine (peptide-YY, PYY). The major physiologically relevant PGDPs are the C-terminally amidated 30-amino-acid peptide GLP-1 and the 33-amino-acid peptide GLP-2.

The major stimulant to glucagon release is hypoglycemia. Glucagon is also released in response to amino acids, catecholamines (stress), vagal stimulation, and several hormones. Glucagon release is inhibited by hyperglycemia, hyperinsulinemia, and high circulating FFAs. Since the α-cell is located on

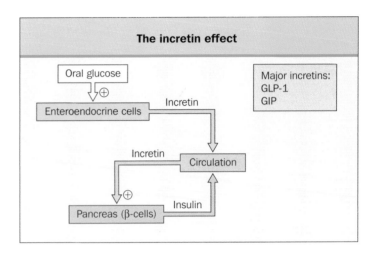

Figure 31.8 The incretin effect. GLP, glucagon-like peptide; GIP, glucose-dependent insulinotropic polypeptide.

the periphery of the islets of Langerhans, it is under paracrine inhibition by insulin from centrally located β-cells. GLP-1 inhibits glucagon secretion indirectly through stimulation of local somatostatin release. GLP-1 is released after ingestion of a meal, with GLP-1 (7–36) amide being the major released form. GLP-1, the most potent incretin known (**Fig. 31.8**), is released in response to oral but not intravenous glucose. GLP-1 release is also stimulated by ingestion of mixed fats and triglyceride, by bile acids, and by protein hydrosylates (peptones). Insulin and somatostatin inhibit, while epinephrine and β agonists stimulate, GLP-1 secretion.

Glucagon, acting on hepatocytes inhibits glycogen synthesis and stimulates glycogenolysis, gluconeogenesis, and ketogenesis. Glucagon has a lipolytic effect on adipocytes. In the heart, glucagon has positive inotropic and chronotropic effects (hence its clinical use in the treatment of beta-blocker poisoning) while it has a diuretic effect on the kidney and a spasmolytic effect on the intestine (hence its use in gastrointestinal imaging). GLP-1 is the major hormone responsible for the incretin effect. The GLP-1 receptor antagonist, exendin 9–39 (derived from the venom of the *Gila* monster), reduces the insulin response to intestinal glucose. The effects of GLP-1 on glucagon and insulin secretion are glucose-dependent, with little effect observed at low glucose levels. Exogenous GLP-1 can normalize blood glucose levels in type-2 diabetes mellitus and is being explored as a potential therapeutic agent in this condition. Unfortunately, exogenous GLP-1 has a half-life of only 4min intravenously and 20–30min subcutaneously. GLP-1 is an enterogastrone (**Fig. 31.5**). It also inhibits pancreatic exocrine secretion and almost completely inhibits vagally mediated gastric acid secretion. GLP-1 may contribute to the ileal brake effect, i.e. endocrine inhibition of upper gastrointestinal motility and secretion elicited by the presence of unabsorbed nutrients in the distal small intestine and colon (**Fig. 31.9**). This may occur in combination with PYY, co-stored with GLP-1 in some L-cells. GLP-2 is an important growth factor in the intestine and may find a role in the treatment of patients with short bowel or with damage to the intestinal epithelium.

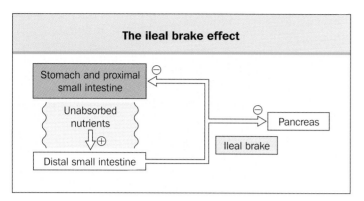

Figure 31.9 The ileal brake effect.

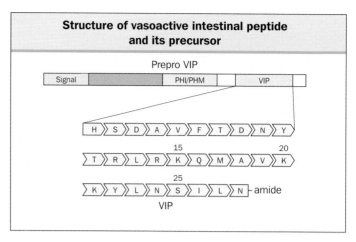

Figure 31.10 The structure of vasoactive intestinal peptide (VIP) and its precursor. PHI, peptide-histidine-isoleucine; PHM, peptide-histidine-methionine.

Vasoactive intestinal peptide and related peptides

Vasoactive intestinal peptide (VIP) is a 28-amino-acid peptide (**Fig. 31.10**). It belongs to a group of related peptides: PHM, peptide-histidine-valine (PHV), and PACAP. PHM and its C-terminally-extended form, PHV, are derived from the same precursor as VIP, preproVIP (**Fig. 31.10**). VIP is an inhibitory neurotransmitter found in intrinsic neural elements throughout the gastrointestinal tract from the esophagus to the rectum, and also in salivary glands and the pancreas. VIP is also found throughout the CNS, the lung, the urogenital tract, and in immune cells. PACAP and PHM are also neurotransmitters/ neuromodulators in the enteric nervous system. In the gut, VIP and PACAP have been localized to the same neurons in humans. VIP is usually undetectable in plasma and any detected is likely to represent spillover from local nerve terminals. VIP's inhibitory actions include the induction of relaxation of the lower esophageal sphincter, the sphincter of Oddi, and the anal sphincter. It mediates the descending relaxation of the peristaltic reflex and may be involved in reflex vasodilatation in the small intestine. VIP potently stimulates intestinal secretion by inhibiting sodium reabsorption and stimulating chloride secretion, secretion of bicarbonate in the pancreas and liver, and insulin and glucagon release from pancreatic islets. PACAP appears to have similar actions to VIP in the gut.

PANCREATIC POLYPEPTIDE FAMILY

The pancreatic polypeptide family (**Fig. 31.11**) includes pancreatic polypeptide (PP), PYY, and neuropeptide-tyrosine (NPY). All three peptides are composed of 36 amino acids and have a C-terminal amide that is essential for biologic activity. The 'Y' designation refers to the presence of tyrosine (Y) residues at the carboxyl and amino terminus of PYY and NPY.

Pancreatic polypeptide (PP)

Pancreatic polypeptide (PP) is synthesized by F cells, found mainly in the islets of Langerhans but also throughout the exocrine pancreas. PP, found as a dimer in plasma, is released into the circulation in a biphasic manner. The first and rapid phase is mainly under vagal control while the second and longer-lasting phase is caused by stimulation by ingested nutrients. This phase occurs through pathways that form the enteropancreatic reflex. Gut distention, CCK, gastrin, and motilin stimulate PP secretion, whereas somatostatin is inhibitory. PP is also released

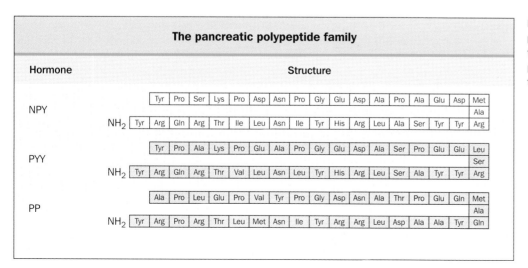

Figure 31.11 The pancreatic polypeptide family. NPY, neuropeptide tyrosine (neuropeptide Y); PP, pancreatic polypeptide; PYY, peptide-tyrosine-tyrosine.

in response to insulin-induced hypoglycemia. The inhibition of pancreatic exocrine secretion by PP appears to be its most physiologic effect. Plasma PP may be raised in several gastro-enteropancreatic neuroendocrine tumors, in which it may be a useful tumor marker.

Peptide YY

Peptide YY has a similar distribution to GLP-1, and the two peptides can be co-localized in L-cells. The main physiologic stimulus to PYY release is the ingestion of a meal, particularly fat. PYY levels rise at least 50-fold after consumption of a meal and remain elevated for several hours thereafter, the plasma level achieved being proportional to meal size. PYY is an entero-gastrone (**Fig. 31.5**). It reduces intestinal motility, gallbladder contraction, and pancreatic exocrine secretion (a pancreatone). It is a potent inhibitor of intestinal fluid and electrolyte secretion. PYY is also a mediator of the ileal brake (**Fig. 31.9**).

Neuropeptide Y

Neuropeptide Y has a widespread distribution in the central and peripheral nervous systems. In the gut, NPY is a neurotransmitter expressed in the enteric nervous system and in extrinsic sympathetic neurons. NPY neurons are also found in the pancreas. Any NPY detected in the circulation, for instance in patients with pheochromocytomas, is likely to be due to neuronal spillover into the plasma. NPY is a powerful vasoconstrictor, depending on the experimental system used. It attenuates epithelial anion and fluid secretion in the small intestine and descending colon *in vitro*. NPY is inhibitory to gastrointestinal motility.

OTHER HORMONES AND NEUROPEPTIDES

Motilin

Motilin is a 22-amino-acid peptide found in M cells, which are most dense in the epithelium of the duodenum and proximal jejunum. Motilin immunoreactivity is also found in the muscle layers of the intestine and has been detected in the large intestine, with the exception of the cecum, and in the gallbladder and the biliary tract. Motilin release is stimulated by ingestion of a meal but also occurs cyclically between meals. Motilin induces phase III contractions of the migrating motor complex in the stomach and associated events such as lower esophageal sphincter contraction, sphincter of Oddi and gallbladder contraction, and inhibition of gastric and pancreatic enzyme secretion. Macrolide antibiotics (e.g. erythromycin) are motilin-receptor agonists, which explains their side effects of diarrhea and abdominal cramps.

Somatostatin

In the gastrointestinal tract, somatostatin occurs as a 14-amino-acid peptide (somatostatin-14, S-14) and a 28-amino-acid peptide (somatostatin-28, S-28); both have an identical carboxy-terminal sequence, which is the biologically active region (**Fig. 31.12**). Somatostatin is secreted by specific endocrine D cells in the gastric and intestinal mucosa, and in pancreatic islets. It is also found in the extrinsic and intrinsic neurons of the intestinal myenteric and submucosal plexuses. S-14 predominates in gastric and pancreatic D cells, while the N-terminally-extended S-28 predominates in intestinal mucosal

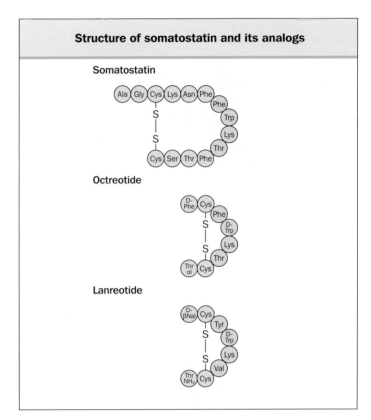

Figure 31.12 Structure of somatostatin and its analogs.

cells. Somatostatin functions as a hormone and paracrine agent, and as a neurotransmitter. It is released in response to a mixed meal. Somatostatin is a universal inhibitor of a wide range of hormones and other factors (**Table 31.2**). Somatostatin analogs (**Fig. 31.12**) are used therapeutically in the treatment of acromegaly, gastroenteropancreatic neuroendocrine tumors, portal hypertension and several other conditions.

Neurotensin

Neurotensin is a 13-amino-acid peptide that is produced by the N cells of the ileal mucosa but is also found in enteric nerves. Neurotensin release is potently stimulated by the ingestion of fat. The biologic actions attributed to neurotensin include: vasodilatation, inhibition of gastric motility and gastric acid secretion, stimulation of the exocrine and endocrine pancreas, effects on intestinal motility and secretion, increased histamine release from mast cells, and inhibition of blood flow to adipose tissue. Neurotensin may have growth regulatory functions in the pancreas and colon.

Calcitonin-gene-related peptide

Calcitonin-gene related peptide (CGRP) is a 37-amino-acid C-terminally-amidated neuropeptide that is the product of tissue-specific differential splicing of the calcitonin/CGRP mRNA. Several actions have been attributed to CGRP, including effects on gut motility (muscle relaxation), secretion (inhibition of gastric acid secretion via somatostatin; inhibition of pancreatic exocrine secretion), and blood flow (vasodilator). CGRP may have an important protective role in the mucosal response to injurious stimuli.

Inhibitory actions of somatostatin		
Endocrine		**Exocrine**
Gastrointestinal Tract	**Pituitary**	
Inhibits secretion of: Gastrin Cholecystokinin (CCK) Secretin Vasoactive intestinal peptide (VIP) Glucose-dependent insulinotropic polypeptide (GIP) Motilin Proglucagon-derived peptides Pancreatic polypeptide (PP) Insulin Somatostatin (autocrine)	Inhibits secretion of: Growth hormone (GH) Thyroid-stimulating hormone (TSH)	Inhbits: Gastric acid secretion and emptying Pancreatic secretion Gallbladder contraction Intestinal nutrient absorption Intestinal motility Splanchnic blood flow

Table 31.2 Inhibitory actions of somatostatin.

The tachykinins

The tachykinins include substance P and the neurokinins A and B. These peptides are vasoactive. They can either stimulate or inhibit motility in the gut depending on the type and site of activated tachykinin receptors. Extrinsic afferent neurons expressing substance P are sensitive to tissue irritation, inflammation, and injury and may participate in several reflexes involved in the gastrointestinal motor response to injury.

METHODS IN GASTROINTESTINAL ENDOCRINOLOGY

An understanding of gastrointestinal endocrinology has relied upon peptide hormone measurement by radioimmunoassay. Radioimmunoassay allows measurement of peptide levels, which are often as low as 10pmol/L in circulation and tissue. Although different antisera are used by different laboratories, thus preventing standardization of results, there is consistency in the magnitude of hormone levels. Peptide assay is clinically most important in the diagnosis of gut-hormone-secreting tumors. The elevation in circulating hormone levels is usually great, but a variety of gastrointestinal disorders and other conditions (**Table 31.3**) may be associated with more modest elevations.

In the normal gastrointestinal tract, immunocytochemistry is useful to determine the architecture of endocrine cells and the peptide hormone that is produced by individual cells. Electron microscopy allows identification of secretory granules, which are often characteristic of a particular hormone (**Fig. 31.13**). *In situ* hybridization, which detects hormone mRNA, is useful for identification of poorly granulated cells.

The histologic features of gut-hormone-secreting tumors on light microscopy are a solid trabecular, glandular, or mixed pattern. The techniques used to study normal cells can also be used to identify the peptides synthesized by tumors (**Fig. 31.14**). In nonsecretory tumors, nonspecific markers such as neuron-specific enolase and chromogranins can be used to demonstrate the endocrine nature of the tumor. Unfortunately, the biologic behavior of gastroenteropancreatic neuroendocrine tumors cannot be predicted reliably from the histologic or other features of the primary tumor, except in a minority of poorly differentiated tumors, which behave aggressively.

GUT HORMONES IN GASTROINTESTINAL DISEASE

The changes in gut hormones in gastrointestinal disease are usually the result of decreased hormone secretion from the affected region and of compensatory elevation of other peptides that assist the adaptation of the gastrointestinal tract to loss of absorptive surface. Occasionally, the elevation in levels of gut peptide may contribute to the disease process.

Nontumorous causes of elevated gut hormone levels					
Gastrin	**Vasoactive intestinal polypeptide (VIP)**	**Glucagon**	**Somatostatin**	**Pancreatic polypeptide (PP)**	**Neurotensin**

Chronic renal failure
Hypercalcemia
H$_2$ blockers and
  proton-pump inhibitors
Nonfasting sample
Pernicious anemia
	Bowel ischemia
	Hepatic cirrhosis
		Renal or hepatic failure
		Stress
		Prolonged fasting
		Gonadotropin-release inhibitors,
		  e.g. danazol
		Oral contraceptives
		Familial hyperglucagonemia
			Non-fasting sample	Nonfasting sample
				Elderly
				Pernicious anemia
					Nonfasting sample

Table 31.3 Nontumorous causes of elevated gut hormone levels.

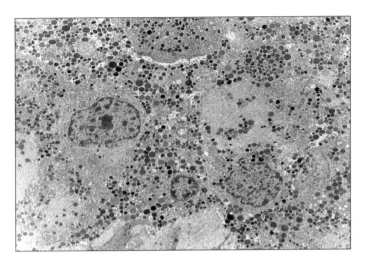

Figure 31.13 Electron micrograph of a somatostatinoma with typical electron-dense granules.

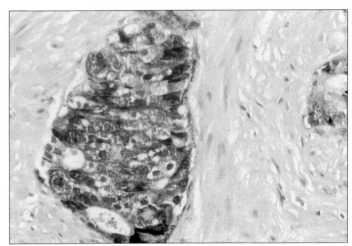

Figure 31.14 A duodenal endocrine tumor showing dense immunoreactivity for somatostatin.

Gastric pathology

Gastrin levels are elevated in a variety of gastric disorders. Usually, gastrin is secreted in response to a diminished output of gastric acid, as in atrophic gastritis (which is associated with achlorhydria) and following vagotomy. If the antrum is retained following surgery, gastrin-secreting cells are no longer exposed to gastric acid and so hypersecrete gastrin. G-cell hyperplasia results in gastrin excess despite normal or elevated acid output. The most common cause of elevated plasma gastrin levels is the powerful acid-antisecretory drugs such as the proton-pump inhibitors (PPIs).

In the postgastrectomy dumping syndrome, there is a gross exaggeration in the postprandial rise of VIP, PYY, enteroglucagon, and neurotensin levels, and a decrease in motilin levels. These changes may contribute to the impaired neural control of gastric emptying in this condition.

Surgery

Following partial ileal resection, gastrin, enteroglucagon, PP, motilin, and PYY levels are all elevated (**Fig. 31.15**), leading to hypertrophy of the remaining small intestine and delayed intestinal transit and thus creating more area and time for nutrient absorption. Similar changes occur in association with colonic resection, when the levels of gastrin and PP, but not of the principally colonic hormones, are elevated.

Jejunoileal bypass is an operation that was performed for gross obesity. It resulted in almost complete loss of the postprandial rise in GIP, which is secreted by the bypassed segment, but the elevation of hormones from other segments (**Fig. 31.15**) led to compensatory hypertrophy of the remaining bowel so that the effect of the operation was ultimately negated.

Malabsorption

In chronic pancreatitis, the pancreatic endocrine cells are often affected to some extent, and decreased levels of PP reflect this. The excess of nutrients passing into the colon as a result of the steatorrhea causes elevation of enteroglucagon, PYY, and neurotensin (**Fig. 31.16**). The gut adaptation resulting from these hormonal changes may explain the improvement in absorptive function seen with age in patients with cystic fibrosis.

Celiac disease is associated with reduced secretion of hormones from the affected duodenum and jejunum, such as secretin, CCK, and GIP. This in turn leads to impaired pancreatic exocrine secretion, thus exacerbating the malabsorption. There is gross elevation of other hormones to compensate for the malabsorption, particularly neurotensin and proglucagon-derived peptides (**Fig. 31.16**). Similar changes occur in tropical sprue. Following successful treatment of these malabsorptive conditions, gut hormone levels return to normal.

Acute diarrhea

There is a great elevation in motilin and PGDP levels in acute infective diarrhea (**Fig. 31.17**). These peptides may help in the repair process or may contribute to the altered motility, particularly motilin. In Crohn's disease there is an elevation of PP levels with a lesser increase in GIP, motilin and enteroglucagon levels; in ulcerative colitis there is a moderate elevation in PP, gastrin, GIP and motilin levels.

Neuropathic disease

In conditions in which local enteric nerves are destroyed, such as Hirschsprung's and Chagas' disease, there is a loss of local neuropeptides such as substance P, VIP, and somatostatin. These peptides are unaffected by diseases that affect distant neural gut innervation, such as the Shy–Drager syndrome.

GASTROENTEROPANCREATIC NEUROENDOCRINE TUMORS

Despite the large number of peptides in the gut, only a few, when secreted in excess by gastroenteropancreatic neuroendocrine tumors, result in clinical syndromes (**Fig. 31.18**). The majority of gut-hormone-secreting tumors originate in pancreatic islet cells, with the exception of carcinoid tumors, which usually occur in the midgut. Gastrointestinal neuroendocrine tumors are rare and often slow-growing. These tumors can be broadly classified as functioning and nonfunctioning tumors. Functioning tumors include carcinoid tumors (resulting in the carcinoid syndrome), insulinomas, gastrinomas, VIPomas, glucagonomas,

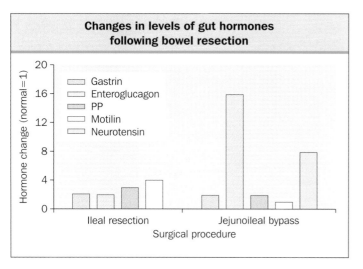

Figure 31.15 Changes in levels of gut hormones following bowel resection. PP, pancreatic polypeptide.

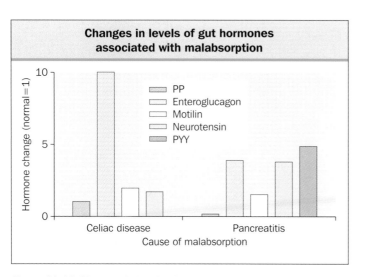

Figure 31.16 Changes in levels of gut hormones associated with malabsorption. PYY, peptide-tyrosine-tyrosine.

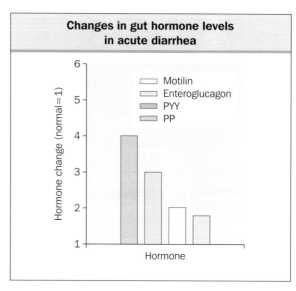

Figure 31.17 Changes in gut hormone levels in acute diarrhea. PP, pancreatic polypeptide; PYY, peptide-tyrosine-tyrosine.

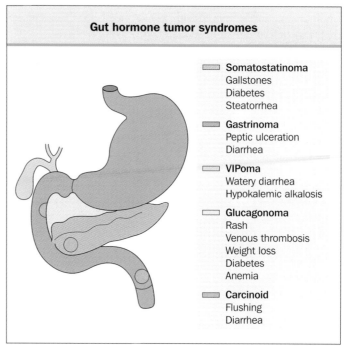

Figure 31.18 Gut hormone tumor syndromes.

and somatostatinomas. The clinical manifestations of functioning tumors are caused by excess peptide hormone (also serotonin in carcinoids) secretion. The hormone secreted may be eutopic (from a tumor of the tissue from which the hormone is secreted normally – e.g. glucagon or somatostatin) or ectopic (e.g. VIP or gastrin). The tumors may produce other hormones during the course of the disease or after treatment (e.g. surgery to reduce tumor bulk), giving rise to secondary hormone syndromes. Such secondary syndromes occur in approximately 5% of cases; therefore, all patients should have their plasma peptide levels screened at least yearly to identify such cases. Some 50% of pancreatic islet cell tumors are nonfunctioning. Nonfunctioning tumors have a worse prognosis (5-year survival chance of less than 50%) and present with local pressure symptoms and/or symptoms such as anorexia and weight loss. Gastroenteropancreatic neuroendocrine tumors may also

secrete parathyroid-hormone-related peptide (PTH-rp), resulting in hypercalcemia, growth-hormone-releasing hormone (GHRH), resulting in acromegaly, and corticotropin-releasing factor (CRF) or ACTH, resulting in Cushing's syndrome.

Approximately 25% of islet cell tumors, particularly gastrinomas and nonfunctioning tumors, may be associated with the autosomal dominant syndrome of multiple endocrine neoplasia type 1 (MEN-1), with features of parathyroid disease, pituitary and pancreatic tumors, and sometimes adrenocortical nodules or tumors (see Chapter 30). Some 70% of sporadic islet cell tumors and 45% of those associated with MEN-1 are malignant.

The most common sites for metastases are the liver and regional lymph nodes, although they may occur in bone, the adrenals, the brain, and the lungs, where they carry a much worse prognosis. Metastases are usually slow-growing, so that prolonged survival is often possible, particularly if treatment can minimize the effects of hormone excess. Since these tumors and their associated syndromes are rare, there is often a delay in diagnosis following the onset of symptoms, averaging 3 years. Following diagnosis, there is a 50% chance of survival of around 6 years for those with sporadic tumors, and of 15 years for those with MEN-1.

Carcinoid tumors

Carcinoid tumors have an annual incidence of 1 in 150,000 (comparable to acromegaly), with an average age at presentation of around 50 years. They account for up to 35% of small-bowel tumors. Carcinoid tumors are classically subdivided into foregut (from thyroid, bronchus, stomach, proximal duodenum, gallbladder), midgut (the remainder of the small intestine to mid-transverse colon) and hindgut (from distal colon and rectum) tumors. The most common site of carcinoid tumors is the appendix, followed by the ileum and rectum (**Table 31.4**). Appendiceal and rectal carcinoids are usually incidental surgical findings and rarely metastasize, while small-bowel carcinoids metastasize to the liver in some 50% of cases.

Midgut carcinoids release the monoamine serotonin (5-hydroxytryptamine, 5-HT), while foregut carcinoids may release serotonin, ACTH, gastrin, histamine, and calcitonin. Hindgut carcinoids never produce serotonin but may produce somatostatin and peptide YY. The clinical manifestations of carcinoid tumors are varied and are often determined by the site of the tumor. The term carcinoid is the preferred name for midgut tumors located outside the appendix that result in the carcinoid syndrome, which occurs in about 10% of patients and consists of flushing, diarrhea, carcinoid heart disease (mainly associated with fibrosis of valves on the right side of the heart), and bronchial constriction. The diarrhea is secretory (**Table 31.5**) and may be profuse, with passage of several liters per day, and occasionally there are associated electrolyte disturbances. It may also be associated with cramping abdominal pain. The flushing is paroxysmal and usually unprovoked, although it may occur in association with exertion or with ingestion of food or alcohol. It usually affects the face and upper thorax (**Fig. 31.19**) and may be associated with palpitations and postural hypotension, and rarely lacrimation and facial edema. When flushing occurs over a prolonged period, patients often develop a permanent plethoric, cyanotic facial appearance (**Fig. 31.20**). This latter feature is more common in those with foregut tumors. Paroxysmal wheezing occurs in a small number of patients, attacks often occurring in association with flushing. Around 20% of patients have cardiac valve abnormalities, usually affecting the right side of the heart (tricuspid incompetence and pulmonary stenosis). These valve abnormalities may precipitate right-sided heart failure, which carries a poor prognosis. Rare left-sided valve lesions may occur in the presence of right to left shunts or in association with bronchial carcinoids. Pellagra may occur with nicotinamide deficiency resulting from the increased conversion of 5-hydroxytryptophan into serotonin (**Fig. 31.21**). Occasionally, a carcinoid crisis occurs, with severe hypotension and hemodynamic instability requiring fluid and inotropic support.

Sites of carcinoid tumors	
Site	**Incidence (%)**
Appendix	40
Small bowel	25
Rectum	15
Bronchus	10
Colon	5
Stomach	<5
Duodenum	
Pancreas	
Ovary	<1
Testis	

Table 31.4 Sites of carcinoid tumors.

Differential diagnosis for secretory diarrhea	
Gastroenteropancreatic neuroendocrine tumours	Carcinoid VIPoma Gastrinoma Medullary carcinoma of thyroid
Infections	Cholera *Escherichia coli*
Drugs	Laxatives
Congenital	Structural abnormalities Congenital dysautonomia Congenital chloridorrhoea Immunoglobulin A deficiency
Other	Idiopathic Systemic mastocytosis Basophilic leukemia

Table 31.5 Differential diagnosis for secretory diarrhea.

With midgut tumors, the syndrome only occurs in the presence of liver metastases. The diarrhea is probably secondary to serotonin secretion, while flushing is likely to be due to excess tachykinin secretion. Growth factors released from the tumor may contribute to the cardiac fibrosis. Apart from the carcinoid syndrome, gastrointestinal carcinoid tumors may present with bowel obstruction, bleeding and intussusception. Surgery is therefore recommended to prevent such complications.

The carcinoid syndrome is associated with elevated urinary 5-hydroxyindoleacetic acid (5-HIAA), a metabolite of serotonin. 5-HIAA accounts for over 95% of the urinary excretion of serotonin (**Fig. 31.21**). The biochemical screening for the carcinoid syndrome requires demonstration of elevated urinary 5-HIAA collected on at least three occasions, since secretion from the tumor may be intermittent. Patients are advised to avoid avocados, bananas, pineapples, plums, eggplant (aubergines), and walnuts, since these may elevate 5-HIAA levels. Elevated plasma chromogranin A has been suggested as an early sensitive, but nonspecific, tumor marker for carcinoid tumors. Flushing may be precipitated by pentagastrin but this test is not routinely carried out.

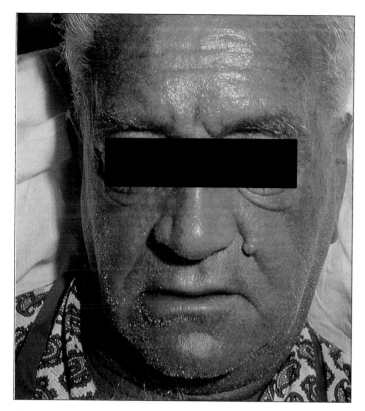

Figure 31.19 Carcinoid syndrome. Acute flushing can be seen.

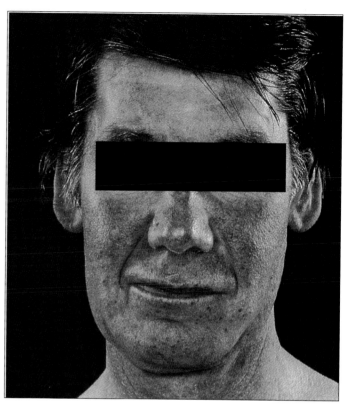

Figure 31.20 Carcinoid syndrome. The patient has a plethoric, cyanosed facies.

Gastrinoma (Zollinger–Ellison syndrome)

Gastrin-producing tumors have an annual incidence of 1 per 1,000,000. The mean age at the onset of symptoms is 50 years, with a male preponderance. Up to one third of gastrinomas are associated with MEN-1 while up to a half of MEN-1 patients develop gastrinomas. The majority of gastrinomas arise in the gastrinoma triangle, an area containing the duodenum, the pancreatic head, and the hepatoduodenal ligament. Gastrinomas mainly occur in the pancreas but approximately 20% of patients will have microadenomas (< 1cm in diameter) in the duodenum, particularly those with MEN-1. Patients with MEN-1 may also develop gastric carcinoids because of the proliferative action of gastrin on ECL cells. Rarely, gastrinomas may be found in the stomach or ovary. At presentation, up to 50% of patients with gastrinoma have metastases, mainly to the liver. The 5-year survival of patients with liver metastases is 20%, compared to 81% in those without metastases.

The gastrinoma syndrome was first described by Zollinger and Ellison, with the triad of fulminating ulcer diathesis, recurrent ulceration despite medical and surgical therapy, and a non-β-cell pancreatic islet tumor. The diagnosis of gastrinoma has been complicated to some extent by the widespread use of powerful acid-antisecretory drugs. Patients less commonly present with the complications of peptic ulcer disease (hemorrhage, perforation, or pyloric stenosis) but may present with ordinary-looking ulcers that fail to respond to standard therapy (including the eradication of *Helicobacter pylori*) or with gastric mucosal hypertrophy. Esophagitis and diarrhea are now more common but do not distinguish gastrinoma from other more common conditions.

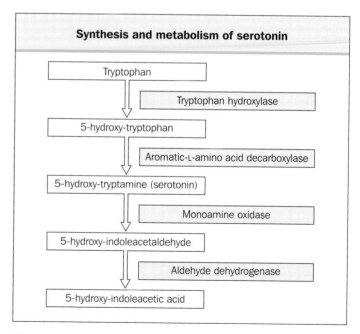

Figure 31.21 Synthesis and metabolism of serotonin.

The diarrhea is caused by increased acid secretion, secondary to elevated gastrin levels, neutralizing digestive enzymes and damaging the intestinal mucosa. Diarrhea that persists in spite of fasting and that is relieved by acid-antisecretory drugs is suggestive of a gastrinoma.

Biochemically, gastrinoma is diagnosed by the demonstration of high levels of fasting serum gastrin in the face of high basal gastric acid secretion (> 15mmol/h). Several conditions can result in raised gastrin levels (**Fig. 31.15**) and it is important to note that there is no absolute cutoff level of plasma gastrin that is diagnostic of gastrinoma. H_2-blockers should be discontinued for at least 72 hours, and proton-pump inhibitors for at least 14 days, before fasting plasma gastrin is measured. Since hypercalcemia raises gastrin levels, hyperparathyroidism should be excluded in patients with MEN-1. The secretin provocation test is carried out when gastrin levels are borderline and acid secretion results equivocal. In this test, fasting plasma gastrin concentrations are assessed at 15 and 2min before and 0, 2, 5, 10 and 20min after an intravenous bolus injection of secretin (2U/kg body weight). Up to 87% of patients will demonstrate a positive response to secretin (gastrin levels paradoxically increase by at least twofold from baseline).

VIPoma (Verner–Morrison syndrome)

VIPomas have an annual incidence of 1 per 10,000,000, the mean age at presentation being 49 years. About 90% of VIPomas are pancreatic. VIPomas are usually large and solitary, with 37–68% having metastasized at the time of diagnosis, usually to the liver and regional lymph nodes. Extrapancreatic tumors usually occur in children and arise in neural crest tissue as ganglioneuromas, ganglioneuroblastomas, or neuroblastomas. Extrapancreatic VIPomas in the retroperitoneum, lungs, jejunum, liver, and adrenal gland have also been described.

The VIPoma syndrome, caused by elevated circulating VIP, results in secretory diarrhea (initially intermittent, but later continuous; **Table 31.5**) with fluid, chloride, bicarbonate, potassium, and magnesium loss from the small intestine. Hypochlorhydria occurs in 73% of cases. Stool volumes can be as high as 20L/day, despite fasting, and potassium losses greater than 400mmol/day. The stool is otherwise normal. Stool volume of less than 700mL/day excludes the diagnosis but it is important to note that the diarrhea may be intermittent. The severe hypokalemia is frequently accompanied by a metabolic acidosis and hypomagnesemia caused by stool losses. Other features of the syndrome are hypercalcemia, glucose intolerance, and mild diabetes mellitus. In up to 20% of patients, flushing of the head and trunk may occur in association with a patchy erythematous rash.

The diagnosis of VIPoma requires the demonstration of secretory diarrhea associated with elevated plasma VIP levels. The plasma levels of PHM, PP, and neurotensin may also be elevated.

Glucagonoma

The glucagonoma syndrome has an annual incidence of 1 per 20,000,000, and over 99% of cases result from pancreatic tumors that secrete glucagon and other proglucagon-derived peptides (**Fig. 31.2**). Over 75% of glucagonomas are malignant and over 50% of patients have metastases at the time of diagnosis. The median age at presentation is 62 years. The diagnosis of glucagonoma can be delayed for up to 10 years. The cardinal feature of the syndrome is the necrolytic migratory erythematous rash (**Fig. 31.22**). This usually starts in the groins, with erythematous blotches that become eroded and then heal, leaving indurated pigmented areas. The rash migrates to the perineum, buttocks, and distal extremities. The underlying cause of the rash is unknown but several factors such as direct action of glucagon on the skin, amino acid and fatty acid deficiency, and zinc deficiency have been implicated in its etiology. Mucosal

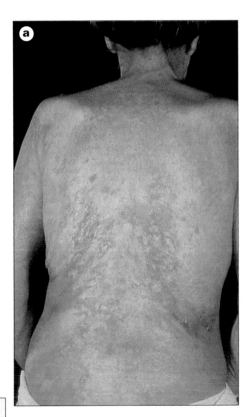

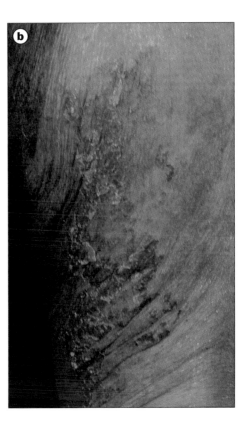

Figure 31.22 Glucagonoma syndrome: necrolytic migratory erythema.

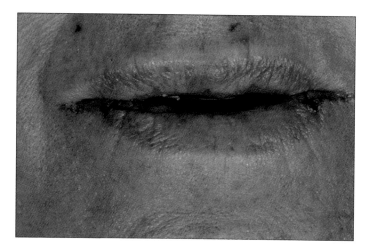

Figure 31.23 Glucagonoma syndrome: cheilitis.

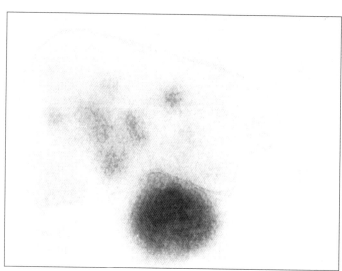

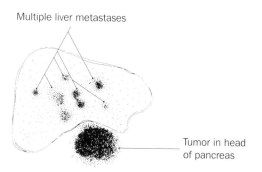

Figure 31.24 Indium-labeled octreotide scan showing a pancreatic tumor and hepatic metastases.

involvement also occurs resulting in stomatitis, cheilitis (**Fig. 31.23**) and glossitis. Other manifestations include cachexia (which may be extreme), impaired glucose tolerance, normocytic anemia, nail dystrophy, diarrhea, tendency to venous thrombosis and life-threatening pulmonary embolism, and neuropsychiatric disorders (such as slow mentation, psychosis, or depression).

Glucagonoma is biochemically diagnosed by highly elevated fasting plasma glucagon levels. Plasma glucagon may be elevated in other conditions, but these are easily distinguishable from glucagonoma. Elevated plasma gastrin, insulin, pancreatic polypeptide, VIP, and urinary 5-HIAA levels have all been observed with glucagonoma.

Somatostatinoma

Somatostatinomas are very rare tumors (annual incidence of 1 in 40,000,000). Some 50% arise in the pancreas, with 90% of these being malignant. The remaining 50% arise from the duodenum and over half of these occur in association with neurofibromatosis type 1. Duodenal tumors usually present early as a result of intestinal obstruction, obstructive jaundice, or gastrointestinal hemorrhage; they are rarely associated with the somatostatinoma syndrome and rarely metastasize. The somatostatinoma syndrome is characterized by the triad of gallstones, steatorrhea, and diabetes. Occasionally, hypoglycemia may occur, as a result of greater inhibition of counterregulatory hormones than of insulin. Postprandial fullness, weight loss, and anemia have also been described. Highly elevated plasma somatostatin levels confirm the diagnosis.

Tumor localization

Tumor localization is necessary to identify patients who benefit from curative resection of the tumor. Most gastroenteropancreatic neuroendocrine tumors can usually be localized using radiolabeled somatostatin receptor scintigraphy, which is the imaging modality of choice to localize primary tumors and to determine the extent of metastatic disease (**Fig. 31.24**). This technique also allows identification of patients who are most likely to

respond to treatment with somatostatin analogs. Some tumors may also be visualized with ^{123m}iodobenzylguanidine (MIBG) and some patients respond to therapy with ^{131}I-labeled MIBG. Macroadenomas (> 1cm), such as the majority of VIPomas and glucagonomas, can be easily localized by ultrasound, CT (**Figs 31.25–27**) and radiolabeled somatostatin receptor scintigraphy. In the case of small microadenomas (< 1cm), CT, MRI, and ultrasound have only up to 40% sensitivity. Therefore, for these tumors, such as microgastrinomas, more invasive localization techniques may be required. The techniques used depend on local expertise, the possibility of MEN-1 (multiple microgastrinomas), and the location of tumor (pancreatic or duodenal). The initial investigation is radiolabeled somatostatin analog imaging, which can identify up to 60% of tumors. Up to 80% of small tumors may be detected with endoscopic ultrasound, particularly tumors in the pancreatic head. Selective arterial angiography can localize 30–90% of tumors (**Fig. 31.28**). Intraarterial secretin or calcium injection at the time of angiography may further aid localization by precipitating secretion of the target hormone. Surgical exploration, in conjunction with intraoperative ultrasound, duodenal transillumination, with sensitivity of greater than 80%, may be necessary to localize and treat small tumors.

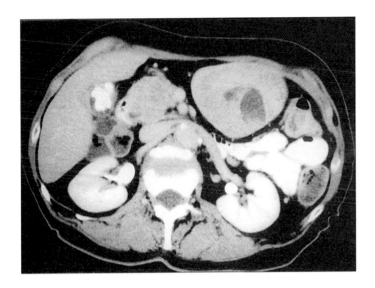

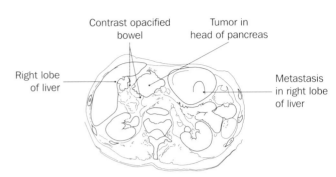

Figure 31.25 VIPoma syndrome showing a pancreatic tumor with liver metastasis.

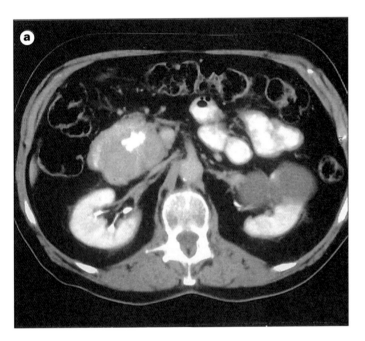

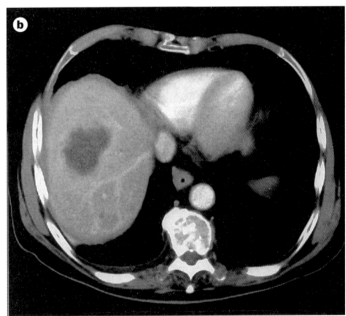

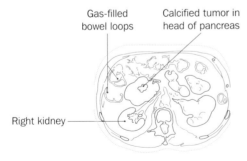

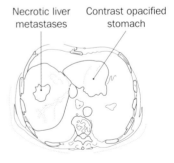

Figure 31.26 Glucagonoma syndrome. (a) Calcified pancreatic tumor. (b) Necrotic liver metastasis following hepatic embolization. (Same patient as shown in Fig. 31.24.)

Treatment

Surgery

Surgery is used for curative resection of gastrointestinal tumors, for debulking of tumors (thus reducing hormone output and pressure symptoms), and to prevent local complications such as intestinal obstruction. Surgical excision offers the only chance of cure for patients with gut-hormone-secreting tumors and should always be undertaken, if possible, when a primary tumor

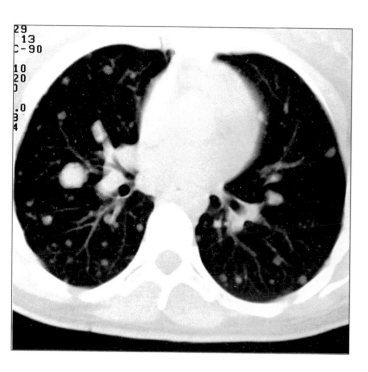

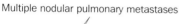

Multiple nodular pulmonary metastases

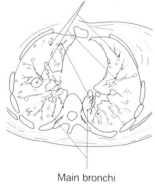

Main bronchi

Figure 31.27 Nonfunctioning pancreatic endocrine tumor with lung metastases shown on CT scan of lungs.

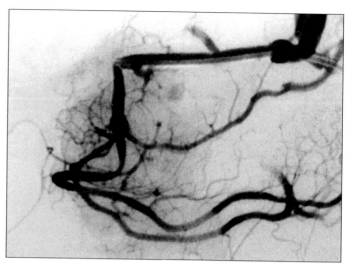

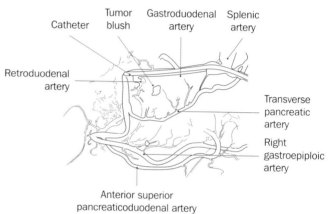

Catheter — Tumor blush — Gastroduodenal artery — Splenic artery

Retroduodenal artery

Transverse pancreatic artery

Right gastroepiploic artery

Anterior superior pancreaticoduodenal artery

Figure 31.28 Gastroduodenal arteriogram showing a gastrinoma blush in pancreatic head.

is identified that has not obviously metastasized. Such an approach is commonly of benefit only in gastrinomas or VIPomas, since other tumor types have usually metastasized by the time of diagnosis. Gastrinomas without diffuse hepatic metastases or MEN-1 should be surgically explored with the aim of curing the patient. In patients with MEN-1 and gastrinoma, studies show that over 90% of patients cannot be cured by surgical resection. The role of liver transplantation for metastatic gastrointestinal tumors remains to be determined. For tumors that cannot be cured surgically, noncurative tumor debulking can provide excellent palliation, reducing hormone levels and morbidity from local effects.

Somatostatin analogs

Somatostatin is used to reduce peptide secretion from the tumor and metastases. Somatostatin analogs (**Fig. 31.12**) are the mainstay of treatment in carcinoid syndrome, being used to control diarrhea, flushing, and bronchoconstriction. These analogs are also used in the treatment of diarrhea caused by excess VIP, in the treatment of the glucagonoma rash, and for the control of gastrinomas. Five different somatostatin receptors (sst) have been cloned. The somatostatin analogs in clinical use bind with high affinity to sst_2 and sst_5 receptors. Because somatostatin has a half-life of less than 3 minutes, longer-acting analogs have been developed (**Fig. 31.12**).

The octapeptide octreotide is usually administered subcutaneously three times a day, since its effects last between 6 and 8 hours. A slow-release depot form of octreotide is available and is administered intramuscularly every 4 weeks. Lanreotide is another cyclic octapeptide; it can be given subcutaneously, intravenously, or as a slow-release depot form (administered once every 2 weeks).

Although treatment with longer-acting preparations of somatostatin analogs are likely to be used increasingly, patients may still require unmodified octreotide injections for breakthrough symptoms and some patients may respond better to one longer-acting preparation than the other. Side effects of treatment with somatostatin analogs include nausea, abdominal cramps, flatulence, and malabsorption. Long-term treatment results in the formation of cholesterol gallstones and biliary sludge, which are not symptomatic in the majority of patients. Tachyphylaxis to the actions of somatostatin analogs may occur, requiring the use of increasing doses and/or hepatic tumor embolization and surgery to reduce the tumor bulk. The role of radiolabeled somatostatin analogs in the treatment of gastrointestinal neuroendocrine tumors remains to be determined.

Cytotoxic chemotherapy

Cytotoxic chemotherapy of gastrointestinal neuroendocrine tumors has been disappointing except in tumors secreting vasoactive intestinal peptide (VIPomas). However, chemotherapy has a role in reducing hormone secretion by widespread tumors. One commonly used regimen is streptozotocin with 5-fluorouracil (**Table 31.6**), although CCNU (lomastin) is sometimes used instead of streptozotocin. Alpha-interferon has been used in symptom control (such as the diarrhea of carcinoid syndrome) and in attempts to arrest tumor growth but is limited by its side effects, such as flu-like symptoms and bone marrow suppression.

Hepatic tumor embolization

Hepatic tumor embolization takes advantage of the fact that the liver parenchyma derives its blood supply from both the portal and systemic circulations while hepatic metastases are particularly dependent on blood supply from the hepatic artery (**Figs 31.29 & 31.30**). Injection of inert microspheres into branches of the hepatic artery supplying the tumor results in tumor infarction and regression while leaving the artery itself patent. This is superior to occlusion of the hepatic artery branches, which cannot be repeated. Hepatic embolization can provide good palliation in over 50% of patients with symptomatic hepatic metastases, and the procedure can be repeated when symptoms recur. If more than 50% of the liver parenchyma

Cytotoxic chemotherapy for gut hormone tumors		
	Response rate (%)	
Regimen	Islet cell tumors	Carcinoid tumors
Single agent		
Streptozotocin	30–40	10
Chlorozotocin	30–40	–
Dacarbazine	25–50	15
Doxorubicin	20	20
5-fluorouracil (5-FU)	–	25
Combination		
Streptozotocin + 5-FU	45–65	15–33
Streptozotocin + doxorubicin	69	–
Chlorozotocin + 5-FU	32	–

Table 31.6 Cytotoxic chemotherapy for gut hormone tumors.

is replaced by tumor, then embolization is contraindicated, as fulminant hepatic failure may occur. The somatostatin analog octreotide and aprotinin are administered intravenously to counter the effects of massive hormone release following embolization, and broad-spectrum antibiotic prophylaxis is recommended. The procedure may result in fever, malaise, nausea, vomiting, abdominal pain, and paralytic ileus. Persistent fever necessitates exclusion of a hepatic abscess by abdominal ultrasound. Chemoembolization, using agents such as doxorubicin, has been advocated in the treatment of metastatic neuroendocrine tumors and may have less morbidity than cytotoxic chemotherapy or embolization alone.

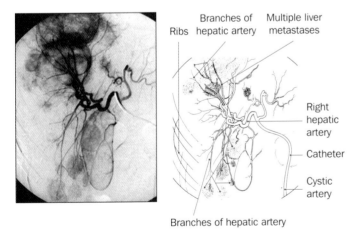

Figure 31.29 Arteriogram of the right hepatic artery showing multiple liver metastases.

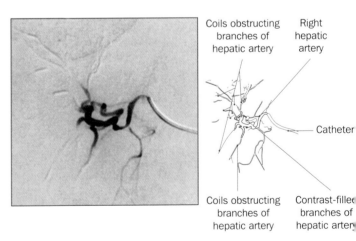

Figure 31.30 Arteriogram showing branches of hepatic artery (as in Fig. 31.29) occluded by coils.

Other treatments

Patients with the carcinoid syndrome are advised to avoid alcohol. Niacin supplements are given for pellagra-like skin symptoms. Agents second line to somatostatin analogs include H_1 and H_2 antagonists, α-receptor blockers, phenothiazines, α-interferon and glucocorticoids for flushing and serotonin antagonists (ondansetron), loperamide and α-interferon for diarrhea. In the treatment of gastrinoma, PPIs, at dosages titrated to the patient's response and aimed at reducing gastric acid secretion to less than 10mmol/hour for the hour prior to the next dose of the drug, have extended life expectancy by reducing the complications of hyperacidity. When high doses are required, patients benefit from the PPI dose being given twice a day rather than once a day. With metastatic gastrinoma, symptoms are controlled well with PPIs for many years but when symptoms become difficult to control or the tumor behaves more malignantly, then additional treatment modalities are employed.

The initial treatment of VIPoma requires restoration of fluid, electrolyte, and acid–base balance. Specific treatment involves somatostatin analogs. Other agents used include glucocorticoids, indometacin, lithium carbonate, loperamide, and phenothiazines but are rarely necessary. The glucagonoma rash responds well to oral and topical zinc, and to somatostatin analogs. Warfarin is used for prevention of thromboembolic episodes and insulin for diabetes mellitus. Tumors co-secreting PTH-rp may result in severe hypercalcemia, requiring vigorous rehydration of the patient followed by treatment with bisphosphonates. Cytoreductive surgery and hepatic tumor embolization may then be used to reduce the secretion of PTH-rp.

FURTHER READING

Bloom SR, Long RG. Radioimmunoassay of gut regulatory peptides. London:WB Saunders;1982.

Bloom SR, Polak JM. Glucagonoma syndrome. Am J Med. 1987;82:25–36.

Hammond PJ, Jackson JA, Bloom SR. Localization of pancreatic endocrine tumors. Clin Endocrinol. 1994;40:3–14.

Holst JJ. Enteroglucagon. Annu Rev Physiol. 1997;59:257–71.

Jensen RT. Management of the Zollinger–Ellison syndrome in patients with multiple endocrine neoplasia type 1. J Intern Med. 1998;243:477–88.

Kulke MH, Mayer R. Carcinoid tumors. N Engl J Med. 1999;340:858–68.

Modlin IM, Tang LH. Approaches to the diagnosis of gut neuroendocrine tumors: the last word (today). Gastroenterology 1997;112:583–90.

Norton-JA, Fraker-DL, Alexander-HR, et al. Surgery to cure the Zollinger–Ellison syndrome. N Engl J Med. 1999;341:635–44.

Frankton S, Bloom SR. Gastrointestinal endocrine tumours. Baillière's Clin Gastroenterol. 1996;10697–705.

Taheri S, Meeran K. Islet cell tumours: diagnosis and medical management. Hosp Med. 2000;61:824–9.

Taheri S, Ghatei MA, Bloom SR. Cholecystokinin. In: Creighton TE, ed. Encyclopedia of molecular medicine. New York: John Wiley, 2001.

Taheri S, Ghatei MA, Bloom SR. Proglucagon-derived peptides. In Creighton TE, ed. Encyclopedia of molecular medicine. New York: John Wiley,2001.

Taheri S, Ghatei MA, Bloom SR. Vasoactive intestinal peptide. In Creighton TE, ed. Encyclopedia of molecular medicine. New York: John Wiley, 2001.

Termanini B, Gibril F, Reynolds JC, et al. Value of somatostatin receptor scintigraphy: a prospective study in gastrinoma of its effect on clinical management. Gastroenterology 1997;112:335–47.

Walsh JH, Dockray GJ. Gut peptides. New York:Raven Press, 1994.

Yu F, Venzon DJ, Serrano J, et al. Prospective study of the clinical course, prognostic factors, causes of death, and survival in patients with long-standing Zollinger–Ellison syndrome. J Clin Oncol. 1999;17:615–30.

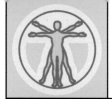
Chapter 32

Lipids and Lipoproteins

Alan Chait and John D Brunzell

CLINICAL SIGNIFICANCE OF LIPIDS AND LIPOPROTEINS

Hyperlipidemia, defined as an increase in levels of plasma cholesterol or triglyceride, or of both, is one of the most common metabolic disorders that occurs in industrialized societies. It results from genetic and/or acquired derangements in the metabolism of plasma lipoproteins. The major significance of hyperlipidemia, particularly hypercholesterolemia, is that it is one of the main modifiable risk factors for the development of premature atherosclerotic complications (**Table 32.1**), with the principal lipoprotein-related cardiovascular risk factors being increased levels of low-density lipoproteins (LDL) and low levels of high-density lipoproteins (HDL). Hypertriglyceridemia also can be a marker for cardiovascular risk. The constellation of high triglycerides, low HDL, and the presence of compositional changes in LDL (see later) is termed dyslipidemia. Recognition and treatment of the atherogenic disorders of lipoprotein metabolism can be of value in the primary prevention of atherosclerosis. Treatment of hyperlipidemia or dyslipidemia in patients with established cardiovascular disease can slow progression of lesions, in some cases can even result in regression of established lesions, and can reduce the recurrence of clinical events. Treatment of individuals with established atherosclerotic disease is termed secondary prevention. The diagnosis and management of disorders of lipoproteins requires an understanding of lipoprotein structure, function, and metabolism.

LIPOPROTEIN PHYSIOLOGY

Lipoprotein structure

Lipoproteins are composed of a central core in which the more lipophilic components, cholesteryl esters and triglycerides, are sequestered from the aqueous environment of plasma by a surface comprised of unesterified (free) cholesterol, phospholipids, and apolipoproteins (**Fig. 32.1**). These components exist in distinct proportions in the different lipoprotein classes, thereby permitting their separation by operational means such as ultracentrifugation and electrophoresis. There is, however, considerable heterogeneity within each lipoprotein class (**Fig. 32.2**). Several apolipoproteins are found in the different lipoprotein classes (**Fig. 32.2**), each having one of three major functions: structural; as ligands for receptors; and as enzyme cofactors.

Table 32.1 Major cardiovascular risk factors.

Major cardiovascular risk factors		
Modifiable	Nonmodifiable	Emerging
Lipid-associated		
Hypercholesterolemia	Age	Homocystine
Hypertriglyceridemia*	Male gender	Inflammatory markers
Low high-density lipoprotein*	Family history of premature cardiovascular disease	Infectious agents
Increased Lp (a)		Oxidative stress
Increased apolipoprotein B*		
Atherogenic diet		
Physical inactivity		
Nonlipid		
Hypertension*		
Cigarette smoking		
Diabetes*		
*Often associated with central obesity and insulin resistance.		

Lipoprotein function

As can be deduced from their structure, lipoproteins sequester lipids during their transport through plasma. Triglycerides are transported from sites of synthesis and absorption to sites of utilization and storage. Cholesterol is transported to cells of the body where it forms part of critical structural components of cell membranes (all cells), or is used for bile acid synthesis (liver), for steroidogenesis (adrenals, gonads), and as a precursor for vitamin D (skin). These functions are achieved by the exogenous and endogenous metabolic pathways of lipoprotein metabolism and by the metabolism of HDL.

Lipoprotein metabolism

Exogenous pathway

Chylomicrons are formed by the intestines after ingestion of dietary fat. These large, triglyceride-rich lipoproteins enter the plasma via the thoracic duct. In adipose tissue and muscle part of this triglyceride component is hydrolyzed by the enzyme lipoprotein lipase (LPL). LPL is synthesized by adipocytes and myocytes and attaches to heparin on the luminal side of capillary endothelium in these tissues, where it hydrolyzes the triglycerides in chylomicrons (and very-low-density lipoprotein – VLDL – see below). Apolipoprotein (apo) CII activates and apo CIII may inhibit LPL activity (**Fig. 32.3**). Hydrolysis of the triglycerides in chylomicrons leads to the formation of partially triglyceride-depleted chylomicron remnants (**Fig. 32.4**). Free fatty acids that are liberated by the action of LPL are taken up and re-esterified for storage as triglycerides in adipose tissue or utilized for energy by muscle (**Fig. 32.3**).

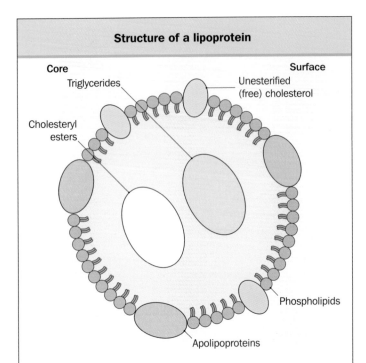

Structure of a lipoprotein

Figure 32.1 Structure of a lipoprotein. The central core contains the more lipophilic components – triglycerides and cholesteryl esters – which are sequestered from the aqueous environment of plasma by a surface layer of free cholesterol, phospholipids, and apolipoproteins.

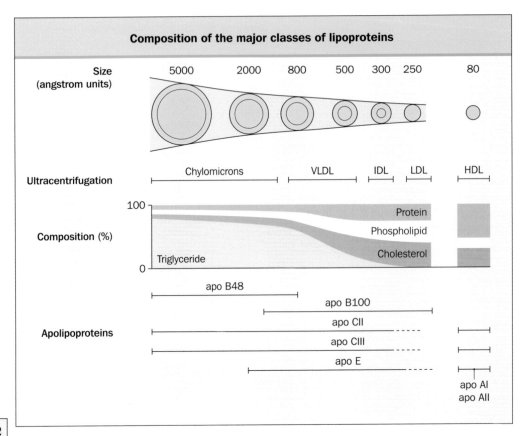

Figure 32.2 Composition of the major classes of lipoproteins. Although each of the lipoproteins is distinct with respect to its relative proportions of cholesterol, triglycerides, phospholipids, and apolipoproteins, considerable heterogeneity exists within each lipoprotein class. Lipoproteins are graded according to their density: very low (VLDL), low (LDL), intermediate (IDL) or high (HDL). Clinical measures of LDL include both LDL and IDL.

The function of lipoprotein lipase

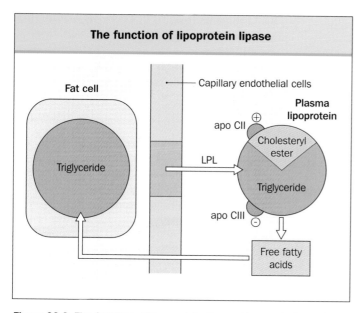

Figure 32.3 The function of lipoprotein lipase. Lipoprotein lipase (LPL) works on the luminal side of endothelial cells, where it hydrolyzes triglycerides in chylomicrons and very-low-density lipoprotein particles. The free fatty acids that are liberated are translocated into adipocytes where they are re-esterified to form fat droplets, or are used by muscles for energy.

The chylomicron remnants lose apo CII and acquire apo E, which is shuttled to and from HDL (see below). Apo E mediates the binding of chylomicron remnants to receptors on the liver. The remnants then deliver cholesterol to the hepatocyte for synthesis of bile acid and very low-density lipoproteins (VLDL). Chylomicrons are not further metabolized to LDL.

Endogenous pathway

In the liver, VLDL particles are formed using triglyceride that is synthesized from circulating free fatty acids or from fatty acids that are newly formed from glucose by lipogenesis. VLDL-cholesterol is derived largely from cholesterol that is delivered in chylomicron remnants. These lipids combine with apo B100, their major structural apolipoprotein, and are subsequently secreted into plasma (**Fig. 32.5**). There they acquire apo CII, undergo hydrolysis of their triglycerides by LPL (**Fig. 32.3**), and become remnant particles, which acquire apo E in a manner similar to that described in the exogenous pathway. Some VLDL remnants are taken up and can be degraded by the liver after their apo E component binds to the LDL receptor (rather than to the chylomicron remnant receptor as occurs with chylomicron remnants). Other VLDL remnants are converted into LDL (see **Fig. 32.4**). Hepatic lipase contributes to hepatic remnant lipoprotein recognition. Hepatic lipase also determines the size and density of the circulating LDL particle by removing

Exogenous and endogenous pathway of lipoprotein metabolism

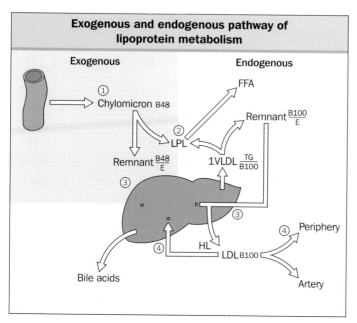

Figure 32.4 Exogenous and endogenous pathway of lipoprotein metabolism. Chylomicrons [containing apolipoprotein (apo) B48] are formed in response to the consumption of dietary fat. They subsequently enter plasma where their triglyceride component is hydrolyzed by lipoprotein lipase (LPL). The triglyceride-depleted chylomicron remnant is taken up by receptors on the liver, which recognize apo E. Very-low-density lipoprotein (VLDL) particles (containing apo B100) enter plasma after being secreted by the liver, and triglycerides are hydrolyzed by LPL. Some VLDL remnants are taken up and degraded by the liver, while others are converted into low-density lipoproteins (LDL). LDL is remodeled by hepatic lipase (HL). The major site of LDL uptake is the liver: LDL also supplies cholesterol to peripheral tissues. FFA, free fatty acids.

The formation of high-density lipoprotein

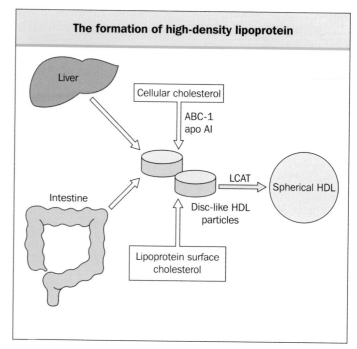

Figure 32.5 The formation of high-density lipoprotein. Lipids shed from the surface of the triglyceride-rich lipoprotein during its catabolism can be taken up by disc-like high-density lipoprotein (HDL) particles that are secreted from the liver and intestine. Cholesteryl esters that are formed as a result of lecithin-cholesterol acyltransferase (LCAT) activity enter the core of HDL particles, which then become spherical. Disk-like HDL particles containing unesterified cholesterol, phospholipids and apo AI also are generated by cells such as macrophages, when they become laden with excess cholesterol. Movement of cholesterol out of cells requires a transporter, adenosine-triphosphate-binding cassette-A1 (ABC-A1).

LDL lipids. A single molecule of apo B100 is present in each particle in this metabolic cascade. The apo B in LDL binds to LDL receptors on cells throughout the body, thereby supplying them with cholesterol when required. The major site of LDL catabolism is the liver, where the level of expression of LDL receptors largely determines the rate of removal of plasma LDL.

High-density lipoprotein metabolism

Nascent HDL is synthesized in the liver and intestines and secreted as bilayers of apo AI, apo AII and phospholipid. HDL also can be generated by the uptake of free cholesterol from peripheral cells, especially macrophages, by lipid-poor apo AI. The transport of free cholesterol out of cells by this apolipoprotein-mediated pathway is facilitated by a protein, adenosine-triphosphate-binding cassette-A1 (ABC-A1). In addition to acquiring excess cholesterol secreted from cells, HDL also acquires cholesterol from lipoprotein surface components that become redundant as lipoprotein particles decrease in size through loss of core lipids. The free cholesterol in HDL is subsequently esterified by the enzyme lecithin-cholesterol acyltransferase (LCAT). The hydrophobic cholesteryl ester that results moves into the core of the HDL particle, leading to the formation of a spherical particle (**Fig. 32.5**). cholesteryl ester transfer protein (CETP) mediates transfer of cholesteryl esters to lower density lipoproteins (VLDL and LDL), which can then acquire apo E from HDL. Apo E is a ligand for hepatic lipoprotein receptors, which allows cholesterol to be delivered to the liver from where it can be secreted. These processes are known as reverse cholesterol transport (**Fig. 32.6**). Cholesteryl esters in HDL (and in lower density lipoproteins also) can be selectively taken up, independently of uptake of the whole lipoprotein particle, by a liver receptor, scavenger receptor B1 (SR-B1). HDL apolipoproteins can be taken up and degraded by receptors in the kidney. In addition, apolipoproteins are shuttled between HDL and the triglyceride-rich lipoproteins in response to metabolic needs. Thus, the nascent triglyceride-rich lipoproteins acquire apo CII and apo CIII from HDL to form mature triglyceride-rich lipoproteins. Following LPL-mediated hydrolysis of triglycerides, apo CII, which is no longer required by the remnant lipoprotein, transfers back to HDL, which then donates the apo E required for hepatic remnant uptake (**Fig. 32.7**).

PATHOPHYSIOLOGY

Acquired and genetic forms of hyperlipidemia can occur as a result of disturbances at four main sites in the endogenous pathway: (1) increased input of VLDL and (2) impaired LPL-mediated triglyceride removal can cause hypertriglyceridemia; (3) impaired remnant removal results in a combined elevation of cholesterol and triglyceride levels of approximately equal magnitude; and (4) accumulation of LDL due to impaired LDL receptor-mediated clearance leads to hypercholesterolemia.

Acquired (secondary) hyperlipidemia

Several underlying disorders or drugs also lead to disturbances at these four major sites of regulation of lipoprotein metabolism. Acquired hyperlipidemia tends to manifest either as hypertriglyceridemia alone or as combined elevations of cholesterol and triglyceride (**Table 32.2**). Acquired hyperlipidemia usually responds to treatment of the underlying condition, where possible, or to discontinuation of the responsible drug.

Genetic forms of hyperlipidemia
Very-low-density lipoprotein overproduction

Two major genetic forms of hyperlipidemia result from increased VLDL secretion: familial hypertriglyceridemia and familial combined hyperlipidemia. In the former, the VLDL particles that enter plasma are large and triglyceride-enriched, while in the latter they are smaller and less rich in triglycerides.

The primary defect in familial hypertriglyceridemia is probably a defect in small intestinal bile acid reabsorption. This leads to overproduction of cholic acid, which is related to increased

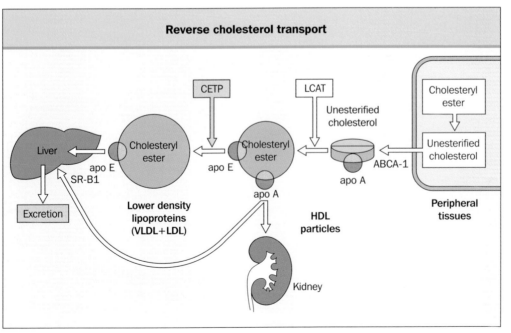

Figure 32.6 Reverse cholesterol transport. Excess unesterified cholesterol from cells is picked up by high-density lipoprotein (HDL) particles and esterified by lecithin-cholesterol acyltransferase (LCAT). The cholesteryl esters in HDL are transferred to lower-density lipoproteins (VLDL and LDL) by cholesteryl ester transfer protein (CETP). These lipoproteins deliver cholesterol by apolipoprotein (apo)-E-mediated mechanisms to the liver, from where they can be excreted. SR-B1, scavenger receptor B1.

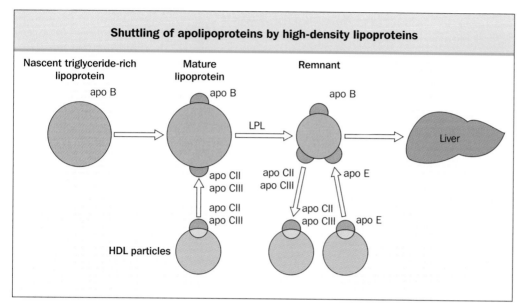

Shuttling of apolipoproteins by high-density lipoproteins

Figure 32.7 Shuttling of apolipoproteins by high-density lipoproteins. Nascent high-density lipoprotein (HDL) particles mature after acquiring apolipoprotein (apo) CII from HDL. Apo CII then activates lipoprotein lipase (LPL) and is subsequently shuttled back to HDL. Apo E, which is then shuttled from HDL to remnant lipoproteins, is used for remnant uptake by hepatic receptors.

Acquired forms of hyperlipidemia		
VLDL	**VLDL + LDL**	**LDL**
Diabetes	Hypothyrodism	Anorexia Nervosa
Uraemia	Nephrotic syndrome	Fibrates
Beta-blockers	Diuretics	
Alcohol	Glucocorticoids	
Estrogens	Cyclosporin	
Retinoids		
Resins		

Table 32.2 Acquired forms of hyperlipidemia. LDL, low-density lipoprotein; VLDL, very low-density lipoprotein.

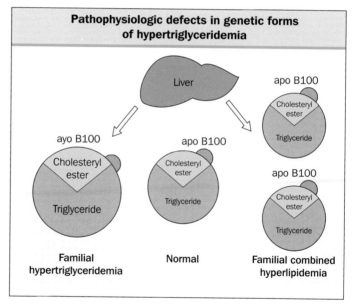

Pathophysiologic defects in genetic forms of hypertriglyceridemia

Figure 32.8 Pathophysiologic defects in genetic forms of hypertriglyceridemia. Familial hypertriglyceridemia is primarily due to overproduction of triglycerides, whereas familial combined hyperlipidemia is primarily characterized by increased production of apolipoprotein (apo) B. Both lead to an increased input of very-low-density lipoprotein (VLDL) into plasma, although the composition of the VLDL particles differs in the two disorders.

hepatic triglyceride synthesis. In familial combined hyperlipidemia the precise cause is unknown, although the disorder is characterized by overproduction of apo B (**Fig. 32.8**): apo B is overproduced in VLDL, leading primarily to hypertriglyceridemia; occasionally in LDL, leading primarily to hypercholesterolemia; and often in both VLDL and LDL, leading to combined elevations of cholesterol and triglyceride. Individuals with familial combined hyperlipidemia may be centrally obese or have mild defects in LPL. Affected family members with familial hypertriglyceridemia all have hypertriglyceridemia, whereas affected individuals from families with familial combined hyperlipidemia may have hypercholesterolemia alone, hypertriglyceridemia alone, or elevations of cholesterol and triglyceride level. The lipoprotein pattern in an individual with familial combined hyperlipidemia can frequently change.

Individuals with familial hypertriglyceridemia have increased risk of atherosclerosis at older ages. Conversely, familial combined hyperlipidemia markedly increases cardiovascular risk in middle age. Both disorders may be heterogeneous; further classification must await a better understanding of their pathogenetic mechanisms.

A common population trait is associated with LDL particles that are small and dense (phenotype B), which is distinct from phenotype A, where the particles are larger and more buoyant (**Fig. 32.9**). Small, dense LDL particles are found in association with central obesity and high-to-normal plasma triglyceride levels, increased levels of remnant lipoproteins, and reduced levels of a subclass of HDL. Individuals with this atherogenic-lipoprotein phenotype also are frequently insulin-resistant. The trait for small, dense LDL may interact with the other genes that raise levels of lipids and apo B, to cause familial combined hyperlipidemia.

Particle size distribution of low-density lipoproteins

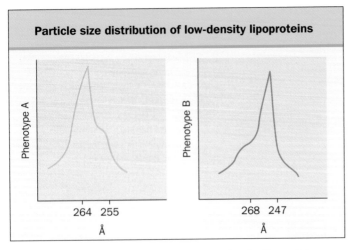

Figure 32.9 Particle size distribution of low-density lipoproteins (LDL). LDL particle size and density have been measured by nondenaturing gradient gel electrophoresis. Particle size distribution falls into two major patterns; large, buoyant LDL particles are characteristic of phenotype A, while smaller, more dense particles are characteristic of phenotype B.

The small, dense LDL phenotype also occurs in the insulin-resistant states, particularly type 2 diabetes.

Lipoprotein lipase defects

Multiple mutations have now been described that impair the action of LPL. These include mutations in which there is no functional protein, defects that result in the production of non-functional enzyme, and mutations that result in the formation of an enzyme that does not bind normally to heparin on endothelial cells (the normal site of action of LPL). Rarely, defective LPL function results from a mutation in the gene for apo CII, which is a necessary cofactor for LPL (see **Fig. 32.3**). These defects usually result in marked hypertriglyceridemia in early childhood because of the inability to hydrolyze triglycerides absorbed from ingested meals. Occasionally, affected individuals present for the first time in adult life.

Genetic defects in LPL or apo CII result in grossly impaired clearance of exogenous and endogenous triglycerides and the features of the chylomicronemia syndrome (see later).

Remnant removal disease

Genetic defects in remnant catabolism are uncommon and result from mutations in the apoE gene. Multiple mutations have been described, although arginine–cysteine substitution at residue 158 of the gene is the most common. Most of the mutations described result in a charge change that can be detected by the isoelectric focusing. Polymerize chain reaction (PCR) techniques have also been used to characterize defects in apoE.

Although most cases of remnant removal disease result from inheritance of an abnormal gene from both parents, autosomal dominant forms of apoE defects also have been described. Remnant removal disease occurs as a result of a combination of a defect in the apoE gene, leading to a defect in apo E structure, and an abnormality leading to VLDL overproduction (e.g. familial combined hyperlipidemia or occasionally diabetes mellitus; **Fig. 32.10**). The disorder is also known as broad-beta disease because of the electrophoretic appearance of the remnant accumulation, dysbetalipoproteinemia, and type III hyperlipoproteinemia. Very rarely, a total absence of apo E will result in remnant removal disease.

Low-density-lipoprotein cholesterol removal

Genetic defects of LDL-cholesterol removal are relatively common, occurring in approximately 1 in 500 of the population. Many mutations have been described at the LDL-receptor gene locus, leading to the clinical manifestations of familial hypercholesterolemia. These mutations, when inherited from one parent, result in approximately a 50% reduction in LDL-receptor activity, and is known as heterozygous familial hypercholesterolemia. Very occasionally (roughly 1 in 1,000,000), an individual inherits an abnormal gene for the LDL receptor from both parents, leading to homozygous familial hypercholesterolemia, in which there are essentially no functional LDL receptors. This situation is associated with very high levels of LDL and very accelerated atherosclerotic complications.

A genetic mutation of apoB, at residue 3500 of apoB, also results in defective removal of LDL via the LDL-receptor pathway. This genetic defect of apo B, termed familial defective apo B, occurs less commonly than the mutations in the LDL receptor leading to familial hypercholesterolemia. ApoB mutations result in an identical clinical picture to that seen in heterozygous familial hypercholesterolemia. In both these conditions, LDL

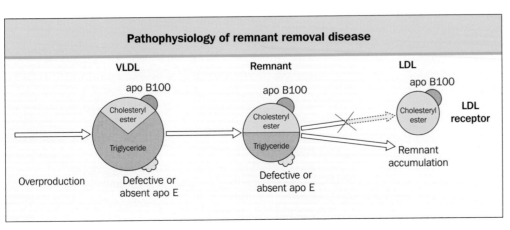

Figure 32.10 Pathophysiology of remnant removal disease. For hyperlipidemia to occur, there must be overproduction of very-low-density lipoprotein (VLDL), and the apolipoprotein (apo) E structure must be structurally defective or absent. LDL, low-density lipoprotein.

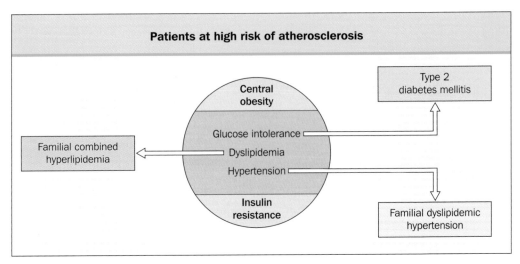

Figure 32.11 Patients at high risk of atherosclerosis. The figure illustrates glucose intolerance, dyslipidemia, and hypertension relationships in individuals at high risk of atherosclerosis. A feature common to all of these conditions is the presence of central obesity and insulin resistance.

particles tend to be large and buoyant. Cardiovascular disease risk is increased in both these disorders.

Hyper-apolipoprotein B

Several genetic disorders can lead to increased levels of plasma apo B (apo B100), which can now be measured by immunochemical techniques. Such disorders include familial hypercholesterolemia, familial defective apo B, and familial combined hyperlipidemia.

Small, dense LDL particles are often found, together with high-to-normal triglyceride levels, modest increases in remnant lipoproteins, decreased levels of HDL, and elevated levels of apo B. This 'dyslipidemic' pattern is quite common and occurs in association with central obesity and often with hypertension and insulin-resistance-type diabetes to yield a very atherogenic risk profile (**Fig. 32.11**). Apo B levels can also be increased as a result of excessive levels of Lp(a), a lipoprotein that consists of apo (a) in disulfide linkage with LDL (**Fig. 32.12**). The source, fate, and precise function of Lp(a) are not yet known, although the primary determinant of Lp(a) levels appears to be genetic. Apo (a) has considerable structural homology with plasminogen. Lp(a) may therefore play a physiologic role in modulating fibrinolysis; high levels are associated with an increased risk of atherosclerosis.

Genetic and acquired forms of hyperlipidemia

Occasionally, genetic and acquired forms of hyperlipidemia coexist in the same patient, thereby resulting in hyperlipidemia of a greater degree than would result from each alone. This is particularly important with respect to the several common genetic and acquired conditions that can affect triglyceride secretion and removal from plasma. The coexistence of genetic and acquired disorders at these sites can saturate LPL-mediated plasma triglyceride removal. The removal of further chylomicrons that enter plasma is thereby impaired, resulting in extremely elevated triglyceride levels with unique consequences (see below).

CLINICAL MANIFESTATIONS OF HYPERLIPIDEMIA

There are three main clinical manifestations of hyperlipidemia: clinical consequences of atherosclerosis; cutaneous manifestations of hyperlipidemia (xanthomata); and the chylomicronemia syndrome that can occur when chylomicrons accumulate chronically.

Increased risk of cardiovascular disease

There is consensus that elevated plasma LDL levels and reduced HDL levels are associated with an increased atherosclerosis risk. The role of hypertriglyceridemia as a cardiovascular risk factor is more complex. Hypertriglyceridemia may be a marker for other lipoprotein abnormalities – such as increased levels of LDL, the presence of an LDL subclass phenotype B, low levels of HDL, or remnant accumulation – that are part of the dyslipidemic

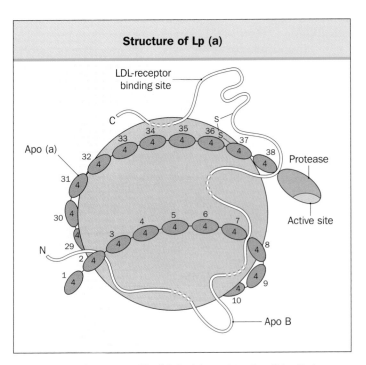

Figure 32.12 Structure of Lp (a). Lp (a) consists of particles that resemble low-density lipoprotein (LDL) in structure and composition but have an additional apolipoprotein, apo (a), attached to apo B by a disulfide bond.

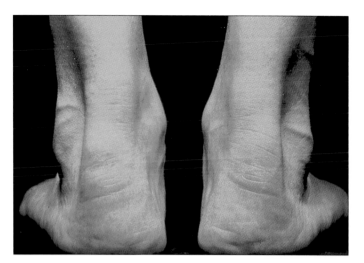

Figure 32.13 Achilles tendon xanthomata.

Oxidized low-density lipoprotein and atherogenesis

Cytotoxicity

Stimulation of monocyte adhesion to endothelium

Stimulation of monocyte chemotaxis

Stimulation of colony-stimulating factor expression

Stimulation of matrix expression

Foam cell formation

Modulation of growth factor and cytokine expression

Inhibition of endothelial-derived-relaxation-factor-mediated vasodilatation

Stimulation of tissue-factor expression

Stimulation of metalloproteinase expression

Table 32.3 Oxidized low-density lipoprotein (LDL) and atherogenesis. The table lists the biologic effects of oxidized low-density lipoprotein that may affect atherogenesis.

pattern associated with the familial combined hyperlipidemia, type 2 diabetes mellitus, and the insulin resistance syndrome. In these situations, hypertriglyceridemia is a predictor of increased premature cardiovascular risk. However, other forms of hypertriglyceridemia may not be associated with increased cardiovascular risk.

The precise mechanisms whereby increased levels of LDL result in increased atherosclerosis risk is unclear. Both very high levels of large, buoyant LDL, such as occurs in familial hypercholesterolemia and familial defective apo B, and the presence of more moderate levels of small, dense LDL, are associated with an increased risk of cardiovascular disease. Recent studies have suggested that LDL needs to be modified, before it becomes atherogenic. Modifications of LDL that may increase their atherogenicity include oxidation and aggregation. Oxidized LDL has many biologic properties that may cause it to become atherogenic (**Table 32.3**). The atherogenicity of small, dense LDL may be due to its being more able to enter the arterial intima, be retained by matrix molecules, and undergo oxidation more readily than bigger, more buoyant LDL. The antiatherogenic properties of HDL are probably related to its role in reverse cholesterol transport.

Xanthomata and other external manifestations

Xanthomata, when present, give important clinical clues to the nature of the underlying pathophysiologic defect. Thus, tendon xanthomata typically occur in familial hypercholesterolemia and in familial defective apo B. Their presence in the Achilles tendons (**Fig. 32.13**) or the extensor tendons of the hand (**Fig. 32.14**) is pathognomonic of genetic defects in interactions of LDL with its receptor. Occasionally, xanthomata are seen on the patellar tendon. Since xanthomata are often subtle, careful examination of these sites is required for their detection.

Eruptive xanthomata (**Fig. 32.15**) are indicative of chronic and longstanding chylomicronemia. They occur most frequently on the buttocks and the extensor surfaces of the upper limb,

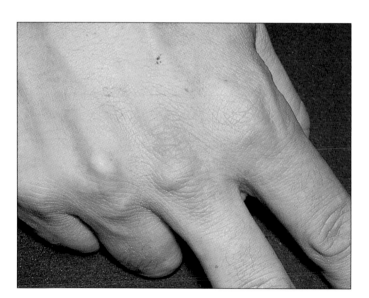

Figure 32.14 Xanthomata on the extensor tendons of the hands.

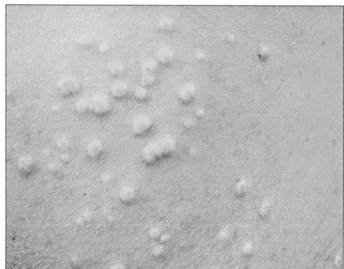

Figure 32.15 Eruptive xanthomata on the buttocks. Note the erythematous base around the raised xanthomata.

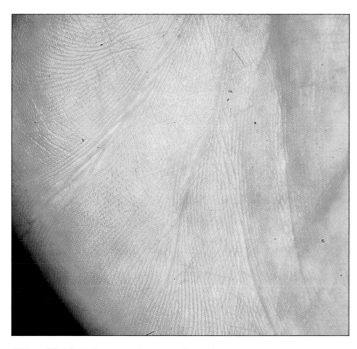

Figure 32.16 Palmar or planar xanthomata

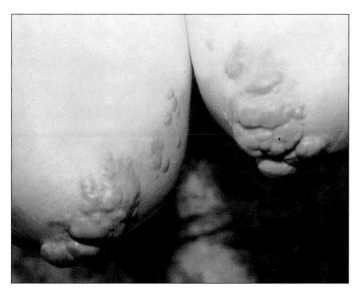

Figure 32.17 Tuberoeruptive xanthomata of the elbow. The pink color of these xanthomata is characteristically seen in remnant removal disease.

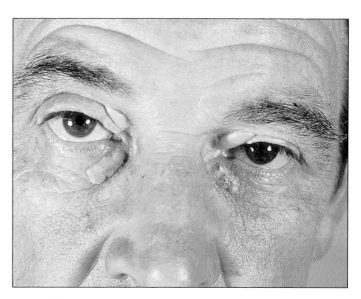

Figure 32.18 Xanthelasma.

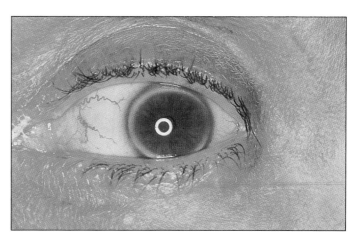

Figure 32.19 Extensive corneal arcus. Early corneal arcus is characterized by deposition of cholesterol at the superior and inferior aspects of the cornea. With time, the arcus may become totally circumferential, as illustrated.

only rarely being found on the face, soles, and palms. Palmar or planar xanthomata (**Fig. 32.16**) are pathognomonic for remnant removal disease, which can also manifest with tuberoeruptive xanthomata (**Fig. 32.17**). Palmar xanthomata may be difficult to see and should be carefully sought using good lighting.

Several other external manifestations of hyperlipidemia are more nonspecific but should, nonetheless, alert the clinician to the possibility that disorders of lipoprotein metabolism may be present. These include the presence of xanthelasma and corneal arcus. Xanthelasma (**Fig. 32.18**) can occur in familial hyper-cholesterolemia, diabetes, and chronic obstructive liver disease,

and may even signify more subtle abnormalities of plasma lipoproteins, such as those seen with the apo E2 variant or hyper-apo B. Early corneal arcus is seen superiorly and inferiorly in the eyes and later becomes totally circumferential (**Fig. 32.19**). Arcus occurs fairly frequently in the elderly (arcus senilis). Its presence before the age of 50 warrants evaluation of plasma lipids and lipoproteins.

Chylomicronemia syndrome

A constellation of signs and symptoms, the chylomicronemia syndrome, occurs in association with long-standing chylomicronemia (**Table 32.4**). The most important consequence is pancreatitis, which is often acute and recurrent. Pancreatitis is believed to be due to the release of free fatty acids and lysolecithin from chylomicrons in the capillaries of the pancreas by pancreatic lipase (**Fig. 32.20**). More chronic abdominal pain can result from expansion of the liver capsule by hepatic fatty infiltration, which often accompanies the chylomicronemia.

Manifestations of the chylomicronemia syndrome

Abdominal pain/acute pancreatis

Eruptive xanthomata

Reversible memory loss/mental confusion

Peripheral neuropathy

Lipemia retinalis

Table 32.4 Manifestations of the chylomicronemia syndrome.

Proposed mechanism of pancreatitis in chylomicronemia

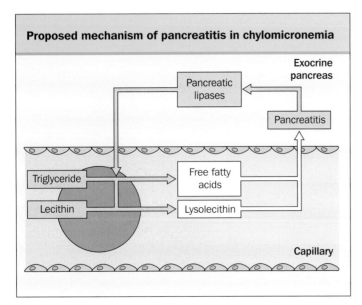

Figure 32.20 Proposed mechanism of pancreatitis in chylomicronemia. Pancreatic lipase hydrolyzes chylomicron triglycerides and phospholipids (lecithin) to free fatty acids and lysolecithin, respectively. Both the latter can cause chemical pancreatitis. Pancreatitis leads to the release of additional lipase, which leads to more free fatty acids and lysolecithin, and so the cycle continues.

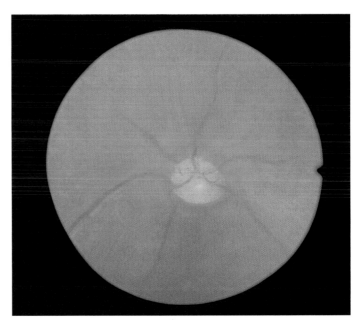

Figure 32.21 Lipemia retinalis seen in association with marked hypertriglyceridemia. Note the pale color of the retinal vessels (due to circulating chylomicrons) against the pink background of the retina.

Genetic and acquired forms of hypertriglyceridemia	
Genetic	Acquired
Familial hypertriglyceridemia	**Various disorders**
Familial combined hypertriglyceridemia	Diabetes mellitus
	Hypothyroidism
	Uremia
	Obesity (central)
	Drugs
	Alcohol
	Estrogens
	Glucocorticoids
	Beta-blockers
	Diuretics

Table 32.5 Genetic and acquired forms of hypertriglyceridemia.
These can lead to marked hypertriglyceridemia when present concurrently.

Eruptive xanthomata are frequently present, and the retinal vessels occasionally demonstrate lipemia retinalis (**Fig. 32.21**). A reversible loss of memory, particularly for recent events, and peripheral neuropathy, which sometimes mimics the carpal tunnel syndrome, also occur. These clinical manifestations can be prevented or reversed by keeping the triglyceride level below approximately 15mmol/L. Eruptive xanthomata resolve after 6–12 weeks of lower triglyceride levels. Acute pancreatitis can be fatal and is often recurrent until low triglyceride levels are maintained permanently.

The chylomicronemia syndrome occasionally occurs when LPL is inactive as a result of a genetic defect in the enzyme or its cofactor, apo CII. Much more commonly, it is due to saturation of the capacity of LPL to remove triglyceride, a result of the coexistence of a genetic form of hypertriglyceridemia with an acquired disorder of plasma triglyceride metabolism. The latter may be caused by one or more diseases, or by drugs (**Table 32.5**).

ASSESSMENT OF HYPERLIPIDEMIC PATIENTS

Hyperlipidemia may present to the clinician in several ways. Unfortunately, the first manifestation is often a cardiovascular event, such as myocardial infarction. Lipids and lipoproteins should be evaluated within 24 hours of the onset of chest pain. After that, they should not be evaluated for about 3 months following a major illness such as a myocardial infarction or surgery, since they can be markedly altered by these clinical events. As routine screening for hyperlipidemia becomes more commonplace, asymptomatic cases are being detected

Assessment of hyperlipidemic patients
Confirm hyperlipidemia
Exclude secondary causes
Evaluate family history for genetic causes
Decide whether to treat
Decide how to treat
• Diet alone
• Diet and drugs

Table 32.6 Assessment of hyperlipidemic patients.

Recent secondary prevention lipid-lowering trials		
Acronym	**Intervention**	**Outcome**
POSCH	Surgical	↓ nonfatal MI and CV mortality
4S	Simvastatin	↓ CV events, ↓ CV mortality
CARE	Pravastatin	↓ CV events, ↓ CV mortality
LIPID	Pravastatin	↓ CV events, ↓ CV mortality
VA-HIT	Gemfibrozil	↓ nonfatal MI and CV mortality
BIP	Bezafibrate	No significant benefit

Table 32.7 Recent secondary prevention lipid-lowering trials. CV, cardiovascular; MI, myocardial infarction.

more frequently. It is particularly important to screen young and middle-aged adult relatives of individuals who have presented with manifestations of premature cardiovascular disease. Occasionally, individuals present with cutaneous manifestations or with signs and symptoms of the chylomicronemia syndrome.

Once hyperlipidemia has been discovered, it should be confirmed (**Table 32.6**), and lipoproteins should be evaluated by using appropriate methods (see below). Acquired forms of hyperlipidemia need to be excluded, and genetic forms should be sought by careful evaluation of the family history. Special emphasis should be placed on the mother's side of the family, since atherosclerotic complications manifest later in females. Information concerning the mother's male siblings and parents may therefore prove valuable in arriving at a genetic diagnosis.

The decision will then need to be made as to whether to treat the condition. The objective of treatment is prevention of atherosclerosis or of features of the chylomicronemia syndrome. With respect to atherosclerosis, guidelines for the detection, evaluation, and treatment of hyperlipidemia have been provided by major organizations, such as the Adult Treatment Panel of the National Cholesterol Education Program in the USA, and the European Atherosclerosis Society in Western Europe. These guidelines are updated every few years. Therapeutic decisions in current guidelines are based primarily on LDL cholesterol levels, since reduction of LDL cholesterol has been shown to reduce risk of clinical events. Despite some differences in approach, the US and European guidelines essentially target the same patients for therapy. Other risk factors (see **Fig. 32.1**) should be taken into account when considering whether, and how aggressively, to treat. As a result of clinical trials that have shown that the rate of recurrent clinical events can be markedly reduced by lipid-lowering drugs, particularly statins, in individuals with prior evidence of cardiovascular disease, there is widespread consensus that aggressive lipid lowering is appropriate for secondary prevention (**Table 32.7**) Because individuals with type 2 diabetes who have not had a prior myocardial infarction have the same risk of cardiovascular disease morbidity and mortality as non-diabetic individuals with established cardiovascular disease, patients with type 2 diabetes should be treated as aggressively as for secondary prevention. A LDL goal of less than 2.6mmol/L, which is agreed upon by most authorities, usually requires the use of statins. The approach

to primary prevention, i.e. treatment of hyperlipidemic or dyslipidemic individuals prior to the onset of clinical disease, is more controversial. Although recent clinical trials also have shown the benefit of statins, primary prevention is less cost-effective and drug therapy should be reserved for those at the highest risk of developing clinical events. Diet is advocated initially; however, if compliance with the lipid-lowering diet fails to yield the desired goals, drug therapy may also need to be initiated. Several approaches have been recommended to target those at highest risk. The presence of multiple cardiovascular risk factors and a strongly positive family history of premature cardiovascular disease, taken in conjunction with the LDL-cholesterol level, are factors that favor the use of drugs for primary prevention. Treatment of chylomicronemia is geared towards prevention of the features of the chylomicronemia syndrome and is discussed below.

LABORATORY TESTS

A detailed description of the various laboratory tests that are available is beyond the scope of this chapter. Generally, however, therapeutic decisions aimed at atherosclerosis prevention are based on determination of LDL and HDL levels. Estimation of LDL levels using a formula (**Fig. 32.22**) is adequate when triglyceride levels are below about 5mmol/L. When they are higher, however, ultracentrifugation of plasma is necessary to accurately determine LDL levels. There is no place in routine practice for lipoprotein electrophoresis.

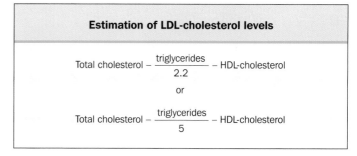

Estimation of LDL-cholesterol levels

$$\text{Total cholesterol} - \frac{\text{triglycerides}}{2.2} - \text{HDL-cholesterol}$$

or

$$\text{Total cholesterol} - \frac{\text{triglycerides}}{5} - \text{HDL-cholesterol}$$

Figure 32.22. Estimation of low-density-lipoprotein (LDL)-cholesterol levels. The estimation requires the use of a plasma sample taken from a fasted patient. It is valid for triglyceride levels of less than 5mmol/L.

Diagnosis of remnant removal disease requires ultracentrifugation for assessment to determine the apo E phenotype or DNA studies for genotype. As measurements of apolipoproteins become better standardized, their use will no doubt become widespread. Methods to measure apo B will soon be widely available and may be useful diagnostic tools, particularly in detecting at-risk individuals with increased levels of small, dense LDL and an atherogenic lipoprotein phenotype. Measurement of apo B, however, will not enable distinction of the several causes of elevation of this apolipoprotein. Measurement of Lp(a) also can be a useful addendum in assessing cardiovascular risk. At present, a high level of Lp(a) might best be considered as an additional risk factor when considering therapy of the hyperlipidemia. At present, assessment of the size of the LDL particle remains a research tool. The value of measures such as homocysteine and various inflammatory markers in deciding who to treat awaits further evaluation.

A simple test that can be used to diagnose marked hypertriglyceridemia is inspection of the plasma. A milky or creamy appearance is indicative of extreme elevations of triglyceride levels (**Fig. 32.23**).

TREATMENT

Dietary treatment

A diet low in saturated fat and cholesterol (both of which suppress LDL-receptor activity) will reduce elevated cholesterol levels substantially in most cases. Reductions of 5–15% can be achieved by long-term compliance with this type of diet, although the response will, to some extent, be determined by

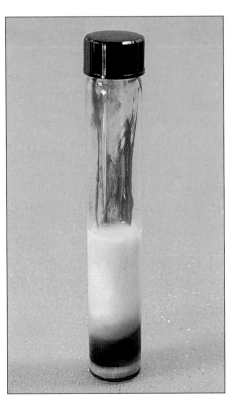

Figure 32.23 Milky appearance of plasma from a patient with marked hypertriglyceridemia.

patients' baseline diet and their degree of compliance. Compliance can be markedly enhanced if patients are offered counseling by a qualified dietitian or nutritionist, who should try to make the meal plan as appetizing as possible and tailor it to the taste of individual patients. Lack of adequate compliance is the most common cause of failure of diet therapy. The American Heart Association has recommended two diets for the treatment of hypercholesterolemia. Treatment should commence with a Step I diet, in which less than 10% of calories are derived from saturated fat and cholesterol consumption is less than 300 mg/day. If the desired response is not obtained after an adequate period of good compliance, the Step II diet should be applied, whereby saturated fats should provide less than 7% of calories, and cholesterol consumption should be less than 200mg/day. Similar diets have been recommended by many other organizations. Overall, however, the diets should be nutritionally sound and appetizing, and should contain abundant fruits, vegetables, grains, pasta, and legumes. Attention should also be given to weight control since obesity, particularly central obesity, is associated with many cardiovascular risk factors. Weight control often requires increased emphasis on restriction of dietary fat and on physical activity.

Drug therapy

Drug therapy may need to be initiated when target lipid levels are not achieved with diet alone. Most patients with a genetic form of hyperlipidemia or who have a history of clinical cardiovascular disease will need to take drugs in addition to following a diet. The effects of diet and drugs are independent and additive; consumption of an appropriate diet can reduce the dose of drug required. **Table 32.8** shows the available lipid-lowering drugs and their indications, dosages, and side effects. An understanding of their mechanisms of action provides important insights into their use.

As discussed earlier, LDL-cholesterol levels are a result of the relative rates of input and removal of this class of lipoprotein from plasma. Removal of LDL occurs primarily via LDL receptors in the liver. Hepatocytes derive their cholesterol from exogenous sources via the LDL receptor and by endogenous synthesis from HMG CoA. A major use of cholesterol by the liver is for the synthesis of bile acids, which undergo enterohepatic circulation after secretion into the intestinal tract (**Fig. 32.24**, left panel). HMG CoA reductase inhibitors (statins) inhibit endogenous cholesterol synthesis by blocking the rate-limiting step in cholesterol synthesis. This results in a compensatory increase in hepatic LDL-receptors (**Fig. 32.24**, center left panel) to permit adequate bile acid secretion. Bile-acid-binding resins can interrupt the enterohepatic circulation of bile acids, leading to a compensatory increase in both LDL receptors and cholesterol synthesis (**Fig. 32.24**, center right panel). Combined use of statins and bile acid resins leads to a marked increase in LDL-receptor activity (**Fig. 32.24**, right panel).

Niacin (nicotinic acid) has a different mechanism of action. Its major effects are to reduce the production of the apo-B-containing lipoproteins and to inhibit the mobilization of free fatty acids from adipose tissue (**Fig. 32.25**). Use of niacin leads to a reduction in VLDL and LDL levels and is also associated with an increase in HDL-cholesterol levels.

Major lipid-lowering drugs

Group	Drug	Usual daily dose	Major effect	Other effects on lipoproteins	Side effects	Comments
Bile-acid binding resins	Cholestyramine Colestipol	8–32g 10–40g	↓ LDL	slightly ↑ HDL, ↑ TG	Constipation, interferes with absorption of drugs	Hypertriglyceridemia is a relative contraindication; take other drugs 1 hour before or 4 hours after resin
Nicotinic acid (niacin)	Nicotinic acid Niaspan	1.5–6g 750mg-2g	↓ TG, ↓ LDL, ↑ HDL	↓ apo B	Flushing, itching, ↑ insulin resistance, liver function abnormalities	Need to increase dose slowly, take with food, avoid hot drinks
HMG CoA reductase inhibitors	Lovastatin Pravastatin Simvastatin Atorvastatin Fluvastatin	20–80mg 10–40mg 5–80mg 10–80mg 20–80mg	↓ LDL	Slightly ↓ TG, slightly ↑ HDL	Occasional liver function test abnormalities, occasional myopathy especially when used in combination with cyclosporin, fibrates	
Fibric acid derivatives	Gemfibrozil Fenofibrate Bezafibrate Clofibrate	600mg twice per day 60–200mg per day 200mg three times per day 1g twice per day	↑ TG, ↑ HDL	Slightly ↓ LDL, sometimes ↑ LDL	Gallstones, gastrointestinal symptoms, myopathy	

Table 32.8 Major lipid-lowering drugs. apo, apolipoprotein; HDL, high-density lipoprotein; LDL, low-density lipoprotein; TG, triglycerides.

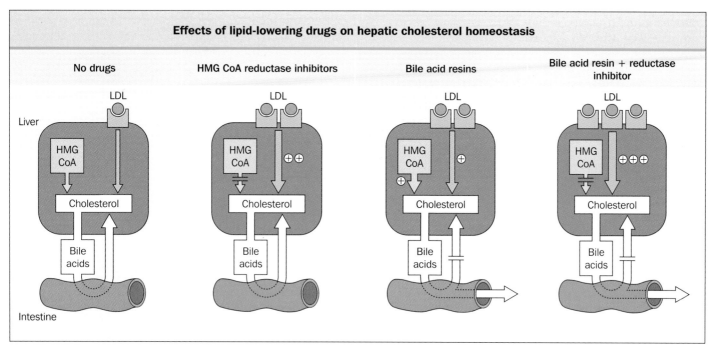

Figure 32.24 Effects of lipid-lowering drugs on hepatic cholesterol homeostasis. (Left panel) The hepatocyte derives cholesterol for bile acid synthesis via the low-density lipoprotein (LDL) receptor and by endogenous synthesis from HMGCoA. Bile acids enter the intestinal tract from where they are reabsorbed for reuse. (Center left panel) HMG CoA reductase inhibitors inhibit cholesterol synthesis and are associated with an increase in hepatic LDL receptors. (Center right panel) Interruption of the enterohepatic circulation by bile-acid-binding resins leads to an increase in LDL receptor activity and cholesterol synthesis. (Right panel) The combined use of a bile acid resin and HMG CoA reductase inhibitor leads to a marked increase in LDL-receptor levels by inhibiting the increase in cholesterol synthesis that occurs when resins are used alone.

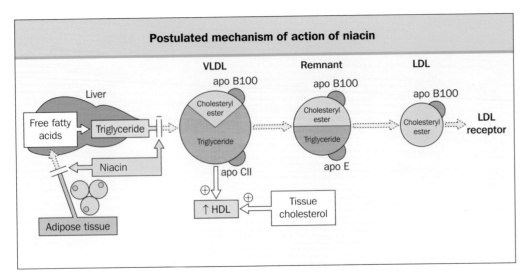

Postulated mechanism of action of niacin

Figure 32.25 Postulated mechanism of action of niacin. The primary effect of niacin is to reduce the production of the apolipoprotein (apo) B lipoproteins. HDL, high-density lipoprotein; LDL, low-density lipoprotein; VLDL, very-low-density lipoprotein.

The fibric acid derivatives (fibrates) primarily affect VLDL metabolism, whereby VLDL input is reduced and removal is enhanced. Their major use, therefore, is for the treatment of hypertriglyceridemia, in which they also increase HDL levels.

Other cardiovascular risk factors

Atherosclerosis is a multifactorial disease for which hyperlipidemia is but one of several important risk factors. Other risk factors should therefore also be evaluated and treated in their own right. In particular, cigarette smoking should be discouraged in the strongest possible terms. Smoking cessation is also associated with an increase in HDL-cholesterol levels. Hypertension should be treated when indicated, although it should be noted that use of diuretics and beta-adrenergic blocking agents may aggravate hyperlipidemia. Lipid-neutral antihypertensive agents may therefore be more appropriate.

Chylomicronemia syndrome

Management of the chylomicronemia syndrome requires special consideration. Since marked hypertriglyceridemia usually results from a combination of genetic and acquired causes of hypertriglyceridemia, identification and therapy of treatable secondary causes are essential. Furthermore, administration of triglyceride-raising drugs should be discontinued where possible and a trial of alcohol restriction should be attempted. If triglyceride levels remain elevated, fibric acid derivatives should be used to lower them. Symptoms of the chylomicronemia syndrome and risk of recurrence of pancreatitis can be prevented by maintaining triglyceride levels below 20mmol/L and 10mmol/L, respectively.

FURTHER READING

Breslow JL. Familial disorders of high-density lipoprotein metabolism. In: Scriver CR, Beaudet AL, Sly WS, Valle D, eds. Metabolic basis of inherited diseases, 6th edn. New York: McGraw-Hill, 1989:1251-66.

Brunzell JD. The hyperlipoproteinemias. In: Wyngaarden JD, Smith LH, Bennett JC, eds. Cecil textbook of medicine, 19th edn. Philadelphia: WB Saunders, 1992: 1082-90.

Chait A. Hyperlipidemia. In: Rakel RE, ed. Conn's current therapy. Philadelphia: WB Saunders; 1992:504-9.

Chait A, Brunzell JD. Chylomicronemia syndrome. Adv Int Med. 1991; 37:249-73.

Goldstein JL, Brown MS. Familial hypercholesterolemia. In: Scriver CR, Beaudet AL, Sly WS, Valle D, eds. Metabolic basis of inherited diseases, 6th edn. New York: McGraw-Hill, 1989:1215-60.

LaRosa JC. Disorders of lipid metabolism. Endocrinol Metab Clin N Am. 1991;19:211-467.

Study Group, European Atherosclerosis Society. The recognition and management of hyperlipidaemia in adults: A policy statement of the European Atherosclerosis Society. Eur Heart J. 1988;9:571-600.

The Expert Panel. Report of the National Cholesterol Education Program Expert Panel on detection, evaluation, and treatment of high blood cholesterol in adults. Arch Int Med. 1988; 18:36-69.

Thompson GR. A handbook of hyperlipidaemia. London: Current Science; 1989.

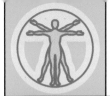

Chapter 33 Cardiovascular Hormones

Miriam T Rademaker and Eric A Espiner

INTRODUCTION

Blood pressure and body fluid volume regulation, pivotal in sustaining organ perfusion and function, are maintained in health by the integrated actions of many systems, including those of a complex series of interlocking neurohumoral (endocrine) responses. Traditionally the endocrine regulation of body fluid volume has focused on the renal–adrenal axis (renin–angiotensin–aldosterone system), nonosmotic release of vasopressin from the neurohypophysis, and changes in local (and possibly circulatory) levels of norepinephrine under the influence of the sympathetic nervous system. However, discoveries over the past 20 years have made it clear that both cardiac and vascular tissues have the ability to synthesize hormones and local peptides and regulatory hormones with important local and humoral actions affecting pressure and body fluid volume and distribution. While a large number of peptides with potent hemodynamic effects have been identified within vascular tissues, this chapter is confined to a description of the natriuretic peptide family (atrial natriuretic peptide, ANP; brain natriuretic peptide, BNP; and C-type natriuretic peptide, CNP), endothelins, and adrenomedullin. In contrast to ANP and BNP, which have clearly defined physiologic roles as circulating hormones, the systemic contribution of CNP, the endothelins, and adrenomedullin is controversial.

NATRIURETIC PEPTIDES

The natriuretic peptide family consists of three peptides – atrial, brain, and C-type natriuretic peptide – the actions of which are largely directed towards the regulation of blood pressure and fluid homeostasis. Whereas both ANP and BNP are true circulating hormones secreted predominantly by the atria and ventricles of the heart respectively, CNP is largely a product of the vascular endothelium and appears to act locally within the vessel wall and other organ systems including the brain and kidney.

Natriuretic peptide synthesis, structure, and regulation

In humans, the two genes encoding ANP and BNP are arranged in tandem on the short arm of chromosome 1. Transcription yields similar polypeptide precursors, which are further processed to the mature (circulating) forms (**Fig. 33.1**).

ANP is synthesized in numerous tissues but most abundantly in the atria of the normal adult heart, where it is stored in specific granules within the muscle cells (myocytes) as a 126 amino acid polypeptide (pro-ANP). Subsequent cleavage during release into the circulation yields the biologically active C-terminal peptide – ANP_{99-126} (ANP-28; **Fig. 33.2**) and the N-terminal fragment ANP_{1-98}. While the major determinant of ANP secretion is atrial stretch, many other factors contribute to its regulation

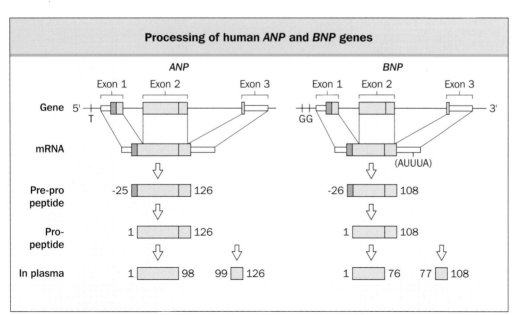

Figure 33.1 Processing of human ANP and BNP genes. The figure shows the structure of human ANP and BNP genes (located on chromosome 1 in region p36) and subsequent steps through to the mature processed products found in plasma. Blue sections are those that ultimately constitute the mature active peptides. Pink areas are those from which the amino terminal fragments are derived. Red sections represent the region coding for the signal peptide and the signal peptide itself. T indicates the location of the TATAAA sequence upstream from the transcription initiation site of ANP, while GG is the location of the two GATAAA sequences (potential TATAAA sequences) on the BNP gene.

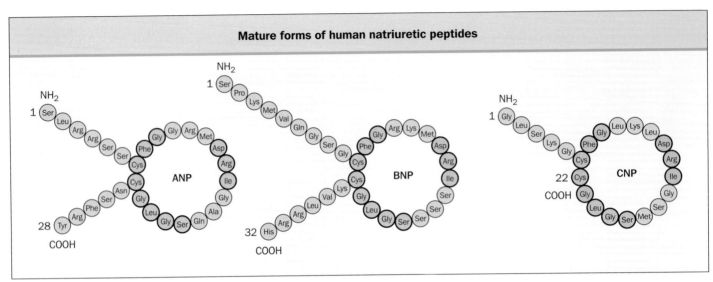

Figure 33.2 Mature forms of human natriuretic peptides. ANP, atrial natriuretic peptide; BNP, brain natriuretic peptide; CNP, C-type natriuretic peptide. Blue circles are amino acids common to the three human hormones. The mature forms shown are ANP, BNP-32, CNP-22.

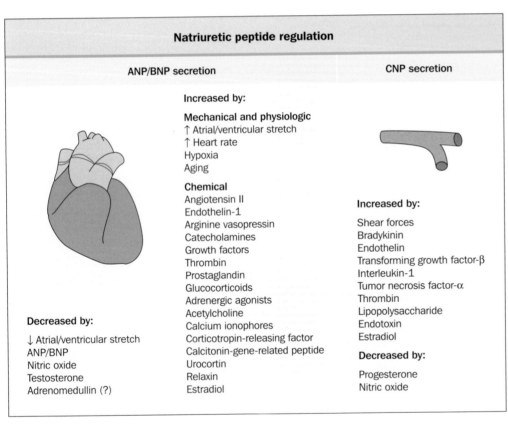

Figure 33.3 Natriuretic peptide regulation. The figure illustrates factors regulating the secretion of atrial and brain natriuretic peptide (ANP and BNP) from the heart and C-type natriuretic peptide (CNP) from the vasculature.

(Fig. 33.3). In health, approximately 95% of the total ANP secreted arises from the cardiac atria, whereas in pathologic states such as congestive heart failure and ventricular hypertrophy the ventricle becomes an important source of circulating ANP. BNP is primarily a ventricular hormone, which is synthesized and secreted directly from the myocytes in response to increased ventricular pressure and work. Small amounts are also co-stored and secreted from atrial granules with ANP. In humans, both the bioactive 32 amino acid form BNP_{77-108} (or BNP-32; Fig. 33.2) and the N-terminal BNP_{1-76} form circulate in plasma, together with a higher molecular weight component, probably the prohormone (BNP_{1-108}). Although BNP secretion appears to be regulated in a similar fashion to that of ANP, proportionately greater increases in BNP concentrations are reported after acute myocardial infarction, and in patients with congestive heart failure and hypertrophic cardiomyopathy. However, BNP is less responsive

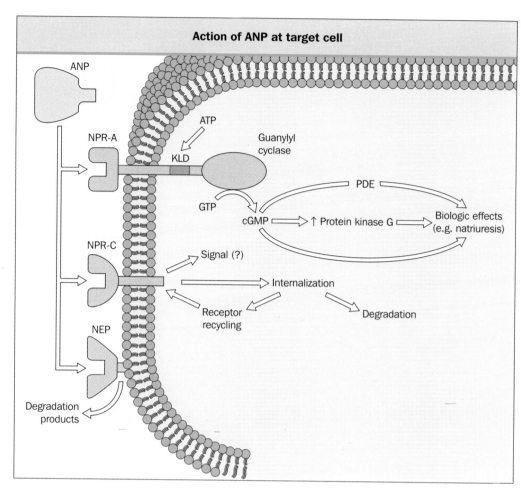

Action of ANP at target cell

ANP

NPR-A

ATP

KLD

Guanylyl cyclase

GTP

cGMP ⟹ ↑ Protein kinase G ⟹ Biologic effects (e.g. natriuresis)

PDE

NPR-C

Signal (?)

Internalization

Receptor recycling

Degradation

NEP

Degradation products

Figure 33.4 Action of atrial natriuretic peptide (ANP) at target cell. ANP (and brain natriuretic peptide, BNP) bind to natriuretic peptide receptor A (NPR-A) and, in an ATP-dependent fashion that requires the kinase-like domain (KLD), stimulate the intrinsic guanylyl cyclase activity of the receptor. Cyclic guanosine monophosphate (cGMP) exerts its biologic effects indirectly through cGMP-dependent protein kinase G or one or more phosphodiesterases (PDE). The natriuretic peptide receptor B (NPR-B; not shown) is activated in a similar fashion by C-type natriuretic peptide. ANP (and BNP) also bind to the NPR-C, after which they are internalized and degraded. The NPR-C may also have independent signaling functions. ANP (and BNP) are also degraded by extracellular neutral endopeptidase EC 24.11 (NEP). GTP, guanosine triphosphate. (Modified with permission from Levin ER, Gardner DG, Samson WK. Mechanisms of disease: natriuretic peptides. N Engl J Med. 1998;339: 321–8 © 1998 Massachusetts Medical Society.)

than ANP to acute changes in intracardiac pressure such as occur during exercise and acute volume loading – maneuvers that distend the atria but may not affect intraventricular pressure to the same degree.

Distinct from the ANP and BNP genes, the gene encoding CNP is located on chromosome 2 in humans and is expressed predominantly in the central nervous system and within vascular endothelial and smooth muscle tissues. Two mature forms of CNP have been isolated – CNP_{51-103} (CNP-53) and CNP_{82-103} (CNP-22; **Fig. 33.2**) – both of which have been detected in central nervous tissue and in plasma. CNP-53 is the main form in the vascular endothelium. The vascular CNP system appears to be regulated by a variety of factors affecting vascular tone and cell growth (**Fig. 33.3**). Although CNP is not considered to be primarily a product of cardiac secretion, concentrations in ventricular myocardium are reported to increase some threefold in severe cardiac failure – suggesting a local (paracrine) action within the heart.

Receptors and metabolism

To date, three different natriuretic peptide receptors (NPR) have been identified. Two of these, NPR-A and NPR-B, are coupled to particulate guanylate cyclase and appear to mediate most of the actions of the natriuretic peptides through the production of the second messenger, cyclic guanosine monophosphate (cGMP; **Fig. 33.4**). The NPR-A receptor selectively binds

both ANP and BNP (with preference for ANP), while the NPR-B is highly specific for CNP. The third (and most prevalent) receptor subtype, NPR-C, is not coupled to guanylate cyclase and binds all three natriuretic peptides. The NPR-C is thought to act as a 'clearance' receptor by internalizing the peptides for lysosomal degradation (**Fig. 33.4**). In addition, some reports suggest that the receptor may be linked to the phosphoinositol system, inhibit adenyl cyclase, and transduce some of the antimitogenic effects of the natriuretic peptides. The second metabolic pathway of the natriuretic peptides is cleavage by membrane-bound neutral endopeptidase (NEP) 24.11 (**Fig. 33.4**), an enzyme with a broad substrate specificity and wide tissue distribution (particularly concentrated in the proximal tubule of the kidney and in the lung). In humans, BNP is much more resistant to hydrolysis by NEP than either ANP or CNP. Together with its lower affinity for the NPR-C in humans, these findings may explain in part the prolonged plasma half-life of BNP (approximately 22min) compared to ANP or CNP (both 2–4min).

Biologic actions

The natriuretic peptides exhibit a wide spectrum of biologic effects at virtually all the multiple sites affecting sodium and blood pressure homeostasis (**Fig. 33.5**). Many of these actions, particularly those within the kidney, are influenced by a variety of physiologic variables, including resting arterial pressure,

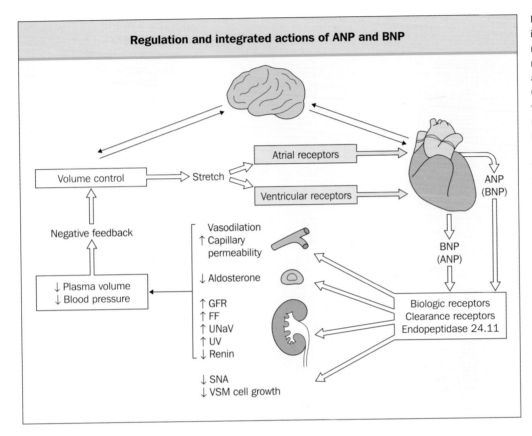

Regulation and integrated actions of ANP and BNP

Figure 33.5 Regulation and integrated actions of atrial natriuretic peptide (ANP) and brain natriuretic peptide (BNP). Paracrine actions of the natriuretic peptides (also C-type natriuretic peptide, CNP) on vessel wall, kidney, etc. are omitted for reasons of clarity. Arrows to and from the brain refer to the central actions of the natriuretic peptides and the effects of the peptides synthesized within neural tissues. FF, filtration fraction; GFR, glomerular filtration rate; SNA, sympathetic nervous activity; UV, urine volume; UNaV, urine sodium excretion; VSM, vascular smooth muscle. (Modified with permission from Rademaker MT, Espiner EA. The endocrine heart. In: Becker K, ed. Principles and practice of endocrinology and metabolism, 3rd edn. Baltimore, MD:Lippincott, Williams & Wilkins; 2001.)

sodium status, and the degree of neurohormonal activation. All the tissue effects of the natriuretic peptides appear to oppose those of angiotensin II, excepting within renal efferent arterioles, where both systems are vasoconstricting. N-terminal forms of ANP and BNP are currently viewed as biologically inactive.

ANP acts within the kidney to promote the excretion of sodium and water by inhibiting sodium transport in the inner medullary collecting duct, increasing renal blood flow and enhancing glomerular filtration rate (GFR), and – to a lesser degree – inhibiting the tubular actions of angiotensin II, arginine vasopressin, and aldosterone. In addition to its renal effects, ANP induces various cardiovascular, endocrine, and neural responses directed towards the reduction of vascular volume and tone (**Fig. 33.5**). These actions include arterial vasodilation, increased vascular permeability (and consequently plasma volume contraction), suppression of sympathetic nerve activity, and inhibition of renin, aldosterone, arginine vasopressin, and endothelin-1 secretion. In addition, ANP inhibits the vasopressor responses to angiotensin II and endothelin. Intracerebroventricular ANP is reported to reduce systemic blood pressure and heart rate, suppress basal, dehydration-induced, and angiotensin II-induced drinking, reduce salt appetite, and attenuate the pressor action of central angiotensin II.

The effects of infused ANP in health vary according to dose and duration of administration but generally include natriuresis and consequent falls in systolic arterial pressure, peripheral vascular resistance, plasma volume, and central filling pressure, without activation of heart rate, sympathetic nervous activity, or renin–angiotensin–aldosterone. The responses to ANP in hypertensive states are largely similar to those observed in normal

subjects, although increased renal perfusion pressure (as may occur in volume expanded states accompanying some forms of hypertension) augments the natriuretic effect of ANP (**Fig. 33.6**). In keeping with the reduced renal perfusion pressure and augmented neurohormonal stimulation as the heart fails, the renal response to the natriuretic peptides is diminished in severe congestive heart failure, yet cardiac output increases as preload falls.

ANP exhibits growth inhibitory effects in a wide range of cell types and tissues, including vascular smooth muscle cells (VSMC) and endothelial cells, and cardiac fibroblasts. ANP has also been shown to induce apoptosis in neonatal rat cardiac myocytes as well as to stimulate the growth of osteoblasts.

The effects of BNP are largely identical to those of ANP. In contrast, CNP has limited natriuretic and diuretic effects and displays minimal antagonism of the renin–angiotensin–aldosterone system. CNP is, however, a potent venodilator and inhibitor of vascular cell growth and is also reported to suppress the secretion of endothelin-1 and arginine vasopressin. The central effects of CNP, which is the most abundant of the three natriuretic peptides in the tissues of the central nervous system, include stimulation of drinking and reduction of blood pressure and adrenocortical activity.

Role in physiology and pathophysiology

The cardiac natriuretic peptides appear to play a critical role in circulatory homeostasis and participate as local regulators of vascular and ventricular remodeling (**Table 33.1**). While information on the physiologic and pathophysiologic role of CNP is relatively limited, it appears that this peptide is likely to play a lesser part than that of ANP and BNP in sodium and blood

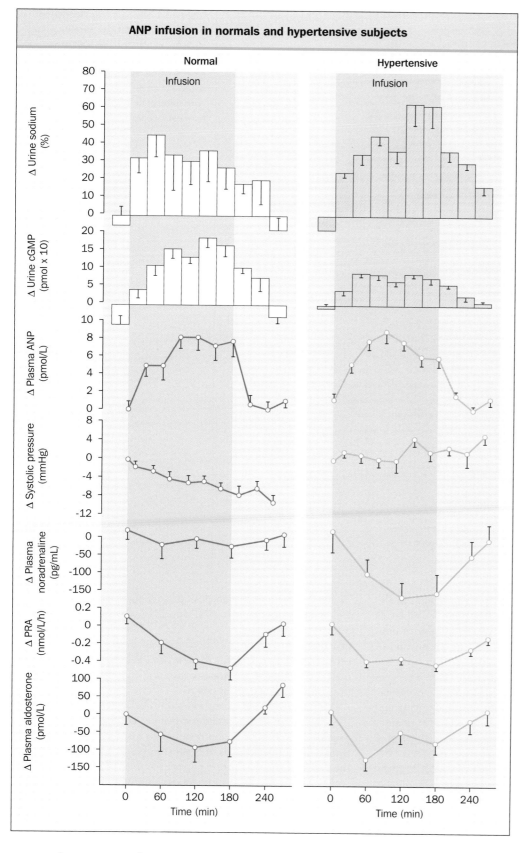

Figure 33.6 Atrial natriuretic peptide (ANP) infusion in normals and hypertensive subjects. Response to intravenous ANP (2.25ng/kg/min for 180min) in six normotensive subjects (left panel) and six hypertensive subjects (right panel) equilibrated on a daily sodium intake of 150mmol. Values (mean ± SEM) are plotted as change (Δ) from time-matched levels on control day. Change in urine sodium excretion is expressed as percentage change from baseline (mean of first three collection periods before infusions = 100%). Change in systolic blood pressure is shown relative to values integrated for 30min immediately before infusions. cGMP, cyclic guanosine monophosphate; PRA, plasma renin activity. (Modified with permission from Espiner EA, Richards AM. Atrial natriuretic peptide. An important factor in sodium and blood pressure regulation. Lancet. 1989;1:707–10 © The Lancet Ltd.)

pressure homeostasis in humans. Current evidence suggests that CNP acts as a local autocrine/paracrine factor in a 'vascular CNP system' concerned largely with the regulation of vasomotor tone and vascular cell growth.

In healthy humans, plasma venous levels of ANP range from 5 to 25pmol/L, whereas BNP levels are consistently lower at 0.3–10pmol/L. Plasma levels of the cardiac natriuretic peptides are elevated when blood volume increases. The most striking

Biologic significance of the cardiac natriuretic peptides

Natriuretic peptide administration (at physiologically relevant doses)		↑ sodium excretion – 'left shift' in pressure natriuresis curve
		↓ peripheral vascular resistance and systolic arterial pressure
		↓ plasma volume and central filling pressure
		↓ sympathetic nervous activity
		↓ renin–angiotensin–aldosterone activity
Natriuretic peptide blockade		↓ sodium excretion and glomerular filtration rate
		↑ systemic vascular resistance and blood pressure
		↓ ventricular relaxation and coronary blood flow
		↑ cardiac filling pressure
		↑ plasma renin–angiotensin–aldosterone
		↑ plasma endothelin and catecholamines
		↑ accelerated development of hypertension and heart failure
Transgenic mice		
Gain of function	ANP/BNP overexpression	↑ plasma ANP/BNP and cGMP levels
		↓ blood pressure
		↑ protection from hypoxia-induced pulmonary hypertension
		↑ bone turnover (skeletal overgrowth)
	NPR-C knockout	↑ plasma ANP half-life (by two thirds)
		↓ blood pressure
		↓ urine concentration (progressive; become volume-depleted)
		↑ bone turnover (skeletal overgrowth)
Loss of function	ANP/BNP knockout	No circulating ANP/BNP
		↑ peripheral resistance and blood pressure
		↑ cardiac fibrosis
		↓ natriuretic and diuretic response to acute volume expansion
	NPR-A knockout	↑ cardiac hypertrophy, dilatation, interstitial fibrosis
		↑ blood pressure
		↑ incidence of sudden death (in males)
		↓ natriuretic response to exogenous ANP and volume expansion
	CNP knockout	↓ endochondral ossification resulting in severe dwarfism

Table 33.1 Biologic significance of the cardiac natriuretic peptides. ANP, atrial natriuretic peptide; BNP, brain natriuretic peptide; cGMP, cyclic guanosine monophosphate; CNP, C-type natriuretic peptide; NPR-A, natriuretic peptide receptor type A; NPR-C, natriuretic peptide receptor type C.

increases occur in heart failure (**Fig. 33.7**) in proportion to the severity of cardiac dysfunction. These increases in plasma levels are largely due to augmented ventricular secretion of both peptides and are characterized by an increase in the proportion of prohormone forms. Plasma ANP and BNP concentrations are also elevated soon after myocardial infarction (**Fig. 33.7**), in which case they correlate with infarct size and increase in cardiac filling pressure, as well as in patients with unstable angina and severe chronic obstructive pulmonary disease, where hypoxia is likely to be an additional stimulus for secretion. Raised levels of both hormones are also observed in a variety of noncardiac edematous states – including nephrosis and cirrhosis, where central blood volume may be increased. The increased concentrations of ANP and BNP observed in chronic renal failure may also be related to 'volume overload', since levels fall after dialysis, ANP more than BNP (**Fig. 33.7**). Significant but smaller increases in both ANP and BNP levels occur in hypertension (**Fig. 33.7**) and correlate with severity of blood pressure elevation and presence of left ventricular hypertrophy. A variety of tachyarrhythmias may also increase plasma hormone levels in humans, ANP more than BNP.

CNP is present at very low plasma concentrations in health and, in strong contrast to ANP and BNP, levels are not altered in human hypertension or severe heart failure. However, marked elevations in plasma CNP are observed in patients with severe sepsis as well as in chronic renal failure. Whether these increases reflect a response to specific stimuli, endothelial damage, or impaired clearance is unknown.

With the possible exception of familial open-angle glaucoma, there are no reports of validated primary disorders of natriuretic peptide secretion or action resulting in disease. By analogy with transgenic animal studies, it is conceivable that polymorphism in the genes of the natriuretic peptides and/or their receptors may contribute or predispose to the development of some forms of hypertension. Indeed, a number of studies have reported that mutations in the human *ANP* (exons 1 and 3, and intron 2), *NPR-B* and *NPR-C* genes are associated with the development of hypertension. A further study in hypertension-prone men proposes that deficient ANP production during sodium loading predicts the subsequent development of systemic hypertension, while inappropriately low basal circulating ANP has been reported in offspring of hypertensive families. These findings raise the

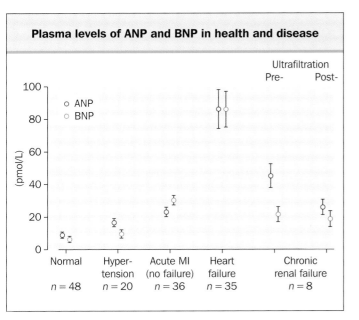

Figure 33.7 Plasma levels of atrial natriuretic peptide (ANP) and brain natriuretic peptide (BNP) in health and disease. The figure shows levels of venous plasma ANP (blue circles) and concurrent BNP (red circles) in normal subjects and patients with circulatory disorders. Values are mean ± SEM. *n* is the number of subjects in each group. All samples were assayed in the same laboratory (Endocrine Department, Christchurch Hospital, New Zealand) using previously published techniques. Hypertensive patients showed no evidence of significant end-organ disease (Modified with permission from Rademaker MT, Espiner EA. The endocrine heart. In: Becker K, ed. Principles and practice of endocrinology and metabolism, 3rd edn. Baltimore, MD:Lippincott, Williams & Wilkins; 2001.)

possibility that ANP secretion may be impaired in the early phase of the disorder.

Clinical applications

Diagnosis

The close relationship linking natriuretic peptide plasma levels with 'cardiac overloading' has led to applications in clinical practice. Raised plasma levels of ANP, and in particular BNP and its N-terminal fragment (NT-proBNP), are useful for detecting symptomless left ventricular dysfunction, heart failure based on diastolic dysfunction (which is difficult to diagnose and constitutes a third of all clinical cardiac failure), increased left ventricular mass in patients with essential hypertension, and unstable angina, and in distinguishing acute dyspnea of cardiac origin from that due to primary lung disease. The measurement of plasma BNP concentrations by primary care physicians also provides a useful screening test for the selection of patients for further cardiac investigation – a test both cheaper and more available than echocardiogram or radionuclide ventriculography.

Prognosis

Measurement of plasma natriuretic peptides may be useful in clinical prognosis. The prognosis for patients with established heart failure or after acute myocardial infarction (**Fig. 33.8**) is predicted by levels of the cardiac natriuretic peptides. Indeed, these cardiac peptides appear to be independent of, and superior to, other neurohormones (as well as more conventional indicators such as ejection fraction) in identifying patients at risk of developing left ventricular dysfunction, progressive heart failure, or death, and thus those who require aggressive treatment.

Optimizing/guiding therapy

The natriuretic peptides may also be a useful tool for monitoring the effectiveness of antifailure therapy since plasma levels decrease following hemodynamic and cardiac improvement. Measurement of natriuretic peptide levels in the assessment of 'volume' status in noncardiac disorders is also a possibility. Assay of plasma ANP has already proved helpful in assessing the adequacy of mineralocorticoid replacement in patients with Addison's disease and may prove to be a useful marker (along with aldosterone and renin) of the hyperexpanded state associated with primary hyperaldosteronism.

Treatment

Their recognized actions make the natriuretic peptides attractive therapeutic agents in a variety of cardiovascular and hypervolemic disorders. Early studies suggest that the administration of ANP and BNP has salutary effects in patients with hypertension and heart failure. Natriuretic peptide administration may also prove beneficial in reperfusion therapy for acute myocardial infarction as the hormones inhibit reperfusion-induced ventricular arrhythmias and preserve ATP content in the ischemic myocardium. ANP has also been shown to improve myocardial perfusion to areas of ischemia by dilating coronary resistance and epicardial collateral vessels – without inducing reflex tachycardia and tachyphylaxis – while both peptides suppress hyperventilation-induced variant angina by preventing coronary spasm. In acute renal failure, ANP administration significantly improved glomerular function and reduced the need for dialysis, while in patients with cor pulmonale, BNP produced pulmonary vasodilation without worsening oxygen saturation. The use of NEP inhibitors (which enhance endogenous levels of the peptides through inhibition of their enzymatic breakdown) in hypertension and heart failure have beneficial effects that mimic those of exogenous ANP and BNP. In chronic renal failure, NEP inhibition is reported to induce pronounced natriuresis at a stage when loop diuretics would have little effect. Long-term NEP inhibition is also reported to reduce intraocular pressure and may have a place in the management of glaucoma. The development of drug combinations with both NEP and angiotensin-converting enzyme inhibitory activity shows particular promise. The use of such compounds also has important longer-term actions in reducing cardiac hypertrophy and endothelial and vascular smooth muscle proliferation.

ENDOTHELIN

The endothelin (ET) family of 21-amino-acid-residue peptides, designated ET-1, ET-2, and ET-3, is best viewed as a paracrine regulator in multiple tissue systems participating in the maintenance of circulatory pressure and tissue blood flow. ET-1, a powerful vasoconstrictor, is the major isoform generated in the human vasculature and is considered to be the most important functionally in regulating local vascular tone. As already shown for angiotensin II, ET and the natriuretic peptides appear to be mutually opposing forces in many tissues and cellular pathways.

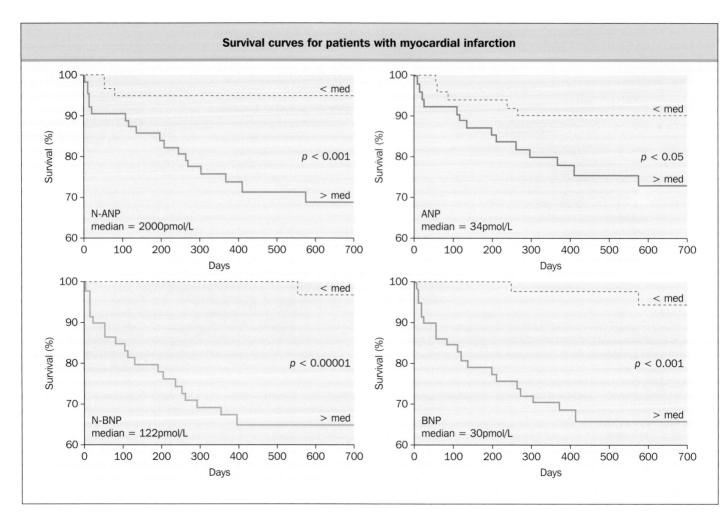

Figure 33.8 Survival curves for patients with myocardial infarction. A total of 121 patients were divided into two subgroups with early postinfarction plasma natriuretic peptide concentrations – atrial natriuretic peptide (ANP), NT-ANP (N-ANP), brain natriuretic peptide (BNP), NT-BNP (N-BNP) – above (solid line) and below (dashed line) the group median. Venous blood was drawn between 24 and 96 hours after the onset of symptoms. Inclusion criteria included age less than 80 years, absence of cardiogenic shock, and survival for at least 24 hours after myocardial infarction. Probability values refer to significance values between the two groups. (Modified with permission from Richards AM, Nicholls MG, Yandle TG, et al. Plasma N-terminal pro-brain natriuretic peptide and adrenomedullin: new neurohormonal predictors of left ventricular function and prognosis after myocardial infarction. Circulation 1998;97:1921–9.)

Synthesis, structure and regulation

In humans, the genes that encode ET-1, ET-2, and ET-3 are located on chromosomes 6, 1, and 20 respectively. Transcription and processing of the ET genes yields the mature bioactive peptides (**Figs 33.9** & **33.10**).

The main site of ET-1 synthesis is the vascular endothelium but the gene is also expressed in epithelial and VSMCs, heart, lung, kidney, pancreas, placenta, endometrium, and central nervous system. ET-2 is detected in the kidneys and intestines, as well as the heart, placenta, and uterus, whereas ET-3 is present predominantly in the central nervous system but also located throughout the gastrointestinal tract, lung, and kidney. ET-3 is not present in endothelial cells. Secretion of the peptides appear to be largely constitutive and occurs in response to a variety of mechanical and chemical stimuli (**Fig. 33.10**).

Receptors and metabolism

Two ET receptors have been identified, ET_A and ET_B, both of which are G-protein-coupled. The ET_A receptor, highly selective for ET-1 (ET-1>ET-2>>ET-3), is found most abundantly in VSMCs, cardiac myocytes, fibroblasts, and renal glomeruli and vasculature. This receptor largely mediates the vasoconstrictor action of ET (through activation of phospholipase C) as well as mitogenesis and the stimulation of aldosterone secretion. The ET_B is the preferred receptor for ET-3 and is expressed predominantly in endothelial cells and to a lesser extent in VSMCs, brain, lung, and kidney. Endothelial ET_B receptor activation is characterized by transient vasodilation (through stimulation of nitric oxide and prostacyclin), although vasoconstrictor effects are also reported in some tissues, including the coronary arteries and the renal vasculature. The ET_B receptor also mediates inhibition of apoptosis and platelet aggregation. In addition, the ET_B receptor plays a major role in the clearance of ET-1 through the binding and internalization of the peptide in numerous vascular beds (primarily in the lungs and kidneys). Enzymatic degradation by endopeptidases (particularly NEP 24.11) also contributes to the degradation of ET-1.

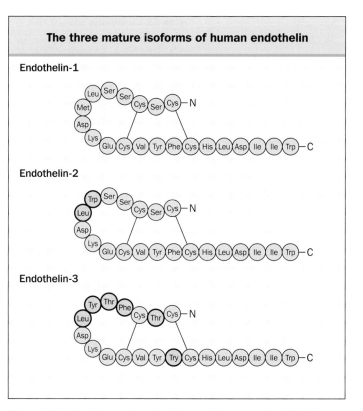

Figure 33.9 The three mature isoforms of human endothelin. Blue circles represent amino acids different from those of endothelin-1.

Biologic actions

Endothelin-1 induces various cardiovascular, renal, and endocrine responses, directed largely towards the increase of vascular volume and tone (**Fig. 33.11**). These actions include powerful smooth muscle contraction (particularly of resistance vessels and veins), which is slow both to develop and reverse, positive effects on cardiac contractility, stimulation of both the secretion and actions angiotensin II and catecholamines, augmentation of aldosterone secretion, and enhancement of peripheral as well as central sympathetic activity. The renal circulation is especially sensitive to the vasoconstrictor effects of ET-1 (via the ET_A receptor), where it acts to reduce renal plasma flow, GFR, and the glomerular capillary ultrafiltration coefficient. However, tubular actions of ET-1 (ET_B- receptor-mediated) actually inhibit sodium reabsorption in the proximal tubules and collecting ducts. Water reabsorption in the collecting duct is also inhibited by ET-1 via inhibition of vasopressin. ET-1 also inhibits renin release. Other effects of ET-1 include the stimulation of ANP, BNP, histamine, estrogen, prostaglandin, growth hormone, thyrotropin, and luteinizing and follicle-stimulating hormone secretion, and inhibition of prolactin. The physiologic importance of these actions in humans remains to be assessed.

Endothelin-1 also constricts nonvascular smooth muscle in numerous tissues (including those of the airways, intestine, bladder, myometrium, mesangium, prostate, and vas deferens) and has been implicated in the stimulation of uterine contractions during labor and closure of the umbilical vessels and ductus arteriosus after birth.

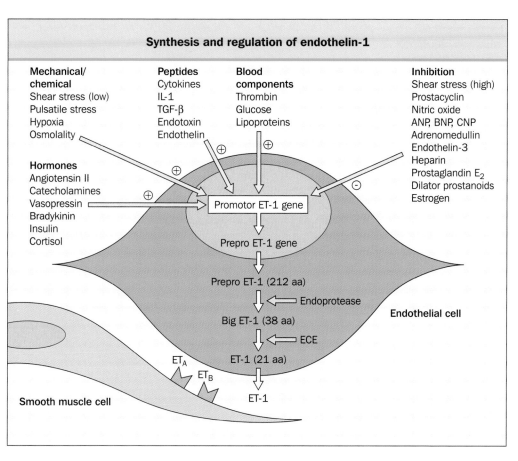

Figure 33.10 Synthesis and regulation of endothelin-1 (ET-1). ANP, atrial natriuretic peptide; BNP, brain natriuretic peptide; CNP, C-type natriuretic peptide; ECE, endothelin converting enzyme; IL-1, interleukin-1; TGF-β, transforming growth factor-β. ET_A and ET_B are ET receptors. (Modified with permission from Rademaker MT, Espiner EA. Hormones of the cardiovascular system. In: Degroot LJ & Jameson JL, eds. Endocrinology, 4th edn. Philadelphia, PA:WB Saunders Company; 2001.)

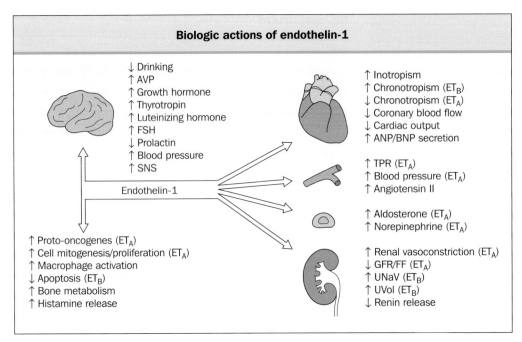

Biologic actions of endothelin-1

↓ Drinking
↑ AVP
↑ Growth hormone
↑ Thyrotropin
↑ Luteinizing hormone
↑ FSH
↓ Prolactin
↑ Blood pressure
↑ SNS

Endothelin-1

↑ Proto-oncogenes (ET$_A$)
↑ Cell mitogenesis/proliferation (ET$_A$)
↑ Macrophage activation
↓ Apoptosis (ET$_B$)
↑ Bone metabolism
↑ Histamine release

↑ Inotropism
↑ Chronotropism (ET$_B$)
↓ Chronotropism (ET$_A$)
↓ Coronary blood flow
↓ Cardiac output
↑ ANP/BNP secretion

↑ TPR (ET$_A$)
↑ Blood pressure (ET$_A$)
↑ Angiotensin II

↑ Aldosterone (ET$_A$)
↑ Norepinephrine (ET$_A$)

↑ Renal vasoconstriction (ET$_A$)
↓ GFR/FF (ET$_A$)
↑ UNaV (ET$_B$)
↑ UVol (ET$_B$)
↓ Renin release

Figure 33.11 Biologic actions of endothelin-1. Receptors (ET$_A$ / ET$_B$) mediating actions (if known) are shown in brackets. ANP, atrial natriuretic peptide; AVP, arginine vasopressin; BNP, brain natriuretic peptide; FF, filtration fraction; FSH, follicle-stimulating hormone; GFR, glomerular filtration rate; TPR, total peripheral resistance; UNa.V, urine sodium excretion; Uvol, urine volume; SNS, sympathetic nervous system.

Endothelin-1 is a potent mitogen in a wide variety of cell types (including VSMCs, cardiac myocytes, fibroblasts, glomerular mesangial cells, and bronchial smooth muscle cells), as well as being a powerful activator of macrophages and other inflammatory cells.

Role in physiology and pathophysiology

A substantial body of evidence indicates that there is sufficient endogenous (local) generation of ET for the peptide to play a physiologic role in control of vascular tone and blood pressure. Blockade of the ET system through the use of endothelin-converting enzyme (ECE) inhibitors or receptor antagonist produces systemic vasodilation and reductions in arterial pressure in normal humans. ET blockade is also reported to cause vasodilation in numerous vascular beds, including the renal and pulmonary vasculature, and to reduce the growth promoting effects of ET in various organs and tissues. A key role for the ET system is further supported by findings in transgenic models, where overexpression of ET-1 causes systemic hypertension as well as the development of renal lesions and cysts, interstitial fibrosis, and glomerulosclerosis (largely through activation of the ET$_A$ receptor). On the other hand, rodents lacking the ET$_B$ receptor gene exhibit salt-sensitive hypertension.

Endothelin immunoreactivity is present in normal human plasma at levels usually less than 3pmol/L and constitutes big ET-1 (about 60%), ET-1 (about 30%) and ET-3 (about 10%). ET-2 has not been detected. Increased levels of circulating ET-1 occur in a variety of disease states, including heart failure (**Fig. 33.12**), myocardial infarction, atherosclerosis, pulmonary hypertension, renal failure, septic shock, diabetes, systemic sclerosis, and possibly essential hypertension. Higher than normal concentrations have also been reported in patients with coronary artery spasm, preeclampsia, hyperlipoproteinemia, cirrhosis with ascites, Crohn's disease and ulcerative colitis, biliary atresia, sickle cell disease (particularly those in acute vaso-occlusive crisis), subarachnoid hemorrhage, and ischemic stroke. While the source and

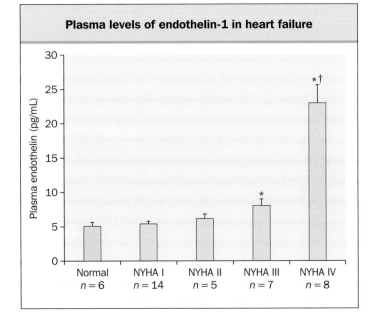

Plasma levels of endothelin-1 in heart failure

| | Normal $n = 6$ | NYHA I $n = 14$ | NYHA II $n = 5$ | NYHA III $n = 7$ | NYHA IV $n = 8$ |

Figure 33.12 Plasma levels of endothelin-1 in heart failure. The figure shows venous plasma endothelin levels in normal subjects and patients with increasing degrees of congestive heart failure. Values are mean ± SEM; *n* is the number of subjects in each group. NYHA indicates the New York Heart Association grading of heart failure (I–IV).
*$p < 0.05$ vs normal; †$p < 0.05$ vs NYHA III. (Modified with permission from Wei CM, Lerman A, Rodeheffer RJ, et al. Endothelin in human congestive heart failure. Circulation 1994;89:1580–6.)

significance of elevated levels in many of these disorders are unclear, it is now recognized that ET-1 – through its actions to increase vascular tone, activate the angiotensin–aldosterone and sympathetic nervous systems, and augment mitogenesis – may contribute significantly to their pathogenesis, end-organ damage, and morbidity. Obvious examples include states of sustained vasoconstriction (as occurs in a range of cardiovascular diseases), intermittent vasospasm, and other vasospastic states such as may occur in stroke and brain injury. ET-1 is also implicated in the development of a variety of lung disorders, including asthma, primary pulmonary hypertension, and pulmonary fibrosis, and in the kidney has extensive renovascular and parenchymal effects. However, a direct causal connection between increased circulating levels of ET-1 and hypertension appears to have been established only in malignant hemangioendothelioma. In addition, in patients with essential hypertension there is a strong correlation between diastolic blood pressure and a polymorphism in the *ET-1* gene. Possible racial differences in ET-1 activity are also suggested by the threefold higher plasma ET concentrations reported in hypertensive African-Americans compared to Caucasians. Furthermore, mutations in the ET_B and *ET-3* (and possibly *ECE-1*) genes are implicated in Hirschsprung's disease. Other associations have been found in allergic disorders; for example, polymorphisms in the *ET-1* gene were found to be significantly linked in patients with both asthma and rhinitis.

Clinical and therapeutic applications

As shown for the natriuretic peptides, measurement of plasma ET may provide useful diagnostic and prognostic information in heart failure. For example, in patients with (moderate to severe) congestive heart failure, circulating ET-1 concentrations correlate with the severity of left ventricular dysfunction, are inversely associated with prognosis and predict mortality, and are lowered by drug treatment known to reduce mortality. Following myocardial infarction, plasma levels 3 days after infarction predict 1-year mortality. In addition, in patients with atherosclerosis, a significant correlation exists between circulating ET-1 levels and number of atherosclerotic sites.

Blockade of the ET system (through the use of receptor antagonists or ECE inhibitors) may yield novel therapeutic options for a wide range of disorders associated with increased expression of ET-1, vasoconstriction, and vascular dysfunction. In clinical studies, administration of bosentan (a combined ET_A/ET_B receptor antagonist) decreases the 24-hour ambulatory diastolic blood pressure in patients with essential hypertension, increases coronary diameter in patients with coronary artery disease, and induces sustained peripheral, pulmonary, and venous vasodilation in association with improved cardiac performance in patients with severe congestive heart failure. In chronic renal failure, ET blockade reduces blood pressure and renal vascular resistance while maintaining GFR.

ADRENOMEDULLIN

Adrenomedullin (AM) is a potent vasodilator 52-amino-acid residue peptide found widely in tissues and organs where it may function as a local autocrine/paracrine rather than endocrine factor. It has multifunctional biologic properties, many of which are involved in the regulation of circulation and body fluid volume. While many of the effects of AM are similar to those of the natriuretic peptides, the modes of action differ.

Synthesis, structure and regulation

The transcription and processing of the *AM* gene, situated on chromosome 11 in humans, yields two biologically active

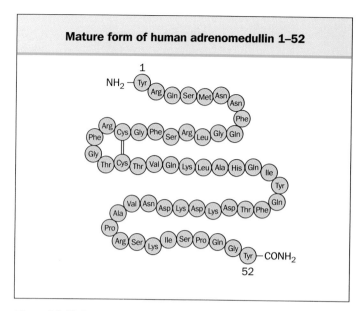

Figure 33.13 Mature form of human adrenomedullin 1–52.

hormones – the 52-amino-acid AM peptide, containing a six-residue ring structure and a C-terminal amide group (essential for its bioactivity), and the 20-residue proadrenomedullin N-terminal peptide (PAMP) (**Figs 33.13 & 33.14**).

AM immunoreactivity is detectable in high concentrations in the adrenal medulla, with lower levels found in tissues such as the heart, lung, kidney, brain, and vasculature. Both endothelial cells and VSMCs actively synthesize and secrete AM, current evidence pointing to vascular tissue as the probable major source of circulating AM in health. As shown in **Figure 33.14**, AM secretion from vascular tissues is subject to regulation by multiple local and circulating factors.

Receptors and metabolism

The exact number and specificity of receptors that interact with AM remains unclear and may vary according to species, tissue type, and experimental setting. To date, at least three types of AM receptors have been described. While one of these is reported to be specific for AM, the other two receptors – the orphan receptor RDC-1 and the calcitonin-gene-related peptide (CGRP) receptor 1, are reported to bind both AM and CGRP. Although cyclic adenosine monophosphate (cAMP) is considered to be the major second messenger for AM, alternative signal transduction pathways have also been reported – including nitric oxide, prostaglandins, intracellular calcium mobilization, and activation of the inositol phosphate pathway. In addition, AM's antiproliferative activity may be mediated at least partly by inhibiting the mitogen-activated protein-kinase pathway.

Little is yet understood about the mechanisms of clearance of AM from plasma. Estimates in humans indicate a half-life approximating 22min. Sites of clearance include the lungs and possibly the kidney.

Biologic actions

Identified initially as a vasoactive peptide, AM has multiple actions, the net effect of which is to promote reduction of blood

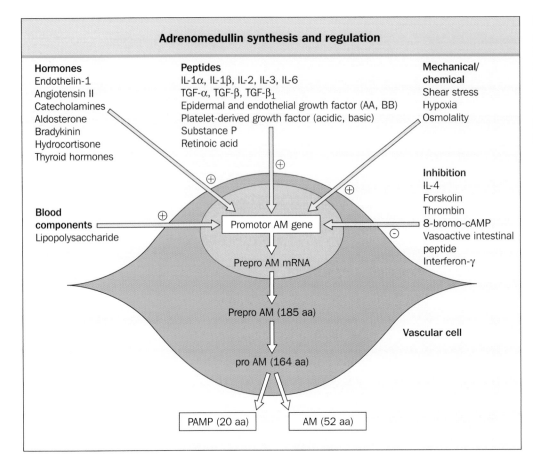

Adrenomedullin synthesis and regulation

Hormones
Endothelin-1
Angiotensin II
Catecholamines
Aldosterone
Bradykinin
Hydrocortisone
Thyroid hormones

Peptides
IL-1α, IL-1β, IL-2, IL-3, IL-6
TGF-α, TGF-β, TGF-β$_1$
Epidermal and endothelial growth factor (AA, BB)
Platelet-derived growth factor (acidic, basic)
Substance P
Retinoic acid

Mechanical/chemical
Shear stress
Hypoxia
Osmolality

Inhibition
IL-4
Forskolin
Thrombin
8-bromo-cAMP
Vasoactive intestinal peptide
Interferon-γ

Blood components
Lipopolysaccharide

Promotor AM gene

Prepro AM mRNA

Prepro AM (185 aa)

pro AM (164 aa)

Vascular cell

PAMP (20 aa)   AM (52 aa)

Figure 33.14 Adrenomedullin synthesis and regulation. The figure illustrates the synthesis and regulation of adrenomedullin (AM) and pro-adrenomedullin N-terminal 20 peptide (PAMP) within vascular tissue. cAMP, cyclic adenosine monophosphate; IL, interleukin; TGF, transforming growth factor.

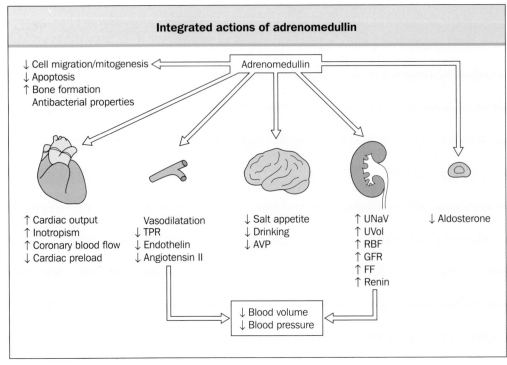

Integrated actions of adrenomedullin

Adrenomedullin

↓ Cell migration/mitogenesis
↓ Apoptosis
↑ Bone formation
  Antibacterial properties

↑ Cardiac output
↑ Inotropism
↑ Coronary blood flow
↓ Cardiac preload

  Vasodilatation
↓ TPR
↓ Endothelin
↓ Angiotensin II

↓ Salt appetite
↓ Drinking
↓ AVP

↑ UNaV
↑ UVol
↑ RBF
↑ GFR
↑ FF
↑ Renin

↓ Aldosterone

↓ Blood volume
↓ Blood pressure

Figure 33.15 Integrated actions of adrenomedullin. AVP, arginine vasopressin; FF, filtration fraction; GFR, glomerular filtration rate; RBF, renal blood flow; TPR, total peripheral resistance; UNaV, urine sodium excretion; UVol, urine volume.

volume and pressure (**Fig. 33.15**). These actions include vasodilation of resistance vessels (largely the result of the generation of nitric oxide within the vessel wall), as well as inhibitory actions on procontractile factors such as ET-1, angiotensin II, and norepinephrine. In addition, AM may desensitize the baroreceptor reflex. In the kidney, AM exerts potent natriuretic and diuretic effects through its actions to increase renal blood flow and to decrease tubular sodium reabsorption. In addition,

AM increases osmotic permeability of the inner medullary collecting duct, and at higher doses, increases GFR and filtration fraction. These renal effects of AM are complemented by adrenal actions to inhibit aldosterone secretion and effects within the central nervous system to inhibit vasopressin release, salt-appetite, and angiotensin-II-induced drinking. Administration of AM at larger doses is associated with reductions in cardiac preload and rise in heart rate and cardiac output. These latter effects may be due in part to the powerful positive inotropic actions of AM.

In contrast to its inhibitory actions on angiotensin II and aldosterone secretion, AM directly stimulates renin production. Other effects of AM include an increase of plasma oxytocin levels, reduction of plasma ACTH and cortisol levels, inhibition of gastric acid secretion and regulation of insulin secretion. The effect of AM on the natriuretic peptide system remains unclear. AM exhibits a variety of cell growth inhibitory actions including the suppression of cytokine-induced neutrophil chemoattractant secretion (a key mediator of neutrophil migration in inflammatory sites), and migration and mitogenesis of VSMCs and cardiomyocytes. Less is known concerning the range of actions of PAMP. However, like AM it lowers blood pressure and inhibits the secretion of aldosterone, epinephrine, and ACTH, and may complement the actions of AM.

Role in physiology and pathophysiology

The multitude of actions induced by AM in a wide variety of tissues provide strong circumstantial evidence supporting a central role for this peptide in pressure/volume homeostasis. Further evidence of its physiologic importance is provided by preliminary reports in transgenic mice overexpressing AM. These mice exhibit reduced blood pressure, an enhanced hypertensive response to false substrates for nitric oxide synthase, and increased survival following lipopolysaccharide administration. These findings suggest that AM is protective against circulatory collapse.

Circulating levels of AM (and PAMP) in health are typically low, in the 2–8pmol/L range, and do not appear to be increased by either acute or chronic salt-loading in humans, but may rise with severe exercise. Elevated levels have been observed in normal pregnancy. Significant increases in plasma AM concentrations have been described in numerous human disease states, with the most striking increases (12-fold) reported in patients with acute sepsis, where levels correlate with severity and predict survival. Significant but smaller increases are reported in patients with hemorrhagic and cardiogenic shock, Addison's disease, chronic renal failure (**Fig. 33.16**), acute asthma, chronic obstructive pulmonary disease, and primary aldosteronism. Increases observed with type 1 diabetes mellitus correlate with duration of disease and renal impairment. AM is reported to be raised in a range of other disorders, including hepatic insufficiency with ascites, hyperthyroidism, subarachnoid hemorrhage, and gastrointestinal and pulmonary neoplasms. In several of these situations AM elevation is reported to correlate with increases in C-reactive protein, a marker of acute inflammation. Small but still significant increases in plasma AM are observed in a number of cardiovascular disorders, including congestive heart failure and left ventricular dysfunction after myocardial infarction (**Fig. 33.16**), where levels correlate with the severity of cardiac dysfunction

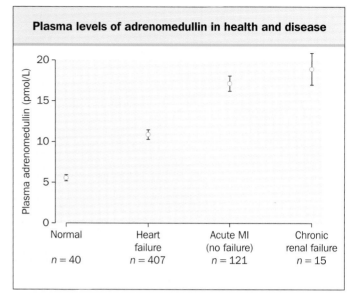

Figure 33.16 Plasma levels of adrenomedullin in health and disease. Venous plasma AM levels in normal subjects and patients with circulatory disorders are illustrated. Values are mean ± SEM. *n* is the number of subjects in each group. All samples were assayed in the same laboratory (Endocrine Department, Christchurch Hospital, New Zealand) using previously published techniques. Heart failure was due to coronary artery disease, New York Heart Association heart failure functional class I–III (ejection fraction less than 45%). Patients with acute (uncomplicated) myocardial infarction (MI) had blood drawn within 24 hours of admission (data from Foy et al. Eur Heart J. 1995;16:770–9). Patients with chronic renal failure were all receiving maintenance hemodialysis. (Modified with permission from Rademaker MT, Espiner EA. Hormones of the cardiovascular system. In: DeGroot LJ & Jameson JL, eds. Endocrinology, 4th edn. Philadelphia, PA:WB Saunders Company; 2001.)

and other markers of cardiac impairment. In essential hypertension, increases in circulating AM appear to relate positively with blood pressure and negatively with GFR. Greater rises are observed in both renovascular and malignant hypertension. In heart failure and hypertension, plasma AM levels decrease following successful antifailure and antihypertensive therapy. As yet, no primary disorder of AM production or action resulting in disease has been reported.

The origin of increased circulating AM levels in many of the above disorders is uncertain. However, in congestive heart failure, there is evidence that the failing ventricle contributes at least in part to the raised levels. In the instance of sepsis, experimental data supports the increased synthesis of AM in multiple tissues. Decreased renal clearance may also be an underlying factor in many disorders, particularly in chronic renal failure. Although plasma concentrations of AM in many clinical disorders are often increased in proportion to severity, it remains unclear whether these pathologic elevations reflect tissue/organ damage or, alternatively, represent an increased production as part of a compensatory mechanism.

Clinical and therapeutic implications

Given its vasodilator, positive inotropic, natriuretic, counter-neurohormonal, and antimitogenic properties, AM may be

Comparative overview of secretion and cardiovascular actions

	ANP (BNP)	CNP	ET-1	Adrenomedullin
Major site of synthesis	Cardiac atrium (cardiac ventricle)	Vascular endothelium/brain	Vascular endothelium	Vascular tissue?
Major stimulus to secretion	Atrial (ventricular) transmural pressure	Multiple local factors	Multiple local factors	Multiple local factors
Normal plasma levels	5–25pmol/L (0.3–10pmol/L)	? very low	<5pmol/L	2–8pmol/L
Plasma half-life	3min (22min)	2–3min	1–1.5min	22min
Main biological receptor	**NPR-A**	**NPR-B**	**ET$_A$** **ET$_B$**	**AM-R, CGRP-R, RDC-1**
Major intracellular mediator	cGMP	cGMP	[Ca] NO	cAMP/NO
Main effects — Vasculature	Dilatation ↓ ET-1/↓ angiotensin II ↑ vascular permeability	Dilatation	Constriction ↑ angiotensin II Dilatation (and constriction)	Dilatation ↓ ET-1/↓ angiotensin II
Heart	Negative inotropism ↑ coronary blood flow	↑ coronary blood flow	Negative chronotropism Positive inotropism ↓ coronary blood flow ↑ ANP/BNP Positive chronotropism	Positive chronotropism Positive inotropism ↑ coronary blood flow
Kidney	Natriuresis ↓ renin	— —	Antinatriuresis ↓ renin Natriuresis	Natriuresis ↑ renin
Adrenal gland	↓ aldosterone	—	↑ aldosterone	↓ aldosterone
Other	Antimitogenesis ↓ Sympathetic nervous activity	Antimitogenesis	Mitogenesis ↑ sympathetic nervous activity	Antimitogenesis ↓ sympathetic nervous activity

Table 33.2 Comparative overview of secretion and cardiovascular actions. The table compares the natriuretic peptides (atrial, brain, and C-type natriuretic peptide: ANP, BNP, and CNP respectively), endothelin-1 (ET-1), and adrenomedullin (AM). Data relating to BNP, if different from ANP, is bracketed. AM-R, adrenomedullin receptor; cAMP, cyclic adenosine monophosphate; cGMP, cyclic guanosine monophosphate; CGRP-R, calcitonin-gene-related peptide receptor; NO, nitric oxide; NPR, natriuretic peptide receptor; RDC-1, orphan receptor. (Reproduced with permission from Rademaker MT, Espiner EA. Hormones of the cardiovascular system. In: DeGroot LJ & Jameson JL, eds. Endocrinology. 4th edn. Philadelphia, PA:WB Saunders Company; 2001.)

clinically useful in the treatment of a variety of cardiovascular disorders associated with volume overload. Indeed, short-term AM administration in patients with heart failure decreases arterial pressure, pulmonary arterial and capillary wedge pressures, and plasma aldosterone, and increases cardiac index, urine volume, and urinary sodium excretion. AM may be a treatment for hypertension in the future. AM is a potent vasodilator of several major vascular beds and has been shown to be protective in ischemic brain injury and vascular reperfusion injury, to induce coronary and renal vasodilation, and improve microcirculation in hepatic cirrhosis.

OVERVIEW

By direct natriuretic effects, vascular relaxation, and inhibition of production and actions of vasoconstrictor peptides, the natriuretic peptide system (both hormonal and paracrine) appears to be a major defense against the threat of volume expansion (hypervolemia). In the longer term – and equally importantly – these hormones reset the sympathetic nervous system (reduce sympathetic nervous activity) and restrain vascular and cardiac cell growth (**Table 33.2**). CNP appears to be uniquely placed within the vascular system, interacting with numerous other peptides and regulatory hormones to reduce vascular tone and

to contribute to vascular remodeling. As noted with the natriuretic peptides, AM also exerts multiple effects on a variety of tissues, the combined actions of which promote reduction in blood volume and pressure (**Table 33.2**). Superficially, this might suggest redundancy. However, differences in their production and effects on tissues suggest otherwise. For example, in contrast to the natriuretic peptides, AM is clearly inotropic and appears to stimulate renin.

Counterbalancing these dilator hormonal systems are the potent vasoconstrictor peptides ET-1 and angiotensin II. ET-1, acting as a local autocrine/paracrine mediator, exerts uniquely sustained vasoconstrictor actions, augments angiotensin II activity, stimulates aldosterone, and at the same time increases sympathetic nervous activity and promotes mitogenesis (**Table 33.2**). Although likely to be important in controlling peripheral resistance, the major role of tissue ET may be to counterbalance other endothelial factors such as nitric oxide, prostacyclin, AM, and CNP, thereby contributing to the maintenance of blood fluidity and tissue perfusion. A remarkable interplay among the natriuretic peptides, AM, endothelins, and angiotensin II (along with prostaglandins) appears to dictate the local actions of these hormones in many tissues. The challenge now is to define the physiologic roles of these many factors at the molecular level and their importance in human disease.

FURTHER READING

Barr CS, Rhodes P, Struthers AD. C-type natriuretic peptide. Peptides 1996;17:1243–51.

Brenner BM, Ballermann BJ, Gunning ME, et al. Diverse biological actions of atrial natriuretic peptide. Physiolog Rev. 1990;70:665–99.

Chao J, Jin L, Lin K, et al. Adrenomedullin gene delivery reduces blood pressure in spontaneously hypertensive rats. Hypertens Res. 1997;20:269–77.

Davis M, Espiner EA, Richards G, et al. Plasma brain natriuretic peptide in the assessment of acute dyspnoea. Lancet 1994;343:440–4.

Ehlenz K, Koch B, Preuss P, et al. High levels of circulating adrenomedullin in severe illness: correlation with C-reactive protein and evidence against the adrenal medulla as site of origin. Exp Clin Endocrinol Diabetes 1997;105:156–62.

Espiner EA, Richards AM. Atrial natriuretic peptide. An important factor in sodium and blood pressure regulation. Lancet 1989;1:707–10.

Haynes WG, Webb DJ. Endothelin as a regulator of cardiovascular function in health and disease. J Hypertens. 1998;16:1081–98.

Hocher B, Thone-Reineke C, Rohmeiss P, et al. Endothelin-1 transgenic mice develop glomerulosclerosis, interstitial fibrosis, and renal cysts but not hypertension. J Clin Invest. 99:1380–9.

Kitashiro S, Sugiura T, Takayama Y, et al. Long-term administration of atrial natriuretic peptide in patients with acute heart failure. J Cardiovasc Pharmacol. 1999;33:948–52.

Nagaya N, Satoh T, Nishikimi T, et al. Hemodynamic, renal and hormonal effects of adrenomedullin in patients with congestive heart failure. Circulation 2000;101:498–503.

Oliver PM, Fox JE, Kim R, et al. Hypertension, cardiac hypertrophy, and sudden death in mice lacking natriuretic peptide receptor A. Proc Nat Acad Sci USA 1997;94:14730–5.

Rademaker MT, Espiner EA. The endocrine heart. In: Becker K, ed. Principles and practice of endocrinology and metabolism, 3rd edn. Baltimore, MD:Lippincott Williams & Wilkins; 2001.

Rademaker MT, Espiner EA. Hormones of the cardiovascular system. In: DeGroot LJ & Jameson JL, eds. Endocrinology, 4th edn. Philadelphia, PA:WB Saunders Company; 2001.

Richards AM, Nicholls MG, Yandle TG, et al. Plasma N-terminal pro-brain natriuretic peptide and adrenomedullin: new neurohormonal predictors of left ventricular function and prognosis after myocardial infarction. Circulation 1998;97:1921–9.

Samson WK. Adrenomedullin and the control of fluid and electrolyte homeostasis. Annu Rev Physiol. 1999;61:363–89.

Sarzani R, Dessi-Fulgheri P, Salvi F, et al. A novel promoter variant of the natriuretic peptide clearance receptor gene is associated with lower atrial natriuretic peptide and higher blood pressure in obese hypertensives. J Hypertens. 1999;17:1301–5.

Shimosawa T, Shiagaki Y, Katoh S, et al. Adrenomedullin knock out mouse study: its lethality and vasculitis. Paper presented at 82nd Endocrinology Meeting, Toronto, Canada, 2000.

Stevens PA, Brown MJ. Genetic variability of the ET-1 and the ET$_A$ receptor genes in essential hypertension. J Cardiovasc Pharmacol. 1995;26:S9–S12.

Troughton RW, Frampton CM, Yandle TG, et al. Treatment of heart failure guided by plasma aminoterminal brain natriuretic peptide (N-BNP) concentrations. Lancet 2000;355:1126–30.

Webb DJ, Strachan FE. Clinical experience with endothelin antagonists. Am J Hypertens. 1998;11:71S–79S.

Wei CM, Lerman A, Rodeheffer RJ, et al. Endothelin in human congestive heart failure. Circulation 1994;89:1580–6.

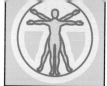

Section 7 General Conditions – Clinical

Chapter 34

Calcium and Common Bone Disorders

Gregory R Mundy and Andrew F Stewart

CALCIUM HOMEOSTASIS

Extracellular fluid calcium or plasma calcium is very carefully controlled by fluxes of calcium, which occur between the extracellular fluid and the skeleton, and between the gut and the kidney (**Fig. 34.1**). These fluxes are regulated by two systemic hormones, parathyroid hormone (PTH) and 1,25-dihydroxyvitamin D. In turn, the production of these hormones by their corresponding cells of origin is regulated either directly or indirectly by changes in the extracellular calcium, so that they all form long negative-feedback loops (**Table 34.1**).

Calcium is one of the most carefully controlled variables in the body. Although the long negative-feedback loops appear to overlap and are therefore redundant, they are probably necessary for such tight control of extracellular fluid calcium. Careful regulation of the latter is necessary for a whole range of cellular functions. Small changes in extracellular fluid calcium have major effects on neuromuscular function, and the symptoms and signs of hypercalcemia and hypocalcemia are accompanied by changes in both central and peripheral neuronal function.

The distribution of calcium in the body is important in considerations of calcium homeostasis. Of all the calcium in the body, 99% is stored in the skeleton (approximately 1.0kg). Calcium, however, is also present in extracellular fluid (approximately 1mmol/L) and intracellularly (about 100nmol/L). Small changes in intracellular calcium have major effects on cell function. Within cells, calcium is bound to a number of proteins. When calcium is bound to proteins it may change their conformation and, as a consequence, their function. Changes in protein conformation lead to changes in cell activation and subsequent cell function.

The extracellular fluid calcium is controlled not only by the homeostatic mechanisms are mediated by long negative-feedback loops but also by a complex blood–bone exchange system that is still poorly understood. Bones contain a specialized fluid, which has a different ionic composition to that of extracellular fluid. This specialized bone fluid, which can be considered to be similar to cerebrospinal fluid, is separated from extracellular fluid by a metabolically active membrane, probably comprising the 'bone-lining' cells that cover bone surfaces. The extracellular fluid is supersaturated with respect to the calcium concentration in the bone fluid and at the bone surface. Small changes in extracellular fluid calcium can be modified by the bone surface taking up this calcium. The bone membrane functions as a barrier to keep calcium out of the bone fluid and in the extracellular fluid.

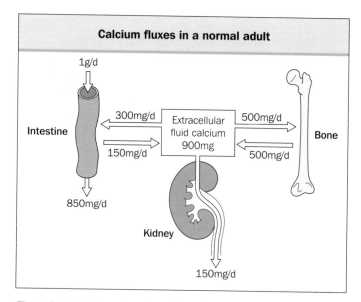

Figure 34.1 Calcium fluxes in a normal adult. The figure shows the calcium fluxes occur between the extracellular fluid and gut, and between the kidney and bone, in a normal adult in zero calcium balance. Note that net calcium absorption (150mg/d) is equal to calcium losses in the urine.

Hormonal regulation of calcium homeostasis

Hormone	Effect	Control
PTH	Calcium ↑ Phosphate ↓	Calcium ions ↓
Calcitonin	Calcium ↓ Phosphate ↓	Calcium ions ↑ Gastrin
Vitamin D metabolites	Calcium ↑ Phosphate ↑	Phosphate ↓ PTH ↑

Table 34.1 Hormonal regulation of calcium homeostasis.

Parathyroid hormone

Parathyroid hormone is a single-gene polypeptide of 84 amino acids and is synthesized by the chief cells of the parathyroid gland. Its synthesis and secretion are primarily controlled by the concentrations of ionized calcium in the extracellular fluid. An inverse relationship exists between the extracellular fluid calcium concentration and PTH synthesis and secretion

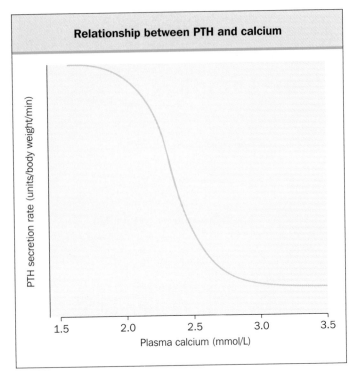

Relationship between PTH and calcium

Figure 34.2 Relationship between parathyroid hormone (PTH) and calcium. There is an inverse relationship between PTH secretion rate and plasma calcium. Note that PTH secretion is not completely suppressible by extracellular calcium.

(Fig. 34.2). As the extracellular fluid calcium concentration decreases, there is an increase in PTH synthesis and secretion. The first 34 amino acids from the amino-terminal part of the molecule are responsible for the biologic effects of PTH and for the binding of PTH to its receptor.

The overall effects of PTH are to increase the extracellular fluid calcium concentration and decrease the extracellular fluid phosphate concentration. It increases reabsorption of calcium in renal tubules, inhibits phosphate reabsorption in renal tubules, and increases bone resorption. In addition, it indirectly increases the absorption of calcium and phosphate from the gastrointestinal tract by its effect of increasing the metabolism of vitamin D precursors – forming the highly active 1,25-dihydroxyvitamin D – in the proximal tubules of the kidney. PTH also activates osteoclastic bone resorption acutely, and over the longer term, stimulates new bone formation. Since the acute effects of PTH favor bone resorption, short-term PTH elevations add calcium to the extracellular fluid from bone. PTH exerts its effects on its target cells both by increasing intracellular cyclic adenosine monophosphate (cAMP), and by increasing intracellular calcium. The cell-surface receptor for PTH has recently been identified and molecularly cloned.

Calcitonin

Calcitonin is a 32 amino-acid peptide that is synthesized and secreted by the parafollicular cells of the thyroid gland. Its synthesis and secretion are controlled by extracellular fluid calcium concentrations and also by hormones from the gastrointestinal tract, predominantly gastrin. The major biologic effect of calcitonin is to inhibit transiently osteoclastic bone resorption, and it does this by inhibiting the formation and activity of bone-resorbing osteoclasts. Calcitonin mediates its effects on target cells by increasing intracellular cAMP. The cell-surface receptor for calcitonin has recently been identified and, surprisingly, seems to be closely related in structure to the PTH receptor. While acute and large doses of calcitonin do influence bone resorption, the precise role of calcitonin in humans is uncertain, since absence (thyroidectomy) or excess (certain thyroid cancers) has no evident effect on serum calcium or the skeleton.

1,25-dihydroxyvitamin D

1,25-dihydroxyvitamin D is the major biologically active metabolite of the vitamin D sterol family. Vitamin D precursor (7-dehydrocholesterol) is either ingested in the diet or synthesized in the skin to form hydroxylated metabolites that are hydroxylated in the liver and kidney to form 1,25-dihydroxyvitamin D. The renal 1-hydroxylase enzyme system is under the control of ambient phosphate concentrations, circulating PTH concentrations, calcium concentrations, and other mechanisms, possibly including circulating sex hormones and prolactin levels. PTH and the ambient phosphate concentration appear to be the primary regulators. The 1-hydroxylase enzyme is present in the proximal tubules of the kidney and is a complex cytochrome P_{450} mitochondrial enzyme system.

1,25-dihydroxyvitamin D increases plasma calcium and phosphate concentrations by increasing the absorption of calcium and phosphate from the gastrointestinal tract. It also increases bone resorption and enhances the capacity for PTH to promote renal tubular calcium reabsorption in the renal tubules. It is a powerful differentiation agent for committed osteoclast precursors, causing their maturation to form multinucleated cells that are capable of resorbing bone. By these actions, 1,25-dihydroxyvitamin D provides a supply of calcium and phosphate available at bone surfaces for the formation of normal mineralized bone. Absence of 1,25-dihydroxyvitamin D leads to hypocalcemia, and to rickets or osteomalacia, bone disorders that are characterized by impaired mineralization of the newly formed proteinaceous bone matrix.

Defenses against hypercalcemia and hypocalcemia

The homeostatic response to increased plasma calcium concentration is controlled predominantly by PTH and 1,25-dihydroxyvitamin D. PTH is most important for short-term regulation of extracellular fluid calcium, and 1,25-dihydroxyvitamin D for more long-term responses. PTH has major effects on the kidney to promote renal tubular calcium reabsorption, and on bone to stimulate bone resorption. 1,25-dihydroxyvitamin D works on the gastrointestinal tract to increase calcium absorption and thereby protect against hypocalcemia. The defenses against hypercalcemia and hypocalcemia are described in **Table 34.2**.

BONE REMODELING AND CHANGES WITH AGE

Types of bone

There are two types of bone; cortical (or compact) and trabecular (or cancellous). Cortical bone is present in long bone shafts of the appendicular skeleton, while trabecular or cancellous bone makes up the flat plates of bone that crisscross the marrow cavity. The latter type of bone is in intimate contact with the

Table 34.2 Defenses against hypocalcemia and hypercalcemia.
PTH, parathyroid hormone.

Defenses against hypocalcemia and hypercalcemia

Protection against decreases in plasma calcium (e.g. dietary deficiency, hormonal deficiency)

Glomerular filtration	Filtration load of calcium decreases with reduced serum calcium
Renal tubules	Hypocalcemia stimulates PTH release, which increases calcium resorption
Gastrointestinal tract	Increased PTH leads to a rise in 1,25-dihydroxyvitamin D, which increases fractional absorption of dietary calcium
Skeletal system	Acute rise in PTH leads to acute rise in osteoclast activity and net entry of calcium into extracellular fluid

Protection against increases in plasma calcium (caused by bone destruction, large dietary calcium load)

Glomerular filtration	Filtration load of calcium increases with increased serum calcium
Renal tubules	PTH suppressed, tubular resorption of calcium decreased
Gastrointestinal tract	Decreased PTH; therefore 1,25-dihydroxyvitamin D suppressed and calcium absorption decreased
Skeletal system	Acute decrease in PTH leads to acute rise in osteoclastic activity with unopposed bone formation leading to net loss of calcium from the extracellular fluid into bone

cells of the marrow cavity and is probably metabolically regulated by these cells and their products. The axial skeleton, the vertebrae, and the ends of long bones are rich in trabecular bone. The skeleton is made up of 80% cortical bone and 20% trabecular bone.

Bone turnover

Bone is cellularly and metabolically active. The cells in bone are present on endosteal surfaces of cancellous bone adjacent to the marrow cavity, and within channels that tunnel through cortical bone known as the haversian systems. These cells are continually restructuring the skeleton. The bone restructuring or remodeling occurs in discrete packets known as bone-remodeling units. The cells involved in the remodeling of bone are osteoclasts and osteoblasts. Osteoclasts are large multinucleated cells that are responsible for breaking down bone, and osteoblasts are small cuboidal cells that are responsible for synthesizing new bone and then mineralizing it. Osteoclasts are unique cells: they are the only cells in the body known to have the capability of resorbing bone.

Bone is remodeled by a specific sequence of cellular events, which always begins with osteoclastic bone resorption, followed by new bone formation (**Fig. 34.3**). This occurs both within the haversian systems and on trabecular bone surfaces. The cellular events are always the same, commencing with osteoclastic resorption and concluding with new bone formation. The bone that is removed by the activity of the osteoclasts is precisely replaced in normal health by the activity of osteoblasts. Thus, there is a balance in normal health between the processes of bone resorption and bone formation.

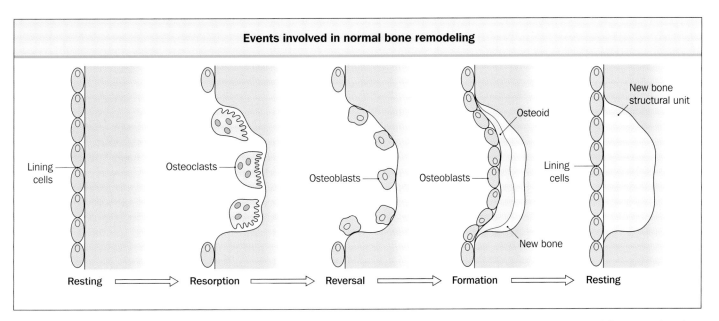

Figure 34.3 Events involved in normal bone remodeling. The figure shows the sequence of events involved in normal bone remodeling on a trabecular bone surface. These remodeling events occur in discrete packets throughout the skeleton, known as bone-remodeling units.

Control of bone turnover

The activity of osteoclasts and osteoblasts is under the control of systemic hormones and local factors. Systemic hormones that control osteoclastic activity are PTH and 1,25-dihydroxyvitamin D. PTH and 1,25-dihydroxyvitamin D stimulate osteoclasts to resorb bone. Local factors produced by bone cells and by immune cells in the marrow cavity are also capable of stimulating osteoclasts; these include cytokines such as interleukin-1 (IL-1), tumor necrosis factor (TNF), and interleukin-6 (IL-6). The activity of osteoblasts is also regulated by factors that stimulate the activity of osteoclasts. The major factors that stimulate osteoblasts to make new bone, however, may be peptide growth factors, which are actually stored within the bone matrix and released as a consequence of bone resorption. These peptide growth factors include transforming growth factor-α (TGFα), the bone morphogenic proteins, and the insulin-like growth factors.

The cellular events of bone remodeling are highly coordinated so that a balance always exists under normal circumstances between the processes of bone formation and bone resorption. When an imbalance occurs between bone formation and bone resorption, such as with aging, osteoporosis, immobilization, and other disorders there is usually more bone lost by the activity of osteoclasts than can be replaced by the activity of osteoblasts.

Changes with age

There are alterations in the rates of bone resorption and bone formation at different stages during life (**Fig. 34.4**). During adolescence, bone formation is relatively greater than bone resorption so that there is an increase in skeletal mass. In young adult life there is a perfect balance between bone resorption and bone formation, and skeletal mass remains constant. After the middle of the third decade, however, there is usually an increase in bone resorption relative to bone formation and bone is progressively lost. In women there is an additional marked acceleration of bone loss at the time of the menopause, which lasts for a period of 10 years. This accelerated phase of bone loss is due to an increase in bone resorption and occurs as a consequence of the effects of withdrawal of estrogen: estrogen deficiency leads to increased bone resorption. In later life, decreased osteoblast activity occurs in men and women, and further progressive decrease in bone formation is seen in advanced age in both sexes. The decline in bone mass that occurs in men and women, but is more pronounced in women, makes the skeleton more fragile in the elderly and is the reason why older people develop fractures of susceptible bones following trivial injuries – a condition known as osteoporosis.

Bone remodeling

Bone physiologists have argued for many years over the primary function of bone remodeling; it may serve a number of purposes. Bone remodeling is presumably necessary to preserve the structural integrity of the skeleton by continually replacing it. It also plays a minor role in calcium homeostasis, since the skeleton is the source of most of the calcium in the body, and bone resorption releases calcium into the extracellular fluid. The skeleton is also a storehouse for minerals and buffers, which may be released when bone is resorbed. This may be important in the maintenance of the acid–base balance, and also

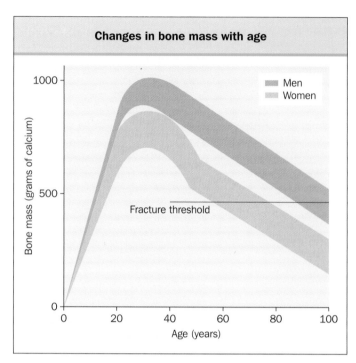

Figure 34.4 Changes in bone mass with age. Note that bone mass increases during growth and adolescence and declines progressively after mid-adult life. Acceleration of bone loss occurs in women for 10 years after menopause.

in supplying minerals such as magnesium and phosphate to the extracellular fluid at times of need.

HYPERCALCEMIA

Hypercalcemia occurs when the total serum calcium, corrected for changes in plasma protein, is >2.55mmol/L (10.2mg/dL). This is now a very common clinical finding, since measurements of total serum calcium have become routine in most patients in whom blood is drawn. Hypercalcemia always indicates serious underlying pathology and should be evaluated carefully. The two most common causes are primary hyperparathyroidism and malignant disease (**Table 34.3**).

Causes

Hypercalcemia occurs when the complex homeostatic mechanism that is responsible for maintaining normal extracellular fluid calcium concentrations is overwhelmed. It usually involves an increase in entry of calcium into the extracellular fluid from two of the major organ systems that control calcium homeostasis. For example, in primary hyperparathyroidism there is an increase in renal tubular calcium reabsorption, an increase in bone resorption, and an increase in calcium absorption from the gastrointestinal tract. There is a marked increase in bone resorption in many patients with malignant disease, together with an increase in renal tubular calcium reabsorption. Since the homeostatic mechanism is so efficient under normal circumstances, hypercalcemia occurs only when there are profound abnormalities in calcium fluxes, and always means severe underlying pathology.

Clinical features

The clinical features of hypercalcemia are listed in **Table 34.4**; they vary considerably from patient to patient and are related both to the absolute concentration of serum calcium and to the rate of rise in serum calcium. In patients who are older, or when serum calcium rises abruptly, symptoms of hypercalcemia may be prominent with relatively small increases in serum calcium concentrations.

Primary hyperparathyroidism

Primary hyperparathyroidism is the most common cause of hypercalcemia; it is responsible for more than 50% of all cases but is more common in the ambulant or outpatient population than it is in the hospitalized patient population. The annual incidence rate is between 50 and 250:1,000,000 population per year. It is most common in elderly female patients, although it can occur at any age.

Pathology

There are three causes of primary hyperparathyroidism. Some 85% of patients have a single benign adenoma of one of the four parathyroid glands. Most of the remainder have hyperplasia of four parathyroid glands. This occurs more commonly in patients with familial hyperparathyroidism syndromes, and particularly in patients with multiple endocrine neoplasia (MEN). Less than 1% of all patients have a carcinoma of one of the four parathyroid glands.

Pathophysiology

In patients with primary hyperparathyroidism, the inverse relationship between serum PTH (and parathyroid cell number) and serum calcium still exists, although the relationship is altered and occurs at a different level of serum calcium. In other words, PTH secretion can be suppressed or kept constant by an increase in extracellular fluid calcium concentration above a critical level, although the sensitivity of the parathyroid glands to changes in serum calcium is altered and set at a different level. This occurs in the majority of patients with parathyroid gland adenomas. In patients with parathyroid hyperplasia, the set point for PTH release may be normal but the mass of parathyroid tissue is increased and so the result is a relatively greater circulating PTH concentration for any serum calcium concentration.

Etiology

The cause of primary hyperparathyroidism is unknown. Since this condition is not one pathologic entity but involves at least two and possibly more conditions, the heterogeneity of pathology probably means heterogeneity of causes. Recent data suggest that in most patients with parathyroid adenomas, there is a monoclonal disorder that arises from an abnormality within a single cell. Activating mutations in cell-cycle genes and inactivating mutations in tumor suppressor genes have been identified in some parathyroid adenomas. However, four-gland hyperplasia may be a polyclonal disorder caused by an external stimulus to parathyroid cell growth, as well as PTH synthesis and secretion.

Another factor that has been implicated in the pathophysiology of primary hyperparathyroidism is external irradiation, since there is some evidence that patients with a history of neck irradiation may be predisposed to the condition.

Biochemical effects

The biochemical effects of primary hyperparathyroidism are depicted in **Table 34.5**. These characteristics are due to the

Clinical manifestations of hypercalcemia	
Neurological	Lethargy, confusion, irritability, stupor, coma
Psychiatric	Depression, hallucinations
Gastrointestinal	Anorexia, nausea, vomiting, constipation
Cardiovascular	Increased myocardial contractility, shortened ventricular systole
Renal	Nephrogenic diabetes insipidus, impaired glomerular filtration, nephrocalcinosis, nephrolithiasis

Table 34.4 Clinical manifestations of hypercalcemia.

Causes of hypercalcemia	
Primary hyperparathyroidism	
Malignant disease	Cancer with bone metastases
	Cancer without bone metastases
	Multiple myeloma
Thyrotoxicosis	
Paget's disease with immobilization	
Immobilization, e.g. spinal cord injury	
Vitamin A intoxication	
Vitamin D intoxication	
Milk–alkali syndrome	
Sarcoidosis and other granulomatous disease (tuberculosis, berylliosis)	
Idiopathic hypercalcemia of infancy	
Hypercalciuria	
Familial hypercalcemia	
Thiazide diuretics	
Diuretic phase of acute renal failure	
Addison's disease	

Table 34.3 Causes of hypercalcemia.

Biochemical effects of PTH excess on calcium homeostasis	
Serum	Urine
Parathyroid hormone ↑	Calcium ↑
Calcium ↑	Phosphorus ↑
Phosphorus ↓	Cyclic adenosine monophosphate ↑
Alkaline phosphatase ↑	
Chloride ↑	
Bicarbonate ↓	

Table 34.5 Biochemical effects of parathyroid hormone excess.

effects of PTH on target cells and on serum calcium and phosphate homeostasis. The characteristic abnormalities are an increase in serum calcium, a decrease in serum phosphate, and an increase in urine calcium.

Clinical features

There has been a changing pattern of presentation of primary hyperparathyroidism in the past 20 years. Original descriptions of the disease suggested that it was a disease of 'bones and stones and abnormal groans associated with psychologic moans'. Modern presentation has been influenced by the advent of the autoanalyser and by routine measurements of serum calcium. Most patients are now diagnosed when they are still asymptomatic, as measurement of serum calcium is routinely carried out in patients who have blood drawn for almost any reason. This has also meant a change in the age and sex incidence. Although primary hyperparathyroidism can occur at any age, it is now most commonly seen in elderly women, the same group of patients who are subject to postmenopausal osteoporosis.

In the past, primary hyperparathyroidism was characterized by presentation with recurrent renal stones due to hypercalciuria, associated with polyuria that occurred as a result of loss of the concentrating ability of the kidney. Some patients developed a peculiar type of bone disease known as osteitis fibrosa, characterized by increased generalized osteoclastic bone resorption, particularly involving the phalanges (causing subperiosteal resorption; **Fig. 34.5**) and the skull (causing the radiologic appearance known as 'salt and pepper' skull; see Chapter 41). This presentation is rarely seen nowadays. Some patients develop a proximal myopathy, and many patients complain of anorexia, nausea, and vomiting due to hypercalcemia, associated with constipation. Acute pancreatitis is seen in some patients, and it has long been debated whether or not the disease is associated with peptic ulceration and with hypertension.

In a small number of patients, primary hyperparathyroidism is associated with other endocrine syndromes. This occurs in two familial syndromes, multiple endocrine neoplasia (MEN) type 1 and MEN type 2. The former type is associated with hypersecretion of hormones of the pituitary (growth hormone or prolactin, usually), islet cells of the pancreas (usually insulin or gastrin secreting), and the parathyroids. MEN1 is due to mutations in the menin gene. In MEN2, patients develop medullary carcinoma of the thyroid associated with pheochromocytoma. MEN2 is caused by mutations in the *ret* proto-oncogene. Primary hyperparathyroidism occurs in a minority of patients. Both these MEN syndromes are inherited as autosomal-dominant conditions but hyperparathyroidism is not expressed in either before the age of 10.

Diagnosis

The diagnosis of primary hyperparathyroidism is best made by consideration of the natural history (most patients will be found to have been hypercalcemic for more than 1 year if records are available) and by measurement of immunoreactive PTH. With improvements in the PTH assay and the availability of two-site assays (using antibodies directed at two different sites of the PTH molecule), intact PTH can be measured accurately and, in the majority of patients with primary hyperparathyroidism, the diagnosis can be made with certainty as long as renal failure is not present. Other characteristic features of primary

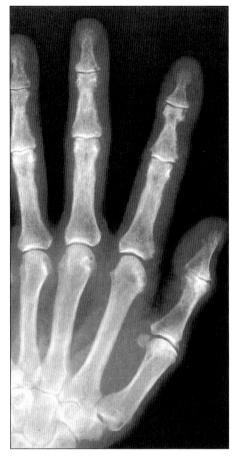

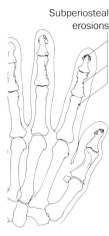

Subperiosteal erosions

Figure 34.5 A hand radiograph in primary hyperparathyroidism. Note the subperiosteal erosions, which are more prominent along the radial border of the phalanges.

hyperparathyroidism that help distinguish it from other types of hypercalcemia include:

- measurements of serum chloride (most patients have mild hyperchloremic acidosis);
- serum phosphate (patients are hypophosphatemic due to renal phosphate wasting);
- urinary cAMP (patients may have increased urinary cAMP because of the effects of PTH on the renal tubules);
- serum 1,25-dihydroxyvitamin D (often found to be normal or slightly elevated in patients);
- urinary calcium excretion (calcium excretion is usually mildly to moderately increased due to an increased filtered load of calcium, despite the effects of PTH to promote renal tubular calcium reabsorption).

Differential diagnosis

The differential diagnosis of hypercalcemia involves the consideration of all other causes of hypercalcemia. In patients who are normocalcemic but present with recurrent renal stones, other causes of recurrent renal stones (such as idiopathic hypercalciuria, oxaluria, urate stones, or cystinuria) should be considered. In patients who present with osteopenia, osteoporosis, osteomalacia, and malignant disease (most notably myeloma) should be excluded.

Management

Most patients with primary hyperparathyroidism are best treated by surgery. If the condition is due to a solitary adenoma,

Malignancies associated with hypercalcemia	
Site	Frequency (%)
Lung	35
Breast	25
Blood (myeloma, lymphoma)	14
Head and neck	6
Renal	3
Prostate	3
Unknown primary	7
Others	7

Table 34.6 Malignancies associated with hypercalcemia. The relative frequencies of different malignancies as causes of hypercalcemia of malignancy are listed.

this should be excised. If the condition is due to four-gland hyperplasia, surgeons remove three-and-a-half parathyroid glands. In patients in whom surgery is contraindicated, medical therapy for hypercalcemia may be necessary if the patient is symptomatic. In many patients who are asymptomatic, and whose serum calcium concentration is only marginally elevated, active therapy may not be indicated.

Other causes of hypercalcemia
Hypercalcemia of malignancy
Hypercalcemia of malignancy is the most common cause of hypercalcemia in hospitalized patients. It is one of the most common paraneoplastic syndromes associated with cancer and is particularly common in patients with breast cancer (30%), lung cancer (15–20%), and myeloma (25%). The relative frequency of different types of malignancy associated with hypercalcemia is shown in **Table 34.6**.

Several mechanisms are responsible for hypercalcemia of malignancy, other than the condition being secondary to multiple lytic secondary deposits (**Fig. 34.6**). In some patients, it is due to one or more factors that are secreted directly by the tumor cells, which are responsible for disrupted calcium homeostasis. One of the most commonly implicated factors is a peptide hormone related to PTH, which is secreted by many squamous cell carcinomas, binds to the PTH receptor, and shares all of the known effects of PTH, on its target organs. This factor is known as PTH-related protein (PTHrP). PTHrP is normally a local autocrine or paracrine factor that regulates growth, cell turnover, differentiation and development in many organs but does not normally enter the systemic circulation. In some patients, hypercalcemia is due caused by local factors that are produced by tumor cells in the bone environment which stimulate osteoclasts. These factors include IL-1, TGF, PTHrP and TNF. In patients with

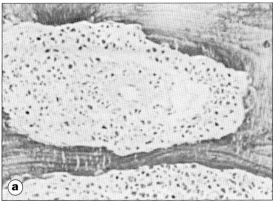
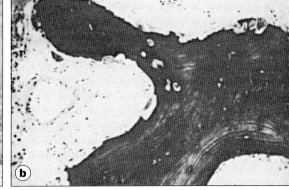
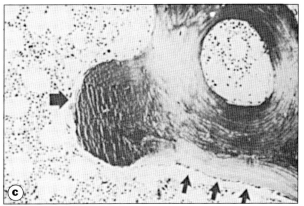

Figure 34.6 Bone biopsy micrographs in hypercalcemia. (a) Local osteolytic hypercalcemia secondary to leukemia. There are leukemic cells in the marrow space and numerous osteoclasts lining the trabecular surface. (With permission from Stewart AF. Parathyroid gland, calciotropic hormones and bone metabolism. In: DeGroot LJ, Jameson JL, eds. Endocrinology, 4th edn. Philadelphia, PA:WB Saunders; 2001:1094.) (b) Hypercalcemia of malignancy secondary to squamous cell carcinoma. There is no tumor in the marrow spaces but numerous active osteoclasts on the trabecular surface; note also the absence of osteoblasts and osteoid. (c) Hyperparathyroidism. Note the abundant osteoclasts (large arrow), osteoblasts (small arrows) and osteoid. (Panels (b) and (c) with permission from Stewart AF, Vignery A, Silverate A, et al. Quantitative bone histomorphometry in humoral hypercalcemia of malignancy: uncoupling of bone cell activity. J Clin Endocrinol Metab. 55:219–27 © 1982 The Endocrine Society.)

myeloma, the myeloma cells secrete osteoclast-activating factors, which are responsible for osteoclast activation. In all patients with hypercalcemia of malignancy, there is an increase in osteoclastic bone resorption and in many there is also an increase in renal tubular calcium reabsorption. Medical therapy is therefore aimed at inhibiting bone resorption and promoting renal calcium excretion.

Sarcoidosis

In sarcoidosis and granulomatous disorders such as histoplasmosis, hypercalcemia occurs together with hyperphosphatemia and impaired renal function, and is responsive to glucocorticoid therapy. Patients have increased plasma 1,25-dihydroxyvitamin D concentrations but normal 25-hydroxyvitamin D concentrations. A likely explanation for these findings is increased 1-hydroxylase activity in the sarcoid granulomas.

Familial hypocalciuric hypercalcemia

Familial hypocalciuric hypercalcemia is an autosomal dominant condition that is frequently found in patients with a history of unsuccessful surgery for primary hyperparathyroidism. This disorder results from activating mutations in the calcium-sensing receptor (see Chapter 30) The characteristics of this condition are a family history in siblings or offspring, low renal excretion of calcium (<100mg/24h up to 2.5mmol/24h) and magnesium, and usually little or no symptomatology. This condition is also referred to as familial benign hypercalcemia. Patients need to be identified, since they have a very poor response to parathyroidectomy. Unlike familial forms of primary hyperparathyroidism, hypercalcemia and hypocalciuria are present from the neonatal period. In contrast, primary hyperparathyroidism associated with MEN syndromes is rarely evident before the age of 10.

Treatment of hypercalcemia

Hypercalcemia of malignancy should be treated by vigorous intravenous hydration with normal saline to ensure that deficits in extracellular fluid volume are corrected. In addition, drug therapy to inhibit osteoclastic bone resorption should be instituted. Currently, the most effective forms of therapy are the new-generation bisphosphonates. These are very effective inhibitors of osteoclastic bone resorption and are successful in the majority of patients. Other forms of calcium-lowering therapy include plicamycin (mithramycin), which is efficacious but more toxic than the bisphosphonates, calcitonin, and corticosteroids (which are most likely to be effective in myeloma). Therapies available for hypercalcemia of malignancy are listed in **Table 34.7**.

HYPOCALCEMIA

Causes

The causes of hypocalcemia are listed in **Table 34.8**; these include hyperparathyroidism, which is associated with decreased PTH secretion from the parathyroid glands as a result of disease or surgical damage to the parathyroids. Pseudohypoparathyroidism is an interesting condition in which there is decreased PTH effectiveness on peripheral tissues because of peripheral tissue resistance. One of the mechanisms for this increase in peripheral tissue resistance may be related to loss of an essential component of the PTH-receptor–adenylate-cyclase complex in the cell membrane (the G-protein or nucleotide regulatory unit). Patients with pseudohypoparathyroidism also have somatic features such as short stature, a short fourth metacarpal, and obesity (**Fig. 34.7**). They show no renal response to exogenous PTH administration, unlike normal individuals or patients with primary hyperparathyroidism, who respond to PTH with increased cAMP excretion and phosphate excretion.

Hypocalcemia also occurs in renal failure, where it is due to 1,25-dihydroxyvitamin D deficiency and phosphate retention, both of which lower serum calcium. Hypocalcemia occurs in magnesium depletion for several reasons: it can be caused by the effects of magnesium deficiency impairing peripheral effects of PTH, and by a decrease in the release of PTH from the parathyroid glands, which may be the most important reason. Patients with hypocalcemia due to magnesium depletion cannot be adequately treated until the magnesium deficiency is corrected.

Patients with acute pancreatitis become hypocalcemic for multiple reasons, the most important of which is the formation of free-fatty-acid–calcium soaps within the peritoneum and retroperitoneum.

Therapy for hypercalcemia of malignancy

Ablation of tumor

Intravenous saline

Furosemide (frusemide)

Bisphosphonates

Calcitonin/glucocorticoids

Plicamycin (mithramycin)

Oral phosphate (with caution)

Table 34.7 Therapy for hypercalcemia of malignancy.

Causes of hypocalcemia

Hypoparathyroidism	Idiopathic
	Postsurgical
Pseudohypoparathyroidism	
Hypocalcemia associated with osteoblastic bone metastases	
Hypomagnesemia	
Toxic shock syndrome	
Neonatal	
Acute pancreatitis	
Renal failure	
Vitamin D deficiency	Dietary
	Malabsorption
	Anticonvulsant therapy
	Chronic liver disease
	Chronic renal disease
	Vitamin-D-dependent rickets

Table 34.8 Causes of hypocalcemia.

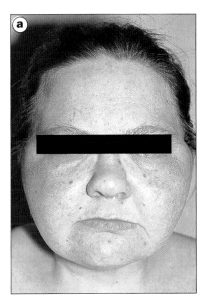

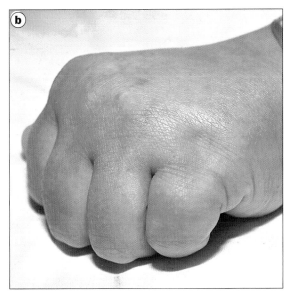

Figure 34.7 A patient with pseudohypoparathyroidism.
(a) Typical round facies characteristic of pseudohypoparathyroidism.
(b) A dimpled knuckle as a result of a shortened fifth metacarpal.

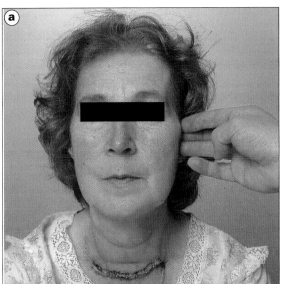

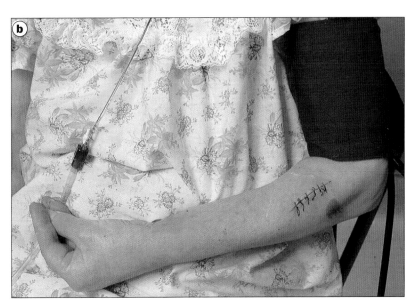

Figure 34.8 The clinical signs of hypocalcemia. (a) Chvostek's sign is elicited by tapping over the facial nerve, producing a contraction of the upper lip muscles. (b) Trousseau's sign is produced when a sphygmomanometer cuff is inflated to above systolic pressure for up to 3min. This patient had four-gland hyperplasia and developed transient postoperative hypocalcemia. All four glands were removed, and pieces from one were autotransplanted into the forearm. The site of the transplantation can be seen clearly.

The vitamin D deficiency syndromes are considered below. Vitamin D deficiency leads to decreased absorption of calcium from the gut, which is responsible for hypocalcemia.

Clinical features

Hypocalcemia is characterized by changes in neuromuscular function. The most common symptoms are paresthesias around the mouth and in the fingers, muscle cramps and seizures. Tetany (involuntary muscle contraction) may occur in the hands, producing the *main d'accoucheur* (obstetrician's hand) or carpopedal spasm. Chronic hypocalcemia causes cataracts and calcification of the basal ganglia of the brain.

Incipient tetany can be predicted by Chvostek's sign. Chvostek's sign is a twitch of the perioral muscle elicited by

tapping the facial nerve immediately after it exits from the auditory canal. Tetany can also be anticipated by Trousseau's sign. To perform this, a blood-pressure cuff is maintained for 3 min at 10mmHg above the systolic pressure. Spasmodic contraction of the small muscles of the hand (carpopedal spasm) occurs in patients with Trousseau's sign. Chvostek's and Trousseau's clinical signs are depicted in **Figure 34.8**.

Diagnosis

The diagnosis of hypocalcemia is usually achieved by careful consideration of the clinical setting, and measurements of serum calcium, magnesium, albumin, ionized calcium, and, where warranted, vitamin D metabolites and circulating PTH concentrations. In patients with suspected pseudohypoparathyroidism,

Treatment of hypocalcemia	
Chronic	Vitamin D metabolite
	Oral calcium
	Parathyroid gland autotransplantation (postoperatively) in a patient with parathyroid gland hyperplasia
Urgent	Intravenous calcium
	Short-acting vitamin D metabolite

Table 34.9 Treatment of hypocalcemia.

measurement of plasma PTH is very useful and has, in most cases, replaced the measurement of responses of target organs to a PTH infusion or injection. Plasma PTH is elevated in pseudohypoparathyroidism.

Treatment

Successful treatment of hypocalcemia (**Table 34.9**) usually requires calcium administered orally or intravenously, depending on the urgency of obtaining a rapid response, and by treatment with a short-acting vitamin D metabolite, most frequently 1,25-dihydroxyvitamin D.

OSTEOPOROSIS

Before discussing osteoporosis, this bone disease will be placed in context with other bone diseases in the aging population that may be confused with osteoporosis and present a similar clinical and radiologic picture. In most cases, osteopenia will be due to osteoporosis. A similar radiologic picture of osteopenia, however, can be produced by osteomalacia, osteitis fibrosa cystica (the bone disease sometimes associated with primary hyperparathyroidism), and the osteopenia associated with myeloma and other malignant diseases.

Osteoporosis is by far the most important of these conditions and affects between 5% and 10% of the population of Western countries. It is between five and eight times as common in women as it is in men, and represents a major public health problem. An estimated 250,000 hip fractures and 500,000 vertebral fractures in the USA each year are attributed to osteoporosis, and the prevalence is rising as the population ages. Hip fracture is the most serious complication since it is a major cause of morbidity and often of mortality in the elderly.

Definition

Osteoporosis is characterized by decreased trabecular bone mass in which both the mineral and the matrix are decreased to the same extent but there is no gross abnormality of bone composition. Although cortical bone is also affected, trabecular bone loss is most striking. Subtle chemical defects in mineral or matrix (bone proteins such as type I collagen) may exist in some patients. This disease accounts for more than 90% of patients with osteopenia.

Classification

There are several different classifications for osteoporosis. For many years it has been separated into primary osteoporosis, in which osteoporosis occurs without association with other diseases, and secondary osteoporosis, which occurs in association with other conditions (**Table 34.10**). A separate classification has been proposed in which primary osteoporosis is subdivided into type I (postmenopausal) and type II (senile). The type I variant predominantly involves trabecular bone, occurs at an earlier age, is much more frequent in women, and is often complicated by vertebral fractures. The type II variant occurs in men and women, is more common in the older age group, and is often complicated by hip fractures. Some workers have suggested that different pathogenic events may be involved in these two forms. Type I may be due primarily to estrogen deficiency, whereas type II may be due to a combination of impaired calcium absorption from the gut and impaired osteoblast function.

Table 34.10 Classification of osteoporosis.

Classification of osteoporosis	
Primary: without associated diseases	Senile or postmenopausal (involutional) (95% of all patients, most frequent in elderly white women)
	Idiopathic (occurring in middle age)
	Juvenile (occurring during adolescence or 20s)
Secondary: associated with other conditions	Cushing's syndrome
	Chronic liver disease
	Turner's syndrome
	Immobilization
	Heparin therapy
	Alcoholism
	Diabetes mellitus
	Malabsorption
	Osteogenesis imperfecta
	Pregnancy and lactation
	Elite female athletes
	Anorexia nervosa

Risk factors for osteoporosis

Female sex

Menopause

Genetics/family history

Race – Blacks and Mexican Americans are protected

Diet – calcium deficiency, phosphate and protein excess

Smoking – Smokers are leaner and have a lower bone mass

Alcohol – alcoholics have less bone than corresponding nondrinking controls

Inactivity

Leanness

Diseases associated with secondary osteoporosis, such as Cushing's syndrome, previous gastric surgery, and hypogonadism in males; the major risk factors in males may be cigarette smoking, alcohol consumption and leanness, which predisposes men to vertebral fractures

Table 34.11 Risk factors for osteoporosis.

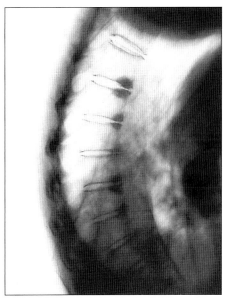
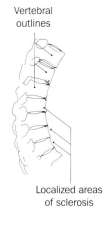

Vertebral outlines

Localized areas of sclerosis

Figure 34.9 Radiographic appearance of osteoporosis. The vertebrae show decreased bone mineral density, and some are clearly compressed.

Risk factors

Since osteoporosis is of such slow onset and is difficult to treat once established, investigators have studied in some detail the risk factors that could predispose patients to later development of the disease. Factors that have been associated with increased risk of later development of osteoporosis are listed in **Table 34.11**.

Clinical features

The clinical features of osteoporosis include pain, which occurs most frequently in association with crush or compression fractures of the lower thoracic, midthoracic, or lumbar spine. Fractures frequently occur spontaneously or with minimal trauma. The most common fractures are those of the vertebral bodies, followed by fractures of the hip. Femoral neck fractures are the most serious because they lead to considerable morbidity and mortality in the elderly population. Other fractures, such as those of the distal forearm following a fall on the outstretched hand, are less common.

The initial compression fractures usually occur in the midthoracic region. As bone is progressively lost, the patient loses height and develops a dorsal kyphosis (hunchback). Compression fractures occur at the lower dorsal–upper lumbar vertebrae. With further bone loss the kyphosis becomes more marked, the lower lumbar vertebrae become compressed as more height is lost, and the thoracic cage may eventually come to rest on the pelvic brim, producing a 'pot-belly' appearance. The radiologic appearance of osteoporosis is shown in **Figure 34.9**.

Abnormalities in calcium homeostasis

There are no detectable abnormalities in calcium or phosphate homeostasis in osteoporosis.

Diagnosis

There have been major advances recently in the development of techniques for monitoring changes in bone mass, and these have received widespread acceptance. The state-of-the-art technique is dual-beam X-ray absorptiometry, in which two X-ray sources are used to allow precise measurements of bone mass in specific and strategic areas of the skeleton, such as the lumbar spine, the neck of the femur, and the forearm bones, or in the total skeleton (**Fig. 34.10**). Other techniques include dual-beam photon absorptiometry, computerized tomography, neutron-activation analysis, skeletal ultrasound, and the previously used method of single-beam photon absorptiometry. These techniques may be used to follow treatment regimens and assess the risk of later development of osteoporosis. Their usefulness is, however, still somewhat controversial.

Treatment

The following approaches have been used in an attempt to increase bone mass in osteoporotic patients.

General symptomatic treatment

Patients with osteoporosis should be advised to avoid alcohol, smoking, caffeine, and a sedentary lifestyle, since all of these factors have been associated with bone loss. Pain should be treated with analgesics. For vertebral fractures, orthopedic support garments, heat, and massage may be helpful. Bed rest should be avoided as far as possible, and patients should be advised to avoid situations where falls are most likely to occur.

Specific medical therapy

Treatment of osteoporosis can be prophylactic treatment or treatment of the established disease. The most useful prophylactic therapy is to avoid risk factors that are associated with osteoporosis where possible: patients at high risk should use estrogen or selective estrogen response modifiers (SERMs) in the years following menopause, unless contraindicated, or an alternative inhibitor of bone resorption such as a bisphosphonate. In patients with established osteoporosis, therapies that are available include drugs that inhibit bone resorption – SERMs, bisphosphonates, calcitonin, and estrogen. All of these drugs are efficacious, although their relative efficacy is fiercely

Dual energy x-ray absorptiometry scan for bone mineral density

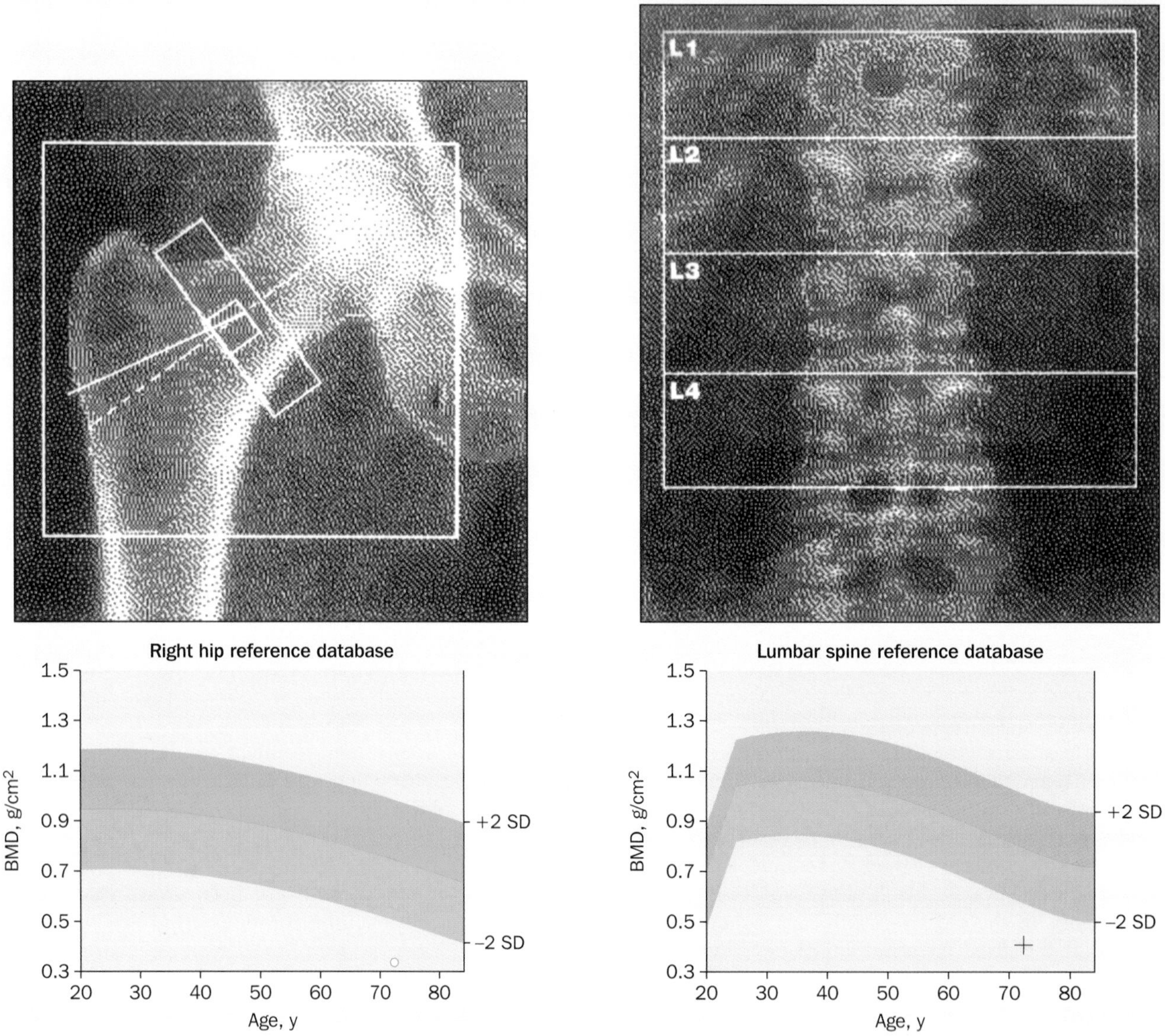

Region	BMD, g/cm²	Peak BMD-Matched T Score	Peak BMD-Matched % of Mean	Age-Matched Z Score	Age-Matched % of Mean
Neck	0.328	–4.69	39	–2.75	52
Trochanter	0.176	–5.22	25	–3.77	32
Intertrochanyeric	0.428	–4.34	39	–2.93	49
Total	0.330	–5.02	35	–3.37	45
Ward Triangle	0.180	–4.74	24	–2.04	43

Region	BMD, g/cm²	Peak BMD-Matched T Score	Peak BMD-Matched % of Mean	Age-Matched Z Score	Age-Matched % of Mean
L1	0.305	–5.63	33	–3.62	43
L2	0.406	–5.66	39	–3.42	52
L3	0.382	–6.38	35	–4.03	46
L4	0.495	–5.65	44	–3.23	58
L1–L4	0.410	–5.79	39	–3.53	51

Figure 34.10 Dual energy x-ray absorptiometry scan for bone mineral density. These two panels are dual energy X-ray absorptiometry (DXA) images, widely used as a measure of bone mineral density (BMD). The panel on the left is a right hip and that on the right is a lumbar spine. The graph in the middle of each panel represents the patient's bone mineral density (the black dot or cross) expressed as a function of the patient's age. The two shaded areas represent two standard deviations (95% confidence limits) above and below the mean age-adjusted BMD. These data are also race and gender adjusted. BMD may be expressed as a 'T-score' in which the patient's BMD is expressed in standard deviation units as compared to peak bone mass, or as a 'Z-score', in which BMD is expressed in standard deviation units above or below age-matched mean BMD. For example, a T-score of –3 means that the patient's BMD at the site in question is three SD below the mean peak BMD in gender and race comparable normals. The bottom table of each panel shows the BMD data expressed per site within the hip or spine, expressed as BMD, T-scores or Z-scores. Osteoporosisis defined variously as having a T-score below –2.0 or –2.5 or greater. (Reproduced with permission from Greenspan SL. A 73-year-old woman with osteoporosis. JAMA 1999;281:1531–40.)

Causes of osteomalacia

Vitamin D deficiency	Dietary lack – rare in industrialized countries because of supplementation of diet with vitamin D; however, may occur in the elderly and alcoholics in association with other mechanisms
	Poor sunlight exposure
	Gut malabsorption (vitamin D is a fat-soluble vitamin) and fat malabsorption (steatorrhea) leads to vitamin D deficiency
	Anticonvulsant therapy (these drugs stimulate liver metabolism of vitamin D to inactive metabolites and cause a decrease in serum 25-hydroxyvitamin D)
	Chronic liver disease, particularly primary biliary cirrhosis
	Chronic renal disease, because of impaired formation of 1,25-dihydroxyvitamin D by the kidneys and because of circulating inhibitors of mineralization found in the uremic state
	Vitamin-D-dependent osteomalacia — Type I – inherited deficiency of the 1-hydroxylase enzyme necessary for conversion of 25-hydroxyvitamin D to 1,25-dihydroxyvitamin D
	— Type II – inherited inability of target organs to respond to vitamin D
Hypophosphatemia	Excess ingestion of aluminum hydroxide gels, which decrease phosphate absorption
	Sex-linked hypophosphatemia (inherited phosphate transport abnormality, with renal phosphate wasting)
	Tumor osteomalacia (some tumors, particularly mesenchymal tumors, produce a humoral factor that causes renal phosphate wasting)
	Other renal tubular disorders, such as Fanconi's syndrome

Table 34.12 Causes of osteomalacia.

debated. Their effects are predominantly on bone resorption. Patients started on long-term glucocorticoid therapy should be cotreated with antiresorptive therapy or a bisphosphonate to prevent development of osteoporosis.

Attempts to stimulate bone formation over prolonged periods in patients with osteoporosis are still experimental. Fluoride increases bone mass, although it may also increase propensity to fracture. Low-dose daily injections of PTH have a marked anabolic effect on the skeleton to increase bone mass. This drug is still investigational.

OSTEOMALACIA

Definition

Osteomalacia is the bone disease that results from impaired mineralization of newly formed bone. The result is excess unmineralized bone matrix (known as osteoid). Osteomalacia is the result of a lack of vitamin D, impairment of vitamin D metabolism, or a lack of calcium or phosphorus at the mineralizing site. Before growth-plate closure, the same condition is referred to as rickets and is characterized by failure of calcification of cartilage at the growth plate (i.e. decreased endochondral ossification). The causes of osteomalacia and rickets are shown in **Table 34.12**.

Pathology

The definitive diagnosis of osteomalacia is made by bone biopsy using undecalcified sections and labeling with tetracycline. A fluorescent antibiotic, tetracycline localizes at sites of mineralization so that, when sequential courses of tetracycline are given before bone biopsy, rates of bone mineralization can be assessed. Other histologic parameters that are quantified in a bone biopsy include the volume of osteoid tissue (i.e. the volume of tissue that is nonmineralized), the relative osteoid surface, and the osteoid seam thickness.

Abnormalities in mineral homeostasis

In the majority of patients with osteomalacia the serum chemistry is abnormal (**Table 34.13**). When there is advanced malabsorption or dietary lack of vitamin D, serum calcium is

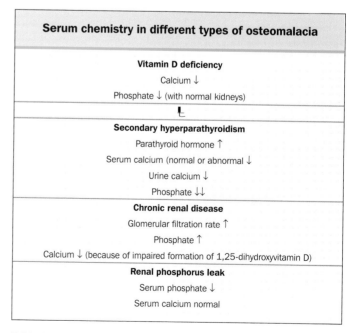

Serum chemistry in different types of osteomalacia

Vitamin D deficiency
Calcium ↓
Phosphate ↓ (with normal kidneys)

Secondary hyperparathyroidism
Parathyroid hormone ↑
Serum calcium (normal or abnormal ↓
Urine calcium ↓
Phosphate ↓↓

Chronic renal disease
Glomerular filtration rate ↑
Phosphate ↑
Calcium ↓ (because of impaired formation of 1,25-dihydroxyvitamin D)

Renal phosphorus leak
Serum phosphate ↓
Serum calcium normal

Table 34.13 Serum chemistry in different types of osteomalacia.

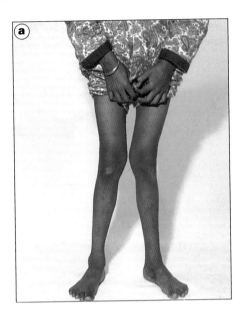

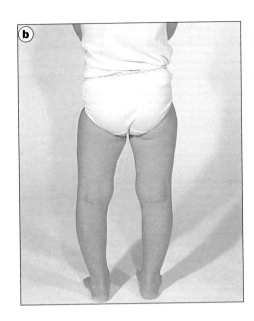

decreased or at the lower limit of normal, serum phosphorus is markedly decreased due to secondary hyperparathyroidism, and urine calcium excretion is also decreased, reflecting a reduced filtered load of calcium and increased tubular calcium reabsorption mediated by PTH. In patients with rickets or osteomalacia caused by chronic renal disease, impairment of glomerular filtration leads to phosphate retention so that serum calcium is low because of impaired formation of 1,25-dihydroxyvitamin D and impaired gut absorption of calcium, but serum phosphorus is high. In patients with rickets or osteomalacia primarily as the result of a renal phosphate leak, serum calcium concentrations may be normal but the serum phosphorus concentration is decreased. A major clue to the presence of osteomalacia or rickets is an elevation in serum alkaline phosphatase.

Clinically, rickets and osteomalacia are characterized by bone pain, occasional fracture, and sometimes deformity, particularly in patients with longstanding osteomalacia resulting from hereditary conditions or chronic renal disease (**Fig. 34.11**). This occurs particularly in children with renal rickets or sex-linked hypophosphatemic rickets, who may have outward bowing of the lower extremities. Patients with osteomalacia also develop muscle weakness and tenderness, particularly affecting the proximal muscles of the lower extremities.

The diagnosis of rickets or osteomalacia may be suspected from the presence of a painful deforming bone disease that is associated with characteristic abnormalities of serum chemistry.

In patients with malabsorption or dietary deficiency of vitamin D, serum 25-hydroxyvitamin D is an important measurement, since it reflects the major transport form of vitamin D in the circulation. It is also a good parameter of gut absorption of vitamin D. X-rays may be characteristic in children with rickets and in some adult patients with osteomalacia who develop pseudofractures. However, pseudofractures are uncommon and, in patients in whom osteomalacia is suspected on clinical or radiologic grounds, it may be necessary to perform a definitive bone biopsy.

Rickets or osteomalacia caused by lack of vitamin D is treated with oral calcium and with vitamin D. The form of vitamin D depends on the nature of defect in vitamin D metabolism. The available vitamin D preparations are shown in **Table 34.14**. Patients with rickets or osteomalacia resulting from hypophosphatemia require oral phosphate and a form of vitamin D, preferably 1,25-dihydroxyvitamin D.

Hypophosphatemic rickets

Hypophosphatemic rickets, also known as phosphate diabetes or vitamin-D-resistant rickets, occurs in two forms, X-linked hypophosphatemic rickets and autosomal dominant hypophosphatemic rickets. These are inherited conditions, in which rickets may develop in early life and is associated with growth retardation and bowing deformities of the legs; it does not respond to vitamin D therapy. Patients have normal serum calcium concentrations with a low serum phosphate concentration

Vitamin D metabolites used in the treatment of hypocalcemia			
Nonproprietary name	Abbreviation	Effective daily dose	Time for reversal of toxic effects (days)
Ergocalciferol	Vitamin D_3	1–10mg	17–60
Calcifediol (calcidiol)	25-$(OH)D_3$	0.05–0.5mg	7–30
Dihydrotachysterol	DHT	0.1–1.0mg	314
Alfacalcidol	1α-$(OH)D_3$	1–2µg	5–10
Calcitriol	1,25-$(OH)_2D_2$	0.5–1.0µg	2–10

Table 34.14 Vitamin D metabolites used in the treatment of hypocalcemia.

due to increased urine phosphate excretion. Serum alkaline phosphatase is usually increased. The plasma 1,25-dihydroxyvitamin D concentration may be decreased or inappropriately normal. (In the presence of hypophosphatemia, it should be increased.) The reason for this failure of increase in 1-hydroxylase activity in the renal tubular cells is unexplained. The basic defect is phosphate depletion resulting from renal tubular dysfunction. The X-linked form of the disorder is due to mutations in an ectoenzyme, phex, and the autosomal dominant form is associated with mutations in fibroblast growth factor 23 (FGF-23). Therapy for this condition involves use of oral phosphate and a vitamin D metabolite. The clinical features of this condition are very similar to those of oncogenic osteomalacia described below.

Oncogenic osteomalacia

Rickets or osteomalacia develops in some patients with tumors. The tumor produces an unknown factor, possibly FGF-23 or phosphotonin, that causes phosphate wasting from the kidneys, because of an impairment of renal tubular phosphate reabsorption. The syndrome of oncogenic osteomalacia mimics hypophosphatemic rickets or osteomalacia very closely. Tumors are usually benign and slow-growing, of the mesenchymal type. This syndrome is reversed when the tumor is successfully removed.

PAGET'S DISEASE OF BONE

Paget's disease of bone is a common disorder of the elderly and is characterized by marked focal increases in bone resorption and bone formation. The consequence is disordered bone architecture. Although the etiology is still unclear, it seems likely that the disease is related to a viral infection involving a virus in the measles family related to the parainfluenza viruses. In the UK, some researchers have linked Paget's disease to dog ownership and have implicated canine distemper virus. The pathophysiology of Paget's disease, however, may also involve abnormal production of cytokines in the bone cell environment. Recently, IL-6 production by cells in the osteoclast lineage has been implicated as an autocrine/paracrine factor. There are often abnormal numbers of hemopoietic precursors in the bone marrow of patients with Paget's disease. This may reflect an increase in the precursors for the osteoclast, since the osteoclast shares its precursor with the mature cells of the blood.

Pathogenesis

The primary abnormality is an increase in osteoclastic bone resorption. The osteoclasts are of enormous size and contain up to 100 nuclei. The osteoclast nuclei contain inclusion bodies that resemble the those seen in viral diseases. The main reason for linking Paget's disease to a viral etiology is the morphologic observation of these inclusion bodies. There is also an increase in new bone formation, which is probably secondary to the osteoclastic bone resorption. The new bone that is formed is immature woven bone. It is disorganized in structure and of irregular pattern. There is also an increase in vascularity of the bone.

Lesions occur most frequently in the vertebrae, skull, pelvis, and axial skeleton, and in the proximal ends of the long bones and the tibia. They can be single ('monoostotic') or multiple ('polyostotic').

Clinical features of Paget's disease	
Focal – unlike other diffuse skeletal disorders	
Pain	Commonly caused by deformities in joints adjacent to affected bones
Deformity	Caused by the abnormal bone architecture
Complications	Fracture
	Nerve entrapment (due to increased bone formation)
	Deafness (due to compression of the VIIIth cranial nerve and to otosclerosis)
	Cardiac failure (due to increased cardiac output)
	Sarcomatous transformation (rarely, there may be development of osteosarcomas, chondrosarcomas, or fibrosarcomas in pagetic bones)

Table 34.15 Clinical features of Paget's disease. Most patients are asymptomatic.

Clinical features

The majority of patients with Paget's disease are asymptomatic. In patients who have symptoms, the most common is pain, which is usually localized to the area of pagetic bone disease. Commonly, bone pain is caused not by Paget's disease but rather by associated degenerative joint disease. Patients also develop characteristic deformities, most frequently an enlargement of the skull or outward bowing of the lower extremities. Furthermore, the disordered bone architecture may occasionally be associated with complications such as pathologic fracture, nerve entrapment syndromes due to increased bone formation, deafness (which may be due to compression of the eighth cranial nerve or to otosclerosis), cardiac failure due to increased cardiac output and increased blood flow through the highly vascularized Pagetic bones, and, rarely, sarcomatous transformation. This last condition is a complication that, although rare, is usually rapidly fatal. The tumors may be osteosarcomas, chondrosarcomas, fibrosarcomas, or mixed mesenchymal tumors.

The clinical features of Paget's disease are listed in **Table 34.15**, and bone deformities of the condition are shown in **Figs 34.12 & 34.13**.

Laboratory evaluation

There is no abnormality in calcium or phosphate homeostasis. There is, however, a marked increase in urinary hydroxyproline (hydroxyproline is an amino acid that is almost unique to collagen, and urinary excretion reflects increased bone turnover) and serum alkaline phosphatase. Alkaline phosphatase is an enzyme that is produced by osteoblasts and its increase reflects increased osteoblastic activity.

Treatment

The main aim of treatment is to inhibit bone resorption. Three drugs that are effective inhibitors of bone resorption have been useful in Paget's disease: bisphosphonates, calcitonin, and plicamycin (mithramycin). More than 70% of patients respond to treatment, and the improvement in their wellbeing is dramatic. Current drugs of choice are the new bisphosphonates.

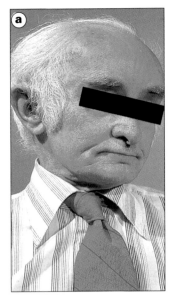

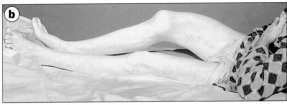

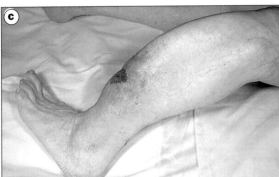

Figure 34.12 Bone deformity in Paget's disease. (a) Marked enlargement of the cranium, with normal facial bones – a hearing aid can be seen. (b) Anterior bowing of the femur. (c) Marked bowing of the tibia with overlying ulceration.

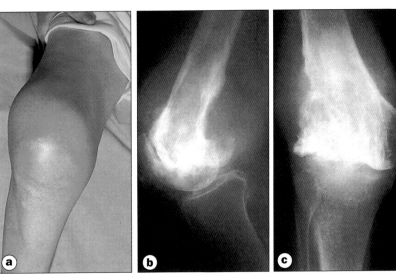

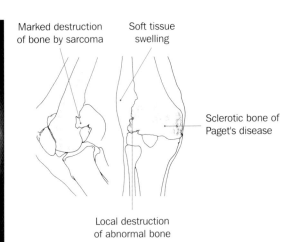

Figure 34.13 Development of osteogenic sarcoma in Paget's disease. Painful swelling developed in the knee of this patient 2 years after the diagnosis of Paget's disease. Marked bone destruction and soft-tissue swelling can be seen on the radiographs.

FURTHER READING

Becker KL, ed. Principles and practice of endocrinology and metabolism, 3rd edn. New York: Lippincott Williams and Wilkins; 2001: 574-586.

Black DM, Thompson DE, Bauer DC, et al. Fracture risk reduction with alendronate in women with osteoporosis: The fracture intervention trial. J Clin Endocrinol Metab. 2000: 85; 4118-4124.

DeGroot L, Jameson LJ, eds. Endocrinology, 4th edn. Philadelphia, PA: WB Saunders; 2001: 1093-1100.

Favus M, ed. The American Society for Bone and Mineral Research primer on metabolic bone diseases and disorders of mineral metabolism, 4th edn. New York: Lippincott Williams and Wilkins; 1999: 238-241.

Guise TA, Mundy GM. Cancer and Bone. Endocrine Reviews 1998: 19;18-54.

McClung MR, Geusens P, Miler SD et al. Effect of risedronate on the risk of hip fracture in elderly women. N Engl J Med. 2001: 344;333-40.

Neer RM, Arnaud CD, Zanchetta JR, et al. Effect of parathyroid hormone (1-34) on fractures and bone mineral density in postmenopausal women with osteoporosis. N Engl J Med. 2000: 344; 1434-41.

Proceedings of the Third International Symposium on Paget's Disease. J Bone Min Res. 1999: 14(Suppl); 1-104.

Recker RR, Davies KM, Dowd RM, Heaney RP. The effect of low dose continuous estrogen and progesterone therapy with calcium and vitamin D on bone in elderly women. Ann Int Med. 1999: 130; 897-904

Rossini M, Gatta D, Isaia G, Sartori L, Braga V, Adami S. Effects of oral alendronate in elderly patients with osteoporosis and mild primary hyperparathyroidism. J Bone Min Res. 2001: 16;113-116.

Silverberg SJ, Shane E, Jacobs TP, Siris E, Bilezikian JP. A 10-year prospective study of primary hypeparathyroidism with or without parathyroid surgery. N Engl J Med. 1999: 341;1249-55.

Siris E. Chines AA, Altman RD et al. Risedronate in the treatment of Paget's disease of bone: an open label multicenter study. J Bone Min Res. 1998: 13; 1032-1038.

Strewler GJ. The physiology of parathyroid hormone-related protein. N Engl J Med. 2000: 342;177-185.

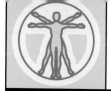

Chapter

35

Ectopic Humoral Syndromes

Klaus von Werder

INTRODUCTION

Patients with malignant tumors present occasionally with symptoms that are not explained by the neoplastic lesion in a specific anatomic site. Thus, a variety of clinical symptoms occur at sites that are distant from the location of the primary tumor and metastases. Manifestations of these paraneoplastic syndromes are either neurologic or metabolic–hormonal. These syndromes that are caused by tumor products can be more dangerous to the patient's health than the tumor mass itself.

The paraneoplastic neurologic symptoms are explained by antibody formation induced by expression of immunoaccessible antigens by various neoplasms. When the neuronal tissue expresses antigens that are also recognized by the antibodies directed against the tumor antigens, characteristic neurologic symptoms can occur, which are not discussed in this chapter. The so-called ectopic humoral syndromes that lead to endocrine or metabolic disturbances are caused by direct secretion of a hormone or biologically active factors like cytokines from a tumor arising from tissue other than the endocrine gland or tissue that normally produces the hormone or the biologically active factor (**Table 35.1**). In fact, this is not strictly correct, since it has been shown that many hormones and cytokines are expressed in low quantities in most tissues. However, it is customary and generally accepted to speak of 'ectopic hormones' whenever they are secreted from these tissues into the bloodstream, where they can be measured in sufficient quantities that they cause clinical syndromes.

Classic endocrine hyperfunction in contrast is due to eutopic hormone secretion from a hyperplastic, adenomatous, or rarely malignant tumorous transformed endocrine gland that normally secretes this hormone. The clinical syndromes caused by ectopic

Pathogenesis of paraneoplastic syndromes

Tumor production and secretion of biologically active peptide hormones

→ Endocrine diseases

Tumor is capable of metabolizing steroids (aromatase activity, vitamin D-hydroxylase)

→ Gynecomastia, hypercalcemia

Tumor production of cytokines

→ weight loss, fever, leucocytosis, hypercalcemia etc.

Tumor stimulation of antibody formation

→ neurological syndrome (Lambert-Eaton, encephalomyelitis, neuropathy etc.)

Table 35.1 Pathogenesis of paraneoplastic syndromes.

hormone secretion are often indistinguishable from the clinical picture of classic endocrine hyperfunction.

Ectopically produced hormones are always peptides or glycoproteins, never steroids, biogenic amines, or thyroid hormones, although occasionally a malignant tumor or inflammatory tissue will be capable of metabolizing steroid or thyroid hormones, leading to alteration of biologic activity and causing clinical syndromes (e.g. hypercalcemia in sarcoid disease; **Fig. 35.1**).

The differential diagnosis between ectopic and eutopic hormone hypersecretion is further complicated by the fact that, in addition to ectopic hormone secretion, the hormone-producing gland may be ectopically located or receptors for hormones that are normally secreted are ectopically expressed in glands that are normally not a target organ for the receptor ligands

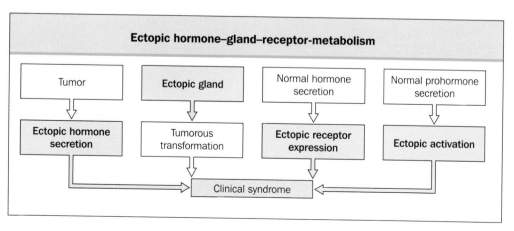

Figure 35.1 Ectopic hormone–gland–receptor-metabolism.

Table 35.2 Summary of ectopic humoral syndromes.

Summary of ectopic humoral syndromes

Clinical syndrome	Tumor	Secreted hormone or substance
Cushing's syndrome	Small cell cancer Carcinoid tumour	Adrenocorticotropic hormone (ACTH)
	Pancreatic islet cell cancer Medullary thyroid cancer Prostate and other cancers Lymphoma	Corticotropic-releasing hormone/ACTH
Acromegaly	Carcinoid tumour Pancreatic islet cell cancer Lymphoma	Growth-hormone-releasing hormone Growth hormone
Hypercalcemia	Lung cancer Renal cancer Breast cancer etc.	Parathyroid-hormone-related peptide Osteoclast activating cytokines (interleukin-1) Transforming growth factor-α
Syndrome of inappropriate ADH (vasopressin) secretion (SIADH)	Lung cancer (usually small-cell)	Vasopressin
Gynecomastia	Trophoblastic tumors Chorioncarcinoma Lung cancer	Human chorionic gonadotropin
Zollinger–Ellison syndrome (gastrinoma)	Pancreatic islet cell adenoma and cancer	Gastrin
Verner–Morrison (WDHA = watery diarrhea, hypokalemia, achlorhydria)	Pancreatic islet cell cancer	Vasoactive intestinal peptide
Hypoglycemia	Mesenchymal tumors (sarcomas, hemangiopericytoma), hepatoma Other cancers	Insulin-like growth factor-2
Polycythemia	Renal cancer Cerebellar haemangioblastoma	Erythropoietin
Cachexia	Often pancreatic cancers	Tumor necrosis factor
Neutrophilia	Lymphoma/leukemia	Granulocyte colony stimulating factor
Leukocytosis	Many cancers	Granulocyte–macrophage colony stimulating factor

Figure 35.2 Diagnosis of ectopic humoral syndromes.

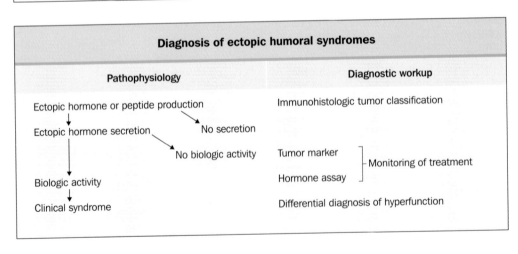

Diagnosis of ectopic humoral syndromes

(Fig. 35.1). Receptors and target organ can also lose their specificity; for example, ectopically produced human chorionic gonadotropin causes hyperthyroidism by activating the TSH receptor (see below). That autoantibodies may stimulate specific hormone receptors explains the pathophysiology of Graves' disease, which is again not a topic discussed in this chapter.

There are certain malignant tumors – endocrine tumors, neuroendocrine tumors, small-cell carcinomas, other cancers, sarcomas, and lymphomas – that are more frequently associated with specific ectopic hormone secretion (Table 35.2). The ectopically produced peptide hormones are not always secreted but remain stored in the tumor cell, where they can help to identify the tumorous cell types (Fig. 35.2). However, when the hormones are secreted, they can lead to early detection of the cancer by inducing symptoms, e.g. gynecomastia in patients with still small cancers secreting human chorionic gonadotropin. Furthermore, these peptides that are secreted from the tumor cells can, even when they are not biologically active, serve as tumor markers

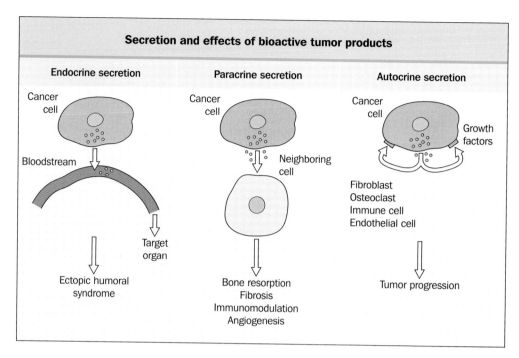

Figure 35.3 Secretion and biological effects of bioactive tumor products. There are three different modes of secretion; only endocrine secretion produces the classical ectopic humoral syndrome. Paracrine secretion of bioactive substances may lead to local effects whereas autocrine secretion is important for the tumor growth itself.

that are helpful for monitoring cancer therapy (**Fig. 35.2**). Since some ectopic hormone syndromes occur rather frequently, they are part of the differential diagnosis of endocrine diseases, e.g. Cushing's syndrome (see below).

CRITERIA FOR ECTOPIC HORMONE PRODUCTION

There are different modes of secretion of bioactive tumor products (**Fig. 35.3**). Only the endocrine type of secretion of tumor products is associated with the ectopic humoral syndrome. The criteria for the latter comprise demonstration of hormone synthesis, storage, and secretion by the tumor using *in situ* hybridization to detect hormone messenger RNA and immunocytochemistry to demonstrate the peptide in the tumor tissue. Furthermore, an arteriovenous gradient in hormone concentration provides important evidence for secretion of the hormone from the tumor, as does the release of hormone into the medium from cultured tumor cells *in vitro* (**Table 35.3**).

Furthermore, successful tumor removal should lead to remission of the ectopic humoral syndrome and tumor recurrence should also lead to recurrence of the clinical picture of the ectopic humoral syndrome (**Table 35.3**). Parallel with the disappearance and reappearance of the syndrome, normalization and return of pathologic hormone levels are observed. The hormone secretion is usually atypically regulated, as demonstrated by the results of endocrine dynamic function tests. In addition, the hormone in circulation appears often in molecular forms atypical of an eutopic but typical of an ectopic source.

HYPOTHESES EXPLAINING THE ORIGIN OF ECTOPIC HORMONE PRODUCTION

A number of hypotheses exist, which may indicate that we know little about why ectopic hormone secretion occurs. The general assumption is that a single event may have led to

Criteria for proof of an ectopic humoral syndrome

- Endocrine or metabolic disturbance in a patient with a nonendocrine tumor
- Remission after successful treatment
- Return of endocrine syndrome with tumor recurrence
- Abnormally regulated elevated blood hormone levels
- Significant gradient between hormone concentration in the venous effluent from the tumor and arterial hormone levels
- Extracts from tumor contain hormone bio- and immunoreactivity
- Relevant hormone mRNA can be identified in tumor tissue
- Synthesis and secretion of relevant hormone by tumor cells *in vitro*

Table 35.3 Criteria for proof of an ectopic humoral syndrome.

production and secretion of different peptide hormones in different tumor types. That these tumors are monoclonal is another assumption, although this is supported by good experimental evidence.

That not only genes of hormones but multiple genes may be expressed 'ectopically' is very probable. The reason why the other ectopically produced peptides are not picked up is because they are either not secreted into the bloodstream or have no biologic activity and we do not have assays to measure them. Some of these tumor products, however, can be measured and serve as tumor markers (e.g. fetal proteins). Nevertheless, we can rightly assume that a large number of proteins are made by the tumor, of which the secreted hormone causing the ectopic syndrome is only one. We know that all cells contain the same genetic information, of which only a fraction is expressed in the normal situation. An important question, which we cannot answer now, is, whether the gene expression for the hormone in question in the ectopic hormone syndrome is turned on before or after neoplastic transformation of the cell.

According to the *derepression hypothesis*, neoplastic transformation leads to a disturbance of cell replication that includes derangement of the inhibition of gene expression. Thus, genes are turned on at random, leading to deregulated expression of hormones. This hypothesis cannot explain why certain tumors produce certain hormones whereas other tumors do not and why certain proteins are never produced and secreted ectopically.

The *dedifferentiation hypothesis* retraces the tumor cell to a precursor, which normally expresses the hormone in question. We know that with the help of differentiation factors progenitor cells for blood cells but also for endocrine cells can differentiate in a stepwise fashion into very specialized cells, e.g. erythrocytes and platelets in bone marrow and gonadotropes and somatotropes in the pituitary gland.

The dedifferentiation hypothesis assumes that this process can be reversed by neoplastic transformation of a differentiated cell that has lost its receptors for differentiating factors. Thus, this cell has become once more capable of expressing hormone genes. This concept would be particularly compatible with the observation that only certain tumors produce specific hormones as the progenitor cells of the neoplastically transformed cells.

The *neuroendocrine cell hypothesis* was put forward by Pearse, who recognized that there are a number of morphologic and cytochemical characteristics of the peptide-hormone-producing tumor cells. In particular, these cells were shown to be capable of amine precursor uptake and decarboxylation (APUD). The characteristics of the APUD cells are that they contain dense-core secretory granules as well as membrane-bound secretory vesicles, a rough and a smooth endoplasmic reticulum, and free ribosomes. According to the proposed theory the APUD cells are derived from the neural crest in the embryo. Hormone-secreting tumors that are most probably derived from neural crest stem cells are the pancreatic neuroendocrine tumors – gastrinomas, insulinomas, glucagonomas, VIPomas, somatostatinomas and GHRHomas, the bronchial and thymic neuroendocrine tumors, such as bronchial and thymic carcinoids (foregut) and small-cell lung carcinomas, and classic carcinoid (midgut) tumors, which when they have metastasized into the liver cause a clinical syndrome with flushing, diarrhea, abdominal pain, asthma and carcinoid heart disease (Chapter 33). However, although many of the ectopic-hormone-secreting tumor cells contain APUD characteristics, the concept that all hormone-producing tumors stem from neural crest tissue is unfounded. Tumor cells of the APUD type can be shown to be very active hormone secretors, although some of the tumors with high malignancy lacking any APUD features are also very actively producing and secreting hormones.

It is clear that neoplastic transformation is closely linked to or caused by the switching on of certain cellular genes that control cell growth. The same mechanism that leads to oncogene overexpression could also turn on hormone production by changing the activity of genes known to regulate the expression of hormone genes. Again, there is little experimental evidence for this theory.

In summary, ectopic hormone production is one example of altered gene expression of neoplastic cells that we still do not understand as many of the events occurring in neoplastic transformation.

GENERAL ASPECTS OF ECTOPIC HORMONE SYNDROMES

There are several patterns of ectopic hormone production and secretion leading to characteristic syndromes. The most common is the production and secretion of peptide hormones by tumors, which are often malignant, derived from neuroendocrine cells (**Table 35.2**). These neuroendocrine cells are widely dispersed throughout the lung, gastrointestinal tract, pancreas, thyroid gland, adrenal medulla, skin, prostate, and breast. The characteristic morphology and ultrastructure, as well as the common neuroendocrine markers, are those of the APUD or enterochromaffin cells and are summarized in **Table 35.4**. The list of hormones produced by tumors derived from members of this group include adrenocorticotropic hormone (ACTH), growth-hormone-releasing hormone (GHRH), gastrin, vasoactive intestinal polypeptide (VIP), calcitonin, somatostatin, and other small peptides.

The second group of hormone-producing cancers is derived from squamous epithelium. These tumors frequently produce parathyroid-hormone-related peptide (PTHrP) but are also capable of producing other peptide hormones (**Table 35.2**). Trophoblastic tumors typically produce human chorionic gonadotropin, whereas mesenchymal tumors may produce insulin-like growth factor (IGF)-2. In addition, lymphoid tissue, which is known to be capable of producing ACTH, growth hormone and prolactin, among other peptides, can, after malignant transformation, overproduce ACTH and growth hormone, leading to the clinically manifested ectopic hormone syndromes. There are actually no common clinical characteristics that may lead to the diagnosis of ectopic hormone secretion. However, in certain patients, we might diagnose lung cancer because of typical symptoms, such as coughing and hemoptysis, which are accompanied by hyponatremia or hypercalcemia suggestive of the syndrome of inappropriate antidiuretic hormone (vasopressin) secretion (SIADH) or humoral hypercalcemia of malignancy.

In most instances the ectopic hormone syndrome presents as a classic endocrine disease such as hypercalcemia, Cushing's syndrome or acromegaly. In this situation ectopic PTHrP or

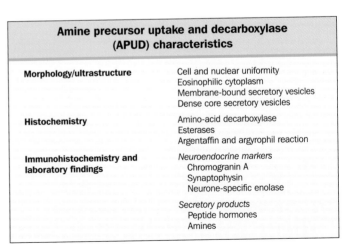

Amine precursor uptake and decarboxylase (APUD) characteristics	
Morphology/ultrastructure	Cell and nuclear uniformity Eosinophilic cytoplasm Membrane-bound secretory vesicles Dense core secretory vesicles
Histochemistry	Amino-acid decarboxylase Esterases Argentaffin and argyrophil reaction
Immunohistochemistry and laboratory findings	*Neuroendocrine markers* Chromogranin A Synaptophysin Neurone-specific enolase *Secretory products* Peptide hormones Amines

Table 35.4 Amine precursor uptake and decarboxylase (APUD) characteristics.

ACTH secretion or somatotrope hyperplasia due to ectopic GHRH secretion belongs to the differential diagnosis of the hypercalcemic state, Cushing's syndrome, or acromegaly. Occasionally the diagnosis of hormone hypersecretion, with its clinical impact, is made simultaneously with the diagnosis of the tumor. This happens in situations where hormone hypersecretion is almost exclusively of ectopic origin. For example, recurrent peptic ulcers lead to the diagnosis of hypergastrinemia with parallel detection of a gastrin-producing tumor within the pancreas with or without liver secondaries. Depending on the severity of the symptoms caused directly by the cancer (respiratory problems, gastrointestinal bleeding, bile obstruction, etc.) or the hormone excess (severe Cushing's syndrome, hyponatremic encephalopathy, or severe hypercalcemia), the patient presents clinically more as a typical patient with malignancy or a patient with a primarily endocrine disease.

In the following examples, the most common ectopic hormone syndromes will be discussed, with emphasis on the clinical and laboratory aspects that allow the differential diagnosis between ectopic and eutopic hormone syndromes.

ECTOPIC ACTH SYNDROME

In 1928, before Cushing's syndrome was defined as a clinical entity caused by hypercortisolemia, a female patient with hirsutism, diabetes, hypertension, adrenal hyperplasia, and a small-cell carcinoma of the lung was described. At that time, no causal relationship between lung cancer and adrenal hyperplasia was inferred. In 1962, Cushing's syndrome due to ectopic ACTH secretion from nonendocrine tumors was definitely proven and described by Liddle and colleagues. Ever since, ectopic ACTH syndrome has been one of the most extensively studied of the ectopic humoral syndromes.

Ectopic ACTH secretion is defined as production and secretion of ACTH and other pro-opiomelanocortin (POMC)-derived peptides from extrapituitary tumors, leading to adrenal hyperplasia, hypercortisolemia, and development of Cushing's syndrome (**Fig. 35.4**). Since ectopic ACTH syndrome accounts for 5–20% of all cases of endogenous Cushing's syndrome, the

differential diagnosis between the two types of ACTH-dependent Cushing's syndrome, i.e. eutopic or ectopic, is of paramount importance (**Fig. 35.4** & **Table 35.5**).

The ectopic production and secretion of corticotropin-releasing hormone (CRH) together with ACTH by an extrapituitary tumor is extremely rare. Even rarer is the isolated production and secretion of CRH by nonpituitary tumors leading to pituitary ACTH hypersecretion due to corticotrope hyperplasia. In most of the patients described in the literature the diagnosis was made post mortem. In none of the patients described so far all the criteria for demonstrating ectopic hormone secretion summarized in **Table 35.3** had been fulfilled. Whether the ectopic production of other peptides that enhance the efficacy of endogenous CRH to stimulate ACTH secretion is a true pathophysiologic phenomenon is not clear yet. In one case with a medullary thyroid carcinoma that produced bombesin in addition to calcitonin but no ACTH, the cause of Cushing's syndrome was thought to be the enhancing effect of bombesin on the action of CRH on the pituitary corticotrope.

Clinical features of the ectopic ACTH syndrome may be indistinguishable from pituitary-dependent Cushing's disease. However, rapid onset with pronounced weight loss, which is usually not observed in Cushing's disease, and very pronounced muscle weakness may raise the suspicion of an ectopic ACTH syndrome (**Table 35.5**). In addition, patients with the ectopic ACTH syndrome usually appear more pigmented. Hypertension and diabetes mellitus, typical for all forms of Cushing's syndrome, do not contribute to the differential diagnosis between eutopic and ectopic hypersecretion.

Laboratory findings

Typically, patients with the ectopic ACTH syndrome have more pronounced hypokalemia than patients with eutopic ACTH secretion and present with hypokalemic alkalosis. The latter is due to the very high cortisol level, which the saturated renal 11β-hydroxysteroid-dehydrogenase enzyme (11β-HSD) is unable to convert into cortisone. This allows the nonmetabolized cortisol inappropriately to gain access to and activate the mineralocorticoid receptor.

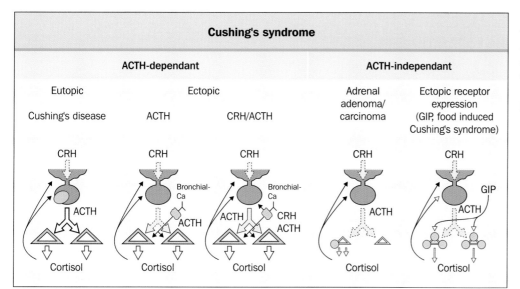

Figure 35.4 Cushing's syndrome. The figure illustrates the difference between adrenocorticotropic hormone (ACTH)-dependent and ACTH-independent Cushing's syndrome. CRH, corticotropin-releasing hormone; GIP, gastric inhibitory peptide.

Table 35.5 Differential diagnosis of ACTH-dependent Cushing's syndrome

	Cushing's disease (pituitary corticotropinoma)	Ectopic ACTH syndrome
Skin pigmentation	+	++
Weight loss	–	–/+
Muscle weakness	+	++
Pituitary adenoma (MRI)	– or +	– seldom + (incidentaloma)
Hypokalemia	–/+	++
ACTH basal level	↑	↑ or ↑↑
Cortisol level	Normal/↑	↑ or ↑↑
Dexamethasone suppression (high dose)	+	–
CRH stimulation	++	–
Desmopressin stimulation	+	–
Inferior petrosal sinus: peripheral blood ACTH ratio	> 2	< 1.7
Octreotide suppression	–	– or +
Octreoscan®	Negative	negative/positive

Table 35.5 Differential diagnosis of adrenocorticotropic hormone (ACTH)-dependent Cushing's syndrome. There are exceptions for all clinical symptoms and also for the laboratory findings. Thus, there are rare patients with ectopic ACTH syndrome in whom cortisol can be suppressed with dexamethasone and ACTH stimulated with corticotropin-releasing hormone (CRH) or desmopressin. Sometimes a pituitary adenoma can be found by MRI in a patient with the ectopic ACTH syndrome. In this situation the pituitary lesion is an incidentaloma, not an ACTH-secreting corticotropinoma. The decisive test in these instances is the ratio between ACTH concentration in the inferior petrosal sinus blood over ACTH in the peripheral blood. MRI, magnetic resonance imaging.

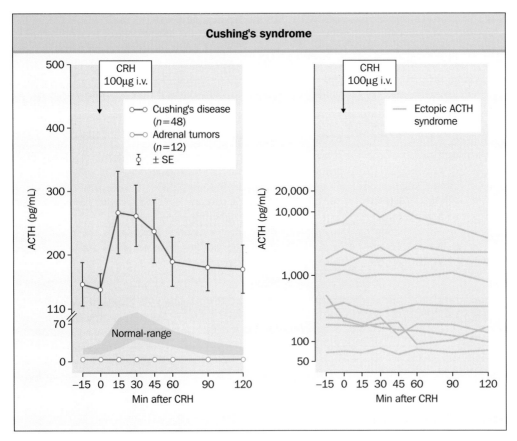

Figure 35.5 Cushing's syndrome. The figure shows the effect of intravenous administration of corticotropin-releasing hormone (CRH) on adrenocorticotropic hormone (ACTH) secretion in (left panel) classic Cushing's disease, cortisol secreting adrenal tumors and (right panel) nine patients with the ectopic ACTH syndrome.

Endocrine investigation

The ACTH dependency of hypercortisolism is documented by measurable, usually elevated ACTH levels, which are usually significantly higher in patients with the ectopic ACTH syndrome although there is an overlap because small carcinoid tumors also have only slightly elevated ACTH levels (**Fig. 35.5**). Typically, the ACTH levels do not rise after stimulation with corticotropin releasing hormone (CRH) in patients with ectopic ACTH syndrome whereas there is usually a dramatic CRH-induced ACTH rise in patients with Cushing's disease (**Fig. 35.5**). This is also true for the synthetic vasopressin analog 1-deamino-8-D-arginine vasopressin (DDAVP or desmopressin), which leads to stimulation of ACTH secretion only in patients with pituitary-dependent Cushing's syndrome.

Cortisol levels in patients with Cushing's disease are not necessarily outside the normal early-morning range but show no circadian rhythm. In patients with ectopic ACTH syndrome the cortisol levels also lack circadian variation but in addition morning cortisol levels are almost always elevated. Furthermore, whereas high doses of dexamethasone lead to suppression of cortisol levels in patients with an eutopic ACTH source, the drug does not affect cortisol levels in patients with ectopic ACTH secretion (**Fig. 35.6**).

However, the results of the stimulation and suppression tests may not be clearcut or may even point in opposite directions. Even the demonstration of a pituitary adenoma by magnetic resonance tomography may be misleading – it could be an endocrine inactive adenoma (coincidentaloma) in a patient with an ectopic ACTH syndrome. For this reason, bilateral inferior petrosal sinus sampling with CRH stimulation is necessary in those patients in whom the differential diagnosis is not clearcut. In fact, many neurosurgeons nowadays ask for a petrosal sinus catheter study routinely and operate by the transsphenoidal route only in those patients in whom the ratio of central to peripheral ACTH concentration is more than 2. In contrast, patients with ectopic ACTH syndrome have always a ratio of less than 1.7. Since inferior petrosal sinus sampling has the greatest diagnostic power in discriminating between Cushing's disease and ectopic ACTH syndrome, this test is definitely indicated in all questionable cases. However, the test is invasive and, considering the vascular fragility of patients with hypercortisolism, should be performed only in centers with experience in this procedure.

Extrapituitary tumors producing ACTH process the *POMC* gene products differently from the pituitary corticotrope. Thus, altered POMC maturation in nonpituitary tumors is reflected by abnormal POMC fragments, which can be detected in peripheral blood of those patients. Though the circulating ACTH from tumor patients has been shown to be identical to pituitary ACTH, partial degradation of ACTH into corticotropin-like intermediate lobe peptide (CLIP) is quite common. However, measurement of POMC-derived peptides in the circulation is only available in highly specialized laboratories and is therefore of no clinical use to differentiate eutopic from ectopic pituitary ACTH secretion.

The differential diagnosis between eutopic and ectopic ACTH syndrome can be complicated further by the fact that occasionally an ectopic pituitary ACTH-secreting tumor mimics occult paraneoplastic ectopic ACTH secretion. Thus, 13 cases have been published in whom the ACTH dynamics in the endocrine function test were comparable to those seen in Cushing's disease although the pituitary tumor was located extrasellar.

After the diagnosis of ectopic ACTH syndrome has been made, it is sometimes difficult to find the tumor, particularly if we are dealing with small carcinoid tumors of the lung. In this situation, when the conventional chest X-ray is completely normal, computerized tomography (CT) of the chest using thin cuts and contrast enhancement X-ray demonstrate the ACTH-producing lesion (**Fig. 35.7**). Recently, multiple microscopic nests of neuroendocrine cells in the lung (pulmonary tumorlets) have been described as producing and secreting ACTH and causing Cushing's syndrome. These small cell conglomerates can also not be detected by conventional chest X-ray but only by high resolution CT of the lungs.

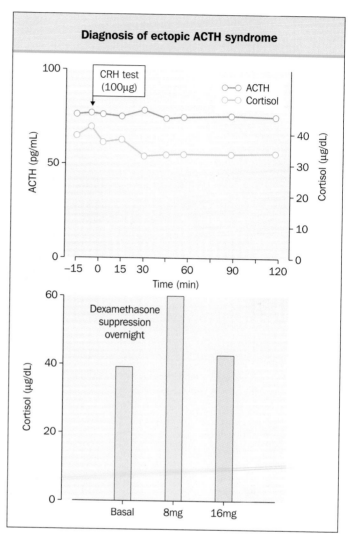

Figure 35.6 Diagnosis of ectopic adrenocorticotropic hormone (ACTH) syndrome. Nonresponsiveness of ACTH and cortisol to corticotropin-releasing hormone (CRH), no suppression after high doses of dexamethasone and a ratio of inferior petrosal sinus to peripheral ACTH of 0.96 are all consistent with a diagnosis of ectopic ACTH syndrome. The low ACTH levels suggest a small occult carcinoid tumor. However, the source of ACTH could not be located using body catheterization, computerized tomography, and octreotide scanning.

Since about 80% of ACTH-producing extrapituitary tumors express somatostatin receptors, somatostatin receptor scintigraphy (Octreoscan®) may be helpful in visualizing the tumor, as in patients with the carcinoid syndrome. Correspondingly, patients who have been demonstrated to have tumors expressing somatostatin receptors will respond with acute suppression of the plasma ACTH level after octreotide administration, which is not observed in patients with pituitary ACTH hypersecretion.

Therapy

Curative therapy in patients with the ectopic ACTH syndrome is only possible in patients with benign or operable malignant ACTH-producing tumors. In all other patients in whom the tumor cannot be found (**Fig. 35.6**) and with disease that is already metastatic, hypercortisolism should be treated because it contributes considerably to the morbidity of these patients. Since 80% of the patients express somatostatin receptors subtypes 2 and 5, treatment with somatostatin receptor ligands (SRL) such as octreotide may be effective. Only when the latter is ineffective adrenolytic medication such as mitotane, metyrapone, etomidate, or ketoconazole is required. The prognosis in respect to life expectancy depends on the type of tumor, the extent of metastatic disease, and the response to chemotherapy.

SYNDROME OF INAPPROPRIATE ANTIDIURETIC HORMONE SECRETION

The syndrome of inappropriate antidiuretic hormone (vasopressin) secretion was suspected to occur in patients with lung cancers who presented with hyponatremia even before 1957, when Bartter and Schwartz described and defined the typical features of this syndrome. SIADH is characterized by dilutional hyponatremia (serum sodium < 135mmol/L) and low plasma osmolality (< 250mosmol/kg). The urinary sodium concentration and urinary osmolality are inappropriately high considering the hyponatremia and the low plasma osmolality. Furthermore, there is persistent urinary sodium excretion (> 20mmol/24h) in the absence of clinically apparent edema (i.e. normal extracellular fluid volume on clinical examination). When plasma vasopressin is detectable or even elevated in patients presenting with the described features, the diagnosis of SIADH is established (Fig. 35.8).

Figure 35.7 Computerized tomography of the chest in a 23-year-old female patient with ectopic adrenocorticotropic hormone syndrome. In this patient conventional chest X-ray did not demonstrate the lesion seen here in the right side of the thorax (shown by arrow).

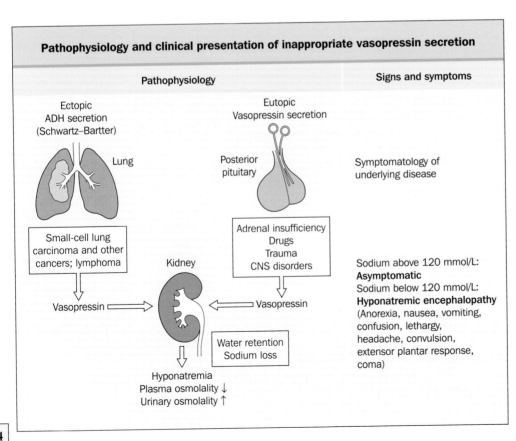

Figure 35.8 Pathophysiology and clinical presentation of inappropriate vasopressin secretion.

Pathophysiology

Small cell lung cancer is probably the most common malignancy associated with SIADH. Arginine vasopressin (AVP) and neurophysin II, which are normally synthesized in the hypothalamus as parts of a common glucopeptide precursor molecule, have also been found in extracts of small-cell lung carcinomas from patients with SIADH. Furthermore, inappropriately elevated plasma levels of bioactive and immunoreactive AVP have been found in patients with SIADH. When in patients with SIADH the plasma osmolality is increased by administering a sodium load, different responses of the plasma AVP level can be observed. Whereas in some patients the AVP level is not influenced by serum osmolality at all, demonstrating autonomous AVP release from the tumor, other patients have a resetting of the vasopressin osmostat; in other words, AVP levels start to rise when plasma osmolality is increased up to a range where AVP levels normally remain undetectable. Since malignant tumors are most probably not osmotically sensitive, this AVP secretion points to inappropriate ADH release from the neuro-hypophysial tract (**Table 35.6**), which can occur in patients with central nervous system (CNS) diseases.

In addition to tumors that produce ADH ectopically and CNS disorders that stimulate ADH release from the posterior pituitary, respiratory diseases, which can accompany malignancies, may cause inappropriate ADH secretion (**Table 35.6**).

Furthermore, drugs, particularly psychotropic and cytotoxic medication, can lead to stimulation of ADH secretion from the posterior pituitary. One important cause of eutopic ADH hypersecretion leading to hyponatremia is secondary or primary adrenal insufficiency. In this situation ADH is hypersecreted from the neurohypophysis because of missing inhibitory feedback of cortisol upon ADH release from the posterior pituitary and coexisting hypovolemia. Replacement with cortisol leads to prompt resolution of hyponatremia.

Clinical presentation of hyponatremia

The symptoms of hyponatremia caused by SIADH relate to:
- the absolute value of serum sodium concentration; and
- the rate of the fall of the serum sodium level.

Moderate hyponatremia, occasionally values even below 120mmol/L, may not cause any symptoms. However, a sudden fall in serum sodium to levels of 120mmol/L can cause seizures as a sign of hyponatremic encephalopathy. Patients with serum sodium levels below 110mmol/L usually all exhibit signs of encephalopathy, with headache, nausea and vomiting, muscle weakness, and later psychotic symptoms and finally seizures and coma. The central nervous symptoms are due to brain edema, which leads to decrease in cerebral blood flow and eventually brain necrosis.

Diagnosis and treatment

First the cause of hyponatremia has to be evaluated. Although SIADH is a very common cause of hyponatremia, hypervolemic hyponatremia in patients with cardiac failure, decompensated cirrhosis of the liver, and other diseases that present clinically with edema and ascites have to be excluded. Furthermore, hypovolemic hyponatremia in patients with salt and water loss due to diarrhea, vomiting, and other salt-wasting syndromes are also not difficult to differentiate from the euvolemic hyponatremia of

Causes of the syndrome of inappropriate antidiuretic hormone secretion

Tumors
Small-cell carcinoma of the lung
Other bronchial carcinomas
Thymoma
Pancreatic and intestinal carcinoma
Bladder carcinoma
Prostatic carcinoma
Lymphoma
Leukemia

Respiratory disorders
Pneumonia
Empyema
Asthma
Positive pressure ventilation

Central nervous system disorders
Meningitis/encephalitis
Brain abscess
Head injury
Brain tumor
Ganglioglioma of the neurohypophysis
Subarachnoid hemorrhage
Sinus thrombosis

Drugs
Cytotoxic therapeutic agents
Phenothiazine
Carbamazepine
Thiazide diuretics
Clofibrate

Endocrine
Adrenal insufficiency
Hypothyroidism

Table 35.6 Causes of the syndrome of inappropriate antidiuretic hormone secretion.

SIADH. The differential diagnosis between eutopic and ectopic ADH secretion has to be made on the basis of the patient's history, drug intake, clinical examination, and diagnostic procedures indicated for the workup of cancer patients.

The treatment of choice for ectopic ADH secretion is complete removal of the tumor. However, in the most common malignancy causing SIADH – small cell lung carcinoma – this is usually not feasible and patients have to be treated with chemotherapy.

Before chemotherapy or surgical therapy is started, hyponatremia has to be treated in those patients who have sodium levels below 120mosmol/L and clinical symptoms. The treatment of choice is to restrict fluid intake to less than 1L per day. Hypertonic saline infusions are only indicated in severely symptomatic patients. Care must be taken that the sodium does not increase more rapidly than 10mmol/L per day in order to avoid central pontine myelinolysis. The treatment of choice would be the administration of V_2-receptor antagonists, which are at present under investigation.

ECTOPIC GROWTH-HORMONE-RELEASING HORMONE/GROWTH HORMONE SECRETION

The typical features of acromegaly include enlargement of hands and feet, thickening of the skin, bulging of the frontal sinuses, enlargement of the mandible, and visceromegaly. Furthermore, patients have soft tissue swelling, carpal tunnel syndrome, and complain about excessive sweating, these latter

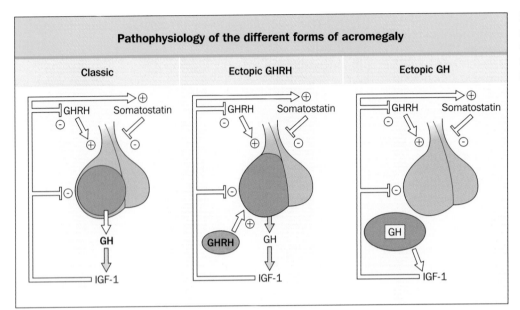

Figure 35.9 Pathophysiology of the different forms acromegaly.
GH, growth hormone; GHRH, growth-hormone-releasing hormone; IGF-1, insulin-like growth factor-1.

Pathophysiology of the different forms of acromegaly

| Classic | Ectopic GHRH | Ectopic GH |

symptoms all indicating active disease. Most patients with acromegaly have hypersecretion of growth hormone as the result of a monoclonal somatotrope adenoma of the pituitary leading to enhanced production and secretion of IGF-1 in peripheral tissues. A few patients (fewer than 0.5%) have polyclonal pituitary somatotrope hyperplasia due to ectopic production and secretion of GHRH (see **Fig. 35.10**). Extremely rare is the ectopic secretion of growth hormone itself, which has been demonstrated unequivocally in only two cases, one patient with a pancreatic islet cell tumor and another patient with a non-Hodgkin's B-cell lymphoma (**Fig. 35.9**). In contrast to ACTH-dependent Cushing's syndrome, in which ectopic ACTH secretion is more common than ectopic CRH/ACTH or CRH secretion, the ectopic production and secretion of the releasing hormone for growth hormone is certainly much more common than the rare production of growth hormone from nonpituitary tumors. Parallel to the situation in Cushing's syndrome, ectopic growth hormone secretion from nonpituitary tumors has to be differentiated from growth hormone hypersecretion caused by an ectopic somatotrope pituitary adenoma.

Morphology and clinical aspects of GHRH-producing tumors

Neuroendocrine tumors, especially of the lung and the gastrointestinal tract, and islet cell tumors are the most frequent tumor types in patients with the ectopic GHRH syndrome, making up about 80% of all cases. Among the other tumors associated with ectopic acromegaly, pheochromocytoma, retroperitoneal paraganglioma, and cystic adenocarcinoma of the lung have been reported. Rarely, hypothalamic tumors such as hamartomas cause somatotrope hyperplasia as a result of eutopic GHRH secretion.

The prevalence and incidence of ectopic acromegaly are unknown. Up to now about 40 cases of ectopic GHRH syndrome have been reported.

Clinically, patients with classic acromegaly do not differ significantly from those with the ectopic GHRH syndrome. In fact,

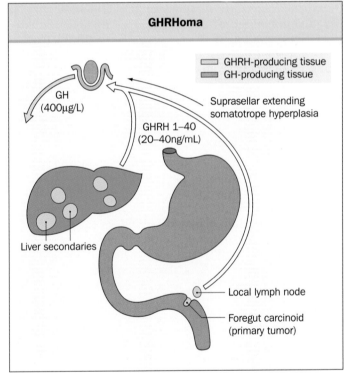

GHRHoma

Figure 35.10 GHRHoma. The mechanism leading to somatotrope hyperplasia and GH-hypersection in the case of a 14-year-old girl with gigantism is illustrated. GH, growth hormone; GHRH, growth-hormone-releasing hormone.

somatotrope hyperplasia may be so pronounced as to lead to suprasellar extension and mimic a pituitary macroadenoma (**Fig. 35.10**). Sometimes there is clinical evidence for a pancreatic or lung tumor in a patient with acromegaly, which should alert the physician to think of ectopic GHRH secretion. Also, in acromegalic patients in whom no pituitary tumor is detectable by magnetic resonance imaging, ectopic acromegaly should be considered.

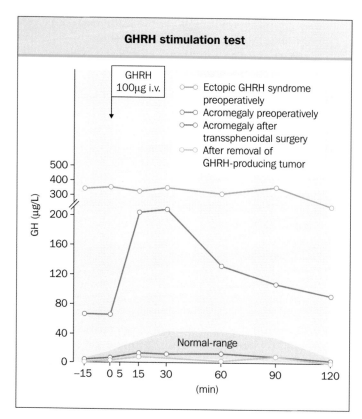

Figure 35.11 Growth-hormone-releasing hormone (GHRH) stimulation test. The results illustrated are from one patient with classic acromegaly and one with the ectopic GHRH syndrome. GH, growth hormone.

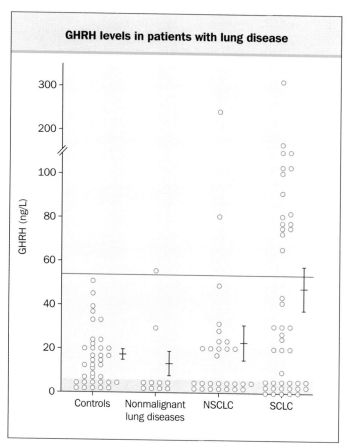

Figure 35.12 Growth-hormone-releasing hormone (GHRH) levels in patients with benign and malignant lung disease. The figure illustrates mean (± SEM) and individual GHRH levels in normal subjects and patients with nonmalignant lung disease, non-small-cell lung carcinoma (NSCLC) and small-cell lung carcinoma (SCLC). The shaded area represents the lower limit of the GHRH assay (< 5ng/L). The horizontal line shows the upper limit of the normal range (mean ± 3SD) of GHRH concentration. Patients with SCLC had significantly higher plasma GHRH levels than all other groups. (Adapted from Schopohl J, Losa M, Frey C, et al. Plasma growth hormone (GH)-releasing hormone levels in patients with lung carcinoma. Clin Endocrinol. 1991;34:463–7.)

Laboratory findings

The diagnosis of acromegaly due to ectopic GHRH secretion is confirmed by documenting the presence of acromegaly, by demonstrating elevated IGF-1 levels, and ectopic GHRH secretion, by documenting elevated GHRH levels in peripheral blood, which are usually above 1ng/mL.

Patients with ectopic GHRH syndrome usually do not respond to exogenous GHRH administration, unlike those with classic acromegaly (**Fig. 35.11**). However, when the endogenous GHRH source is removed, a normal response of growth hormone to the administration of the releasing hormone is reestablished (**Fig. 35.11**).

Patients with the ectopic GHRH syndrome often have elevated prolactin levels because of the prolactin-releasing activity of GHRH. Thus, administration of high dosages of GHRH to normal subjects leads to moderately increased prolactin levels.

Fulfilling the criteria of ectopic hormone production, GHRH messenger RNA as well as GHRH peptides can be demonstrated in tumor tissue. Thus, both natural forms of GHRH, GHRH$_{1-44}$ and GHRH$_{1-40}$, have been detected in tumor tissue. GHRH can also be demonstrated in rather high concentrations in carcinoid tumors of patients who do not suffer from acromegaly. These tumors produce but do not secrete GHRH, or at least not enough to release growth hormone in excess.

Furthermore, patients with small-cell lung cancer can have significantly higher plasma GHRH levels than control patients

and patients with nonmalignant lung disease (**Fig. 35.12**). This shows that these tumors can secrete small amounts of GHRH, which are not sufficient to induce growth hormone hypersecretion leading to clinical acromegaly but may be responsible for the qualitative abnormalities of growth hormone secretion observed in patients with malignancies.

Therapy

The therapy of choice would be the removal of the GHRH-producing tumor. However, since these tumors have often led to metastases (**Fig. 35.10**), medical therapy is indicated. Somatostatin receptor ligands are the therapy of choice since almost all GHRH-producing tumors express somatostatin receptors (**Fig. 35.13**). Thus, growth hormone hypersecretion can be effectively treated by inhibiting GHRH release from the tumor as well as inhibiting growth hormone secretion directly at the pituitary level (**Fig. 35.14**).

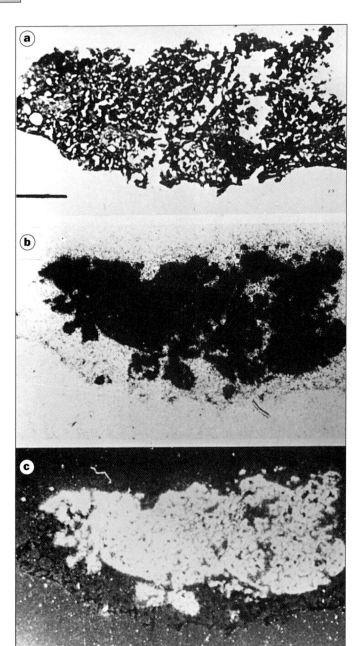

Figure 35.13 Somatostatin receptors demonstrated by autoradiography with a ^{125}I-labeled somatostatin analog of a GHRH-producing foregut carcinoid tumor. (a) Tumor stained conventionally with toluidine-kernechtrot (b) Autoradiograph obtained with the iodinated somatostatin octapeptide analog. (c) Dark-field photograph of a photoemulsion-coated cover slip from the tissue section. The nonhomogenous distribution of somatostatin receptors is clear. (Reproduced with permission from Reubi JC, Maurer R, von Werder K, Torhorst J, Klijn DIG, Lamberts SW. Somatostatin receptors in human endocrine tumors. Cancer Res. 1987;47:551–8.)

HUMORAL HYPERCALCEMIA OF MALIGNANCY

The human body contains about 1kg of calcium, of which 99% is in the skeleton. Only 1g of calcium is found in the extracellular fluid. The plasma calcium clievel is maintained within a narrow range between 2.2 and 2.65mmol/L (8.8–10.6 mg/dL) by the calcium-regulating hormones, of which parathyroid hormone is the most important (**Fig. 35.15**). The excitability of nerve and muscle cells, muscular contraction, intracellular transport, and also endocrine secretion, are very much influenced by the ionized calcium level in the plasma, which represents about half of the total plasma calcium. Thus, the fall of ionized calcium to below the normal range causes tetanic symptoms and later convulsions, whereas hypercalcemia leads to gastrointestinal disturbances, renal diabetes insipidus with polyuria, dehydration, and later decrease in the glomerular filtration rate.

Hypercalcemic patients are depressed and often confused and sleepy, complaining of headaches and irritability. Typical is the shortening of the QT interval in the electrocardiogram. Severe hypercalcemia leads to cardiac arrhythmias, and finally loss of consciousness and coma.

Differential diagnosis

The measurement of intact parathyroid hormone usually allows differentiation between the two most important causes of hypercalcemia – primary hyperparathyroidism and tumorous humoral hypercalcemia of malignancy. High normal or elevated parathyroid hormone (PTH) levels in the presence of hypercalcemia indicate primary hyperparathyroidism whereas suppressed intact PTH levels are compatible with tumoral hypercalcemia (**Fig. 35.15 & Table 35.7**). The latter is most commonly associated with squamous cell cancers of the lung, breast cancer, cancer of the pancreas and urogenital organs, and hematologic diseases such as myeloma and lymphoma. Carcinomas capable of producing and secreting true parathyroid hormone ectopically are extremely rare.

The tumors that cause hypercalcemia without metastases are those usually that secrete PTHrP (**Table 35.8**). This peptide, which is produced almost ubiquitously, is not a physiologic regulator of calcium metabolism but acts in a paracrine fashion in such different tissues as the lactating breast, the wall of blood-vessels, and keratinocytes. When produced and secreted into the blood by malignant tumors, PTHrP acts like a classic hormone. The amino terminal of PTHrP, which is similar to the amino terminal of PTH, binds to the PTH receptor in the target organs, leading to hypercalcemia and hyperphosphaturia in the same way as PTH itself. PTHrP does not crossreact with PTH in the intact PTH radioimmunoassay. Therefore, PTHrP-induced hypercalcemia is associated with circulating levels of PTH that are suppressed by the elevated calcium concentration.

Lymphomas may also cause hypercalcemia by producing 1,25-dihydroxycholecalciferol. 1,25-OH vitamin-D can also be produced by sarcoid or tuberculous granulomas and is occasionally found in other diseases associated with granulomatous changes.

Patients with tumors and bone metastases can have hypercalcemia because of local production of cytokines such as tumor necrosis factor-α (TNFα), interleukin 1 (osteoclast activating factor), and interleukin 6.

Treatment

The treatment of hypercalcemia of malignancy depends on the severity of the hypercalcemia and the underlying condition. Since patients usually become hypercalcemic at a later stage of their disease, sometimes with extensive metastases, it has to be seriously considered whether these patients, who are often

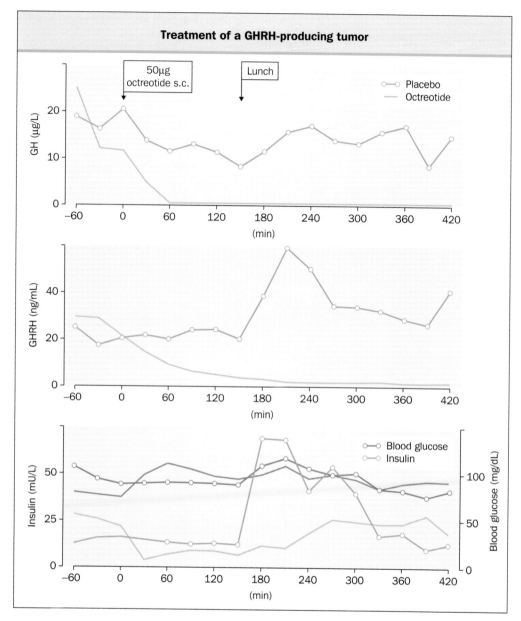

Figure 35.14 Treatment of a growth-hormone-releasing hormone (GHRH)-producing tumor. The figure shows the effect of subcutaneous administration of 50μg of somatostatin analog (octreotide) on levels of growth hormone (GH), growth-hormone-releasing hormone, insulin and blood sugar in a patient with the ectopic GHRH syndrome. Therapy leads to prompt lowering of GH and GHRH levels and suppresses the postprandial rise of insulin. However, there is no change in postprandial blood glucose levels, since growth hormone is suppressed at the same time.

comatose and for whom no other anticancer therapy will be available, should be treated at all. However, when this is not the case or the situation is not clear, treatment has to be instigated immediately because of life-threatening hypercalcemia. Since these patients are dehydrated (elevated calcium levels block the action of ADH at the distal renal tubule), rehydration is mandatory. When the latter has been achieved, antiosteoclastic medication, preferably intravenous bisphosphonates (pamidronate or ibandronate) have to be given. Bisphosphonates are more effective and have fewer side effects than calcitonin. Alternatively, in vitamin-D-mediated hypercalcemia, glucocorticoids can be given. Mithramycin, an inhibitor of RNA synthesis, should be given only when large doses of bisphosphonates are not effective, since its effects are transient.

TUMOR-ASSOCIATED OSTEOMALACIA

Tumor-associated osteomalacia (oncogenic osteomalacia) is a rare syndrome. Approximately 100 cases have been reported

with this syndrome, which is characterized by the classic clinical symptoms of osteomalacia, such as bone pain, muscle weakness, gait disturbances, fractures, and skeletal deformities.

The typical laboratory finding is profound phosphaturia in the presence of a very low serum phosphate level. The alkaline phosphatase is elevated and the level of 1,25-dihydroxycholecalciferol is decreased. When adult patients presenting with these clearcut clinical and laboratory findings also have a tumor of mesenchymal origin, oncogenic osteomalacia is the most likely diagnosis.

The pathogenesis of oncogenic osteomalacia is not understood. There is evidence that these tumors – mostly benign mesenchymal tumors, although the syndrome has also been reported in patients with lung, breast, and prostatic cancer – produce a heat-labile factor that inhibits phosphate reabsorption in the renal tubule. This phosphaturic factor is definitely different from PTH or PTHrP and does not influence phosphate transports through a mechanism dependent on cyclic adenosine monophosphate (cAMP). The low 1,25-dihydroxycholecalciferol level is

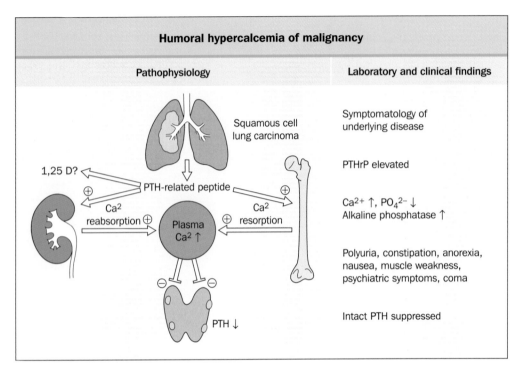

Humoral hypercalcemia of malignancy

Pathophysiology	Laboratory and clinical findings
	Symptomatology of underlying disease
	PTHrP elevated
	$Ca^{2+} \uparrow$, $PO_4^{2-} \downarrow$ Alkaline phosphatase $\uparrow$
	Polyuria, constipation, anorexia, nausea, muscle weakness, psychiatric symptoms, coma
	Intact PTH suppressed

Figure 35.15 Humoral hypercalcemia of malignancy. 1,25 D, 1,25-dihydroxycholecalciferol; PTH, parathyroid hormone; PTHrP, parathyroid-hormone-related peptide.

Differential diagnosis of hypercalcemia

Primary hyperparathyroidism

Humoral hypercalcemia of malignancy (no metastases)

Tumorous hypercalcemia with metastases

Granulomatous disease (sarcoidosis)

Vitamin D intoxication

Vitamin A intoxication

Lithium

Thiazide diuretics

Endocrine diseases (hyperthyroidism and Addison's disease)

Familial hypocalciuric hypercalcemia

Immobilization

Table 35.7 Differential diagnosis of hypercalcemia.

Mediators of tumorous hypercalcemia

Mediators	Tumour type
Parathyroid-hormone-related peptide	Squamous cell carcinoma of the lung, esophagus, larynx, tongue, and uterus Adenocarcinoma (renal, ovary) Transitional cell carcinoma (urogenital)
1,25-dihydroxycholecalciferol	Lymphoma Sarcoidosis
Local cytokines [tumor necrosis factor-α, interleukin-1 (osteoclast-activating factor), interleukin-6]	Metastasizing breast cancer, lymphomas, multiple myeloma

Table 35.8 Mediators of tumorous hypercalcemia.

difficult to explain because PTH, which is a strong stimulator of 1α-hydroxylase, is elevated because of hypophosphatemia in these patients. There is evidence that this phosphaturic factor, which has a molecular mass between 8,000 and 25,000Da, has a direct inhibitory effect on 1α-hydroxylase activity.

Although the oncogenic osteomalacia syndrome is not very well clarified, it fulfills some criteria of an ectopic humoral syndrome. Thus, removal of the tumor results in rapid and dramatic reversal of all clinical and laboratory findings of osteomalacia.

In patients with oncogenic osteomalacia and malignant tumors that cannot be completely removed, treatment with 1,25-dihydroxycholecalciferol and oral phosphate supplementation improves the clinical symptoms, although phosphate levels in serum usually remain low.

NON-ISLET-CELL TUMOROUS HYPOGLYCEMIA

Severe fasting hypoglycemia is usually caused by endogenous hyperinsulinism due to eutopic insulinomas (see Chapter 20). There are sporadic reports of hypoglycemia caused by insulin secretion from non islet cell tumors, obviously an extremely rare event. Recently a small-cell-carcinoma of the cervix producing excessive amounts of insulin has been described. Also rare but more frequently are patients with large retroperitoneal tumors, who present with severe symptomatic hypoglycemia and have low insulin levels (non-islet-cell tumoral hypoglycemia). Most cases of non-islet-cell tumoral hypoglycemia have been associated with mesenchymal tumors such as sarcomas, but hepatomas and other carcinomas, usually located in the abdominal or retroperitoneal region, can also cause hypoglycemia. Like patients with insulinomas, these patients start with adrenergic or neuroglucopenic symptoms of hypoglycemia in the fasting state. The symptoms are usually controlled by supplemental carbohydrates in the beginning, although patients may become later severely hypoglycemic, needing intravenous glucose administration.

Pathophysiology

It is known that IGF-1 and IGF-2 can cause hypoglycemia when given to human subjects. The explanation is that the administered IGF-1 or IGF-2 raises the level of the free IGF not bound to the binding proteins. The free IGF finds access to the insulin receptor, which can cause hypoglycemia.

It has been shown that patients with non-islet-cell tumoral hypoglycemia harbor tumors that are capable of synthesizing and secreting IGF-2 (**Fig. 35.16**), which has different effects on the pituitary, the liver, the endocrine pancreas, and the insulin receptor. At the pituitary level IGF-2 inhibits growth hormone secretion, which leads to a decrease in production and release of IGF-1 and the IGF-binding protein-3 (IGFBP-3) from the liver. The lack of IGFBP-3, which usually forms a complex with IGF-1 or IGF-2, leaves the IGF-2 secreted from the tumor in the free form. Thus, free IGF 2 is ready to bind and activate the insulin receptor, causing hypoglycemia. At the same time, pancreatic insulin and glucagon secretion are suppressed.

Treatment

Since these tumors are often rather large, curative surgery is not possible but debulking of the primary tumor leads to prolonged remission by reducing the amount of IGF-2 secreted. Prednisone may help by antagonizing the insulin-like action of IGF-2. Growth hormone replacement is also helpful, since it stimulates production not only of hepatic IGF-1 but also of IGFBP-3, which is then able to bind and inactivate the excess IGF-2.

ECTOPIC CHORIONIC GONADOTROPIN SECRETION

Trophoblastic tumors, notably chorioncarcinomas of the placenta and testis, are sources of eutopic human chorionic gonadotropin (hCG) secretion. The tumors that cause ectopic hCG secretion are germ cell tumors, which can occur in the pineal gland area, where they can lead to visual and endocrine disturbances, i.e. diabetes insipidus and hypopituitarism. Other tumors associated with ectopic hCG hypersecretion are hepatocellular, gastrointestinal, and lung cancers. Ectopically produced chorionic gonadotropin stimulates secretion of testosterone but also estradiol by testicular Leydig cells. Excess of hCG in young boys may therefore cause precocious puberty. The latter is not observed in females, since hCG has only luteinizing hormone but no follicle stimulating hormone activity, which is needed for follicular maturation and estrogen production, essential for sexual maturation in females. In adult males, elevated hCG leads to gynecomastia resulting from an elevated estradiol:testosterone ratio, whereas in the female menstrual irregularities are common.

The diagnosis of ectopic hCG syndrome is based on the demonstration of a malignant lesion and elevated hCG-β serum levels measured by immunoassay. Whenever gynecomastia is observed and has led to the detection of elevated hCG-β levels, testicular tumors have to be excluded first by clinical examination and ultrasonography, followed by the exclusion of other lesions, particularly in the lung, liver, and gastrointestinal tract.

The hyperthyroid states which have been observed in patients with elevated hCG levels are caused by molecular variants of this hormone that are occasionally secreted by malignant tumors. These hCG variants with altered glycosylation have a high affinity to the TSH receptor. The same mechanism may lead to gestational hyperthyroidism although mutant thyrotropin receptors hypersensitive to hCG have been reported.

Not all cases of male gynecomastia are due to elevated hCG levels (**Table 35.9**). Thus, testicular tumors can cause gynecomastia not by producing hCG but by secreting estrogens directly. Very rarely, male gynecomastia can be caused by tumorous aromatase production, which leads to an elevated estrogen level because of enhanced conversion of testosterone into estradiol. Androgen-deficient males present with hypogonadism and often gynecomastia. Another common cause of gynecomastia is drugs with antiandrogen or estrogenic activity.

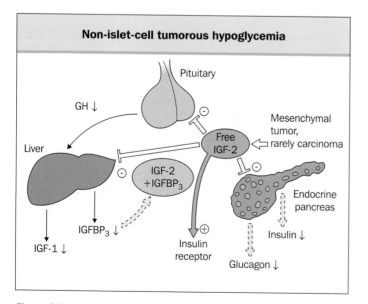

Figure 35.16 Non-islet-cell tumorous hypoglycemia. GH, growth hormone; IGF, insulin-like growth factor; IGFBP, IGF-binding protein.

Pathologic causes of gynecomastia

Human-chorionic-gonadotropin-producing tumors (testis, lung, liver, etc.)

Estrogen-producing tumors (testicular and adrenal)

Tumors with enhanced aromatase activity

Primary hypogonadism (Klinefelter's syndrome, acquired testicular disease, etc.)

Secondary hypogonadism (hypopituitarism, hyperprolactinemia)

Androgen resistance syndrome (testicular feminization, Reifenstein's syndrome, etc.)

Systemic chronic diseases (liver disease, renal disease, starvation)

Drugs (estrogens, antiandrogens, gonadotropins, cytotoxic drugs)

Table 35.9 Pathologic causes of gynecomastia.

ECTOPIC HORMONE PRODUCTION BY PANCREATIC ISLET TUMORS

Pancreatic islet tumors are derived from neuroendocrine cells of the pancreas and belong to the group of gastroenteropancreatic endocrine tumors (see Chapter 33). Since insulin, glucagon, and somatostatin are produced normally by the endocrine pancreas, these tumors do not qualify as producers of the ectopic hormone syndrome. However, since gastrin is normally produced by dispersed cells in the antral mucosa of the stomach and the small intestine, the gastrinoma syndrome could be regarded as an ectopic hormone syndrome or, better, as a result of tumor development from ectopically located gastrin-producing cells in the pancreas. The same is true for the rather rare benign or malignant islet cell tumors, which produce excessive VIP, causing the VIPoma syndrome, i.e. watery diarrhea, achlorhydria, and hypokalemia. These two syndromes are not discussed in this chapter because they are extensively described in Chapter 33. They illustrate, however, that when dealing with ectopic humoral syndromes one has to realize that there is a significant overlap with other classic endocrine syndromes and that the differentiation between eutopic and ectopic is sometimes arbitrary.

ECTOPIC CYTOKINE SYNDROMES

Neoplasms are capable of producing a number of cytokines and growth factors that are biologically active in an individual patient acting in an endocrine, paracrine, or autocrine fashion (Fig. 35.3). They are responsible for the various paraneoplastic symptoms that are often observed in cancer patients such as the granulocytosis syndrome, which is due to the production and release of factors responsible for stimulating myelopoiesis in the bone marrow, e.g. granulocyte-colony-stimulating factor (CSF) and CS macrophage factor.

Erythropoiesis is stimulated by erythropoietin (EPO), a kidney hormone that can be overproduced by renal carcinomas (eutopic) and also hemangioblastomas of the cerebellum, adrenal, ovarian, and liver cancers. Erythrocytosis as a consequence of renal cancers is already quite rare; it is even rarer still in the other tumors. Here it is not even clear that the elevated hemoglobin in patients with adrenal or ovarian cancer is not caused by other factors, such as enhanced androgen production. In contrast to these rare situations, tumor cachexia is often seen in patients with pancreatic cancer. This often dramatic weight loss seems to be mediated by humoral factors such as cachectin or TNFα.

Another aspect of the ectopic humoral syndrome is the laboratory assessment of ectopically produced substances, particularly hormones, that may serve as tumor markers. Although it is very important to measure hormones that cause clinical syndromes in order to make the diagnosis and monitor therapy, measurement of biologically inactive markers has been disappointing in clinical practice. The classic tumor markers – fetal proteins (carcinoembryonic antigen and α-fetoprotein), specific markers for prostatic malignancy (prostate specific antigen), markers for lung cell carcinoma, breast cancer, and pancreatic cancer – their nature, specificity, and clinical importance for monitoring anticancer therapy are discussed in the relevant chapters in textbooks of oncology.

FURTHER READING

Arioglu E, Doppman J, Gomes M, et al. Cushing's syndrome caused by corticotropin secretion by pulmonary tumorlets. N Engl J Med. 1998; 339:883–6.

Baylis PH. Syndrome of inappropriate antidiuretic hormone secretion. In: Sheaves R, Jenkins PJ, Wass JAH, eds. Clinical endocrine oncology. Oxford:Blackwell; 1998:479–83.

Bethge H, Arlt W, Zimmermann U, et al. Cushing's syndrome due to an ectopic ACTH-secreting pituitary tumour mimicking occult paraneoplastic ectopic ACTH production. Clin Endocrinol. 1999; 51:809–14.

Beuschlein F, Strasburger CJ, Siegerstetter V, et al. Acromegaly caused by secretion of growth hormone by a non-Hodgkin's lymphoma. New Engl J Med. 2000; 342:1871–6.

Cai Q, Hodgson S, Kao PC, et al. Brief report: inhibition of renal phosphate transport by a tumor product in a patient with osteogenic osteomalacia. N Engl J Med. 1994; 330:1645–9.

Glass AL. Gynecomastia. Endocrinol Metab Clin North Am. 1994; 23:825–37.

Grill V, Martin TJ. Hypercalcemia of malignancy. In: Grossman A, ed. Clinical Endocrinology. Oxford:Blackwell; 1998:1018–33.

Kulke MH, Mayer RJ. Carcinoid tumors. New Engl J Med. 1999; 340:858–68.

Losa M, von Werder K. Pathophysiology and clinical aspects of the ectopic GH-releasing hormone syndrome. Clin Endocrinol. 1997; 47:123–35.

Losa M, Wolfram G, Mojto J, et al. Presence of growth hormone-releasing hormone-like immunoreactivity in human tumors: characterization of immunological and biological properties. J Clin Endocrinol Metab. 1990; 70:62–8.

Meador CK, Liddle GW, Island DP, et al. Cause of Cushing's syndrome in patients with tumours arising from 'nonendocrine' tissue. J Clin Endocrinol Metab. 1962; 22:693.

Melmed S, Ezrin C, Kovacs K, Goodman RS, Frohman LA. Acromegaly due to secretion of growth hormone by an ectopic pancreatic islet-cell tumor. N Engl J Med. 1985; 312:9–17.

Oldfield EH, Doppman JL, Nieman LK, et al. Petrosal sinus sampling with and without corticotropin-releasing hormone for the differential diagnosis of Cushing's syndrome. N Engl J Med. 1991; 325:897–905.

Pearse AGE. The cytochemistry and ultrastructure of polypeptide hormone-producing cells of the APUD series and the embryologic, physiologic and pathologic implications of the concept. J Histochem Cytochem. 1969; 17:303.

Phillips LS, Robertson DG. Insulin-like growth factors and non-islet cell tumor hypoglycemia. Metabolism 1993; 42:1093–101.

Rodien P, Bremont C, Raffin Sansom M-L, et al. Familal gestational hyperthyroidism caused by a mutant thyrotropin receptor hypersensitive to human chorionic gonadotropin. New England J Med. 1998; 339:1823–6.

Schwartz WB, Bennett W, Curelop S, Bartter FC. A syndrome of renal sodium loss and hyponatremia probably resulting from inappropriate secretion of antidiuretic hormone. Am J Med. 1957; 23:529.

Seckl MJ, Mulholland PJ, Bishop AE, et al. Hypoglycemia due to insulin-secreting small-cell carcinoma of the cervix. New Eng J Med. 1999; 341:733–36.

Ulick S, Wang JZ, Blumenfeld JD, Pickering TG. Cortisol inactivation overload: a mechanism of mineralocorticoid hypertension in the ectopic adrenocorticotropin syndrome. J Clin Endocrinol Metab. 1992; 74:963–7.

Wajchenberg BL, Mendonca BB, Liberman B, et al. Ectopic adrenocorticotropic hormone syndrome. Endocrine Rev. 1994; 15:752–87.

Wilkins GE, Granleese S, Hegele RG, Anderson DW, Bondy GP. Oncogenic osteomalacia. Evidence for a humoral phosphaturic factor. J Clin Endocrinol Metab. 1995; 80:1628–34.

Zapf J, Futto E, Peter M, Froesch ER. Can 'big' insulin-like growth factor II in serum of tumor patients account for the development of extrapancreatic tumor hypoglycemia? J Clin Invest. 1992; 90:2574–84.

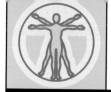

Section 7 General Conditions – Clinical

Chapter 36

Obesity and Satiety

Peter G Kopelman and Stephen O'Rahilly

INTRODUCTION

Obesity has long been the 'Cinderella' of metabolic disorders, largely neglected by mainstream endocrinology, which viewed it as an intractable behavioral problem for which few useful interventions were available. This perception of obesity is changing dramatically. First, obesity is now recognized as a major cause of mortality and morbidity that is increasing dramatically in developed and developing countries. Second, scientific research has brought new and startling insights into the molecular mechanisms involved in the control of bodyweight. Finally, driven by these new discoveries, the pharmaceutical industry is bringing unprecedented resources to the search for novel antiobesity drugs. The next decade will see obesity established as a major area of clinical endocrinology with all the associated diagnostic and therapeutic challenges familiar to endocrinologists.

THE CONTROL OF BODY FAT MASS

Historical perspective

The fact that most adult humans retain a remarkable degree of weight stability over many decades, despite wide variations in day-to-day energy intake and expenditure, suggests the existence of homeostatic mechanisms controlling bodyweight and, in particular, fat mass. Several clinical case reports in the 19th century described the development of intense hyperphagia and obesity in patients with tumors in the region of the hypothalamus, providing the first real clues that this area of the brain was involved in weight homeostasis. In the 1940s, lesioning experiments in rats suggested the existence of both satiety (medial) and feeding (lateral) centers in the hypothalamus. In the 1950s Hervey produced the first evidence for a circulating factor controlling bodyweight when he demonstrated that the induction of obesity through hypothalamic lesioning in one of a pair of rats with artificially joined circulations (parabiosis) produced severe weight loss and suppression of appetite in the other member of the linked pair. Similar experiments undertaken by Coleman in subtypes of genetically obese mice (ob/ob and db/db) suggested that the former lacked this satiety factor and the latter was resistant to it (**Fig. 36.1**). It was not until 1994, however, that the identity of this factor was established by positional cloning.

Leptin as an adipostatic signal

Friedman and colleagues identified in the obese ob/ob mouse a mutation in a previously undescribed gene encoding a secreted cytokine-like protein. They called this protein leptin (**Fig. 36.2**). Leptin appeared to be produced specifically in adipose tissue and, in normal animals, to be increased in states of energy excess and decreased by starvation and weight loss. When leptin was administered in small doses directly into the cerebrospinal fluid of ob/ob animals it completely reversed the abnormalities of appetite and energy balance. Thus, leptin appeared to fulfill characteristics of an endocrine signal between fat and brain (**Fig. 36.3**).

Other roles of leptin

Despite the fact that severe obesity results from an absolute deficiency of leptin it is becoming clear that the primary evolutionary purpose for developing an endocrine signal between fat and brain is not necessarily the prevention of obesity. Flier and colleagues were the first to raise the possibility that leptin might have its most important biologic role in states of undernutrition, in which the reduction in circulating leptin level is largely responsible for the coordinated hypothalamic response to starvation. Thus the administration of leptin to fasted mice ameliorates the hypogonadotropic hypogonadism (low luteinizing and follicle-stimulating hormones and sex steroids), central hypothyroidism (low thyroid-stimulating hormone and thyroxine), and activation of the hypothalamo–pituitary–adrenal (HPA) axis (elevated adrenocorticotropic hormone and corticosterone) associated with nutrient deprivation. The importance of leptin in the control of the human reproductive axis is underlined by the profound hypogonadotropic hypogonadism seen in adults with congenital leptin deficiency and the ability of leptin therapy to facilitate normal puberty in a child with the same condition. Interesting effects of leptin on bone metabolism, immune function, and many other physiologic parameters have also been reported (**Fig. 36.3**).

Central mechanisms of adipostatic signaling

Over the past decade there have been major advances in our understanding of the functional neuroendocrinology of the hypothalamus with respect to control of energy balance. This has included the identification of a large number of hypothalamic neuropeptides that either promote or inhibit feeding (**Table 36.1**). For some peptides, the body of evidence supporting their role is overwhelming (**Fig. 36.4**). Thus, the arcuate nucleus contains the cell bodies of proopiomelanocortin (POMC), neurons whose axons project widely in the hypothalamus and beyond. Leptin directly activates these neurons. Melanocyte-stimulating hormone (MSH) analogs suppress feeding while competitive antagonists increase feeding. Both mice and humans with deleted POMC genes develop hyperphagia and obesity. The melanocortin-4 receptor (MC4R) appears to be the subtype

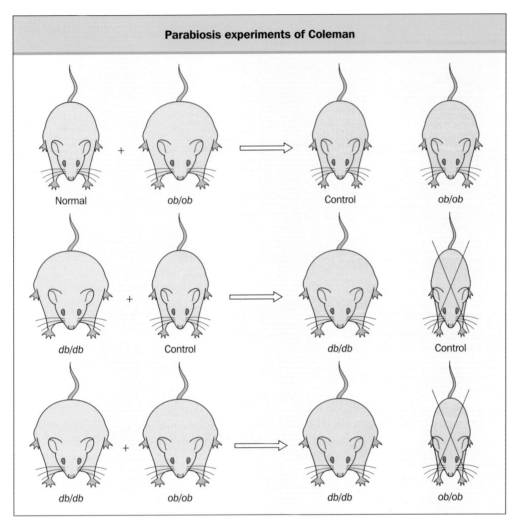

Parabiosis experiments of Coleman

Normal + ob/ob → Control ob/ob

db/db + Control → db/db Control

db/db + ob/ob → db/db ob/ob

Figure 36.1 Parabiosis experiments of Coleman. These provided compelling evidence for the existence of a circulating satiety factor that was absent in the obese ob/ob mouse but was present in very high amounts in the also obese db/db mouse, which was resistant to its actions. Later work found that this circulating factor was the adipocyte hormone leptin. Ob/ob mice have a mutation preventing the formation of leptin and db/db mice have a mutation in the leptin receptor.

responsible for mediating the effects of POMC-derived peptides, as genetic disruption of this receptor in mice and humans results in severe obesity. Neuropeptide Y, when infused centrally in rats, produces persistent hyperphagia and marked obesity. Of note, its expression in the arcuate nucleus is suppressed by leptin. Melanin concentrating hormone (MCH) is found exclusively in the lateral hypothalamus, the traditional feeding center. Consistent with this, central MCH administration increases food intake and transgenic overexpression causes obesity. Moreover, mice rendered null for MCH by gene targeting to ablate the MCH gene have low food intakes and bodyweight.

Signals for meal initiation and satiety

While leptin may be an important adipostatic signal, its levels do not change acutely with meals and it is unlikely to play a direct role in transmitting the sensation of satiety resulting in meal termination. It is clear, however, that in the absence of leptin these signals are ineffective. The precise roles of signals such as gastric distention, cholecystokinin, and other gut-derived peptides in the central control of satiety remain to be established. Recently Ghrelin, the natural ligand for the growth hormone secretagogue receptor, has been identified as being produced mainly in the stomach and appears to have an important impact on increasing food intake.

ETIOLOGY OF OBESITY

Genetic factors

It is well recognized that monogenic disorders, such as Prader–Willi syndrome, Bardet–Biedl syndrome and Cohen's syndrome, are all closely associated with obesity. Apart from the case of mutations in $G_{s\alpha}$ associated with pseudohypoparathyroidism, the molecular bases of these 'syndromic' obesities have yet to be uncovered. In the past 3 years mutations in five different genes have been described as producing severe childhood obesity, some with associated endocrine features, but none with the severe developmental problems seen in the classical named obesity syndromes. The features of those disorders are listed in **Table 36.2**. It should be emphasized that mutations in MC4R are observed in up to 5% of children with severe obesity. Thus, this single condition represents an appreciable burden of disease.

Most cases of human obesity do not have a monogenic basis but there is strong evidence that between 40–70% of interindividual variation in body fat mass are due to inherited factors, be they either multiple (polygenic) gene defects or limited gene defects (oligogenic) in origin. The identification of these polygenes has proved more difficult than in the single gene disorders.

Ribbon diagram of the structure of leptin

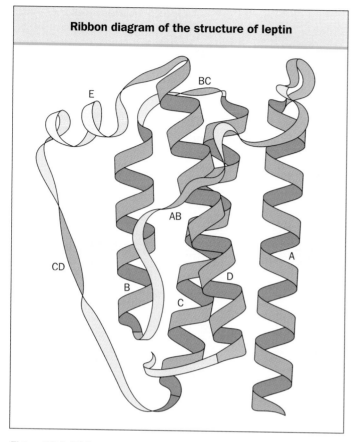

Figure 36.2 Ribbon diagram of the structure of leptin.

Environment

Although genetic factors are clearly important in determining susceptibility to obesity, it is abundantly clear that environmental factors also have a major role. The increase in obesity prevalence in developed countries over the past 20 years has been so rapid that it would be impossible for genetic drift to play a role. While increased energy intake may play a role in some cultures, it appears that in westernized societies the marked reduction in daily energy expenditure over this time period is likely to be the predominant factor.

DEFINITION OF OVERWEIGHT AND OBESITY – BODY MASS INDEX

In clinical practice body fat is most commonly and simply estimated by using a formula that combines weight and height. The formula most frequently used in epidemiologic studies is body mass index (BMI), which is weight in kilograms divided by the square of the height in meters. BMI is strongly correlated with densitometric measurements of fat mass adjusted for height in middle-aged adults. The main limitation of BMI is that it does not readily distinguish fat mass from lean mass. Measurements of body circumference are important because excess visceral (intraabdominal) fat is a potential risk for chronic diseases independent of total adiposity. Waist circumference and the ratio of waist circumference to hip circumference are practical measures for assessing upper body fat distribution, although neither provides a precise estimate of visceral fat. Measurement of skinfold thickness with calipers provides a more precise assessment

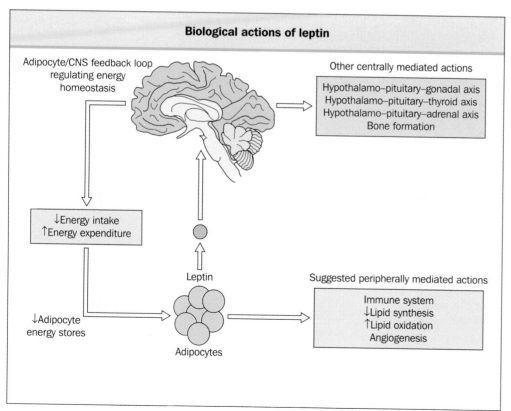

Figure 36.3 Biological actions of leptin. Leptin secretion from adipocytes occurs in proportion to fat mass, but is modulated by other factors such as insulin, glucocorticoids, and sex steroids. Its major effects are central, decreasing appetite and increasing energy expenditure. An increasing number of peripheral actions, as yet of uncertain physiologic significance, are being identified.

Table 36.1 Neuropeptides that affect feeding. The neuropeptides listed are expressed in hypothalamic nuclei and have reproducible effects on feeding after central administration in rodents.

Neuropeptides that affect feeding

Neuropeptides that increase feeding	Neuropeptides that decrease feeding
Neuropeptide Y (NPY)	α-melanocyte-stimulating hormone (αMSH)
Agouti-related protein (AGRP)	Glucagon-like peptide 1 (GLP-1)
Melanin-concentrating hormone (MCH)	Urocortin
Orexin A and B	Corticotropin-releasing hormone (CRH)
β-endorphin	Cocaine- and amphetamine-related transcript (CART)
Galanin	Neuromedin U
Ghrelin	

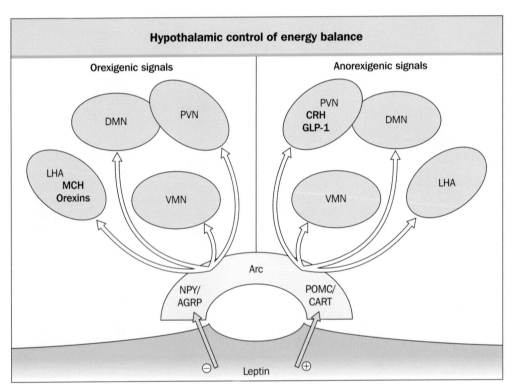

Figure 36.4 Hypothalamic control of energy balance. Neuropeptides expressed in various hypothalamic nuclei have important effects on feeding and satiety. Orexigenic peptides and their main sites of synthesis are shown the left and anorexigenic peptides on the right. In general the expression of the former are reduced by leptin whole the latter are increased. DMN, dorsomedial nucleus; PVN, paraventricular nucleus; LHA, lateral hypothalamus; MCH, melanin concentrating hormone; VMN, ventromedial nucleus; GLP-1, glucagon-like peptide 1; NPY, neuropeptide Y; AGRP, agouti-related protein; Arc, arcuate nucleus; POMC, proopiomelanocortin; CART, cocaine- and amphetamine-related transcript.

of body fat, especially if taken at multiple sites. Skinfolds are useful in the estimation of fatness in children, for whom standards have been published. However, the measurements are more difficult to make in adults (particularly in the very obese), are subject to considerable variation between observers, require accurate calipers, and do not provide any information on abdominal and intramuscular fat. In general they are not superior to simpler measures of height and weight.

Measurement of impedance is based on the principle that lean mass conducts current better than fat mass because it is primarily an electrolyte solution. A measurement of the resistance to a weak current (impedance) applied across the extremities provides an estimate of body fat when combined with height and weight and an empirically derived equation. Although the devices are simple and practical to use, they neither measure fat nor predict biologic outcomes more accurately than the simpler anthropometric measurements. **Table 36.3** lists methods that may be used to quantify obesity.

Body mass index can be used to estimate the prevalence of obesity within a population and the risks associated with it. It does not, however, account for the wide variation in the nature of obesity between different individuals and populations. A World Health Organization Expert Committee has proposed a classification of overweight and obesity that applies to both men and women and to all adult age groups (**Table 36.4**).

Waist circumference correlates with measures of risk for coronary heart disease such as hypertension or blood lipid levels. The choice of cutoff points on the waist circumference continuum involves a trade-off between sensitivity and specificity similar to that for BMI. An expert panel has suggested increased risks if the waist circumference is more than 102cm in men and more than 88cm in women. However, lower cutoff points are associated with two to threefold increase in the relative risk of type 2 diabetes. Gender-specific cutoff points for waist circumference may be of guidance in interpreting values for adults: proposed cut-off levels are shown in **Table 36.5**, level 1 being intended to alert clinicians to potential risk while level 2 should initiate therapeutic action. It is of critical importance to appreciate that these tables reflect knowledge acquired largely from epidemiologic studies in developed countries. Preliminary information from developing

Monogenic causes of human obesity

Syndrome	Locus/mode of inheritance	Obesity characteristics	Other features
Prader–Willi	15q11 Imprinted gene	Feeding difficulties at birth, followed by extreme hyperphagia & weight gain with generalized obesity from age 2–3 years. Short stature	Hypogonadism, hypotonia, small hands and feet, scoliosis, learning difficulties, behavior problems
Bardet–Biedl	16q21, 11q13, 15q22, 3p12 All recessive	Overlap with Lawrence–Moon–Bardet–Biedl (which is characterized by progressive spastic paraparesis and without polydactyly); onset of generalized obesity in first 2 years. Short stature	Retinitis pigmentosa, hypogonadism, learning difficulties, polydactyly
Cohen's	8q22–23 Recessive	Truncal obesity from mid-childhood	Hypogonadism, delayed puberty with or without hypogonadism
Alstrom's	2p12–13 Autosomal recessive	Normal height, truncal obesity from mid-childhood	Hypogonadism, blindness in infancy from retinal degeneration, deafness, insulin resistance, diabetes mellitus, progressive nephropathy
Edwards's			Similar to Alstrom's but with pigmented retinopathy
Klinefelter's	XXY	Adult onset with peripheral distribution. Tall with eunuchoid proportions	Hypogonadal (primary), moderate learning difficulties, gynecomastia with male phenotype
Albright's hereditary osteodystrophy (G$_{s\alpha}$ mutations)	Autosomal recessive	Childhood onset	Round face. Variable hormone resistance including TSH, PTH. Short fourth metacarpal
Congenital leptin deficiency	Autosomal recessive	Childhood onset, generalized obesity, normal stature, marked hyperphagia	Hypogonadal, insulin resistance
Prohormone convertase 1	Autosomal recessive	Childhood onset – one subject described to date	Hypogonadism. Hyperproinsulinemia. Reactive hypoglycemia. Hypoadrenalism
Leptin receptor	Autosomal recessive	Childhood onset – three subjects described to date	Hypogonadism. Short stature. Hypothyroidism
POMC	Autosomal recessive	Childhood onset – two subjects described to date	Hypoadrenalism. Red hair. Pale skin
MC4R	Autosomal dominant	About 10 subjects described to date	None

Table 36.2 Monogenic causes of human obesity. The associated genetic and clinical characteristics are listed.

Practical clinical methods for assessment of an obese subject

Characteristic of obesity measured	Methods
Body composition	Body mass index
	Underwater weighing
	Dual-energy X-ray absorptiometry
	Isotope dilution
	Bioelectrical impedance
	Skinfold thickness
Regional distribution of fat	Waist circumference; waist-to-hip ratio
	Computerized tomography
	Ultrasound
	Magnetic resonance imaging
Energy intake	Dietary recall or record
	'Macronutrient composition' by prospective dietary record or dietary questionnaire
Energy expenditure	Doubly labeled water
	Indirect calorimetry (resting)
	Physical activity level by questionnaire
	Motion detector
	Heart rate monitor

Table 36.3 Practical clinical methods for assessment of an obese subject.

nations indicates that lower cutoff levels for both BMI and waist circumference are necessary for certain populations (e.g. Asian) who are at particular risk from comparatively modest degrees of overweight.

HEALTH CONSEQUENCES OF OBESITY

There is convincing evidence linking increasing bodyweight with important medical complications. A close relationship exists between BMI and the incidence of several chronic conditions caused by excess fat – type 2 diabetes, hypertension, coronary heart disease and cholelithiasis. This relationship is approximately linear for a range of BMI indices less than 30. The risk of hypertension is doubled in both men and women with a BMI of 26. All risks are greatly increased for those subjects with a BMI of more than 29, independent of gender. The Build and Blood Pressure Study has shown that the adverse effects of excess weight tend to be delayed, sometimes for 10 years or longer. Life insurance data and epidemiologic studies confirm that increasing degrees of overweight and obesity are important predictors of decreased longevity.

In the Framingham Heart Study, the risk of death within 26 years increased by 1% for each extra pound (0.45kg) increase in weight between the ages of 30 years and 42 years, and by 2% between the ages of 50 years and 62 years. In the same study, the 26-year incidence of coronary heart disease in women and men was related proportionately to excess weight. In this study the

Table 36.4 Classification of overweight. Cutoff points proposed by a WHO Expert Committee. Body mass index is the weight in kilograms divided by the height in meters.

Classification of overweight		
Body mass index (kg/m²)	WHO classification	Popular description
<18.5	Underweight	Thin
18.5–24.9	–	'Healthy', 'normal', 'acceptable'
25–29.9	Grade 1 overweight	Overweight
30.0–39.9	Grade 2 overweight	Obese
40.0 or greater	Grade 3 overweight	Morbidly obese

Waist measurement and metabolic complications of obesity		
	Risk of obesity-associated metabolic complications	
	Increased	Substantially increased
Men	94cm or greater	102cm or greater
Women	80cm or greater	88cm or greater

Table 36.5 Waist measurement and metabolic complications of obesity. These gender-specific waist circumferences denote 'increased risk' (level 1) and 'substantially increased risk' (level 2) of metabolic complications associated with obesity in Caucasians. Level 1 is intended to alert clinicians to potential risk for coronary heart disease while level 2 should initiate therapeutic action.

Key points when taking a history from an obese patient
Medical history, risk factors, and established complications from obesity – inquire about snoring and daytime somnolence
Bodyweight history (landmarks for weight gain: puberty, employment, marriage, pregnancies, age at menopause, injuries resulting in periods of immobility, etc.)
History of previous treatment(s) for obesity (including successes and failures)
Family history of obesity, related diseases, and risk factors (type 2 diabetes, hypertension, premature coronary heart disease, and gallstones)
Diet history, including usual eating pattern, alcohol intake
Activity and lifestyle, libido
Relevant social history, including cigarette smoking
Drug history – drugs associated with weight gain (e.g. phenothiazines, tricyclic antidepressants, anticonvulsants, lithium, anabolic and glucocorticoid steroids)
In women, menstrual history (irregular menses are associated with polycystic ovary syndrome)

Table 36.6 Key points when taking a history from an obese patient.

incidence of coronary heart disease increased by a factor of 2.4 in obese women and a factor of 2 in obese men under the age of 50 years. Bodyweight, independent of several traditional risk factors, was directly related to the development of congestive cardiac failure in the Framingham Heart Study.

In the Nurses Cohort Study, BMI was the dominant predictor of the risk of diabetes after adjustment for age. Similarly, the risk of diabetes in men increases for all BMI levels of 24 or above. The distribution of fat tissue is also independently associated with diabetes: a waist circumference of more than 40 inches (102cm.) increases the risk of diabetes 3.5-fold, even after controlling for the BMI.

In the Swedish Obese Subjects study, over 50% of men and one third of women with a BMI of more than 35 reported snoring and apnea. In contrast, 15.5% of Swedish men of comparable age were self-reported habitual snorers. A number of groups have reported an increased risk of myocardial infarction and stroke in sleep apnea. Snoring is a strong risk factor for sleep-related strokes while sleep apnea symptoms increase the risk for cerebral infarction.

CLINICAL ASSESSMENT OF THE OBESE PATIENT

Clinical presentation
The majority of adult patients who present to an endocrinologist will not have a readily identifiable and/or easily remediable cause for their obesity. Most referrals to endocrine units result from the patient or the medical practitioner questioning an endocrine or metabolic basis to progressive weight gain or an explanation for the apparently intractable nature of the obesity. The common reasons for referral may be categorized into five groups:
* A direct question about whether the obesity has a metabolic or endocrine basis;
* Menstrual or reproductive abnormalities: progressive weight gain or established obesity associated with irregular menses or infertility – unexplained weight gain with amenorrhea may sometimes be explained by unsuspected pregnancy;
* Specific metabolic disorders accompanying obesity (diabetes mellitus, hyperuricemia and hyperlipidemia);
* Drug-induced causes of obesity: marked weight gain may occasionally coincide with the commencement of certain therapeutic compounds;
* A request for consideration of particular forms of therapy that are not available, or unfamiliar, to general practice.

Clinical history
Table 36.6 outlines the areas of medical history that should be covered at the initial assessment. The history of weight gain should be described in detail to elucidate possible etiologic factors and to assess the patient's insight and understanding of the factors causing weight gain. It is also useful to distinguish childhood-onset obesity from that occurring later in life. A number of syndromes are associated with childhood-onset

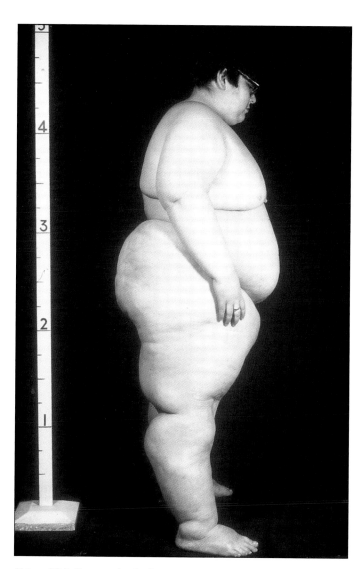

Figure 36.5 Severe obesity in a patient with the Prader–Willi syndrome.

Key points for the examination and investigation of an obese patient
Height, weight – calculate body mass index
Waist circumference
Blood pressure
Neck circumference
Skin – amount of subcutaneous tissue, acanthosis nigricans, hirsutism, abdominal and axillary striae
Any evidence for cardiac valvular disease?
Any evidence for pulmonary hypertension, cor pulmonale or congestive cardiac failure?
External genitalia
Signs of hyperlipidemia
Signs of thyroid disease
Ophthalmic evidence for diabetes or sustained hypertension
Gouty tophi

Table 36.7 Key points for the examination and investigation of an obese patient.

obesity (**Fig. 36.5**). In many, but not all, syndromes the associated clinical features greatly assist diagnosis (**Table 36.2**). Disease involving the hypothalamus can often be distinguished from 'simple' obesity by a shorter duration of weight gain and specific symptoms related to associated endocrine disturbances (**Fig. 36.6**). The identification of the single-gene disorders involving leptin and its signaling pathways are somewhat more difficult to distinguish from simple obesity, but there should be extreme weight gain from early childhood, a positive family history, and the associated clinical features described in **Table 36.2**. The most common single-gene disorder causing obesity, MC4R deficiency, is problematic as there are no pathognomonic features, but the diagnosis should be considered in cases of early-onset familial obesity, usually with a clear dominant inheritance.

Clinical manifestations

An outline of a scheme for the clinical examination is given in **Table 36.7**. Upper-body obesity is a characteristic of Cushing's syndrome and will require a search for other clinical pointers to the diagnosis. An examination of the skin is important: thin, atrophic skin is a feature of corticosteroid excess and there may be associated bruising; acanthosis nigricans (pigmented, 'velvety' skin creases, especially in the axillae; **Fig. 36.7**) suggests insulin resistance and may be associated with hyperandrogenism and/or gonadal dysfunction; severe hirsutism in women is uncommon in simple obesity and may indicate the polycystic ovary syndrome. A buffalo hump and wide violaceous abdominal and axillary striae are uncommon in simple obesity but common in Cushing's syndrome. A neck circumference of more than 43cm (17 inches) indicates a likelihood of obstructive sleep apnea; abnormal external gonadal status accompanied by intellectual impairment may suggest a rare genetic syndrome. Evidence for overt endocrine dysfunction (e.g. hypothyroidism and hypopituitarism), xanthelasma, tendon xanthoma, gouty tophi, and signs of diabetic complications should always be sought. Heat intolerance is common in obesity and makes hypothyroidism unlikely.

ENDOCRINE ALTERATIONS ASSOCIATED WITH OBESITY

Adrenocortical function

Obese subjects have normal circulating serum cortisol levels with a normal circadian rhythm and normal urinary free cortisol but have an accelerated degradation of cortisol, which is compensated by an increased cortisol production rate. It is suggested that enhanced cortisol metabolism by adipose tissue is the primary mechanism behind the changes. If the metabolism of cortisol is increased by adipose tissue in obesity, plasma cortisol will tend to fall, resulting in an increase in pituitary secretion of adrenocorticotropic hormone (ACTH). This in turn causes an increase in adrenal cortisol output to restore plasma cortisol levels to normal. ACTH has been reported to be increased in obesity, and increased ACTH responsiveness to insulin-induced hypoglycemia is associated with increasing bodyweight.

The increase in ACTH secretion stimulates adrenal androgen output and probably accounts for the enhanced androgen

539

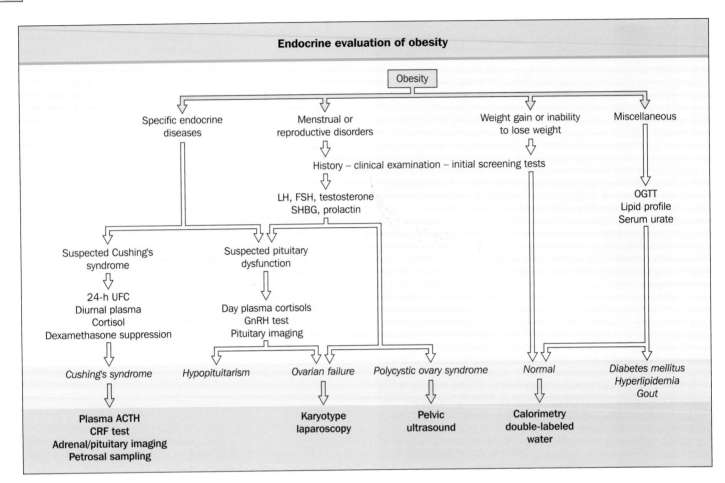

Figure 36.6 Endocrine evaluation of obesity.

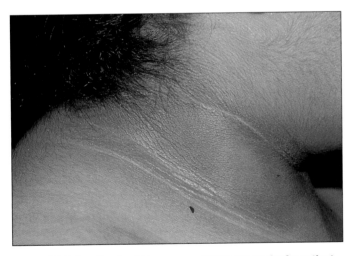

Figure 36.7 Acanthosis nigricans occurring in the neck of a patient with severe insulin resistance associated with obesity.

metabolites, including etiocholananolone, androsterone, dehydroepiandrosterone (DHEA), and its sulfate conjugate DHEAS, often found in obesity. A correlation has been reported between the metabolic clearance of DHEA, androstenedione, and the distribution of fat tissue in the upper body, which suggests that DHEA may have a role in determining adipose tissue deposition.

Furthermore, a positive correlation between bodyweight and changes in DHEA and the DHEA:17-hydroxyprogesterone ratio after the exogenous administration of ACTH has been described.

Prolactin secretion

Two distinct patterns of release to insulin-induced hypoglycemia are seen in obesity. In some obese subjects there is no prolactin response to symptomatic hypoglycemia (prolactin 'nonresponders') while in other equally obese subjects a normal response is seen (prolactin 'responders'). It has been suggested that the impaired prolactin response results from a primary disorder of hypothalamic function because an impaired prolactin response persists in such women despite their subsequent attainment of nearly normal weight. Furthermore, some obese children have been reported to show no prolactin response to hypoglycemia. Jung and colleagues found no significant rise of plasma norepinephrine to hypoglycemia in obese subjects with an impaired prolactin response, although the epinephrine response remained unimpaired. This suggests that the hypothalamic alteration that may occur in those with a propensity for obesity not only involves the control of pituitary but also affects the control of the sympathetic nervous system. Additional evidence for a broader alteration in hypothalamic regulation of prolactin is provided by the finding of a decreased prolactin response to pituitary stimulation by thyrotropin-releasing hormone (TRH) but an increased thyroid-stimulating hormone (TSH) response. The normal circadian rhythm for prolactin secretion, which exists in normal subjects with an increasing number of pulses during the night, is delayed in obesity.

Significant associations are observed between increased insulin secretion and resistance and the prolactin release to insulin-induced hypoglycemia. In addition, an inverse correlation is observed between increasing upper body obesity (as measured by an increasing waist-to-hip ratio) and the prolactin response to hypoglycemia. These findings suggest that hyperinsulinemia may partly explain the impaired prolactin responsiveness seen in some obese subjects.

Growth hormone secretion

Growth hormone (GH) is an important regulator of body mass throughout life. Subcutaneous fat is markedly increased in growth-hormone-deficient children and adults. Moreover, hypopituitary patients have abnormally large amounts of intraabdominal fat, which may be decreased by 30% after 6 months' treatment with growth hormone. Such evidence suggests that relative GH deficiency or insensitivity could play a role in the perpetuation of the obesity.

An impaired GH response to insulin-induced hypoglycemia is found in association with obesity but this seems likely to be a consequence rather than a cause of extreme obesity. Bodyweight gain decreases the GH response to all types of provocative stimuli whereas the GH response significantly increases in obese subjects following weight loss. An input of food in excess of energy expenditure appears to be important because impaired GH responsiveness is not a characteristic of subjects who are overweight as the result of increased musculature induced by vigorous exercise. In this situation, energy expenditure is balanced by an increase in appropriate protein and energy intake whereas 10 days of overfeeding with carbohydrate can produce impaired GH responsiveness without an increase in bodyweight. A significantly reduced GH response to an intravenous bolus of growth-hormone-releasing hormone (GHRH) is also a feature of obesity. This impairment is not dose-dependent because doubling the dose of GHRH in obese subjects does not alter the GH release. Repeated low doses of GHRH will, however, induce improved (but subnormal) GH release in some obese subjects. The explanation for the decreased GH output in obesity has not been fully elucidated. It is not due to an absolute deficiency because the impaired GH response to L-dopa or arginine may be augmented by propranolol or pharmacologic doses of triiodothyronine. Furthermore, in adult obese subjects a comparable rise of free fatty acids to that seen in lean individuals is found after the administration of GH in doses related to bodyweight; obese subjects eating a calorie-restricted diet but treated with injections of GH show raised oxygen consumption, increased weight loss and reduced nitrogen excretion. The evidence suggests a combination of decreased central cholinergic and increased somatostatinergic tone, which influence GH release in obesity. An oral dose of pyridostigmine, an inhibitor of acetylcholinesterase, increases the GH response to GHRH in obese subjects, although this still remains attenuated compared to controls.

It is suggested that altered GH secretion results from alterations in insulin-like growth factor 1 (IGF-1) and its binding proteins. Synthesis of IGF-1 is stimulated by insulin and the hyperinsulinemia of obesity could directly enhance IGF-1 production and

suppress the production of GH from the pituitary by a negative-feedback mechanism. A negative-feedback effect of IGF-1 has been demonstrated in pituitary cells in culture. However, several authors have reported that IGF-1 circulating levels in obese adults are normal. By contrast, IGF binding proteins 1 and 3 (IGFBP-1, IGFBP-3) are both reduced in obesity, with decreased plasma concentrations of IGFBP-1 being inversely related to fasting plasma insulin and increasing upper body obesity.

Thyrotrope and posterior pituitary function

There is no substantial evidence for any clinically significant defect in hypothalamo–pituitary–thyroid function in obesity. Plasma TSH, free thyroxine and free triiodothyronine are normal in obese subjects, although a subnormal TSH response to TRH has been reported in some obese subjects. Starvation or semistarvation will decrease the TSH response to TRH; this underlines the importance of evaluating hypothalamo–pituitary function when subjects are eating adequate amounts of calories. Similarly, basal plasma vasopressin levels are normal in obesity although, after water-loading, arginine vasopressin levels do not suppress normally in obese subjects and water excretion is impaired. Conversely, plasma arginine vasopressin increases erratically after hypertonic saline administration. The arginine vasopressin response to insulin-induced hypoglycemia is normal when adequate symptomatic neuroglycemia occurs. It seems likely that any abnormalities of arginine vasopressin secretion in obesity are minor and of no clinical significance.

Gonadotropins

The association between obesity and abnormalities of reproductive function is well recognized, with decreased libido and impotence commonly seen in extremely overweight men, and an increased incidence of dysfunctional uterine bleeding and amenorrhea being reported in obese women. Subnormal plasma testosterone concentrations and reduced sex-hormone-binding globulin levels occur in massively obese men, with an inverse relationship between plasma testosterone and bodyweight. In these men it has been proposed that elevated plasma estrogens, which result from increased aromatization of androgen precursors by adipose tissue, result in a negative feedback on the hypothalamo–pituitary axis with subnormal luteinizing hormone (LH) and follicle-stimulating hormone (FSH) levels.

In obese women, raised plasma testosterone and androstenedione concentrations are frequently found with reduced sex-hormone-binding globulins and an increased ratio of estrone to estradiol; it is of interest that a similar pattern of changes of sex-steroid concentration and binding are found in women with the polycystic ovary syndrome, many of whom are obese. In contrast to the women with the polycystic ovary syndrome, obese women have a normal LH and FSH response to direct stimulation by gonadotropin-releasing hormone (GnRH) and normal gonadotropin release following the administration of clomiphene, which acts through the hypothalamus. In obese subjects weight loss not only reverses the biochemical changes but frequently results in the reappearance of menses. The precise etiology of these changes is unclear but evidence points to a peripheral effect of adipose tissue on steroid secretion and binding in obesity, which, in turn, influences the release of gonadotropins from the pituitary.

LABORATORY INVESTIGATIONS

It is important to consider the likelihood of an endocrine disorder in an obese patient before embarking upon a series of tests of endocrine function. Such investigations cannot be justified unless there is good historical and clinical evidence to support a diagnosis other than simple obesity.

The initial screening tests for the obese patient should include a full blood count (a raised mean corpuscular volume may be associated with an excessive alcohol intake, an increased packed cell volume may be seen in obstructive sleep apnea and occasionally in Cushing's syndrome), plasma urea and electrolytes (hypokalemia in some cases of Cushing's), fasting blood glucose to exclude diabetes mellitus, and thyroid function tests. The urine should be tested for protein.

Menstrual and reproductive abnormalities

The initial investigations for women with menstrual or reproductive disorders will include the measurement of plasma gonadotropins, serum prolactin, total testosterone, and sex-hormone-binding globulin concentrations. The subsequent investigations will depend upon the results from these initial tests. In men, the finding of primary gonadal failure (decreased testosterone and elevated plasma gonadotropins) will require chromosomal analysis.

Suspected endocrine abnormalities

Possible Cushing's syndrome in an obese patient:

A common clinical problem is excluding Cushing's syndrome in patients with obesity. The usual screening test is the measurement of urinary free cortisol concentration in a 24-hour urine collection. A 1mg overnight dexamethasone suppression test is an alternative but neither is entirely reliable. If the results of the screening tests are positive or equivocal then a formal 'low-dose' dexamethasone suppression test is appropriate (see Chapter 15). In simple obesity the cortisol values should suppress normally.

Possible pituitary dysfunction in an obese patient

Subtle changes in anterior pituitary function may be associated with extreme obesity. Such changes should be taken into account when evaluating the results from anterior pituitary tests. Results from investigations that make pituitary dysfunction unlikely are:

- Absence of physical/clinical signs suggestive of hypopituitarism or a genetic cause for obesity;
- Normal free thyroxine and TSH;
- Normal plasma LH and FSH;
- Normal plasma prolactin.

The hormonal response to GnRH and TRH is within the normal range in obesity. Interpretation of anterior pituitary response to insulin-induced hypoglycemia may be difficult in obesity because:

- It is sometimes difficult to achieve symptomatic hypoglycemia despite the use of larger doses of insulin, because of insulin resistance;
- Growth hormone and prolactin release are commonly diminished in association with obesity.

The measurement of serum leptin is not recommended as a routine but should be undertaken in cases of severe, early-onset obesity as, although rare, congenital leptin deficiency is a potentially treatable disorder.

If pituitary disease is suspected, imaging of the pituitary should be performed either by magnetic resonance imaging or computerized tomography. Remember, however, that magnetic resonance imaging machines will be unable to accommodate the bulk of many severely obese patients.

Diagnostic tests for other possible causes or associations of obesity
These investigations will depend largely on clinical suspicion and may include:

- 75g oral glucose tolerance test with measurement of fasting plasma insulin in acanthosis nigricans;
- Fasting serum lipid profile with measurement of total cholesterol, triglycerides, high-density lipoprotein (HDL) and low-density lipoprotein (LDL) cholesterol;
- serum urate.

Most, if not all, of the abnormalities in endocrine function seen in association with obesity are reversed with substantial weight loss.

TREATMENT

The recommendation to treat overweight and obesity is based on evidence that relates obesity to increased mortality, and on results from randomized controlled trials that demonstrate that weight loss reduces risk factors for other diseases.

Aims for a weight loss program

Any treatment program for overweight and obese patients should place equal importance on the problem of weight reduction and the maintenance of the lowered weight. Obesity may not respond to conventional methods of treatment such as a low calorie diet: its management frequently requires an individually tailored approach.

In the obese patient who smokes, smoking cessation is a major goal for risk management. A major obstacle to smoking cessation is the attendant weight gain. The weight gained with smoking cessation is less likely to produce negative health consequences than continued smoking. For this reason, smoking cessation should initially be strongly advocated combined with prevention of weight gain.

Goals of weight loss

After an initial period of relatively rapid weight reduction, an average continuing loss of anything up to 1kg per week should be considered as acceptable. Assessment of success must take account of the age of the patient, the initial degree of obesity, the presence of indicators of associated risk or complications and previous attempts at weight control. Weight loss goals for overweight and obese patients and weight goals should be tailored to the individual. A weight loss of 5% of the initial bodyweight will result in some improvement while a loss of 10% is of major benefit, with clinically useful changes such as a lowered blood pressure, reduction in plasma total cholesterol and triglycerides, an increase in HDL cholesterol and a significant improvement in diabetic control (**Table 36.8**).

Benefits of weight loss	
Mortality	20–25% fall in total mortality
	30–40% fall in diabetes-related deaths
	40–50% fall in obesity-related cancer deaths
Blood pressure	Fall of approximately 10mmHg in both systolic and diastolic values
Diabetes	Reduces risk of developing diabetes by more than 50%
	Fall of 30–50% in fasting glucose
	Fall of 15% in HbA1c
Lipids	Fall of 10% in total cholesterol
	Fall of 15% in low-density lipoprotein
	Fall of 30% in triglycerides
	Increase of 8% in high-density lipoprotein

Table 36.8 Benefits of weight loss. The potential health benefits are listed that may accrue from the loss of 10kg from the initial bodyweight in those patients with comorbidities. (Adapted from Jung RT, Obesity as a disease. British Medical Bulletin 1997;53:307–21).

Dietary treatment of obesity

Control of diet is the cornerstone for the management of overweight and obese patients and its primary importance must be emphasized. Long-term changes in food choices, eating behavior and lifestyle are needed, rather than a temporary restriction of specific foods. The treatment should be nutritionally sound and aim to promote a healthier diet while moderating energy intake and increasing physical activity. Such a treatment may require a period of supervision for at least 6 months.

Very-low-calorie diets

The use of very-low-calorie diets should only be considered after the failure of determined attempts to lose weight with conventional restriction of normal diets. Such preparations must provide a minimum of 400kcal per day for women and 500kcal per day for men. It must be recognized that these diets do not beneficially alter eating habits or weight loss in the longer term. Very-low-calorie diets may occasionally be useful in the hospital setting for rapid weight loss prior to a surgical procedure. Controlled trials confirm that over the longer term (>1 year) weight loss following very-low-calorie diets is no different from that following low-calorie diets.

Behavior management

Behavior interventions use strategies to facilitate changes in an individual's lifestyle. Behavior weight control programs encourage patients to become more aware of their eating and physical activity, focusing on changing the lifestyle and environmental factors that are controlling their behavior. All dietary regimens should ideally be linked to behavior therapy; such therapy may be incorporated into self-help groups. The key difference between behavioral methods and other forms of treatment for obesity is that they lay particular emphasis on personal responsibility for initiating and maintaining treatment rather than relying on external forces.

Controlled trial evidence suggests that behavior therapy, when used in combination with other weight-loss approaches, provides additional benefits in assisting patients to lose weight in the short term (up to 1 year); extended treatment programs improve long-term weight maintenance.

Exercise and physical activity

When physical activity or exercise alone is used in the treatment of obesity, weight losses are modest and average 2–3kg. This weight loss, although small, exceeds that predicted if direct energy expenditure calculations are performed. For any given weight loss, the loss of fat-free mass is less in exercising versus non-exercising subjects; this is important because fat-free mass is the best predictor of resting metabolic rate, which is the largest contributor to total daily energy expenditure. Physical activity alone in obese adults results in only modest weight loss but increased cardiovascular fitness.

Persuading an obese person to participate in long term exercise programs and to maintain exercise as part of the daily routine is not easy. It is not necessary for the obese patient to increase maximal oxygen uptake by strenuous exercise to derive benefit from exercise: metabolic evidence of improvement in fitness is achieved with less vigorous exercise such as walking increased distances and swimming. The risks from exercise are not great providing it is introduced gradually and other complications such as osteoarthritis and ischemic heart disease are taken into account. One of the most consistent findings in studies of exercise is weight maintenance with maintenance of lost weight being seen in randomized control trials after 2 years from the start of intervention.

Drug treatment

The criteria applied to the use of an antiobesity drug should be similar to those applied to the treatment of other relapsing disorders.

A large number of drugs have been advocated over the years as treatment for obesity. Some of these compounds are effective but many are ineffective. The use of drugs in the management of obesity is bedeviled by the limitations of the available published scientific evidence.

Indications for anti-obesity drug treatment

It may be appropriate to consider drug treatment if, after at least 3 months of supervised diet, exercise, and behavioral management, or at a subsequent review, a patient's BMI is equal to or greater than 30 and weight loss is less than 10% of the presenting weight. In certain clinical circumstances it may also be appropriate to consider antiobesity drug treatment for those patients with established comorbidities whose BMI is 27 or greater if this is permitted by the drug's license.

The initiation of drug treatment will depend on the clinician's judgment about the risks to an individual from continuing obesity: drug treatment may be particularly appropriate for patients with comorbid risk factors or complications from their obesity. A drug should not be considered ineffective because weight loss has stopped, providing the lowered weight is maintained. However, continuation of the drug should depend on the balance between the health benefits of maintained weight and the potential adverse effects of the drug. **Figure 36.8** summarizes recommendations for the appropriate use of an antiobesity drug. A system of regular medical audit should be a prerequisite of a weight management program, with a record of results and audit action.

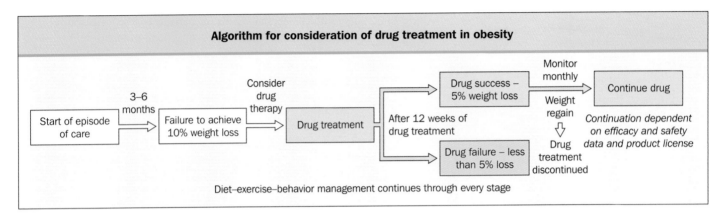

Figure 36.8 Algorithm for consideration of drug treatment in obesity.

Types of drug treatment for obesity

There are currently two categories of antiobesity drug – those that act on the gastrointestinal system (pancreatic lipase inhibitors) and those that act on the central nervous system to suppress appetite.

Drugs acting on the gastrointestinal system

Pancreatic lipase inhibitors

Orlistat inhibits pancreatic and gastric lipases, thereby decreasing ingested triglyceride hydrolysis. It produces a dose-dependent reduction in dietary fat absorption that is near maximum at a dose of 120mg three times daily. These actions lead to weight loss in obese subjects. Adverse effects of orlistat are predominantly related to its gastrointestinal actions owing to fat malabsorption. These include loose or liquid stools, fecal urgency, and oily discharge and can be associated with fat-soluble vitamin malabsorption.

Centrally acting antiobesity drugs

Drugs acting on noradrenergic and serotoninergic pathways

Sibutramine promotes a sense of satiety through its central action as a serotonin and norepinephrine reuptake inhibitor. In addition, it may have an enhancing effect on thermogenesis through stimulation of peripheral noradrenergic receptors. Sibutramine is well absorbed following oral ingestion and undergoes first-pass metabolism in the liver to produce two active metabolites that have long elimination half-lives. This enables sibutramine to be given on a single daily basis at a starting dose of 10mg. Adverse effects include nausea, dry mouth, rhinitis, and constipation. The noradrenergic actions of the drug may cause an increase in blood pressure and heart rate in some patients, or prevent the expected fall in these parameters with weight loss. The drug should be used with caution in hypertensive patients.

Drugs not appropriate for the treatment of obesity

There is no published evidence to suggest that bulk-forming agents (e.g. methyl cellulose) have any beneficial long-term action for weight reduction. Diuretics, human chorionic gonadotropin, amphetamine, dexamphetamine, and thyroxine are not treatments for obesity and should not be used to achieve weight loss. Under no circumstance should thyroxine be prescribed for obesity in the absence of biochemically proven hypothyroidism. Metformin and acarbose may be useful in the management of the obese non-insulin-dependent diabetic patient; they have no proven efficacy for obesity alone and are not licensed for such use.

Surgical treatment of obesity

There are two operative procedures currently used for the surgical treatment of obesity: gastric restriction and gastric bypass.

Gastric restriction involves the creation of a small-capacity compartment (<20ml) by either a combination of vertical stapling and a constrictive band opening or a circumgastric band pinching off a small proximal pouch. A modification of the latter procedure is an inflatable circumgastric band attached to a subcutaneous reservoir, which allows access by an hypodermic syringe to inject or withdraw fluid, thereby tightening or enlarging the band width.

Gastric bypass is performed by stapling shut a vertically oriented pouch of less than 20ml capacity and connecting this pouch to the jejunum, transected 50cm from the ligament of Treitz (Roux-en-Y gastric bypass). Published evidence confirms that this procedure produces greater weight loss but is accompanied by more frequent adverse effects, including 'dumping'. Most antiobesity surgical procedures have been successfully performed laparoscopically, which reduces the requirement for sedating pain medication and facilitates prompt postoperative mobilization.

A review of evidence from controlled trials confirms that surgery for obesity is an option for carefully selected patients with clinically severe obesity (BMI ≥ 40 or BMI ≥ 35 with comorbid conditions) when less invasive methods of weight loss have failed and the patient is at high risk for obesity-associated morbidity and mortality. The nature of the surgical procedures necessitate long-term hospital followup for such patients.

COMPLICATIONS OF OBESITY

Obesity causes or exacerbates a large number of health problems, both independently and in association with other diseases (Table 36.9). In particular, it is associated with the development of diabetes mellitus, coronary heart disease, an increased incidence of certain forms of cancer, obstructive sleep apnea, and osteoarthritis of large and small joints.

Systemic comorbidities associated with obesity

Cardiovascular	Hypertension
	Coronary heart disease
	Cerebrovascular disease varicose veins
	Deep vein thrombosis
Respiratory	Breathlessness
	Sleep-related hypoventilation
	Sleep apnea
	Obesity hypoventilation syndrome
Gastrointestinal	Hiatus hernia
	Gallstones
	Fatty liver & cirrhosis
	Colorectal cancer
Metabolic	Dyslipidemia
	Insulin resistance
	Type 2 diabetes mellitus
	Hyperuricemia
Endocrine	Increased adrenocortical activity
	Altered circulating sex steroids and binding
	Breast cancer
	Polycystic ovary syndrome
	Hirsutism
Locomotor	Osteoarthritis
	Nerve entrapment
Renal	Proteinuria
Genitourinary	Endometrial cancer
	Prostate cancer
	Stress incontinence
Skin	Acanthosis nigricans
	Lymphedema
	Sweat rashes

Table 36.9 Systemic comorbidities associated with obesity.

Obesity and type 2 diabetes mellitus

Obesity is characterized by elevated fasting plasma insulin and an exaggerated insulin response to an oral glucose load. Overall fatness and the distribution of body fat influence glucose metabolism through independent but additive mechanisms. Increasing upper body obesity is accompanied by a progressive increase in the glucose and insulin response to an oral glucose challenge with a positive correlation being observed between increasing upper body obesity and measures of insulin resistance. Posthepatic insulin delivery is increased in upper body obesity, leading to more marked peripheral insulin concentrations that, in turn, lead to peripheral insulin resistance.

Differences in the ability of insulin to suppress lipolysis, and of catecholamines to stimulate lipolysis, also vary according to fat distribution. These factors contribute to an exaggerated release of free fatty acids (FFA) from abdominal adipocytes into the portal system. FFA have a deleterious effect on insulin uptake by the liver and contribute to the increased hepatic gluconeogenesis and hepatic glucose release observed in upper body obesity. Insulin insensitivity is not confined to adipocytes, with the process being accentuated by skeletal muscle insulin resistance.

The elevation in plasma FFA concentration, particularly postprandially when they are usually suppressed by insulin, leads to an inappropriate maintenance of glucose production and an impairment of hepatic glucose utilization (impaired glucose tolerance).

In the initial phases of this process, the pancreas can respond by maintaining a state of compensatory hyperinsulinemia, with gross decompensation of glucose tolerance being prevented. With ever-increasing plasma concentrations of FFA, the insulin-resistant individual cannot continue to maintain this state of compensatory hyperinsulinemia, and hyperglycemia prevails. Hyperinsulinemia and insulin resistance are both significant correlates of a dyslipoproteinemic state and contribute to the characteristic alterations of plasma lipid profile associated with obesity: elevated fasting plasma triglyceride concentration, reduced HDL-cholesterol, marginal elevations of cholesterol and LDL-cholesterol concentrations, and increased number of apoprotein-B-carrying lipoproteins.

Cardiovascular function in obesity

The effects of increased body fatness on cardiovascular function are predictable.

Total body oxygen consumption is increased because of an expanded lean tissue mass as well as the oxidative demands of metabolically active adipose tissue, and this is accompanied by an absolute increase in cardiac output. However, the values are within the normal range when they are normalized to body surface area. The total blood volume in obesity is increased in proportion to bodyweight such that obesity can be regarded as a volume-expanded state. This increase in blood volume contributes to an increase in the left ventricular preload and an increase in resting cardiac output. The increased demand for cardiac output is achieved by an increase in stroke volume while the heart rate remains comparatively unchanged. The obesity-related increase in stroke volume results from an increase in diastolic filling of the left ventricle. The volume expansion and increase in cardiac output lead to structural changes of the heart. The increase in left ventricular filling results in an increase in the left ventricular cavity dimension and an increase in wall stress. As left ventricular dilatation is accompanied by myocardial hypertrophy, the ratio between ventricular cavity radius and wall thickness is preserved. This thickening of the wall with dilatation results in eccentric hypertrophy. Left ventricular mass increases directly in proportion to BMI or the degree of overweight.

The blood pressure is a function of cardiac output and the vascular resistance against which the blood is pumped – systemic vascular resistance. An elevated cardiac output is common with moderate obesity but not all obese patients are hypertensive. However, in those subjects where systemic resistance is increased, the combination of hypertension and obesity results in an increase of ventricular wall dimensions disproportionate to the chamber radius and this leads, in time, to concentric hypertrophy.

The cardiovascular adaptation to the increased intravascular volume of obesity may not completely restore normal hemodynamic function. Marked systolic dysfunction occurs when the ventricle can no longer adapt to volume overload. Dilatation of the left ventricle cavity radius leads to a decline in ventricular contractility. Despite an elevation of cardiac output, obese individuals have been shown to have depressed myocardial contractility proportional to excess weight. With left ventricular hypertrophy, reduced ventricular compliance alters the ability of the chamber to accommodate an increased volume during diastole and this results in diastolic dysfunction. A combination of systolic and diastolic dysfunction progresses to clinically significant heart failure.

In addition to congestive cardiac failure, the presence of left ventricular hypertrophy has been associated with a greater risk of morbidity and mortality from coronary heart disease and sudden death, as well as arrhythmia.

Sleep-breathing abnormalities in obesity

An increased amount of fat in the chest wall and abdomen has a predictable effect on the mechanical properties of the chest and the diaphragm and leads to an alteration of respiratory excursions during inspiration and expiration, reducing lung volume and altering the pattern of ventilation to each region. The increased mass of fat additionally leads to a decrease in compliance of the respiratory system as a whole. All these changes are significantly exaggerated when an obese person lies flat. The mass loading effect of fat requires an increased respiratory muscle force to overcome the excessive elastic recoil and an associated increase in the elastic work of breathing. The obesity-related changes in respiratory function are most important during sleep.

During the rapid-eye-movement (REM) phase of sleep, there are decreases in voluntary muscle tone with reduced arterial oxygen saturation and a rise in carbon dioxide in all individuals, but these are especially marked in obese subjects. Irregular respiration and occasional apneic episodes often occur in lean people during REM sleep but obesity, with its influence on respiratory mechanics, increases their frequency and may result in severe hypoxia with resultant cardiac arrhythmias. Studies of obese men and women have demonstrated that the obstruction occurs in the larynx and is associated with loss of tone of the pharyngeal

and glossal muscles, in particular the genioglossus muscle. Relaxation of the genioglossus allows the base of the tongue to fall back against the posterior pharyngeal wall, occluding the pharynx. This results in a temporary cessation of breathing (apnea) and associated transient hypoxia. It is not uncommon to observe saturation values as low as 6.5kPa during REM sleep in some obese subjects while their awake arterial gases are normal. A minority of obese patients develop a situation characterized by a marked depression in both hypercapnic and hypoxic respiratory drives accompanied by abnormal and irregular pattern of breathing during sleep and (eventually) in the waking state. Characteristically, such individuals show frequent and prolonged episodes of sleep apnea – sleep is disturbed with frequent awakening related to the resumption of breathing following an apneic episode. Daytime somnolence soon intervenes accompanied by persistent hypoxia/hypercapnia, pulmonary hypertension (superimposed upon an increased circulatory volume), and right-sided cardiac failure. Such changes constitute the clinical manifestation of the obesity–hypoventilation syndrome (formerly known as the Pickwickian syndrome).

Other obesity-associated complications

Gallbladder disease is the most common form of digestive disease in obese individuals with a progressive and linear risk from a BMI of 20 upwards. Liver abnormalities are described in obesity, mainly due to fatty infiltration but on occasions associated with fibrosis and/or cirrhosis. Certain forms of cancer are more common in obese subjects: colorectal and prostate in obese men, carcinoma of the gallbladder, breast and endometrium in obese women. Osteoarthritis frequently accompanies obesity, while bone density tends to be increased in obese subjects. As peviously described, obesity in women is also associated with menstrual irregularity and infertility; obesity may be, but is not always, associated with the polycystic ovary syndrome.

FURTHER READING

Clinical management of overweight and obese patients with particular reference to the use of drugs. London:Royal College of Physicians of London; 1998.

De Divitiis O, Fazio S, Petitto M, Maddalena G, Contaldo F, Mancini M. Obesity and cardiac function. Circulation 1981;64:477–82.

Donders SHJ, Pieters GF, Heeval JG, et al. Disparity of thyrotrophin (TSH) and prolactin responses to TSH-releasing hormone in obesity. J Clin Endocrinol Metab. 1985;61:56–9.

Garavaglia GE, Messerli FH, Nunez BD, Schmieder RE, Grossman E. Myocardial contractility and left ventricular function in obese patients with essential hypertension. Am J Cardiol. 1988;62:594–7.

Grunstein RR. Pulmonary function, sleep apnoea and obesity. In: Kopelman PG, Stock MJ, eds. Clinical obesity. Oxford:Blackwell Science; 1998:248–89.

Han TS, van Leer EM, Seidell JC, Lean MEJ. Waist circumference action levels in the identification of cardiovascular risk factors: prevalence study in a random sample. Br Med J. 1995;311:1401–5.

Hubert HB, Feinleib M, McNamara PM, Castelli WP. Obesity as an independent risk factor for cardiovascular disease: a 26-year follow-up of participants in the Framingham heart study. Circulation 1983; 67:968–77.

Jung RT, Campbell RG, James WPT, Callingham BA. Altered hypothalamic sympathetic responses to hypoglycaemia in familial obesity. Lancet 1982;i:1043–6.

Kopelman PG. Effects of obesity on fat topography: metabolic and endocrine determinants. In: Kopelman PG, Stock MJ, eds. Clinical obesity. Oxford:Blackwell Science; 1998:158–75.

Kopelman PG. Obesity as a medical problem. Nature 2000;404:635–43.

Kopelman PG, Albon L. Obesity, non-insulin-dependent diabetes mellitus and the metabolic syndrome. Br Med Bull. 1998;53:322–40.

Manson JE, Willett WC, Stampfer MJ, et al. Body weight and mortality among women. New Engl J Med. 1995;333:677–85.

National Heart, Lung and Blood Institute. Clinical guidelines on the identification, evaluation and treatment of overweight and obesity in adults. 1998.

Scottish Intercollegiate Guidelines Network. The management of obese patients in Scotland – integrating a new approach in primary health care with a national prevention and management strategy. Edinburgh:SIGN; 1996.

Sjostrom L, Narbro K, Sjostrom D. Costs and benefits when treating obesity. Int J Obesity 1995;19(suppl. 6):S9–12.

Society of Actuaries, Build study of the Society of Actuaries. London: Recording and Statistical Corporation; 1980.

Willett WC, Dietz WH, Colditz GA. Guidelines for healthy weight. New Engl J Med. 1999;341:427–33.

World Health Organization Expert Committee. Physical status: the use and interpretation of anthropometry. WHO Technical Report Series no. 854. Geneva:WHO; 1995.

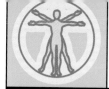

Chapter 37

Psychiatric and Behavioral Changes and Endocrine Function

Ehud Ur

INTRODUCTION

Alterations in mood, behavior and cognition are important features in many endocrine disorders. As a consequence, the study of hormonal influences on neuronal function has accumulated a wealth of data that underscores the biologic basis of mental phenomena. In recent years, the discovery of subtle abnormalities in neuroendocrine function among patients with major psychiatric disorders has been a focus of intense research interest. The demonstration of objective biologic abnormalities in these functional disorders has been used as evidence of the organic nature of these conditions.

This chapter will review the effects of hormones on the neural substrates of behavior, the psychologic manifestations of endocrine conditions, and the hormonal abnormalities found in primary psychiatric disorders.

HORMONAL EFFECTS ON BEHAVIOR

Hypothalamo–pituitary–adrenal axis

The hypothalamo–pituitary–adrenal (HPA) axis plays a central role in the integration of the organism's response to stress (Fig. 37.1). This is achieved through various homeostatic mechanisms controlling intermediary metabolism, blood pressure, and behavior. The neuroendocrine cascade triggered by stress that underlies this process begins with central perception of a stressor, which in turn leads to the release of corticotropin-releasing hormone (CRH), arginine vasopressin (AVP), and other secretagogues for adrenocorticotropic hormone (ACTH). ACTH is released from the corticotropic cells of the anterior pituitary, following posttranslational modification of its parent molecule proopiomelanocortin (POMC), and this peptide promotes the release of glucocorticoids from the adrenal gland.

Stress

Stress represents the principal paradigm for HPA axis activation. Numerous studies have examined cortisol responses to stressful circumstances generated by a wide variety of experimental strategies. Through such studies it is recognized that an individual's psychologic perceptions of a stressor are more important than the physical characteristics of the stress itself in determining adrenocortical responses. Factors that modulate this response can be ascribed to parameters specific to the stimulus or to the individual (Table 37.1). For example, cortisol response to major surgery is larger and of longer duration than that occurring with minor procedures. Studies of cortisol

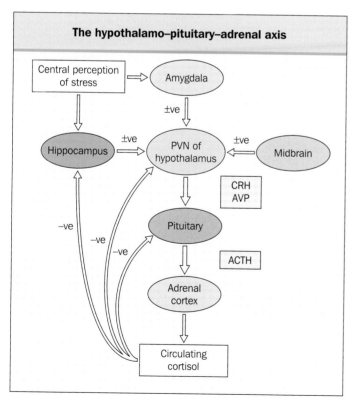

Figure 37.1 The hypothalamo–pituitary–adrenal axis. This schematic diagram shows the response to stress and describes the regulation and negative feedback of cortisol via glucocorticoid receptors. ACTH, adrenocorticotropic hormone; AVP, arginine vasopressin; CRH, corticotropin-releasing hormone; PVN, paraventricular nucleus.

Parameters modulating stress response			
Stimulus	**Physiologic**	**Psychologic**	**Social**
Intensity	Gender	Personality	Hierarchy
Duration	Age	Behavior	
Novelty	Physical fitness	Affect	
Control		Coping mechanisms	
Predictability		Locus of control	

Table 37.1 Parameters modulating stress response.

responses to paradigms of persistent threat or constant high level of demand have generally shown rapid adaptation, such that the individual's baseline response to chronic stimulation shows little if any hormonal difference from the unstimulated state. Psychobiologic stress responses are most intense when the provoking stimulus is a novel one, as shown by classical studies of parachutists and other individuals engaged in similarly dangerous pursuits, where repeated exposures result in rapid diminution of responses.

Individual parameters include gender, age, and the presence of specific personality traits. For example, in males, higher irritability and increased competitiveness are predictive of lower cortisol levels. Social factors are also important. In human and animal studies, it has been shown that individuals with a low level of control over their environment – those who lie at the lower echelons of a social structure – tend to display the most marked adrenocortical responses in reply to a given stimulus.

Corticotropin-releasing hormone

There are several major systems of CRH neurons. The best characterized of these is the paraventricular-nucleus–median-eminence pathway (**Fig. 37.2**), which is responsible for most ACTH regulatory activity. The paraventricular nucleus consists of:

- anterior and medial–dorsal parvicellular CRH neurons with axons projecting to hypophyseal portal capillaries;
- dorsolateral magnocellular vasopressinergic and oxytocinergic neurons projecting to the posterior pituitary;
- autonomic CRH neurons in dorsal, medial ventral, and lateral parvicellular divisions, which project to the brainstem.

Corticotropin-releasing hormone neurons are also found in the limbic system (particularly the amygdala and the nucleus of the stria terminalis) and as scattered interneurons within the cerebral cortex. Acute stress induces release of CRH into the hypophyseal portal circulation, whereas CRH antagonists or antibodies inhibit 70% of the ACTH response to acute stress.

In the rat, direct intracerebroventricular administration of CRH results in activation of the HPA axis as well as of the sympathetic nervous system, with consequent elevation in plasma catecholamines and suppression of the hypothalamo–pituitary–gonadal axis. Using this paradigm, as well as transgenic animals that overexpress the CRH gene, distinct behavioral responses have been observed, including decreased social interaction, feeding, and sexual behavior, and dose-dependent increases in locomotor activity and grooming. Overall there is an increase in arousal, associated with increased exploratory maneuvers, hostility, enhancement of conditioned fear responses, and improved acquisition of the learned response in a visual discrimination task (**Fig. 37.3**). In addition, there are a number of non-behavioral effects, which include increased blood pressure and tachycardia and decreased gastrointestinal activity. These effects are independent of factors at lower levels of the HPA axis since they occur in hypophysectomized and dexamethasone-pretreated animals. In contrast to the effects of the agonist, administration of a CRH antagonist into the cerebrospinal fluid (CSF) of the ventricular system increases exploratory behavior and diminishes the acquisition of conditioned fear responses. In humans, peripheral administration of human CRH has been shown to augment selective attention.

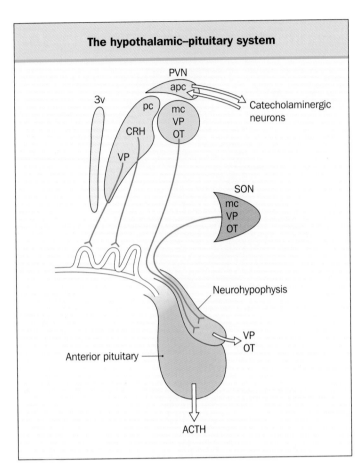

The hypothalamic–pituitary system

Figure 37.2 The hypothalamic–pituitary system. Axons from the parvicellular (pc) paraventricular nucleus (PVN) release corticotropin-releasing hormone (CRH) and vasopressin (VP) into pituitary portal capillaries. Parvicellular neurons project to autonomic catecholaminergic neurons in the brainstem. Axons from the supraoptic nucleus (SON), and magnocellular (mc) division of the paraventricular nucleus and PVN, transport vasopressin and oxytocin (OT) to the neurohypophysis. 3v, third ventricle; ACTH, adrenocorticotropic hormone.

The two receptors for CRH, CRHR1 and CRHR2, are found throughout the central nervous system and periphery. CRH has a higher affinity for CRHR1 than for CRHR2, and urocortin, a CRH-related peptide, is thought to be the endogenous ligand for CRHR2 because it binds with almost 40-fold higher affinity than does CRH. The two receptors share 71% amino-acid sequence similarity and are distinct in their localization within the brain and peripheral tissues. Mice deficient for CRHR2 are hypersensitive to stress and display increased anxiety-like behavior.

Arginine vasopressin

There are several distinct AVP-containing pathways in the hypothalamus (**Fig. 37.2**). A pathway originating in the magnocellular neurons of the paraventricular nucleus and supraoptic nucleus (SON), passing through the zona interna of the median eminence, and concluding at the neurohypophysis is responsible for the circulating peptide with its classical renal and vascular effects. Another pathway originates in the medial parvocellular nucleus of the PVN and passes to the zona externa of the median eminence at the portal capillary plexus. AVP secreted

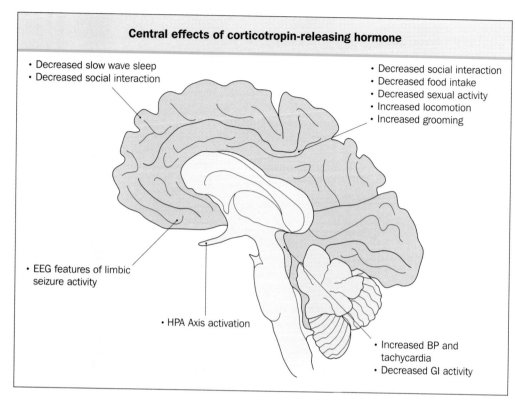

Figure 37.3 Central effects of corticotropin-releasing hormone. BP, blood pressure; EEG, electroencephalogram; GI, gastrointestinal; HPA, hypothalamo–pituitary–adrenal.

Within the figure:

Central effects of corticotropin-releasing hormone

- Decreased slow wave sleep
- Decreased social interaction

- Decreased social interaction
- Decreased food intake
- Decreased sexual activity
- Increased locomotion
- Increased grooming

- EEG features of limbic seizure activity

- HPA Axis activation

- Increased BP and tachycardia
- Decreased GI activity

into the portal blood here acts as a secretagogue for ACTH, potentiating the action of CRH. Apart from its well-known effects on the renal collecting ducts and arteriolar smooth muscle, AVP plays an important role in the control of ACTH release and also manifests significant behavioral effects. There is an extensive literature on the role of vasopressin in memory. This stems from the primary observation that removal of the posterior pituitary from the rat was found to interfere with escape behavior, a deficit that was restored using pitressin. Subsequent studies have shown that AVP and even endocrinologically inactive analogs enhance consolidation and retrieval of memory and that these effects are long-lived, lasting for several days or even weeks. The posterior thalamus, and, in particular, the parafascicular nucleus, appear to be the main site of this action. Bilateral lesions to this area have abolished the behavioral effects of AVP. Interestingly, the effect of AVP on passive avoidance has been shown to be blocked by lesions to the dorsal noradrenergic system made in the locus ceruleus. In human subjects, desmopressin given daily for 1 week has been shown to improve both long- and short-term episodic memory. Studies looking at patients with senile dementia of the Alzheimer type who were given desmopressin show significant enhancement of semantic memory. Therapeutic responses have also been seen in patients with retrograde amnesia and Korsakoff's syndrome.

Adrenocorticotropic hormone and its precursor, proopiomelanocortin

There is substantial evidence showing that peptides derived from proopiomelanocortin (POMC, see Chapter 1) exert neurotropic effects. Hypophysectomized rats, which are thus rendered deficient in ACTH, show impaired acquisition of avoidance conditioning. This can subsequently be restored by the administration of ACTH, or indeed by a number of POMC

fragments including α-melanocyte-stimulating hormone and $ACTH_{4-10}$. $ACTH_{4-10}$ is a fragment of the whole 39-amino-acid-residue ACTH molecule that lacks any steroidogenic activity.

In rats, ACTH delays the extinction of learned responses such as taste aversion induced with lithium and alleviates the amnesia produced by CO_2 inhalation, electroconvulsive shock, or intracerebral administration of puromycin, an inhibitor of protein synthesis. Administration of $ACTH_{4-10}$ to human subjects has been shown to increase selective attention to the exclusion of other environmental clues but does not alter consolidation or retrieval of memory. Such behavioral effects are generally short-lived, lasting from one to four hours. Thus, ACTH and subfragments such as $ACTH_{4-10}$, which lack endocrine capability, appear to exert profound behavioral effects. They do not have a direct effect on memory but accentuate selective attention, allowing the individual to focus on the task in hand and eliminating extraneous influences.

Glucocorticoids

Regulation of the HPA axis occurs mainly through negative feedback of glucocorticoids on pituitary, hypothalamic, and suprahypothalamic sites. The hippocampus is the region of the brain that is richest in glucocorticoid receptors, and plays an important role in maintaining the basal tone of the HPA axis and in terminating the stress response. The hippocampus also plays a critical role in spatial learning and memory tasks. Acute elevations in glucocorticoids, in response to short-term stressors, appear to enhance hippocampal function, for example, strengthening the memory of instrumental responses. In contrast, chronic exposure to glucocorticoids may have a neurotoxic effect on the hippocampus, causing explicit memory deficits.. Thus, in conditions with raised levels of corticosteroids (e.g. Cushing's disease, depression), there are significant impairments in cognitive function. Studies that have used magnetic resonance imaging to image the brain in these conditions have shown hippocampal atrophy (**Fig. 37.4**).

Hypothalamo–pituitary–gonadal axis

Males and females are genetically very similar, except that different hormones enter the brain at different times, promoting changes critical to brain development. The default developmental program in mammals produces female sexual behavior, dependent at least in part on the sequential actions of estradiol and progesterone in the ventromedial nucleus of the hypothalamus. Perinatal administration of testosterone, acting via its neural metabolism to estradiol, decreases female psychosexual function, such as sexual receptive behavior partner preference. The precise features of this are dependent on the species and the dose and duration of testosterone exposure. In males, psychosexual defeminization occurs naturally, in response to perinatal secretion of testosterone by the testes. From then until puberty, the brain's hormonal environment is again very similar in males and females. During sexual maturity, hormone levels of women fluctuate cyclically over a much larger range than those of men. At female menopause, ovarian secretion is terminated. In the aging male, the testes continue to produce testosterone, which is partly converted to estradiol in the brain, but at an increasingly slower rate. At old age the brain's hormonal environment is once again similar in the two sexes.

Testosterone

Testosterone is the principal steroid secreted by mammalian testes during development and in adulthood. Testosterone induces behavioral changes via altered central neurophysiologic functioning of certain neuronal pathways. Testosterone is metabolized by the aromatase enzyme to estradiol and by 5α-reductase into dihydrotestosterone. Aromatase is present in subcortical brain areas, including the preoptic region and the medial amygdala. High levels of neuronal aromatase activity occur perinatally in the hypothalamus and fall by a factor of 10 in adulthood.

In many mammalian species, female sexual behavior is regulated by female sex steroids. As a consequence, the capacity for copulation is limited to the period of ovulation. In humans and other higher primates, testosterone is responsible for female sexual activity, thus promoting intercourse outside the periovulatory period. In women the loss of testosterone after ovariectomy and adrenalectomy may result in a complete loss of libido, which can be restored with adequate substitution.

Estrogen

Estrogens appear to have a significant neuroprotective role, through the modulation of neurotropins, and the regulation of synaptic connectivity. Replacement of estrogen in ovariectomized animals results in an increase in the number and density of dendritic spines and axospinous synapses in hippocampal CA1 pyramidal cells. Estrogens also modulate the secretion of acetylcholine in the hippocampus by their effect on choline acetyltransferase. Thus estrogens play an active organizing role in the developing brain and a maintenance role in the aging brain. They appear to protect neurons against developmental

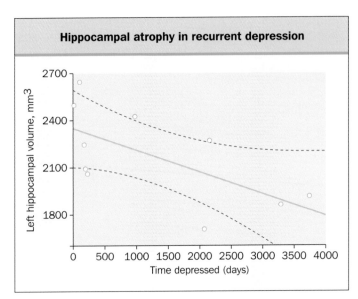

Figure 37.4 Hippocampal atrophy in recurrent depression. The graph shows the correlation between left hippocampal gray matter volume and total days of major depression. (Adapted from Sheline YI, Wang PW, Gado MH, Csernansky JG, Vannier MW. Hippocampal atrophy in recurrent major depression. Proc Natl Acad Sci USA. 1996;93:3908–13 © 1996 National Academy of Sciences, USA.)

dysfunction (e.g. schizophrenia) and degenerative dysfunction (e.g. Alzheimer's disease). The cyclical nature of estrogen activity from puberty to menopause and its subsequent abrupt withdrawal may be a significant factor in the predisposition of women to disorders of mood and anxiety, rendering them inherently more vulnerable to glucocorticoid-induced neurotoxicity.

Prolactin

Prolactin enters the central nervous system via the choroid plexuses, and achieves concentrations in the (CSF) that are about 20% those of plasma. There is also a modest amount of brain synthesis, some of which may be involved in neurotransmission. Prolactin-binding sites have been identified in the hypothalamus and the substantia nigra. Most of the biologic functions of prolactin are associated with metabolic and behavioral adaptation to parenthood and inhibition of reproductive behavior. Hypophysectomized or bromocriptine-treated female rats display delayed onset of maternal behavior, a latency that can be reversed with prolactin. In hamsters, postpartum administration of a single dose of bromocriptine induces eating of the pups by the mothers. Prolactin markedly inhibits sexual behavior, an effect mediated through increased opioid and dopaminergic tones, which suppress the secretion of gonadotropin-releasing hormone. Reduction in pain sensitivity is also probably mediated by opioid pathways.

Growth hormone

Binding sites specific for growth hormone (GH) have been demonstrated in several areas of the central nervous system, including the hypothalamus and the hippocampus. GH binding in the choroid plexus may play a role in the transport of GH across the blood–brain barrier. Treatment with GH has been shown to decrease CSF levels of dopamine metabolites, an effect similar to that found after treatment with tricyclic antidepressants and monoamine oxidase inhibitors. GH is also thought to enhance triiodothyronine (T_3) to thyroxine (T_4) conversion, a change that is considered of clinical relevance for mood.

PSYCHOLOGIC MANIFESTATIONS OF ENDOCRINE DISEASE

Cushing's syndrome

Cushing's syndrome (see Chapter 15) is a complex disorder that results from abnormally high levels of cortisol. The commonest cause is iatrogenic administration of exogenous steroids. Among the endogenous etiologies, adrenal tumors are relatively rare and carcinomas and bilateral nodular adrenal hyperplasia even more so. The majority of ACTH-dependent forms are caused by pituitary microadenomas (Cushing's disease). Macroadenomas, corticotroph hyperplasia, and ectopic ACTH secretion from a tumor of nonpituitary origin are less common.

Regardless of the origin, Cushing's syndrome is characterized by truncal obesity, hypertension, hyperglycemia, proximal muscle atrophy, thinning of the skin, and easy bruising. Since Cushing's original observation, published in 1912, psychiatric disturbances have been recognized as a central feature of hyperadrenocorticalism. Despite the heterogeneous nature of Cushing's syndrome, most investigations of behavioral change in these disorders have made no distinctions between the various etiologies. Mental changes are usually diagnostically nonspecific, although depressive symptoms predominate in Cushing's disease whereas euphoria is generally believed to be more common in exogenous corticosteroid therapy. Risk factors for depression, including an excess of adverse early life events and a family history of suicide and affective disorders, are common in patients with Cushing's disease, prompting the suggestion that psychiatric factors may even be etiologic in pituitary-dependent disease. A meta-analysis of 12 studies involving 330 patients identified depression in 45%. Schizophreniform manifestations were not evident. Major psychiatric disturbances other than mood and anxiety disorders are infrequent in Cushing's syndrome.

It appears that there are no significant differences in depression between patients with pituitary-dependent and pituitary-independent forms of the disease. Depression is significantly associated with older age, female sex, higher pretreatment urinary cortisol levels, relatively more severe clinical features, and absence of demonstrable pituitary adenoma. Symptoms are more prominent in patients with active as compared with inactive disease. Treatment results in a significant fall in the severity of depression as measured by objective rating scales. Half the patients are better by 3 months.

Neuropsychologic testing suggests that over 60% of patients with Cushing's syndrome have evidence of diffuse bilateral cerebral dysfunction, with impairment in nonverbal, visual-memory, and spatial–constructional functions. Difficulties with concentration, poor reasoning abilities, diminished comprehension, and information processing have also been described.

Acute administration of corticosteroids at doses above 30mg prednisone per day is commonly associated with the onset of hyperactivity, hyperphagia, insomnia, and other euphoric symptoms within several days. Their sudden withdrawal may precipitate depressive symptoms.

Addison's disease

Primary hypoadrenocorticalism (Chapter 16) is now most commonly autoimmune in origin, although, in Addison's day, infectious causes like tuberculosis predominated. The occurrence of psychologic symptoms is well recognized, regardless of etiology. In Addison's original study, patients were described as having 'an inability to concentrate, drowsiness, restlessness, insomnia, irritability, apprehension, and disturbed sleep'. Depressive symptoms are prominent in over 50% of patients and can reach psychotic proportions in terms of their severity. Psychiatric symptoms often predate the classic physical signs and can lead to diagnostic delays. Symptomatic improvement is dependent on corticosteroid replacement. An acute self-limiting manic response to treatment with physiologic doses of glucocorticoids has been described, which may be attributable to upregulation of cerebral glucocorticoid receptors as a consequence of prolonged hypocortisolemia.

Glucocorticoid replacement therapy

Patients with primary or secondary adrenal insufficiency require long-term glucocorticoid replacement therapy. Inadequate replacement results in features similar to untreated adrenal failure. Subtle underreplacement may be more difficult to identify, with patients complaining of malaise and a poor response to stress. Conversely, gross overreplacement will lead to Cushingoid manifestations, but even modest excess of glucocorticoid, e.g. too high a dose in the evening, will result in psychologic manifestations such as anxiety and sleep disturbances. Thus monitoring of cortisol replacement therapy using multiple timed blood samples (cortisol day curves) and close attention to physical and psychologic symptoms are warranted.

Hyperprolactinemia and prolactinoma

Patients with hyperprolactinemia (Chapter 6) have a higher than expected incidence of depression, characterized by low mood, loss of interest, decreased libido, and irritability. Sexual dysfunction is present in about 60% of patients but does not correlate with hypoestrogenism. In men with hyperprolactinemia, impairment in sexual function is even more marked but the frequent occurrence of impaired testosterone secretion in these patients means that at least some of the symptoms must be attributable to the direct effects of the latter.

Growth hormone deficiency

Growth hormone deficiency in adults (see Chapter 4) most commonly results from pituitary or parasellar tumors and their treatment. The majority of these are benign pituitary adenomas. Childhood-onset GH deficiency is most commonly idiopathic. In the past 10 years, the availability of recombinant GH has led to intense interest in the clinical features of GH deficiency and the benefits of GH replacement in adults. Much of this work has focused on the psychologic wellbeing and quality of life

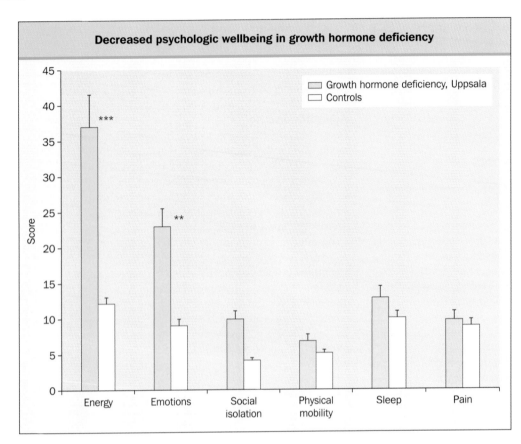

Figure 37.5 Decreased psychologic wellbeing in growth hormone deficiency. Baseline data (mean ± SEM) for the six dimensions of the Nottingham Health Profile in 36 adults with growth hormone deficiency. Healthy age- and sex-matched controls are shown in comparison. *** $p < 0.001$; ** $p < 0.01$. (Adapted from Burman P, Broman JE, Hetta J, et al. Quality of life in adults with growth hormone (GH) deficiency: response to treatment with recombinant human GH in a placebo-controlled 21-month trial. J Clin Endocrinol Metab. 1995;80:3585–90.)

of GH-deficient patients and the effects of GH replacement. Decreased psychologic wellbeing has been reported in hypopituitary patients despite adequate replacement of all hormonal deficiencies except GH. Subjects reported less energy, greater emotional lability, more difficulties with sexual relationships, and a greater sense of social isolation (**Fig. 37.5**). GH replacement is associated with an improvement in mood and energy levels. In studies that assessed general health and wellbeing, using the Nottingham Health Profile, the Psychological and General Well-Being Schedule, and the General Health Questionnaire, patients showed significant improvements in subjective wellbeing and quality of life after 6 months of GH therapy. Other data suggest that GH replacement may result in improved memory (**Fig. 37.6**) and in restoration of abnormal sleep patterns.

Clearly, not all underlying deficiencies in hypopituitary patients can be attributed to lack of GH. Surgical treatment and irradiation of the underlying disorder may be responsible for irreversible brain damage. An inadequate replacement regimen for adrenal and sex steroids or thyroxine may be an issue in some cases, as may the effects of chronic disease.

The combined data from clinical studies of GH therapy suggest beneficial effects on psychosocial capacity. The mechanism behind alterations in quality of life is unclear, and it is not known whether the reported effects of GH on brain dopamine and thyroxine are of relevance for these improvements.

Congenital adrenal hyperplasia

Congenital adrenal hyperplasia, commonly due to a mutation in the gene encoding 21-hydroxylase, results in underproduction of glucocorticoids and mineralocorticoids and overproduction of androgens, which in females causes varying degrees of virilization. Hormone replacement and surgical reconstruction of external genitalia allow most of these women to be assigned to a female gender role. However, when compared to controls, women with congenital adrenal hyperplasia have a higher frequency of homosexual or bisexual activity. Similar psychosexual profiles are evident in women exposed prenatally to diethylstilbestrol at a time when it was thought to reduce the incidence of spontaneous abortion.

Androgen resistance syndrome

Androgen resistance syndrome is caused by mutations in the androgen receptor in genetic males, which result in androgen insensitivity (see Chapters 24A and 25). Despite normal expression of differentiation of testes, affected individuals have female external genitalia. Breasts develop at puberty, in response to estrogens formed through peripheral aromatization of testosterone. Testosterone action in the brain is mainly through estradiol, yet core sexual identity in androgen resistance syndrome subjects is female, and sexual orientation is towards men. This suggests that humans require testosterone to act through the androgen receptor in the central nervous system to complete psychosexual differentiation begun prenatally by the actions of estrogen.

Hyperthyroidism

Hyperthyroidism (Chapter 13) is associated with multiple neurobehavioral and psychologic changes. Typical features include anxiety, insomnia, emotional lability, and in some cases cognitive dysfunction. Difficulty with concentrating may be an early symptom. Motor activity may be increased, with symptoms suggestive of hypomania, although frank psychosis is unusual and

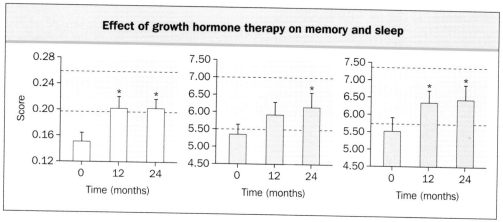

Figure 37.6 Effect of growth hormone therapy on memory and sleep. Mean scores (± SEM) for (left panel) iconic, (b) short-term (associate learning), and (c) long-term (associate recognition) memory tasks at baseline (*n* = 45) and after 12 (*n* = 45) and 24 months (*n* = 43) of growth hormone treatment. Dotted lines represent 95% confidence interval of the mean for the control group (*n* = 41). (Adapted from Deijen JB, Van der Veen EA. The influence of growth hormone (GH) deficiency and GH replacement on quality of life in GH-deficient patients. J Endocrinol Invest. 1999;22(5 Suppl.):127–36.)

occurs typically in patients with a personal or family history of bipolar disorder. Apathetic thyrotoxicosis is an uncommon variant of hyperthyroidism that mimics depression and usually occurs in the elderly. Features include apathy, weight loss, and depressed mood. Absence of the characteristic signs of thyrotoxicosis found in younger patients may lead to delays in diagnosis and treatment. Thyrotoxicosis should also be excluded in patients who present with anxiety states (where the intensity of symptoms tends to vary over time) and panic attacks (where resting pulses are normal and hands are cold and clammy rather than warm and moist).

There have been longstanding suggestions that psychosocial stress may be of etiologic significance in Graves' disease but this is not established. In case-control studies, patients developing Graves' thyrotoxicosis report more negative life events than controls. There is also evidence that stress plays a role in relapses of established Graves' disease. The likeliest mechanism for such effects lies in hormonal, especially HPA axis, modulation of immune function.

Treatment with beta-blockers such as propranolol is effective in controlling the anxiety symptoms associated with thyrotoxicosis. Patients with more florid, or indeed psychotic, symptoms may require treatment with phenothiazines.

Hypothyroidism

Thyroid hypofunction (see Chapter 11) has significant effects on brain function and can irreversibly damage the developing brain. Neonatal screening linked with early treatment has improved the prognosis for children with congenital hypothyroidism. Followup studies have shown that most children with congenital hypothyroidism achieve scores for intelligence within the normal range but those with severe hypothyroidism show significant deficits in mean IQ scores despite early treatment. Impaired motor performance and behavior problems have also been reported in children with congenital hypothyroidism.

In adults, initial features are nonspecific. They may include inattentiveness, poor concentration, and short-term memory loss. With progression, motor function may become slowed, and patients may lose interest in their surroundings. Eventually visual hallucinations and paranoid ideation become manifest. Finally, lethargy gives way to stupor and coma. Early features may be indistinguishable from depression. Objective findings, however, have much in common with organic syndromes of brain dysfunction, and include electroencephalographic changes (predominance of low-voltage q and d-waves) and impaired cognitive function. Some of these abnormalities are nonspecifically related to hypometabolism and circulatory changes (i.e. reductions in cerebral blood flow and oxygen and glucose consumption). High concentrations of T_3 nuclear receptors are found in the amygdala and hippocampus, areas that are important in the regulation of mood and memory.

Since cognitive impairment or pseudodementia is common in elderly patients with affective disorders, routine thyroid screening should be done in all patients over 60 who present with clinical symptoms of depression and cognitive decline. Many of the behavioral changes in hypothyroidism respond to T_4 replacement, although it should be borne in mind that psychotic phenomena may become exacerbated for a while after the initiation of hormone replacement. Phenothiazines may be used, although with great caution, as patients are at high risk for cardiac arrhythmias and, if T_4 replacement is insufficient, myxedema coma. In patients with a strong family history of affective disorder, initiation of hormone replacement may precipitate a manic response, which can be controlled with lithium or a phenothiazine. In most patients, cognitive function improves markedly with treatment, although there is evidence to suggest that combinations of T_3 with T_4 improve responses better than T_4 alone. In some patients, cognitive dysfunction is not always reversed, suggesting that chronic thyroid hormone deficiency may induce irreversible deficits in central nervous system function.

ENDOCRINE ABNORMALITIES IN PRIMARY PSYCHIATRIC DISORDERS

Major depression

Major depression is a diagnostic category characterized by features of depressive mood, altered psychomotor activity, changes in sleep, altered eating behavior, decreased libido, cognitive deficits, and alterations in neuroendocrine function (**Table 37.2**). While measurable features, such as changes in hormonal activities, are not used for diagnostic purposes, they do offer a biologic handle on the disorder and provide the basis for scientific research.

Baseline measures of hypothalamo–pituitary–adrenal axis activity

Approximately 50% of patients with major depression have abnormalities in ACTH and cortisol secretory activity. Studies of secretory patterns over 24 hours show increased numbers of ACTH pulses and increases in the amplitude of cortisol secretion, with preservation of the circadian pattern. Further studies have shown enhanced adrenal sensitivity to exogenous ACTH stimulation, and radiographic evidence of pituitary and adrenal hyperplasia in depressed subjects relative to normal controls.

Dynamic measures of hypothalamo–pituitary–adrenal axis activity

Large numbers of studies have shown that a significant proportion of patients with major depression demonstrate resistance to pituitary adrenal suppression following the administration of dexamethasone, and this phenomenon has been clinically formalized in the psychiatric variant of the dexamethasone suppression test. Although 40–50% of patients diagnosed with major depression escape suppression within 16 hours after the administration of 1–2mg dexamethasone at midnight, the test has not found a use in diagnosis. Dexamethasone nonsuppression after treatment has been found to help identify patients who are at risk of relapse.

Corticotropin-releasing hormone and vasopressin

A number of studies have suggested that the hypercortisolemia of depression is a consequence of excessive hypothalamic CRH

Neuroendocrine abnormalities in depression	
Hypothalamo–pituitary–adrenal axis	
Baseline abnormalities	Increased CRH in CSF
	Increased numbers of ACTH pulses
	Increased amplitude of cortisol secretion
	Reduced glucocorticoid receptors in the hippocampus
Dynamic abnormalities	Dexamethasone nonsuppression
	Attenuated ACTH responses to CRH injection
	Exaggerated ACTH responses to metyrapone
Radiographic abnormalities	Hippocampal atrophy
	Pituitary hyperplasia
	Adrenal hyperplasia
Pituitary–growth-hormone axis	
Daytime GH suppression	
Blunting of sleep-related nocturnal GH surge	
Pituitary–thyroid axis	
Blunted TSH response to TRH stimulation	
Loss of nocturnal TSH rise	

Table 37.2 Neuroendocrine abnormalities in depression. ACTH, adrenocorticotropic hormone; CRH, corticotropin-releasing hormone; CSF, cerebrospinal fluid; GH, growth hormone; TRH, thyrotropin-releasing hormone; TSH, thyroid-stimulating hormone.

drive. Raised levels of immunoreactive CRH were found in the cerebrospinal fluid of depressed subjects and downregulation of CRH receptors in the frontal cortex of suicide victims has also been identified. Studies examining hormonal responses to an intravenous bolus dose of ovine CRH (oCRH) in subjects with major depression have shown attenuated ACTH secretion, although normal cortisol responses were seen (**Fig. 37.7**). In contrast, patients with Cushing's disease have exaggerated

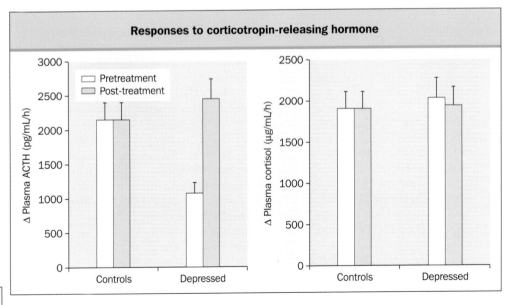

Figure 37.7 Responses to corticotropin-releasing hormone. Mean increases in plasma adrenocorticotropic hormone (left panel) and cortisol (right panel) in 15 controls and nine patients with depression. (Adapted from Gold PW, Chrousos G, Kellner C, et al. Psychiatric implications of basic and clinical studies with corticotropin-releasing factor. Am J Psychiat. 1984;141:619–27.)

ACTH responses. Continuous 24-hour infusions of CRH in normal subjects have resulted in modest hypercortisolemia that shares some of the features of that found in major depression. These include the preservation of circadian rhythms in cortisol and ACTH secretion and an attenuated ACTH response to a further bolus dose of oCRH. Through the abolition of the feedback effect of cortisol using metyrapone, an 11β-hydroxylase inhibitor, hypercortisolemic depressive patients show exaggerated rises in ACTH as compared with normocortisolemic controls (**Fig. 37.8**). There is also evidence that enhanced vasopressin secretion contributes to HPA axis overactivity in major depression. For example, blockade of the vasopressin V_1 receptor subtype inhibits anxiety-related behavior in rats.

Glucocorticoid receptors

One possible explanation for CRH hypersecretion is impaired feedback inhibition by endogenous glucocorticoids. Since glucocorticoid receptors in the HPA axis are a key component of the feedback mechanism, changes in these receptors are of potential etiologic significance in the development of HPA axis hyperactivity. Evidence of abnormalities in glucocorticoid receptors has been shown by post-mortem studies demonstrating reduced glucocorticoid receptor mRNA in the hippocampi of patients with affective disorders. It has also been shown that antidepressants stimulate glucocorticoid receptor mRNA expression in the brain, enhancing HPA autoregulation, although much of these data are from animal and *in vitro* studies. Direct antagonists of glucocorticoid receptors may be a future therapeutic modality in the treatment of affective disorders

Significance of hypothalamo–pituitary–adrenal axis abnormalities

Although the hypercortisolemia in major depression and the underlying CRH overdrive appear to be consistently demonstrable, it remains unclear as to whether these biologic markers reflect primary derangements in neural mechanisms that modulate HPA axis activity or whether they exist purely as a result of changes in the brain as a result of depression. Investigators have shown that fasting and sleep deprivation in normal volunteers will mimic the features of dexamethasone resistance found in depression. On the other hand, animal studies show that central administration of CRH and overexpression of the CRH gene produce behavioral and neuroendocrine changes characteristic of severe stress, many of which are also seen in depression. These include behavioral activation in nonstressful surroundings and anxiogenic-like effects in novel environments that appear to augment the effects of stress.

Pituitary–growth-hormone axis

A number of abnormalities in GH secretion have been identified in patients with major depression. Chief among these is daytime hypersecretion, combined with blunting of the sleep-related nocturnal GH surge. GH is known to be regulated by a number of neurotransmitter and neuropeptide systems, which are thought to be of etiologic significance in depression and are undoubtedly involved in the mechanism of action of a number of antidepressant drugs. As a consequence, GH responses to pharmacologic challenges have been used to identify abnormalities in neuroregulatory pathways in depression. For example, the GH stimulatory effect of insulin-induced hypoglycemia can

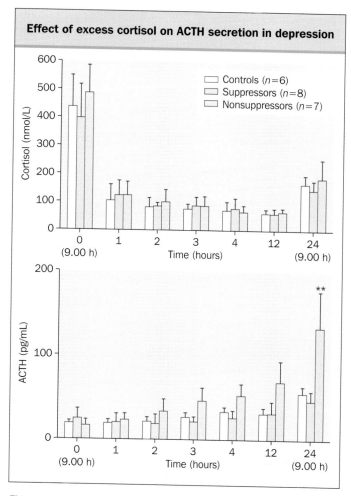

Figure 37.8 Effect of excess cortisol on adrenocorticotropic hormone (ACTH) secretion in depression. The graphs show the mean (± SD) serum cortisol (left panel) and ACTH (right panel) after metyrapone (4.5g/24h) in 15 inpatients with depression (seven dexamethasone suppressors, eight nonsuppressors) and six control subjects. ** p <0.01. (Adapted from Ur E, Dinan TG, O'Keane V, et al. Effect of metyrapone on the pituitary–adrenal axis in depression: relation to dexamethasone suppressor status. Neuroendocrinology 1992;56:533–8.)

be blocked by α_2-adrenergic antagonists, while the GH secretory response to the adrenergic agonist clonidine is blunted. Such data support the view that postsynaptic adrenergic receptors are subsensitive in depression. However, two important confounders must be borne in mind: (1) a number of studies suggest that GH responses to GHRH are blunted in depression, and (2) abnormalities in the HPA axis and in gonadal function may also affect GH axis dynamics. The behavioral consequences of the reported abnormalities in GH remain unclear.

Pituitary–thyroid axis

Most patients with depression have subtle alterations in thyroid function. These include slight elevations in T_4, blunted TSH responses to TRH stimulation, and loss of the nocturnal TSH rise. These changes have been attributed to glucocorticoid activation of the TRH neuron, leading to increased TRH secretion with resultant downregulation of the TRH receptor on the thyrotrope. The finding of elevated CSF concentrations of

TRH would support this hypothesis. Normalization of thyroid function usually occurs after treatment with antidepressants and may result, in part, from inhibition of the TRH neuron. Interestingly, treatment with triiodothyronine has been shown conclusively to augment the efficacy of various antidepressants. Data suggest benefit in about *25%* of patients with resistant depression. The underlying mechanism for this effect is unknown, although there are suggestions that there may be relative cerebral hypothyroidism, coexistent with peripheral euthyroidism.

Chronic fatigue syndrome

Chronic fatigue syndrome has been defined by the Centers for Disease Control and Prevention as the presence of intense fatigue of at least 6 months duration, resulting in a substantial reduction in activity level, associated with any four of the following: recurrent sore throats; tender lymphadenopathy; postexertional malaise; arthralgia; myalgia; unrefreshing sleep; neuropsychologic disturbances; new-onset headaches (**Table 37.3**). Chronic fatigue syndrome has a prevalence of between 0.5% and 2% and, because of its debilitating features, represents an important public health issue. Since many of the symptoms of chronic fatigue syndrome overlap with features of cortisol deficiency states, there has been a compelling rationale for the study of neuroendocrine function in the condition. Studies of the HPA axis in chronic fatigue syndrome show a mild hypocortisolism of central origin, as distinct from the hypercortisolism found in depression. While cortisol and ACTH responses to insulin hypoglycemia and adrenal responses to exogenous ACTH are normal in these patients, more subtle abnormalities such as subnormal responses to CRH and serotoninergic challenges appear to be robust findings. While it is possible that HPA axis underactivity could result from secondary factors, such as sleep disturbances, rather than reflecting primary etiologic features, there is evidence that some patients (approximately 30%) treated with low-dose hydrocortisone (5–10mg) gain clinical benefit, though not necessarily amelioration of the fatigue, with no evidence of suppression of endogenous adrenal function.

Another frequently cited abnormality in chronic fatigue syndrome patients is delayed orthostatic hypotension (evident only after standing for more than 10min), often in association with a subnormal circulating red cell mass. Symptomatic improvement has occurred with treatment with fludrocortisone.

Schizophrenia

Schizophrenia is a psychotic disease characterized by hallucinations, delusions, and disturbed organization of thought, as well as negative features of social withdrawal and loss of motivation. Although there is strong evidence to support a biologic base for the disorder, including genetic and imaging data implicating developmental defects, there is little evidence for consistent endocrine abnormalities. Some of the inconsistencies are due to the variability of the disorder, which may coexist or overlap with affective and anxiety states. Normal 24-hour profiles of ACTH, cortisol, and GH have been shown in patients with schizophrenia, as well as normal ACTH and cortisol responses to CRH. Abnormalities have been shown in nocturnal plasma prolactin, with increased numbers of pulses and greater pulse amplitude.

Diagnostic criteria for chronic fatigue syndrome

Diagnostic criteria

1. Clinically evaluated, medically unexplained fatigue of at least 6 months' duration that is:
- Of new onset
- Not a result of ongoing exertion
- Not substantially alleviated by rest
- A substantial reduction in previous levels of activity.

2. The occurrence of four or more of the following symptoms:
- Subjective memory impairment
- Tender lymph nodes
- Muscle pain
- Joint pain
- Headache
- Unrefreshing sleep
- Postexertional malaise (> 24 hours).

Exclusion criteria

1. Active, unresolved, or suspected disease likely to cause fatigue
2. Psychotic, melancholic, or bipolar depression (but not uncomplicated major depression)
3. Psychotic disorders
4. Dementia
5. Anorexia or bulimia nervosa
6. Alcohol misuse or other substance misuse
7. Severe obesity

Table 37.3 Diagnostic criteria for chronic fatigue syndrome.

Studies that looked at responses to apomorphine showed increased GH levels. Such abnormalities have been cited as hormonal epiphenomena consistent with the dopamine hypothesis of schizophrenia. Treatment with phenothiazines and other dopamine-receptor blockers commonly lead to elevations in prolactin and in some cases disturbances in menstrual function and galactorrhea. Usually, in such cases, antipsychotic treatment takes priority, but if there is significant hypogonadism then estrogen supplementation may be warranted, especially in individuals at risk for osteoporosis. Care must be taken in order to exclude primary pituitary pathology, since schizophrenics are just as likely to have a pituitary tumor as nonschizophrenics. Newer atypical antipsychotics have a more complex pharmacologic profile with multiple effects at different neurotransmitter receptor sites. Significant serotoninergic effects have been cited as the reason why many of these drugs cause marked weight gain.

Anxiety disorders

While anxiety is a component of many psychiatric conditions, anxiety disorders can be defined as those in which excessive anxiety is present in isolation.

Although behavioral studies in animals show that CRH has anxiogenic effects, patients with anxiety disorders do not show signs of HPA axis activation at baseline. Subtle abnormalities such as blunted ACTH responses to CRH have led to suggestions that desensitization of pituitary CRH receptors occurs in these subjects, perhaps as a result of excessive hypothalamic CRH activity, which is normally episodic rather than sustained.

Hypothalamo–pituitary–adrenal axis activation is not evident during experimentally induced panic attacks using lactate infusions. Increased atrial natriuretic peptide activity has been found in such subjects, suggesting that atrial natriuretic peptide (a putative inhibitor of the HPA axis) may mediate the suppression of CRH-induced ACTH and cortisol secretion, which would be expected in such circumstances. This finding is supported by the anxiolytic effect of atrial natriuretic peptide analogs. Blunting of TSH responses to TRH and GH responses to GHRH, analogous to those found in major depression, have also been found in patients with anxiety disorders, although the significance of these remains unclear.

Posttraumatic stress disorder
Posttraumatic stress disorder is another psychiatric condition that is associated with significant alterations in neuroendocrine regulation. The syndrome is characterized by three sets of symptoms:

- recurrent and intrusive recollections of a traumatic event;
- avoidant symptoms (feelings of detachment and estrangement); and
- persistent symptoms of hyperarousal (e.g. hypervigilance, exaggerated startle response).

Evidence of HPA dysregulation in posttraumatic stress disorder patients includes lower mean 24-hour urinary cortisol secretion, lower baseline plasma cortisol concentrations, increased glucocorticoid binding in lymphocytes, increased sensitivity to the HPA-suppressive effects of dexamethasone, and lower levels of pituitary ACTH secretion in response to exogenous challenge with CRH in comparison with normal controls. Taken together, these abnormalities suggest enhanced negative-feedback sensitivity in these patients. There is also evidence for hyperactivity in the sympathetic nervous system. Twenty-four-hour urinary excretion of catecholamines is significantly elevated in patients with posttraumatic stress disorder and this probably underlies observed increases in resting heart rate, systolic blood pressure and conditioned responses. Moreover, catecholamine levels appear to correlate with specifically intrusive posttraumatic stress disorder symptoms such as flashbacks. The mechanisms that underlie these phenomena remain unexplained, although there have been speculations that the development of posttraumatic stress disorder may be facilitated by an atypical biologic response in the immediate aftermath of a traumatic event, which in turn leads to a maladaptive psychologic state.

Postpartum depression
Some 10–15% of women develop syndromal depressions within the first 2–3 months postpartum. Prior history of depression and stressful life events with lack of support are risk factors. Psychotic mood disorders occur after 1–2/1000 deliveries. History of bipolar illness and postpartum psychosis increase the risk considerably. The hormonal events that characterize pregnancy and the postpartum period are obvious etiologic candidates, but careful study has shown that there are no abnormalities in hormone levels in women with postpartum depression. The occurrence of symptoms during withdrawal from gonadal steroids, and their amelioration during a period of

Diagnostic features of eating disorders	
Anorexia nervosa	Body weight willfully maintained below normal level
	Abnormal perception of body morphology
	Intense fear of weight gain
	Amenorrhea
Bulimia nervosa	Large uncontrolled eating binges at least twice weekly
	Inappropriate compensatory behavior (e.g. vomiting, purging)
Binge eating disorder	Large uncontrolled eating binges at least twice weekly
	No regular inappropriate compensatory disorders
	Marked distress about binges

Table 37.4 Diagnostic features of eating disorders.

relative hypogonadism, would suggest that it is the actual withdrawal that is the significant factor. This is supported by the reported efficacy of estrogen in treating or preventing the recurrence of postpartum depression. Given the neuromodulatory effects of gonadal steroids, postpartum depression probably represents a failure to compensate for neuroregulatory changes induced by significant (albeit physiologic) perturbations of gonadal steroid levels.

Premenstrual syndrome
Premenstrual syndrome refers to the cyclic recurrence of mood and behavioral symptoms during the luteal phase of the menstrual cycle. Studies of basal hormone levels in women with premenstrual syndrome have revealed no consistent differences when compared with controls, while dynamic studies have yielded mixed results. These include increased frequency and decreased amplitude of LH pulses and decreased LH responses to Gonadotropin-releasing hormone (GnRH). Treatment with ovarian suppression (e.g. a GnRH agonist), so that gonadal steroid levels are reduced to hypogonadal levels, does not yield a therapeutic response in all patients, suggesting that other factors may play a role. Reinduction of symptoms can be brought about by replacement doses of estrogen or progesterone.

Eating disorders
Anorexia nervosa is a disorder of food intake and body image that is characterized by restriction of food intake and obsessive physical activity aimed at achieving a low body weight. Bulimia nervosa is an eating disorder characterized by episodic bingeing, which may exist alone or in combination with anorexia. Both syndromes occur predominantly in young females, especially in adolescent girls, although there is an increasing incidence in young males. Together, these illnesses affect about 3% of women over their lifetime. Binge eating disorder, a syndrome characterized by eating binges that are not followed by vomiting, is more evenly distributed in terms of gender and age (Table 37.4). The causes of anorexia nervosa and bulimia nervosa are unknown, but cultural and environmental factors are thought to play a key role, since both conditions are much more common in developed than in developing nations. Frequently highlighted among multifactorial etiologies are social pressures to slim, and characteristic family dynamics.

The biologic abnormalities evident in anorexia nervosa are almost certainly a consequence rather than a cause of the disease. Prominent among these abnormalities are activation of the HPA axis when in the underweight state, as manifested by dexamethasone nonsuppression, blunted ACTH responses to CRH, and elevations of CRH in the CSF. It has been suggested that elevation in central CRH, a known anorexigenic factor, may act to sustain the appetite suppression that occurs in these patients.

Amenorrhea is a frequent feature of anorexia nervosa, and sometimes precedes the weight loss. A number of studies suggest that central CRH overactivity inhibits hypothalamic GnRH secretion through an action on β-endorphin at the arcuate nucleus. Low levels of leptin, which are apparent with starvation even before weight loss, are likely to be of even greater importance, since adequate plasma leptin appears to be necessary to facilitate GnRH secretion and reproductive function. Altered menstrual function usually normalizes after correction of weight fluctuations.

Changes in thyroid hormone that occur in anorexia nervosa are characteristic of starvation; with decreased T_3, elevated reverse T_3 and attenuated TSH responses to TRH. Basal GH levels are elevated in anorexia nervosa, with exaggerated GH responses to GHRH, probably because of reduced feedback from IGF-1, which in turn is due to a combination of weight loss and elevated glucocorticoids.

FURTHER READING

Burman P, Deijen JB. Quality of life and cognitive function in patients with pituitary insufficiency. Psychother Psychosom 1998;67:154–67.

Chiovato L, Pinchera. A. Stressful life events and Graves' disease. Eur J Endocrinol. 1996;134:680–2.

Cleare AJ, Heap E, Malhi GS, Wessely S, O'Keane V, Miell J. Low-dose hydrocortisone in chronic fatigue syndrome: a randomised crossover trial. Lancet 1999;353:455–8.

Dorn LD, Burgess ES, Friedman TC, Dubbert B, Gold PW, Chrousos GP. The longitudinal course of psychopathology in Cushing's syndrome after correction of hypercortisolism. J Clin Endocrinol Metab. 1997;82:912–9.

Holsboer F. The corticosteroid receptor hypothesis of depression. Neuropsychopharmacology 2000;23:477–501.

Kelly WF. Psychiatric aspects of Cushing's syndrome. Q J Med. 1996;89:543–51.

Koob GF, Heinrichs SC. A role for corticotropin releasing factor and urocortin in behavioral responses to stressors. Brain Res. 1999;848:141–52.

McGauley G, Cuneo R, Salomon F, Sonksen PH. Growth hormone deficiency and quality of life. Hormone Res. 1996;45:34–7.

Sapoisky RM Glucocorticoids and hippocampal atrophy in neuropsychiatric disorders. Arch Gen Psychiat. 2000;10:925–35.

Simons WF, Fuggle PW, Grant DB, Smith I. Educational progress, behaviour, and motor skills at 10 years in early treated congenital hypothyroidism. Arch Dis Child. 1997;77:219–22.

Walsh BT, Devlin MJ. Eating disorders: progress and problems. Science. 1998;280:1387–90.

Wise PM, Dubal DB, Wilson ME, Rau SW, Liu Y. Estrogens: trophic and protective factors in the adult brain. Front Neuroendocrinol. 2001;22:33–66.

Wong ML Kung MA, Munson PJ, et al. Pronounced and sustained central hypernoradrenergic function in major depression with melancholic features: relation to hypercortisolism and corticotropin-releasing hormone. Proc Natl Acad Sci USA 2000;97:325–30.

Yehuda R Biology of posttraumatic stress disorder. J Clin Psychiat. 2000;61:14–21.

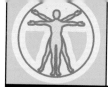

Chapter 38

Endocrinology of the Placenta, Fetus and Pregnancy

Ram K Menon and Mark A Sperling

INTRODUCTION

The placenta is a tissue of largely fetal origin imbedded in the maternal uterine wall to permit exchange of vital nutrients and other elements essential to fetal growth, development, and survival. The trophoblast cell lineage that forms the fetal portion of the placenta is specified by fibroblast growth factor 4 (FGF-4). Placental tissue is capable of steroid and polypeptide synthesis (**Figs 38.1 & 38.2**). Hormonal products and inter-conversions resulting from these synthetic pathways appear to be critically important for ordered fetal growth, development, and the onset of labor. In some instances, notably estradiol (E_2) and estriol (E_3) synthesis, the placenta converts steroids pre-cursors synthesized in the fetal adrenal (**Fig. 38.1**). Thus, the placenta completes a task initiated in the fetal adrenal so that the fetus and the placenta act as a unit, the fetoplacental unit. This chapter presents endocrine aspects of the placenta and fetus during gestation and the immediate newborn and presents selected examples of fetal and perinatal endocrine disorders.

PLACENTA

Steroid synthesis

The most important of the steroids synthesized by the placenta are progesterone and estrogen. The human placenta does not synthesize or secrete glucocorticoids or mineralocorticoids. Cholesterol derived from low-density lipoprotein (LDL-C) serves as the principal precursor for all steroids in the placenta, fetal adrenal, and corpus luteum, each of which possesses membrane-bound receptors for LDL. Apoprotein (Apo) B100, located on the surface of the LDL particle, binds to these spe-cific membrane-bound receptors, enabling endocytic internal-ization of the LDL particle, fusion with acid-lipase-containing lysosomes, and the hydrolytic release of cholesterol esters. The cell's requirement for cholesterol regulates the number of low-capacity-high affinity LDL receptors.

Progesterone

In the first trimester, the maternal corpus luteum secretes large amounts of progesterone, which is essential for maintaining

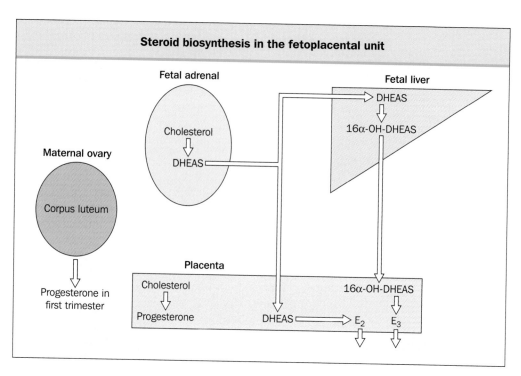

Figure 38.1 Steroid biosynthesis in the fetoplacental unit. See text for details. DHEAS, dehydroepiandrosterone sulfate; E_2, estradiol; E_3, estriol.

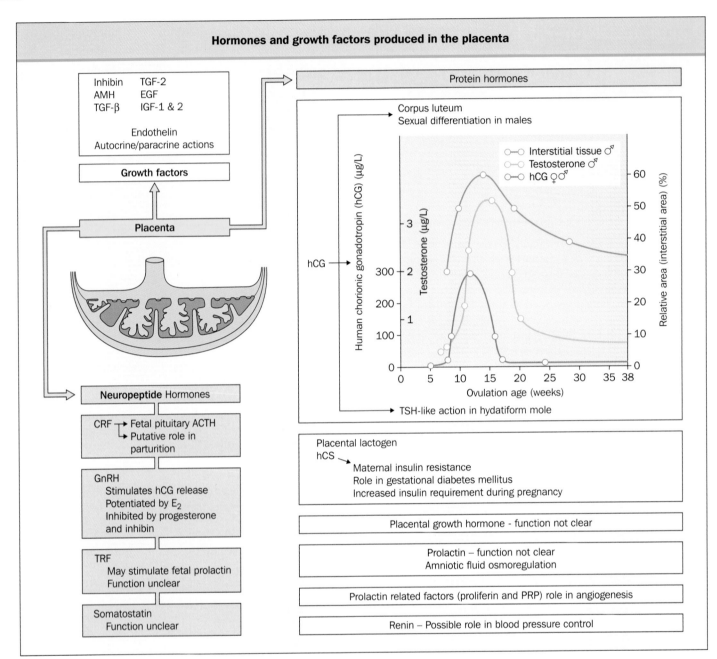

Figure 38.2 Hormones and growth factors produced in the placenta. See text for some proposed functions. ACTH, adrenocorticotropic hormone; AMH, Anti-Müllerian hormone; CRF, corticotropin-releasing factor; E_2, estradiol; EGF, epidermal growth factor; GnRH, gonadotropin-releasing hormone; hCS, human chorionic somatomammotropin; hCG, human chorionic gonadotropin; IGF, insulin-like growth factor; PRP, proliferin-related protein; TGF, transforming growth factor; TRF, thyrotropin-releasing factor; TSH, thyroid-stimulating hormone.

pregnancy via suppression of uterine contractions. At about the onset of the second trimester, progesterone synthesis by the corpus luteum is replaced by placental synthesis, the 'luteoplacental shift'. Thus, ovariectomy or disruption of the ovarian synthesis or action of progesterone (e.g. by administration of a receptor-blocking drug, RU486) results in first trimester abortion. The placenta does not use the steroid acute regulatory protein, StAR, for progesterone synthesis but does require P450$_{scc}$ (**Fig. 38.3** and **Table 38.1**). Hence, P450$_{scc}$ deficiency in the fetus is incompatible with survival, causing second trimester abortion from the lack of placental progesterone to suppress uterine contractility.

At term, the placenta secretes about 250mg of progesterone per day. In contrast with estrogens, the fetus does not contribute to progesterone formation by the placenta. The rate of incorporation of radio-labeled acetate into cholesterol is low as is the activity of the enzyme HMG-CoA reductase, indicating that the rate of *de novo* synthesis of cholesterol in the placenta is low. In cultured human trophoblasts and choriocarcinoma cells, LDL is the principal source of cholesterol, whereas cholesterol esters are absent. Generally, the uptake of LDL in tissue increases the formation of cholesterol esters by stimulating acyl-CoA:cholesterol acyl-transferase (ACAT) activity. This ACAT activity is almost completely inhibited by progesterone at concentrations found in

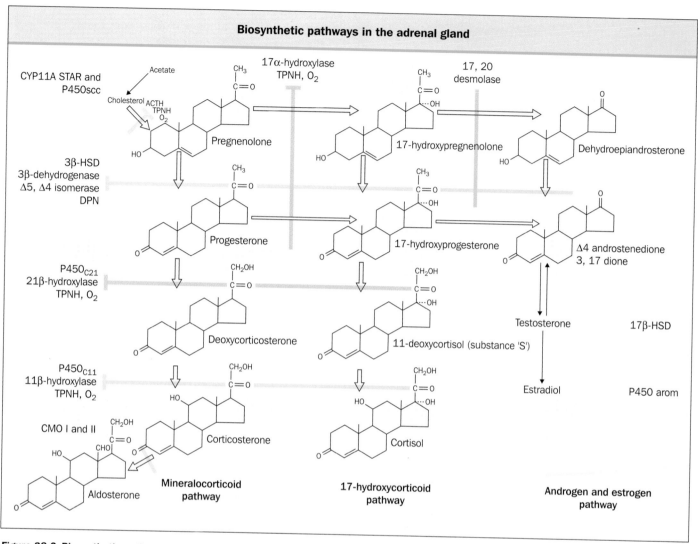

Figure 38.3 Biosynthetic pathways in the adrenal gland. The figure shows the structure of the major steroids. The shaded lines indicate the potential site of a block in the appropriate enzymatic step. See text and Table 38.1 for details. Note: $P450_{c11}$ catalyzes 11-hydroxylase as well as 18-hydroxylas and 18-oxidase activity. $P450_{c17}$ catalyzes both 17-hydroxylase and 17-20 desmolase (lyase) activity. StAR, steroidogenic acute regulatory protein. (Modified from Sperling MA. Ontogeny of adrenal function. In: Tuchinsky D, Little AB, eds. Maternal–fetal endocrinology. Philadelphia, PA: WB Saunders; 1994.)

trophoblastic cells. Therefore, ACAT activity is inhibited in the human placenta, preventing sequestration of cholesterol as cholesterol esters. This mechanism allows for a continuous supply of cholesterol for progesterone biosynthesis; amino acids derived from the hydrolysis of the protein component of the LDL molecule serve as the source of the essential amino acids for the fetus.

Estrogen

After the first 3–4 weeks of gestation, nearly all the estrogen produced is synthesized in the trophoblasts by a unique mechanism. Because the human placenta is devoid of 17α-hydroxylase/17-lyase activity (**Fig. 38.3** and **Table 38.1**), there is very little conversion of C21 to C19 steroids and progesterone is not metabolized within the placenta to any significant extent. However, the human placenta has a remarkable capacity for aromatization of C19 steroids and depends on circulating C19 precursors for estrogen synthesis (**Fig. 38.1**). The principal precursor for placental estradiol (E_2) is circulating dehydroepiandrosterone sulfate (DHEAS); for estriol (E_3), it is

plasma 16α-hydroxy dehydroepiandrosterone sulfate (16-OH DHEAS). Near term, the source of the E_2 synthesized by the placenta is equally divided between precursors in the maternal and the fetal circulation. On the other hand placental E_3 production derives mostly from the 16-OH DHEAS originating in the fetal compartment and requires the action of a sulfatase to permit subsequent aromatization of 16α-dehydroepiandrosterone (DHEA). Placental sulfatase deficiency is an X-linked syndrome associated with ichthyosis; absence of hydrolysis of DHEAS or 16-OH DHEAS results in deficiency of placental estrogen production. Therefore, low levels of estriol in the maternal plasma and urine during pregnancy may mistakenly lead to consideration of severe placental insufficiency, fetal adrenal disease, or a spurious diagnosis of fetal compromise or death. The large capacity for aromatization of C19 steroids by the placenta results in the conversion of androgen such as DHEAS, DHEA, androstenedione, and testosterone to estrogens, resulting in minimal transfer of androgens from the maternal to the fetal circulation. This mechanism affords relative

Genes and gene products involved in glucocorticoid, mineralocorticoid and sex hormone biosynthesis and action

Gene	Chromosome	Product	Function	Deficiency state
SLOS	7q32.1	7-dehydrocholesterol reductase	7-dehydrocholesterol → cholesterol	Smith–Lemli–Opitz syndrome
StAR	8p11.2	StAR	Transporter	Lipoid congenital adrenal hyperplasia (CAH)
CYP11A	15q23–q24	P450$_{scc}$	Cholesterol → pregnenolone	–
HSD3B2	1p13.1	3β-hydroxysteroid dehydrogenase	Pregnenolone → progesterone	Male and female pseudohermaphroditism
CYP17	10q24.3	17α-hydroxylase 17,20-lyase	17α-hydroxypregnenolone → 17α-hydroxyprogesterone Dehydroepiandrosterone → androstenedione Pregnenolone → 17α-hydroxypregnenolone Progesterone → 17α-hydroxyprogesterone 17α-hydroxypregnenolone → dehydroepiandrosterone 17α-hydroxyprogesterone → androstenedione	Male pseudohermaphroditism Female infantilism Hypertension
CYP21	6p21.3	P450$_{c21}$	Progesterone → desoxycorticosterone 17α-hydroxyprogesterone → deoxycortisol	CAH: classical and nonclassical
CYP11B1	8q21	P450$_{c11}$	Deoxycortisol → cortisol	CAH: hypertensive form
CYP11B2	8q21	18-hydroxylase (CMO 1) Aldosterone reductase (CMO II)	Corticosterone → 18-OH-corticosterone → aldosterone	Isolated aldosterone deficiency
HSD17B3	9q22	17β-hydroxysteroid dehydrogenase	Androstenedione → Testosterone	Male pseudohermaphroditism
SRD5A2	2p23	Steroid 5α-reductase type 2	Testosterone → dihydrotestosterone	Pseudovaginal perineal hypospadias
AR	Xq11-q12	Transcription factor	Transmits effect of androgens on gene expression	Androgen insensitivity: complete/partial/mild
CYP19	15q21.1	P450$_{arom}$	Aromatizes androgens to estrogens	Female pseudohermaphroditism
ESR	6q25.1	Transcription factor	Transmits effects of estrogens on gene expression	Male: osteopenia, delayed skeletal maturation

Table 38.1 Genes and gene products involved in glucocorticoid, mineralocorticoid and sex hormone biosynthesis and action. SLOS, Smith–Lemli–Opitz syndrome; StAR, steroidogenic acute regulatory protein. (Adapted from Root AW. Genetic errors of sexual differentiation. Adv Pediatr. 1999;46:67–97.)

protection to the fetus from the virilizing effects of maternal androgens, unless aromatase deficiency exists.

Likewise, aromatase deficiency can lead to significant virilization of the mother and female fetus. **Table 38.2** summarizes the values of several steroids, including DHEAS, progesterone, and cortisol, in the fetal and maternal circulations at term and postnatally. Although the concept of a fetoplacental unit in steroidogenesis is generally accepted, its precise significance is less clear because development appears to proceed normally with congenital absence of the adrenals, placental sulfatase deficiency, or anencephaly with adrenocorticotropic hormone (ACTH) deficiency.

FETAL ADRENAL

The adrenal glands of the human fetus at term are as large as the adult gland but morphologically the fetal adrenal undergoes significant changes during development. The fetal adrenal gland is composed principally of an inner fetal zone, which forms 85% of the gland, whereas the outer cortex (neocortex) that ultimately develops into the adult adrenal cortex accounts for less than 15% of the gland. The fetal zone is deficient in 3β-OH-steroid dehydrogenase (3β-HSD) activity but can convert progesterone to cortisol so that the other key enzymatic steps in steroidogenesis are operative and functional (**Fig. 38.3**). In the definitive zone, 3β-HSD is more active, but this zone has fewer LDL-binding sites, less cholesterol synthesis, less sulfokinase, and less aldosterone, suggesting decreased 18-hydroxylase activity. Near term, the fetal adrenal gland secretes 100–200mg of steroid per day and its principal secretory products are DHEAS and pregnenolone sulfate. About 50–70% of the steroids secreted by the fetal adrenal are derived from circulating LDL cholesterol and

the remainder from cholesterol synthesized *de novo* in the adrenal gland. High-density lipoprotein (HDL) is less of a source and very-low-density lipoprotein (VLDL) is not used by the fetal adrenal. Because of the paucity of adipose tissue in the human fetus prior to 36 weeks gestation, the major source of the LDL in the fetus is hydrolysis of VLDL in the fetal lungs by lipoprotein lipase, the activity of which is stimulated by prolactin. Hence, it has been proposed that prolactin may be an indirect trophic agent for the fetal adrenal, acting via the regulation of the availability of precursors for steroidogenesis. Other peptide growth factors implicated in fetal adrenal growth and function include insulin-like growth factor 1 (IGF-1), transforming growth factor β (TGF-β), tumor necrosis factor α (TNF-α), IGF-2, epithelial growth factor (EGF), and fibroblast growth factor (FGF) (**Fig. 38.2**). Of the placental steroids synthesized, most enter the maternal circulation and only a minor fraction enters the fetal compartment. Thus, more than 85–90% of the E_2, E_3 and progesterone synthesized by the trophoblasts enters the maternal compartment.

A key mitochondrial protein, termed steroidogenic acute regulatory protein (StAR), enables steroidogenesis by permitting contact sites between the outer and inner mitochondrial membranes. Mutations in this protein cause congenital adrenal lipoid hyperplasia (see below), because StAR is expressed in the adrenal and gonads but not in the placenta. Thus, placental steroidogenesis remains normal in patients with this condition, whereas adrenal and gonadal steroidogenesis is abnormal.

Defects in fetal adrenal steroidogenesis

Figure 38.3 outlines potential sites of the defects in steroidogenesis leading to deficient cortisol, deficient aldosterone, and

Plasma corticosteroids in normal newborn infants

Source/time	Corticosterone (µg/dL)	Deoxycorticosterone (µg/dL)	Progesterone (µg/dL)	Hydroxyprogesterone (µg/dL)	Cortisol (µg/dL)	Cortisone (µg/dL)	11-desoxycortisone compound-S (ng/dL)	Aldosterone (ng/dL)	DHEAS (µg/dL)
MV	3.6	0.29	12.0	1.1	54.8	6.1	6.20	0.40	100
UV	1.1	0.63	27.1	3.3	7.0	13.8	5.41	0.37	130–250
2 hours	0.9	0.55	5.7	0.89	10.4	8.3	8.12	0.17	130–250
4 hours	0.3	0.45	6.8	0.60	4.9	8.7	–	–	130–250
6 hours	0.28	0.30	4.6	0.40	2.8	7.5	4.20	0.19	130–250
12 hours	0.52	0.12	2.4	0.20	7.6	5.7	3.88	0.20	130–250
24 hours	0.08	0.12	1.25	0.09	2.7	4.1	3.33	0.17	130–250
4 days	0.19	0.01	0.09	0.08	5.7	2.3	2.94	0.16	130–250
7 days	0.25	0.01	0.05	0.12	3.5	2.2	1.83	0.06	2–100

Table 38.2 Plasma corticosteroids in newborn infants. DHEAS, dehydroepiandrosterone sulfate; MV, maternal vein; UV, umbilical vein. All other samples from peripheral blood. (From Sperling MA. Newborn adaptation: adrenocortical hormones and adrenocorticotropic hormone. In: Tuchinsky D, Little AB, eds. Maternal–fetal endocrinology, 2nd edn. Philadelphia, PA: WB Saunders; 1994.)

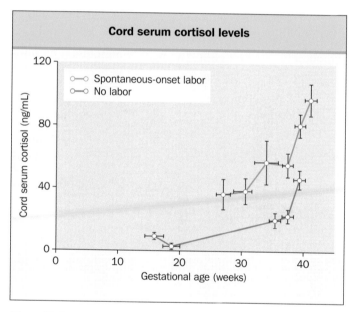

Figure 38.4 Cord serum cortisol levels. The figure shows cord serum cortisol levels in infants born with or without active labor. (Adapted from Murphy BEP, Branchaud CL. The fetal adrenal. In: Tuchinsky D, Little AB, eds. Maternal–fetal endocrinology, 2nd edn. Philadelphia, PA: WB Saunders; 1994: 281.)

Clinical manifestations of adrenal insufficiency in infancy

Cortisol deficiency	Hypoglycemia
	Inability to withstand stress
	Vasomotor collapse
	Hyperpigmentation (adrenocorticotropic hormone excess)
	Apneic spells
	Seizure
Adolesterone deficiency	Vomiting
	Hyponatremia
	Urinary salt wasting
	Hyperkalemia
	Failure to thrive
	Volume depletion
	Hypotension
	Dehydration
	Cyanosis
	Shock
Androgen excess or deficiency	Ambiguous genitalia

Table 38.3 Clinical manifestations of adrenal insufficiency in infancy. (From Sperling MA. Newborn adaptation: adrenocortical hormones and adrenocorticotropic hormone. In: Tuchinsky D, Little AB, eds. Maternal–fetal endocrinology, 2nd edn. Philadelphia, PA: WB Saunders; 1994.)

deficient or excess androgen production. The deficiency of cortisol in these syndromes (as well as congenital adrenal hypoplasia/aplasia, discussed below) is largely compensated by adequate transfer of cortisol from the maternal to fetal compartment where most is converted to cortisone by the action of C11-hydroxysteroid dehydrogenase, active in placenta and most fetal tissues. These small amounts of cortisol are sufficient to allow normal development of systems dependent on cortisol, including maturation of enzymes essential for extrauterine survival, glycogen accumulation, development of the adrenal medulla, thyroid function, and lung maturation and differentiation, including surfactant synthesis.

Normally, endogenous fetal adrenal cortisol synthesis is low; fetal total cortisol levels are 5–12ng/mL from 15–30 weeks, rise to approximately 20ng/mL by 38 weeks and 40–50ng/mL at term in the absence of labor and twice as high with active labor (**Fig. 38.4**). However, with defects in steroidogenesis affecting cortisol, the lower cortisol levels are inadequate to regulate the hypothalamo–pituitary–adrenal axis resulting in overproduction of endogenous ACTH. The consequences of glucocorticoid and mineralocorticoid deficiencies become apparent only after birth (**Table 38.3**). In the same way, mild defects may have progressive

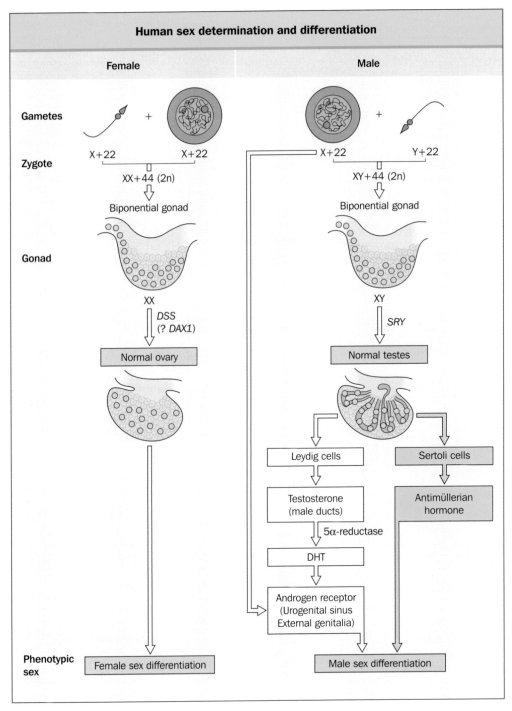

Human sex determination and differentiation

| Female | Male |

Gametes

Zygote
X+22   X+22   X+22   Y+22

XX+44 (2n)   XY+44 (2n)

Biponential gonad   Biponential gonad

Gonad

XX   XY

DSS
(? DAX1)   SRY

Normal ovary   Normal testes

Leydig cells   Sertoli cells

Testosterone
(male ducts)   Antimüllerian
                         hormone
5α-reductase

DHT

Androgen receptor
(Urogenital sinus
External genitalia)

Phenotypic
sex   Female sex differentiation   Male sex differentiation

Figure 38.5 Human sex determination and differentiation. Intrinsic or extrinsic factors adversely affecting any stage of these processes can lead to anomalies of sex. (From Grumbach MM, Conti FA. Sex differentiation. In: Wilson JD, Foster DW, Kronenberg HM, Larsen PR, eds. Williams textbook of endocrinology, 9th edn. Philadelphia, PA:WB Saunders; 1998:1239.)

consequences in postnatal virilization not apparent at birth. **Table 38.1** summarizes the syndromes resulting from defects in steroid biosynthesis or action in terms of enzyme defects, their responsible genes and chromosomal location. Reference to **Figure 38.3** permits delineation of the consequences of a particular enzyme defect.

Figures 38.5, 38.6 and **38.7** illustrate key factors involved in the differentiation of male or female internal and external genitalia. Note that only the external genitalia are affected by defects in steroid biosynthesis; ambiguous genitalia are separately discussed below.

Specific defects in steroidogenesis
Defects proximal to pregnenolone
Side-chain cleavage of cholesterol requires the enzymatic action of P450$_{scc}$, preceded by the action of StAR. The StAR protein facilitates the transfer of cholesterol from the outer to the inner mitochondrial membrane and is the rate-limiting step for steroidogenesis. The placenta does not utilize StAR but requires P450$_{scc}$. Hence, deficiency of P450$_{scc}$ is incompatible with fetal survival, as outlined above. Thus, defects proximal to pregnenolone are restricted to defects in StAR.

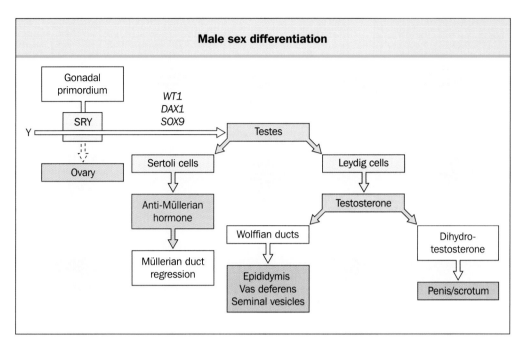

Figure 38.6 Male sex differentiation.

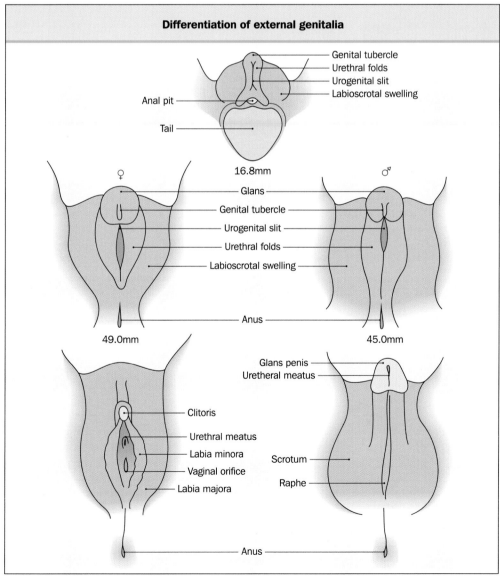

Figure 38.7 Differentiation of external genitalia. The figure illustrates the differentiation of male and female external genitalia from indifferent primordia. Male development occurs only in the presence of androgenic stimulation during the first 12 fetal weeks. (From Grumbach MM, Conti FA. Sex differentiation. In: Wilson JD, Foster DW, Kronenberg HM, Larsen PR, eds. Williams textbook of endocrinology, 9th edn. Philadelphia, PA:WB Saunders; 1998:1325.)

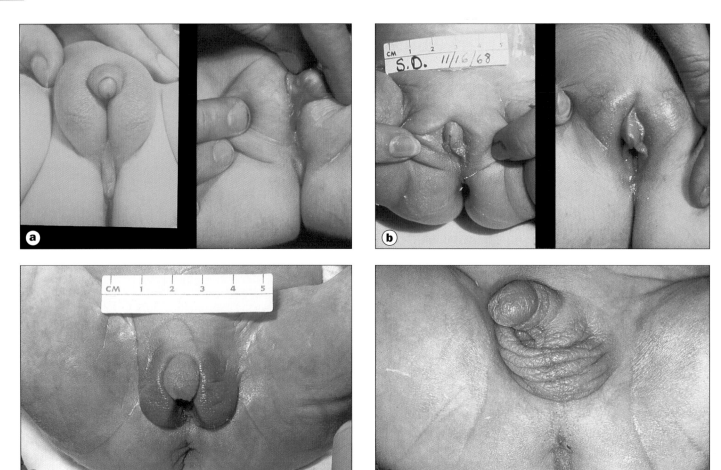

Figure 38.8 Virilization in fetal adrenal steroidogenesis defects. (a & b) 3β-hydroxysteroid dehydrogenase deficiency in a male (a) and a female (b). Note the bifid scrotum and third-degree hypospadias in the male and the clitoral hypertrophy with pubic hair development in the female. (c) Moderately severe virilization in a genetic female infant with 21-hydroxylase deficiency. Clitoral hypertrophy is prominent, with some fusion of the labioscrotal folds. Note the hyperpigmentation of the labia, indicating excessive adrenocorticotropic hormone with its inherent melanocyte-stimulating-hormone-like activity. (d) Complete virilization in a genetic female infant with 21-hydroxylase deficiency. The labia have completely fused to simulate a scrotum in which no gonads were palpable. The clitoris is enlarged to simulate a small phallus, which has undergone circumcision. The infant had vascular collapse, hyponatremia, and hyperkalemia.

Because these defects are shared by the adrenal and gonad and occur early in steroidogenesis, genetic males will have ambiguous genitalia or be phenotypically female. In genetic males, ultrasound shows no uterus and may show enlarged, lipid-laden adrenal glands. Postnatal salt wasting is severe, survival depending upon early diagnosis and appropriate replacement with glucocorticoid and mineralocorticoid. Laboratory tests show virtual absence of all plasma steroids, as also occurs in congenital adrenal hypoplasia. The latter is distinguished by absence of adrenal glands on ultrasonography. After an index case has been identified, antenatal diagnosis of future pregnancies is aided by monitoring maternal estriol and by molecular genetic typing of amniocentesis samples.

Beta-hydroxysteroid dehydrogenase deficiency

This enzyme defect also includes an isomerase function converting Δ5 to Δ4 steroids and there are separate isoforms for placental and adrenal/gonadal function. This early defect affects glucocorticoid, mineralocorticoid, and sex steroid pathways in various graduations in both adrenal and gonads. Excessive accumulations of DHEA, a weak androgen, and defective conversion to the potent androgens result in 'partial' virilization in both females and males. Females have labial fusion, clitoral hypertrophy, and modest hirsutism, which may progress. Males have hypospadias, bifid scrotum, and a small phallus (**Fig. 38.8**).

P450$_{C17}$ deficiency

This enzyme possesses both 17α-hydroxylase and 17,20-lyase activity, the latter permitting formation of DHEA or androstenedione from respectively 17-OH pregnenolone and 17-OH progesterone (**Fig. 38.3**). Genotypic males appear as complete phenotypic females or have ambiguous genitalia with a small or rudimentary phallus, hypospadias, cryptorchidism, and the appearance of a shallow vagina. Genetic females have no ambiguity at birth but fail to feminize at puberty. Mineralocorticoid formation is normal so that postnatal salt loss does not occur. The molecular basis for the differing clinical and biochemical abnormalities affecting predominantly 17α-hydroxylase or 17,20-lyase activity are reviewed elsewhere.

Clinical and biochemical features in newborn adrenal insufficiency

	Electrolyte disturbance	Ambiguous genitalia		Cortisol	Aldosterone	Serum			Urine	
		Virilized female	Incomplete male			17-hydroxy-progesterone	Dehydroepi-androsterone	17-hydroxy-corticosteroids	17-keto-steroids	Pregnanetriol
Hypoplasia	Severe	No	No	Decrease	Decrease	Decrease	Decrease	Decrease	Decrease	Decrease
Hemorrhage	Moderate–severe	No	No	Decrease	Decrease	Decrease	Decrease	Decrease	Decrease	Decrease
Desmolase (20.22)	Severe	No	Yes	Decrease	Decrease	Decrease	Decrease	Decrease	Decrease	Decrease
3β-HSD	Severe	Yes	Yes	Decrease	Decrease	Decrease	Increase	Decrease	Increase	Decrease
21-hydroxylase	Moderate–Severe	Yes	No	Decrease	Decrease	Increase	Increase	Decrease	Increase	Increase
Aldosterone synthesis block*	Severe	No	No	Normal	Normal	Normal	Normal	Normal	Normal	Normal
Pseudohypoaldosteronism	Severe	No	No	Normal	Increase	Normal	Normal	Normal	Normal	Normal
11-hydroxylase	None	Yes	No	Decrease	Decrease	Normal–slight increase	Normal	Increase	Increase	Normal–slight increase
17-hydroxylase	None	No	Yes	Decrease	Normal–decrease	Decrease	Decrease	Decrease	Decrease	Decrease
Unresponsiveness to ACTH	None	No	No	Decrease	Normal–low	Normal	Normal	Decrease	Decrease	Decrease

* Mediated by P450$_{c11}$, which catalyzes 18-hydroxylase and 18-oxidase activity as well as 11-hydroxylase activity. 17-hydroxylase (P450$_{c17}$) also catalyses 17–20 desmolase (lyase) activity.

Table 38.4 Clinical and biochemical features in newborn adrenal insufficiency. ACTH, adrenocorticotropic hormone; HSD, hydroxysteroid dehydrogenase. (From Sperling MA. Newborn adaptation: adrenocortical hormones and adrenocorticotropic hormone. In: Tuchinsky D, Little AB, eds. Maternal–fetal endocrinology, 2nd edn. Philadelphia, PA: WB Saunders; 1994.)

P450$_{C21}$ (21-hydroxylase) deficiency

This is the most common and prototypic variant of congenital adrenal hyperplasia. Because the androgenic pathway is not affected, the fetus is exposed to excessive androgens from about the third month of intrauterine life (**Fig. 38.3**). Therefore, genetic females show variable degrees of masculinization of the external genitalia, ranging from mild clitoral hypertrophy to simulation of completely normal male genitalia but without palpable testes (**Fig. 38.8**). Ultrasound shows a uterus and provides a rapid means of detecting genetic females. The heterogeneic manifestations of this syndrome include life-threatening salt loss, hyponatremia, hyperkalemia, and hypo-glycemia from deficiency of aldosterone and cortisol in severe cases, or progressive virilization with minimal salt loss in mildly affected individuals (**Fig. 38.3**). The relative frequency of this disorder, about 1:10,000 live births, has prompted neonatal screening programs using the measurement of 17-OH proges-terone in filter paper blood spots. The heterogeneic clinical manifestations and their biochemical and molecular basis are extensively reviewed elsewhere.

P450$_{C11}$ (11-hydroxylase) deficiency

This enzyme activity includes hydroxylation at C11 as well as the 18-oxido-reductase pathway (**Fig. 38.3**). With primary 11-OH deficiency, external virilization will occur in genetic females similar to that described above but without postnatal salt-losing crises. With 18-oxido-reductase deficiency there is no ambiguity of external genitalia but aldosterone deficiency may manifest postnatally as salt loss. **Table 38.4** summarizes the clinical and biochemical features in newborns with adrenal insufficiency syndromes.

Congenital adrenal hypoplasia/aplasia – X-linked

Congenital adrenal hypoplasia/aplasia is caused by mutations in the DAX1 nuclear receptor, whose gene is on Xp-21. Deletion of contiguous loci in this region are also associated with Duchenne muscular dystrophy and glycerol kinase deficiency. There are no fetal manifestations of this disorder, which is potentially life-threatening postnatally. The gene is expressed in the hypothalamic–pituitary–gonadal axis as well as in the adre-nal and may affect Sertoli cell function. Whereas mutations or deletions in DAX1 cause adrenal hypoplasia and hypogonado-tropic hypogonadism, duplications or overexpression cause XY sex reversal, suggesting that DAX1 acts in part as a repressor of testis development.

PROTEIN HORMONES

Several of the major placental protein hormones produced are illustrated in **Figure 38.2**. While the physiology of some of these is well characterized, others, such as ACTH or corti-cotropin-releasing hormone (CRH), remain intriguing but not completely delineated – including the role of CRH in labor and parturition.

Human chorionic gonadotropin

Human chorionic gonadotropin is a glycoprotein that has a virtually identical α subunit to that of luteinizing hormone (LH), follicle-stimulating hormone (FSH) and thyroid-stimulating hormone but only about two-thirds homology in amino-acid composition to the β subunit of LH. This difference is adequate to enable assays that reliably distinguish between the two hormones. Further glycosyolation modulates the biologic action of hCG by increasing its half-life. It is proposed that gonadotropin-releasing hormone (GnRH) stimulates production of hCG and that factors such as cyclic adenosine monophosphate (cAMP), interleukin (IL)-6, TNF-α, activin, and inhibin are other regulators of placental hCG production. hCG may be important for the maintenance of the corpus luteum of pregnancy and may be the key factor in the sexual differentiation of the male fetus by stimulating testosterone production in the fetal testis prior to the onset of LH secretion by the fetal pituitary (**Fig. 38.2**). Therefore, males with congenital hypopituitarism or gonadotropin deficiency do not have ambiguous genitalia, since adequate testosterone production was present during early fetal life to masculinize the internal and external genitalia. However, there may be a microphallus with a small undescended testis, reflecting the important input of pituitary gonadotropins in the third trimester of pregnancy.

Placental lactogen/human chorionic somatomammotropin

This protein is a product of genes located within the GH/CS gene cluster on the long arm of chromosome 17 q-22–24. The cluster consists of two growth hormone (GH) genes (*GH1* and *GH2*) and three placental lactogen genes (*CSP*, *CS1* and *CS2*). *GH1*, also termed *GHN*, is expressed in the pituitary and is the source of circulating growth hormone, whereas *GH2*, also termed *hGHV*, is expressed only in the placenta and specifies a gene product that differs by 13 of the 191 amino acids encoded by *GH1*.

Human placental lactogen (hPL) is produced by two genes, *CS1* and *CS2*; the *CSP* gene is considered to be a pseudogene because it contains a nucleotide substitution (G to A at the splice site of intron 2) that predicts absence of normal splicing and hence absence of a product. In terms of amino acids, hPL has over 80% and 60% homology with respectively human growth hormone and prolactin. The production and secretion of hPL by the placenta begins at the time of nidation and progressively increases during pregnancy in proportion to placental mass. The maximum daily production of human chorionic somatomammotropin (hCS)/hPL is estimated to be 1g or more, the largest mass of protein hormone produced in the human. hPL has both lactogenic and somatotropic actions that are much weaker than that of pituitary growth hormone, with about 1% equivalent potency per unit mass. The growth-hormone-like actions of hPL may induce resistance to insulin action and unmask latent diabetes during pregnancy if genetic or acquired defects in insulin secretion limit compensatory hyperinsulinemia. Thus, hPL may be responsible for some cases of gestational diabetes mellitus with its deleterious effects on fetal growth and development in the third trimester. Likewise, hPL contributes to the increase in insulin requirement in women with type 1 diabetes as their pregnancy progresses.

Proliferin and proliferin-related protein (PRP) have been implicated as potent regulators of angiogenesis controlling the start and cessation of placental neovascularization (**Fig. 38.2**).

Renin

The placenta also produces renin, suggesting that it may be involved in regulating maternal blood pressure, blood flow, and vascular resistance in the uteroplacental circulation; there is no direct evidence for this in humans.

Inhibin

Because inhibin suppresses the secretion of FSH, it has been proposed that placental inhibin prevents ovulation during pregnancy. Inhibin also may modulate the production of hCG by the trophoblasts via a paracrine action.

HYPOTHALAMIC PEPTIDES

Several of the major hypothalamic peptides produced by the placenta are illustrated in **Figure 38.2**. They are similar or identical to those produced by the hypothalamus. However, their physiologic role is debatable. Placental GnRH acting via cognate receptors present on trophoblasts stimulates hCG production and release by the placenta. Inhibin, activin, progesterone, estrogen, vasoactive intestinal peptide (VIP), insulin, prostaglandins, and epinephrine modulate the release of hCG by regulating placental GnRH production or action.

Placental CRH has identical bioactivity and immunoactivity to hypothalamic CRH. CRH concentrations in maternal plasma and amniotic fluid rise significantly during the last 5 weeks of pregnancy but do not evoke an increase in maternal ACTH, probably because of CRH-binding proteins in maternal plasma. By contrast, it is proposed that the fetal pituitary does respond to increased placental CRH, in turn responding with ACTH that stimulates adrenal steroidogenesis. In addition, glucocorticoids have a positive regulatory effect on the expression of CRH mRNA, and CRH released by the placenta. This regulatory loop has been implicated in the mechanisms responsible for labor and parturition. This evidence is strong in sheep and less clear in primates. Thus, the length of gestation in anencephalic infants and infants with X-linked adrenal aplasia is not significantly different from that in the control population. Moreover, it does not appear that human fetal adrenal cortisol metabolism plays an essential role in determining the duration of gestation, the onset of parturition, or various other fetal developmental aspects, since all appear to be normal in the human with congenital adrenal insufficiency of various etiologies.

ONTOGENY OF THE PITUITARY GLAND

The hypothalamus develops from the caudal portion of the neutral tube termed the prosencephalon and by 34 days the primitive hypothalamus derived from the diencephalon can be discerned. The primitive neurohypophysis is recognized by 37 days, the supraoptic–hypophyseal tract by 60 days, and the hypothalamic nuclei are differentiated by 100 days. All the classic hypothalamic peptides are synthesized by neurons in the prosencephalon with the exception of the neurons that secrete GnRH, which develop from the epithelium of the medial olfactory pit. These neurons then migrate along the olfactory-nerve–lamina-terminalis complex to reach the developing hypothalamus. GnRH-containing neurons are detectable by 9 weeks; a functional pulse generator that directs pulsatile secretion of GnRH is active by midgestation. The olfactory origins of the GnRH neurons are reflected in Kallmann's syndrome, characterized by the association of hypogonadotropic hypogonadism with anosmia. The X-linked variety of this genotypic heterogenous disorder is caused by the function of the *KAL* gene located on the Xp 22.3 region, a gene encoding a glycoprotein that acts as an extracellular adhesion molecule. Loss of function of this gene arrests the migration of GnRH neurons as well as aplasia/hypoplasia of the olfactory bulbs, resulting in the Kallmann complex.

Adenohypophysis

The precursor of the adenohypophysis, Rathke's pouch, develops as an ectodermal diverticulum of the primitive foregut. Rathke's pouch is apparent by 22 days post conception and by 35 days it is separated from the foregut and the posterior elements come into contact with the structures destined to become the neurohypophysis. The anterior wall of Rathke's pouch forms the adenohypophysis and the posterior wall forms the intermediate lobe and pars tuberalis of the pituitary gland. Cellular differentiation of the anterior pituitary takes place after the 40th day in cell cords that populate the anterior lobe of the primitive pituitary gland and continue to differentiate. Basophils containing ACTH are apparent by the 8th or 9th week and acidophils appear soon thereafter, so that by 14–15 weeks postconception the pituitary gland has achieved its adult organization.

Molecular events regulating the development of the anterior pituitary

The five cell types of the anterior pituitary – gonadotrophs, thyrotrophs, somatotrophs, lactotrophs, and corticotrophs – all develop from a common progenitor cell. Transcripts of the hormones produced can be detected as early as 16–17 days postconception. There is both a cell-type specificity and a spatial specificity within the pituitary such that each cell type develops within a specific glandular area. Three major transcription factors orchestrate the embryologic development of the anterior pituitary and defects in them result in hypopituitarism. These three transcription factors are Pit-1, Prop-1, and HSX-1. Pit-1, also known as GHF-1, is a member of the POU family (Pit-1; Oct-1 and Oct-2; Unc-86) of transcription factors. Pit-1 is pituitary specific and essential for the transcriptional activation of the GH, prolactin, and TSH-β genes in mammals. Abnormalities in Pit-1 structure and/or function result in phenotypic alteration such that mutant Pit-1 protein may not be able to bind to the appropriate DNA response element or the mutant Pit-1 may act as a dominant negative element interfering with the function of the wild-type molecule. Mutant Pit-1 molecules may interact with and alter the action of the DNA-binding protein, including Oct-1 or retinoic acid receptor. The function of this family of transcription factors, including Prop-1 and HSX-1, are detailed elsewhere. They are helpful in the diagnosis of familial causes of hypopituitarism and their specific hormonal defects.

Growth hormone

Growth hormone is detectable in fetal plasma by the 70th day of gestation, increases to a peak of 150ng/mL at midgestation,

and subsequently declines to levels of 30–50ng/mL in cord blood at term. The secretion of GH is primarily under the stimulatory control of growth-hormone-releasing hormone (GHRH) and the inhibitory control of somatostatin. Decreased activity of somatostatin inhibitory control early in gestation, resulting from lack of somatostatin receptors, allows unrestrained stimulation of GHRH and secretion of the high levels of fetal growth hormone. Thus, during early fetal life, unrestrained action of GHRH results in elevated levels of growth hormone; progressive decline in GH levels occurs with the maturation of the somatostatin–somatostatin-receptor axis. Whereas GHRH effects are mediated by a stimulatory G-protein, somatostatin uses an inhibitory G-protein pathway.

Growth hormone receptors are poorly expressed in fetal life and mature postnatally, thereby limiting short-loop inhibition by GH of its own secretion. Likewise, neurotransmitter-mediated regulation of GH secretion and/or nutrient regulation of GH secretion is poorly developed in fetal life. For example, glucose is relatively ineffective in suppressing growth hormone until 1 month postnatally, whereas sleep-associated increments in GH do not occur until about 3 months postnatally. By contrast, the stress response appears early and even at midgestation fetal delivery is associated with increased GH secretion. GH appears to play only a minor role, if any, in regulating fetal growth, probably because GH receptors are poorly expressed. Thus, congenital growth hormone deficiency and anencephaly are associated with near-normal birth length, and transgenic mice overexpressing GH are not large at birth. Some metabolic effects of GH are apparent earlier; GH is important for normal islet development, insulin secretion, and glycogen deposition. Neonates with growth hormone deficiency rapidly develop hypoglycemia. Some key manifestations and causes of hypopituitarism at birth are summarized in **Table 38.5**.

Prolactin

Prolactin is detectable in fetal plasma by 12 weeks but remains relatively low at approximately 20ng/mL until 30 weeks when it rises exponentially until term to values of approximately 150ng/mL. Estrogens enhance prolactin and thyrotropin-releasing hormone (TRH) stimulates it as well as thyroid-stimulating hormone (TSH), whereas dopamine inhibits prolactin. Placental TRH may cross the placenta to stimulate fetal prolactin release. Prolactin is also present in amniotic fluid in high concentrations of as much as 1300ng/mL at midgestation, falling progressively thereafter. Its probable source is the placenta and it has been proposed that it may have a role in regulating amniotic fluid volume, osmolality, and perinatal sodium homeostasis; however, none of these actions are proven in humans.

Insulin-like growth factors and insulin-like-growth-factor-binding proteins

Insulin-like growth factors appear to play a role in fetal development. Almost all fetal tissues express IGF-1 and IGF-2, as does the placenta. Mutations in the genes for IGF-1 result in embryonic growth retardation in animal models; a mutation in the human *IGF-1* gene was associated with intrauterine growth retardation and postnatal growth delay. Both IGF-1 and IGF-2 circulate in low concentrations in the human fetus but IGF-1 rises late in gestation. In large part, total IGF-1 reflects nutritional balance, with glucose availability and insulin secretion,

Some manifestations and causes of hypopituitarism at birth		
Manifestation		**Causes**
Hypoglycemia	Jitteriness	Breech delivery
	Seizures	Perinatal hypoxia
	Apneic spells	
	Blood glucose <40mg/dL	*Pit-1* gene mutations
Prolonged direct hyperbilirubinemia	Cholestasis	Central nervous system defects
	Giant cell hepatitis	Hypoplastic/dysgenetic pituitary stalk
Micropenis/small testis		Septo-optic dysplasia
Pendular nystagmus		Holoprosencephaly
Midline facial cleft defects		Kallmann's syndrome
Excessive urination/dehydration		

Table 38.5 Some manifestations and causes of hypopituitarism at birth.

although growth hormone exerts some influence on IGF-1 since IGF-1 levels are lower at term in the syndrome of complete end-organ resistance to growth hormone (Laron's syndrome). In contrast to transgenic mice overexpressing growth hormone, those overexpressing IGF-1 are larger at birth.

ENDOCRINE REGULATION OF FETAL GROWTH

Endocrine regulation of fetal growth is more closely related to insulin secretion and action, including their impact on IGF-1 secretion, than on the GH family and sex steroids. Whereas GH deficiency is not generally associated with significant reduction of fetal length or weight, deficiency or excess of insulin secretion has profound effects on fetal growth. Thus, the infant of the poorly controlled diabetic mother develops hyperinsulinemia and is macrosomic at birth. The impact of this fetal environmental on other developmental aspects is summarized in **Figure 38.9**. Likewise, fetal hyperinsulinemia resulting from mutations in the genes regulating the SUR–KIR6.2 system are associated with macrosomia at birth but without the other deleterious effects on development seen in the infant of the diabetic mother. By contrast, neonatal diabetes mellitus, whether transient or permanent, including pancreatic agenesis resulting from homozygous mutations in the transcription factor PDX-1, is associated with intrauterine growth retardation. Such infants are not only small at birth but have postnatal delay in normal growth and manifest polyuria and polydipsia. Offspring who have inherited a mutation in the glucokinase gene, which acts as a glucose sensor for insulin secretion, are also relatively smaller at birth than those who have not inherited this mutation.

The Rabson–Mendenhall syndrome and leprechaunism represent examples of intrauterine growth retardation and defective postnatal growth that result from insulin-receptor defects limiting the tyrosine-kinase/MAP-kinase growth signaling cascade. This growth-promoting signaling cascade is functional earlier *in utero* than the system coupled to glucose homeostasis and glycogen synthesis. As indicated above, mutations in the *IGF-1* gene are associated with intrauterine growth retardation as well. Finally, under normal circumstances, insulin secretion is a function of maternal nutritional state and maternal placental size, including hCS/hPL secretion, so that nutrient availability and transfer dictate insulin/IGF-1 concentrations and hence fetal size.

Management of the infant of the diabetic mother and of an infant with hypoglycemia are discussed in the section below dealing with disorders of carbohydrate metabolism.

A synopsis of factors involved in regulating fetal growth is shown in **Table 38.6**. Note that insulin and its receptors are more commonly associated with disorders of fetal growth regulation than are growth hormone or the insulin-like growth factors.

GONADOTROPINS

In the fetus, gonadotropin activity is initially attributed to hCG (**Fig. 38.2**) and only later to fetal pituitary LH and FSH. The pattern of fetal circulating hCG, which reaches its peak at 12 weeks and declines to a nadir at 18–20 weeks, is linked to the production of testosterone by the fetal testis during the critical period of differentiation of the Wolffian ducts and the urogenital sinus, and masculinization of the external genitalia (**Fig. 38.2**). Endogenous FSH and LH become significant in the third trimester when they continue stimulating testicular development. Because sexual differentiation is complete by the time FSH and LH exert significant effects, their insufficiency in the male is characterized by the presence of micropenis and undescended testes but not by sexual ambiguity.

Both LH and FSH can be detected in the fetal pituitary gland by 10 weeks of gestation, with LH reaching a peak by 27 weeks and remaining unchanged thereafter. Similar patterns exist for pituitary FSH content. There is sexual dimorphism in FSH and LH such that these pituitary hormones are higher in females than males. In general, the levels of circulating LH and FSH follow patterns similar to the profile of pituitary content. Gonadotropins are detectable in the fetal circulation at around 100 days of gestation but reach a peak at midgestation and decline thereafter to reach a nadir at birth. The sexual dimorphism of FSH and LH noted in the pituitary content is also apparent in the circulation. Plasma FSH is high, but higher in females, and plasma LH is higher in males at midgestation. At term, both FSH and LH levels are low, although LH levels tend to remain higher in males. **Figure 38.10** summarizes the ontogeny of these systems in males and females.

Fetal gonadotropin secretion is regulated by fetal GnRH secreted from the hypothalamus into the hypophyseal portal system; both the amount of GnRH and, more significantly, its

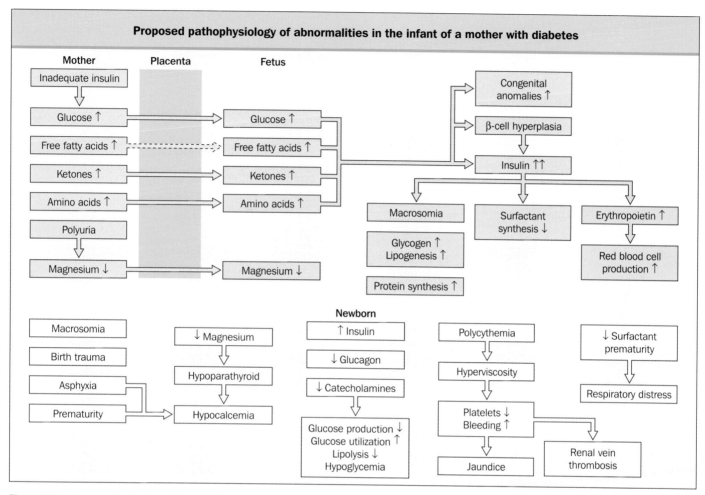

Figure 38.9 Proposed pathophysiology of abnormalities in the infant of a mother with diabetes. (Redrawn from Devaskar S, Sperling MA. Infants of diabetic mothers. In: Kelly, VC, ed. Practice of pediatrics, vol. 6. New York:Harper & Rowe; 1987:3.)

Hormonal factors involved in regulating fetal growth

Major			
Insulin	*Hyperinsulinemia* is associated with excessive fetal growth	Infant of mother with diabetes	
		Persistent hyperinsulinemic hypoglycemia of infancy	*SUR–KIR6.2* mutations
			Activating glucokinase mutations
	Hypoinsulinemia is associated with intrauterine growth retardation	Pancreatic agenesis – homozygous *PDX1* mutation	
		Congenital diabetes mellitus	Paternal uniparental isodisomy of chromosome 6
			Other differentiation, transcription and growth factor mutations
		Inactivating mutations in glucokinase	
	Insulin-receptor defects are associated with intrauterine growth retardation	Leprechaunism	
		Rabson–Mendenhall syndrome	
Insulin-like growth factors (IGF) 1 and 2	*High IGF-1* in most nutritional/insulin overgrowth syndromes		
	High IGF-2 in Beckwith–Wiedemann syndrome		
	Transgenic mice overexpressing IGF-1 are large at birth, whereas mice overexpressing growth hormone are not		
Minor			
Growth hormone	Congenital deficiency of secretion or action (Laron's syndrome) has minimal effects on length/size at birth		
	Growth factors – EGF, TGF, and PDGF – may have a role but precise function is unknown		

Table 38.6 Hormonal factors involved in regulating fetal growth. EGF, epithelial growth factor; PDGF, platelet-derived growth factor; TGF, transforming growth factor.

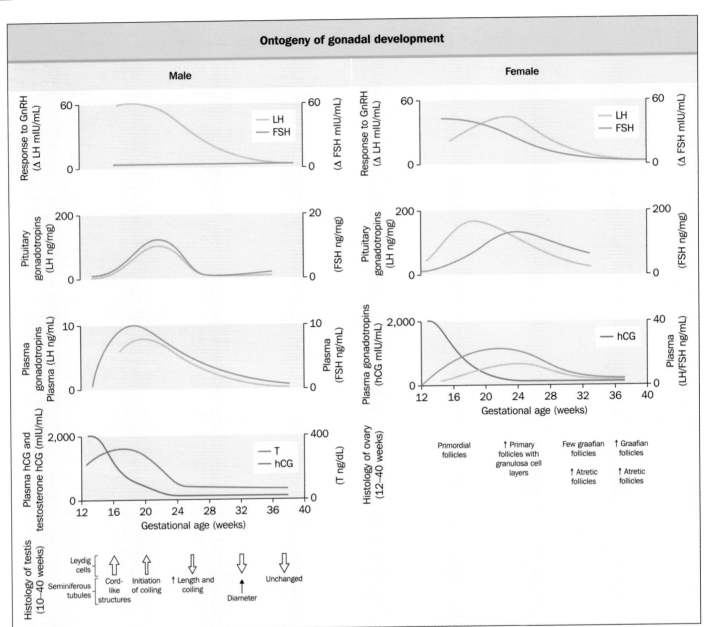

Figure 38.10 Ontogeny of gonadal development. The figure compares the ontogeny of male (left panel) and female (right panel) gonadal development in relation to pituitary responsiveness to gonadotropin-releasing hormone (GnRH), pituitary follicle-stimulating hormone (FSH)/luteinizing hormone (LH) content, plasma circulating levels of FSH and LH, and the critical early role of hCG and testosterone in male genital development. hCG, human chorionic gonadotropin; T, testosterone. (Modified from Grumbach MM, Conti FA. Sex differentiation. In: Wilson JD, Foster DW, Kronenberg HM, Larsen PR, eds. Williams textbook of endocrinology, 9th edn. Philadelphia, PA:WB Saunders; 1998:1536.)

pulsatile nature affect pituitary gonadotropin secretion. GnRH is detectable in fetal hypothalamic extracts by the 10th week of gestation and its pulsatile secretion has been demonstrated in the midgestation human fetus both *in vivo* and *in vitro*. The profile of circulating gonadotropins in the fetus, high in midgestation with decline thereafter, is attributed to the maturation of negative feedback mechanisms involving sex steroids and inhibitory central-nervous-system influences. Thus, the initial unrestrained pulsatile release of GnRH in midgestation progressively matures into inhibition of GnRH released from the hypothalamus (**Fig. 38.11**).

INHIBIN AND ACTIVIN

Inhibin is present in both male and female fetal gonads but is higher in the testis than ovary at mid-gestation thereby contributing to the sexual dimorphism of circulating FSH at this time. The placenta also is a source of synthesis and secretion of inhibin, which circulates in high concentrations in maternal serum from 10 weeks gestation through term. Umbilical-cord inhibin concentrations are high by radioimmunoassay but of low bioactivity and the inhibin is probably of placental origin. Serum levels of inhibin are high throughout the third trimester in the human fetus, declining modestly toward term.

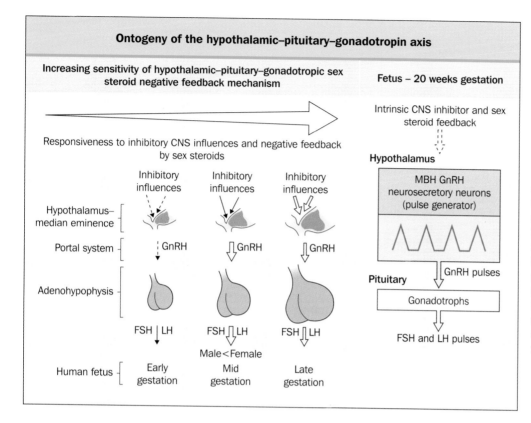

Figure 38.11 Ontogeny of the hypothalamic–pituitary–gonadotropin axis. The gonadotropin-releasing hormone (GnRH) pulse generator is highly functional by midterm (right panel), resulting in significant follicle-stimulating hormone (FSH) and luteinizing hormone (LH) secretion. Responsiveness to inhibitory central nervous system (CNS) signals and negative feedback by sex steroids develops later. (Left panel modified from Grumbach MM, Kaplan SL. In: Gluck L, ed. Modern perinatal medicine. Chicago, IL: Year Book Medical Publishers; 1974:247, and right panel from Grumbach MM, Styne DM. Puberty: ontogeny, neuroendocrinology, physiology, and disorders. In: Wilson JD, Foster DW, Kronenberg HM, Larsen PR, eds. Williams textbook of endocrinology, 9th edn. Philadelphia, PA:WB Saunders; 1998:1542.)

ADAPTATIONS IN THE GONADOTROPIN–GONADAL AXIS AT BIRTH

There are remarkable neonatal changes in the hypothalamic–pituitary–gonadal axis in males, but not females, immediately after birth. In males, the hypothalamic GnRH pulse generator is active on day 1 of life, resulting in a pulsatile pattern of LH and a surge of testosterone to adult levels within hours of birth. This process becomes quiescent by the end of the first week, as reflected in low testosterone values, only to be reactivated in a month and persist for the initial 3–6 months of life. During this neonatal time frame, plasma testosterone in males is equivalent to that of healthy young adults and GnRH evokes a 'pubertal' gonadotropin response. After 6 months to 1 year of life, the entire hypothalamic–pituitary–gonadal axis becomes inhibited until its reactivation at puberty. In females, FSH rises after the first week of life, reaching a peak by 3–4 months at levels comparable to menopausal concentrations. FSH then declines over 2–3 years, remaining low until puberty. In female infants, GnRH elicits a response of FSH that is log-order greater than in the male.

ADRENOCORTICOTROPIC HORMONE

The corticotroph is the first pituitary cell type to differentiate and ACTH is detectable in the pituitary at 9 weeks and in fetal serum at 12 weeks gestation. Fetal serum concentrations rise progressively until 34 weeks gestation and then decline but remain higher than in adults. ACTH rises during the stress of labor and the fetal hypothalamic–pituitary–adrenal axis is operative from about 3 months, as is evident from the consequences

of defects in steroidogenesis discussed earlier. Both hypothalamic CRH and arginine vasopressin synergistically stimulate ACTH release in the human fetal pituitary. Administration of potent glucocorticoids such as betamethasone or dexamethasone to mothers during pregnancy suppresses the hypothalamic–pituitary–adrenal axis in the fetus, resulting in lower cortisol and DHEA levels in cord blood.

HYPOPITUITARISM AT BIRTH

Table 38.5 describes the manifestations of hypopituitarism at birth and some of its major causes. The combined effects of ACTH/cortisol and GH deficiency manifest as neonatal hypoglycemia. In males, FSH/LH deficiency manifests as a micropenis, often with small undescended testes, and the usual surge of testosterone does not occur. Polyuria, often associated with dehydration, provides the clue to diabetes insipidus. Growth hormone levels are low, less than 5–10ng/mL, compared to the normally high levels in the normal newborn of 40–50ng/mL. Thus, stimulation tests for GH are not usually necessary in the newborn period. Prolactin levels are also low in cases of primary pituitary pathology; when it is secondary to hypothalamic hypopituitarism, with its disconnection of the inhibitory influence of dopamine, prolactin levels may be high. Early clues to congenital hypopituitarism include low maternal estriol during pregnancy, and recognizable midline cleft malformations of the central nervous system and face, including palate and lip, in the fetus/baby. In early neonatal life, prolonged direct hyperbilirubinemia resulting from hepatic cholestasis and giant-cell hepatitis provide clues. Pendular nystagmus is seen in the syndrome of septo-optic dysplasia. Treatment requires replacement with

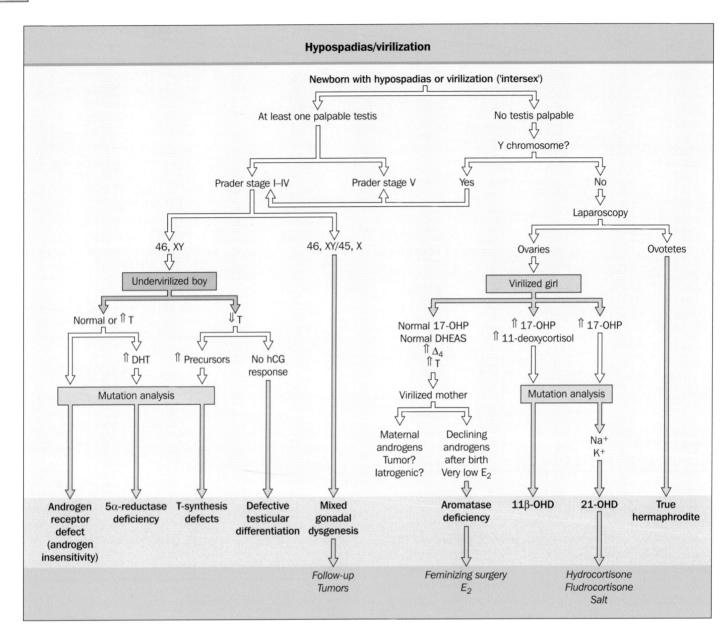

Figure 38.12 Hypospadias/virilization. The figure provides a schematic approach to the diagnosis and management of ambiguous genitalia in the newborn. Δ_4, androstenedione; DHEAS, dehydroepiandrosterone sulfate; DHT, dihydrotestosterone; E_2, estradiol; hCG, human chorionic gonadotropin; OHD, hydroxysteroid dehydrogenase; OHP, hydroxyprogesterone. (Modified from Hochberg Z, ed. Practical algorithms in pediatric endocrinology. Basel: Karger; 1999.)

cortisol at a dose of 15–20mg/m²/day; thyroxine 25–50µg/day; growth hormone 0.15–0.3mg/kg/week subcutaneously divided into seven nightly injections; and management of diabetes insipidus by judicious and cautious use of desmopressin and fluid replacement or restriction.

AMBIGUOUS GENITALIA

Ambiguous genitalia result from defects in the synthesis or action of androgens in males, from the lack of antimüllerian hormone in males, and from excessive androgens that virilize the external genitalia in females. Major pathways and manifestations have been delineated in **Figures 38.5–38.8** and in

Table 38.1. **Figure 38.12** provides a schematic approach to the diagnosis and management of ambiguous genitalia in the newborn.

CARBOHYDRATE METABOLISM IN THE FETUS

The fetus receives its glucose supply from the mother by placental transfer involving a non-insulin-dependent glucose transporter. Fetal glucose concentration is proportional to maternal glucose concentration, and fetal glucose production or gluconeogenesis is minimal until shortly before term. Thus, maternal hypoglycemia is associated with fetal hypoglycemia and hypoinsulinemia with little evidence of autoregulation or compensation by endogenous

Stigmata of infants of mothers with diabetes and their possible causes.	
Problem	**Mechanism/cause**
Fetal death	Placental insufficiency Hyperglycemia Hypoxia?
Macrosomia	Hyperinsulinism
Respiratory distress syndrome type 1 (hyaline membrane disease)	Insulin antagonism of surfactant synthesis
Respiratory distress syndrome type 2 (wet lung disease)	Cesarean section
Hypoglycemia	Hyperinsulinism (↓ glucose and fat mobilization)
Polycythemia	↑ erythropoietin Fetal hypoxia HBA1c – ↓ O_2 delivery to fetus?
Hypocalcemia	↑ parathyroid hormone Hypomagnesemia ↑ calcitonin?
Hyperbilirubinemia	Erythropoietic mass Bilirubin production Immature hepatic conjugation? Oxytocin administration
Congenital malformations	Hyperglycemia? Genetic linkage? Insulin? Vascular accident?
Renal vein thrombosis	Polycythemia Dehydration
Neonatal small left colon syndrome	Immature gastrointestinal motility
Cardiomyopathy	Septal hypertrophy

Table 38.7 Stigmata of infants of mothers with diabetes and their possible causes.

Management of the infant of a mother with diabetes	
Problem	**Management**
Congenital malformations	Early detection Supportive measures Specific corrective treatment
Birth asphyxia	Supportive measures (including ventilatory support)
Birth trauma	Early detection (clinical examination, X-ray studies) Specific and supportive measures
Macrosomia	Avoid birth trauma
Cardiomyopathy	Confirmation by echocardiography Supportive measures
Hypoglycemia	Intravenous glucose Rarely, glucagon/epinephrine
Respiratory distress syndrome	Prevention (avoid prematurity; corticosteroids; surfactant therapy) Supportive and ventilatory therapy
Hypocalcemia	Calcium and magnesium supplementation
Hyperbilirubinemia	Phototherapy Exchange transfusion
Polycythemia	Hydration Partial exchange transfusion
Renal vein thrombosis	Supportive measures Heparin? Nephrectomy?
Long-term problems:	
Increased incidence of type 1 diabetes mellitus	
Increased incidence of obesity	

Table 38.8 Management of the infant of a mother with diabetes.

fetal glucose production. Hypoxia, or the direct infusion of catecholamines, raises fetal glucose, indicating the existence of appropriate receptors that are coupled to their effector systems. By contrast, the dose-response effects of glucagon infusion on glucose levels are blunted in the fetus relative to the adult, suggesting a deficiency of glucagon receptors coupled to their respective effector systems. Maternal hyperglycemia is associated with fetal hyperglycemia and hyperinsulinemia (**Fig. 38.9**). Glycogen deposits increase exponentially in the third trimester and fetal gluconeogenesis is evident close to term and is inducible by cortisol.

At birth, with the abrupt curtailment of nutrient supply following placental separation, a series of integrated signals involving hormones and their receptors mobilizes endogenous glucose via glycogenolysis and gluconeogenesis. Insulin, glucagon, catecholamines, growth hormone, and their receptors are pivotal in these adaptations. These normal adaptive events permit a rational framework for understanding the relatively frequent disturbances of glucose homeostasis in the newborn. The role of insulin as a

fetal growth factor has been discussed above and is summarized in **Table 38.6**. Tables **38.7** and **38.8** summarize the manifestations of the infant of the mother with diabetes, their mechanisms or cause, and their management. **Figure 38.13** depicts the typical appearance of the large macrosomic infant of the mother with diabetes. Such a macrosomic infant at birth, in the absence of diabetes mellitus in the mother, suggests a genetic defect in insulin secretion resulting in persistent hyperinsulinemic hypoglycemia of infancy, as summarized in **Tables 38.9** and **38.10**. Whereas manifestations in the infant of the diabetic mother are transitory, generally resolving over the first week of life, those of persistent hyperinsulinemic hypoglycemia are permanent and generally require surgical intervention for subtotal pancreatectomy in diffuse lesions and localized resection in the focal-adenomatous types. An algorithmic approach to management of neonatal hypoglycemia is summarized in **Figure 38.14**. Neonatal diabetes mellitus is rare and may be transitory or permanent, as a result of several genetic defects in pancreatic development and/or insulin action.

Classification of genetic forms of hyperinsulinemic hypoglycemia of infancy

K$_{ATP}$ Channel defects	*SUR* mutations
	KIR6.2 mutations
	Loss of heterozygosity
Glucokinase-activating mutation	
Glutamate-dehydrogenase-activating mutation	
Undefined	Autosomal dominant
	Autosomal recessive
	Sporadic
Beckwith–Wiedemann syndrome	

Table 38.9 Classification of genetic forms of hyperinsulinemic hypoglycemia of infancy. K$_{ATP}$, ATP-dependent potassium channel.

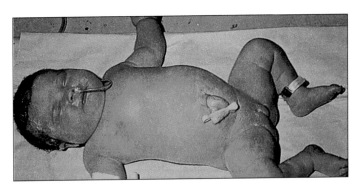

Figure 38.13 Infant of mother with diabetes. Note large size and plethoric appearance.

THYROID FUNCTION IN THE FETUS AND NEWBORN

Thyroid disorders are relatively common in the newborn (**Table 38.11**), reflecting their relative importance in fetal/neonatal endocrinology.

The placenta acts both as a source of molecules that influence fetal thyroid function and also as a barrier protecting the fetus from the influence of maternal thyroid hormones (**Fig. 38.15**). However, in general, the fetal thyroid unit develops independently of maternal influences. Although placental TRH contributes to circulating fetal TRH levels (**Fig. 38.15**) the role of placentally derived TRH in regulating fetal thyroid function remains unclear. The TSH molecule does not cross the placenta: there is no significant effect of maternal TSH on fetal thyroid function. However, placentally derived hCG does enter the fetal circulation and may have TSH-like activity resulting from the partial homology between the β subunits. This results in a relative potency of only 0.01% of TSH-like activity in the hCG molecule. Normally, it is not a significant influence on the maternal thyroid function. However, in hydatidiform moles, the extraordinarily high levels of hCG can result in some manifestations of maternal hyperthyroidism.

The human placenta is also relatively impermeable to maternally derived iodothyronines, in part because of the activity of placental monoiodinase, which converts biologically active thyroxine (T$_4$) and triiodothyronine (T$_3$) to their inactive metabolites reverse triiodothyronine (rT$_3$) and diiodothyronine (T$_2$). Some degree of placental transfer of maternal iodothyronines must occur in the first trimester and in the hypothyroid human fetus (**Fig. 38.15**). It has been postulated that this transferred iodothyronine may play a role in modulating some of the potentially deleterious effects of hypothyroidism on fetal organs whose development is particularly sensitive to the thyroid status. For example, the intellectual development of infants born to mothers whose TSH was elevated in the first trimester is less that

Correlation of clinical features with molecular defect in persistent hyperinsulinemic hypoglycemia of infancy

	Macrosomia	Hypoglycemia/ hyperinsulinemia, FH	Molecular defect	Response to medical management	Prognosis
Sporadic	Present at birth	Moderate/severe, negative FH	?SUR/KIR6.2	Generally poor	Partial Px – excellent, total Px – poor
Autosomal recessive	Present at birth	Severe – first days/weeks, positive FH	SUR/KIR6.2	Poor	Guarded
Autosomal dominant	Unusual	Moderate – post 6 months, positive FH	Glucokinase-activating	Very good/excellent	Excellent
Autosomal dominant	Unusual	Moderate – post 6 months, positive FH	Glutamate dehydrogenase	Very good/excellent	Excellent
Beckwith–Wiedeman syndrome	Present at birth	Moderate, resolves post 6 months, negative FH	Duplication/imprinting 11p15.1	Good	Excellent

Table 38.10 Correlation of clinical features with molecular defect in persistent hyperinsulinemic hypoglycemia of infancy. FH, family history.

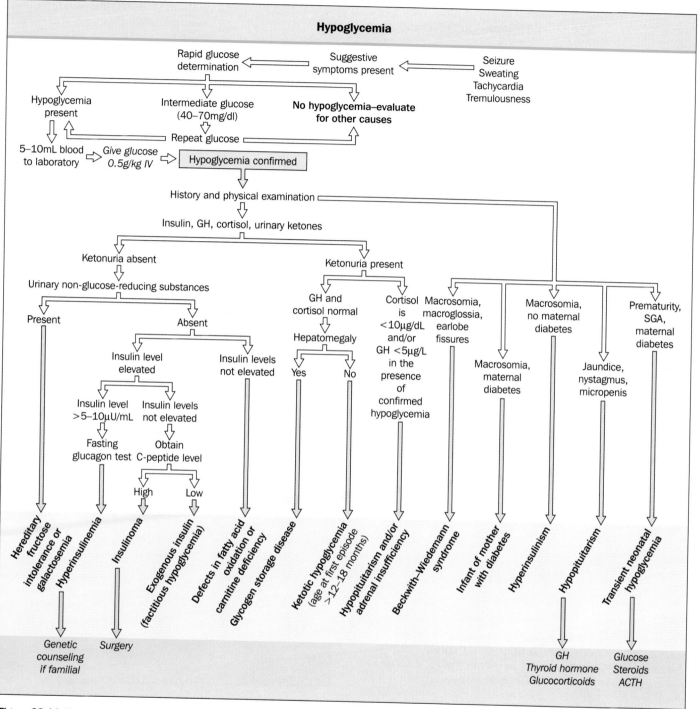

Figure 38.14 Hypoglycemia. The figure provides a schematic approach to the diagnosis and management of hypoglycemia in the newborn. GH, growth hormone. (Modified from Hochberg Z, ed. Practical algorithms in pediatric endocrinology. Basel: Karger; 1999.)

that of appropriate controls. And, there is a wide spectrum in clinical manifestations of congenital hypothyroidism despite similar biochemical abnormalities in thyroid function postnatally.

The human placenta is permeable to iodide and the fetal thyroid sensitive to its inhibitory effects. The effect of the exogenous iodide on fetal thyroid function is usually evident only after 70–75 days of gestation when this aspect of gland function achieves maturity. Moreover, autoregulation of iodide transport into the thyroid follicular cells, which normally compensates for iodide excess or deficiency, does not mature in the fetal gland until close to term. In addition, the placenta is also permeable to the thiourea group of antithyroid drugs, including propylthiouracil (PTU).

Table 38.11 Thyroid disorders in the neonatal period

	Disorder	Approximate prevalence
Thyroid dysgenesis	Agenesis	1:4000
	Hypogenesis	
	Ectopia	
Thyroid dyshormonogenesis	TSH unresponsiveness	1:40,000
	Iodide trapping defect	
	Organification defect	
	Defect in thyroglobulin	
	Iodotyrosine deiodinase deficiency	
Hypothalamic–pituitary hypothyroidism	Hypothalamic–pituitary anomaly	1:100,000
	Panhypopituitarism	
	Isolated TSH deficiency	
	Thyroid hormone resistance	
Transient hypothyroidism	Drug-induced	1:40,000
	Maternal-antibody-induced	
	Idiopathic	

Table 38.11 Thyroid disorders in the neonatal period. TSH, thyroid-stimulating hormone. (From Fisher DA. Disorders of the thyroid in the newborn and infant. In: Sperling MA, ed. Pediatric endocrinology. Philadelphia, PA: WB Saunders; 1996:51–70.)

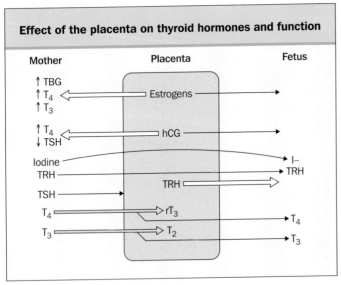

Figure 38.15 Effect of the placenta on thyroid hormones and function. hCG, human chorionic gonadotropin; rT3, reverse triiodothyronine; T_2, diiodothyronine; T_3, triiodothyronine; T_4, thyroxine; TBG, thyroxine-binding globulin; TRH, thyrotropin-releasing hormone; TSH, thyroid-stimulating hormone. (From Fisher DA. Disorders of the thyroid in the newborn and infant. In: Sperling MA, ed. Pediatric endocrinology. Philadelphia, PA: WB Saunders; 1996:51–70.)

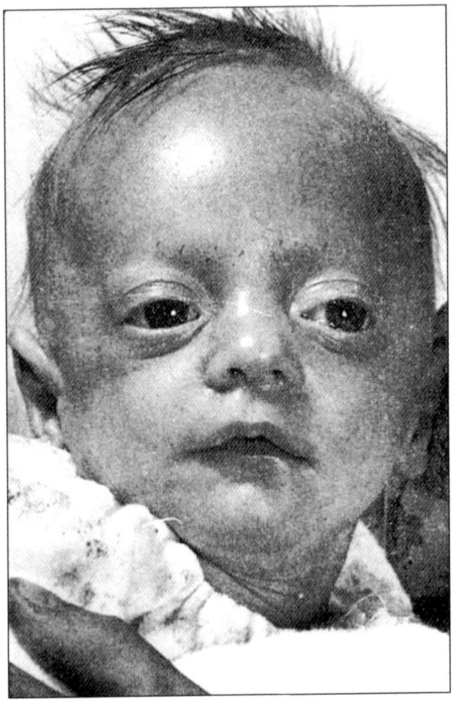

Figure 38.16 Newborn with neonatal thyrotoxicosis. Note 'stare'; the infant had tachycardia, failure to thrive and irritability. The mother had had a partial thyroidectomy for Graves' disease before pregnancy. The infant was treated with a beta-blocker and low doses of propylthiouracil (2–3mg/kg daily for 6 weeks), by which time the clinical symptoms were controlled and the influence of transplacentally derived thyroid-stimulating globulins was waning.

Hence, administration of these drugs to the mother for management of hyperthyroidism can result in alterations in fetal thyroid function, causing goiter and transient hypothyroidism that spontaneously resolves over 1–2 weeks as the effects of the PTU wear off. Caution is necessary in interpreting newborn thyroid function tests in this setting. Finally, immunoglobulins of the IgG class, present in the maternal circulation, cross the placenta into the fetal compartment. Hence, the function of the fetal thyroid gland can be modulated by the transfer of maternal IgG, most commonly directed against the TSH receptor. The precise clinical effect of these antibodies will depend upon whether they are stimulatory or blocking in nature, producing respectively neonatal thyrotoxicosis or occasional hypothyroidism with goiter. Here, the biochemical abnormalities will take several weeks to normalize because of the half-life of IgG. **Figure 38.16** represents a newborn with thyrotoxicosis as a result of maternal transfer of thyroid-stimulating immunoglobulins.

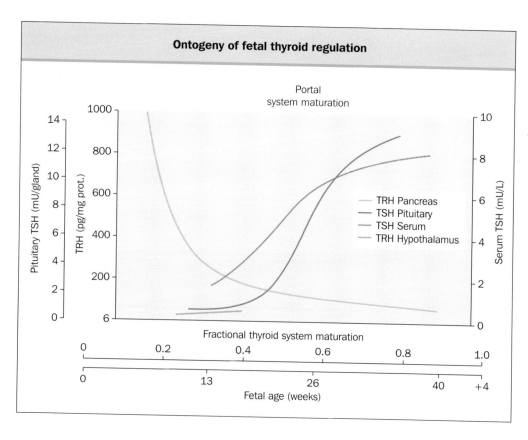

Figure 38.17 Ontogeny of fetal thyroid regulation. TRH, thyrotropin-releasing hormone; TSH, thyroid-stimulating hormone. (From Fisher DA. Disorders of the thyroid in the newborn and infant. In: Sperling MA, ed. Pediatric endocrinology. Philadelphia, PA: WB Saunders; 1996:51–70.)

Embryology of the thyroid gland development

The thyroid gland originates from the primitive buccopharyngeal cavity by a fusion of the median and lateral endodermal anlage. The anlage originate from the ultimobranchial bodies, which come from the fourth branchial pouch. The process occurs early and fusion is complete by the 24th day. Several key genes are involved in this process, of which the three most important are those for thyroid transcription factors (*TTF1, TTF2*) and *pax-8*, whose gene products are expressed in the thyroid follicular cell.

Thyroid hormone production and metabolism

Key steps in the synthesis and metabolism of thyroid hormones are reviewed elsewhere (Chapter 10). Various defects in these processes have been described that result in alterations of fetal thyroid function. Key among these in the ontogeny of thyroid function is the process of deiodination. Three types of mono-deiodinase (MDI) regulate the process of deiodination of iodotyrosines formed in the thyroid gland. Two of these act on the outer ring and the third acts on the inner ring of the iodothyronine molecule. Whereas removal of the outer ring of the iodothyronine molecule converts T_4 to its active metabolite

T_3, removal of iodine from the inner ring converts T_4 and T_3 to rT_3 and diiodothyronine (DIT), respectively, both of which are inactive metabolites. The inner ring MDI, type 3 MDI, is widely distributed in fetal tissues, including the placenta, and is responsible for the elevated levels of rT_3 during fetal life. The ontogeny of fetal thyroid regulation via TRH and TSH is illustrated in **Figure 38.17**. The ontogeny of fetal thyroxine-binding globulin, total T_4, total T_3, TSH, free T_4 and free T_3 is summarized in **Figure 38.18**.

Parturition is associated with a series of dramatic changes in the profile of thyroid hormones (**Fig. 38.19**). The first is a surge in the level of TSH, which peaks by 30min at between 70 and 100mIU/mL, and rapidly declines thereafter to reach basal levels within 2–3 days of life. The surge in TSH is followed by subsequent rises in T_3 and T_4 levels that peak by 36–48 hours of life and then gradually decline over the subsequent 4–6 weeks. However, it is important to emphasize that values of T_4 and T_3 are considerably higher in newborns than they are in adults and that appropriate age-specific standards are necessary for appropriate interpretation of newborn infantile and thyroid function tests. **Table 38.12** summarizes values of T_3, free T_4, free T_3 and rT_3 from cord blood through to adulthood.

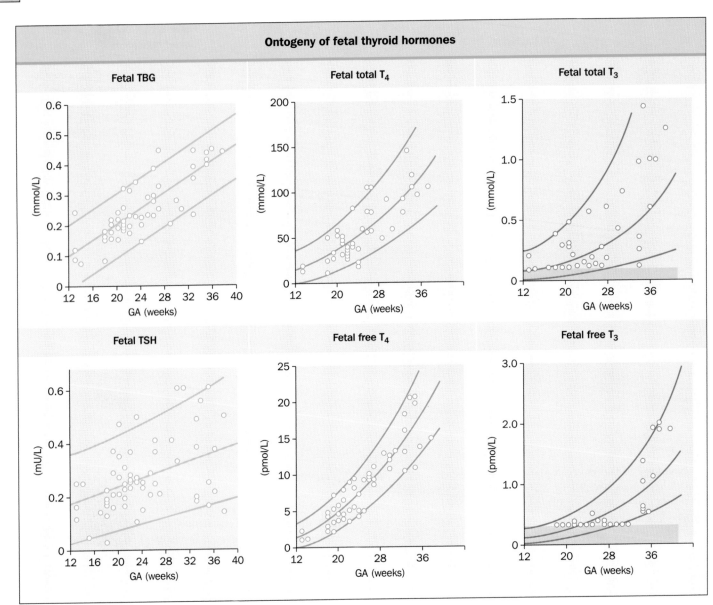

Figure 38.18 Ontogeny of fetal thyroid hormones. GA, gestational age; T_3, triiodothyronine; T_4, thyroxine; TBG, thyroxine-binding globulin; TSH, thyroid-stimulating hormone. (From Fisher DA. Disorders of the thyroid in the newborn and infant. In: Sperling MA, ed. Pediatric endocrinology. Philadelphia, PA: WB Saunders; 1996:51–70.)

Newborn screening programs for congenital hypothyroidism take advantage of these normal adaptive events by measuring T_4 in newborn (heelstick) blood on day 2–3 of life. Sample values 3 standard deviations below the mean of the appropriate gestational age control have immediate TSH measurements performed; values 2 standard deviations below the mean are repeated and, if confirmed, TSH is also measured. If TSH is elevated, primary hypothyroidism is confirmed and thyroid replacement is begun in a dose of approximately $10\mu g/kg/day$, usually within 2–3 weeks of life. Long-term intellectual outcome is usually excellent, but not universally so.

Primary hypothyroidism is common, occurring in about 1:4,000 live births most due to thyroid dysgenesis so that no goiter is evident (**Table 38.11**). A defect in thyroid hormone synthesis, thyroid dyshormonogenesis, is less common, occurring about 1:40,000 live births (**Table 38.11**). These may be manifest by the presence of a goiter. Likewise, transient hypothyroidism from the maternal transfer of drugs or antibodies also may be associated with a goiter and has an incidence of about 1:40,000 live births. Finally, hypothalamic–pituitary hypothyroidism is least common occurring in about 1:100,000 live births. Most cases of thyroid dysgenesis are sporadic and, in the familial cases, *TTF1*, *TTF2* and *pax-2* mutations are being increasingly found. **Table 38.13** summarizes the characteristics of inborn abnormalities of thyroid hormone metabolism and **Table 38.14** thyroid hormone-binding abnormalities.

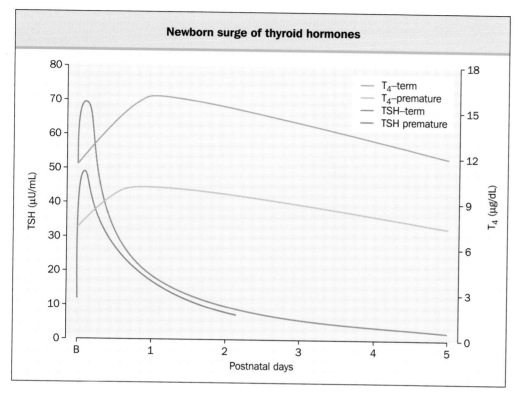

Figure 38.19 Newborn surge of thyroid hormones. The figure compares the newborn surge of thyroxine (T₄) and thyroid-stimulating hormone (TSH) in full-term and healthy premature infants. Note that values are lower in healthy premature newborns; this must be taken into account for the appropriate interpretation of newborn screening thyroid function tests.

Changes with age in serum concentrations of thyroid hormones

	T₃* (ng/dL)	rT₃* (ng/dL)	Free T₄† (pg/mL)	Free T₃ (pg/mL)
Cord blood	50 (14–86)	224 (100–501)	13.8 (±3.5)	1.9 (1.1)
4–7 days	186 (36–316)	146 (34–258)	22.3 (3.9)	3.7 (1.2)
1–4 weeks	225 (105–345)	90 (26–290)		
1–12 months	125 (105–245)	40 (11–129)		
1–5 years	168 (105–269)	33 (15–71)	11.4 (2.0)	4.9 (1.0)
6–10 years	150 (94–241)	36 (17–79)	11.4 (2.0)	4.9 (1.0)
11–15 years	133 (83–213)	41 (19–88)	10.8 (0.0)	4.3 (0.9)
16–20 years	130 (80–210)	41 (25–80)	10.8 (0.0)	4.3 (0.9)
21–50 years	123 (70–204)	42 (30–80)	10.3 (3.1)	3.7 (0.6)

*Geometric mean and range. † Mean and standard deviation.

Table 38.12 Changes with age in serum concentrations of thyroid hormones. (From Fisher DA. Disorders of the thyroid in the newborn and infant. In: Sperling MA, ed. Pediatric endocrinology. Philadelphia, PA: WB Saunders; 1996:51–70.)

Figure 38.20 shows a newborn with classical characteristics of congenital hypothyroidism. Such classical characteristics are present only in the minority of patients; the majority are detected by thyroid screening programs in the newborn because clinical manifestations may be subtle or entirely inapparent. **Figure 38.21** describes an algorithmic approach to management of a positive screening test in a newborn infant. It should be emphasized that premature infants have lower values in all of the newborn thyroid function tests (**Fig. 38.19**). In addition, they are often complicated by the euthyroid sick syndrome. The use of supplemental T₄ or T₃ in the premature infant with or without euthyroid sick syndrome remains controversial.

Inborn abnormalities of thyroid hormone metabolism

Abnormality	Prevalence	Inheritance	CH	Goiter	T$_4$	TSH	Tg	RAIU	Other	Molecular abnormality
Familial TSH deficiency	Rare	AR	Yes	No	↓	↓	↓	↓	Absent TSH response to TRH	TSHβ gene mutations
Pit-1 deficiency hypopituitarism	Not yet clear	AR	Yes	No	↓	N or ↓	↓	↓	GH and prolactin deficiencies	pit-1 gene mutations
TSH unresponsiveness	Rare	AR	Yes	No	↓	↑	↓	N	No RAIU, T$_4$ or Tg response to TSH	TSH receptor gene mutations
Iodine transport defect	Rare	AR	Yes	Yes	↓	↑	↑	↓	Salivary and gastric tissues also fail to concentrate iodide. Hypothyroid state responds to iodide administration	Defect not characterized
Organification defects	1:40,000 newborns	AR	Yes	Yes	↓	↑	↑	↑	Positive perchlorate discharge test	Thyroid peroxidase gene mutations. Defective H$_2$O$_2$ generation
Pendred's syndrome	1:50,000 children	AR	Variable	Yes	N,↑	↑	↑	↑	Deaf mutism; positive perchlorate discharge	Thyroid defect not clear. Cochlear defect
Thyroglobulin defects	1:40,000 newborns	AR	Yes	Yes	↓	↑	↓↑	↑	Usually low Tg with no Tg response to TSH	Tg gene mutations (absent or defective Tg); hyposialylated Tg due to sialyltransferase defect
Iodotyrosine deiodinase defect	Rare	AR	Yes	Yes	↓	↑	↑	↑	High RAIU with early discharge: high serum MIT, DIT; failure to deiodinate IV dose of labeled DIT (excretion intact)	Presumed iodotyrosine deiodinase gene mutation
Thyroid hormone resistance	1:100,000 newborns?	Autosomal dominant or sporadic	Variable	Yes	↑	N,↑	↑	↑	Generalized resistance, TSH normal or ↑; peripheral resistance TSH ↑; pituitary resistance TSH ↑ (patient hyperthyroid)	Thyroid nuclear receptor gene mutations (TRβ; TRα)
Autosomal dominant hyperthyroidism	Rare	Autosomal dominant	No, hyper	Yes	↑	↓	↑	↑	Absence of thyroid autoimmunity	Activating TSH receptor gene mutations

Table 38.13 Inborn abnormalities of thyroid hormone metabolism. AR, autosomal recessive; CHI, congenital hypothyroidism; DIT, diiodotyrosine; GH, growth hormone; IV, intravenous; MIT, monoiodotyrosine; RAIU, thyroid radioactive iodine uptake; T4, thyroxine; Tg, serum thyroglobulin; TRH, thyrotropin-releasing hormone; TSH, thyroid-stimulating hormone. (From Fisher DA. Disorders of the thyroid in the newborn and infant. In: Sperling MA, ed. Pediatric endocrinology. Philadelphia, PA: WB Saunders; 1996:51–70.)

Thyroid hormone binding protein abnormalities

Abnormality	Prevalence	Inheritance	T$_4$	T$_3$	T$_3$RU	fT$_4$	Protein level	Other	Molecular abnormality
Complete TBG deficiency	1:15,000 newborns	X-linked	Low	↓	↑	N	TBG <0.5mg/dL	TBG absent or decreased immunoreactivity; decreased binding affinity	TBG gene mutations
Partial TBG deficiency	1:4000–12,000 newborns	X-linked	↓	↓	↑	N	↓	TBG decreased immunoreactivity or decreased stability; decreased binding affinity	TBG gene mutations
TBG excess	1:25,000 newborns	X-linked	↑	↑	↓	N	TBG ↑ 3.0–4.5 ×	Defect not yet clear	
TTR variants	Rare	Autosomal dominant	↑	N	N	N	N	Increased T$_4$-binding affinity*	TTR gene mutations
			↓	N	N	N	N	Decreased T$_4$-binding affinity†	TTR gene mutations
Familial dysalbuminemic hyperthyroxinemia	1:100 newborns?	Autosomal dominant	↑	N	N	N	N	Increased T$_4$-binding affinity	Genetic polymorphism?

*Manifest in heterozygotes. † Manifest in heterozygotes or homozygotes depending on mutation.

Table 38.14 Thyroid hormone binding protein abnormalities. fT$_4$, free thyroxine; N, normal; T$_3$, triiodothyronine, T$_3$RU, T$_3$ Resin uptake; T$_4$, thyroxine; TBG, thyroxine-binding globulin; TTR, transthyretin. (From Fisher DA. Disorders of the thyroid in the newborn and infant. In: Sperling MA, ed. Pediatric endocrinology. Philadelphia, PA: WB Saunders; 1996:51–70.)

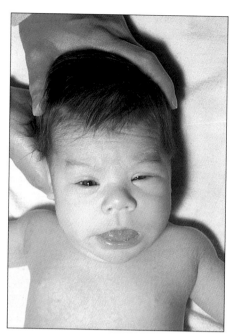

Figure 38.20 Infant with typical stigmata of severe congenital hypothyroidism. Note coarse features, periorbital edema, flattened bridge of nose, and large protruding tongue. Not seen in the picture are umbilical hernia, cutis marmorata, and cold extremities. The infant had a hoarse cry, somnolence, and constipation. Such typical stigmata are rare; the majority of hypothyroid newborns identified in newborn screening programs are not clinically suspected.

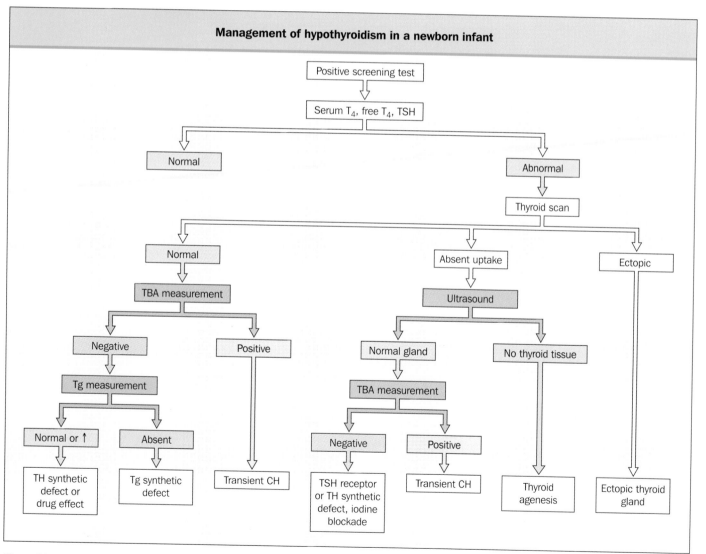

Figure 38.21 Management of hypothyroidism in a newborn infant. CH, congenital hypothyroidism; T4, thyroxine; TBA, thyroid-stimulating hormone receptor-blocking antibody; Tg, thyroglobulin; TH, thyroid hormone; TSH, thyroid-stimulating hormone. (From Fisher DA. Disorders of the thyroid in the newborn and infant. In: Sperling MA, ed. Pediatric endocrinology. Philadelphia, PA: WB Saunders; 1996:51–70.)

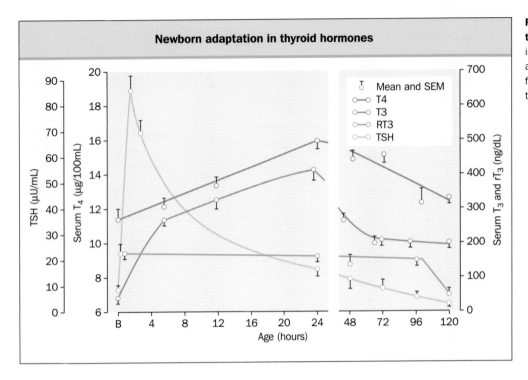

Figure 38.22 Newborn adaptation in thyroid hormones. Note the rapid surge in thyroid-stimulating hormone (TSH) after cutting of the umbilical cord, followed by rises in thyroxine (T$_4$) and triiodothyronine (T$_3$).

FURTHER READING

Acherman JC, Meeks JJ, James JL. X-linked adrenal hypoplasia congenita and DAX-1. Endocrinologist 2000;10:289–99.

Bauer MK, et al. Fetal growth and placental function. Molec Cell Endocrinol. 1998;140:115–20.

Burrow GN, Fisher DA, Larsen PR. Maternal and fetal thyroid function. N Engl J Med. 1994;331:1072–8.

Casey ML, MacDonald PC. Endocrine changes of pregnancy. In: William JD, Foster DW, Kronenberg HM, Larsen PR, eds. Williams textbook of endocrinology. Philadelphia, PA:WB Saunders; 1998:1259–71.

Damante G, Tell G, DiLauro R. A unique combination of transcription factors controls differentiation of thyroid cells. Prog Nucleic Acid Res Molec Biol. 2000;66:307–56.

Fisher DA. Disorders of the thyroid in the newborn and infant. In: Sperling MA, ed. Pediatric endocrinology. Philadelphia, PA:WB Saunders; 1996:51–70.

Fisher DA. Endocrinology of fetal development. In: William JD, Foster DW, Kronenberg HM, Larsen PR, eds. Williams textbook of endocrinology. Philadelphia, PA:WB Saunders; 1998:1273–301.

Grumbach M, Gluckman PD. The human fetal hypothalamus and pituitary gland: the maturation of neuroendocrine mechanisms controlling the secretion of fetal pituitary growth hormone, prolactin, gonadotropins, andenocorticotropin-related peptides and thyrotropin. In: Tulchinsky D, Little B, eds. Maternal-fetal endocrinology, 2nd edn. Philadelphia, PA:WB Saunders; 1994:193–261.

Jackson D, Volpert OV, Bouck N, Linzer DIH. Stimulation and inhibition of angiogenesis by placental proliferin and proliferin-related protein. Science 1994;266:1581–4.

Menon RK, Sperling MA. Developmental endocrinology in the fetal-placental unit. In: Cowett RM, ed. Principles of perinatal-neonatal metabolism, 2nd edn. New York:Springer; 1998:425–36.

Menon RK, Sperling MA. Insulin as a growth factor. Endocrinol Metab Clin North Am. 1996;25:633–48.

Miller WL. Steroid hormone biosynthesis and actions in the materno-fetoplacental unit. Clin Perinatol. 1998;25:799–817.

Root AW. Genetic errors of sexual differentiation. Adv Pediatr. 1999;46:67–97.

Sperling MA, ed. Pediatric endocrinology. Philadelphia, PA:WB Saunders; 2002.

Sperling MA, Menon RK. Hyperinsulinemic hypoglycemia of infancy. Endocrinol Metab Clin North Am. 1999;28:695–708.

Sperling MA, Menon RK. Infant of the diabetic mother. In: Defronzo RA, ed. Current therapy of diabetes mellitus. St Louis, MO:Mosby; 1998:237–41.

Sperling MA. Newborn adaption: adrenocortical hormones and adreno-corticotropic hormone. In: Tulchinsky D, Little B, eds. Maternal-fetal endocrinology, 2nd edn. Philadelphia, PA:WB Saunders; 1994:419–42.

Styne DM. Fetal growth. Clin Perinatol. 1998;25:917–38.

Takimoto E, et al. Hypertension induced in pregnant mice by placental renin and maternal angiotensinogen. Science 1996;274:995–8.

Tanaka S, Kunath T, Hadjantonakis AK, Nagy A, Rossant J. Promotion of trophoblast stem cell proliferation by FGF4. Science 1998;282:2072–5.

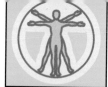

Chapter 39

The Breast: Gynecomastia and Benign Breast Disease in Women

Richard J. Santen, Lisa A Cerilli, and Jennifer A Harvey

GYNECOMASTIA

Introduction

Stimulatory and inhibitory hormones control the growth and differentiation of mammary tissue in the male (**Fig. 39.1**). Estradiol binds to estrogen receptors and stimulates glandular cells whereas testosterone exerts a generalized inhibitory action on growth and differentiation. The balance between stimulatory and inhibitory hormones controls the development and maintenance of breast tissue. Growth hormone, insulin, insulin-like growth factor 1 (IGF-1), and cortisol act permissively, exerting no specific effects but are required for the activity of other hormones. Regulatory hormones modulate the effects of other factors, which, in turn, influence breast growth and differentiation. Thyroxine increases the level of testosterone–estradiol-binding globulin (TeBG). Cortisol and prolactin lower circulating testosterone levels through hypothalamic effects. The application of these physiologic principles provides a framework for evaluation of gynecomastia on a pathophysiologic basis.

Causes

Physiologic forms of gynecomastia

Newborn

The high levels of estradiol, progesterone and prolactin during fetal life stimulate newborn breast tissue that persists for several weeks after birth in boys.

Pubertal

Beginning at age 11, approximately 30% of normal boys develop detectable gynecomastia (i.e. glandular tissue >0.5cm in diameter). By age 14, gynecomastia is detectable in 65%. While usually bilateral, gynecomastia is unilateral in 20% of cases. Spontaneous regression occurs in the majority of boys after 1 year. Hormonal alterations in pubertal boys with gynecomastia are not found consistently and are variably reported as low free testosterone, increased estradiol, elevated estradiol/testosterone ratio, elevated testosterone/dihydrotestosterone ratio, and increased TeBG levels.

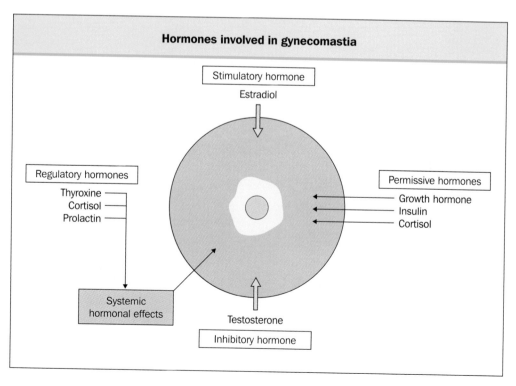

Figure 39.1 Hormones involved in gynecomastia. The figure indicates the hormones that affect breast tissue growth and differentiation in patients with gynecomastia. This diagram provides a framework for the logical assessment of disorders causing gynecomastia.

Adult

A careful physical examination frequently detects palpable breast tissue in normal volunteers and in hospitalized patients. One third of normal military recruits have between 2cm and 4cm of palpable glandular tissue. This percentage gradually increases with age, from 17% in men less than 19 years old to 41% between ages 40 and 44. These men are not usually aware that they have palpable breast tissue. The prevalence of gynecomastia is not overestimated on physical examination, given that autopsy-proven gynecomastia in hospitalized patients approaches 57% in men between the ages of 45 and 59.

Breast tissue diameter does not exceed 5cm in 83% of hospitalized men with gynecomastia. The etiology of this form of physiologic gynecomastia is not clear but evidence suggests increased aromatase activity converting androgens to estrogens. The total amount of aromatase activity in the body increases as a function of body fat. The percentage of patients with gynecomastia (**Fig. 39.2**) and its diameter (**Fig. 39.3**) appear to increase as a function of body mass index.

Pathologic forms of gynecomastia

Two subtypes of gynecomastia can be distinguished histologically. Glandular predominance occurs in 5–9% of adult patients and represents the early phase of gynecomastia with recent hormonal stimulation of glandular elements. Stromal tissue predominates in 32–48% of adults with gynecomastia and reflects the aftermath of a prior hormonal imbalance with spontaneous resolution.

Diagnosis

The distinction between physiologic and pathologic gynecomastia in adult men presents a challenge because of the common presence of breast enlargement in normal men and its association with obesity. An operational definition of pathologic

gynecomastia is useful to the clinician, who must decide upon the need for and extent of evaluation. Accordingly, pathologic gynecomastia is arbitrarily defined as palpable tissue more than 4cm in diameter, palpable tissue greater than 2cm that is tender, or palpable tissue greater than 2cm demonstrated to be gradually increasing in diameter on followup. Often the physician detects palpable tissue less than 4cm in diameter but the patient is unaware of this finding. Under these circumstances, followup in 6 months without any other testing is warranted. True gynecomastia should be distinguished from pseudogynecomastia—fat tissue present underneath the nipple. Mammography may occasionally be necessary to make this distinction, particularly in obese patients (**Fig. 39.4**). Ultrasonography can also be used but is not considered as sensitive as mammography.

Differential diagnosis

A logical approach to the differential diagnosis is based on the physiologic framework represented in **Figure 39.1** and **Table 39.1**. An excess of estradiol, a deficiency of testosterone, an imbalance in the ratio of estradiol to testosterone, and abnormalities of regulatory hormones may be responsible for non-drug-related gynecomastia. A multitude of drugs, which interact at each of these levels, can also cause gynecomastia. The remainder of causes remain largely idiopathic or uncertain.

Excess of estradiol

Tumors

Adenomas or carcinomas of the adrenal may produce large amounts of estradiol or, alternatively, estrogen precursors such as androstenedione, dehydroepiandrosterone (DHEA), and DHEA sulfate (DHEAS). Patients harboring these tumors generally exhibit a rapid onset of gynecomastia in association with hypertension, elevated ketosteroids, elevated DHEA and DHEAS levels, and an adrenal mass.

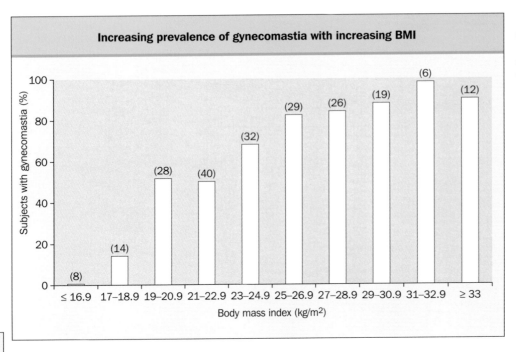

Figure 39.2 Increasing prevalence of gynecomastia with increasing body mass index (BMI). The graph shows the correlation of percentage of subjects with gynecomastia and body mass index. (With permission from Niewoehner CB, Nuttal FQ. Gynecomastia in a hospitalized male population. Am J Med. 1984;77:633.)

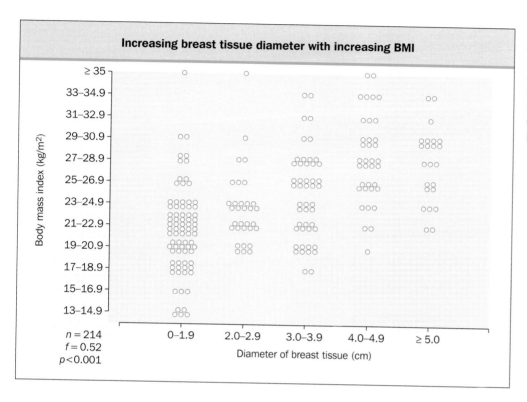

Figure 39.3 Increasing breast tissue
diameter with body mass index (BMI).
The correlation coefficient was
determined by the method of least
squares. (With permission from
Niewoehner CB, Nuttal FQ.
Gynecomastia in a hospitalized male
population. Am J Med. 1984;77:633.)

Testicular tumors of germ, sex cord, Leydig cell, or Sertoli cell origin (**Fig. 39.5**) secrete either an excess of estrogen or estrogen precursors. Tumors are large enough to be palpated in approximately half of patients whereas the remainder require detection by testicular ultrasound (**Fig. 39.5**). Choriocarcinomas of the testis may produce human chorionic gonadotropin (hCG) *in situ* and stimulate production of both estradiol and testosterone. Ectopic production of hCG by lung, kidney, liver, and gastric carcinomas can also stimulate estradiol production and cause gynecomastia.

Aromatase excess
Overexpression of the aromatase enzyme may be a unifying feature of several clinical causes of gynecomastia (**Table 39.2**). Familial gynecomastia with early onset as the cardinal clinical feature is associated with aromatase excess. Interestingly, a kindred of familial gynecomastia from the time of the 18th dynasty in Egypt involving King Tutankhamun, his brother Smenkhare, his grandfather Amenophis III and his uncle Akhenaton (**Fig. 39.6**) could potentially represent aromatase excess as the causal mechanism.

Idiopathic gynecomastia may also reflect a sporadic increase in aromatase activity. Bulard et al. detected an increase in peripheral aromatase activity in subsets of patients with idiopathic gynecomastia. Sasano recently provided additional evidence by demonstrating that 11 of 30 cases of gynecomastia had aromatase excess as evidenced by immunochemical assessment of biopsy tissue using a monospecific antiaromatase antibody.

Excess secretion of precursors of aromatase
Congenital adrenal hyperplasia, as well as adrenal tumors, may produce gynecomastia through excess production of aromatizable androgens.

Administration of estrogen
Several medications or topical creams provide estrogen or estrogenic substances for absorption and systemic action. Synthetic or natural estrogens given to patients with prostatic carcinoma or given illegally to cattle to increase meat yield produce gynecomastia with high frequency. Inadvertent ingestion by boys of oral contraceptives from their mother's medicine bottles or industrial exposure to oral contraceptives during the manufacturing process also cause gynecomastia. Other drugs such as digitoxin may have intrinsic estrogenic properties and stimulate breast enlargement.

Environmental toxins such as embalming fluid may be estrogenic and produce gynecomastia. Unintended exposure to estrogen can occur from coital exposure to women using vaginal estrogen cream or from women using estrogen-containing cosmetics. In France, estrogen cream is distributed over large portions of the body as a means of transdermal estrogen delivery in postmenopausal women. Gynecomastia in their male partners could occur via body contact in this instance as well.

Administration of estrogen precursors
Certain androgens such as testosterone enanthate and cypionate can be converted into estrogens through aromatization and are a common cause of gynecomastia. This is most common in hypogonadal boys during testosterone treatment, but adult athletes using anabolic steroids and men receiving testosterone as a contraceptive also experience this problem. hCG given exogenously to hypogonadal patients raises both testosterone and estradiol levels and may be associated with gynecomastia, but usually for a transient period of several months.

Androgen deficiency
Clinical conditions associated with normal estradiol secretion but low levels of testosterone are uncommon. Hypogonadotropic

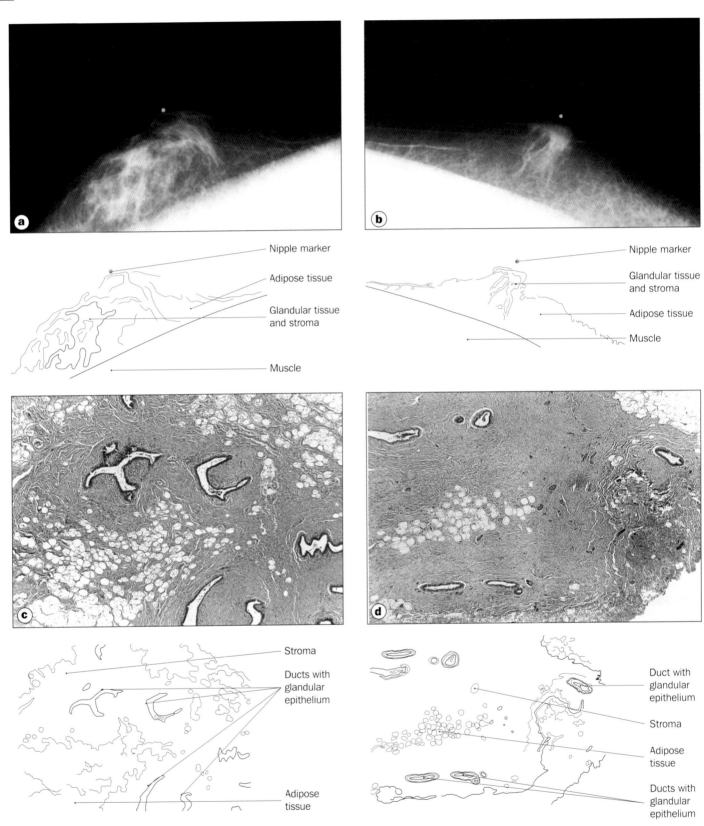

Figure 39.4 Bilateral persistent pubertal gynecomastia. (a, b) Mammograms of right and left breasts in a 27-year-old male patient with bilateral persistent pubertal gynecomastia. The white circles represent the nipple markers. The glandular elements are apparent as radio-opaque areas within the breast tissue. (c, d) Histologic appearance of the tissue excised from the right and left breasts during reduction mammoplasty. (c) illustrates ductal tissue interspersed with stroma and a minimal amount of fat tissue. (d) contains a predominance of stroma.

Causes of pathologic gynecomastia			
Estradiol excess	Estradiol secretion	Adrenal tumors Sporadic testicular tumors (sex cord, Sertoli cell, germ cell, Leydig cell) Testicular tumors associated with familial syndromes (Peutz–Jeghers, Carney complex) Hepatic tumor with aromatase Increased aromatase activity (see Table 39.2)	
	Exogenous estrogens or estrogenic substances	Drug therapy with estrogens Estrogen creams and lotions Occupational exposure to various estrogenic substances Cannabinoids Estrogen analogs: digitoxin	
	Elevated estrogen precursors: aromatizable androgens	Human chorionic gonadotropin (hCG) excess (eutopic or ectopic)	
		Exogenous hormones	Testosterone enanthate; testosterone propionate; anabolic steroids; hCG administration
Testosterone deficiency	Anorchia		
	Hypogonadotropic syndromes		
	Drugs or exogenous substances		Ketoconazole; heroin; methadone; alcohol
Estradiol/testosterone imbalance	Hypergonadotropic syndromes		
	Hypogonadotropic hypogonadism syndromes		
	Primary gonadal diseases		
	Drugs	Cytotoxic drug-induced hypogonadism from:	Busulfan; vincristine; nitrosourea; vincristine; combination chemotherapy; steroid synthesis inhibitory drugs
	Androgen resistance	Complete testicular feminization Partial: Reifenstein, Lubbs, Rosewater, and Dreyfus syndromes	
	Androgen antagonists	Cimetidine; spironolactone; flutamide; bicalutamide; cyproterone acetate	
	Blockers of 5α-reductase	Finasteride	
	Tumor-related: hCG-producing tumors (testis, lung, gastrointestinal tract, etc.)		
Regulatory hormone excess	Hypogonadotropic syndromes		
	Isolated gonadotropin deficiency, particularly 'fertile eunuch syndrome'		
	Panhypopituitarism		
	Systemic illnesses		
	Renal disease		
	Severe liver disease		
	Hyperthyroidism		
	Hypothyroidism		
	Pituitary tumor		
	Drug therapy with:	Catecholamine antagonists or depleters; sulpiride; metoclopramide; phenothiazines; reserpine; domperidone; tricyclic antidepressants; methyldopa; haloperidol	
	Cushing's syndrome		
	Primary breast tumor		
	Other causes	Local trauma; hip spica cast; chest injury; herpes zoster of chest wall; post thoracotomy; spinal cord injury	
	Uncertain causes		
	Other chronic illnesses	Renal failure; pulmonary tuberculosis; HIV; diabetes mellitus; leprosy; refeeding; gynecomastia	
	Persistent pubertal macromastia		
	Idiopathic		
	Drugs associated with gynecomastia with strong relationship of effect	Amiodarone Calcium channel blockers	

Table 39.1 Causes of pathologic gynecomastia.

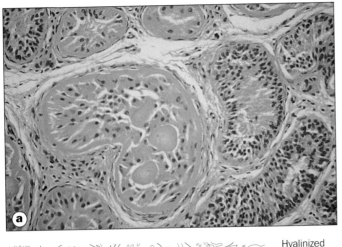

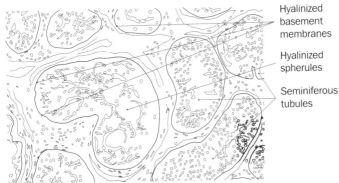

Hyalinized basement membranes

Hyalinized spherules

Seminiferous tubules

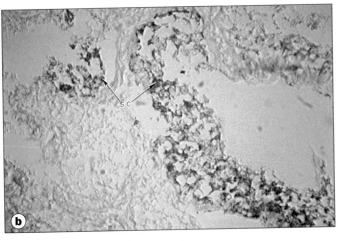

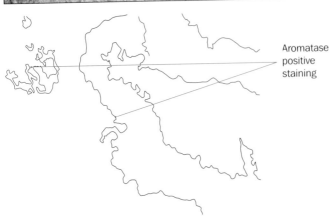

Aromatase positive staining

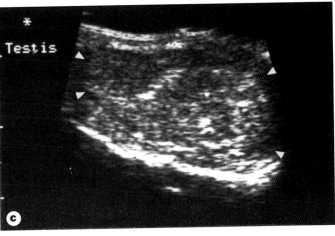

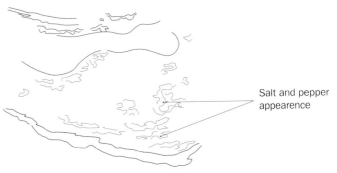

Salt and pepper appearence

Figure 39.5 (a) Histologic examination of a Sertoli cell tumor with annular tubules in a patient with Peutz–Jeghers syndrome. (b) Immuno-histochemical stain for aromatase in this tumor showing large amounts of this enzyme. (c) Ultrasound of the testis in this patient illustrating the 'salt and pepper' findings consistent with a testicular tumor. SC, Sertoli cells with annular sex chords. (With permission from Coen P et al. An aromatase-producing sex-cord tumor resulting in prepubertal gynecomastia. N Engl J Med. 1991;324:317–22.)

patients may have incomplete gonadotropin deficiency and relatively preserved follicle-stimulating hormone (FSH) secretion. Under these circumstances, androgen secretion may be impaired to a greater extent than that of estrogen, with resulting gynecomastia. More commonly this occurs in the 'fertile eunuch syndrome', which is characterized by incomplete gonadotropin deficiency, but patients with panhypopituitarism may also experience this condition. Some 50% of anorchic patients also have gynecomastia, perhaps based upon absence of testicular androgens but also upon adrenal secretion of aromatizable precursors of estrogen.

Androgen/estrogen imbalance
Hypogonadism
Primary gonadal disease is associated with a relative deficiency of androgen secretion and reflex rises in luteinizing hormone (LH) and FSH. The hypergonadotropism stimulates the testes to secrete an excess of estradiol. The resulting alteration of the estradiol:testosterone ratio is causative in producing gynecomastia. Klinefelter's syndrome, with an 85% prevalence of

Aromatase-associated causes of gynecomastia

I. Increased amount of aromatase enzyme	A. Increased activity in normal tissue	1. Obesity		
		2. Aging and its associated increase in percentage fat		
	B. Aromatase dysregulation	1. Aromatase excess syndrome	a. Familial	
			b. Sporadic	
	C. Neoplasms	1. Eutopic production	a. Sertoli cell tumors	i. Isolated
				ii. Peutz–Jeghers syndrome
				iii. Carney complex
			b. Trophoblastic tumors	
		2. Ectopic production	a. Feminizing adrenocortical neoplasms	
			b. Hepatocellular carcinoma	
II. Mechanism unknown	A. Idiopathic gynecomastia			
	B. Thyrotoxicosis			

Table 39.2 Aromatase-associated causes of gynecomastia.

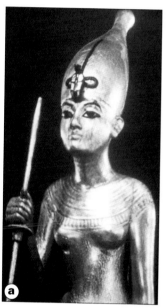

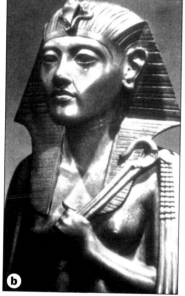

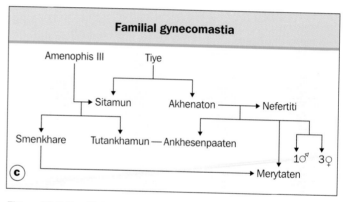

Figure 39.6 Familial gynecomastia (a) King Tutankhamun and (b) his brother Smenkhare are both depicted by contemporary artists as having gynecomastia. (c) The family tree of the royal dynasty. Amenophis III and Akhenaton are also represented in art as having gynecomastia. (From Santen RJ. Gynecomastia. In: DeGroot LJ, Jameson JL, Burger H, et al., eds. Endocrinology, 4th edn. Philadelphia, PA:WB Saunders; 2001:2335–43.)

gynecomastia, is typical of this condition. Patients with this syndrome exhibit reductions in total, and to a greater extent free, testosterone and increases in plasma estradiol, LH, and FSH. All other forms of primary testicular disease, including mumps orchitis, may be associated with gynecomastia on the same basis. Cytotoxic chemotherapeutic drugs or irradiation frequently produce transient or permanent testicular dysfunction and associated gynecomastia.

Compromise of androgen secretion on an enzymatic basis alters testosterone:estradiol ratios. Patients with congenital deficiency of 17-ketoreductase, C_{21} hydroxylase, or 3β-OL dehydrogenase/Δ_5- to Δ_4-isomerase may experience gynecomastia. Drugs inhibiting testosterone biosynthesis, such as the C_{17-20} lyase inhibitor ketoconazole, also commonly produce this finding.

Androgen resistance

A number of disorders and drugs result in a lack of tissue responsiveness to androgen. Since androgens are generally inhibitory to breast development, these conditions are associated with gynecomastia. The degree of breast enlargement varies depending upon the severity of insensitivity to androgen. In the most extreme instance, *complete androgen resistance* results in the development of normal to greater than normal breast tissue in a genetic male with the phenotypic appearance of a female (i.e. testicular feminization syndrome). The pathophysiology of this condition is based upon the fact that the negative-feedback control of LH is dual in males and involves the separate effects of both androgen and estrogen. Consequently, resistance to androgens at hypothalamic and pituitary levels results in hypersecretion of LH, stimulation of the testis to produce increased amounts of testosterone, and aromatization to its metabolic product estradiol. The combination of estrogen excess and androgen resistance results in substantial breast development. Androgen resistance prevents the development of male external genitalia. Together, these effects result in the clinical appearance of a phenotypic female. In syndromes of *partial androgen resistance*, a lesser degree of gynecomastia occurs from similar mechanisms. Cloning and sequencing of the androgen receptor have enabled the detection of specific molecular defects in patients with these disorders.

Another form of androgen resistance is the *Kennedy syndrome*, in which the diagnosis is usually delayed until the third to fifth decade. Features include gynecomastia, androgen resistance, androgen receptor mutations, and neurodegenerative findings including symmetric muscular atrophy, weakness, and fasciculations of the bulbar, facial, and proximal muscles of the extremities.

Cimetidine, spironolactone, flutamide, and cyproterone acetate are capable of blocking tissue effects of androgens on the breast by binding to the androgen receptor. They also interrupt negative feedback and increase the levels of LH, testosterone, and its aromatized product estradiol. Androgen resistance induced by the blockade of conversion of testosterone to dihydrotestosterone can by itself also cause gynecomastia.

Systemic illness

Several systemic illnesses produce gynecomastia through an endocrine mechanism. Patients with chronic renal failure manifest hypogonadal signs and symptoms related to high prolactin levels, moderate elevations of LH and FSH, reductions in testosterone levels, and increments in estradiol. The clinical spectrum of chronic liver diseases, ranging from end-stage cirrhosis to chronic hepatitis, produces gynecomastia through a number of mechanisms. Increased aromatization of androgens to estrogens occurs in the liver. Alcohol ingestion damages testicular steroidogenic capacity, and a state of hypergonadotropic hypogonadism can ensue. Acute alterations in nutritional state and ingestion of drugs such as spironolactone can further contribute to the gynecomastia. Even though liver disease is commonly believed to cause gynecomastia, a carefully conducted study found gynecomastia as frequently in hospitalized patients without liver disease as in those with severe hepatic dysfunction.

Regulatory hormone abnormalities

Prolactin secretion is modulated by central aminergic neuronal pathways, particularly of the dopaminergic variety. A wide range of drugs with catecholamine antagonistic or depleting actions can stimulate prolactin release. It is unlikely that prolactin alone causes gynecomastia, since many men with very high prolactin levels are unaffected. Prolactin elevations, however, result in reductions of gonadotropin-releasing hormone (GnRH), LH, and testosterone, thereby altering the balance between testosterone and estradiol, and causing gynecomastia.. While these putative mechanisms are not fully substantiated, a number of drugs with catecholamine-related properties are associated with gynecomastia (see **Table 39.1**).

Underlying structural disorders of the thyroid may also be associated with gynecomastia. In hypothyroidism, a reduction in serum thyroxine results in increased thyrotropin-releasing hormone (TRH) and thyroid-stimulating hormone (TSH) secretion. If sufficiently high, TRH can stimulate prolactin as well as TSH secretion through its 'cross-talk' properties. Patients with hyperthyroidism may present with gynecomastia and/or breast tenderness based upon several mechanisms. Thyroxine stimulates the production of testosterone–estrogen-binding globulin (TEBG), which binds plasma testosterone and estradiol and increases total serum levels. Because the affinity of TEBG for estradiol is less than that for testosterone, increased estradiol may be available to tissue as one mechanism of gynecomastia. An alternate explanation is that thyroxine increases TEBG and reduces free testosterone. This results in an increased LH level, which then stimulates the testes to increase the production of estradiol. Increased aromatization of androgens to estrogens also occurs as a mechanism for increased estradiol levels.

Several additional endocrine disorders are associated with gynecomastia on the basis of abnormalities of regulatory hormone dysfunction. Pituitary tumors that produce either prolactin, growth hormone, or both may be associated with gynecomastia. In acromegaly, partial gonadotropin deficiency with reductions in bioavailable testosterone is frequently present. Cushing's syndrome causes gynecomastia by directly interfering with testosterone synthesis and inducing a state of relative hypogonadism.

Drug-induced

A number of drugs are reported to cause gynecomastia. Documentation does not always involve drug rechallenge and the causative nature of these associations is not always valid. This review lists several drugs as falling into specific pathophysiologic categories and others whose mechanism is not known (see **Tables 39.1 & 39.2**).

Local trauma

Traumatic gynecomastia has been reported following thoracotomy, in army recruits wearing military packs, in patients with hip spica casts irritating the chest wall, following herpes zoster infection of the chest wall, and following local chest wall irradiation. The recent observation that macrophages contain high levels of aromatase may provide an explanation for this finding. Spinal cord injuries may also be associated with gynecomastia.

Primary breast tumors

Carcinoma of the breast occurs in men with 1/100th the frequency observed in women. The firm, irregular, and unilateral nature of the lesion raises suspicion of this diagnosis and warrants an aggressive approach to diagnosis if present. Ultrasonography, mammography, and fine-needle aspiration or core biopsy provide the means to make the diagnosis if suspected. The frequency of breast cancer is increased in patients with Klinefelter's syndrome and gynecomastia and in men harboring the *BRCA2* mutation. A benign tumor of the breast, myofibroblastoma, has been also been reported in association with bilateral gynecomastia.

Uncertain causes

Following World War II, starved prisoners developed gynecomastia upon refeeding. Starvation suppresses gonadotropin production, and refeeding allows return to normal function. The recovery phase mimics the changes that occur during early puberty. The gynecomastia that ensues is probably also similar to pubertal gynecomastia. This form of gynecomastia is quite frequent and affects patients recovering from chronic illnesses associated with undernutrition. This mechanism probably accounts for the gynecomastia observed in certain patients with diabetes mellitus, tuberculosis, and perhaps also those with

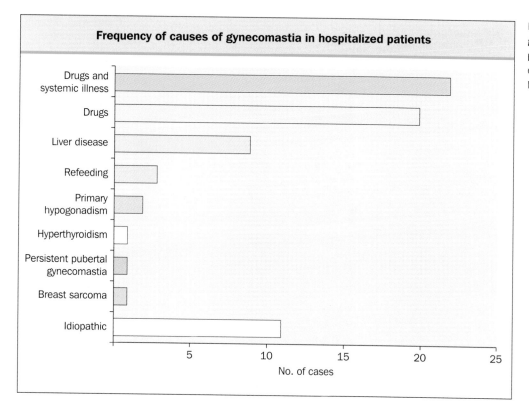

Figure 39.7 Frequency of causes of gynecomastia in hospitalized patients. (From Carlson HE. Current concepts: gynecomastia. N Engl J Med. 1980;303:795.)

leprosy. The finding of gynecomastia in patients with a human immunodeficiency virus (HIV) infection may also fall into this category. Men with diabetes mellitus occasionally develop gynecomastia associated with a fibrous inflammatory reaction. Its histopathologic characteristics are a marked chronic periductal and perivascular mastitis with a predominance of B-lymphocytes, focal fibrosis, and 'epithelioid stromal fibrosis'.

Pubertal macromastia

Gynecomastia occurring normally at puberty is usually mild to moderate in degree (i.e. Tanner grade II) and resolves spontaneously. Boys with more substantial pubertal gynecomastia (i.e. Tanner grades III, IV, and V) experience persistence after puberty (see Chapter 24 for definitions of Tanner stages). Extensive evaluation usually reveals a lack of hormonal abnormalities and surgical therapy is usually required. A recent report describes an extensive evaluation of 60 boys with this condition and provides a guide to the frequency of findings. Of the 60 patients, 45 were found to have idiopathic gynecomastia, eight to have underlying medical disorders (5 neurologic) and 7 to have an endocrine abnormality including the XXY and XY forms of Klinefelter's syndrome, primary testicular failure, partial androgen insensitivity, hepatocellular carcinoma, and increased aromatase activity.

Idiopathic

The majority of patients referred to an endocrinologist on an outpatient basis will fall into the idiopathic category after careful endocrinologic evaluation (personal experience of author). Whether these patients have increased local aromatization of androgens to estrogens in breast tissue, as suggested by Bulard et al., or other causes remains unknown.

Frequency of diagnoses in hospitalized patients

The study of Carlson, which evaluated 68 patients at the Wadsworth Veterans Administration Hospital, provides a guide to expected findings on an inpatient consultation service (**Fig. 39.7**). In this population, drugs in conjunction with other illnesses were implicated in 33% and drugs alone in 30%. Other associated conditions included liver disease in 13%, refeeding in 4%, hypogonadism in 3%, and other miscellaneous disorders (male climacteric, sarcoma, hyperthyroidism, and persistent pubertal gynecomastia) in 7%. Some 10% of patients were considered to have idiopathic gynecomastia.

Diagnostic procedures

The clinician must decide when and how extensively to evaluate men with gynecomastia (**Table 39.3, Figs 39.8 & 39.9**). Clear indications for extensive hormonal evaluation include breast tenderness, rapid breast enlargement, and lesions greater than 4cm in diameter. Eccentric, hard, or irregular masses require fine-needle or core biopsy and possible repeat biopsy if the initial biopsy is not diagnostic. Asymptomatic, stable gynecomastia less than 5cm in diameter, particularly in obese patients, probably requires only a careful history and physical examination for evaluation. In lean subjects, gynecomastia with a breast diameter of 2–4cm should probably be evaluated more extensively.

Key elements of the history, physical examination, and algorithmic approach to diagnosis are provided in **Table 39.3** and in **Figures 39.8 & 39.9**.

Treatment

Management of gynecomastia depends upon the clinical circumstances involved, the severity and presence of pain, and the degree of psychologic discomfort. Boys with *pubertal*

Aspects of the history and physical examination in gynecomastia

Patient history

- Time of onset, rate of progression, degree of pain associated with gynecomastia
- Symptoms of androgen deficiency
- Use of specific medications
- Presence of diabetes, renal, hepatic, cardiac, or pulmonary disease and associated malnutrition
- Symptoms of underlying malignancy, especially testicular
- Symptoms of estradiol, prolactin, growth hormone, cortisol, or thyroxine excess
- History of chest wall trauma
- Family history of gynecomastia

Physical examination

- Distinguish pseudo- from true gynecomastia (see **Fig. 39.8**)
- Determine degree of obesity (calculate body mass index)
- Evaluate for signs of hypogonadism
- Quantify testis size and evaluate consistency
- Evaluate for signs of renal or hepatic disease
- Evaluate for evidence of Cushing's syndrome, hyperthyroidism, and hypogonadism

Table 39.3 Aspects of the history and physical examination in gynecomastia.

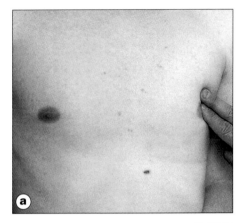

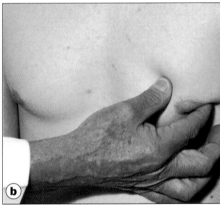

Figure 39.8 Method of examination to detect gynecomastia. Palpation by pressing down on tissue beneath the nipple in a supine patient is an insensitive method for detecting gynecomastia and is considered incorrect. Squeezing of tissue between the thumb and forefinger in a sitting patient is a more sensitive technique and is considered correct. The examiner should try to 'flip an edge' between normal fat tissue and glandular tissue to distinguish the outer limits of the gynecomastia.

gynecomastia can be reassured that regression usually occurs after 1 year and at most after 3 years. Medical therapy may be considered as a temporizing maneuver if the circumstances warrant. A reduction in size of palpable breast tissue occurs in a substantial fraction of patients. Three nonrandomized studies reported a greater than 20% decrease in size associated with use of the antiestrogen clomiphene citrate in 39 of 53 (74%) patients. Two studies reported that the nonaromatizable androgen dihydrotestosterone produced a reduction in 28 of 34 (82%) of subjects. One study examined the effect of danazol in 11 subjects and noted marked or moderate reduction of breast tissue in 10. Finally, the use of the aromatase inhibitor testololactone was associated with reduction in mean breast diameter from 4.4cm to 1.7cm in 20 of 22 subjects. While the results of these studies were consistent, cautious interpretation is required since pubertal gynecomastia resolves spontaneously and placebo controls were not used.

A prudent approach in *pubertal gynecomastia* is to observe the patient for regression and regard medical therapy as a temporizing measure for individuals with substantial gynecomastia, pain, or a preference for some type of therapy. On the other hand, when the diameter of breast tissue is greater than 5.0cm and persists for more than 3 years (persistent pubertal gynecomastia), the only effective therapeutic option in our opinion is surgical excision. The surgical procedure involves a periareolar incision with removal of the palpable breast tissue. For obese patients, liposuction of subdermal chest wall fat may aid in achieving satisfactory recontouring of the chest wall.

In adult men with gynecomastia, the first principle is to stop potentially causative drugs and treat any specific abnormality amenable to therapy. Medical therapy can be considered, based upon available data from randomized studies and observational experience. Two randomized studies compared tamoxifen with placebo and detected a reduction in size in 62% of men receiving drug and 6% with placebo. Pain relief occurred in 90% on tamoxifen and 10% with placebo.. The impeded androgen danazol serves as an alternative to tamoxifen and produced beneficial results in the same proportion. However, a comparative trial involving 68 men with idiopathic adult gynecomastia found a 78% response to tamoxifen versus a 40% response to danazol. Only the early phase of gynecomastia characterized by glandular predominance would be expected to respond to hormonal therapies. The later phase of gynecomastia, which appears to consist predominantly of dense stroma histologically, is no longer hormonally responsive. Thus, a trial of tamoxifen may be warranted in adult patients with recent-onset idiopathic gynecomastia. With persistence of glandular enlargement or pain, reduction mammoplasty is occasionally necessary. A highly experienced surgeon should be asked to perform this procedure because of the precise sculpturing necessary to produce the desired cosmetic effect.

BENIGN BREAST DISORDERS IN WOMEN

Introduction

Breast physiology in women

The female breast is an endocrine target tissue that responds acutely to hormones and growth factors with changes in rate of cellular proliferation and alterations in differentiated function. During the early, middle, and late reproductive periods, and after the menopause, changes in breast structure and function

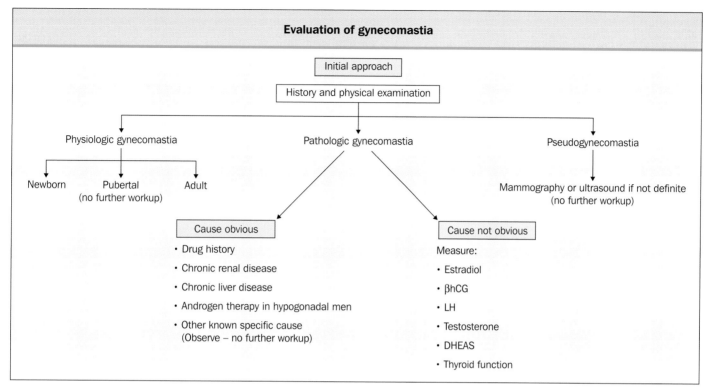

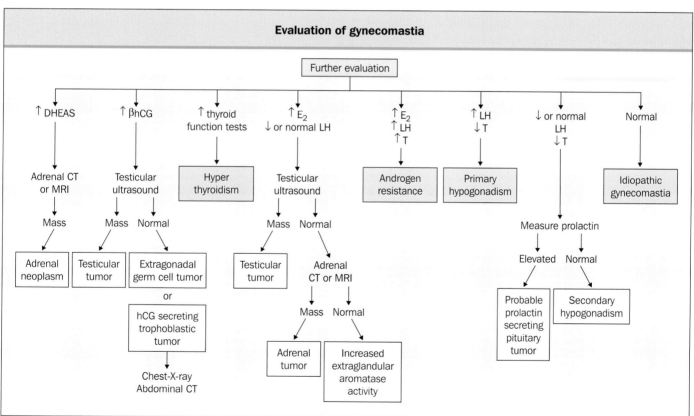

Figure 39.9 Evaluation of gynecomastia. Adapted from the approach outlined by Braunstein et al (Braunstein GD. Aromatase and gynecomastia. Endocr Rel Cancer 1999;6:315–24 and Gynecomastia. N Engl J Med. 1993;328:490–5). CT; computerized tomography; DHEAS, dehydroepiandrosterone sulfate; E_2, estradiol; hCG, human chorionic gonadotropin; LH, luteinizing hormone; MRI, magnetic resonance imaging; T, testosterone.

occur in response to hormonal stimuli. The mature breast undergoes cyclic changes during the menstrual cycle. Estrogen increases breast cell proliferation and progesterone enhances this effect. As a consequence, cell proliferation increases during the follicular phase and is enhanced further during the luteal phase (**Fig. 39.10**). Acute deprivation of these hormones causes an increase in cell death or apoptosis, a process that is maximum during the time of menstrual bleeding. As a result of these cyclic changes, the breast may increase in size by up to 10–15% during the late luteal phase. These changes are associated with mild breast tenderness, swelling, pain, or lumpiness in 60% of normal women and moderate to severe symptoms in another 10%.

Causes

Classification of benign breast disorders

Clinicians traditionally consider benign breast disorders to be part of the spectrum of fibrocystic disease. Clinical studies report a prevalence of 8.8% of fibrocystic disease while autopsy series report this finding in 50–60% of women. The frequency increases from the time of menarche to peak at 40–44 years of age. Clinicians in the USA prefer the term 'fibrocystic changes' rather than fibrocystic disease because of the frequency of this problem in the normal population. European investigators, on the other hand, have introduced the term ANDI, 'aberrations of normal development and involution', to describe a spectrum of histologic changes encountered in women. This classification has been modified to eliminate the poorly substantiated concept of involution and to focus on lesions that can be considered 'disease'. In this schema (**Fig. 39.11**), we separately consider reproductive period and specific histologic change present in stroma, ductal, and glandular tissue. A schematic diagram illustrates the anatomy of the changes to be described (**Fig. 39.12**).

Early reproductive period

Glandular components of the breast may respond to cyclic hormonal stimuli in an exaggerated fashion with the development of single fibroadenomas (**Figs 39.11 & 39.12**). These consist of lobular units that grow to larger than normal size and contain both epithelial and stromal elements. Fibroadenomas range in size from slightly larger than a normal single lobular unit to larger, more discrete palpable lesions. The incidence of fibroadenoma peaks at age 20–24 (**Fig. 39.13**). The prevalence on physical examination in young women is 2% but it is 15–23% when evaluated prospectively at autopsy. When fibroadenomas are giant (>5cm) or multiple, they are considered part of a disease process. Giant fibroadenomas are almost always seen in puberty or pregnancy.

The other components of breast tissue are involved much less commonly in the early reproductive period. **Ductal** abnormalities are exceedingly rare. **Stromal** hyperplasia may occur and produces juvenile breast hypertrophy or, rarely, the more significant problems of unilateral or bilateral macromastia (enlargement of breast tissue beyond what is considered normal).

Middle reproductive years

Glandular breast tissue continues to undergo changes in response to cyclic increments in plasma levels of estradiol and progesterone. The process may progress to an aberrant and then to a disease state depending upon the degree of pain, tenderness,

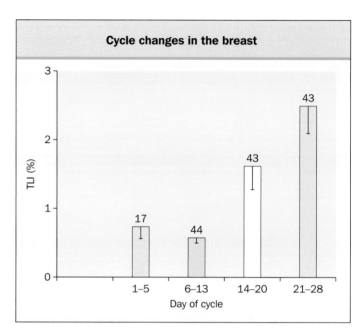

Figure 39.10 Cycle changes in the breast. The figure illustrates the influence of cycle phase on breast total labeling index (TLI) of women less than 34 years of age. (Redrawn from Going JJ, Anderson TJ, Battersby S, et al. Proliferative and secretory activity in human breast during natural and artificial menstrual cycles. Am J Pathol. 1988;130:193–204.)

and nodularity. Some have termed this process of glandular change 'adenosis'. **Ductal** changes remain uncommon in the middle reproductive period. **Stromal** hyperplasia may occur, which results in areas of ill-defined fullness ('lumpy–bumpy' consistency) on physical examination or in firm areas requiring biopsy.

Late reproductive period

Glandular tissue may become hyperplastic, with sclerosing adenosis (**Fig. 39.12**) or lobular hyperplasia. The hyperplastic glandular lesions may progress to palpable or mammographically detectable abnormalities requiring biopsy. Lobular carcinoma-*in-situ* (LCIS) may be found incidentally when these lesions are biopsied. LCIS is typically not palpable and is rarely (5%) associated with calcifications on mammogram.

Ductal tissue also may undergo hyperplastic change, with an increase in the number of ductal cells but without changes in their appearance. With progression, atypical ductal hyperplasia or ductal carcinoma-*in-situ* (DCIS) may ensue. A current theory of carcinogenesis suggests an ordered sequence whereby normal breast tissue progresses to typical and atypical hyperplasia, then to DCIS, and finally to invasive and metastatic cancer. This orderly progression depends upon the number of acquired genetic mutations accumulated by clonal cells in the breast.

Another process, not associated with cancer, involves duct *ectasia*. This is characterized by distention of subareolar ducts and presence within them of yellowish-orange material (**Fig. 39.14**). Histologically, crystalline oval and round structures thought to be lipid in origin are present (**Fig. 39.14**). Penetration of the duct wall by this material produces acute inflammatory changes in the surrounding tissues. Spontaneous resolution may occur but

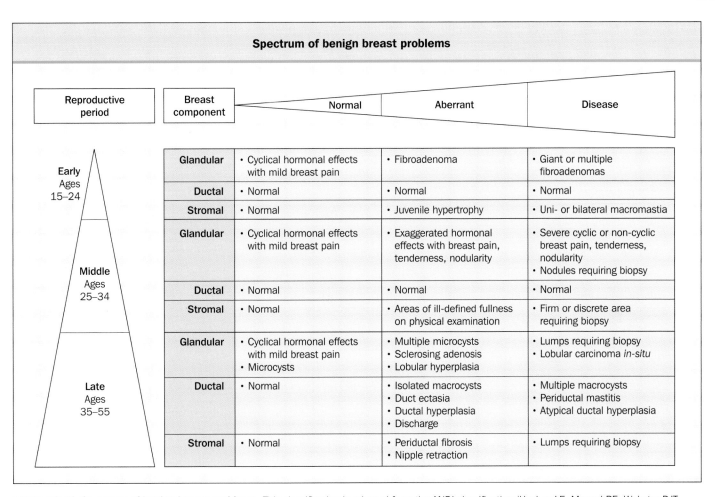

Figure 39.11 Spectrum of benign breast problems. This classification is adapted from the ANDI classification (Hughes LE, Mansel RE, Webster DJT. Aberrations of normal development and involution (ANDI): a new perspective on pathogenesis and nomenclature of benign breast disorders. Lancet 1987;2:1316–9).

residual periductal fibrosis and nodule formation often persist. Periductal mastitis, a condition thought to be more frequent in cigarette smokers, represents a more chronic and extensive inflammatory process. Abnormalities of ductal secretion may result in discharge of clear, cloudy, blue, green, or black aqueous material. Finally, **stromal** hyperplasia can result in nipple retraction or in palpable lesions requiring biopsy to distinguish from breast carcinoma. Histologically, the tissue may contain fibroblasts nearly exclusively, predominantly fibroblasts with admixture of glandular epithelium, or the classic appearance of a radial scar (**Fig. 39.14**). Some degree of stromal hyperplasia may occur in 50–60% of normal women, particularly those in their middle and late reproductive periods.

Menopause
Glandular tissue undergoes atrophic change following the menopause and a greater percentage of the total breast is made up of stroma and fatty tissue (approximately 97%) than prior to menopause. With use of estrogens alone or estrogens plus progestins as postmenopausal hormone replacement therapy (HRT), ductal and lobular tissue persists and the range of lesions observed during the menopause parallels those seen during the late reproductive period.

Overall perspective
This classification regarding early, mid- and late reproductive years emphasizes that fibrocystic type changes are minimal in young women and increase in frequency with age. Fibro-adenomas are more common in younger women, peaking at age 20–24 years (**Fig. 39.13**). Cysts occur most commonly, but not exclusively, in the perimenopausal period. All of these changes improve spontaneously at menopause unless HRT is used. Other lesions (**Table 39.4**) may also be present, such as diabetic mastitis, which are well recognized but rare.

Etiology of benign breast disorders
Increments in estradiol and progesterone during the luteal phase of the menstrual cycle enhance the number of cells undergoing cell division. This and associated effects on cellular function probably result in the mild cyclic breast pain experienced by 60% of normal women.

Ductal proliferation is associated with genetic abnormalities. Loss of heterozygosity in hyperplastic lesions and the nonrandom inactivation of the X chromosome demonstrate that hyperplasias are clonal neoplasms and perhaps indicate the need for more appropriate terminology (i.e. *typical* and *atypical mammary adenomas*). The multicentric nature of hyperplastic

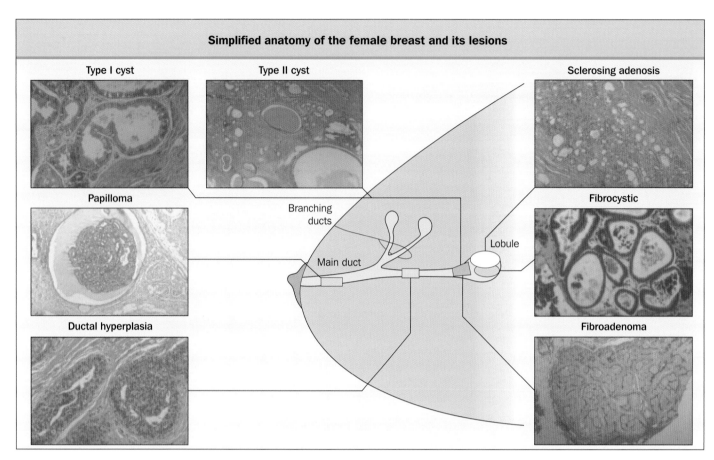

Figure 39.12 Simplified anatomy of the female breast illustrating the major structural components and corresponding sites of origin of potential lesions.

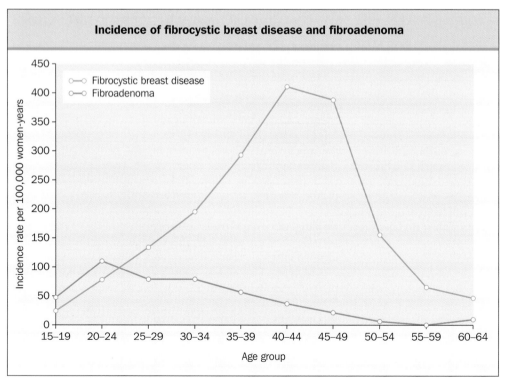

Figure 39.13 Incidence of fibrocystic breast disease and fibroadenoma. (From Goehring C, Morabia A. Epidemiology of benign breast disease, with special attention to histologic types. Epidemiol Rev. 1997;19:310–27, by permission of Oxford University Press.)

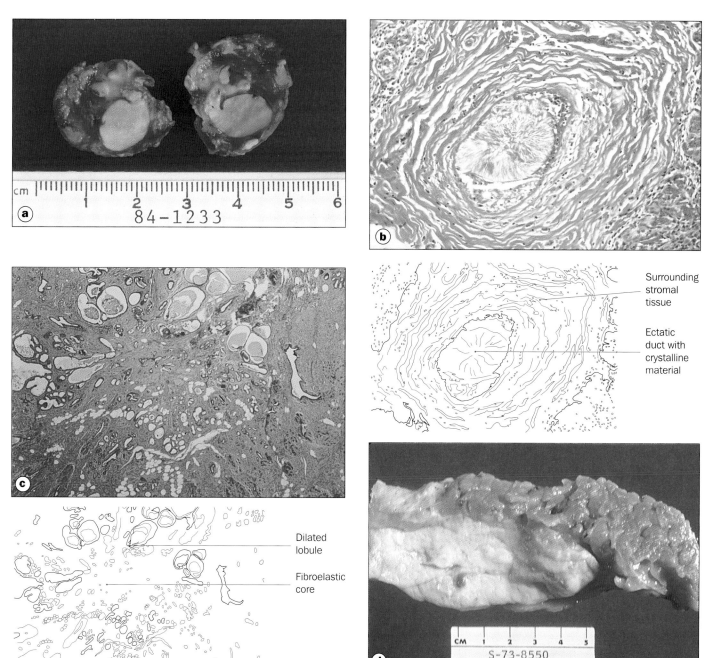

Figure 39.14 Appearances of benign breast disease. (a) Gross appearance of duct ectasia showing a single duct dilated by homogeneous yellow-orange fluid, probably lipid in composition. (b) Histologic appearance of duct ectasia showing the characteristic crystalline formation of the intraluminal contents. (c) Radial scar demonstrating a central fibroelastic core and peripherally radiating lobules, some of which are typically dilated, as in this example. (d) Gross changes with fibrocystic disease showing marked fibrosis and scattered cysts. An area of normal breast tissue is shown in the upper right hand portion of the breast.

ductal lesions suggests that an underlying abnormality or *field defect* is present as an etiologic factor in some women. Multifocality of the associated benign hyperplastic lesions is most apparent in breast tissue from women with cancer. Examination of tissue adjacent to an invasive breast cancer or in the contralateral breast reveals one or more additional hyperplastic lesions in 40% of patients. The nature of the field defect has not been specifically identified but hypothetically could represent a single mutation of a gene controlling local estrogen production, cellular proliferation, DNA repair, metabolism of procarcinogens to carcinogens, or other cellular events. Preliminary data support these concepts since 80–90% of hyperplastic lesions contain DNA mutations similar to those in the contiguous tumors. Extensive molecular genetic studies have now described progression of abnormalities in the spectrum of breast lesions (**Fig. 39.15**).

Classification of common breast disorders in women				
Pain	Nonbreast pain	Chest wall pain		*Tietze's syndrome* or costochondritis *Localized lateral* chest wall pain *Diffuse lateral* chest wall pain *Radicular* pain from cervical arthritis
		Non-chest wall pain		Gallbladder disease Ischemic heart disease
	Breast pain	Noncyclic		Stretching of Cooper's ligaments Pressure from a brassiere Fat necrosis from trauma Hydradenitis suppurativa Focal mastitis Cyst Mondor's disease (thrombophlebitis of breast veins)
Discharge	Worrisome	Spontaneous bloody or serous discharge from single duct		Papilloma Ductal carcinoma-*in-situ* Paget's disease (carcinoma)
		Milky discharge from single or multiple ducts		Hyperprolactinemia from pituitary tumor, hypothyroidism, or drugs
	Reassuring	Green, blue, yellow, black or clear discharge		Fibrocystic changes
Lumps	Cyst(s)	Fat necrosis		Lipoma
	Fibroadenoma	Invasive cancer		Leiomyomas
	Ductal hyperplasia	Fibrocystic changes		Neurofibromas
	Atypical ductal hyperplasia	Duct ectasia (± rupture of wall)		Adenomyoepitheliomas
	DCIS	Granuloma		Mucocele-like lesions
	Lobular hyperplasia	Factitial abscess		Foreign body reaction
	Atypical lobular hyperplasia	Sclerosing adenosis		Sarcoidosis
	Hamartoma	Papilloma		Diabetic mastopathy
	Hematoma	Fibromatosis		

Table 39.4 Classification of common breast disorders in women. DCIS, ductal carcinoma-*in-situ*.

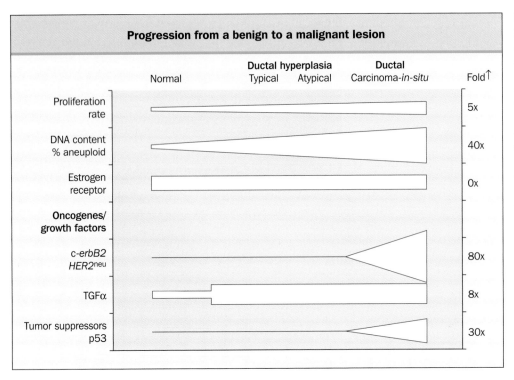

Figure 39.15 Progression from a benign to a malignant lesion. This probably represents the accumulation of an increasing number of genetic mutations. The proliferation rate increases fivefold when comparing benign breast tissue with carcinoma-*in-situ*. The percentage of aneuploid cells (i.e. DNA with greater or less DNA than expected for the presence of 46 chromosomes) increases 40-fold between normal breast tissue and carcinoma-in-situ. Estrogen-receptor status remains stable. Transforming growth factor-α (TGFα) increases concomitantly with the appearance of hyperplasia. Finally, c-*erbB2/HER2*neu and *p53* mutations increase only in ductal carcinoma-*in-situ*. (Compiled from Berardo MD, O'Connell P, Allred DC. Biologic characteristics of premalignant and preinvasive breast disease. In: Pasqualini JR, Katzenellenbogen BS, eds. Hormone dependent cancer. New York:Marcel Dekker; 1996.)

Clinical manifestations

Clinical presentations of benign breast disease are divided into those with pain, lumps, or breast discharge (**Table 39.4**).

Breast pain

A recent study in 1171 healthy American women indicated the presence of moderate to severe cyclic mastalgia in 11% and mild breast pain (mastalgia) in another 58%. Cyclic pain is at its worst during the luteal phase, peaks the day or two before menses, and abates completely during menses. Mastalgia interferes with usual sexual activity in 48% of women and with physical (37%), social (12%), and school (8%) activity in others. The types of pain are listed in **Table 39.4**. The method to distinguish between breast and nonbreast pain by careful physical examination is illustrated in **Figure 39.16**.

Breast nodule

Patients often present with the finding of a new breast nodule on self-examination or are found to have a lump by their health-care provider. Some 90% of these new nodules in

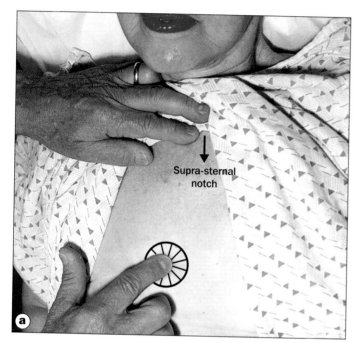

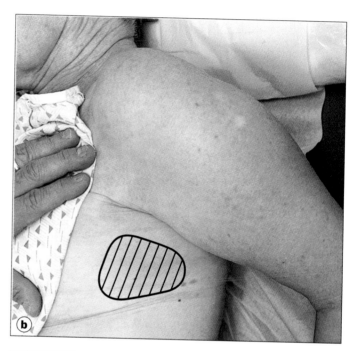

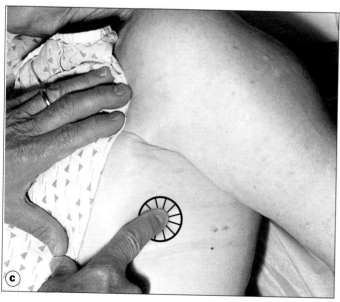

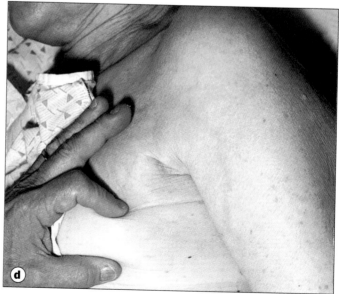

Figure 39.16 Physical examination to detect types of chest wall pain. (a) Detection of pain to palpation over the costochondral junctions to elicit the pain of Tietze's syndrome. To provide anatomic orientation, the suprasternal notch is indicated by an arrow. (b) The area encircled in black indicates an area of diffuse lateral chest wall pain. The patient is examined while lying at 90° on her side. (c) Demonstration by palpation of focal lateral chest wall. The area of pain is encircled in black. (d). Squeezing of breast tissue between the fingers does not elicit pain in the area where the patient complains of pain. This demonstrates to the patient that her pain is chest-wall in origin (see focal area encircled in black in c) rather than in the breast itself.

premenopausal women are benign and usually represent fibro-adenomas in the early reproductive period (**Figs 39.12, 39.13, & 39.17**). In the middle reproductive period, focal areas of fibrosis, hyperplasia, or cyst formation are more likely.

In the later reproductive period, hyperplasia, cysts, and carcinoma-*in-situ* are more common (**Fig. 39.17**). Some lesions present with symptoms suggesting the cause. With *duct ectasia*, penetration of the duct wall by lipid material may be associated

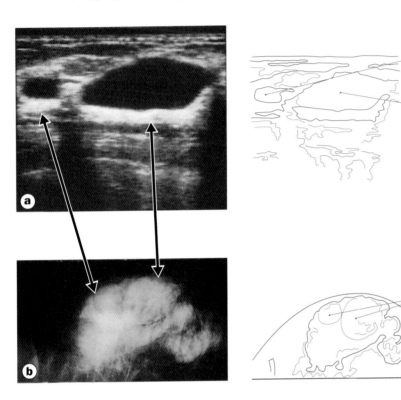

Figure 39.17 (a) Ultrasound and (b) mammographic appearance of two simple cysts. Arrows indicate areas of correspondence between ultrasound and mammogram. (c) Mammographic and (d) ultrasonographic appearance of a fibroadenoma. The arrow shows the correspondence between the lesion on the ultrasound and that on the mammogram.

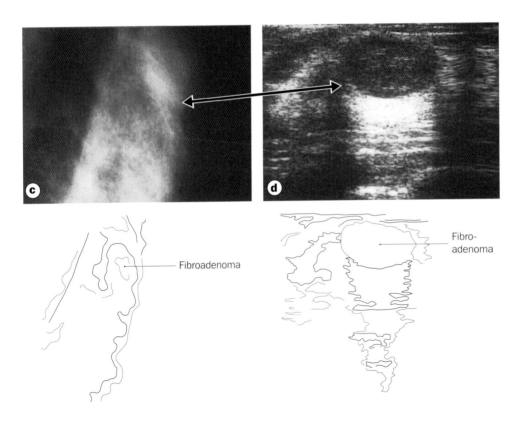

with a nodule exhibiting acute redness and causing pain, and fever; after resolution a subareolar nodule persists (**Fig. 39.14**). All discrete palpable nodules not characteristic of simple cysts or fibroadenomas on ultrasound require biopsy, whether or not the mammogram and ultrasound are negative.

Breast discharge

A careful history characterizes breast discharge as either spontaneous or expressible. On examination, one can detect by careful inspection whether the discharge emanates from a single or multiple ducts. Nipple discharge can be divided into physiologic and pathologic types. Characteristics of physiologic discharge include nonspontaneous, multiple duct, bilateral, and nonbloody. Pathologic discharge is characterized as spontaneous, serous or bloody, usually unilateral and usually single-duct. Reassuring characteristics are that it must be expressed; is green yellow, brown or milky; is bilateral and involves multiple ducts. Spontaneous discharge, whether serous or bloody, requires careful evaluation. A hemoccult card or urine dipstick can be used to test for occult blood if the discharge is spontaneous, unilateral, and from one duct. It should be noted that discharge may be falsely heme-positive because of lactoferrin. Milky discharge (galactorrhea) should be evaluated with measurement of a serum prolactin level (Chapter 6).

If the discharge is physiologic and the patient is under 35, only reassurance is necessary. Screening mammogram is recommended for patients over 35 with physiologic discharge.

Pathologic discharge requires diagnostic mammogram, galactography (**Fig. 39.18**), and referral to a surgeon. The presence of crusting, scaling, and flaking of the nipple could be a manifestation of Paget's disease of breast and underlying cancer or of dermatologic problems. The approach is to obtain a history of other dermatologic problems, or a history of change in soap or clothing. If absent, a diagnostic mammogram should be obtained if the patient is over 35. In a large recent series of 1251 patients with nipple discharge, 433 had unilateral discharge and 194 had no breast lump in association with this symptom. Of these, the lesions found included solitary papilloma ($n = 49$), minimal breast cancer ($n = 20$), fibrocystic disease($n = 11$), papillomatosis ($n = 7$),lobular cancer ($n = 5$) and duct ectasia ($n = 2$).

For women with bloody discharge from a single duct, galactography is warranted. Filling defects can be due to intraductal papilloma, intraductal carcinoma, papillomatosis, debris, or air bubbles.

Diagnostic procedures

Ideally a team including a radiologist experienced in mammography, ultrasound, and core needle biopsy as well as an internist, gynecologist, or surgeon with expertise in breast diseases should be involved in the evaluation of patients with breast disorders. Algorithms for evaluation and treatment of each of these problems are presented in **Figures 39.19–39.25** and **Table 39.5**. Information to be obtained by a focused history and physical examination is outlined in **Table 39.6**. The method of documenting whether breast pain is cyclic or noncyclic is illustrated in **Figure 39.26**. Imaging has become an integral part of the management of benign breast disorders. The key elements to be understood regarding imaging are detailed in the paragraph below and in **Table 39.7**.

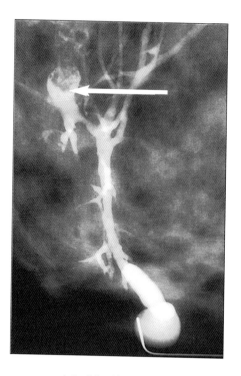

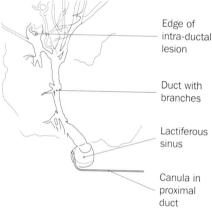

Edge of intra-ductal lesion

Duct with branches

Lactiferous sinus

Canula in proximal duct

Figure 39.18 Galactogram illustrating a space-occupying lesion. On biopsy this was shown to be a solitary papilloma. The lesion is indicated by an arrow.

Imaging studies

Mammography is useful for evaluation of palpable lesions, particularly in those over 35. Ultrasound is often used as initial evaluation of a palpable mass in women under age 35. If a simple cyst is present, no further evaluation is necessary. If not, mammography may also be necessary to fully evaluate the lump. If the mass has findings suggestive of a fibroadenoma by ultrasound and mammography, short-term followup and reimaging can be considered (usually performed in 6 months).

Fibrocystic change typically presents on mammogram as round or oval, well-defined masses that can be subsequently shown to represent cysts on ultrasound (**Fig. 39.17**). Diffusely scattered dystrophic calcifications may also be on the mammogram. Consequently, the goal of mammographic evaluation is to provide reassurance to the patient and physician that the risk of neoplasm is low. Aspiration of cysts is usually necessary only in those cases

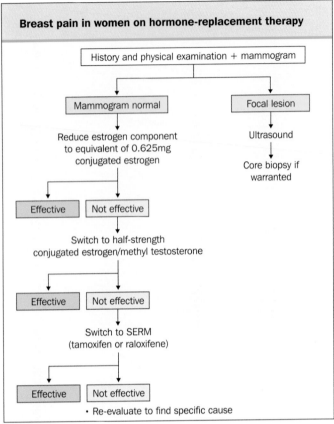

Figure 39.19 Breast pain in women on hormone-replacement therapy (HRT). Algorithm for evaluation and treatment of postmenopausal women on HRT. SERM, selective estrogen receptor modulator.

where the mass does not fulfill all criteria for a simple cyst or if the cyst is painful. Biopsy may be necessary to confirm the benign nature of calcifications, particularly if clustered, linear, or variously shaped.

For round masses or round calcifications on a first mammogram, the risk of cancer is less than 2%, and repeat mammography in 6 months is recommended. These lesions are termed 'probably benign' using the lexicon terminology required in the USA by the Mammography Quality Standards Act. If the risk is believed to be greater, core biopsy is recommended. Stereotactically directed core biopsy is ideal for evaluation of calcifications and provides highly discriminatory information regarding the presence or absence of malignancy. If this technique is not available, insertion of a wire into the lesion radiographically followed by surgical excision or mere removal of a palpable lesion is warranted.

Treatment of benign breast disease in women

Several well-designed, randomized, controlled double-blind crossover trials have validated the efficacy of medical therapy for cyclic mastalgia. Based upon these studies, we categorize therapies as definitely effective, definitely ineffective, possibly effective, and insufficiently studied. For classification as definitely effective, two or more randomized trails are required. For the category possibly effective, one randomized trial must be positive in some respect but others may be negative. For the category definitely ineffective, prospective trials must be uniformly negative. In the category insufficiently studied, only one randomized trial, either negative or positive, is available. Danazol, bromocriptine, linoleic acid (oil of evening primrose), and tamoxifen have been proved to be effective. Vitamin E

Figure 39.20 Breast pain in women on birth control pill. Algorithm for evaluation and treatment of breast pain in premenopausal women on birth control pills.

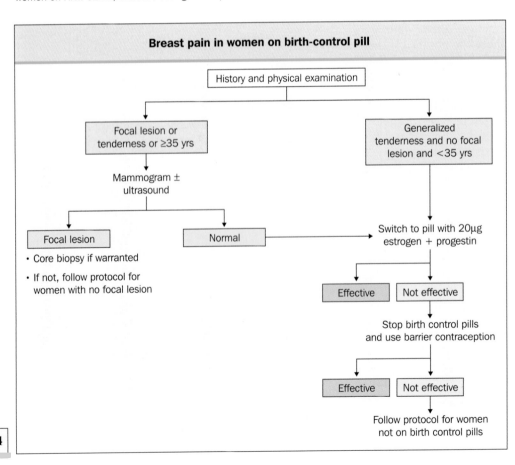

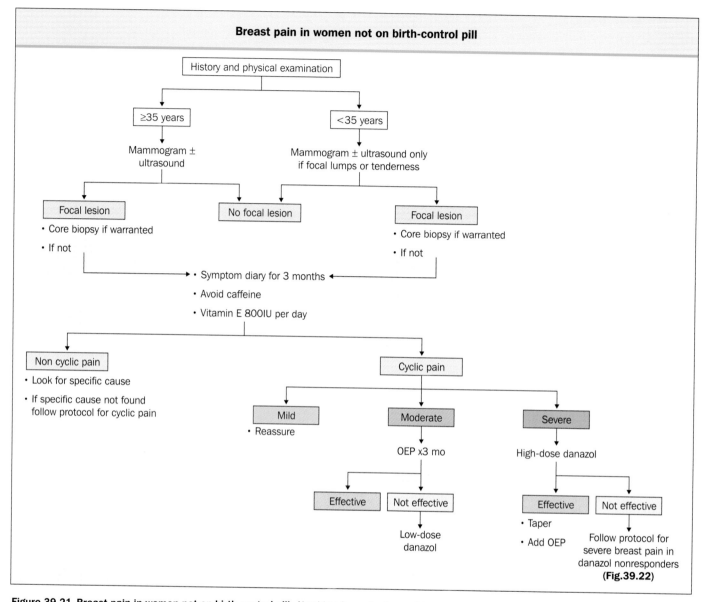

Figure 39.21 Breast pain in women not on birth control pill. Algorithm for evaluation and treatment of breast pain in premenopausal women not on birth control pills. Avoidance of caffeine and use of Vitamin E are suggested even though these strategies have not been proved to be effective. Vitamin E probably acts as a placebo, which is 30% effective in this setting. Avoidance of caffeine may benefit some patients according to anecdotal reports and is not harmful. OEP, oil of evening primrose.

is considered definitely ineffective and iodine and vaginal progesterone possibly effective. Medroxyprogesterone acetate, caffeine avoidance, and progesterone have not been sufficiently studied. Several other therapies have not been examined in randomized controlled trials but are likely to be beneficial since they are based upon physiologic principles. For example, precise fitting of a bra to provide support for pendulous breasts has been

reported to relieve pain in observational studies. GnRH agonist analogues are used to lower LH, FSH, and estradiol levels and to create a temporary postmenopausal state. Onset of menopause is known to reduce the frequency of breast pain. Reduction of the dosage of estrogens in postmenopausal women or addition of an androgen to estrogen replacement therapy appears to be beneficial in reducing breast pain (personal observation of author).

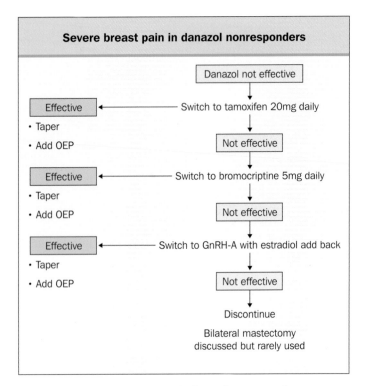

Figure 39.22 Severe breast pain in danazol nonresponders.
Algorithm for evaluation and treatment. GnRH-A, gonadotropin-releasing hormone agonist; OEP, oil of evening primrose.

Relative efficacy of effective therapies

No large, randomized, controlled studies have compared the relative efficacy of danazol, bromocriptine, oil of evening primrose and tamoxifen. **Figure 39.27** ranks them according to efficacy on the basis of data from individual reports. Minimal data are available from clinical trials that involve direct head to head comparisons. It should be noted that overall responses to danazol, bromocriptine, and oil of evening primrose are lower in those with noncyclic pain than in those with cyclic pain. However, not all studies have carefully excluded patients with nonbreast pain and therefore conclusions regarding noncyclic pan should be considered tentative.

Practical treatment strategies for benign breast problems

A series of algorithms, based upon published reports and the authors' experience are presented in **Figures 39.19–39.26** to outline treatment strategies.

Women at high risk for breast cancer

A major consideration for women who present with breast problems is whether they have a higher than normal risk of developing breast cancer. Certain breast lesions, such as fibrocystic changes, are associated with no increased risk of subsequent breast cancer (**Fig. 39.28**). A 1.5–2-fold greater risk of development of breast cancer over a 20-year period of followup occurs with proliferative lesions, including ductal hyperplasia, lobular hyperplasia without atypia, sclerosing adenosis, diffuse

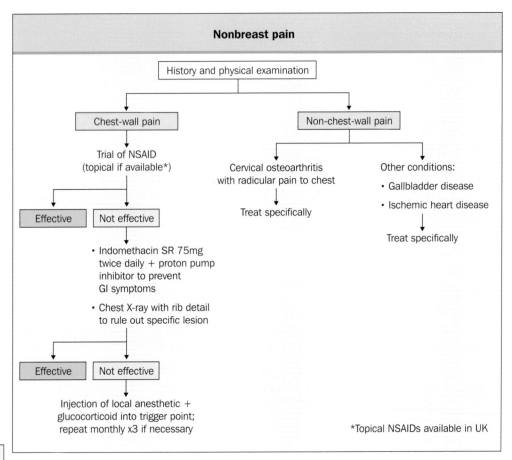

Figure 39.23 Nonbreast pain.
Algorithm for evaluation and treatment of nonbreast pain involving the chest wall, or abnormalities in other structures with pain referred to the breast area. GI, gastrointestinal; NSAID, nonsteroidal antiinflammatory drug.

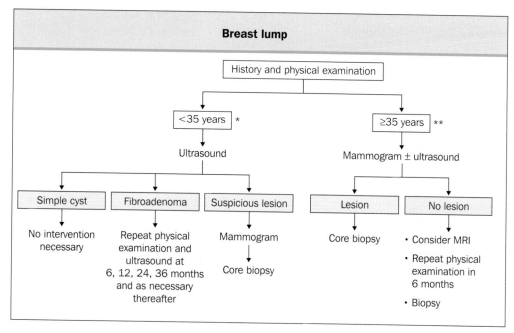

Figure 39.24 Breast lump. Algorithm for evaluation and treatment. * With a family history of breast cancer that increases risk, a mammogram ± ultrasound should be performed and biopsy considered even with a negative imaging study. ** Palpable lesions require biopsy even with negative imaging studies. Neoplasms such as invasive lobular carcinoma may be palpable but not seen on mammography or ultrasound. MRI, magnetic resonance imaging.

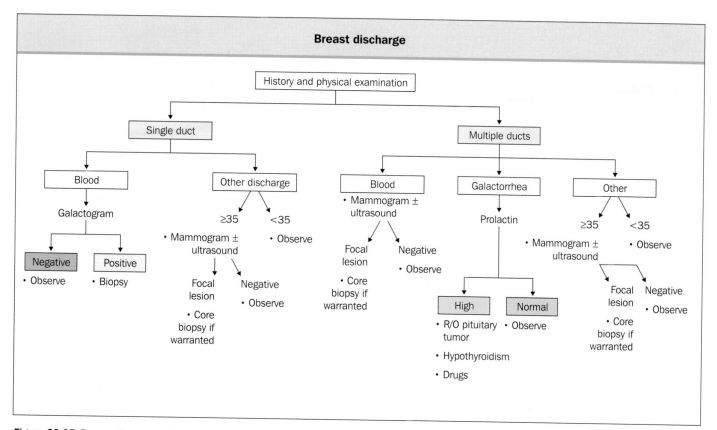

Figure 39.25 Breast discharge. Algorithm for evaluation and treatment. R/O, rule out.

Regimens for the treatment of breast pain	
Oil of evening primrose	500–1000mg three times daily
Low-dose danazol	100mg daily for 2 months, then: Taper 100mg, days 10–25, for 2 months then stop; or 100mg every other day for 2 months then stop
High-dose danazol	200mg daily for 2 months, then: Taper to 100mg daily for 2 months Taper further to 100mg, days 10–25, for 2 months then stop; or 100mg every other day for 2 months then stop

Table 39.5 Regimens for the treatment of breast pain.

Evaluation of breast pain, breast discharge, or breast lumps	
History	Amount of caffeinated drinks per day Smoking history List of all medications Current or previous use of postmenopausal hormone replacement therapy or oral contraceptives Age of onset of menarche Age at first live birth Number of first degree relatives with breast cancer History of prior breast biopsies Diagnosis of atypical ductal hyperplasia on prior breast biopsy History of breast feeding Age of menopause (last menstrual period) if relevant Circumstances under which breast lump detected Severity of breast pain on analog scale of 0–10 Characterize nature, location and precipitating factors for pain Relationship of breast pain to menstrual cycle Presence or absence of breast discharge; whether discharge is spontaneous or elicited only by pressure; whether discharge is bloody, greenish, brownish, blood tinged, or milk History of breast trauma
Physical examination	Characterize and measure discrete lumps and indicate location according to 12-hour clock and number of centimeters from nipple Determine if discharge is from single or multiple ducts Test if occult blood if indicated Determine if pain is from chest wall or breast tissue Examine for evidence of cervical arthritis as it may cause pain referred to breast

Table 39.6 Evaluation of breast pain, breast discharge, or breast lumps. The figure shows the key elements of the history and physical examination for women with these signs and symptoms.

papillomatosis, and complex fibroadenomas. A recent report also suggested that radial scars increase relative risk by a factor of 1.8.

A higher risk of breast cancer is associated with atypical ductal hyperplasia, which imparts a fourfold increased risk of breast cancer if sporadic and a sixfold greater risk in patients with a strong family history of breast cancer. Lobular tissue may also undergo atypical hyperplasia, which imparts an increased risk of subsequent breast cancer although the magnitude is not as precisely defined as for atypical ductal hyperplasia (ADH). When the degree of atypia progresses even further, the lesions are no longer called benign but are classified as carcinoma-*in-situ*. The relative risk of development of invasive cancer when DCIS and LCIS are present is increased 10–12-fold (**Fig. 39.28**). While currently called lobular carcinoma-*in-situ*, this lesion is not generally considered to have reached the neoplastic stage but to be analogous to atypical ductal hyperplasia.

Recent emphasis has been directed toward identification of molecular genetic markers that could predict which patients are at increased risk of developing breast cancer. In a recent study, presence of aberrant p53 protein increased the relative risk of breast cancer by a factor of 2.55 whereas the presence of

c-ErbB2/HER2^{neu} was associated with no increased risk. Aneuploidy on flow cytometry has also been suggested as a marker of increased risk.

The presence of dense breast tissue on mammography has also been reported to be a predictor of increased incidence of breast cancer (**Fig. 39.29**). Ranked according to the categories of density, the increase in breast cancer risk from lowest to highest breast density has been reported to be as high as sevenfold. Two components of this finding must be considered: the presence of high breast density makes it more difficult to read mammograms and decreases the sensitivity of finding breast cancer; and there is an increased risk of breast cancer associated with increased breast density.

Another risk factor is use of hormone replacement therapy. Current data, while exclusively retrospective in nature, suggest an 1% increase in relative risk of breast cancer per year of use of estrogen alone and an 8% increase per year with estrogen plus a progestin (**Fig. 39.30**). These increments in risk appear to apply exclusively to thin women with a body mass index of less than 24kg/m^2.

To aid in assessing breast cancer risk, a questionnaire developed by Gail uses the answers to seven questions to calculate the 5-year

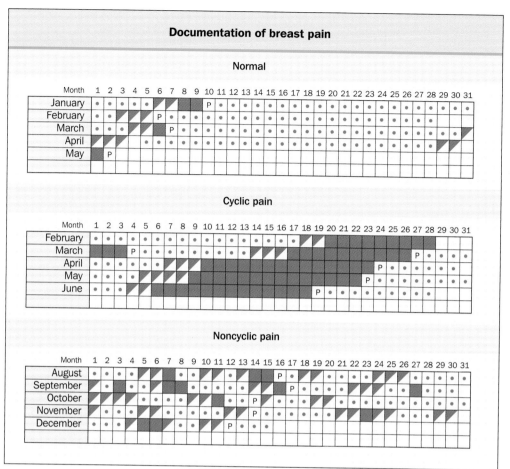

Figure 39.26 Documentation of breast pain. The figure shows examples of breast pain illustrated with a diary developed by Professor Robert Mansell. The cyclicity and severity of breast pain is best documented by using a prospective pain diary that correlates severity of pain with phase of the menstrual cycle. Noncyclic breast pain is diagnosed by lack of cyclicity on pain diary and exclusion of Tietze's syndrome, lateral chest wall pain, and cervical arthritis by physical examination. As shown in the top panel, normal women experience pain of short duration for 3–4 days before the onset of menses. The middle panel reflects cyclic breast pain and the lower panel noncyclic pain. P, menses onset.

Key aspects of imaging studies	
Mammography	Useful for evaluation of suspicious palpable lesions, particularly in those over 35. Microcalcifications suggest cancer, when small, numerous, clustered, and linearly shaped. Dystrophic calcifications are larger, scattered and nonlinear and occur in the presence of fibrocystic disease but are not suspicious for cancer Repeat mammography in 6 months is recommended if the risk of cancer is felt to be less than 2%.
Ultrasonography	Ultrasound may be sufficient to diagnose fibroadenoma in women under 35 Ultrasonography in conjunction with mammography allows discrimination of solid from cystic lesions. Needle aspiration under ultrasound guidance further documents the cystic nature of the lesion and may provide evidence of suspicious cells lining its wall. If the risk is believed to be greater, core biopsy is recommended. Radiographically or ultrasonically directed core biopsy provides highly discriminative information regarding the presence or absence of malignancy.
Excisional biopsy	If core biopsy is not available, insertion of a wire into the lesion radiographically followed by surgical excision or mere removal of clearly palpable lesions is appropriate.
Magnetic resonance imaging and digital mammography	The exact role of these modalities in evaluating breast lesions is currently being determined.

Table 39.7 Key aspects of imaging studies.

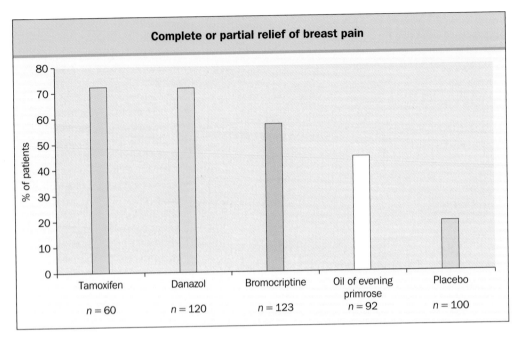

Complete or partial relief of breast pain

Tamoxifen n = 60
Danazol n = 120
Bromocriptine n = 123
Oil of evening primrose n = 92
Placebo n = 100

Figure 39.27 Complete or partial relief of breast pain. The graph shows clinically reported comparative responses to various hormonal therapies for breast pain. Only a limited number of controlled trials have compared one therapy with another. Consequently, the data in this figure represent comparative experience with danazol, oil of evening primrose, and bromocriptine in a large clinic using similar evaluative techniques and subjects for each agent. The data regarding tamoxifen come from another large clinic specializing in benign breast disorders and using similar evaluation methodology. (References to individual trials are contained in Santen RJ, Pinkerton JA. Benign breast disorders. In: DeGroot LJ, Jameson JL, Burger H, et al., eds. Endocrinology, 4th edn. Philadelphia, PA:WB Saunders; 2001:2189–98.)

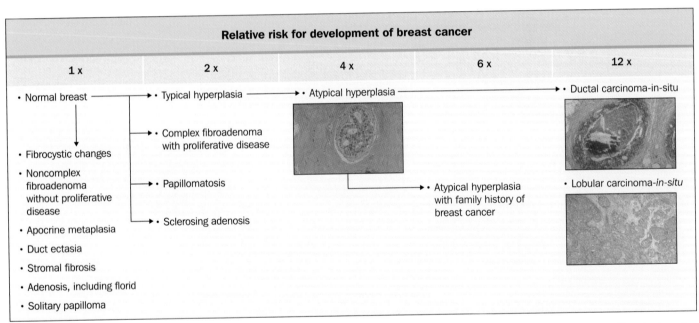

Relative risk for development of breast cancer

1 x — • Normal breast
2 x — • Typical hyperplasia
4 x — • Atypical hyperplasia
6 x
12 x — • Ductal carcinoma-in-situ

• Fibrocystic changes
• Noncomplex fibroadenoma without proliferative disease
• Apocrine metaplasia
• Duct ectasia
• Stromal fibrosis
• Adenosis, including florid
• Solitary papilloma

• Complex fibroadenoma with proliferative disease
• Papillomatosis
• Sclerosing adenosis

• Atypical hyperplasia with family history of breast cancer

• Lobular carcinoma-in-situ

Figure 39.28 Relative risk for development of breast cancer. The figure illustrates the relative risk for the subsequent development of invasive breast cancer in patients with various proliferative breast lesions and carcinoma-in-situ. Interestingly, with each of these lesions, the breast cancer that develops many years later usually involves a different area of the breast from the initial lesion.

and lifetime risk of developing breast cancer (**Fig. 39.31**). This model has recognized deficiencies in that it does not consider second-degree relatives with breast cancer, proliferative lesions of breast other than ADH, alcohol intake, obesity, or birth control pill and HRT use. Nonetheless, the Gail model has been prospectively validated in over 6000 women followed for an average of 4.5 years. It is used only in those without a personal history of breast cancer.

Women with more than a 1.7% chance of developing breast cancer over 5 years, as assessed by the Gail model, are considered for therapy with tamoxifen to prevent breast cancer. Factors favoring use of this agent include: older age; prior surgical removal of the uterus; no prior history of thromboembolic events such as deep vein thrombosis, pulmonary embolism, or CVA (cerebrovascular accident); no incipient cataract; and dense breast tissue on mammogram. For women with low bone density and a high risk of breast cancer, raloxifene may be considered as an agent that enhances bone density, reduces fracture rate, and, at the least, does not increase the risk of breast cancer. Women at substantial risk of breast cancer should be referred to a high-risk breast cancer clinic for followup and referral to a genetics clinic. Criteria for genetics clinic referral are included in **Table 39.8**.

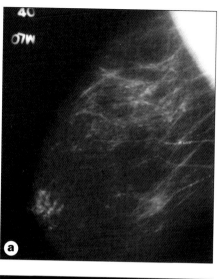

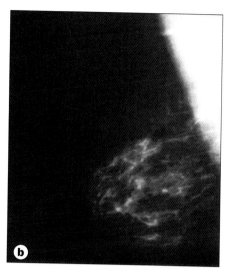

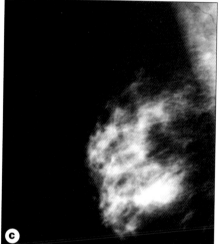

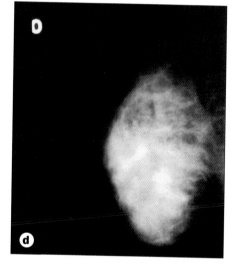

Figure 39.29 Mammographic density. The mammograms illustrate varying degrees of breast density according to the BIRADS (Breast Imaging Reporting and Data System) classification. (a) I: Predominantly fatty. (b) II: Scattered fibroglandular tissue; minimally dense. (c) III: Heterogeneously moderately dense. (d) IV: Extremely dense.

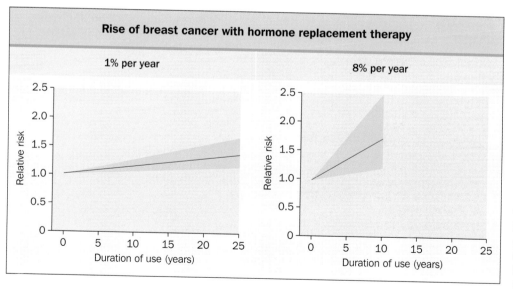

Figure 39.30 Risk of breast cancer with hormone replacement therapy. The graphs illustrate the relative risk of breast cancer with duration of use of estrogen alone (left panel) and estrogen plus a progestin (right panel). The solid line represents the mean and the shaded area the 95% confidence limits. Original data from Schairer C, Lubin J, Troisi R et al. Menopausal estrogen and estrogen–progestin replacement therapy and breast cancer risk. JAMA. 2000;283:485–91. (With permission from Santen RJ, Pinkerton J, McCartney C, Petroni GR. Risk of breast cancer with progestins in combination with estrogen as hormone replacement therapy. J Clin Endocrinol Metab. 2001;86:16–23 © The Endocrine Society.)

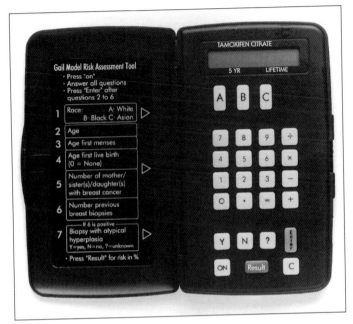

Criteria for referral to a genetics clinic

Family history of known *BRCA1* or *BRCA2* gene

Family history of breast and ovarian cancer

Two or more family members under age 50 with breast cancer

Family history of male breast cancer

One or more family members with breast cancer plus Ashkenazi Jewish ancestry

Ovarian cancer plus Ashkenazi Jewish ancestry

Table 39.8 Criteria for referral to a genetics clinic.

Figure 39.31 The Gail Model for estimating cancer risk. The photograph shows the hand-held calculator used to determine breast cancer risk based upon the model developed by Dr Mitchell Gail (the 'Gail Model'; Costantino JP, Gail MH, Pee D, et al. Validation studies for models projecting the risk of invasive and total breast cancer incidence. J Natl Cancer Inst. 1999;91:1541–8).

FURTHER READING

Ader DN, Browne MW. Prevalence and impact of cyclic mastalgia in a United States clinic-based sample. Am J Obstet Gynecol. 1997;177:126–32.

Boyd NF, Byng JW, Jong RA, et al. Quantitative classification of mammographic densities and breast cancer risk: results from the Canadian national breast screening study. J Natl Cancer Inst. 1995;87:670–5.

Bulun SE, Noble LS, Takayama K, et al. Endocrine disorders associated with inappropriately high aromatase expression. J Steroid Biochem Molec Biol. 1997;61:133–39.

Collaborative Group on Hormone Factors in Breast Cancer. Breast cancer and hormone replacement therapy: collaborative reanalysis of data from 51 epidemiological studies of 52,705 women with breast cancer and 108,411 women without breast cancer. Lancet. 1997;350:1047–59.

Dupont WD, Page DL. Relative risk of breast cancer varies with time since diagnosis of atypical hyperplasia. Hum Pathol. 1989;20:723–5.

Gateley CA, Miers M, Mansel RE, Hughes LE. Drug treatments for mastalgia: 17 years experience in the Cardiff mastalgia clinic. J Roy Soc Med. 1992;85:12–5.

Goehring C, Morabia A. Epidemiology of benign breast disease, with special attention to histologic types. Epidemiol Rev. 1997;19:310–27.

Hughes LE, Mansel RE, Webster DJT. Aberrations of normal development and involution (ANDI): a new perspective on pathogenesis and nomenclature of benign breast disorders. Lancet 1987;2:1316–9.

London SJ, Connolly JL, Schnitt SJ, Colditz GA. A prospective study of benign breast disease and the risk of breast cancer. JAMA. 1992;267:941–4.

O'Connell P, Pekkel V, Fuqua SA, Osborne CK, Clark GM, Allred DC. Analysis of loss of heterozygosity in 399 premalignant breast lesions at 15 genetic loci. J Natl Cancer Inst. 1998;90:697–703.

Russo J, Santen RJ, Russo IM. Hormonal control of breast development. In: DeGroot LJ, Jameson JL, Burger H, et al., eds. Endocrinology, 4th ed. Philadelphia, PA:WB Saunders; 2001:2181–8.

Santen RJ, Pinkerton JA. Benign breast disorders. In: DeGroot LJ, Jameson JL, Burger H, et al., eds. Endocrinology, 4th ed. Philadelphia, PA:WB Saunders; 2001a:2189–98.

Santen RJ. Gynecomastia. In: DeGroot LJ, Jameson JL, Burger H, et al., eds. Endocrinology, 4th ed. Philadelphia, PA:WB Saunders; 2001b:2335–43.

Santen RJ, Pinkerton J, McCartney C, Petroni GR. Risk of breast cancer with progestins in combination with estrogen as hormone replacement therapy. J Clin Endocrinol Metab. 2001;86:16–23.

Thompson DF, Carter JR. Drug induced gynecomastia. Pharmacotherapy 1993;13:37–45.

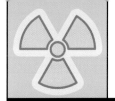

Section 8 Imaging

Chapter 40

Neuroradiology and Endocrine Disease

Todd Peebles and Victor M Haughton

INTRODUCTION

Magnetic resonance imaging (MR) has become the primary modality for imaging the pituitary and hypothalamus. Computerized tomography (CT) can be used in patients who have contraindications to the use of MR, such as a cardiac pacemaker, cochlear implants or ferromagnetic implants in the skull or the body, or marked claustrophobia. Positive-contrast cisternography and pneumoencephalography have now only historical interest.

Magnetic resonance imaging

Since its introduction, magnetic resonance imaging has had a major role in imaging the sella and hypothalamus. Its multiplanar capability and superior tissue contrast differentiation make it the preferred initial modality for patients with pituitary dysfunction or visual field defects.

Magnetic resonance images reflect the proton density and relaxation times, T1 and T2, of tissue. T1 depends on the time the protons take to regain their alignment with the magnetic field and T2 depends on the time the protons take to dephase. Contrast in an MR image is due to the T1 and T2 relaxation properties of tissue, the proton density of tissue, and the imaging parameters chosen for the study. Routinely, T1-weighted images are obtained before and after intravenous contrast administration of a gadolinium chelate (i.e. gadopentetate dimeglumine). T2-weighted images are obtained in studies of the sella when further delineation or characterization is felt necessary. For imaging the sella and hypothalamus, images are acquired in the coronal and sagittal planes predominantly.

Computerized tomography

Computerized tomography was considered for many years to be the standard for imaging the pituitary and hypothalamus because of its high resolution and potential for obtaining images in multiple planes with three-dimensional software programs. CT still provides the means to image the sella quickly and effectively.

Computerized tomography is indicated in patients who are unable to undergo an MR examination because of a cardiac pacemaker, claustrophobia, aneurysm clips that are not MR-compatible, dental devices, etc. In these patients, CT still provides excellent evaluation of the sellar region. CT also provides useful information about the osseous structure of the sphenoid bone, hemorrhage, and tumor calcifications in some cases. A lateral localizer image is used to select contiguous coronal images, with a slice thickness of about 1.5mm. Intravenous contrast medium (containing 30–40mg of iodine per milliliter) is administered immediately prior to the scan to improve the conspicuousness of the pituitary gland, infundibulum, and cavernous sinuses. Patients with a contrast allergy need to be premedicated with corticosteroids for 24 hours prior to the study.

ANATOMY

The pituitary rests in the sella turcica, a shallow impression in the posterior sphenoid (**Fig. 40.1**). The anterior pituitary (adenohypophysis), which accounts for about 75% of the gland when viewed in the sagittal plane, has the same intensity as gray matter on T1-weighted images. The posterior lobe appears as a

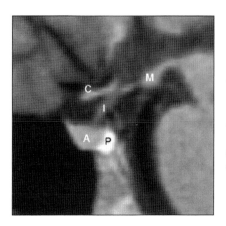

Figure 40.1 Normal pituitary fossa: magnetic resonance imaging. Unenhanced sagittal T1-weighted magnetic resonance image shows a normal anterior pituitary lobe (A), posterior sella 'bright spot' (P), infundibulum (I), optic chiasm (C), and mammillary bodies (M).

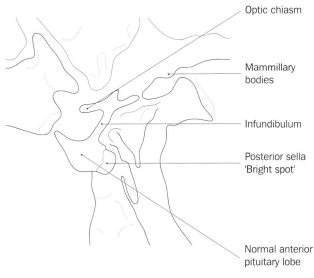

Optic chiasm

Mammillary bodies

Infundibulum

Posterior sella 'Bright spot'

Normal anterior pituitary lobe

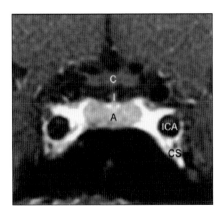

Figure 40.2 Normal sella: magnetic resonance imaging. Coronal T1-weighted magnetic resonance image following contrast administration. Normal anatomic structures include the anterior pituitary (A), cavernous sinus (CS), intracavernous carotid artery (ICA), infundibulum (I), and optic chiasm (C).

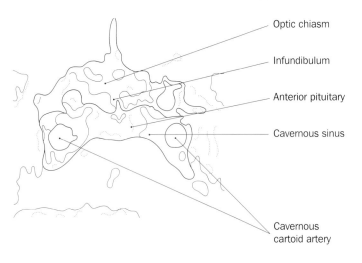

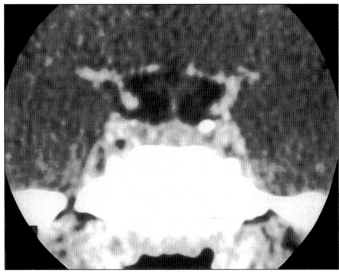

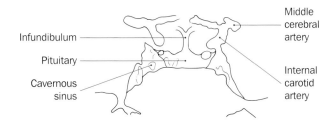

Figure 40.3 Normal sella: computerized tomography. Normal anatomic structures include the pituitary gland, infundibulum, optic chiasm, cavernous sinus, internal carotid artery, and middle cerebral artery.

'bright spot' on T1-weighted images. The source of this bright signal is phospholipids and/or hormones in the posterior gland (neurohypophysis) or tissue adjacent to the gland. The infundibulum can be seen extending from the tuber cinereum of the hypothalamus to the superior surface of the gland through the diaphragma sellae. It shows markedly increased signal intensity ('contrast enhancement') on the contrast-enhanced images because it lacks tight junctions in its capillary endothelium and has therefore no 'blood–brain barrier'. The tuber cinereum can be identified posterior to the optic chiasm and anterior to the mammillary bodies. The third ventricle lies in the midline immediately above the optic chiasm and the tuber cinereum (**Fig. 40.2**).

In the coronal plane (**Figs 40.1 & 40.3**), the sella is bordered laterally by the dural reflection of the cavernous sinuses. Cranial nerves III (oculomotor), IV (trochlear), and V2 (maxillary) course along the lateral wall of the cavernous sinus. Cranial nerve V1 (abducens) courses more medially along the sinus trabeculae. The pituitary stalk normally reaches the pituitary gland in the midline. However, the pituitary stalk has a paramidline insertion into the gland in up to 40% of the normal population. The gland usually measures 4–8mm in vertical dimension, with a flat or concave superior border. Mild superior glandular convexity may be seen at puberty or in lactating women (**Fig. 40.4**).

EMPTY SELLA

Defects in the diaphragma sellae may allow passage of cerebrospinal fluid (CSF) from the suprasellar cistern into the sella turcica. This condition, termed 'empty sella', is usually an incidental finding, although it may be found in patients with the constellation of headache, endocrine dysfunction, and visual disturbances. Empty sella may be simulated by an intra- or suprasellar cyst. These cysts, however, displace the infundibulum from its normal location, which an empty sella does not (**Fig. 40.5**).

ADENOMAS

The most common intrasellar tumor is the pituitary adenoma. They are classified as microadenomas if the maximum diameter is 10mm or less and macroadenomas if they are over 10mm in diameter. Microadenomas are usually associated with symptoms of excess hormone secretion (i.e. prolactin, adrenocorticotropic hormone, or growth hormone). Microadenomas are detected as regions of diminished contrast enhancement within the pituitary gland, usually to one side of the midline (**Fig. 40.6**). The gland may have a convex upper border and increased vertical dimension. It may appear as a region of diminished signal

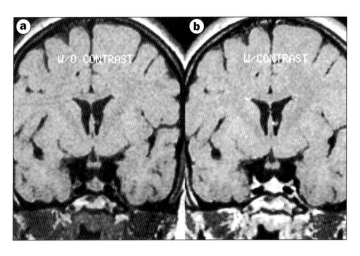

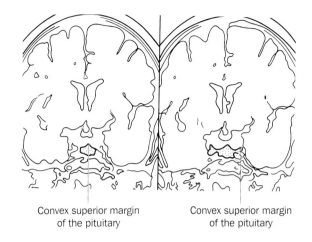

Convex superior margin of the pituitary   Convex superior margin of the pituitary

Figure 40.4 Normal anatomic variant: magnetic resonance imaging. T1-weighted coronal images of the sella before contrast administration (a) and after contrast administration (b), show a convex superior margin of the pituitary, a normal variant in adolescent and lactating women.

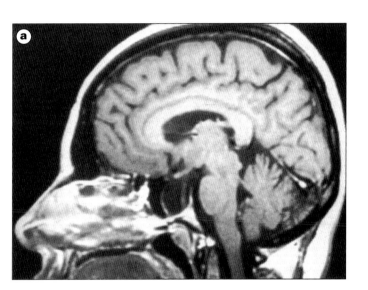

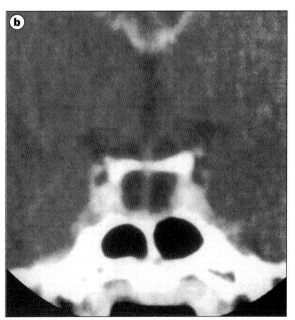

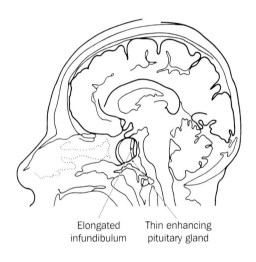

Elongated infundibulum   Thin enhancing pituitary gland

Elongated infundibulum

Pituitary

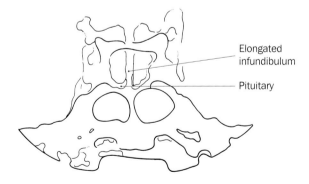

Figure 40.5 Empty sella. (a) Sagittal T1-weighted post-contrast magnetic resonance image showing a large 'empty sella' with an elongated infundibulum inserting into a thin, enhancing pituitary gland. (b) Coronal computerized tomography in a different patient showing insertion of the infundibulum into a thin pituitary.

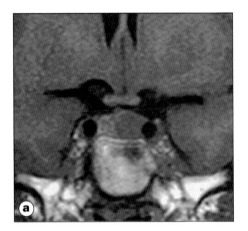

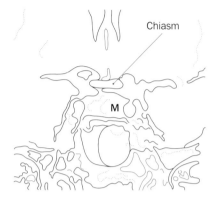

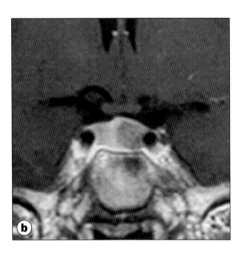

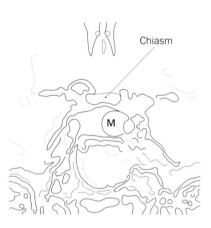

Figure 40.6 Microadenoma. (a) T1-weighted coronal unenhanced magnetic resonance image showing a hypointense microadenoma (M) in the left side of the pituitary. The mass causes a convex superior margin of the gland and displacement of the infundibulum to the right. (b) Contrast-enhanced coronal T1-weighted image in the same patient shows the microadenoma (M) enhancing less intensely than surrounding anterior pituitary.

intensity compared with the normal pituitary on T1-weighted images. Uncommonly, they may have increased signal intensity on the T1-weighted images because of the presence of blood or other T1-shortening substances within them. On T2-weighted images, if they are obtained, they typically have increased signal intensity.

Microadenomas must be differentiated from small incidental cysts in the pars intermedia. These cysts have low signal intensity on T1-weighted images, high signal intensity on T2-weighted images, but no enhancement after intravenous contrast medium.

The timing of the enhanced scan is critical for the detection of the microadenoma. The adenoma increases in signal intensity more slowly than the adjacent gland after the administration of intravenous contrast medium, but when the enhancement of the sinus plateaus, at about 5min after injection, the contrast between the gland and the adenoma diminishes. For about 5min after the administration of contrast medium, the microadenoma has diminished signal intensity compared to the gland but after 5min the contrast begins to diminish and eventually a 'crossover' point occurs when enhancement of the normal gland and microadenoma are equal. Thirty minutes or more after the administration of the contrast medium, a microadenoma may appear hyperintense to the normal adjacent gland (**Fig. 40.7**).

Macroadenomas usually present clinically with signs and symptoms associated with the displacement of the optic chiasm, cavernous sinus, and hypothalamus. These tumors may, like microadenomas, have homogeneous low intensity on T1-weighted images and homogenous enhancement after contrast administration that is less intense than the enhancement in the adjacent pituitary gland (**Fig. 40.8**). Macroadenomas may be heterogeneous in appearance as a result of necrosis, cystic degeneration, or hemorrhage. Necrotic areas appear as regions of lower signal than the surrounding tumor on T1-weighted images. Areas that progress to cystic degeneration have a signal that is similar to CSF (i.e. low on T1-weighted images and high on T2-weighted images; **Fig. 40.9**). Hemorrhage in the subacute or the chronic phase appears as a region of increased signal intensity on T1-weighted images or diminished signal intensity on T2-weighted images within the tumor. Acute hemorrhage (less than 3 days of age) in these tumors may only be detected on CT as regions of high density. Macroadenomas may be inhomogeneous (**Fig. 40.12**) because of hemorrhage, necrosis, liquefaction, and sedimentation of heavy molecules within cavities. The occasional calcifications within pituitary adenomas are sometimes identified as regions of low signal intensity on MR and more often as regions of high density on CT.

Extrasellar extension of a macroadenoma has important clinical and surgical implications. Suprasellar extension may produce a tumor with a 'waist' caused by compression by the diaphragma sellae (**Fig. 40.10(a)**). The tumor may extend inferiorly to invade

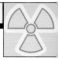

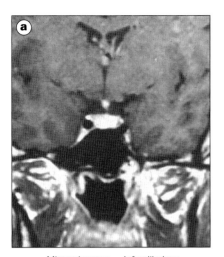

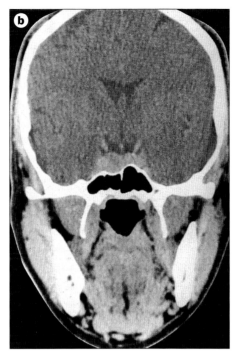

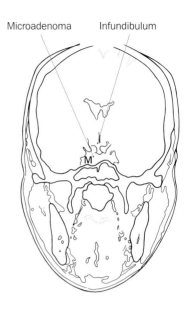

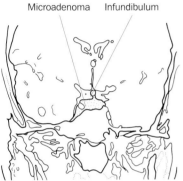

Microadenoma   Infundibulum

Figure 40.7 Enhancing microadenoma: magnetic resonance imaging. (a) Contrast-enhanced T1-weighted coronal magnetic resonance image showing a microadenoma in the right side of the pituitary. The infundibulum is displaced to the left. (b) Coronal computerized tomography in a different patient with a microadenoma in the right side of the pituitary displacing the infundibulum to the left.

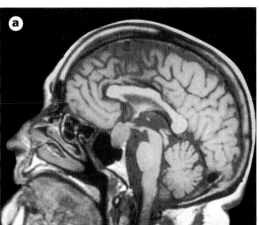

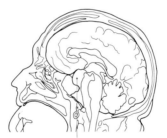

Large sellar/suprasellar macroadenoma

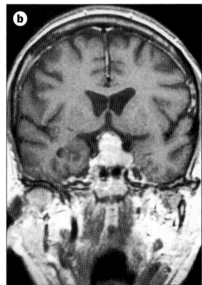

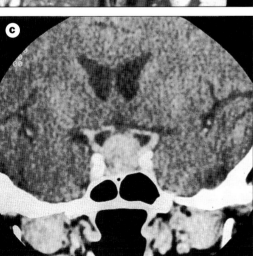

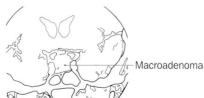

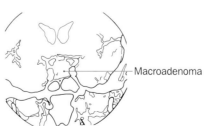

Macroadenoma

Displaced optic chiasm

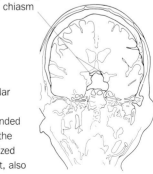

Figure 40.8 Macroadenoma. (a) Sagittal T1-weighted magnetic resonance image showing a large sellar/suprasellar macroadenoma. (b) Coronal image following contrast administration shows a diffuse homogeneous mass surrounded by enhancing pituitary gland with upward displacement of the optic chiasm more clearly identified. (c) Coronal computerized tomography scan of a macroadenoma in a different patient, also demonstrating diffuse homogeneous density.

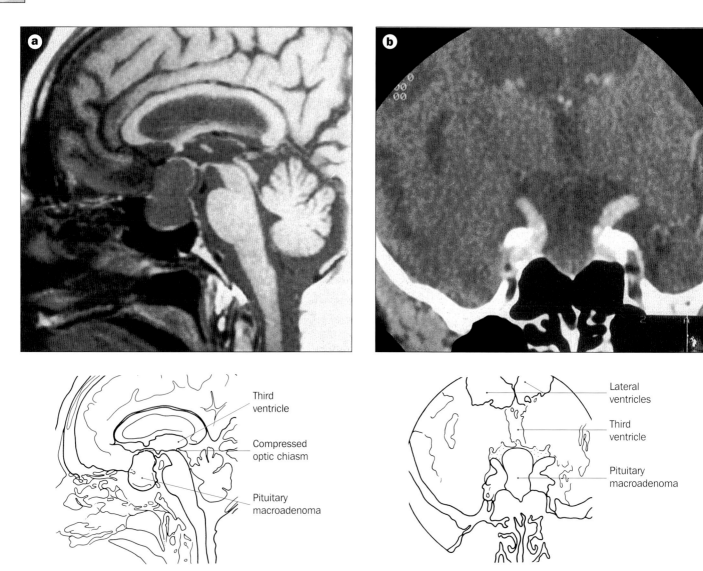

Figure 40.9 Cystic macroadenoma. (a) Sagittal T1-weighted magnetic resonance image showing a large pituitary macroadenoma with suprasellar extension, compressing the optic chiasm. The low-signal-intensity region within the mass, similar in intensity to cerebrospinal fluid (CSF) in the third ventricle, is a fluid-containing cyst. (b) A coronal computerized tomography scan in the same patient shows the mass to have low density, like the CSF in the lateral ventricles and third ventricle.

the sphenoid sinus. CT may show erosion of the sella floor; MR may identify the tumor mass within the sinus. Extension of the tumor into the cavernous sinus may be difficult to evaluate with CT or MR. Encasement of the carotid artery and distortion of the lateral margins of the cavernous sinus are the most reliable signs (**Fig. 40.10 (b–d)**).

Pituitary infarction

Postpartum pituitary hemorrhagic infarction may lead to hypopituitarism (Sheehan's syndrome). In the acute phase, T1-weighted MR images show a high signal intensity within the pituitary gland, suggesting the presence of hemorrhage. The gland rapidly diminishes in size until the sella has the appearance of the empty sella. On CT, the pituitary gland in a patient with Sheehan's syndrome may show high density, indicating the presence of clotted blood (**Fig. 40.11**).

Pituitary apoplexy

Hemorrhage into pituitary adenomas is easily recognized in MR as cavitations within the gland that contains evidence of a paramagnetic effect due to deoxyhemoglobin or methemoglobin. The hemorrhage results in a characteristic high signal intensity on T1-weighted images and/or low signal intensity on T2-weighted images (**Fig. 40.12**). Clinically, the syndrome is manifested by the triad of sudden headache, hypotension, and visual disturbance.

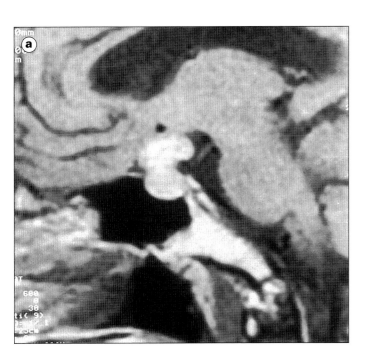

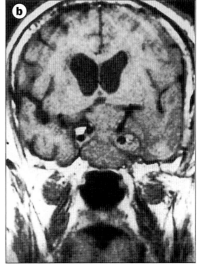

Suprasellar extension
of macroadenoma

Left cavernous
sinus extension of
macroadenoma

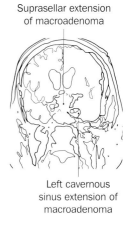

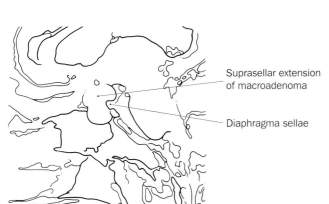

Suprasellar extension
of macroadenoma

Diaphragma sellae

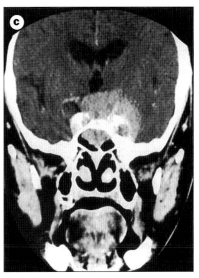

Suprasellar
extension

Cavernous
sinus extension
of macroadenoma

Sphenoid sinus
extension of
macroadenoma

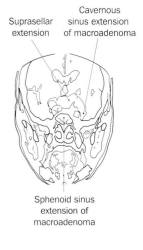

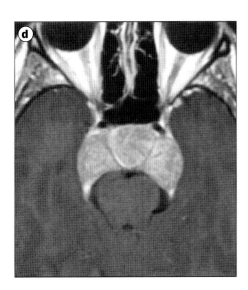

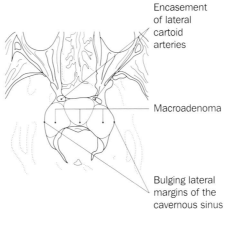

Encasement
of lateral
cartoid
arteries

Macroadenoma

Bulging lateral
margins of the
cavernous sinus

Figure 40.10 Extrasellar extension of macroadenomas. (a) Sagittal T1-weighted magnetic resonance image showing suprasellar extension with a 'waist' caused by the diaphragma sellae. (b) Coronal T1-weighted magnetic resonance image demonstrating suprasellar and left cavernous sinus extension, encasing the left cavernous carotid artery. (c) Coronal computerized tomography image showing suprasellar, cavernous sinus, and sphenoid sinus extension. (d) Axial T1-weighted magnetic resonance image showing bilateral cavernous sinus extension of an enhancing macroadenoma causing encasement of the internal carotid arteries and bulging of the lateral margins of the cavernous sinus.

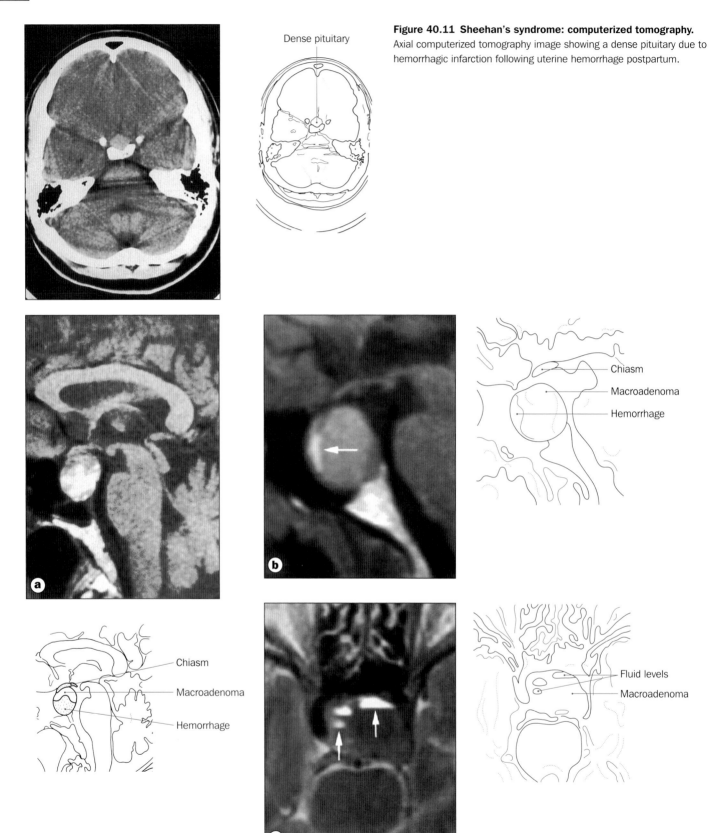

Dense pituitary

Figure 40.11 Sheehan's syndrome: computerized tomography. Axial computerized tomography image showing a dense pituitary due to hemorrhagic infarction following uterine hemorrhage postpartum.

Chiasm
Macroadenoma
Hemorrhage

Chiasm
Macroadenoma
Hemorrhage

Fluid levels
Macroadenoma

Figure 40.12 Pituitary apoplexy: magnetic resonance imaging. (a) T1-weighted sagittal magnetic resonance image showing hemorrhage in a macroadenoma which compresses the optic chiasm. (b) Sagittal T1-weighted magnetic resonance image and (c) axial T2-weighted image in a different patient with sudden onset of headache and hypotension show fluid level (arrows) within a macroadenoma, due to layering of fluid and blood products, which contain methemoglobin from recent hemorrhage into the macroadenoma.

MENINGIOMA

Meningiomas are the second most common tumor in the sellar region. These tumors may arise from dural surfaces such as the diaphragma sellae, tuberculum sellae, or cavernous sinuses. They may project into the suprasellar space and rarely arise within the sella. Meningiomas are usually isointense with gray matter on T1- and T2-weighted images and show dense uniform enhancement following contrast administration. Differentiation from an adenoma with suprasellar extension may be difficult. Imaging findings that may help distinguish meningioma from adenoma include the presence of a thickened dura in the region of the meningioma ('dural tail sign'), bony hyperostosis adjacent to the lesion, and normal sellar dimensions (**Fig. 40.13**). When meningiomas involve the cavernous sinus they frequently cause encasement and narrowing of the internal carotid artery. Coronal images are also very helpful in distinguishing the purely suprasellar location of the meningioma from the intrasellar and suprasellar location of the adenoma. Angiography shows more vascularity and staining in a meningioma than in a pituitary adenoma.

ANEURYSMS

Magnetic resonance imaging usually shows a characteristic 'signal void' in aneurysms of the intracavernous or supraclinoid carotid artery. The signal void is often associated with regions of high signal intensity on T1-weighted images suggesting blood, regions with signal intensity similar to brain tissue suggesting the presence of thrombus, and low-signal regions due to calcification. They appear as dense sellar or juxtasellar masses on CT imaging, with enhancement following contrast administration. Additional MR imaging features that may aid in distinguishing these lesions from parasellar tumors include flow-related artifacts in the phase-encoding direction of the MR image. MR angiography and CT angiography are additional techniques that can be used to characterize and identify aneurysms (**Figs 40.14 & 40.15**).

GLIOMAS

Gliomas occurring in the sellar region primarily involve the hypothalamus and optic chiasm. Hypothalamic gliomas, which typically are tumors of childhood and adolescence, usually involve the chiasm and/or optic nerve and may extend into the suprasellar cistern. Gliomas of the optic chiasm or nerves have a strong association with neurofibromatosis type I in children. They appear as sharply marginated homogeneous suprasellar masses, clearly separate from the pituitary gland. They are also usually hypointense or isointense with gray matter and may or may not enhance (**Fig. 40.16**).

CHORDOMAS

Chordomas are neoplasms that develop from intraosseous vestigial remnants of the notochord. About 15% of chordomas involve the clivus, from which they may project into the sellar or suprasellar regions. MR and CT techniques are both important in the differential diagnosis of these tumors. MR imaging best shows tumor infiltration and tumor origin in the clivus. The characteristic tumoral calcifications are better identified with CT imaging than with MR. These tumors are often slightly hypointense on T1-weighted MR images and intensely enhanced following contrast administration (**Fig. 40.17**). Chondrosarcomas of the clivus may have an identical appearance on CT and MR studies.

HYPOTHALAMIC HAMARTOMA

Hypothalamic hamartoma is a slowly growing congenital lesion that arises in the region of the tuber cinereum. Patients most commonly present during early childhood with signs of precocious puberty or with epileptic seizures and hyperactivity. Hypothalamic hamartomas are not neoplastic but are composed of disorganized neural tissue. This composition is reflected in the MR imaging appearance, which typically shows a sessile mass isointense to gray matter on T1-weighted images and isointense or slightly hyperintense on T2-weighted images. Hypothalamic hamartomas do not demonstrate enhancement with intravenous contrast medium administration (**Fig. 40.18**). Computerized tomography may be insensitive for detecting these small lesions. Hamartomas of the hypothalamus are most often treated medically but surgical resection may be curative in the setting of intractable seizures.

ARACHNOID CYST

Intracranial arachnoid cysts are a common incidental finding on brain CT or MR imaging. They occur most commonly in the middle cranial fossa and less commonly in the suprasellar cistern The membrane of Lillequist, a diaphanous structure that separates the interpeduncular and chiasmatic cisterns, normally transmits flow of CSF. When the membrane fails to transmit CSF, either because it is congenitally imperforate or because it becomes obstructed, then an upwardly directed diverticulum forms as the result of the pressure on the membrane. This is the cause of the arachnoid cysts in the suprasellar region. They may compress the optic chiasm, hypothalamus, or third ventricle. On MR images these lesions have the signal intensity of CSF in all pulse sequences, including diffusion-weighted images (DWI) and fluid attenuating inversion recovery (FLAIR). They are detected because of their effect on the brainstem rather than because of their signal characteristics. DWI may be useful to distinguish arachnoid cysts from epidermoid cysts, which have much higher signal intensity than CSF on DWI. The arachnoid cysts do not show enhancement with contrast medium administration (**Fig. 40.19**). On axial images suprasellar arachnoid cysts may be misinterpreted as enlargement of the third ventricle.

ECTOPIC POSTERIOR PITUITARY BRIGHT SPOT

A high signal intensity in the posterior pituitary gland is a normal finding in 90% of normal children and most adults. The variability of this finding in normal subjects may reflect variation in their state of hydration. The presence and absence of the posterior sellar bright spot may have some diagnostic significance. It may be found in an ectopic location. An ectopic bright spot, thought to have a developmental cause, is frequently associated with short stature due to growth hormone deficiency or multiple

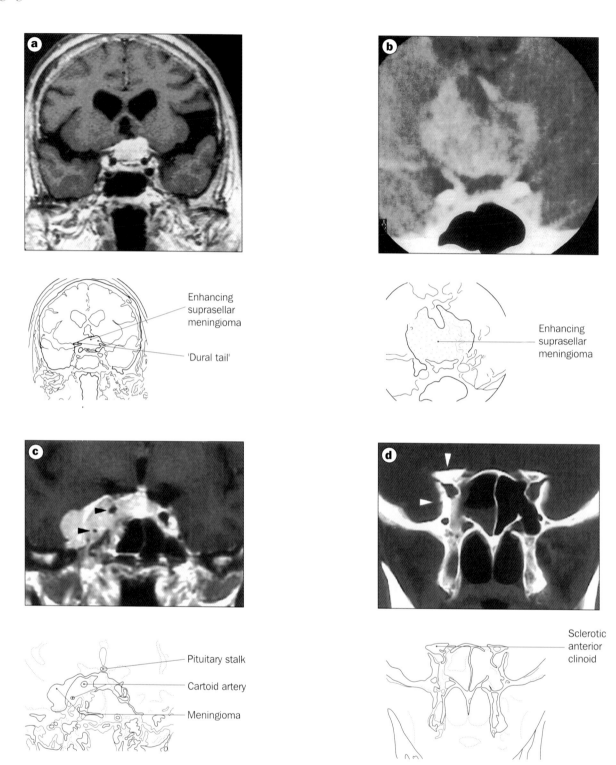

Figure 40.13 Meningioma. (a) Contrast-enhanced, T1-weighted coronal magnetic resonance image demonstrating an enhancing suprasellar meningioma with adjacent 'dural tail'. (b) Coronal computerized tomography image in a different patient also demonstrating an enhancing suprasellar meningioma. (c) Coronal T1-weighted magnetic resonance in a third patient shows a uniformly enhancing meningioma arising in the cavernous sinus, encasing and narrowing the internal carotid artery (arrowheads), with invasion into the sella and sphenoid sinus. (d) Coronal computerized tomography scan of the same patient shows hyperostosis of the right lateral sphenoid sinus wall and anterior clinoid process (arrowheads).

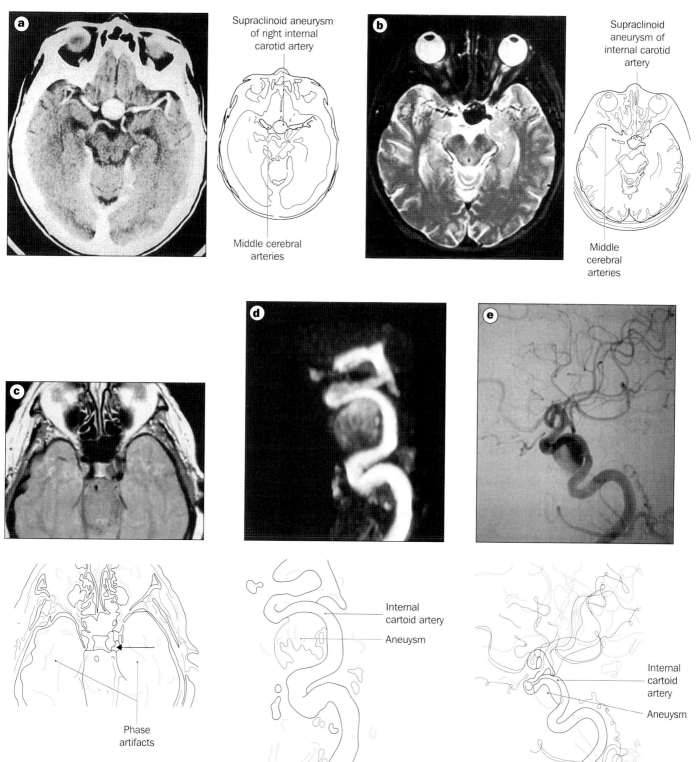

Figure 40.14 Parasellar aneurysms. A supraclinoid aneurysm of the right internal carotid artery is shown in an enhanced computerized tomography image (a) as a densely enhancing circumscribed structure and in a T2-weighted magnetic resonance image (b) as a black void ('flow void') within the aneurysm sac. (c) An axial proton-density-weighted scan in a different patient shows a phase-encoding artifact (arrowheads) related to flow within a left cavernous segment internal carotid artery aneurysm. (d) Lateral oblique magnetic resonance angiogram and (e) digital subtraction angiogram show the cavernous carotid aneurysm.

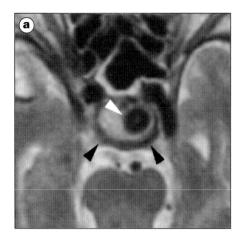

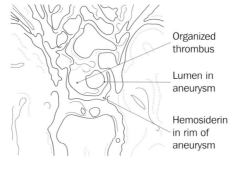

Organized
thrombus

Lumen in
aneurysm

Hemosiderin
in rim of
aneurysm

Figure 40.15 Intrasellar aneurysm.
(a) Axial T2-weighted image showing an
intrasellar mass with hemosiderin-ladened
rim (black arrowheads) and eccentric flow
void (white arrowhead). (b) Sagittal T1-
weighted image without contrast showing
laminated high-signal-intensity mural
thrombus within the aneurysm sac.

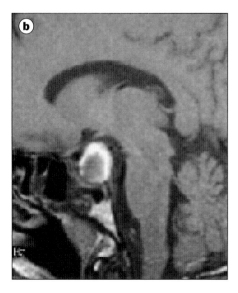

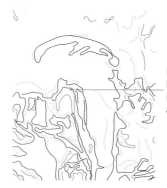

Paramagnetic
blood products
in rim of
aneurysm

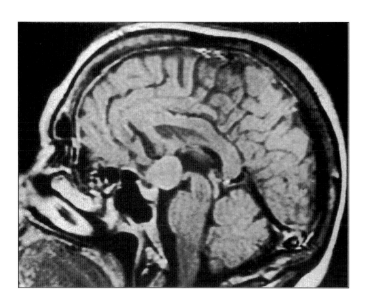

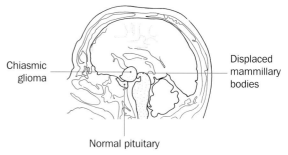

Chiasmic
glioma

Displaced
mammillary
bodies

Normal pituitary

Figure 40.16 Chiasmal glioma: magnetic resonance imaging.
T1-weighted sagittal magnetic resonance image shows a chiasmal glioma
displacing the mammillary bodies posteriorly. Note the normal pituitary
gland.

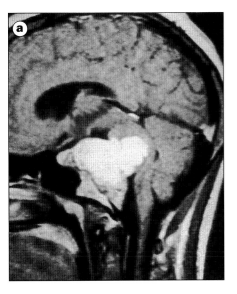

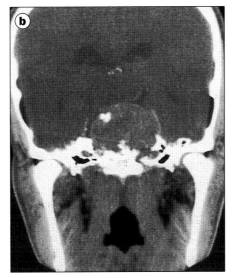

Figure 40.17 Clival chordoma. (a) Contrast-enhanced T1-weighted sagittal magnetic resonance image showing an intensely enhancing large clival chordoma. The tumor compresses and displaces the pons posteriorly. (b) Coronal computerized tomography image in the same patient demonstrates globular calcification within the mass and bone destruction within the clivus.

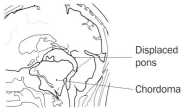

Displaced pons

Chordoma

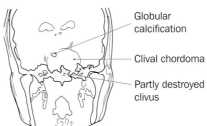

Globular calcification

Clival chordoma

Partly destroyed clivus

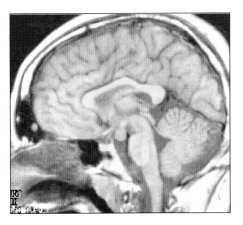

Figure 40.18 Hypothalamic hamartoma. Sagittal postcontrast T1-weighted image shows a sessile nonenhancing mass arising from the tuber cinereum, which is isointense to adjacent brain parenchyma.

pituitary hormone deficiencies. The characteristic MR imaging appearance is an intrinsically bright T1 focus located in the median eminence of the hypothalamus with a small sella turcica, small pituitary gland, and small or absent infundibulum (**Fig. 40.20**). Patients with the full spectrum of findings are more likely to have multiple pituitary hormone deficiencies. An ectopic bright spot may be acquired secondary to traumatic stalk transection, surgical resection of the neurohypophysis, or compression of the neurohypophysis by a pituitary tumor.

CYSTIC EPITHELIAL LESIONS

Epidermoid and dermoid tumors together with craniopharyngioma and Rathke cleft cysts are proposed to be part a single spectrum of intracranial cystic epithelial lesions. This proposal is based on overlapping histologic appearances and embryologic data that support a common ectodermal origin of these lesions.

Epidermoid and dermoid tumors

Epidermoid and dermoid tumors are slowly growing lesions that infiltrate surrounding neurovascular structures. These lesions cause symptoms because of local mass effect on the optic chiasm, cranial nerves, or the hypothalamus and third ventricle. Symptoms of meningism may be associated with rupture of a dermoid cyst. Epidermoid tumors are composed primarily of keratinaceous material and cholesterol, which is produced by a stratified squamous epithelial cyst lining. In contrast, dermoid tumors contain dermal elements that produce lipid contents. Dystrophic calcification is a frequent finding in both tumors.

On MR images epidermoid tumors tend to be isointense to slightly hyperintense to CSF on conventional T1, T2, and proton-density pulse sequences, making distinction from arachnoid cyst difficult. However, the FLAIR and diffusion-weighted sequences show the epidermoid tumors to have high signal intensity, while

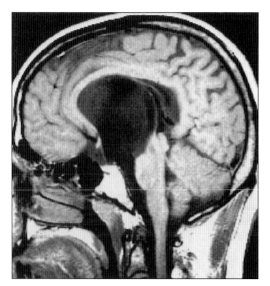

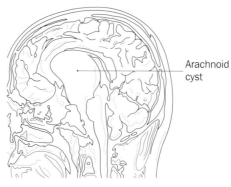

Figure 40.19 Arachnoid cyst. Unenhanced sagittal T1-weighted image showing a large suprasellar cyst with fluid signal intensity compressing the third ventricle and midbrain.

Arachnoid cyst

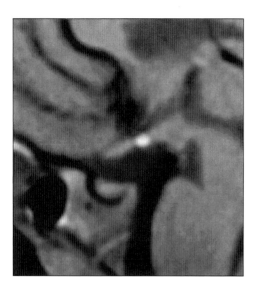

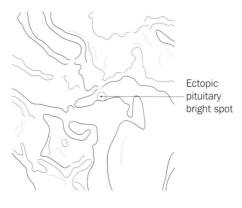

Figure 40.20 Congenital ectopic posterior pituitary bright spot. Sagittal T1-weighted image shows an ectopically located posterior pituitary bright spot in the floor of the third ventricle. Note absence of the normal pituitary bright spot, infundibulum, and diminutive size of the sella turcica.

Ectopic pituitary bright spot

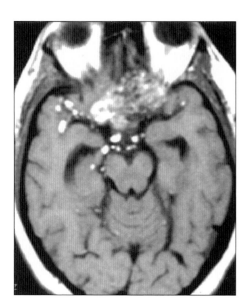

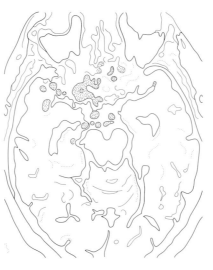

Figure 40.21 Ruptured suprasellar dermoid tumor. Axial T1-weighted image without contrast shows a heterogeneous suprasellar mass. Note numerous globules of high-intensity material representing lipid contents in the cyst and extruded into the subarachnoid space (shown by dark shading in line drawing).

the arachnoid cyst does not. Dermoid tumors appear as heterogeneous circumscribed lesions containing high T1 signal intensity on precontrast images because of their lipid content. Because calcification appears as a signal void in MR, MR is less sensitive than CT for its detection within these lesions (**Fig. 40.21**).

Rathke cleft cyst

Rathke cleft cyst is a cystic epithelial lesion that may arise anywhere along the course of the craniopharyngeal duct, the pathway of ascent of Rathke's pouch from the posterior nasopharynx to the floor of the third ventricle. The intrasellar Rathke's pouch cyst characteristically occurs in the pars intermedia. When located in the suprasellar region, Rathke cysts are seen anterior to the infundibulum. These nonneoplastic lesions are fairly common findings in unselected autopsy populations and are usually discovered incidentally on brain imaging studies performed for other indications. Rarely, Rathke cysts may cause symptoms because of compression of the optic chiasm, pituitary gland, or third ventricle, in which case they may be clinically indistinguishable from other parasellar mass lesions. The cyst is composed of a thin epithelial lining and typically contains serous or mucoid fluid. The cysts are well circumscribed, round to oval lesions with a thin or imperceptible wall and show no enhancement with contrast.

Owing to the variable protein content of the cyst fluid, the MR signal intensity of Rathke cysts may vary greatly. Serous-fluid-containing cysts follow CSF signal intensity on T1- and T2-weighted pulse sequences. Proteinaceous contents may be intrinsically bright on T1- and low-signal on T2-weighted scans (**Fig. 40.22**). There may be significant overlap of imaging findings with other lesions such as craniopharyngioma, which may decrease the specificity of imaging findings. However, some Rathke cysts contain a nonenhancing intracystic proteinaceous nodule that is thought to be indicative of the diagnosis.

Craniopharyngioma

Craniopharyngiomas are usually benign neoplasms that may arise from epithelial remnants of Rathke's pouch. They are the most frequent neoplasm in the sellar region in children and young adults. A second peak also occurs in adults at around

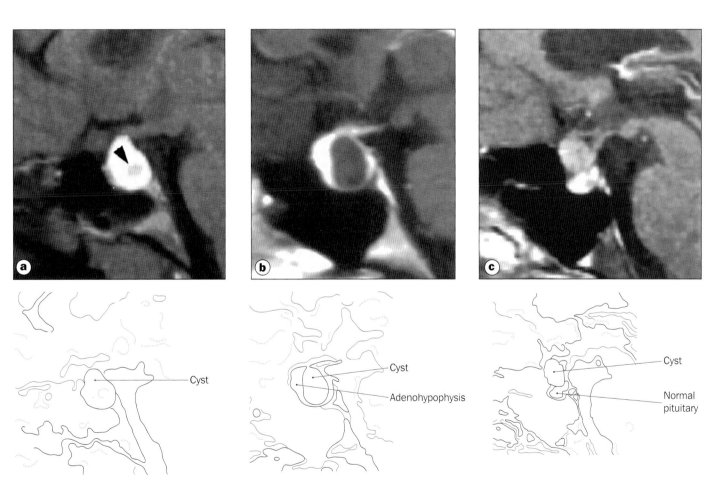

Figure 40.22 Rathke cleft cyst: various MR imaging appearances in three patients. (a) Sagittal T1-weighted unenhanced image showing a high-signal-intensity intrasellar mass with a small intracystic nodule (arrowhead). Intracystic nodules are thought to be specific for the diagnosis of Rathke cyst. (b) A sagittal T1-weighted image with contrast shows a low-signal-intensity cyst in the pars intermedia displacing the normally enhancing adenohypophysis anteriorly and the neurohypophysis posteriorly. (c) A sagittal T1-weighted image with contrast shows an entirely suprasellar high-signal-intensity Rathke cyst.

the fifth decade. These tumors usually arise in the suprasellar region; however, they may be both suprasellar and intrasellar, or entirely intrasellar. Craniopharyngiomas are heterogeneous in appearance, often containing cysts and globular calcification (**Fig. 40.23**). The cystic portions of the mass may appear hypointense on T1-weighted MR images, and hyperintense on T2-weighted images. Craniopharyngiomas may also exhibit both iso- and hyperintense components. The solid portions of the mass, and the periphery of the cystic components often enhance following contrast administration.

Magnetic resonance imaging best shows the anatomic relationship of the mass and the pituitary gland and therefore helps to differentiate the mass from an adenoma. The calcification that occurs in about half of craniopharyngiomas and is best detected on CT may be useful in its differentiation from other masses. Less commonly, these tumors may appear entirely solid or demonstrate ring calcification surrounding a cystic component (**Fig. 40.24**).

METASTASES TO THE PITUITARY GLAND

Symptomatic metastases to the pituitary–hypothalamic axis are rare. Symptoms are usually manifest by diabetes insipidus or panhypopituitarism. Breast and lung carcinoma are the commonest tumors to metastasize to the pituitary gland. Because of the direct arterial supply of the hypothalamus and

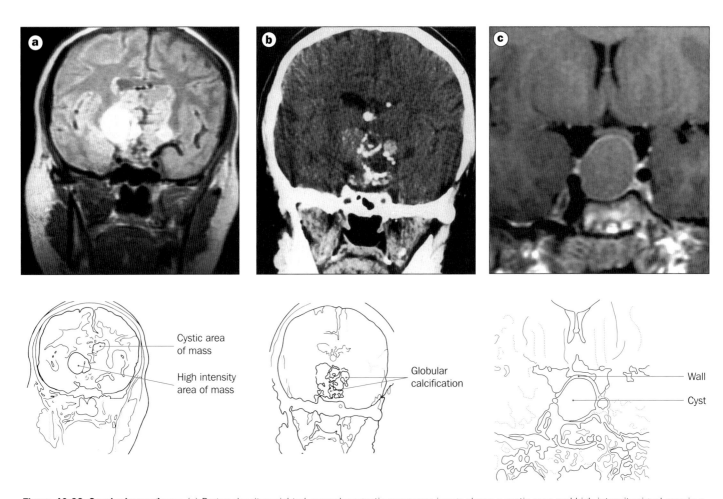

Figure 40.23 Craniopharyngioma. (a) Proton-density-weighted coronal magnetic resonance image shows a cystic area and high-intensity-signal area in a large sellar/suprasellar mass, typical of craniopharyngiomas. Characteristic globular calcification is easier to identify on a coronal computerized tomography image (b) of the same patient. (c) Coronal T1-weighted image of a different patient shows an intrasellar craniopharyngioma with a cyst that has intermediate-signal-intensity contents and a wall that enhances with intravenous contrast medium.

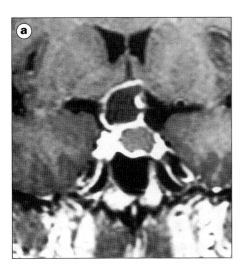

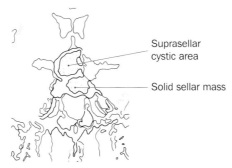

Suprasellar cystic area

Solid sellar mass

Figure 40.24 Atypical craniopharyngioma.
(a) Coronal T1-weighted magnetic resonance image following contrast administration shows enhancement of a solid sellar mass with a ring-enhancing suprasellar cystic component.
(b) An axial computerized tomography image of the same patient shows a ring of calcification around the cystic portion of the mass.

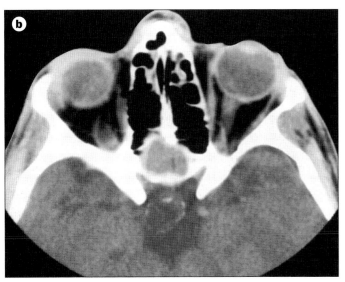

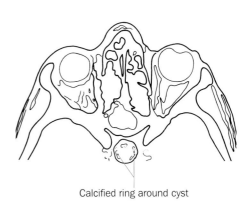

Calcified ring around cyst

neurohypophysis by the superior and inferior hypophysial vessels, hematogenous metastases occur more commonly in the floor of the third ventricle and neural lobe and less often in the adenohypophysis, which is supplied by a rete mirabile of the hypophysial portal system. Other intracranial tumors, such as germ cell neoplasms and primitive neuroectodermal tumors, have a propensity for spread via the CSF, which may also result in metastases to the hypothalamic–pituitary axis (**Fig. 40.25**).

INFLAMMATORY DISEASE

Tuberculosis and sarcoidosis may involve the CNS, producing suprasellar masses or thickening of the infundibulum or optic chiasm. These granulomatous lesions are usually isointense with gray matter on T1-weighted MR images. Enhancement of the parenchymal lesions, as well as leptomeningeal enhancement, is seen following contrast administration (**Fig. 40.26**). Other causes of infundibular thickening include lymphoma, metastatic carcinoma, and Langerhans cell histiocytosis (histiocytosis X; **Fig. 40.27**).

EXOPHTHALMOS

There are many causes of exophthalmos; however, the majority of cases in adults are due to Graves' disease. MR provides optimal imaging of the orbits, with coronal and axial planes obtained with the patient's head in the neutral position. CT can also be used for orbital imaging by using thin slices (3mm) in the axial and direct coronal planes.

The most common presentation is bilateral and symmetric ocular muscle enlargement with preference for the inferior and medial rectus. Bilateral asymmetric and occasionally unilateral involvement can also occur (**Fig. 40.28**). Idiopathic inflammation or 'inflammatory pseudotumor' is another frequent cause of exophthalmos, which often causes ocular muscle enlargement. Involvement is usually unilateral and tends to involve the muscles' tendinous insertion into the globe or may even present as an orbital mass. Other causes for exophthalmos are usually unilateral and include benign and malignant tumors (**Fig. 40.29**), vascular malformations, carotid–cavernous fistula, or cavernous sinus thrombosis.

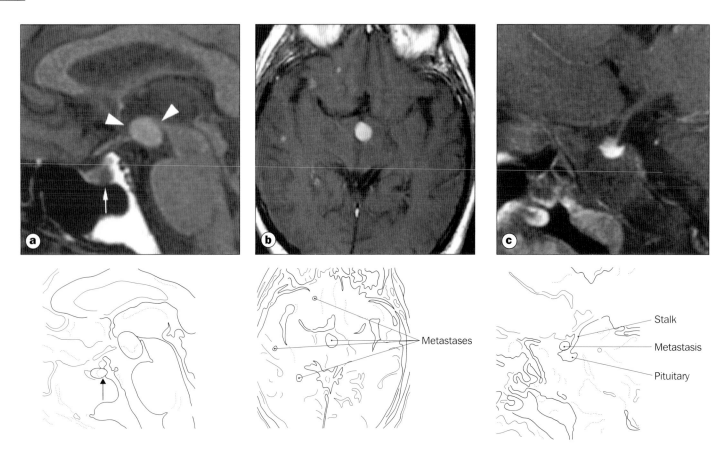

Figure 40.25 Metastasis to the hypothalamus. (a) Sagittal T1-weighted unenhanced image shows a circumscribed intrinsically bright mass in the floor of the third ventricle that proved to be a hematogenous melanoma metastasis (arrowheads). An incidental pars intermedia cyst is also seen (arrow). (b) An axial enhanced T1-weighted image of the same patient shows enhancement of the hypothalamic lesion and several additional punctate hematogenous metastases. (c) Parasagittal T1-weighted scan with contrast of a different patient showing an enhancing mass superior to the adenohypophysis and anterior to the infundibulum representing a metastatic deposit from germ cell tumor spread via the cerebrospinal fluid.

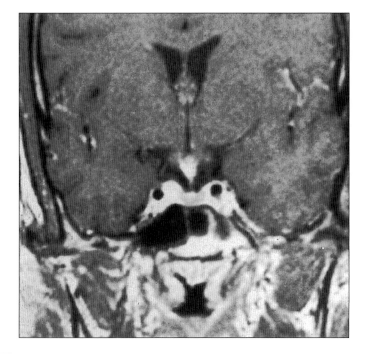

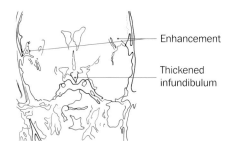

Figure 40.26 Sarcoidosis: magnetic resonance imaging. Coronal T1-weighted image following contrast administration shows a thickened, enhancing infundibulum typical of granulomatous disease. Enhancement in the sylvian fissure on the left and near the inner table on the right identifies leptomeningeal involvement.

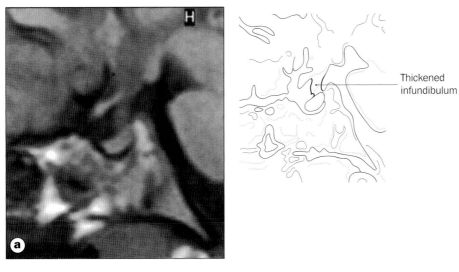

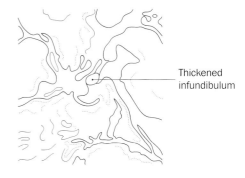

Figure 40.27 Langerhans cell histiocytosis: magnetic resonance imaging. Sagittal T1-weighted (a) non-enhanced and (b) enhanced magnetic resonance images showing a thickened enhancing infundibulum from known histiocytosis.

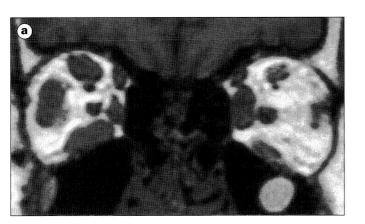

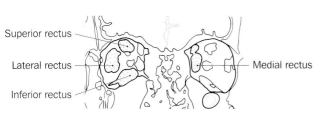

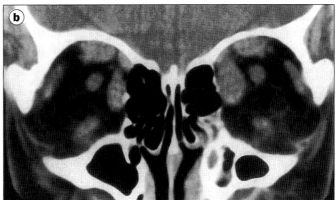

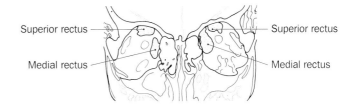

Figure 40.28 Graves' ophthalmopathy. (a) Coronal T1-weighted magnetic resonance image showing extraocular muscle enlargement of the superior rectus, lateral rectus, and inferior rectus of the right orbit. Enlargement of the medial rectus in the left orbit is also present. (b) Coronal computerized tomography in a different patient with enlargement of the medial rectus and superior rectus of both orbits.

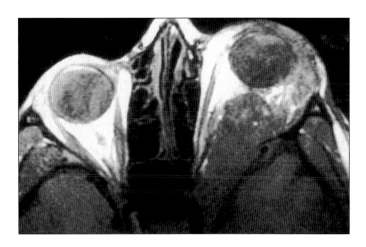

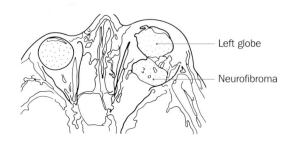

Figure 40.29 Neurofibroma: magnetic resonance imaging. Large neurofibroma of the left orbit causing exophthalmos of the left globe.

FURTHER READING

Boyko OB, Curnes JT, Oakes WJ, Burger PC. Hamartomas of the tuber cinereum: CT, MR and pathologic findings. Am J Neuroradiol. 1991;12:309–14.

Byun WM, Oh LK, Kim DS. MR imaging findings of Rathke's cleft cysts: significance of intracystic nodules. Am J Neuroradiol. 2000;21:485.

Dejager S, Gerber S, Foubert L, Turpin G Sheehan's syndrome: differential diagnosis in the acute phase. J Intern Med. 1998;244:261–6.

Gammal TE, Brooks BS, Hoffman WH. MR imaging of ectopic bright signal of posterior pituitary regeneration. Am J Neuroradiol. 1989;10:323–8.

Gentry LR, Smoker WRK, Turski PA, et al. Suprasellar arachnoid cysts: 1. CT recognition. Am J Neuroradiol. 1986;7:79–86.

Harrison MJ, Morgello S, Post KD. Epithelial cystic lesions of the sellar and parasellar region: a continuum of ectodermal derivatives? J Neurosurg, 1994;80:1018–25.

Kurojwa T, Okabe Y, Hasuo K, et al. MR imaging of pituitary dwarfism. Am J Neuroradiol. 1991;12:161–4.

Schubiger O, Haller D. Metastases to the pituitary-hypothalamic axis. An MR study of 7 symptomatic patients. Neuroradiology 1992;34:131–4.

Triulzi F, Scotti G, di Natale B, et al. Evidence of a congenital midline brain anomaly in pituitary dwarfs: a MRI study in 101 patients. Pediatrics 1994;93:409–16.

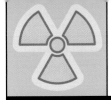

Section 8 Imaging

Chapter 41

General Radiology of Endocrine Disease

Rodney H Reznek and Janet E Dacie

INTRODUCTION

The challenge for the radiologist in imaging patients with disease of the endocrine system usually lies in the anatomic localization of the abnormality leading to the disorder. Despite the development in recent years of high-resolution cross-sectional imaging modalities, identifying the source of such a disorder remains a daunting task for several reasons. The responsible lesion is often small and difficult to identify and the conduct of the technique is therefore crucial. Failure to perform the test adequately can easily result in a small lesion such as an islet cell tumor or bronchial carcinoid being missed. Also, the degree of endocrine abnormality does not necessarily correlate with the size of the lesion and the distinction between a coincidental lesion and a functioning abnormality is frequently impossible without correlation with radionuclide imaging and venous sampling.

For these reasons, perhaps even more than in other disciplines, close collaboration between the endocrinologist and interested radiologist is essential. The imaging studies need to be tailored to the patient's specific problem so that the chances of identifying a source are optimized. The correct interpretation of a finding will also require a clear understanding of its relevance in the clinical context.

Modern cross-sectional imaging techniques have evolved rapidly. Many are expensive, and all have their strengths and weaknesses. Compared with computerized tomography (CT) and magnetic resonance imaging (MRI), ultrasound is relatively cheap but is highly operator-dependent and requires close proximity of the transducer to the target organ for optimal visualization. Like ultrasound, high-resolution CT is widely available but is expensive and involves ionizing radiation. Attention to the technical details and to the conduct of the examination is essential in order to obtain maximum information. MRI is also expensive but, compared with CT, is less readily available. MRI does, however, have several distinct advantages. No ionizing radiation is involved and images can be acquired easily in any plane. Although the spatial resolution of the scans is less with MRI than with CT, soft tissue characterization is better and functional information can be obtained using chemical-shift imaging techniques. The role of radionuclide imaging in endocrine disease is discussed in Chapter 42.

The effective use of this wide range of imaging modalities requires an intimate understanding of the advantages and limitations of the techniques available. Advances in computer technology continue to evolve and knowledge regarding the relative merits of the various cross-sectional imaging modalities in the investigation of endocrine disease continues to expand.

In this chapter we demonstrate the common appearances on cross-sectional imaging of both functioning and nonfunctioning pathology of the endocrine system and we highlight the current approach to the use of these techniques to localize the source of biochemical disturbance. Although the importance of plain radiographs in endocrine disease is appreciated less nowadays than previously, in some clinical circumstances plain films remain essential in the investigation of the patient. Plain radiographic abnormalities can indeed, on occasion, alert the clinician to the presence of endocrine disease. We therefore include examples of the typical plain film appearances of various endocrine conditions as they relate to the patient's condition or where they may provide a clue as to its cause. The illustrations are accompanied by line drawings, and the figure legends contain a brief description of the appearances together with relevant clinical information and comment. The following subjects are included:

- Acromegaly
- Adrenal
  - Normal appearances
  - Cushing's syndrome (including 'occult' ectopic production of adrenocorticotropic hormone (ACTH))
  - Conn's syndrome
  - Pheochromocytoma (also extra-adrenal pheochromocytomas)
  - Congenital adrenal hyperplasia
  - Addison's disease
  - Tuberculosis
  - Nonhyperfunctioning cortical adenoma
  - Spontaneous adrenal hemorrhage
  - Metastases
  - Myelolipoma
  - Cyst
- Islet cell tumors of the pancreas (functioning and nonfunctioning)
- Carcinoid tumor
- Thyroid disease
- Pseudohypoparathyroidism
- Primary hyperparathyroidism
- Renal rickets and renal osteodystrophy
- Nutritional rickets and osteomalacia
- McCune–Albright syndrome
- Gonadal dysgenesis (Turner's syndrome)
- Ovarian cystic disease and tumors.

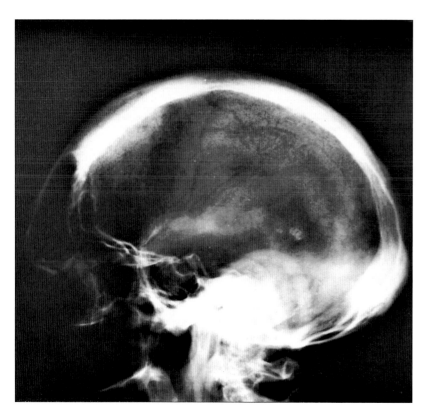

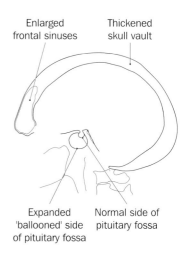

Enlarged frontal sinuses

Thickened skull vault

Expanded 'ballooned' side of pituitary fossa

Normal side of pituitary fossa

Figure 41.1 Acromegaly: lateral skull film showing vault changes and a 'ballooned' pituitary fossa. The main role of radiology in the assessment of acromegaly is to confirm the presence of a pituitary tumor and to provide information necessary for treatment and followup (see Chapter 5 for a discussion of acromegaly and Chapter 40 for pituitary tumors in general). Certain characteristic systemic changes do, however, occur in acromegaly and this lateral skull film demonstrates typical diffuse hyperostosis of the calvarium and abnormally large frontal sinuses. A double floor to the pituitary fossa can be seen. One side is of normal caliber and the other is grossly expanded, i.e. 'ballooned' (see **Fig. 41.3** for details).

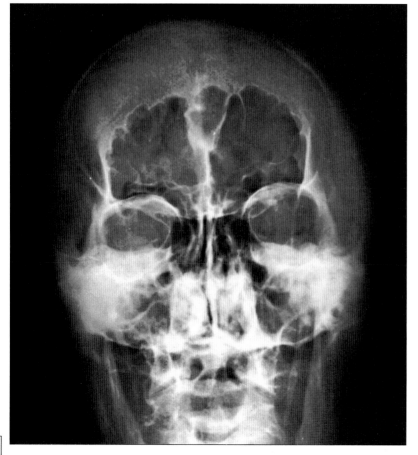

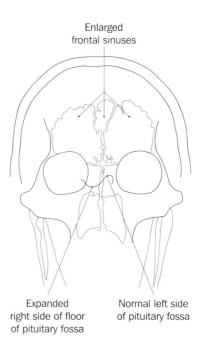

Enlarged frontal sinuses

Expanded right side of floor of pituitary fossa

Normal left side of pituitary fossa

Figure 41.2 Acromegaly: posteroanterior (PA) skull film showing enlarged frontal sinuses. This PA skull film of the same patient as in **Figure 41.1** demonstrates the marked enlargement of the frontal sinuses. The floor of the pituitary fossa is seen to be grossly enlarged on the right side by a large but asymmetric pituitary tumor.

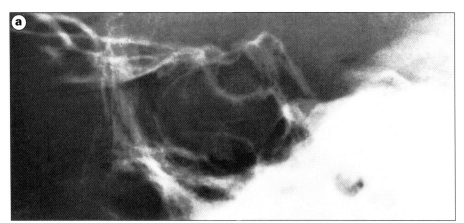

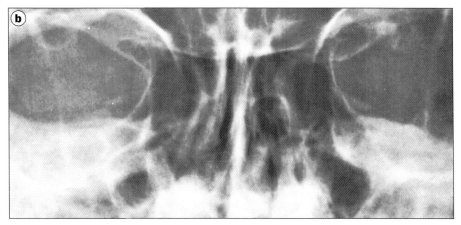

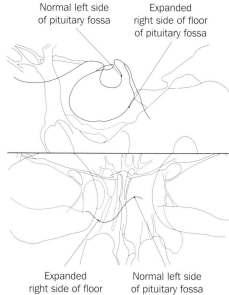

Normal left side of pituitary fossa

Expanded right side of floor of pituitary fossa

Expanded right side of floor of pituitary fossa

Normal left side of pituitary fossa

Figure 41.3 Acromegaly: coned views of 'ballooned' pituitary fossa. These coned lateral (a) and posteroanterior (b) views of the pituitary fossa are of the same patient as in **Figures 41.1** and **41.2**. They demonstrate more clearly the gross asymmetric expansion of the right side of the floor of the pituitary fossa.

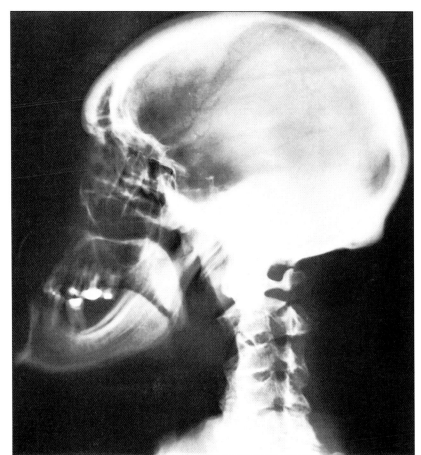

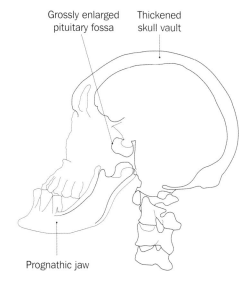

Grossly enlarged pituitary fossa

Thickened skull vault

Prognathic jaw

Figure 41.4 Acromegaly: prognathic jaw. The lateral skull film of another patient shows characteristic prognathism with increase in the normal angle of the mandible. The pituitary fossa is grossly enlarged and the skull vault is markedly thickened, particularly anteriorly, although in this patient the frontal sinuses are not enlarged.

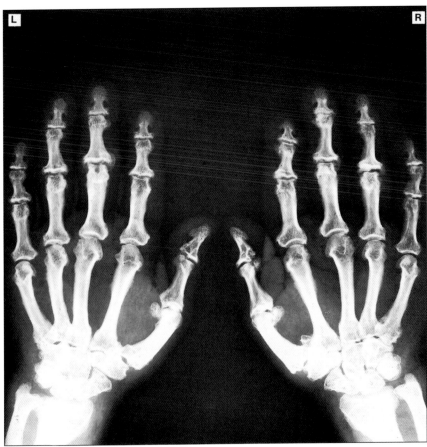

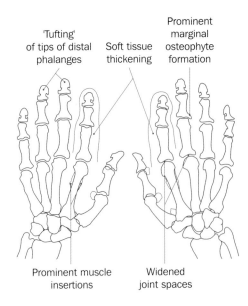

Figure 41.5 Acromegaly: hands. In acromegaly the hands are large and the classic radiologic features include generalized soft tissue thickening, widening of the joint spaces due to hypertrophy of the articular cartilages, prominent muscle insertions, particularly along the metacarpal shafts, tufting of the tips of the terminal phalanges, and prominent osteophyte formation. In addition, in this patient, degenerative cysts are present in some of the carpal bones, particularly in the right carpus.

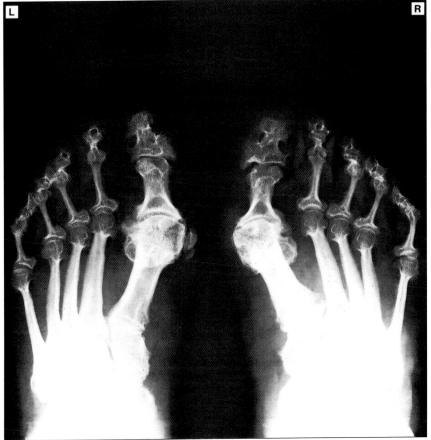

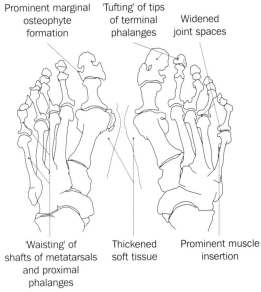

Figure 41.6 Acromegaly: feet. The radiologic changes in the hands in acromegaly are also seen in the feet but, in addition to new bone formation, bone resorption occurs, giving rise to typically thinned metatarsals. Thinning of the shafts of the phalanges may also occur, as in this patient.

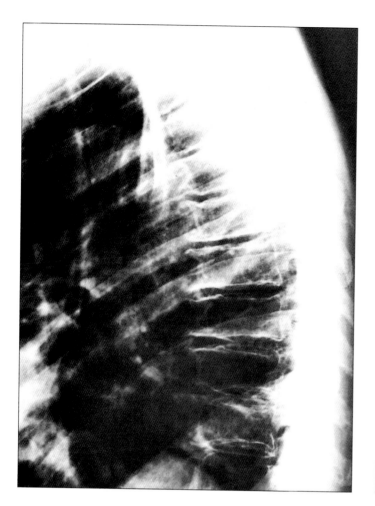

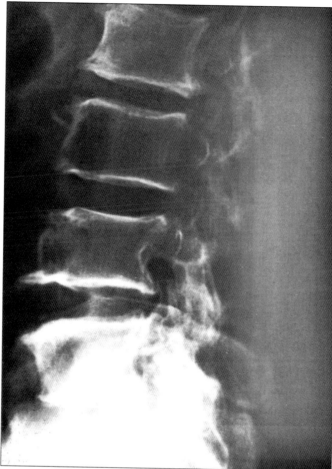

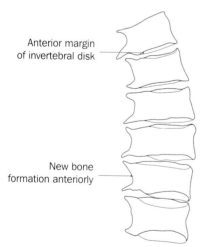

Anterior margin
of invertebral disk

New bone
formation anteriorly

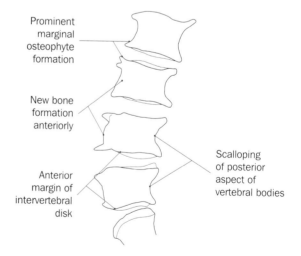

Prominent
marginal
osteophyte
formation

New bone
formation
anteriorly

Anterior
margin of
intervertebral
disk

Scalloping
of posterior
aspect of
vertebral bodies

Figure 41.7 Acromegaly: lateral dorsal spine. In acromegaly new bone formation may occur around the vertebral bodies. This lateral view of the dorsal spine shows such changes at the anterior margins of the vertebrae. The anterior edge of the intervertebral discs can be clearly identified and the vertebral bodies are increased in their anteroposterior diameter. The new bone formation is usually more marked in the dorsal than in the lumbar spine.

Figure 41.8 Acromegaly: lateral lumbar spine. In addition to new bone formation anteriorly this lateral view of the lumbar spine shows prominent marginal osteophyte formation and characteristic scalloping of the posterior margins of the vertebral bodies. Although such scalloping may be seen in the dorsal spine, the lumbar spine is most commonly affected.

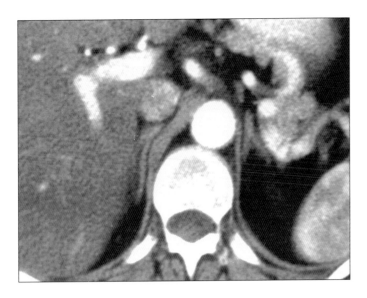

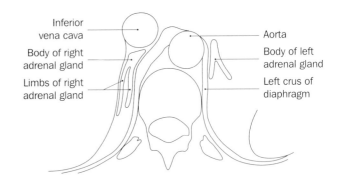

Figure 41.9 Normal adrenal glands on computerized tomography (CT). The normal adrenal glands as seen in cross-section have an arrowhead configuration with a body and medial and lateral limbs. The normal adrenal glands extend 2–4cm in the craniocaudal direction. The thickness of the normal adrenal body does not exceed 10mm and that of the limbs does not exceed 5–6mm.

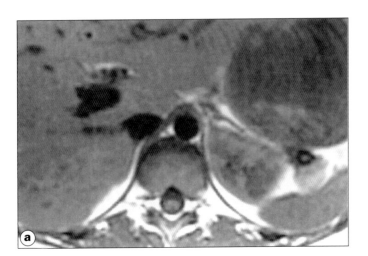

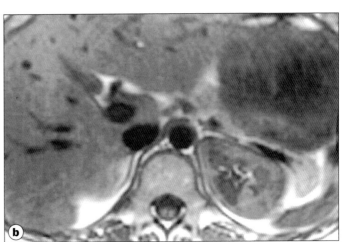

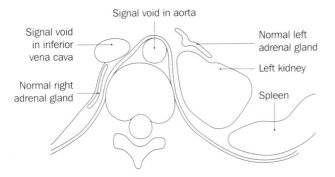

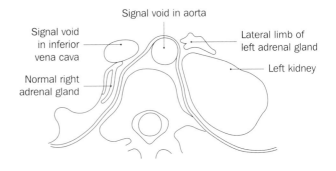

Figure 41.10 Normal adrenal glands on magnetic resonance imaging (MRI). These T1-weighted spin-echo magnetic resonance images were obtained in the axial plain at slightly different levels. They demonstrate the appearance of normal adrenal glands. MRI offers an alternative method for imaging the adrenal gland and can now achieve spatial resolution close to that of computerized tomography. Imaging protocols usually consist of axial T1- and T2-weighted sequences. Imaging in the coronal and sagittal planes helps to identify invasion into adjacent structures by large mass lesions. Chemical shift imaging sequences may be helpful to differentiate between benign and malignant adrenal mass lesions. Intravenous contrast medium (gadolinium DTPA) is administered to differentiate between solid and cystic lesions and to assess the vascularity of the mass.

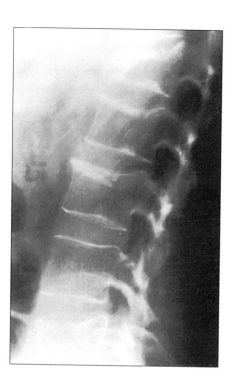

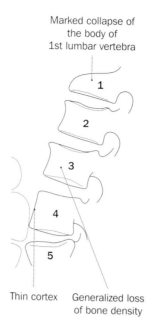

Marked collapse of the body of 1st lumbar vertebra

Thin cortex

Generalized loss of bone density

Figure 41.11 Cushing's syndrome: osteoporosis and vertebral fractures. Cushing's syndrome, when severe, results in generalized osteoporosis and this lateral film of the lumbar spine shows the typical appearance. The bone density is reduced and the cortical margins of the bones are thin. There is marked collapse of the body of the first lumbar vertebra, with marginal condensation of the superior borders of the bodies of the second and third. In the dorsal spine multiple vertebral fractures may lead to a pronounced kyphosis. It should be noted that the radiologic appearances of osteoporosis affecting the spine are similar whatever the cause.

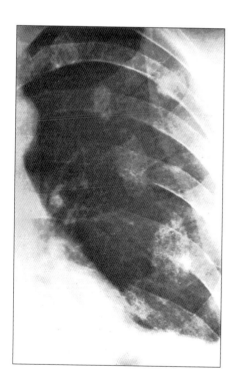

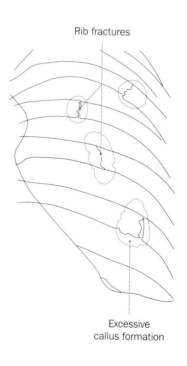

Rib fractures

Excessive callus formation

Figure 41.12 Cushing's syndrome: rib fracture. Spontaneous asymptomatic rib fractures are characteristic of Cushing's syndrome and this coned view shows the typical appearance. Multiple rib fractures are surrounded by excessive callus formation. In some patients, in addition to obvious rib fractures, characteristic widening of the anterior ends of the ribs resulting from numerous stress infractions may be seen.

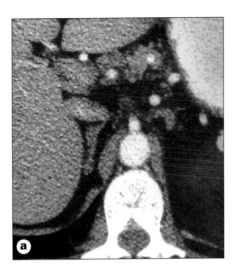

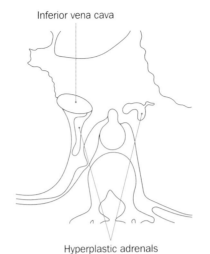

Inferior vena cava

Hyperplastic adrenals

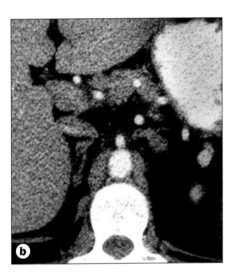

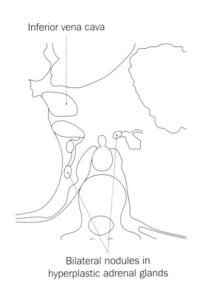

Inferior vena cava

Bilateral nodules in
hyperplastic adrenal glands

Figure 41.13 Nodular hyperplasia of the adrenal glands on CT in Cushing's disease. In adrenocorticotropic hormone (ACTH)-dependent Cushing's syndrome, the adrenal glands appear normal on CT in 30% of cases. In the remaining 70%, the glands appear hyperplastic (a, b) with the contours either smooth or nodular. In nodular hyperplasia, the nodules can become extremely large, reaching a size of 3–4cm. The largest glands are seen usually in patients with 'occult' ectopic ACTH production. (See Chapter 15 for a discussion of venous sampling in Cushing's syndrome.)

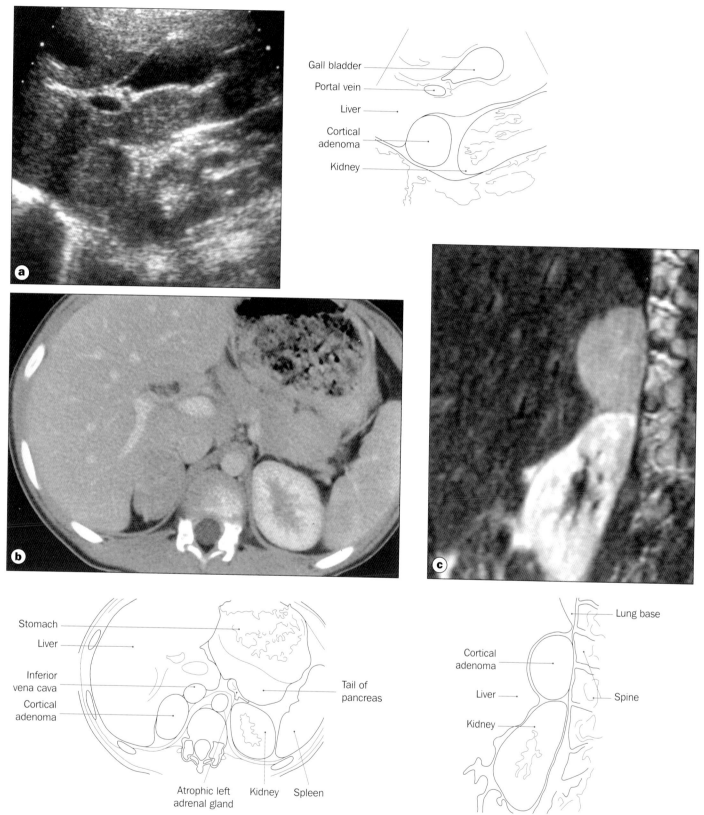

Figure 41.14 Benign cortical adenoma causing Cushing's syndrome. Adrenocortical adenomas account for 10–20% of cases of Cushing's syndrome. Functioning adrenal cortical adenomas responsible for Cushing's syndrome are usually larger than 2cm in diameter. The contralateral gland is usually normal but is occasionally atrophic. On ultrasound (a) the adenoma has a typical appearance of a solid, uniformly echogenic mass, clearly defined from the adjacent liver and kidney. On a post-contrast CT scan (b) the mass is of homogeneous soft tissue density, enhancing slightly following intravenous injection of contrast medium but to a lesser extent than normal renal parenchyma. The contralateral gland is atrophic. The sagittal T2-weighted MR scan (c) shows the typical appearance of a functioning cortical adenoma, uniformly of high signal intensity relative to the adjacent liver. The sensitivity of MRI for the detection of functional adrenal cortical adenomas is equal to that of CT.

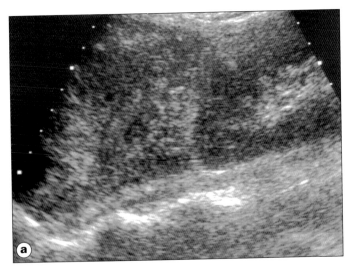

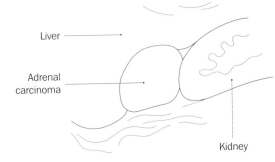

Liver

Adrenal
carcinoma

Kidney

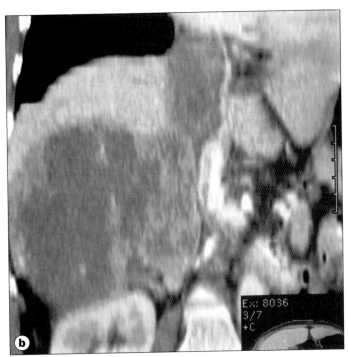

Diaphragm Lung

Tumor
thrombus
in inferior
vena cava

Liver

Adrenal
carcinoma

Loops
of bowel

Kidney

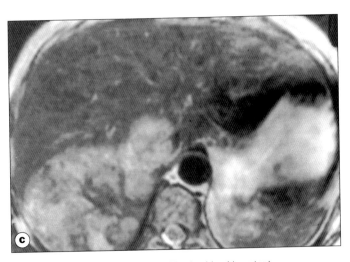

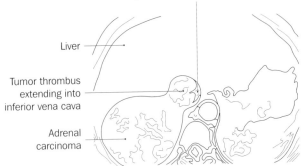

Flowing blood in patent
portion of inferior vena cava

Liver

Tumor thrombus
extending into
inferior vena cava

Adrenal
carcinoma

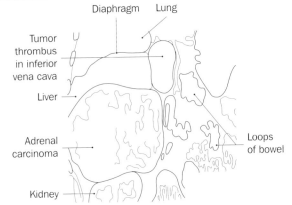

Figure 41.15 Adrenal carcinoma demonstrated on ultrasound, CT and MRI. Most adrenal carcinomas exceed 6cm at the time of presentation and are readily detected on ultrasound. Only about 15% of carcinomas are less than 6cm and then may resemble adenomas. (a) This longitudinal ultrasound scan shows the typical appearance of a large suprarenal mass of mixed, inhomogeneous reflectivity, with high- and low-level echoes. A clear plane can be seen between the mass and the kidney. (b) Postcontrast spiral CT with the axial images reformatted to obtain a coronal projection very clearly shows the relationship of the mass to the adjacent structures. The mass is displacing the kidney inferiorly, is separate from the liver, and tumor thrombus extends into the inferior vena cava. Critically for surgical planning, the upper limit of the thrombus lies above the level of the diaphragm. The mass itself has a typically inhomogeneous appearance. Areas of necrosis and calcification are frequently seen on CT within adrenal carcinomas. (c) Axial T2-weighted MR image also shows the large adrenal mass of inhomogeneous signal intensity with areas of both high and low signal intensity. The normal signal void due to flowing blood has been lost within the inferior vena cava (IVC) as it is infiltrated with high-signal-intensity tumor. Only a small area of patent IVC is seen. Both CT and MRI are extremely accurate in demonstrating the size and extent of adrenal carcinomas, infiltration of adjacent viscera, and invasion of the renal vein and inferior vena cava.

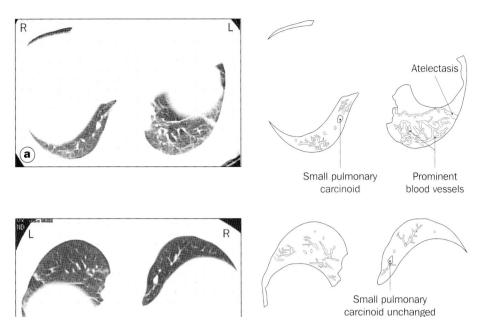

Figure 41.16 Small bronchial carcinoid producing adrenocorticotropic hormone (ACTH). (a) CT scan through the lung bases with the patient supine shows a 4mm nodule in the posterior basal segment of the right lower lobe. The presence of 'gravity-dependent' perfusion and minimal atelectasis (best seen at the left base) can obscure small basal lesions. The patient was therefore rescanned while lying in the prone position (b). This confirms the presence of a small basal lesion, which proved to be a small bronchial carcinoid. As the source of 'occult' ectopic ACTH production is most commonly a small bronchial carcinoid tumor, it is essential that imaging of the lung be conducted with the utmost care.

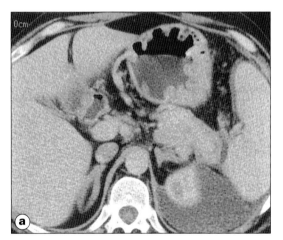

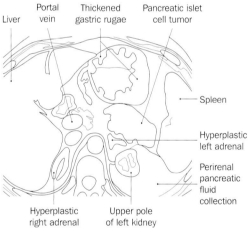

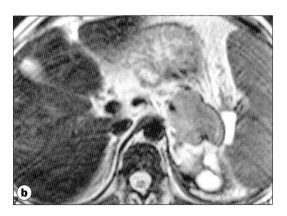

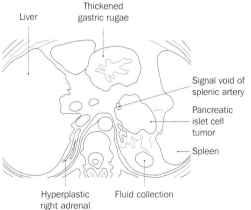

Figure 41.17 'Occult' ectopic adrenocorticotropic hormone (ACTH) production due to a pancreatic gastrinoma. (a) Contrast-enhanced CT scan in a patient with Cushing's syndrome shows bilateral smooth adrenal hyperplasia due to excess ACTH. A large enhancing mass is demonstrated within the tail of the pancreas consistent with an islet cell tumor. The fluid collection in the left perirenal space had an extremely high amylase content and was caused by a bout of pancreatitis at the time of presentation. Although the scan was performed following intravenous administration of hyoscine-N-butyl bromide, the gastric rugae are thickened, consistent with Zollinger–Ellison syndrome. (b) T2-weighted MR scan also shows the mass in the tail of the pancreas, of higher signal intensity than the normal liver. Encasement of the splenic artery (seen as a signal void within the mass) was substantiated at surgery. The gastric rugal hypertrophy and high-signal-intensity perirenal fluid collections are also demonstrated.

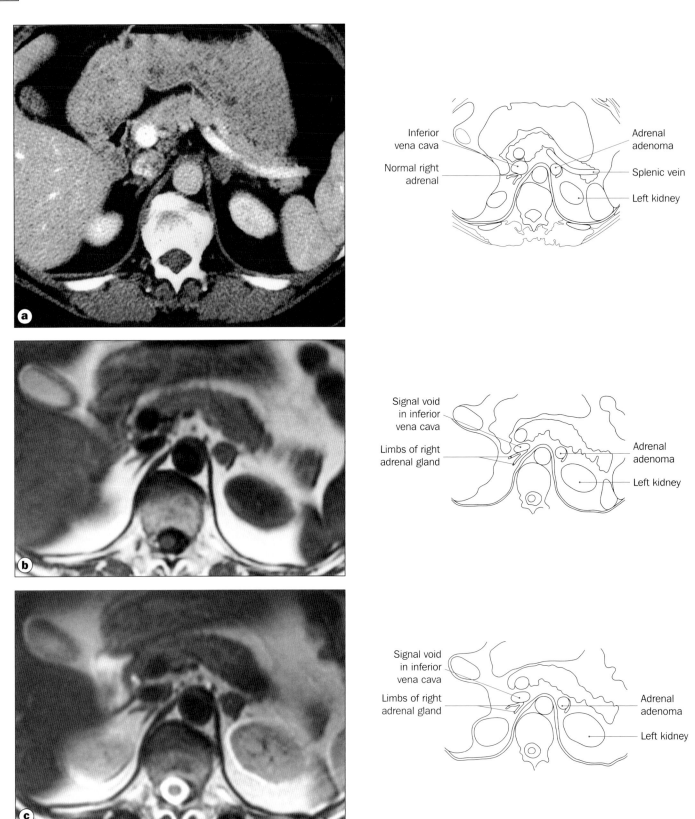

Figure 41.18 Conn's syndrome due to small adrenocortical adenoma. (a) Contrast-enhanced CT scan shows a typical, small, low-density, aldosterone-producing adenoma. On CT, these tumors tend to be small, with an average size of approximately 1.6–1.8cm, of low density (usually less than 10 Hounsfield units), do not enhance significantly after intravenous injection of contrast medium, and rarely calcify. (b) Axial T1-weighted and (c) T2-weighted MR scans show a normal right-sided adrenal gland and a small mass in the left adrenal gland. Typically, on both sequences, the nodule is isointense with the liver parenchyma. The sensitivity of CT in detecting adenomas is 70–90% and the specificity exceeds 90%. MRI is as sensitive and as specific as CT for the detection of these small adenomas.

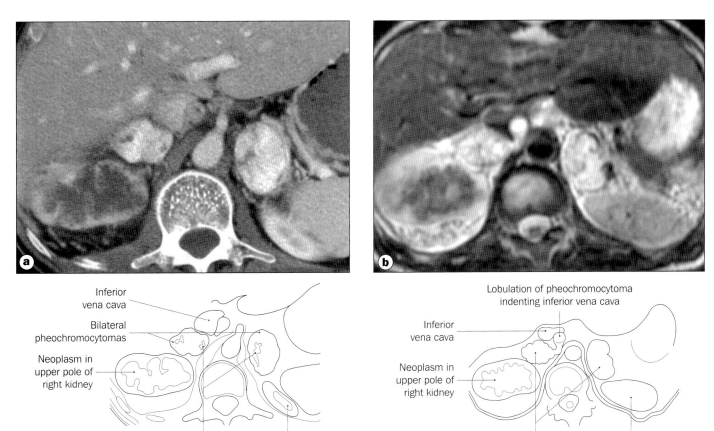

Figure 41.19 Bilateral pheochromocytomas. (a) The contrast-enhanced CT scan shows bilateral pheochromocytomas in a patient presenting with a right renal cell carcinoma. As seen here, pheochromocytomas show intense enhancement following intravenous injection of contrast medium, have areas of necrosis, and in sporadic cases tend to be large. The overall accuracy of CT in detecting adrenal pheochromocytomas is very high, with a sensitivity of 93–100% and a positive predictive value greater than 90%. (b) The T2-weighted MR scan shows the bilateral pheochromocytomas, typically of very high signal intensity. The combination of bilateral pheochromocytomas in a patient presenting with a renal cell carcinoma suggested a diagnosis of von Hippel–Lindau disease, proven genotypically.

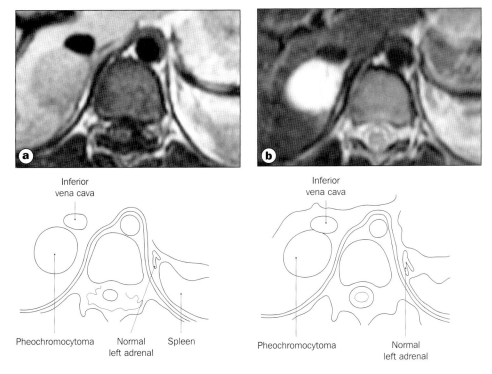

Figure 41.20 Adrenal pheochromocytoma. MR scans of the son of the patient demonstrated in **Figure 41.19**. (a) The axial T1-weighted scan shows a typical large mass of lower signal intensity than the adjacent liver. (b) The T2-weighted scan shows the typical high signal intensity. Although this appearance on T2 weighting is typical it is not specific as there is some similarity in appearance with edematous or necrotic adrenal metastases. Atypical signal intensity is seen in 35% of pheochromocytomas.

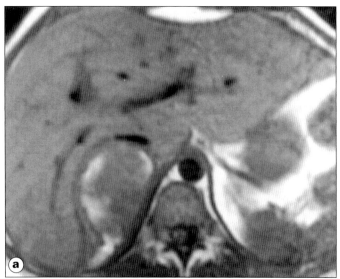

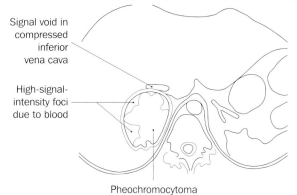

Signal void in
compressed
inferior
vena cava

High-signal-
intensity foci
due to blood

Pheochromocytoma

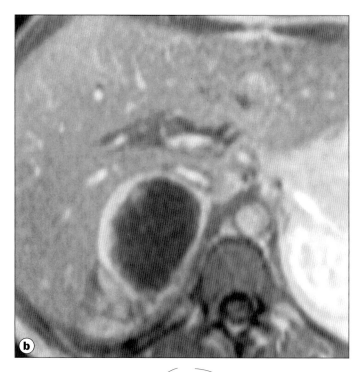

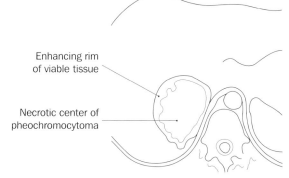

Enhancing rim
of viable tissue

Necrotic center of
pheochromocytoma

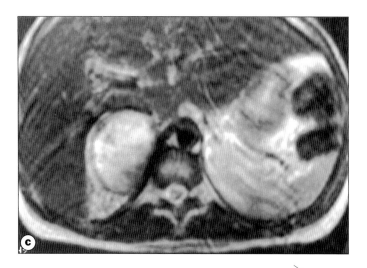

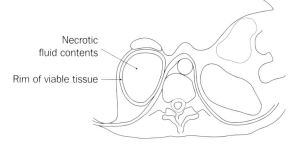

Necrotic
fluid contents

Rim of viable tissue

Figure 41.21 Atypical pheochromocytoma: MR appearances. This
patient presented with right upper quadrant pain. (a) The T1-weighted scan
shows a large right adrenal mass, compressing the inferior vena cava and
containing foci of high signal intensity because of the presence of blood.
(Fat and highly proteinaceous material are also of high signal intensity on a
T1-weighted sequence.) (b) The fat-suppressed axial T1-weighted scan
following intravenous injection of gadolinium-DTPA shows enhancement of
the remaining active tissue located only on the periphery of the mass. The
central component, consisting of hemorrhagic and necrotic material, does
not take up the contrast medium. (c) The axial T2-weighted scan shows
the central high-signal-intensity component of the mass resulting from the
necrotic fluid. On occasion the central necrosis may be so marked that the
mass may resemble a cyst. CT and MRI have equal accuracy in the
detection of adrenal pheochromocytomas.

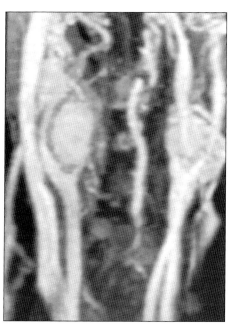

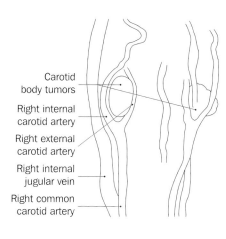

Carotid
body tumors

Right internal
carotid artery

Right external
carotid artery

Right internal
jugular vein

Right common
carotid artery

Figure 41.22 Extra-adrenal pheochromocytomas: bilateral carotid body tumors. The multiplanar capacity of MRI makes it slightly more accurate than CT for the detection of extra-adrenal pheochromocytomas. Several relatively noninvasive magnetic resonance techniques are applied to visualizing the vasculature. On this sequence, 15ml of gadolinium-DTPA has been injected via the median cubital vein and rapid sequential images acquired. This magnetic resonance angiography image shows bilateral vascular tumors at the carotid bifurcation, resulting in splaying of the internal and external carotid arteries producing the so-called 'lyre' sign.

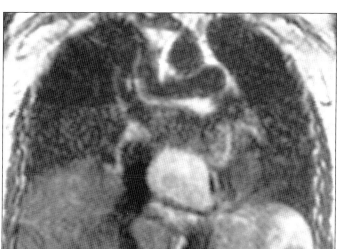

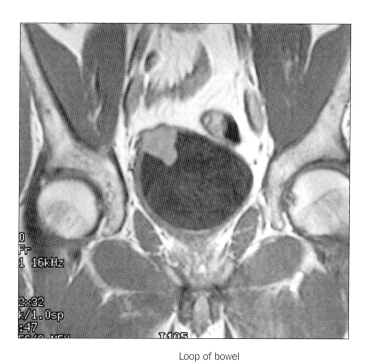

Signal void
within aorta

Signal void within
pulmonary artery

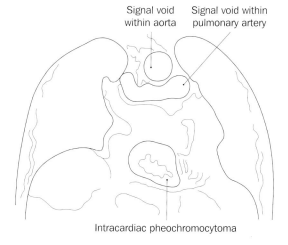

Intracardiac pheochromocytoma

Loop of bowel

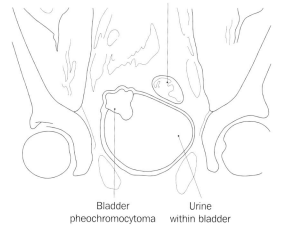

Bladder
pheochromocytoma

Urine
within bladder

Figure 41.23 Extraadrenal intracardiac pheochromocytoma. This coronal T2-weighted scan in a 36-year-old female patient shows a large, high-signal-intensity mass within the left atrium. At surgery, the pheochromocytoma was shown to be within the interatrial septum extending predominantly into the left atrium.

Figure 41.24 Extraadrenal pheochromocytoma within the bladder. This coronal T1-weighted MR scan shows a lobulated mass arising within the wall of the bladder and extending into the lumen. Unlike CT, the coronal sequence clearly depicts the relationship of the mass to the bladder wall and the absence of extravesical spread.

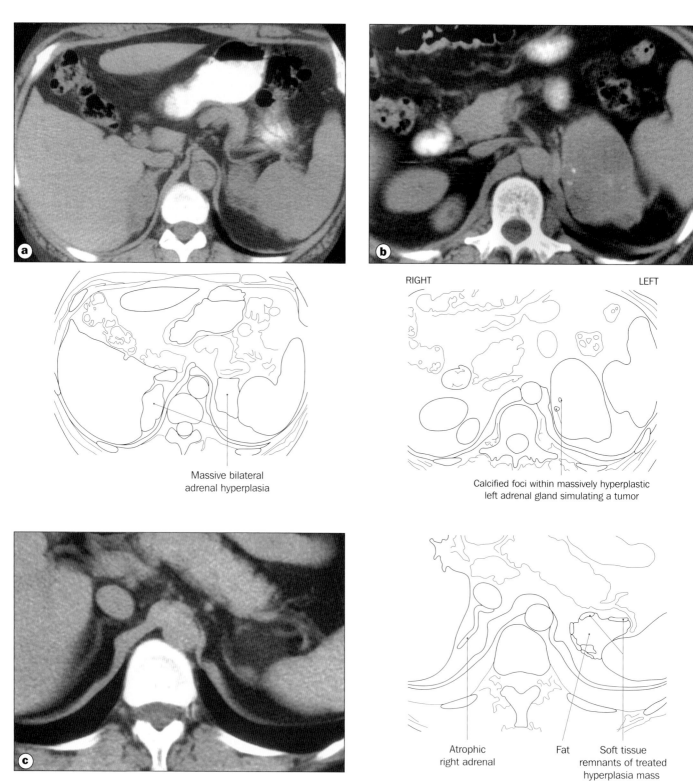

Figure 41.25 Congenital adrenal hyperplasia. (a, b) Unenhanced axial CT scans in a 50-year-old male patient with previously untreated congenital adrenal hyperplasia show that both adrenal glands are massively enlarged and that the normal contour of the glands has been lost. On the left particularly, an inhomogeneous mass-like lesion has resulted and contains foci of calcium. Such severe hyperplasia can, as in this case, simulate the appearance of adrenal carcinomas. (c) The unenhanced CT scan in the same patient following treatment shows that the right adrenal gland now appears atrophic and that the left adrenal gland cannot be identified. The large mass lesion demonstrated on (b) has been replaced by fat.

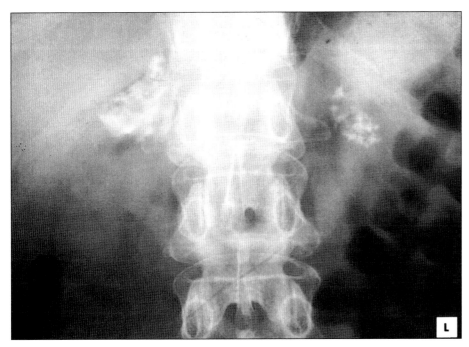

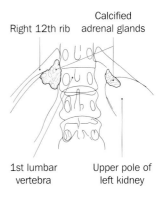

Figure 41.26 Addison's disease: calcified adrenal glands. This coned anteroposterior film of the upper abdomen demonstrates calcified adrenal glands, seen in some patients with Addison's disease. An identical appearance, however, may be found incidentally in patients without evidence of adrenal disease (the so-called 'idiopathic' calcification of the adrenals).

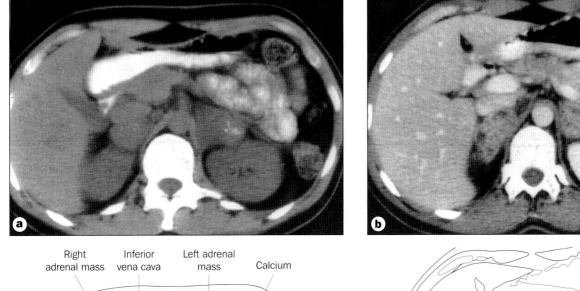

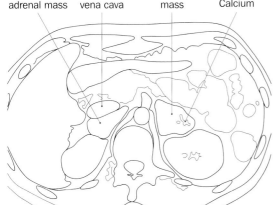

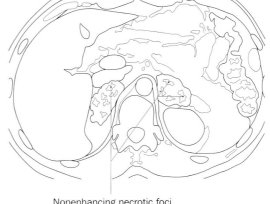

Figure 41.27 Tuberculosis of the adrenal glands. (a) The unenhanced CT scan through the adrenal glands shows marked bilateral enlargement with loss of the normal adrenal outline. Speckled calcification is demonstrated within the left adrenal mass. (b) The postcontrast CT scan shows inhomogeneous enhancement of the enlarged glands. The small, nonenhancing foci correspond with areas of caseous necrosis. This appearance is typical of active infection; long-standing infection results in atrophy. Calcification may be seen in the acute phase or during healing.

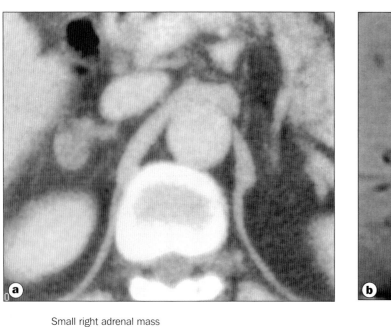

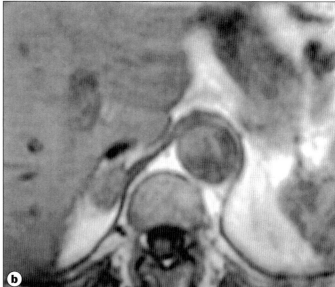

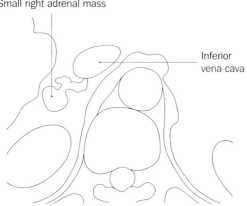

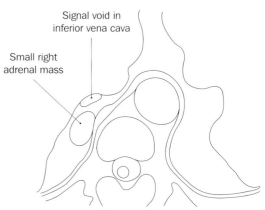

Figure 41.28 (a & b) Incidentally-detected adrenocortical mass: characterization by MRI. Adrenal masses are discovered in about 2% of patients undergoing CT for an indication unrelated to adrenal pathology. Any biochemical abnormality will dictate further management. In the absence of any biochemical abnormality, characterization of the mass is based on the detection of intracellular lipid because the most likely cause is a benign nonhyperfunctioning cortical adenoma, which usually contains a high amount of lipid. Chemical shift imaging on MRI is capable of detecting intracellular lipid. (a) The CT scan shows a small (1.4cm) low-density adrenal mass in a patient scanned following abdominal trauma. (b) An axial spin-echo T1-weighted scan demonstrates the same mass.

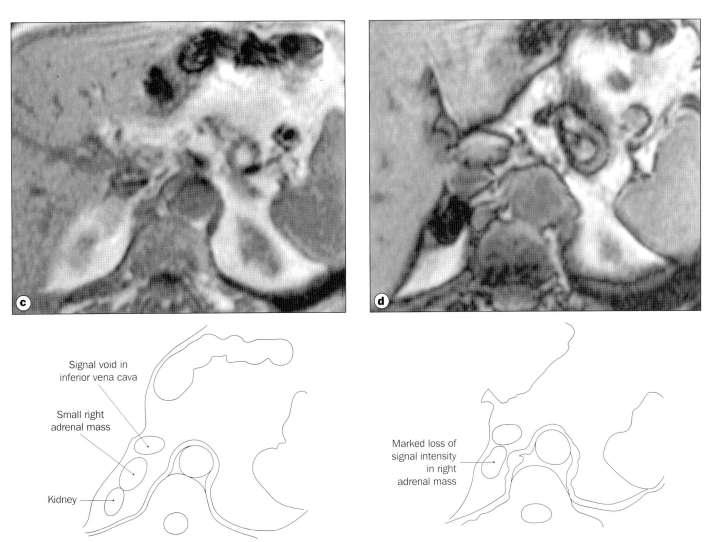

Figure 41.28 (c & d) Incidentally-detected adrenocortical mass: characterization by MRI. Using chemical shift MRI, the gradient-echo T1-weighted in-phase scan (c) is compared with the axial gradient-echo T1-weighted out-of-phase scan (d). The latter shows marked loss of signal intensity. This loss of signal intensity indicates that there is a substantial amount of intracellular lipid within the lesion. Chemical shift MRI has a high specificity for the detection of benign adenomas.

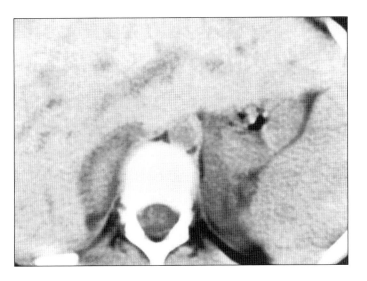

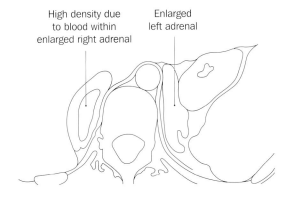

Figure 41.29 Spontaneous adrenal hemorrhage. The axial noncontrast CT scan shows bilateral adrenal enlargement with high density in the right adrenal gland due to a fresh bleed. Approximately 80% of spontaneous adrenal hemorrhages are unilateral, most commonly on the right side.

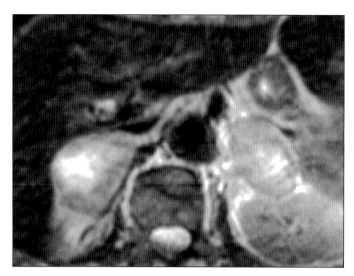

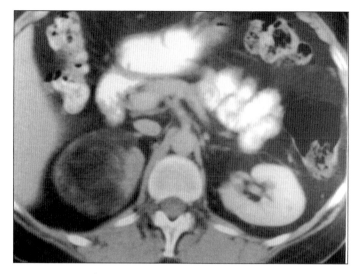

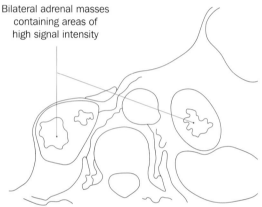

Bilateral adrenal masses
containing areas of
high signal intensity

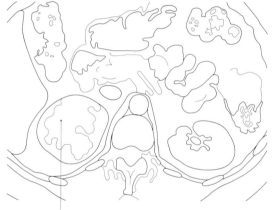

Fat within large adrenal mass

Figure 41.30 Adrenal metastases. This axial T2-weighted MR scan shows large bilateral adrenal masses of inhomogeneous signal intensity due to metastases from a primary bronchial carcinoma. Adrenal metastases are most commonly from tumors of the lung, kidney, melanoma, breast, gastrointestinal tract, and ovary, and are more commonly bilateral than unilateral.

Figure 41.31 Adrenal myelolipoma. This axial CT scan shows a large right adrenal mass made up almost entirely of fat of similar density to the surrounding intraabdominal fat. Adrenal myelolipomas are rare benign neoplasms composed of fat and bone marrow tissue in varying proportions; most are asymptomatic and nonfunctioning and identified incidentally. Hemorrhage or necrosis within the tumor may cause pain. The diagnosis is based on the demonstration of fat within an adrenal mass.

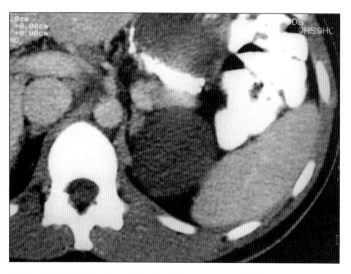

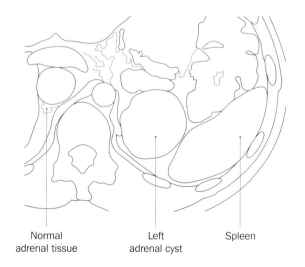

Normal   Left   Spleen
adrenal tissue   adrenal cyst

Figure 41.32 Adrenal cyst. This axial postcontrast CT shows the typical CT appearance of an adrenal cyst – a well-defined, thin-walled structure, uniformly of water density, which exhibits no enhancement following intravenous injection of contrast medium. Adrenal cysts are usually unilateral, most commonly endothelial or epithelial, but rarely may be pseudocysts as a result of previous hemorrhage.

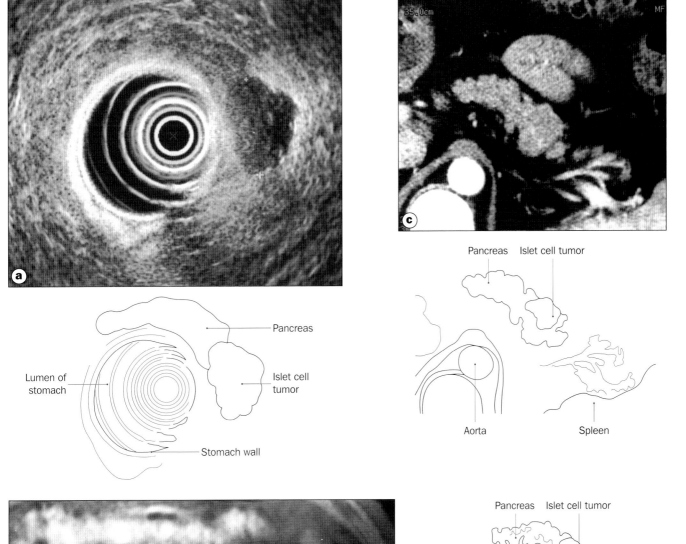

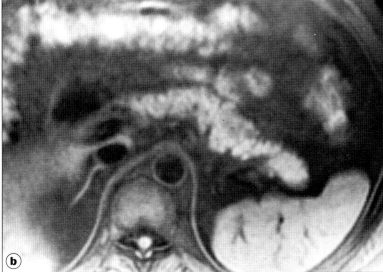

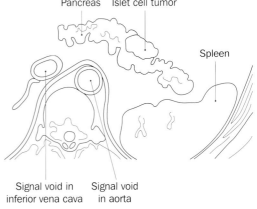

Figure 41.33 Insulinoma: ultrasound, CT and MRI appearances. (a) This endoscopic ultrasound (EUS) image shows an area of low reflectivity corresponding to an insulinoma within the tail of the pancreas. A high-frequency probe (7.5–12MHz) has been placed in close proximity to the duodenum and pancreas. In experienced hands, EUS has proved sensitive in detecting tumors of the pancreatic head but less successful for lesions of the distal tail. It is possible to detect gastrinomas within the duodenal wall. (b) The axial fat-suppressed T1-weighted MR scan shows the same mass, of low signal intensity, within the tail of the pancreas. This sequence is the optimal MRI technique for the documentation of pancreatic islet cell tumors. (c) The axial contrast-enhanced CT scan shows the same islet cell tumor as in (a) and (b). The mass is of similar vascularity to the normal pancreas but is less well demonstrated than on the MR scan. On both MRI and CT insulinomas are typically hypervascular. MRI has a greater sensitivity than CT for the detection of these tumors, particularly when small.

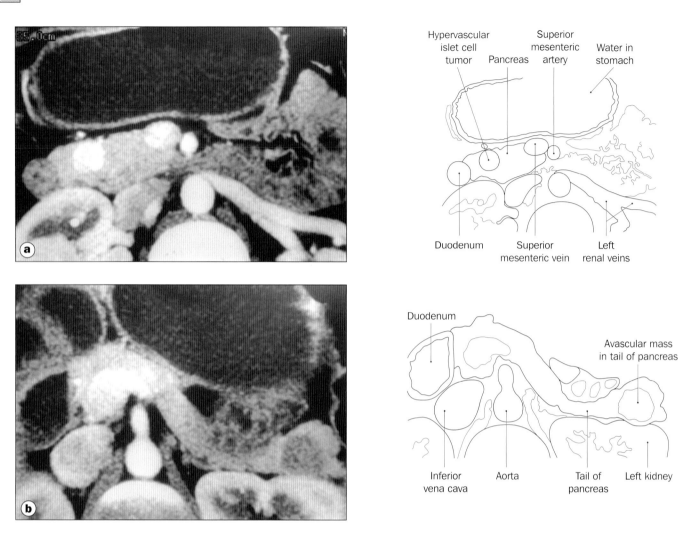

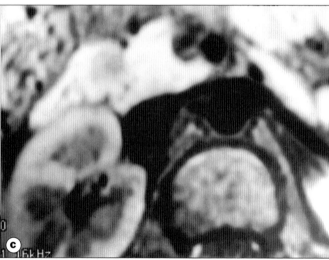

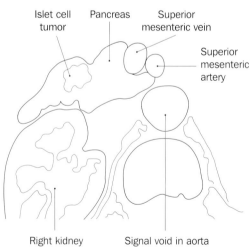

Figure 41.34 (a, b & c) Functioning insulinoma and nonfunctioning islet cell tumor of the pancreas. In this patient suspected of having an insulinoma, axial CT scans of the upper abdomen (a, b) were obtained 30s after the intravenous injection of contrast medium. Prior distention of the stomach with water had been undertaken and hyoscine-*n*-butyl bromide had been injected intravenously. (a) A typical 1cm, rounded lesion is demonstrated within the head of the pancreas. Note that this has been optimally demonstrated by obtaining the scan shortly after contrast medium injection and the mass is of the same density as the superior mesenteric vessels. (b) A further 1.2cm mass is demonstrated in the tail of the pancreas on a scan obtained slightly higher than (a) at the same time. The characteristics of this latter mass are atypical for an islet cell tumor as it is avascular. On contrast-enhanced CT, islet cell tumors are generally seen as hypervascular small rounded masses although they can occasionally be hypovascular. (c) On the axial fat-suppressed T1-weighted MR scan a mass of low signal intensity is present within the head of the pancreas corresponding to that documented on CT.

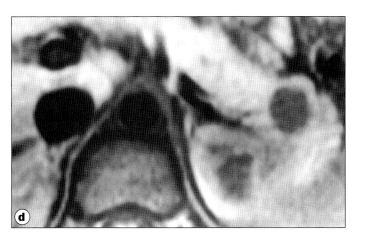

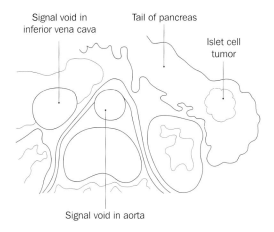

Signal void in inferior vena cava

Tail of pancreas

Islet cell tumor

Signal void in aorta

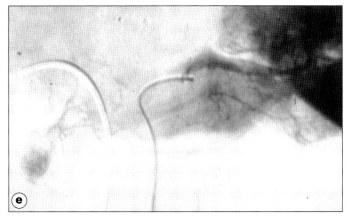

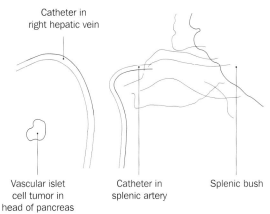

Catheter in right hepatic vein

Vascular islet cell tumor in head of pancreas

Catheter in splenic artery

Splenic bush

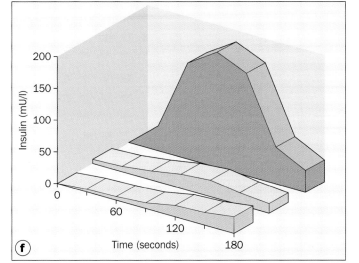

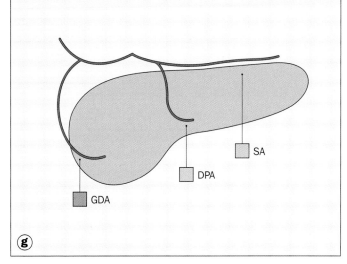

Figure 41.34 (d, e, f & g) Functioning insulinoma and nonfunctioning islet cell tumor of the pancreas. In this patient suspected of having an insulinoma, axial CT scans of the upper abdomen (a, b) were obtained 30s after the intravenous injection of contrast medium. Prior distention of the stomach with water had been undertaken and hyoscine-*n*-butyl bromide had been injected intravenously. (d) The fat-suppressed T1-weighted MR scan shows the mass in the tail of the pancreas. MRI is increasingly being used in the localization of islet cell tumors. The development of fast spin-echo, fat saturation, and dynamic contrast-enhanced imaging has greatly improved imaging for pancreatic lesions. In general, as demonstrated here, islet cell tumors are of lower signal intensity than the normal pancreas on T1-weighted images. As on CT, lesions tend to enhance following intravenous administration of contrast agents such as gadolinium-DTPA. (e) The arteriogram was obtained immediately prior to venous sampling from the right hepatic vein to measure insulin and glucose levels following selective pancreatic stimulation with calcium gluconate. The vascular insulinoma in the head of the pancreas is seen because contrast medium has refluxed back from the splenic artery into the hepatic artery during the procedure. The mass in the tail of the pancreas has not opacified. (f) The time–density curves illustrate the changes in insulin levels in the hepatic vein following the selective injection of calcium gluconate into the splenic (SA), dorsal pancreatic (DPA) and gastroduodenal (GDA) arteries, the injection sites being diagrammatically shown in (g). The time density curves indicate that only the islet cell tumor in the head of the pancreas was functioning. This was confirmed histologically following surgical excision of both masses.

Imaging

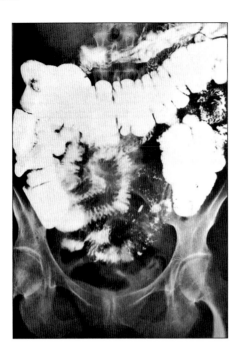

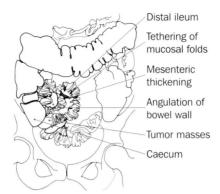

Distal ileum

Tethering of
mucosal folds

Mesenteric
thickening

Angulation of
bowel wall

Tumor masses

Caecum

Figure 41.35 Carcinoid tumor: distal ileal involvement. This 80-minute follow-through film shows an abnormal distal ileum with mesenteric thickening, nodular masses invading the bowel wall, and angulation and tethering of mucosal folds. These appearances are characteristic of carcinoid tumor and reflect invasion by the tumor with an extensive fibroblastic response. Metastatic carcinoma to the mesentery can cause a similar appearance. (Carcinoid tumor producing adrenocorticotropic hormone: see **Fig. 41.16.**)

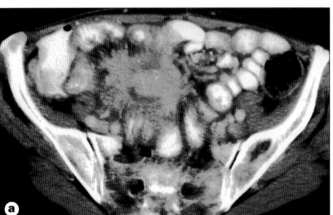

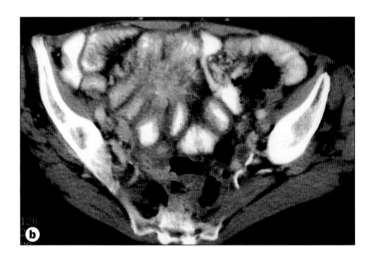

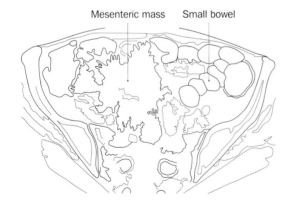

Mesenteric mass   Small bowel

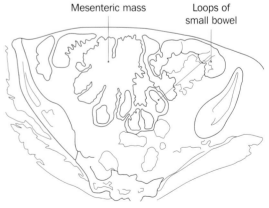

Mesenteric mass   Loops of
small bowel

Figure 41.36 Mesenteric involvement due to a carcinoid tumor: CT appearances. (a) The typical CT appearance of an irregular spiculated stellate mass within the small bowel mesentery is caused by a desmoplastic response, producing fibrous tissue, excited by spread from a carcinoid tumor. (b) A scan taken a few centimeters more inferiorly shows the characteristic tethering of the small bowel loops. There is also thickening of the small bowel wall. Gastrointestinal carcinoids are found most frequently in the appendix (45%), the small bowel (25%), and the colorectum (25%).

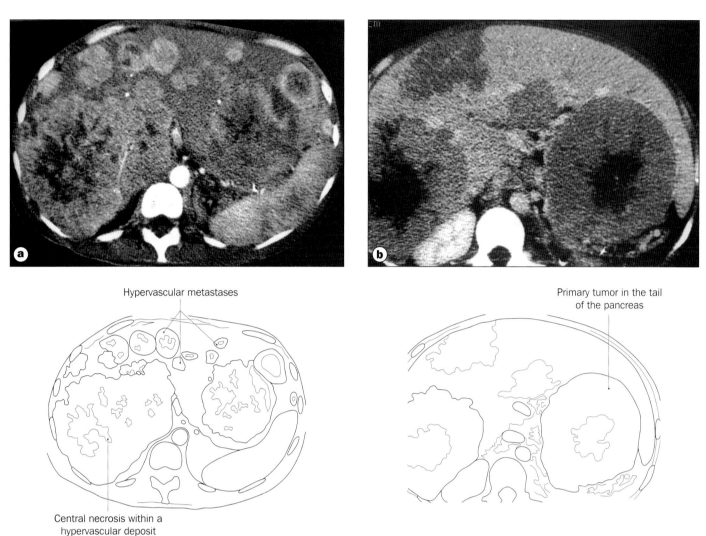

Hypervascular metastases

Central necrosis within a
hypervascular deposit

Primary tumor in the tail
of the pancreas

Figure 41.37 Liver metastases from a primary pancreatic carcinoid tumor: CT appearances. (a) The CT scan performed at 25s following intravenous injection of contrast medium ('arterial' phase) shows typical hypervascular carcinoid liver metastases. The larger lesion in the right lobe shows central necrosis. (b) The CT scan performed at 75s following intravenous injection of contrast medium ('portal venous' phase) shows that the vascular lesions have now become isodense with the normal liver parenchyma. The primary tumor in the tail of the pancreas is also clearly seen. As depicted here, carcinoid hepatic metastases are typically hypervascular and are optimally depicted during the arterial phase of a contrast-enhanced CT or MR scan as they are isoattenuating when compared with adjacent hepatic parenchyma during the portal venous phase of enhancement.

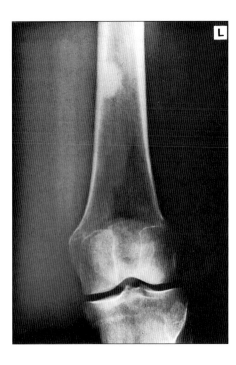

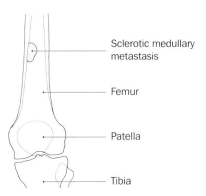

Sclerotic medullary metastasis

Femur

Patella

Tibia

Figure 41.38 Carcinoid tumor: sclerotic bony metastasis. Bony metastases from malignant carcinoid tumors are characteristically densely sclerotic. This anteroposterior film of the distal femur and knee shows the typical appearance of such an intramedullary lesion. The primary tumor was in the rectum.

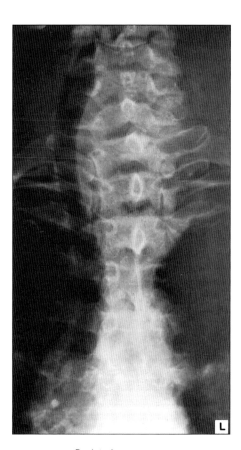

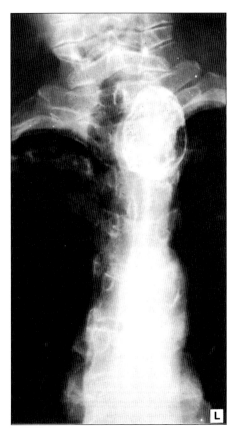

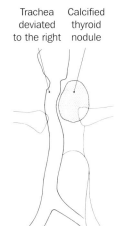

Trachea deviated to the right   Calcified thyroid nodule

Figure 41.39 Goiter: calcified thyroid nodule. This anteroposterior film of the thoracic inlet shows the typical appearance of a large calcified thyroid nodule, which is slightly displacing the trachea to the right side. Most goiters, however, do not show calcification. Calcified goiters are usually benign, but may be malignant.

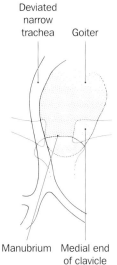

Deviated narrow trachea   Goiter

Manubrium   Medial end of clavicle

Figure 41.40 Goiter: deviation and narrowing of the trachea. This anteroposterior (AP) view of the thoracic inlet shows marked displacement of the trachea to the right by a large left-sided goiter that extends inferiorly to just below the sternal notch. The trachea is slightly narrowed in its transverse diameter just above the level of the thoracic inlet. No calcification can be seen within the goiter. Although any displacement or narrowing of the trachea in the AP plane can be readily assessed on a lateral view of the thoracic inlet, it may be difficult to determine whether or not there is any significant extension of a cervical goiter into the mediastinum.

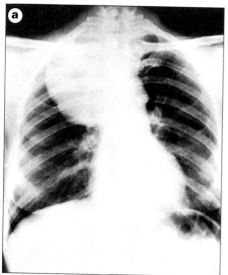 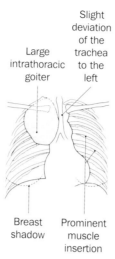

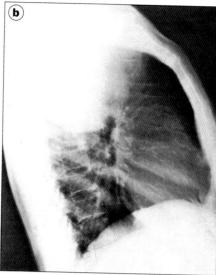 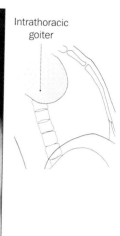

Figure 41.41 Intrathoracic goiter in acromegaly. (a) The posteroanterior (PA) chest film shows a large mass in the right upper chest that is confluent with the mediastinum medially and has a well-defined lateral margin. The mass does not contain any obvious calcification and is only slightly displacing the trachea to the left. (b) The right lateral view shows a clearly defined mass lying posteriorly. The patient had presented with a goiter and had noticed some enlargement of the hands and feet. There were no symptoms of dysphagia or of thyrotoxicosis. The mass in the chest was subsequently shown on radionuclide and CT scans to be in continuity with the cervical goiter. The patient was also found to have a pituitary tumor and acromegaly. Prominent muscle insertions can be seen on the PA chest film at the lower borders of the ribs but no bony changes of acromegaly are present in the dorsal spine (see **Fig. 41.7**). At the combined surgical approach of cervical incision and a right posterolateral thoracotomy, the large mass in the right side of the mediastinum was confirmed to be continuous with an enlarged right lobe of the thyroid gland and was removed. Histologic examination showed that the mass was a large colloid goiter.

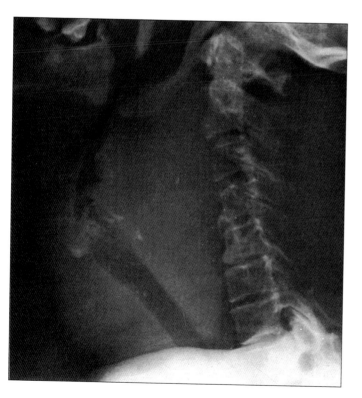 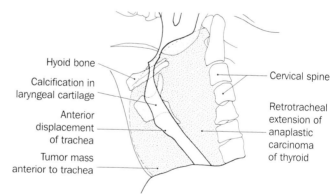

Figure 41.42 Carcinoma of the thyroid: retrotracheal extension of tumor. This lateral view of the neck shows massive soft tissue swelling with marked anterior displacement of the trachea, which is compressed in its anteroposterior diameter. The displacement is caused by gross retrotracheal extension of the thyroid and is indicative of malignancy. This patient had an anaplastic carcinoma of the thyroid.

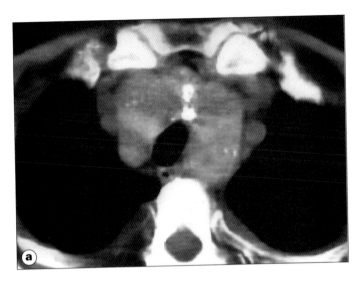

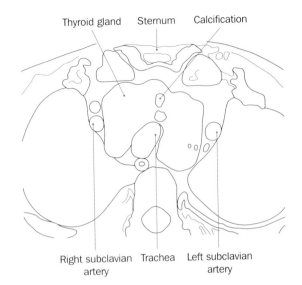

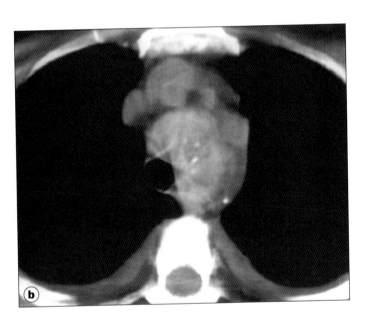

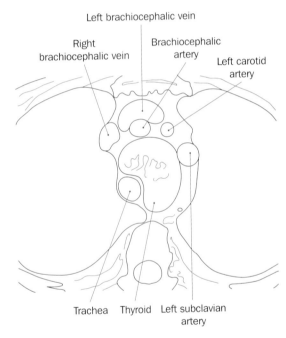

Figure 41.43 Multinodular goiter: retrosternal extension. (a) The unenhanced CT scan shows the enlarged thyroid gland extending retrosternally, encasing much of the trachea and displacing the vessels bilaterally. (b) The CT scan obtained at an inferior level shows the enlarged thyroid gland extending into the middle mediastinum and displacing the trachea to the right. CT has a limited role in the evaluation of thyroid disease. It is occasionally used to demonstrate the extent of local invasion or local recurrence of thyroid malignancy, and to detect the presence of retrosternal and retrotracheal extension of thyroid enlargement.

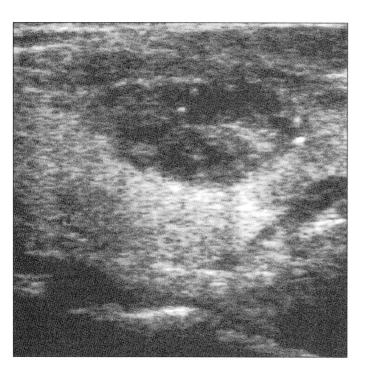

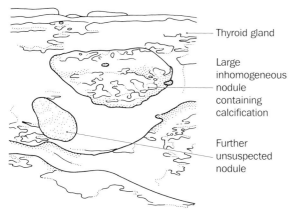

— Thyroid gland

Large
inhomogeneous
nodule
containing
calcification

Further
unsuspected
nodule

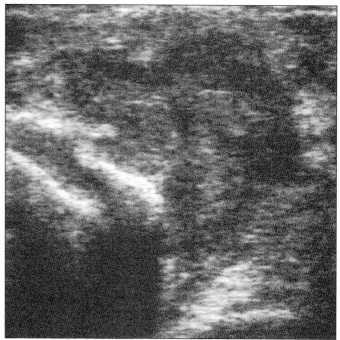

Irregular
inhomogeneous
carcinoma

Trachea

Figure 41.44 Multinodular goiter: ultrasound scan. This longitudinal scan shows a large nodule containing specks of calcium, which was 'cold' on radionuclide scanning (see Chapter 42, **Fig. 42.4**). Ultrasound revealed further nodules, consistent with a multinodular goiter. Fine-needle aspiration confirmed the benign nature of the 'cold' nodule. In patients who appear to have a solitary thyroid nodule clinically, which is 'cold' on radionuclide scanning, neck ultrasound can be of value. It will show if the nodule is cystic or solid. Solitary solid thyroid lesions need further investigation because they may be malignant. The presence of unsuspected further nodules, however, usually indicates a multinodular goiter.

Figure 41.45 Thyroid carcinoma: ultrasound scan. This transverse scan shows an irregular, hypoechoic mass in the left lobe of the thyroid in a patient with metastatic disease but no known primary. Ultrasound-guided fine-needle aspiration yielded abnormal cells consistent with an anaplastic carcinoma.

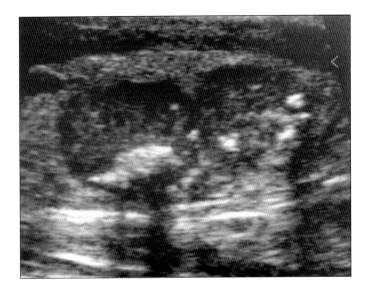

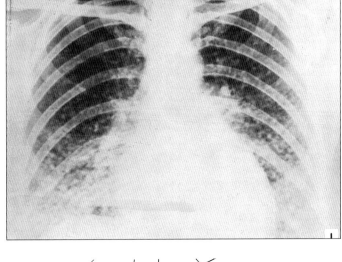

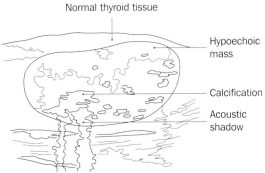

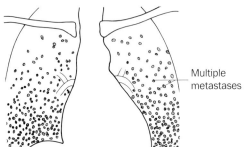

Figure 41.46 Medullary carcinoma of the thyroid: ultrasound scan.
This longitudinal ultrasound scan through the right lobe of the thyroid gland
shows a large hypoechoic mass containing flecks of calcium. Ultrasound
cannot reliably distinguish between benign and malignant thyroid nodules
but is extremely effective in distinguishing between solid and cystic lesions.
As in this patient, certain ultrasound features increase the likelihood of
malignancy of a thyroid nodule. Microcalcification smaller than 2mm in
diameter with acoustic shadowing suggests malignancy, as it is observed in
about 60% of carcinomas but only 2% of benign nodules.

**Figure 41.47 Carcinoma of the thyroid: 'snowstorm' appearance of
pulmonary metastases.** This posteroanterior chest film shows multiple
small nodular opacities throughout both lungs, most marked at the bases,
the characteristic 'snowstorm' appearance of pulmonary metastases from
carcinoma of the thyroid. Such metastatic deposits may remain unchanged
over a long period of time because of very low-grade malignancy and may
take up and be treated with [131]I.

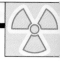

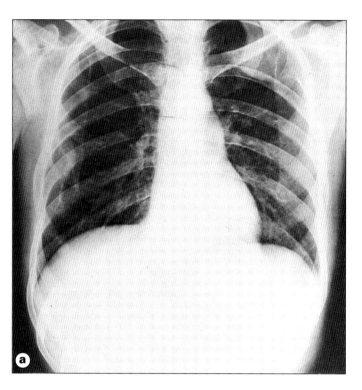

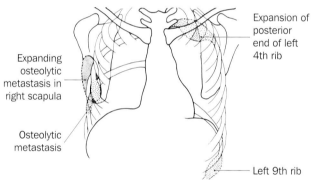

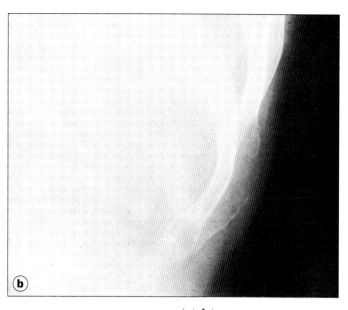

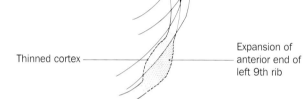

Figure 41.48 Carcinoma of the thyroid: expanded bony metastases.
(a) Posteroanterior chest film showing multiple osteolytic bony metastases.
Those involving the right scapula and the left fourth and ninth ribs show
marked expansion of bone. (b) Coned view of the left ninth rib more clearly
showing the medullary destruction and expansion with thinning of the
overlying cortex. Carcinoma of the thyroid characteristically gives rise to
osteolytic metastases, sometimes accompanied by marked expansion of
bone, as in this patient. The appearance is, however, not diagnostic
because metastatic renal cell carcinoma, multiple myeloma, and
occasionally metastatic carcinoma of the breast may also cause similar
bone expansion. Such thyroid carcinoma metastases may, but do not
necessarily, show up on routine radionuclide bone scanning.

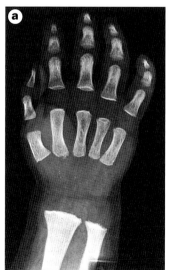

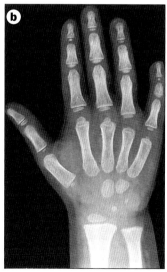

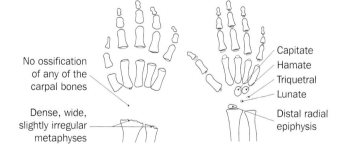

**Figure 41.49 Hypothyroidism in childhood: delay in skeletal
maturation (with normal hand for comparison).** (a) Posteroanterior film
of the hand of a 3-year-old hypothyroid boy demonstrating the
characteristic retardation of skeletal growth. The bones of the hand are
smaller than normal, reflecting the generalized delay in growth that occurs,
and ossification has not yet started in any of the carpal bones or
secondary epiphyses. Irregularity and increased density of the metaphyses
occurs and, in this view, these changes are best seen in the distal radius
and ulna. The appearances should be compared with those of the hand of
a normal boy of similar age (b).

663

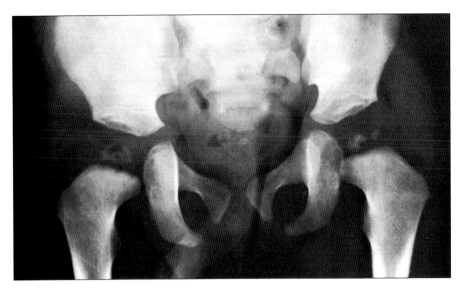

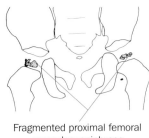

Fragmented proximal femoral
secondary epiphyses

Figure 41.50 Hypothyroidism in childhood: fragmentation of the femoral capital epiphyses. This anteroposterior view of the pelvis shows delay in ossification, with fragmentation and hypoplasia of the femoral capital epiphyses. Fragmentation of the ossification centers of the femoral heads might suggest the diagnosis of bilateral Perthes' disease; however, symmetric involvement would be excessively rare in that condition.

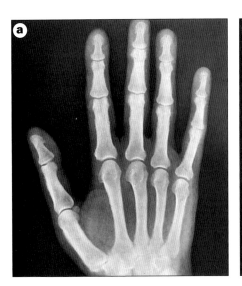

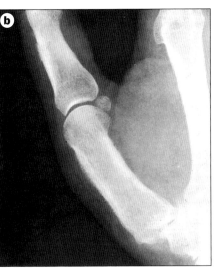

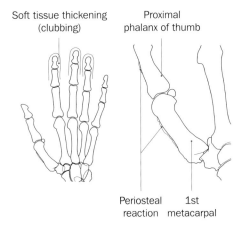

Soft tissue thickening
(clubbing)

Proximal
phalanx of thumb

Periosteal   1st
reaction   metacarpal

Figure 41.51 Thyroid acropachy: hand radiograph showing periosteal reaction and clubbing. Thyroid acropachy occurs as part of Graves' disease and consists of clubbing of the fingers and toes, usually associated with exophthalmos and pretibial myxedema. Bone changes are not necessarily part of the syndrome although they are frequently present. (a) Posteroanterior film of a hand showing the characteristic periosteal reaction of thyroid acropachy along the radial aspect of the shaft of the first metacarpal, the typical site. Soft tissue thickening is evident around some of the distal phalanges. (b) The coned view of the thumb and first metacarpal better demonstrates the characteristic lace-like appearance of the periosteal reaction. Besides the typical involvement of the first metacarpal, periosteal new bone formation may also occur along the shafts of other metacarpals and the proximal phalanges. In this patient a slight periosteal reaction is also present along the shaft of the proximal phalanx of the thumb.

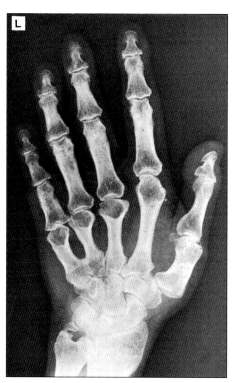

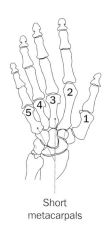

Figure 41.52 Pseudohypoparathyroidism: short metacarpals. This posteroanterior view of the hand shows short, rather broad metacarpals, an appearance seen in pseudohypoparathyroidism. In this patient, all the metacarpals except the second are rather short, but the number involved may be variable.

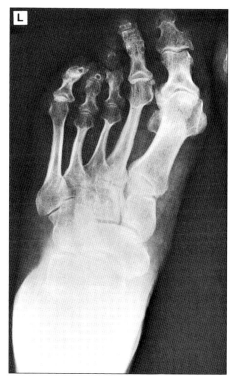

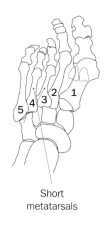

Figure 41.53 Pseudohypoparathyroidism: short metatarsals. This anteroposterior view of the foot shows a similar appearance to that of the hand, with shortening of the third and fourth metatarsals.

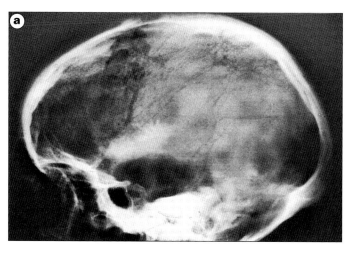

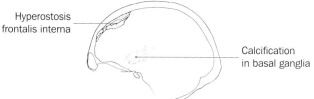

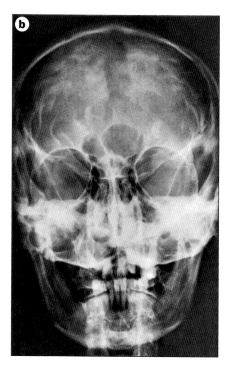

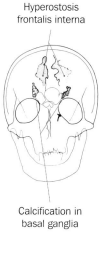

Figure 41.54 Pseudohypoparathyroidism: calcification in the basal ganglia. In pseudohypoparathyroidism, heterotopic deposits of calcium phosphate occur in the soft tissues and most commonly affect the basal ganglia. The lateral (a) and posteroanterior (b) skull films show characteristic symmetric punctate calcification in the basal ganglia. Similar calcification, however, also occurs in hypoparathyroidism. In this patient, slight hyperostosis frontalis interna is also present.

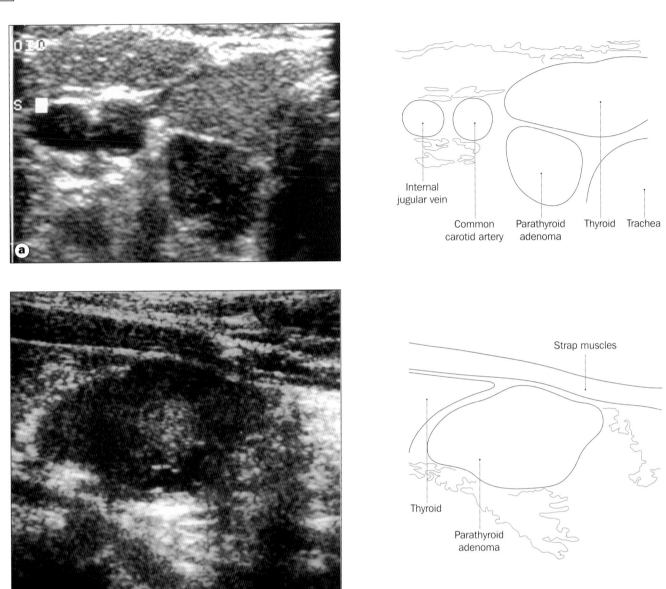

Figure 41.55 Parathyroid tumor: demonstration by ultrasound. (a) Transverse ultrasound scan showing a 1cm parathyroid adenoma, typically of lower reflectivity than the adjacent lower pole thyroid gland. (b) The longitudinal ultrasound scan shows the same adenoma lying adjacent to, but separate from, the lower pole of the thyroid gland. Although ultrasound is relatively sensitive in the localization of parathyroid adenomas that exceed 1cm in diameter, several problems persist. Retropharyngeal, retroesophageal, and mediastinal parathyroids, which account for 5–15% of all glands, are inaccessible. Occasionally in primary hyperplasia, one gland may predominate, simulating a solitary parathyroid adenoma. An exophytic thyroid nodule may also be indistinguishable from a parathyroid nodule. Hyperplastic lymph nodes, prominent longus colli muscles, and sympathetic ganglia can also cause confusion.

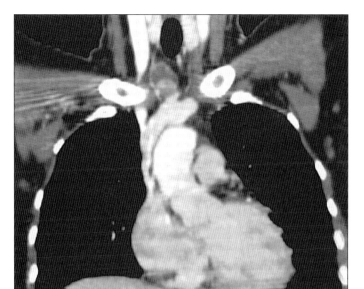

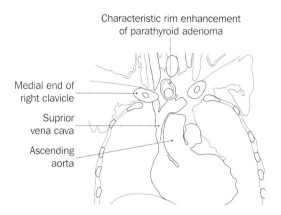

Characteristic rim enhancement
of parathyroid adenoma

Medial end of
right clavicle

Suprior
vena cava

Ascending
aorta

Figure 41.56 Mediastinal parathyroid adenoma. This coronal reformat of a multislice spiral CT scan shows a retrosternal mass due to a parathyroid adenoma. CT (and MRI) are of value before reoperation for persistent hyperparathyroidism and is usually successful at identifying low cervical and mediastinal adenomas. The use of thin-section (2–3mm), contrast-medium-enhanced CT maximizes the chances of locating an adenoma, which often (as in this case) show rim enhancement.

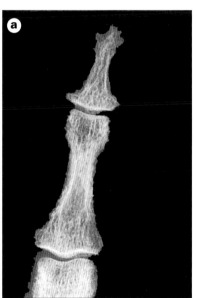

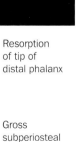

Resorption
of tip of
distal phalanx

Gross
subperiosteal
bone resorption

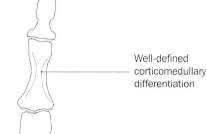

Well-defined
corticomedullary
differentiation

Figure 41.57 Primary hyperparathyroidism: phalanges showing gross subperiosteal bone resorption (with appearance after healing for comparison). Bony changes are now evident radiologically in a minority of patients with primary hyperparathyroidism. Subperiosteal bone resorption is the earliest radiologic sign and is specific for hyperparathyroidism. Generalized skeletal demineralization is a late finding. (a) The film of the middle and distal phalanges of the index finger shows gross subperiosteal bone resorption of the shafts of the phalanges and also of the tip of the distal phalanx. The bone density is decreased and the texture of the cortex shows a 'basketwork' pattern with loss of definition of the normal corticomedullary junction. These appearances of gross hyperparathyroidism should be compared with those in (b), where healing has occurred following removal of a parathyroid adenoma. Although subperiosteal bone resorption classically involves the phalanges, it may also occur at many other sites. These include the outer ends and undersurface of the clavicles, the metaphyseal regions of the growing ends of the long bones, the ischial tuberosities, the pubic bones at the symphysis, the sacroiliac joints, and the inner wall of the dorsum sellae.

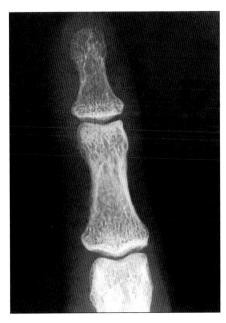

Poor definition
of cortical line
around tip of
distal phalanx

Slight subperiosteal
bone resorption

Figure 41.58 Primary hyperparathyroidism: magnification film of the index finger showing early subperiosteal bone resorption. This magnified film of the middle and distal phalanges of the index finger shows the early bony changes of hyperparathyroidism. Slight subperiosteal bone resorption is present along the radial aspect of the middle phalanx, the characteristic site for early change. There is also poor definition of the cortical outline of the tip of the distal phalanx. The technique of magnification radiography using a fine-focus X-ray tube is helpful in identifying these subtle appearances.

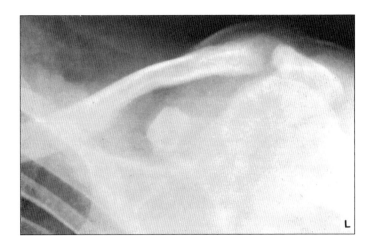

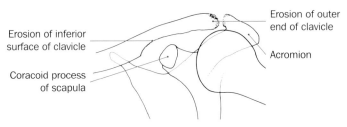

Erosion of inferior
surface of clavicle

Coracoid process
of scapula

Erosion of outer
end of clavicle

Acromion

Figure 41.59 Primary hyperparathyroidism: erosion of the outer end of the clavicle. This coned anteroposterior view of the lateral half of the left clavicle shows subperiosteal bone resorption of the outer end of the clavicle with slight widening of the acromioclavicular joint. There is also erosion of the undersurface of the clavicle above the coracoid process of the scapula.

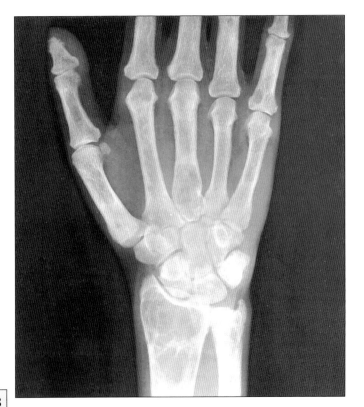

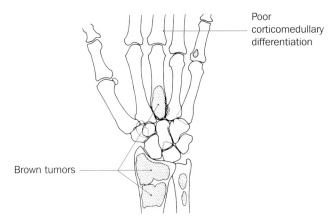

Poor
corticomedullary
differentiation

Brown tumors

Figure 41.60 Primary hyperparathyroidism: brown tumors. Brown tumors sometimes occur in primary hyperparathyroidism but are relatively uncommon in secondary hyperparathyroidism. This posteroanterior film of the wrist shows the typical appearance of brown tumors. Osteolucent bony defects are present in the distal radius and ulna, the base of the third metacarpal, and the proximal phalanx of the little finger. The bone density is generally decreased. After parathyroidectomy brown tumors fill slowly with new bone from the periphery. Incomplete healing results in an appearance that may closely resemble that of fibrous dysplasia.

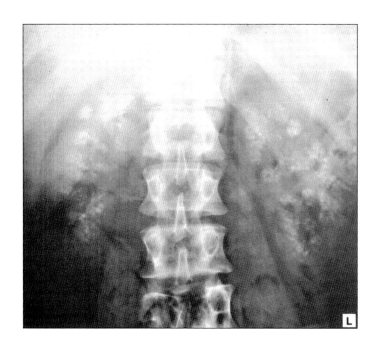

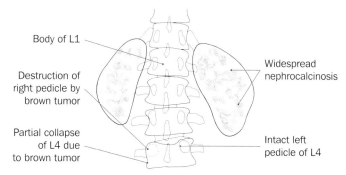

Body of L1

Destruction of
right pedicle by
brown tumor

Partial collapse
of L4 due
to brown tumor

Widespread
nephrocalcinosis

Intact left
pedicle of L4

Figure 41.61 Primary hyperparathyroidism: nephrocalcinosis and a brown tumor. Although pathologically about 60% of patients with primary hyperparathyroidism have renal calculi or nephrocalcinosis, the radiologic demonstration of such abnormalities is far less common. This coned abdominal film shows extensive nephrocalcinosis of the fine type seen in primary hyperparathyroidism. Generalized loss of bone density is present and a brown tumor has resulted in the partial collapse of the body of the fourth lumbar vertebra.

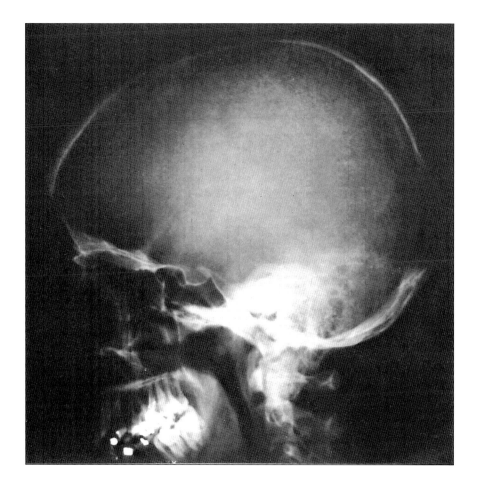

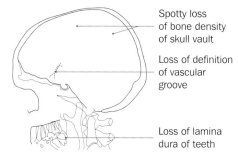

Spotty loss
of bone density
of skull vault

Loss of definition
of vascular
groove

Loss of lamina
dura of teeth

Figure 41.62 Primary hyperparathyroidism: 'pepperpot' skull. This lateral film shows the classical changes in the skull vault of primary hyperparathyroidism. Generalized skeletal demineralization is reflected by diffuse porotic mottling of the calvarium, giving a granular or 'pepperpot' appearance. The vascular grooves are poorly defined and there is absence of the lamina dura of the teeth. The latter appearance is, however, not specific because it may occur in other demineralizing disorders such as osteoporosis and osteomalacia. In some patients with primary hyperparathyroidism the dorsum sellae may be eroded and in those with polyglandular adenomatosis and an associated pituitary tumor there may be enlargement of the pituitary fossa.

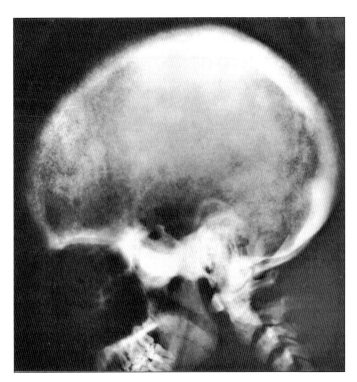

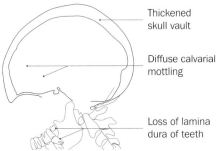

Thickened
skull vault

Diffuse calvarial
mottling

Loss of lamina
dura of teeth

Figure 41.63 Renal osteodystrophy: skull changes. The radiologic
appearances of renal osteodystrophy consist of areas of both
demineralization and sclerosis. These changes are thought to be due to a
combination of osteomalacia, secondary hyperparathyroidism, and a
calcitonin effect. This lateral film of the skull of a 17-year-old girl with
chronic renal failure shows marked calvarial thickening with considerable
mottling. Sometimes such change may resemble Paget's disease. The
skull base and the cervical spine are dense and there is loss of the lamina
dura of the teeth.

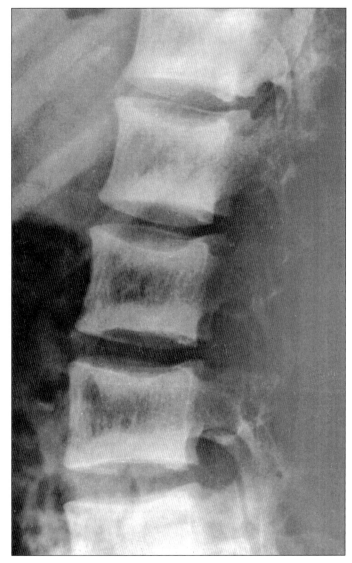

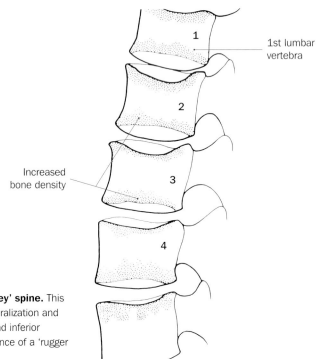

1st lumbar
vertebra

Increased
bone density

Figure 41.64 Renal osteodystrophy: 'rugger jersey' spine. This
lateral film of the lumbar spine shows central demineralization and
linear bands of subarticular density at the superior and inferior
margins of the vertebral bodies – the classic appearance of a 'rugger
jersey' spine.

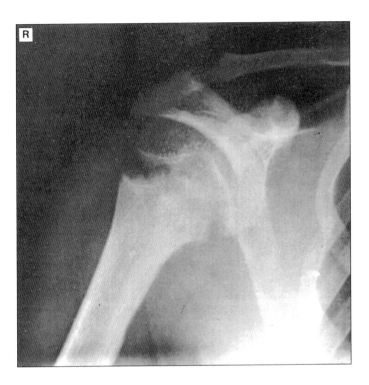

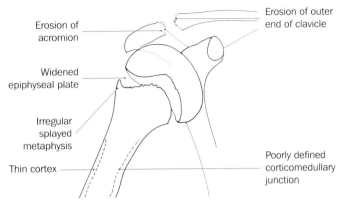

Figure 41.65 Renal rickets: characteristic radiologic appearance of the shoulder. This anteroposterior view of the right shoulder of a 16-year-old boy with chronic renal failure shows marked widening of the epiphyseal plate of the humerus with irregularity and splaying of the metaphysis, characteristic features of rickets. Subperiosteal erosion of the outer end of the clavicle and of the acromion with widening of the acromioclavicular joint indicates secondary hyperparathyroidism. The bone density is generally decreased and the humeral shaft in particular demonstrates thinning of the cortex and poor definition of the corticomedullary junction. The bone age is delayed.

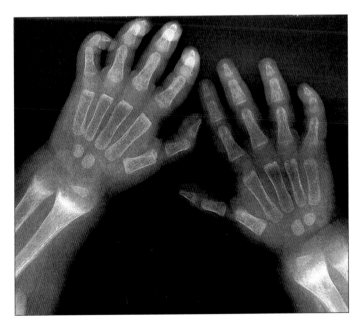

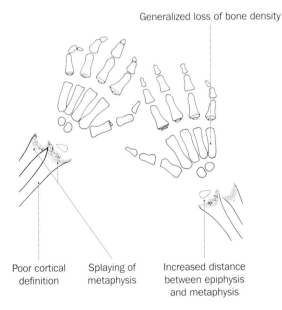

Figure 41.66 Nutritional rickets: characteristic radiologic appearance of the hands. Rickets is the term used when inadequate osteoid mineralization affects the growing skeleton. This posteroanterior film of the hands of a 2-year-old boy illustrates the characteristic appearance of nutritional rickets. Gross demineralization of the bones is present and ossification of the secondary epiphyseal centers is delayed. Wide bands of translucency in the metaphyses and irregularity of the metaphyseal margins are characteristic. The distal radial metaphyses are cupped or splayed because of the effects of weightbearing (i.e. crawling) on the weakened bones.

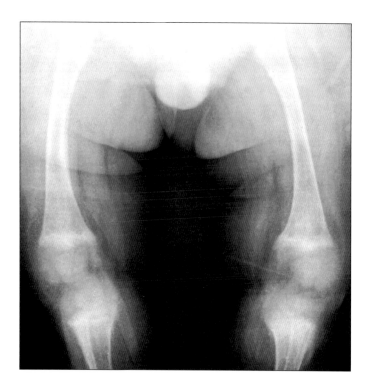

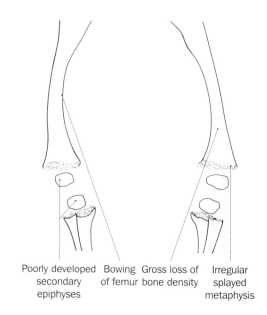

Poorly developed secondary epiphyses | Bowing of femur | Gross loss of bone density | Irregular splayed metaphysis

Figure 41.67 Nutritional rickets: bowing of the femora and genu vara. Gross demineralization of the bones is seen in this anteroposterior film of the femora and knees of the same child as in **Figure 41.66**. Bowing of the femora and genu vara result from the effects of weightbearing on the weakened bones. The film also shows typical splaying and irregularity of the metaphyses and poorly ossified epiphyseal centers.

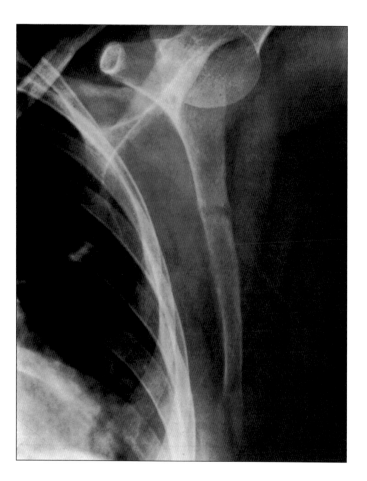

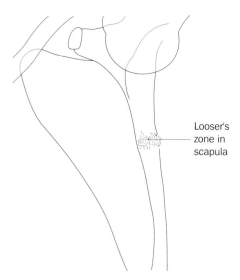

Looser's zone in scapula

Figure 41.68 Osteomalacia: Looser's zone in the scapula. Osteomalacia is the term used to describe inadequate osteoid mineralization in the adult. Stress fractures of the weakened bones are common and the resultant seams of osteoid are known as Looser's zones. This film of the left scapula of a woman with vitamin D deficiency illustrates the typical appearance of a Looser's zone. There is little or no evidence of healing. Because Looser's zones are caused by stress induced by normal activity they tend to occur at constant, symmetric sites: these include the ribs, the scapulae, the obturator rings of the pelvis, the metatarsal shafts, and the femoral necks (see **Fig. 41.69**). Osteomalacia results in generalized demineralization of the bones but this may be evident radiologically only when the disease is severe. When gross osteomalacia is present, deformities of the weakened bones may occur: these include triradiate pelvis, kyphosis, bowing of the limbs, 'hourglass'-shaped thoracic cage, and basilar invagination of the skull.

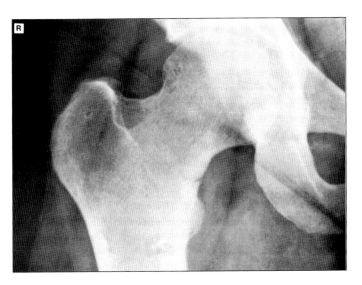

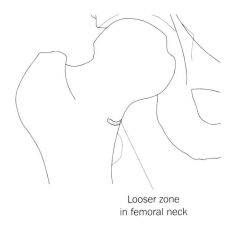

Looser zone
in femoral neck

Figure 41.69 Osteomalacia: Looser's zone in the femoral neck. This coned anteroposterior view of the upper part of the right femur shows a linear lucency in the medial aspect of the femoral neck, a typical site for a Looser's zone.

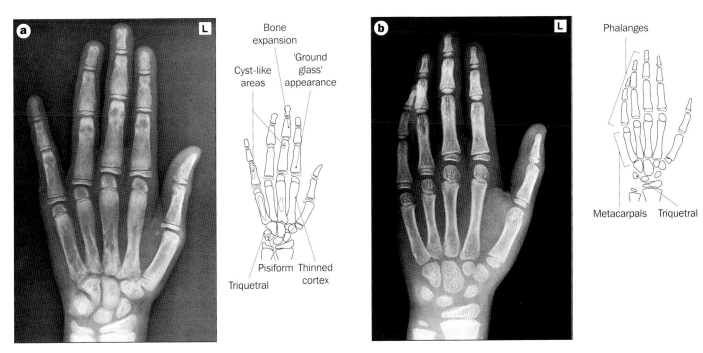

Figure 41.70 McCune–Albright syndrome: hand with normal for comparison. (a) Posteroanterior film of the hand of a 6-year-old girl with skin pigmentation and precocious puberty showing the characteristic appearances of polyostotic fibrous dysplasia. Both bone replacement and new bone formation are evident. The affected spongiosa has an amorphous appearance resembling that of 'ground glass' and the bones show areas of expansion with thinning of the overlying cortex. Small cyst-like lesions are also present, with reactive sclerosis around some of their margins. The carpal bones and secondary epiphyses are well developed and the pisiform bone, which normally starts to ossify at about 9 years in the female, is seen superimposed on the triquetral. The bone age is advanced to 10 years and this film should be compared with (b), that of a normal 6-year-old girl, which shows the degree of bony development that is usual for that age.

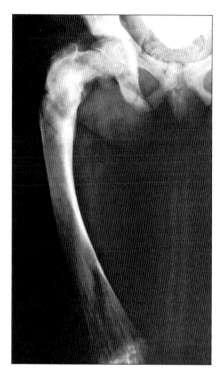
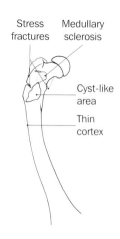

Figure 41.71 McCune–Albright syndrome: deformity of the femur.
This anteroposterior film shows marked coxa vara and bowing of the shaft.
The cyst-like lesions and areas of medullary sclerosis are typical of fibrous
dysplasia. The cortex is thin, particularly at the lateral margin, and stress
fractures are present in the proximal femoral shaft. Such changes often
progress and may result in a 'shepherd's crook' deformity of the upper
femur.

**Figure 41.72 McCune–Albright syndrome: skull showing leontiasis
ossea.** Involvement of the skull by fibrous dysplasia usually manifests by
extensive new bone formation and this lateral film of the same girl as in
Figure 41.70 shows the characteristic appearance of leontiasis ossea.
The convexity of the calvarium is thickened and there is considerable
sclerosis of the floor of the anterior fossae, the base of the skull, the
maxillae, and the frontal bones, making the radiograph features indistinct.

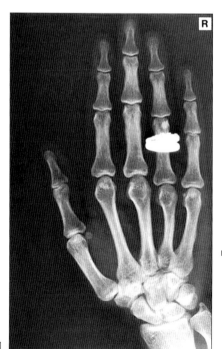
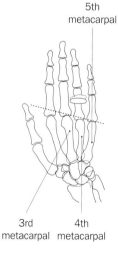

**Figure 41.73 Gonadal dysgenesis (Turner's syndrome): short fourth
metacarpal.** The fourth metacarpal is often short in gonadal dysgenesis,
as in this patient. Normally, a line tangential to the distal ends of the third
and fifth metacarpals will transect the head of the fourth. If the fourth
metacarpal is short, it will touch or lie below such a line. In gonadal
dysgenesis the fifth metacarpal is often also short and occasionally the
third metacarpal may be similarly affected. Premature fusion of the
ossification centers of the involved metacarpals may be seen in young
patients.

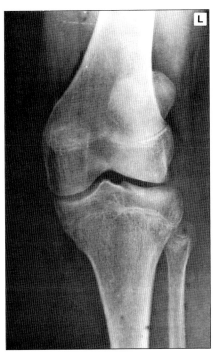
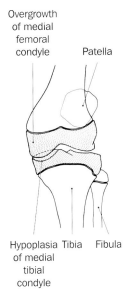

Overgrowth of medial femoral condyle
Patella
Hypoplasia of medial tibial condyle
Tibia
Fibula

Figure 41.74 Gonadal dysgenesis (Turner's syndrome): impaired development of the medial tibial condyle. This anteroposterior film of the knee shows hypoplasia of the medial tibial condyle, which is often a feature of gonadal dysgenesis. The medial tibial condyle appears depressed and there is corresponding overgrowth of the medial femoral condyle.

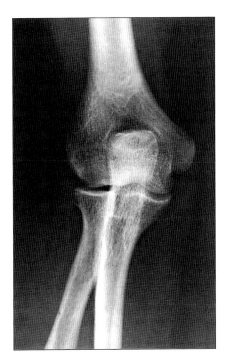
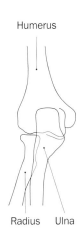

Humerus
Radius
Ulna

Figure 41.75 Gonadal dysgenesis (Turner's syndrome): cubitus valgus. Bilateral cubitus valgus is frequently present in gonadal dysgenesis and this anteroposterior film of the elbow demonstrates the increase in the carrying angle, as shown by lateral deviation of the radius and ulna.

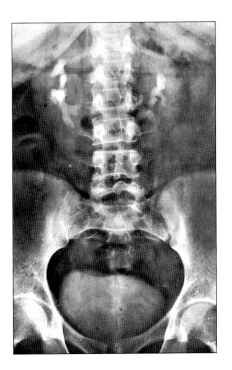
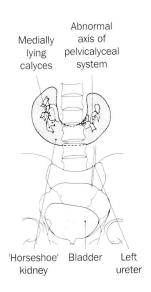

Medially lying calyces
Abnormal axis of pelvicalyceal system
'Horseshoe' kidney
Bladder
Left ureter

Figure 41.76 Gonadal dysgenesis (Turner's syndrome): fused or 'horseshoe' kidney. This full-length film of an intravenous urogram shows a fused or 'horseshoe' kidney, one of the commonest associated anomalies in gonadal dysgenesis. The lower poles of the kidneys are joined in the midline and this results in abnormal orientation of the pelvicalyceal systems and medially lying calyces. Other renal anomalies, in particular those involving rotation and ectopia, are also common in gonadal dysgenesis.

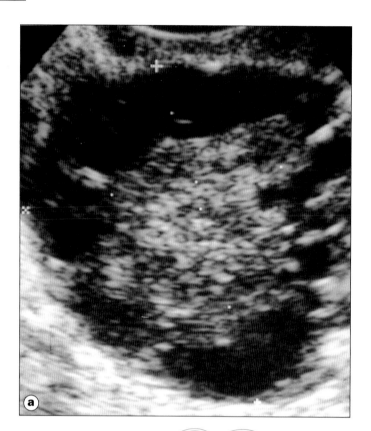

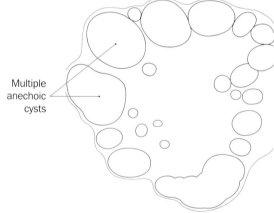

Multiple anechoic cysts

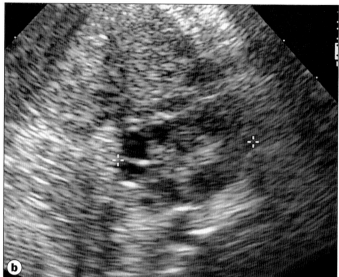

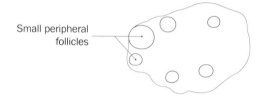

Small peripheral follicles

Figure 41.77 Polycystic ovary syndrome: transvaginal ultrasound appearance with normal for comparison. (a) Transvaginal ultrasound (TVUS) image showing the typical appearance of a polycystic ovary. The ovary is enlarged and multiple anechoic cysts are present. The contralateral ovary (not shown) demonstrated a similar appearance. Polycystic ovaries are best demonstrated on TVUS, which in 50% of cases shows bilateral enlarged ovaries of two to five times normal volume with multiple cysts in a subcortical position, each measuring less than 1cm. A third of patients have normal ovarian volumes, and a quarter will show no cyst formation. (b) TVUS image showing the appearance of a normal ovary for comparison. A few small anechoic foci due to normal-appearing follicles are seen on the periphery. On ultrasound the normal ovary in a premenopausal woman measures up to 3 × 2 × 1cm.

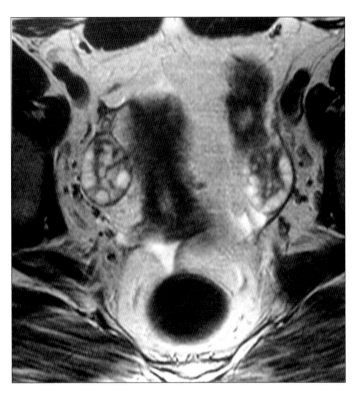

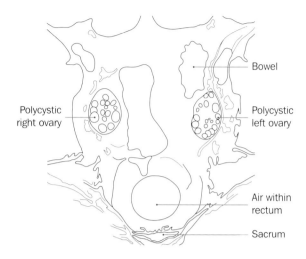

Figure 41.78 Polycystic ovary syndrome: MRI appearance. This axial T2-weighted MRI scan shows the same characteristics of polycystic ovary syndrome demonstrated on ultrasound (**Fig. 41.77**a). The central stromal region of the ovary exhibits low signal intensity on all sequences and, as on ultrasound, more than 10 high-signal-intensity cysts are arranged peripherally.

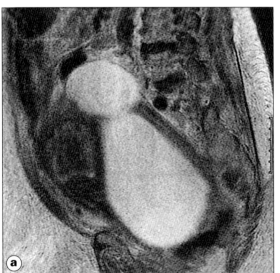

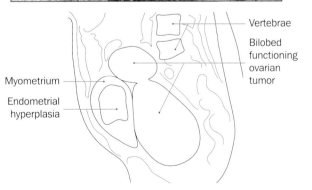

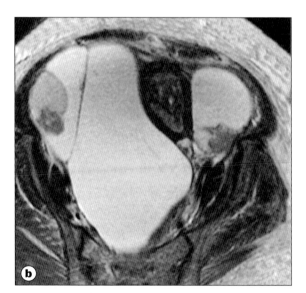

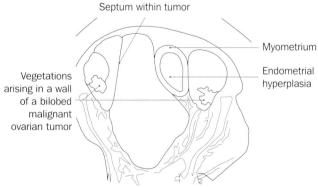

Figure 41.79 Functioning ovarian neoplasm on MRI. These sagittal (a) and axial (b) T2-weighted MRI scans show a large, predominantly cystic, complex ovarian mass subsequently proved to be a granulosa cell tumor. Solid elements (vegetations) within the cystic mass are strongly suggestive of a neoplasm. The endometrial hyperplasia caused by an excess of estrogen produced from this tumor resulted in the patient presenting with postmenopausal bleeding.

FURTHER READING

Francis IR, Gross MD, Shapiro B, Korobkin M, Quint LE. Integrated imaging of adrenal disease. Radiology 1992;184:1–13.

Kawashima A, Sandler CM, Fishman EK, et al. Spectrum of CT findings in nonmalignant disease of the adrenal gland. Radiographics 1998;18:393–412.

King CM, Reznek RH, Dacie JE, Wass JA. Imaging islet cell tumours. Clin Radiol. 1994;49:295–303.

Kohri K, Ishikawa Y, Kodama M, et al. Comparison of imaging methods for localization of parathyroid tumors. Am J Surg. 1992;164:140–5.

Korobkin M, Brodeur FJ, Yutzy GG, et al. Differentiation of adrenal adenomas from nonadenomas using CT attenuation values. AJR. 1996;166:531–6.

Loevner LA. Imaging of the thyroid gland. Semin Ultrasound CT MR. 1996;17:539–62.

Outwater EK, Siegelman ES, Radecki PD, Piccoli CW, Mitchell DG. Distinction between benign and malignant adrenal masses: value of T1-weighted chemical-shift MR imaging. AJR. 1995;165:579–83.

Owen NJ, Sohaib SA, Peppercorn PD, et al. MRI of pancreatic endocrine tumours. BJR. 2001;74:1–8.

Pelage JP, Soyer P, Boudiaf M, et al. Carcinoid tumors of the abdomen: CT features. Abdominal Imaging 1999;24:240–5.

Peppercorn PD, Grossman AB, Reznek RH. Imaging of incidentally discovered adrenal masses. Clin Endocrinol. 1998;48:379–88.

Peppercorn PD, Reznek RH. State-of-the-art CT and MRI of the adrenal gland. Eur Radiol. 1997;7:822–36.

Vincent JM, Trainer PJ, Reznek RH, et al. The radiological investigation of occult ectopic ACTH-dependent Cushing's syndrome. Clin Radiol. 1993;48:11–7.

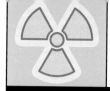

Chapter 42

Nuclear Medicine in Endocrine Disease

Keith E Britton

INTRODUCTION

Nuclear medicine relates to physiology as radiology relates to anatomy. For imaging in endocrinology, an agent is chosen whose uptake or metabolism relates to the function of the particular endocrine system. The agent is radiolabeled with a gamma-ray-emitting radionuclide so that, after its intravenous administration, it can be detected externally and noninvasively by imaging with a gamma camera. If the same agent is radiolabeled with a beta-particle-emitting radionuclide, which deposits considerable energy into tissue, then it can be used for internal targeted radionuclide therapy.

Nuclear medicine techniques may also characterize the tissue by its receptor or antigen expression in ways complementary to radiologic and biochemical techniques. It enables the source of a serum or urinary marker to be determined. It enables the receptor status of a particular neuroendocrine tumor to be demonstrated. The absence of the appropriate receptor is usually related to a failure of therapy with an unlabeled or radiolabeled receptor binding analog. Ultimately, it enables the cancer cell to be demonstrated as different from the normal cell because of features of its essential 'cancerousness'. Unlike radiology, it does not depend directly on the physical size of the tumor and, for a tumor under 1.5cm diameter, its uptake depends on the number of binding sites. In principle, a radioactive pinhead is detectable if it has a sufficient number of binding sites for the radiolabeled agent. Nuclear medicine allows the *in vivo* assessment of aspects of clinical physiology and pathophysiology and is usually very sensitive to metabolic disorders. Stimulation and suppression techniques can be used to enhance its specificity.

The absorbed radiation dose equivalent to the patient from diagnostic tests is of the same order as that from X-ray studies, typically about 4mSv. Natural background radiation from cosmic rays, body potassium, radon, etc. is in the UK and USA on average about 2mSv, but may be as high as 10mSv annually in some locations. These tests give absorbed doses that are considered to be of negligible risk to members of the public. A user of nuclear medicine techniques must be in possession of a license for administration of radioactive substances. In Europe, under the Ionizing Radiation Regulations and the Ionizing Radiations Medical Exposure Regulations, a requestor now has the formal responsibility to provide sufficient information on a signed request form so that the nuclear medicine practitioner can see that the test is justified. Under the same regulations, any medical doctor using ionizing radiation, e.g. for screening a patient during a procedure or for injecting radioactive materials, must have had training in the radiation safety aspects of the use of ionizing radiation.

For therapy the destructive properties of the beta-particle (electron)-emitting radionuclide are used so that radiation therapy can be targeted by the chosen carrier agent to the site of the disorder or cancer. This facilitates delivery of therapeutic levels of radiation even more selectively than is possible by an external beam. Such beta-emitting radionuclides have different energies and different half-lives: iodine-131 (^{131}I) 0.6MeV, half-life 8 days; yttrium-90 (^{90}Y) 2.3MeV, half-life 2.6 days; phosphorus-32 (^{32}P) 1.8MeV, half life 14 days. Thus nuclear medicine techniques are able both to find cancer and to treat cancer.

THYROID

Imaging the thyroid is shown in **Figures 42.1–42.5.** Thyroid cancer is shown as a defect in uptake, which is solitary and in association usually with a palpable nodule in the otherwise normal thyroid gland using technetium-99m pertechnetate (^{99m}Tc), iodine-123 (^{123}I), or iodine-131 (^{131}I); or else as a dominant 'cold' nodule in a multinodular goiter. Once thyroid cancer has been established by histologic examination after surgery, the thyroid remnant (left to protect the parathyroid glands and recurrent laryngeal nerve) is ablated with a high dose of beta-emitting ^{131}I (typically 3GBq (80mCi), range, 1.5–4GBq). Some 3–4 days after the ablation dose a whole-body image is taken of the patient to determine if there are sites of uptake indicating possible metastases. Traditionally, thyroid imaging with a ^{131}I tracer is repeated at 6-monthly, yearly, and then 2-yearly intervals during the follow-up of the patient, together with thyroglobulin (Tg) levels to determine if any iodine-avid recurrence occurs.

To optimize the imaging with such a tracer dose, an administered dose of 400MBq (10mCi) would be preferred. However this and the 200MBq doses usually used have been shown to cause 'stunning', i.e. a prevention or diminution of uptake of a subsequent ^{131}I therapy dose. Thus an 80MBq (2mCi) administered dose is recommended. However, the count rate from this dose is very low. Some patients with a negative ^{131}I tracer scan, but with a raised Tg, who have been given an ^{131}I therapy dose of 5.5GBq (150mCi) may show uptake in recurrent thyroid cancer. This is the problem of a low count rate reducing detectability by an ^{131}I tracer dose. To overcome this it has been proposed that ^{123}I, which gives approximately 20 times the count rate of ^{131}I for the same administered activity, should be used instead. A dose of 185MBq (5mCi) of ^{123}I is therefore equivalent in count rate to therapy with approximately 3.7GBq (100mCi) of ^{131}I. In an initial study it has been shown that this accurately predicts the presence or absence of iodine-avid metastases in the presence of

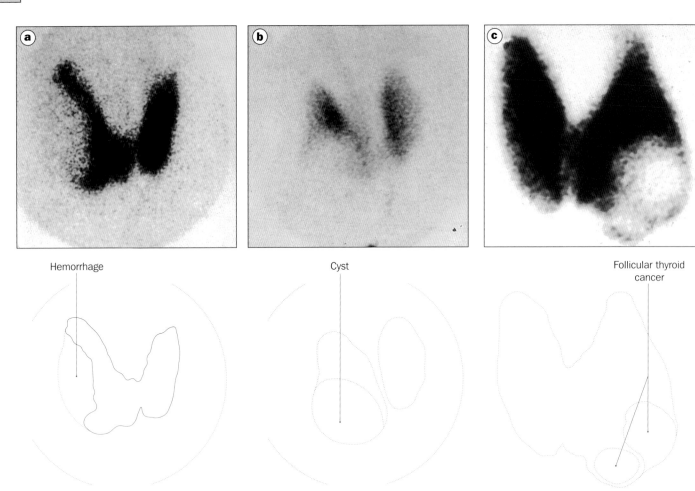

Hemorrhage

Cyst

Follicular thyroid
cancer

Figure 42.1 Thyroid images in patients with palpable solitary nodules in their thyroid glands. You will note that the appearances of the scans are similar, each showing an area of deficient or reduced uptake while the rest of the gland shows a homogenous normal uptake. It is not possible to distinguish between the causes of a solitary nodule: (a) a hemorrhage, (b) a cyst, (c) a follicular thyroid cancer. Ultrasound should be combined with thyroid imaging to demonstrate the simple cyst for aspiration cytology and to enable fine-needle biopsy for the echogenic (solid) nodule, which is nonfunctional in a thyroid scan. If the mass in the gland is solitary and solid, about 12% of these cases prove to be malignant (see Chapter 12).

a raised Tg and thus its use would save unnecessary administration of ^{131}I therapy in patients with noniodine avid thyroid cancer (**Fig. 42.6**). When a therapy dose is given, imaging is undertaken 4 days later to demonstrate the presence of iodine avid metastases, as in **Figure 42.7**.

Medullary carcinoma of the thyroid

This used to be imaged with ^{99m}Tc dimercaptosuccinic acid (DMSA-V), an alkaline version of the agent used for renal imaging, which shows some tumor uptake, particularly in medullary carcinoma of the thyroid. However, its use has been superseded by imaging with iodine-111 (^{111}In) octreotide. This analog of the pharmaceutical octreotide, which is used for treating some neuroendocrine tumors, binds to the somatostatin receptors frequently seen in medullary carcinoma of the thyroid (**Fig. 42.8**).

PARATHYROID IMAGING

The advance in parathyroid imaging has been the use of ^{99m}Tc methoxyisobutyl isonitrile (MIBI) instead of thallium-201 (**Fig. 42.9**).

ADRENAL IMAGING

The adrenal cortex may be demonstrated using selenium-75 (^{75}Se) selenocholesterol in both Conn's and Cushing's syndromes (**Fig. 42.10**) but the technique is less frequently used because of improvement in radiologic imaging of the adrenals. Nevertheless, an incidental adrenal mass may pose a problem (**Fig. 42.11**).

The adrenal medulla and neural crest tumors and some neuroendocrine tumors may be imaged using ^{123}I metaiodobenzylguanidine (MIBG). Several drugs can interfere with MIBG uptake and therapy; these are listed in **Figure 42.12**. In order to be sure that any negative images after MIBG are true negatives, it is always worth imaging the salivary glands since an inhibitor of MIBG uptake will reduce or prevent salivary gland imaging (**Fig. 42.13**).

Imaging of pheochromocytomas and paragangliomas are shown in **Figure 42.12**. In malignant neural crest and/or neuroendocrine tumors, ^{123}I MIBG uptake is used to assess whether ^{131}I MIBG therapy would be appropriate or not, e.g. in malignant paraganglioma (**Fig. 42.14**), in neuroblastoma (**Fig. 42.15**), or in

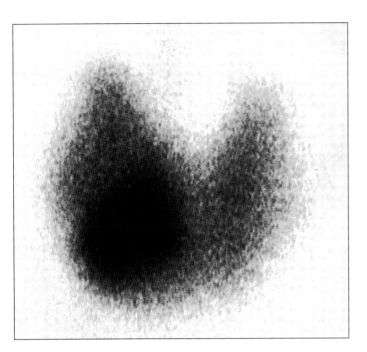

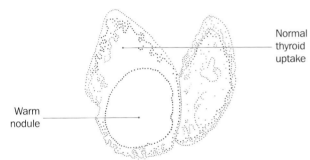

Figure 42.2 A 'warm' nodule imaged using ⁹⁹ᵐTc pertechnetate. Uptake in the inferior pole of the enlarged right lobe of the thyroid is greater than that in the surrounding gland and corresponds to the site of a palpable nodule. The study should be repeated using ¹²³I; see scheme in Figure 42.3.

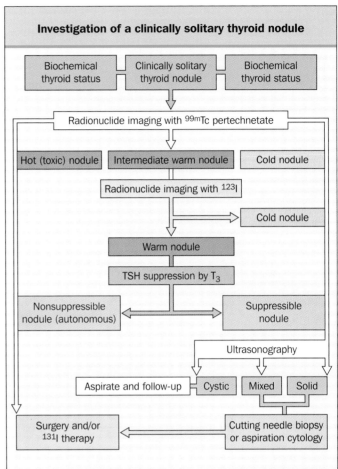

Figure 42.3 Investigation of a clinically solitary thyroid nodule. It should be noted that the cytopathologist can identify anaplastic, papillary, and medullary carcinoma and lymphoma on aspiration biopsy. It is not possible on cytologic smears to differentiate follicular adenomas from follicular carcinomas, since the latter require identification of vascular invasion for diagnosis (see Chapter 12).

carcinoid tumors. Only about 30% of bronchial carcinoids and 50% of abdominal carcinoids show binding of MIBG. This binding is dependent on the reuptake mechanism into chromaffin granules, which may or may not be present in neuroendocrine tumors or indeed may be present in some metastases but not others. Some tumors are MIBG-negative/¹¹¹In octreotide-positive and some are the opposite. Some show uptake of both and some neither of these agents. Only about 30% of medullary carcinomas of the thyroid show MIBG avidity and MIBG therapy is not particularly successful in this tumor.

NEUROENDOCRINE TUMORS

Labelled somatostatin analogs are used to image neuroendocrine tumors. There are at least five types of somatostatin receptor on cells and the distribution of these receptors differs from one cell type to another and from malignant derivative of a cell type to another.

The imaging agent of choice is currently ¹¹¹In octreotide. However, ⁹⁹ᵐTc analogs of octreotide are in the process of development. ¹¹¹In octreotide is the appropriate imaging agent for pituitary adenoma, medullary carcinoma of the thyroid, carcinoid tumors, and neuroendocrine tumors related to the pancreas: insulinoma, glucagonoma, VIPoma, gastrinoma. While typically located in relation to the pancreas, these tumors may be found anywhere in the upper abdomen. Examples are given in **Figures 42.16–42.18.**

New therapeutic peptides that are analogs of octreotide are becoming available such as ⁹⁰Y DOTATOC. It is clear that for therapy with such agents to be likely to be successful, there needs to be demonstration in the tumor of the appropriate receptors for these agents by diagnostic imaging with ¹¹¹In octreotide or ¹¹¹In lanreotide. **Table 42.1** sets out an interpretation of the current receptor binding situation of octreotide analogs. **Figure 42.19** shows a proposed scheme of investigation of neural crest and neuroendocrine tumors leading to appropriate therapy.

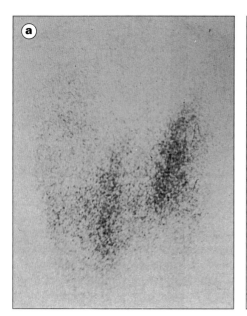

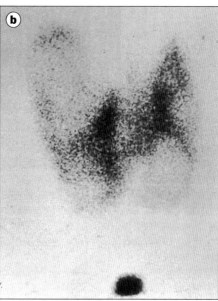

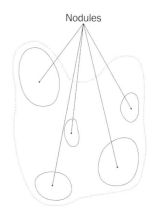

Figure 42.4 Thyroid imaging in a patient with a multinodular goiter. (a) Using 80MBq ^{99m}Tc pertechnetate and (b) using 20MBq ^{123}I sodium iodide. The typical mix of areas of reduced uptake and normal uptake is seen, corresponding to the palpable nodules. The incidence of cancer in such a thyroid is low. However, a dominant nonfunctional nodule should be evaluated as a solitary 'cold' nodule.

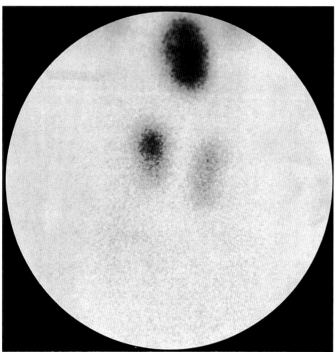

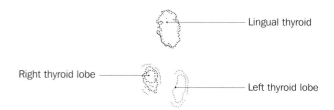

Figure 42.5 Thyroid images in sublingual thyroid. The 77-year-old woman presented with a mass at the back of her tongue. Thyroid ^{99m}Tc pertechnetate imaging shows this to be a source of high uptake. Relatively reduced uptake is seen in the normal thyroid position. Thyroid scanning is an important method for evaluating lumps at the back of the tongue and in the center of the neck. If there is a doubt about pertechnetate uptake, which vascular lesions can mimic, then ^{123}I should be used. A typical thyroglossal cyst is nonfunctional on a thyroid scan.

DIABETES MELLITUS

Nuclear medicine is able to make general and specific contributions to the management of patients with diabetes mellitus (DM) and the evaluation of many of its consequences. Biochemically, the action of insulin on muscle and fat is often emphasized. However, when ^{123}I-radiolabeled insulin is used for imaging and dynamic studies, the uptake of insulin is predominantly by the liver and also by the kidneys. Muscle and fat are not imaged at all.

Insulin-dependent diabetes mellitus (IDDM, type 1) is caused by insulin deficiency consequent on the destruction of pancreatic β cells, which is mediated by an autoimmune process involving activated lymphocyte mononuclear cells. The destructive process precedes the onset of clinical DM by months. This 'insulitis' may now be characterized by imaging the potential diabetic patient with ^{123}I- or ^{99m}Tc-labeled interleukin 2, a cytokine bound by the activated lymphocytes that characterize an autoimmune disease. Initial experimental work in the nonobese diabetic (NOD) mouse demonstrating increased pancreatic uptake of ^{123}I interleukin 2 has been confirmed in the prediabetic offspring of diabetic parents with ^{99m}Tc interleukin 2 (**Fig. 42.20**). The preclinical identification of insulitis may allow therapy of this disease to be instituted before β-cell destruction and thus prevent the clinical onset of the disease.

Non-insulin-dependent diabetes mellitus (NIDDM, type 2) shows insulin-resistant disease that is often related to obesity but is also precipitated by excess growth hormone or excess steroid hormones. The former, due to an eosinophil adenoma of

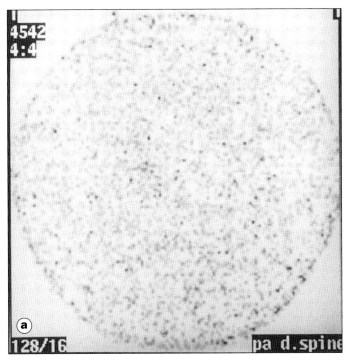

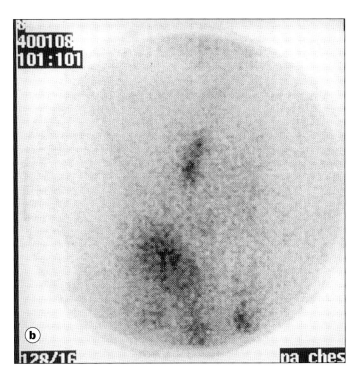

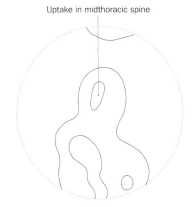

Uptake in midthoracic spine

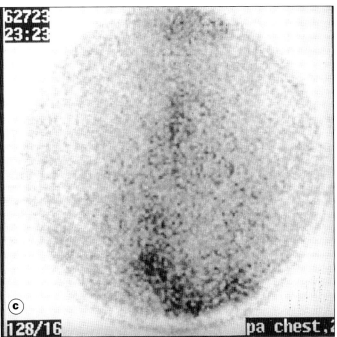

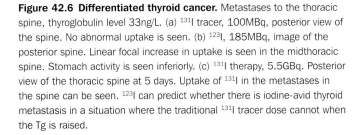

Figure 42.6 Differentiated thyroid cancer. Metastases to the thoracic spine, thyroglobulin level 33ng/L. (a) [131]I tracer, 100MBq, posterior view of the spine. No abnormal uptake is seen. (b) [123]I, 185MBq, image of the posterior spine. Linear focal increase in uptake is seen in the midthoracic spine. Stomach activity is seen inferiorly. (c) [131]I therapy, 5.5GBq. Posterior view of the thoracic spine at 5 days. Uptake of ^{131}I in the metastases in the spine can be seen. [123]I can predict whether there is iodine-avid thyroid metastasis in a situation where the traditional ^{131}I tracer dose cannot when the Tg is raised.

Uptake in metastases in the spine

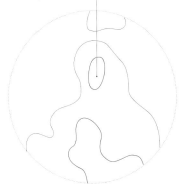

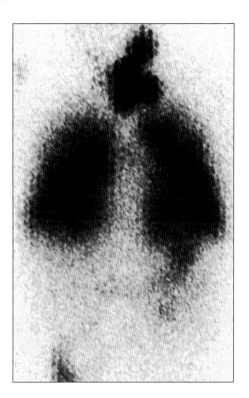

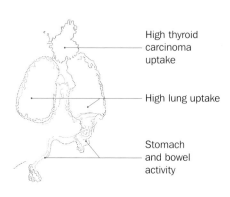

High thyroid
carcinoma
uptake

High lung uptake

Stomach
and bowel
activity

Figure 42.7 Functionally significant thyroid carcinoma imaged 3 days after ^{131}**I therapy (5.5GBq/150mCi).** In this case, imaging shows irregular increased uptake in the superior mediastinum, in the paratracheal and supraclavicular nodes, and diffuse high lung uptake. Such uptake may occur rarely when there is a normal chest X-ray, but is usually associated with miliary lung metastases and shows a good response to ^{131}I therapy. High lung uptake may be followed by radiation fibrosis if the dose administered is too great. Indications for ^{131}I therapy are biopsy-proven papillary or follicular carcinoma and known or suspected incomplete surgical excision. Differentiated tumors concentrate ^{131}I better than undifferentiated and Hürthle cell cancers. Thyroid carcinoma tissue, which at first appears to take up ^{131}I poorly, may show significant uptake of tracer when all higher-avidity normal gland has been ablated (see Chapter 12).

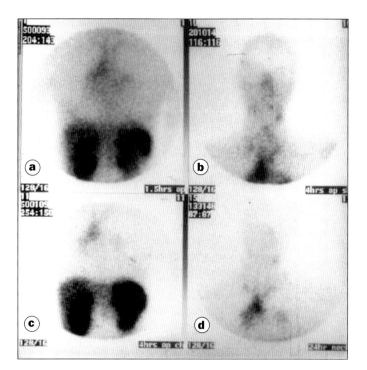

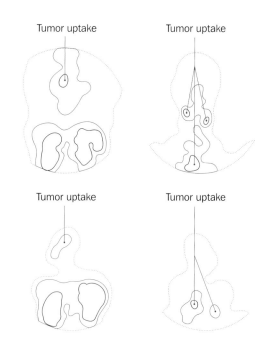

Tumor uptake

Tumor uptake

Tumor uptake

Tumor uptake

Figure 42.8 Medullary carcinoma of the thyroid recurrences. ^{111}In octreotide anterior images of the head and chest. (a) 1.5 hours. (b & c) 4 hours. (d) 24 hours. Irregularly increased uptake in the upper mediastinum centrally and to the left and separately to the right side are sites of metastatic medullary carcinoma. ^{111}In octreotide imaging is more reliable than ^{99m}Tc DMSA (V).

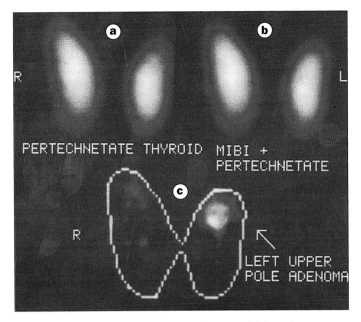

Figure 42.9 Imaging of a parathyroid adenoma. (a) Pertechnetate thyroid scan obtained conventionally 10–20min after the intravenous injection of ^{99m}Tc pertechnetate through an indwelling needle. (b) Without the patient moving, ^{99m}Tc methoxyisobutylisonitrile (MIBI) is injected and a further series of images is taken. ^{99m}Tc MIBI is taken up both by the parathyroid adenoma and by normal thyroid so that a combined composite image is seen. Using a change detection algorithm, the change between the two images is determined and the statistical degree of that difference is plotted as a probability. (c) The high red and orange in the upper pole of the left lobe of the thyroid indicates a change between the two images with a significance of over 1 in 1000. This is the site of the upper-pole parathyroid adenoma. The outline of the thyroid is also shown. A small area of increased probability of change is also seen in the upper pole of the right lobe of the thyroid. Subsequently, a left upper-pole thyroid adenoma was removed and a right upper-pole hyperplastic gland (100mg) was also removed. Prior to imaging, it is important biochemically to confirm that hypercalcemia is due to hyperparathyroidism. Imaging of the parathyroid is intended to localize the site of adenomas or hyperplastic glands. Visualization of a gland depends upon its size. A normal parathyroid gland of less than 20mg will not be visualized by this technique. Earlier attempts to image parathyroid glands using thallium in a similar way have proved less successful than the use of MIBI.

the pituitary, may be imaged with radio-labeled octreotide analogs (**Figs 42.16** & **42.17**). Positive uptake by the tumor means that therapy with subcutaneous 'cold' octreotide would be likely to be beneficial and lack of uptake correlates with a lack of response.

Cushing's syndrome may be associated with bilateral adrenal hyperplasia or adrenal cortical adenoma. Both may be imaged with ^{75}Se selenocholesterol (**Fig. 42.10**).

Carcinoma of the pancreas may be distinguished from chronic pancreatitis by the use of fluorine-18 deoxyglucose (^{18}F DG) positron emission tomography (PET).

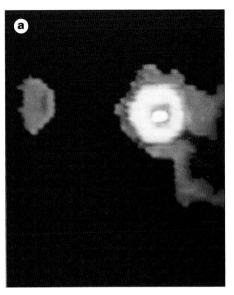

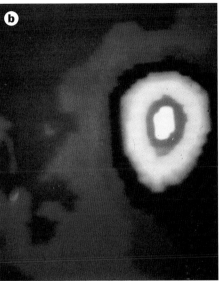

Figure 42.10 ^{75}Se selenocholesterol adrenocortical imaging in Conn's syndrome and Cushing's syndrome. (a) Posterior view of the abdomen in a patient with Conn's syndrome (primary aldosteronism). It reveals high uptake of ^{75}Se selenocholesterol in the right adrenal cortex, shown in red and yellow, as compared to the normal uptake in the left adrenal cortex, shown in blue. Production of aldosterone by a Conn's adenoma does not suppress the uptake of ^{75}Se selenocholesterol by the normal adrenal. The purpose of adrenal cortical imaging is to localize an adenoma or demonstrate bilateral hyperplasia once a positive diagnosis has been made of Conn's or Cushing's syndrome, clinically and biochemically. A second use is to demonstrate whether an adrenal mass, seen incidentally during CT imaging of the abdomen, has a functionally significant abnormality. (b) Posterior view of the abdomen in a patient with Cushing's syndrome due to a solitary cortisol-secreting adenoma. A high uptake of ^{75}Se selenocholesterol is seen in the adenoma. In this case, the left adrenal is not visualized because of suppression of adrenocorticotropic hormone by the high cortisol level, thus reducing the normal uptake of ^{75}Se selenocholesterol.

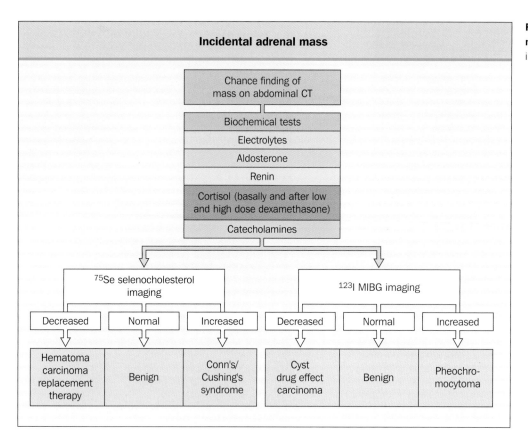

Figure 42.11 Incidental adrenal mass. The figure illustrates a scheme for investigation and diagnosis.

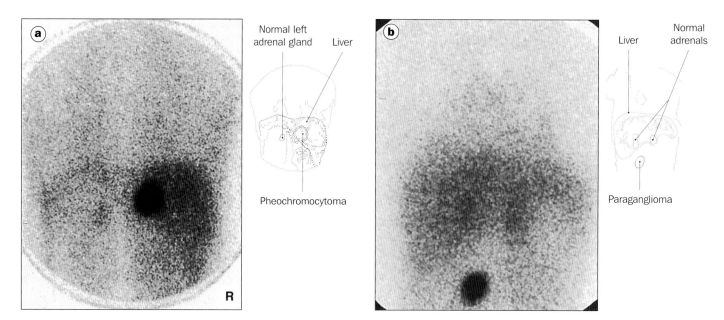

Figure 42.12 **¹²³I metaiodobenzylguanidine (MIBG) imaging in a patient with pheochromocytoma and a patient with ganglioma.** (a) Focally increased uptake is seen in the right adrenal region (pheochromocytoma) and normal uptake in the left adrenal gland. Note that the high levels of circulating epinephrine and norepinephrine have not suppressed the uptake and storage of MIBG by the normal adrenal medulla but cardiac uptake is reduced. (b) High uptake is seen focally in an area in the upper abdomen, inferior to the liver. Uptake in the two normal adrenal medullas is also seen. This technique is 95% accurate in the localization of paraganglioma and pheochromocytoma.

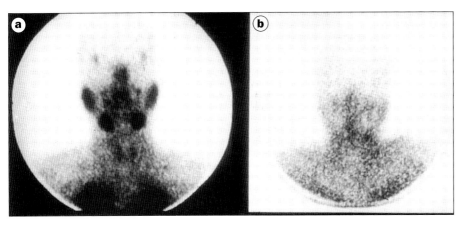

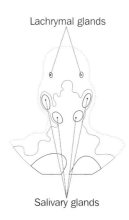

Figure 42.13 Normal ¹²³I metaiodobenzylguanidine (MIBG) images of the face. (a) Normal lachrymal and salivary gland uptake. (b) A normal patient who is taking a drug interfering with MIBG uptake. Note the absent lachrymal glands and a reduced salivary gland uptake. In such a situation a negative MIBG scan may be the result of drug interference and not of absence of a norepinephrine-secreting tumor. (Reproduced with permission from Solanki KK, Bomanji J, Moyes J, Mather SJ, Trainer PJ, Britton KE. A pharmacological guide to medicines which interfere with the biodistribution of radiolabeled metacodobenzyl guanidine (MIBG). Nucl Med Commun. 1992;13:513–2.)

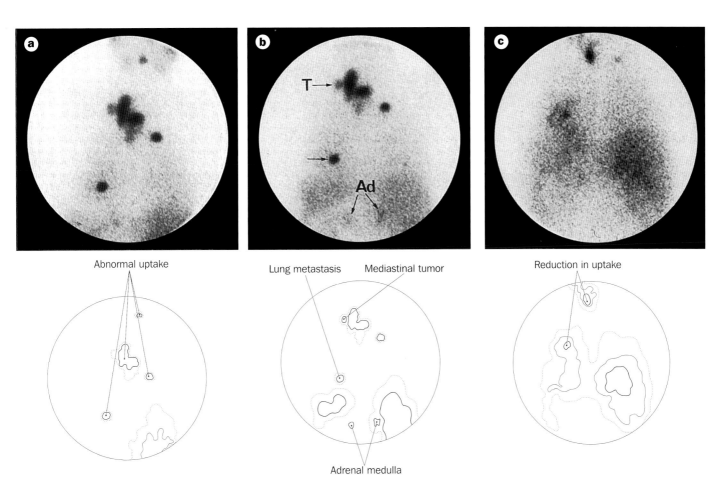

Figure 42.14 Therapy of malignant paraganglioma with ¹³¹I metaiodobenzylguanidine (MIBG). (a) Anterior view of the thorax shows multiple sites of abnormal uptake in the upper mediastinum before therapy. (b) During a course of therapy, 6 months after a total of two doses of 8.9GBq (240mCi) of ¹³¹I MIBG. Arrow, lung metastasis; AD, adrenal medulla; T, mediastinal tumor. (c) 5 years after a total of approximately 37GBq (1Ci) of ¹³¹I MIBG. The reduction in uptake is evident. Before therapy, this patient was incapacitated with symptoms and could not work. After therapy, he resumed full-time work, was taken off all drugs and has fathered three healthy children. In malignant pheochromocytoma, paraganglioma and some metastatic carcinoids, a good clinical and biochemical response is seen after ¹³¹I MIBG therapy. There is usually reduction of active tumor mass observed on computerized tomography. There may be residual sites of uptake seen even although the patient is asymptomatic and catecholamine levels are normal. As the cell turnover in such tumors is slow, so is the interval to response. Thus, benefit may not be clearly established until more than 9 months have passed and, therefore, a course of treatment must be planned.

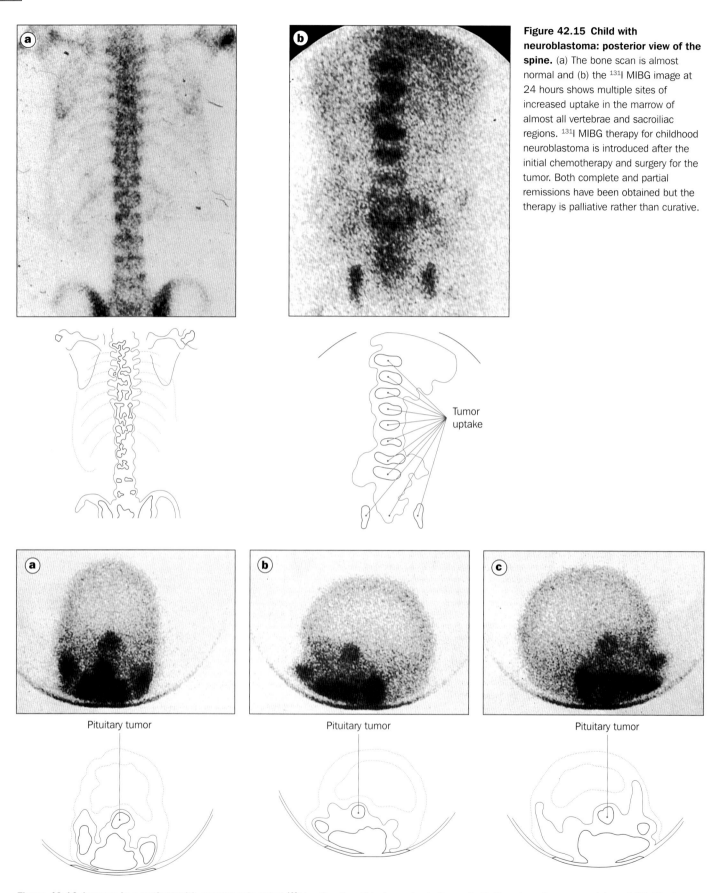

Figure 42.15 Child with neuroblastoma: posterior view of the spine. (a) The bone scan is almost normal and (b) the ^{131}I MIBG image at 24 hours shows multiple sites of increased uptake in the marrow of almost all vertebrae and sacroiliac regions. ^{131}I MIBG therapy for childhood neuroblastoma is introduced after the initial chemotherapy and surgery for the tumor. Both complete and partial remissions have been obtained but the therapy is palliative rather than curative.

Tumor uptake

Pituitary tumor

Pituitary tumor

Pituitary tumor

Figure 42.16 Images in a patient with acromegaly using ^{123}I tyr-3-octreotide (somatostatin analog). The planar images are taken at 10–20min after injection. (a) Anterior view. (b) Left lateral view. (c) Right lateral image of the head. There is intense focally increased uptake in the pituitary region because of the presence of somatostatin receptors on the cells of the tumor, which are labeled. Such patients respond to therapeutic octreotide, with reduction in circulating growth hormone. Indium (^{111}In)-labeled octreotide analog may also be used for imaging.

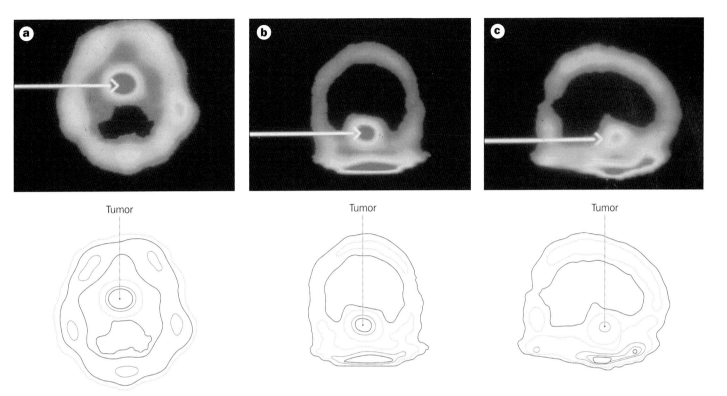

Figure 42.17 Images of acromegaly taken with single photon emission tomography (SPET) using ¹²³I octreotide. (a) Transaxial image through the pituitary adenoma, shown in red. (b) Coronal section. (c) Sagittal section, also showing the pituitary adenoma (arrow).

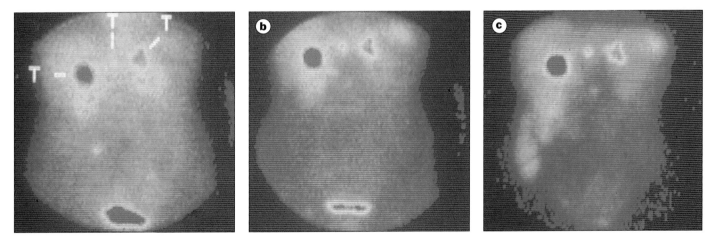

Figure 42.18 Metastatic carcinoid tumor. Indium (¹¹¹In)-labeled octreotide scans taken at (a) 10min, (b) 4 hours, and (c) 21 hours show uptake in the metastases (T). Excreted activity is seen in the urinary bladder in the lower part of (a) and (b). Note that on the delayed images the target-to-background ratio improves.

Postulated somatostatin receptor uptake clinically					
	Octreotide*	¹¹¹In octreotide†	¹¹¹In lanreotide	⁹⁹ᵐTc NeoSpect	⁹⁹ᵐTc H-DOTATOC‡
SSTr1	−	−	+	+	−
SSTr2	+++	+++	++	+	+++
SSTr3	+	+	+	+++	+
SSTr4	−	−	+	++	−
SSTr5	++	+	+++	++	++

* Also ¹²³I tyr-3 octreotide. † Noncompetitive with octreotide in carcinoid. ‡ ⁹⁹ᵐTc HYNIC-DOTATOC, a new agent developed in the author's department.

Table 42.1 Postulated somatostatin receptor uptake clinically. There is disagreement between different workers on the binding to different receptors of these agents experimentally. SSTr2 is typical of neuroendocrine tumors, SSTr3 of adenocarcinoma and lymphoma, SSTr5 of some adenocarcinoma and some neuroendocrine tumors.

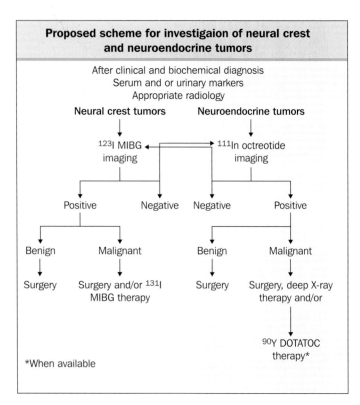

Figure 42.19 Proposed scheme for investigation of neural crest and neuroendocrine tumors.

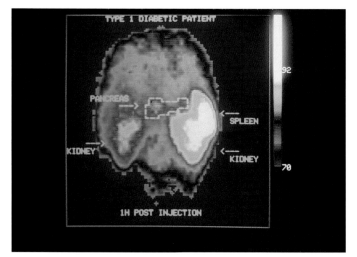

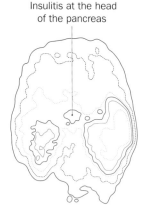

Insulitis at the head of the pancreas

Figure 42.20 Child with early diabetes mellitus whose parents have diabetes. ¹²³I interleukin-2 imaging of insulitis. The pancreas has been outlined using computerized tomography scan section. The area of increased uptake fits the head of the pancreas. Uptake is also seen in the kidneys and spleen.
¹²³I interleukin-2 demonstrates activated T cells participating in the autoimmune destruction of the islets. (Courtesy of Alberto Signore, La Sapienza University, Rome.)

Consequences of diabetes

Diabetes mellitus is a major risk factor for coronary heart disease, for which the stress/rest myocardial perfusion study with thallium-201 (²⁰¹Tl), ⁹⁹ᵐTc MIBI or ⁹⁹ᵐTc tetrofosmin are routine as a prelude to coronary angiography. Diabetes mellitus is also a cause of microangiopathy of the heart and a common reason for cardiac syndrome X. This is a combination of angina, a positive exercise electrocardiogram and normal coronary angiography. Syndrome X accounts for most of the 10% so called 'false-positive' myocardial perfusion studies where coronary angiography is normal. The patient symptoms and a positive myocardial perfusion study show that there is diabetic heart disease even if the exercise electrocardiogram is not positive.

Cardiac single photon emission tomography (SPET) imaging acquired by rotating the camera around the patient with ¹²³I MIBG has provided evidence of diabetic myocardial involvement. With SPET imaging sections of the distribution of radioactivity are obtained. A reduction of the inferior-to-anterior wall count ratio is closely associated with the severity of diabetic cardiac autonomic neuropathy. Prolonged retention of ¹²³I MIBG in the lungs is also a feature of diabetes mellitus and is thought to be related to autonomic neuropathy.

Microangiopathy of the eye is a typical feature of advancing diabetes. The use of a radiolabeled antibody that binds to endothelial receptors in neovascularization is being investigated with the possibility of targeted therapy that would be more specific and less destructive than laser treatment. The antigen is on the ED/B sequence of fibronectin.

The increased tendency to stroke in diabetes mellitus is well recognized and defects may be shown with the conventional ^{99m}Tc hexamethyl propylene amine oxime (HMPAO, a lipophilic agent) SPET imaging. This may also demonstrate abnormalities of regional cerebral blood flow in patients with no history of cerebrovascular disease.

Diabetes mellitus typically causes a progressive microangiopathic nephropathy characterized by proteinuria and loss of renal function. There is often a stage of nephrotic syndrome during this progression. The role of nuclear medicine is in the regular assessment of renal function, typically using the chromium-51 (^{51}Cr) ethylene diamine tetraacetate (EDTA) single-shot clearance technique to measure the glomerular filtration rate. Since the change in renal function is slow, the most accurate clearance method is required. Generally the poorer the renal function and the fewer the blood samples, the greater the error on the estimate of clearance. Thus a technique with a minimum of four blood samples, e.g. at 3, 4, 5, and 6 hours, also at 24 hours if there is edema or impaired renal function, is recommended.

The second area of concern is the attempts to halt progression. This may be assessed by a reduction in proteinuria (as evidence of the degree of microangiopathy) in response to therapy such as that with angiotensin-converting enzyme (ACE) inhibitors. A concern with these drugs is whether detriment will be caused. The benefits/detriment relationship may be evaluated with the captopril renal radionuclide study. The ACE inhibitor captopril improves renal blood flow in essential hypertension and reduces further renal blood flow and glomerular filtration rate in patients with renovascular hypertension. It is also used to evaluate renovascular disorder in diabetes, which has a common association with hypertension. Normally radionuclide studies cannot distinguish small-vessel from large-vessel disease. However, symmetry of renograms is usual in small-vessel disease and asymmetry in functionally significant renal artery stenosis.

Gastroparesis is a feature of diabetic autonomic neuropathy. Gastric emptying may be measured using ^{99m}Tc-labeled liquid and ^{111}In-labeled solids. Both liquid and solid emptying may be affected. Small intestinal and colonic transit times may also be measured.

Because patients with diabetes mellitus are aware that impotence may be a consequence of their disease, impotence should not be assumed to be arteriopathic and may be psychologic. The distinction may be assisted using the ^{99m}Tc or autologous red-cell techniques of Siraj, either with direct pharmacologically induced penile erection or by assessing the pulsatile activity at rest and after intravenous vasodilator stress (**Fig. 42.21**).

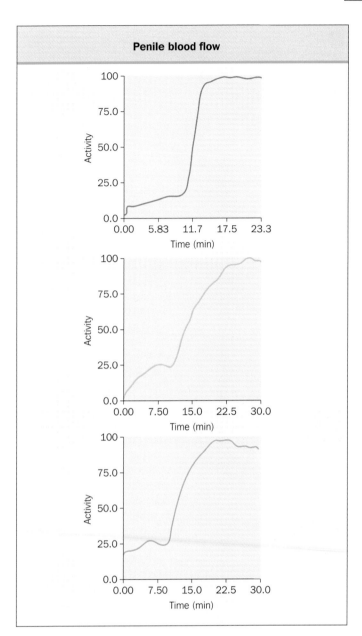

Figure 42.21 Penile blood flow measured with ^{99m}Tc albumin after injection of prostaglandin E into the corpus cavernosum. (Top panel) In the normal patient there is a steep rise to a plateau. (Center panel) In arterial insufficiency there is a slow rise and the plateau is not reached. (Bottom panel) In venous insufficiency there is a slow rise followed by a fall. (Modified with permission from Siraj QH, Bomanji J, Akhtar MA, Rana MH, Sadiq M, Ahmed M. Quantitation of pharmacologically-induced penile erections. Nucl Med Commun. 1990;11:445–58.)

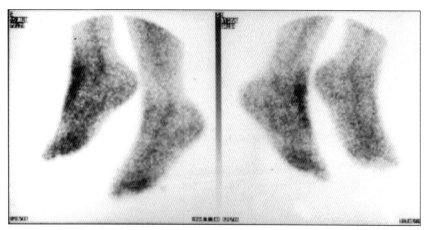

Figure 42.22 Diabetes mellitus: infection of the skin of the foot, imaged with ^{99m}Tc Infecton, a ciprofloxacin antibiotic derivative. Skin uptake is seen in the right foot in the left and right lateral views. The bone is clearly not involved, nor the ankle joint. Infection was confirmed microbiologically.

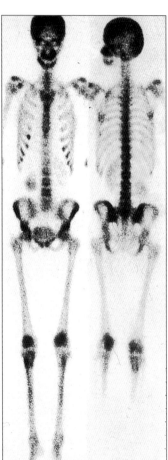

Figure 42.23 Bone scan in hyperparathyroidism. Images were acquired 3 hours after injection of ^{99m}Tc methylene diphosphonate (MDP). The bone scan shows increased uptake in the skull, spine, and long bones. There is also osteomalacia, as shown by the symmetrically increased costochondral uptake. Bone scans with the use of ^{99m}Tc-labeled diphosphonates provide a functional display of skeletal metabolic activity. They may be used in conditions such as osteomalacia, renal osteodystrophy, hyperparathyroidism, and osteoporosis, to identify focal lesions, e.g. pseudofractures, vertebral collapse, avascular necrosis, and generalized increase in bone activity.

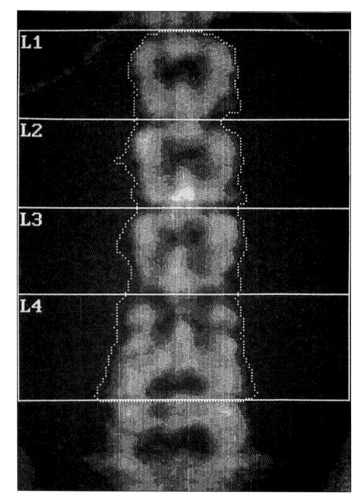

Figure 42.24 Bone mineral densitometry measurement of the lumbar spine using dual-energy X-ray absorptiometry. The method is based on measurement of the radiation transmission of two separate X-ray energies through a medium consisting primarily of two different materials, bone and soft tissue. The total bone mineral content of L2–L4 is measured in grams of hydroxyapatite equivalent (gHA) and expressed as gHA/cm². The normal range depends on age, sex, weight and ethnic origin. Bone mineral measurements from the lumbar spine, femoral neck, and radius are used to assess the bone mass and predict the risk of fractures at these sites.

The high sugar content of blood makes the diabetic prone to skin infections, particularly fungal infections, boils, and abscesses. These are most disabling in the legs and feet where there is a combination of a peripheral neuropathy and arteriopathy. Foot ulcers present a particular problem as to whether the underlying bone is involved as well as the skin. The ankle joint may be neuropathic – a Charcot joint – or infected and the distinction is important. Clinical examination, plain radiography, gallium-67 (^{67}Ga) citrate imaging are nonspecific, but the latter has good sensitivity. ^{111}I and ^{99m}Tc HMPAO or antibody-radiolabeled leukocytes have good sensitivity and specificity. However inflammatory arthropathy and Charcot joints may also show white cell uptake. ^{111}I IgG also has a sensitivity of 86% but has the same disadvantage.

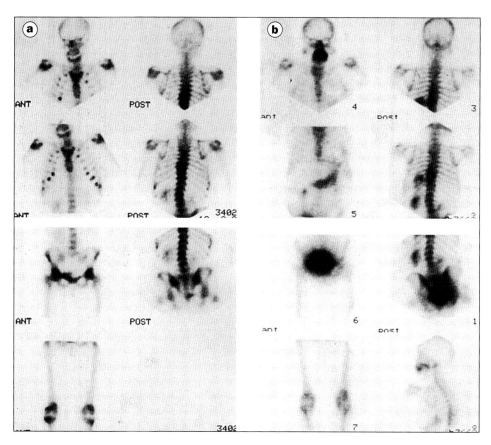

Figure 42.25 Bone scan in osteomalacia.
Bone scans before and after overtreatment with vitamin D derivatives. The set of images (a) shows the following features of osteomalacia: the rickety rosary, symmetrically increased uptake in the costochondral junctions, increased periarticular uptake and increased uptake in the right superior pubic ramus (a pseudofracture). The set of images (b) show that overtreatment has returned all the above features to normal but there is hypercalcemia, a feature of which is intense uptake of the bone imaging agent in the stomach. Renal uptake is also more intense.

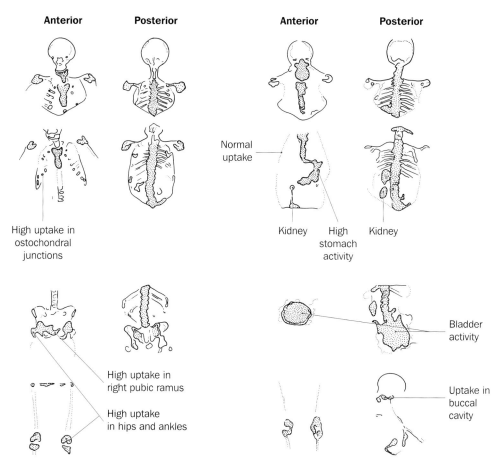

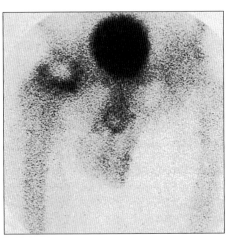

Bladder and penile activity

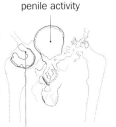

Increased uptake around focal defect in right femoral head

Figure 42.26 Bone scan in avascular necrosis. There is high uptake around a central defect in the head of the right femur. Activity in the bladder and penis is seen centrally. The result is typical of an avascular necrosis of the head of the femur due to prolonged corticosteroid therapy.

The ^{99m}Tc-labeled derivative of the antibiotic ciprofloxacin, Infecton, is a small molecule with good penetration of inflammatory and infected sites. In inflammatory arthropathy and in Charcot joints, this diffusibility means that nonspecific uptake will be seen during the first 4 hours. At 24 hours the uptake fades with the clearance of the Infecton from the blood through the kidneys. Its specific uptake by living bacteria through binding to the DNA gyrase enzyme means that infection can be distinguished from inflammation, since in an infected joint uptake persists at 24 hours. An infected ulcer is imaged positively, as is the associated osteomyelitis if present. Imaging is able to distinguish skin from bone uptake (**Fig. 42.22**). Generally, Infecton has a high sensitivity and specificity for bacterial infection. However a formal study in the diabetic foot has not yet been undertaken.

Infecton studies are positive in infections with acquired antibiotic resistance and conversion to a negative scan appears to correlate with successful treatment, but a formal study is awaited.

In the management of patients with diabetes, it can be seen that nuclear medicine is able to play an important role. It offers the possibility in the future of the preclinical diagnosis of IDDM, of providing therapy for diabetic microangiopathy, and of making a specific evaluation of the presence or absence of bacterial infection.

METABOLIC BONE DISEASE

Osteoporosis is characterized by a tendency to compression fractures, which are seen as linear areas of increased uptake in vertebrae on the bone scan; or else as focal areas of increased uptake in the ribs representing fractures due to trivial trauma or coughing.

Osteomalacia is characterized by focally symmetrically increased uptake at the costochondral junctions as an early finding. Linear uptake at the site of Looser's zones in the scapula, lesser trochanter, or pubic rami occurs later. In hyperparathyroidism it is the long bones that characteristically show increased uptake whereas in osteomalacia the joints often show symmetrically increased uptake. A bone scan may be helpful in hyperparathyroidism and in osteomalacia (**Fig. 42.23**). Dual-energy X-ray absorptiometry is the method of choice for diagnosing osteoporosis (**Fig. 42.24**).

Paget's disease is characterized by increased uptake affecting whole segments of a bone uniformly (**Fig. 42.25**), unlike fibrous dysplasia, which shows irregular uptake in long bones. In Paget's disease the lamina of the vertebrae and the spinous process all show increased uptake, giving a trefoil appearance unlike that seen in osteoarthritis or metastases.

Avascular necrosis, e.g. following steroid therapy, is seen as a characteristic focal defect surrounded by increased uptake, e.g. in the head of the femur (**Fig. 42.26**).

FURTHER READING

Britton KE, Foley RR, Siddiqui A, et al. ^{123}I imaging for the prediction of ^{131}I therapy for recurrent differentiated thyroid cancer, RDTC, when ^{131}I tracer is negative but raised thyroglobulin, Tg. Eur J Nucl Med. 1999;26:1013.

Britton KE, Imaging the adrenal cortex: why and wherefore? Nucl Med Commun. 1992;13:485–7.

Chesser AMS, Carroll MC, Lightowler C, McDougal IC, Britton KE. Technetium-99m methoxyisobutyl isonitrile (MIBI) imaging of the parathyroid glands in patients with renal failure. Nephrol Dialysis Transplant. 1997;12:97–100.

Datseris IE, Sonmezoglu K, Siraj QH, et al. Predictive value of Captopril transit renography in essential hypertension and diabetic nephropathy. Nucl Med Commun. 1995;16:4–9.

Johnston LB, Carroll MC, Britton KE, et al. The accuracy of parathyroid localization in primary hyperparathyroidism using Sestamibi radionuclide imaging. J Clin Endodrinol Metab. 1996;81:346–52.

Krenning EP, Kwekkeboom DJ, Bakkar L, et al. Somatostatin receptor scintigraphy with In-111-DTPA-D-Phe and I-123-Tyr 3-Octreotide: the Rotterdam experience with more than 1000 patients. Eur J Nucl Med. 1993;20:716–31.

Oyen WJG, Netten PM, Lemmens AM, et al. Evaluation of infectious diabetic foot complications with ^{111}I labelled human non specific immunoglobulin G. J Nucl Med. 1992;33:1330–6.

Siraj QH, Hilson AJW. Diagnostic value of radionuclide phallography with intravenous vasodilator stress in the evaluation of arteriogenic impotence. Eur J Nucl Med. 1994;21:651–75.

Solanki KK, Bomanji J, Moyes J, Mather SJ, Trainer PJ, Britton KE. A pharmacological guide to medicines which interfere with the biodistribution of radiolabeled metacodobenzyl guanidine (MIBG). Nucl Med Commun. 1992;13:513–2.

Vinjamuri S, Hall AV, Solanki KK, et al. Comparison of ^{99m}Tc Infecton imaging with radiolabelled white cell imaging in the evaluation of bacterial infection. Lancet 1996;347:233–5.

Zinny M, Bares R, Fass J, et al. Fluorine-18, fluorodeoxyglucose positron emission tomography in the differential diagnosis of pancreatic carcinoma: a report of 106 cases. Eur J Nucl Med. 1997;24:678–82.

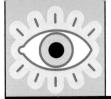
Chapter 43

Patient Perspectives on Endocrine Diseases – Representatives of Patient Support Groups for:

Thyroid Disease

Lora Hammer

I noticed the first symptoms of Graves' disease in June 1973, when I was 27 years old. The only thing I identified as a problem was a constant irritation in my eyes, as if there was sand in them. Soon after, they became swollen, inflamed, and itchy too. The notion that this might be a symptom of a thyroid disorder never entered my mind – I considered it an eye problem and consulted an eye doctor for treatment. The eye doctor, who probably knew little more about thyroid-associated eye changes than I did, diagnosed the problem as a viral infection and treated it as such. I went to another eye doctor when my eyes didn't improve, who said my eyes hurt because my eyelashes were too long and curled inward. He proceeded to cut all of my eyelashes off! Of course, the problem did not go away, and my eyes fluctuated over the course of the summer.

I was experiencing other symptoms, too, but I didn't question them. I lost 15 pounds (7kg) during the summer and was so delighted I didn't think to ask why. I seemed to feel the heat very badly, but it was a hot summer and I worked in a hospital ward without air-conditioning – everyone felt the heat. I certainly never thought to connect my eye problems with anything else in my body.

Near the end of the summer my symptoms became more severe. My eyes bulged and the lids retracted, so that it became difficult to fully close my eyes when I slept. I was constantly on edge and very irritable, and had trouble sleeping. My heart was constantly racing and pounding, and my legs became rubbery and weak after even the slightest exercise. Still I failed to connect these symptoms with each other, or with my eye problems.

I am fortunate to have a brother-in-law who is a doctor. When he came to visit my husband and me at the end of the summer, he took one look at me and immediately diagnosed Graves' disease. He told me that it was crucial to find a good endocrinologist who specialized in thyroid disease because I needed to be treated and followed for the rest of my life. I must say that it was almost a relief to find out that there was a reason for my not feeling well. All of my symptoms suddenly made sense: my husband and others were not deliberately trying to irritate me, my eyes were not suddenly deteriorating for no reason, my insomnia and pounding heart were, although not normal, at least understandable. The symptoms of irritability and nervous excitement, however, made it difficult to cope with my disease because I could not calmly sit down and think things out rationally. I was always too jumpy or too edgy. I knew my irritability was hurting those around me, but I felt there was nothing I could do. It was

also at this point that the heat and frustration at work became so great that I decided to leave until I felt better and could get my life back in control.

Fortunately, my brother-in-law had a friend in Boston who was a thyroid specialist and I was able to see him right away. After having blood tests and a thyroid scan, I was officially diagnosed with Graves' disease.

Although Graves' disease can be difficult to deal with, luckily it is treatable. My physician explained the three choices of treatment for Graves' disease and made his recommendations. One treatment was antithyroid drugs, which act to prevent the thyroid from making thyroid hormone. He explained that once there was less thyroid hormone being made I would probably start to feel better within 2 weeks and be well in about 6–8 weeks. He also explained that he didn't want me to be on these drugs for more than 1–2 years. Also, there was a risk of the Graves' disease coming back once I went off the medication. The second choice of treatment was radioactive iodine. It is a clear liquid that you drink, which then goes into the thyroid gland and destroys the thyroid tissue within 3–6 months. Today, some regard it as the treatment of choice for Graves' disease and it is considered very safe. The only downside is that often patients become hypothyroid after drinking the radioactive iodine. The third choice of treatment is surgery, where about 90% of the thyroid is removed. Again, the patient will probably become hypothyroid.

In my case, which treatment to use was decided by other circumstances in my life. I was 27 and my husband and I wanted to start a family right away. I didn't want to take the antithyroid drugs for a long period of time. I personally was adamant that I never wanted the risk of my Graves' disease coming back, once I went off of the drugs.

At the time, in 1973, there was no guarantee that radioactive iodine might not have serious long-term effects on an unborn child and I felt very uneasy about using this treatment. I also knew that if I used it I would have to wait 6 months to a year to become pregnant and I just didn't want to wait that long. My choice of treatment was, therefore, surgery. I don't know how easy this option would be today, but in 1973 my doctor agreed that surgery would probably be the best one for a woman who was trying to get pregnant.

I was started on methimazole, an antithyroid drug, and a beta-blocker to slow down my heart rate until my surgery could be scheduled.

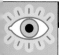
My next challenge was to find the best surgeon in the Boston area. After consulting with him, he convinced me to also see a thyroid physician and ophthalmologist so that they could work together. I was shown how to put ointment in my eyes and tape them shut while sleeping at night. Much of the irritation was relieved simply by sleeping with my eyes fully closed, and I was very grateful to find a way to relieve some of the discomfort.

After being on methimazole for a few months my thyroid hormone levels returned to normal and I was in remission and my thyroid surgery was scheduled 6 months after the diagnosis was made. I was admitted to hospital the day before the operation was scheduled but in the evening my surgeon decided to postpone my thyroidectomy. After consulting my endocrinologist and ophthalmologist, the three doctors had agreed that my eyes were too unstable for surgery. They were afraid that they would get worse and felt I should wait another month to see if my eyes would stabilize. I was devastated by the postponement but knew deep in my heart that they were doing this because they were truly concerned about my welfare and the condition of my eyes.

When I finally had my thyroid surgery, I can honestly say that the surgery was not bad at all. I had some discomfort in my neck and it felt stiff when I tried to lift my head up off of the pillow, but I do not remember any pain. My incision was very small and healed very quickly. I was put on thyroid hormone replacement after my thyroidectomy because, even though a small amount of my thyroid was left, I had become hypothyroid. I was told that I would be on this medication for the rest of my life and that it would be necessary to have my blood thyroid levels checked at least once a year.

Unfortunately, I did have problems with my eyes. Right after the thyroidectomy I developed an ulcer on my cornea and had to be transferred to an eye hospital, where I stayed for 5 days. My eyes were very painful and it was necessary to sew them shut. Every morning the surgeon would untie the threads holding them shut to see how they were healing. It was very frightening to not be able to see, but my ulcer healed quickly because my eyes were closed all the time. When I was discharged I was sent home on corticosteroid pills, which I had to stay on for a month and a half to reduce the inflammation in my eyes. I think this was the most difficult time for me. My vision was very blurred and my eyes were swollen and inflamed. Also my lids were very retracted. Besides the pain, I was very frightened that I might not ever see clearly again. I also had to deal with the fact that my appearance had greatly changed. It is hard to hide your eyes and I felt very self-conscious about how I looked.

After about 6 weeks I was able to go off of the corticosteroid pills and my vision did improve somewhat, but my eyes were still very inflamed and they still protruded. The realization that I might have permanent eye problems was very hard to accept. Gradually, over the next few months, things started to calm down and my thyroid levels became stabilized. In June, my endocrinologist finally told me that I could try to become pregnant and by August I was! My pregnancy was totally normal, but I was followed very closely by my endocrinologist, as well as by my obstetrician. I had my blood levels checked frequently to adjust my medication because the amount of thyroid hormone I needed

increased as the baby developed. It was during my pregnancy that I noticed that my eyes were slowly getting better. I still had to tape them shut at night, but they were not as inflamed and they didn't seem to protrude as much. My lids seemed to be less retracted, also. Almost 2 years after my initial diagnosis, I gave birth to a beautiful baby boy. My husband and I were so thrilled that we finally had a child, and that he was healthy and normal.

When my son was 3 years old I became pregnant again – and I had a beautiful and healthy baby girl. Again, my pregnancy was followed very closely by my endocrinologist and obstetrician, and it and my delivery were completely normal. At that stage of my life I was still putting ointment in my eyes and taping them shut at night, but they were continuing to improve and I had reached a point where I was not embarrassed about my appearance. Since my diagnosis, I felt that whenever I met new people I had to explain why I looked the way I did. Now, for the first time, when I told people about my Graves' disease, they said they didn't even notice that there was anything wrong with my eyes. After a few more years, I stopped taping my eyes at bedtime. To this day, I still put ointment in them at night to protect them in case I don't close them all the way when I sleep, and I put hypoallergenic drops in them every morning to clear out the ointment and to moisten them. Although I don't feel that I look the same as I did before, I am confident that my eyes look normal now.

Graves' disease is an autoimmune disease that tends to run in families. There are also other autoimmune diseases that tend to occur more frequently in Graves' disease patients and their families. Type 1 diabetes, or insulin-dependent diabetes, is one of those autoimmune diseases. I learned from my parents that my paternal grandmother had had insulin-dependent diabetes and that my father's sister had had Graves' disease. My daughter developed type 1 diabetes soon after her 12th birthday. It was a very difficult adjustment for all of us, but my daughter has done very well and continues to stay in excellent control. Her illness has made me very aware of the importance of my children being periodically tested for thyroid disease.

When my daughter was 6 years old I decided that I would like to go back to work part time. I mentioned it to my endocrinologist, who told me he wanted to start a nonprofit organization specifically for the education and support of thyroid patients. He asked me if I was interested in working with him and of course I was. The Thyroid Foundation of America, Inc. was founded in 1985 and he has been its President and Medical Director since its inception. I have worked as the Assistant Director for Membership for the past 15 years and I have found it very rewarding and fulfilling. We get thousands of phone calls and letters per year from thyroid patients and health professionals who request free information about thyroid disorders, and we are there to educate and support them. We also have a membership of about 4,500 people who receive our newsletter four times a year with articles written by leading thyroid specialists about different thyroid problems. We have a website at www.allthyroid.org, which is very informative and links to other thyroid-related websites. Similar organizations exist in other countries.

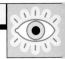

I know that when I was first diagnosed with Graves' disease I was frightened and confused. It would have been so helpful to have an organization to turn to to help me understand what was happening to my body and to help me through the emotional and physical problems I was experiencing. That is one of the main reasons I get such satisfaction from speaking to other thyroid patients who are newly diagnosed. I know that by telling them that my eyes have almost fully recovered and that I have been basically on the same dosage of thyroid hormone replacement since my children were born 25 years ago, I have given them hope and the realization that they will get better, too.

- The Thyroid Foundation of America, Inc., 410 Stuart Street, Boston, MA 02116 USA. Tel: (+1) 800–832–8321 or 617–534–1500; Fax: (+1) 617–534–1515; E-mail: info@allthyroid.org
- The Thyroid Federation International (our worldwide contact), 96 Mack Street, Kingston, Ontario K7L 1N9 Canada. Tel: (+1) 613–544–8364; Fax: (+1) 613–544–9731; E-mail: tfi@on.aibn.com
- British Thyroid Foundation, P.O. Box 97, Clifford, Wetherby, West Yorkshire, L523 6XD, UK

Thyroid Eye Disease   Julian Britton

In all areas of human contact one of the most important factors is the first impression. It is well known that upon meeting someone for the first time we evaluate, categorize, and impress in our psyche our perception of this person in only just 3 seconds! Amazing, isn't it? We store the judgment of this person in our memory along with our feelings for them. Many things contribute to this – what they wear, how they hold themselves, a smile or a frown – but eye contact is the most important.

Sufferers with thyroid eye disease have a double burden to bear. Not only have they a thyroid imbalance that makes them feel ill most of the time but, in addition to this, their appearance, especially their faces, change. So they are reluctant to make eye contact with strangers or even with people who knew them before the illness struck.

In severe cases, when the eyes become proptotic, this has the effect of making the person seem aggressive to outsiders, who are likely to react with equal aggression.

But, first things first. Before a patient gets to know what is wrong, there has to be a diagnosis. Time and time again we hear the same story. The patient has a thyroid condition, and then begins to have eye problems. The first port of call is the family doctor (primary care physician, general practitioner (GP)), who may not be familiar with thyroid eye disease, as it is not a common condition. If the GP picks up the symptoms then the procedure is fairly simple: a referral to an ophthalmologist and/or endocrinologist, who can explain just what is going on and what treatment is available.

However, a great many of our patient members relate a different tale. Because of the huge pressure on resources they may have to wait a long time before they get a blood test, which, because of the nature of the condition and the inherent problems with the present blood tests, may give a negative result. The GP reports to the patient, who is still feeling terrible, that there is nothing wrong. It is at this stage that anger generally sets in.

The patient may be prescribed artificial tears, tranquilizers or, if a woman of a certain age, hormone replacement therapy. None of these help the condition and this situation can go on for years.

This is a typical story written by one of our members for our newsletter.

One morning, a few years ago I awoke with one eye red and swollen. It looked starey and frightening. I had not been feeling well for some time. Sometimes I had felt hot and my heart would race. Sometimes I had woken in the night feeling so weak and faint that I thought I was slowly passing away. I was referred to the hospital eye department where the consultant tested me for thyroid disease. To his surprise the result was normal. After more visits to the GP I was told there was nothing wrong with me and, being a busy mother, I accepted his verdict. But my illness continued and I was very depressed. After another year I paid to see a consultant privately. I was told not to 'worry about myself' and that I had 'a very rare eye condition' for which there was no treatment. I was prescribed tranquilizers, which did no good at all. In fact they made me feel worse. The other eye was by now also affected.

I carried on, feeling dreadful and looking ill. I was irritable and difficult to live with, especially with those I loved best. I felt sure there was something wrong. Another 2 years went by.

Eventually this patient got to see an endocrinologist and received treatment.

Once a diagnosis has been made there is still a very long way to go. The most disturbing part of this disease is the effect it has on the whole person, in particular the emotional imbalance resulting in extreme mood swings devastating those closest to them. One of our members was asked by a little girl in the street if she was a witch. It is hardly surprising that such a reaction from strangers makes a sufferer unwilling to face the world.

Double vision may have an effect on the patient's ability to drive and take part in sporting activities and other hobbies.

Social life suffers and the patient becomes withdrawn and isolated, and, if the other family members are not made aware of the mental and emotional problems, there can be conflict within the home. This increases the stress level, which in turn makes the condition worse. Partners who are not aware of the effects of the illness on their loved ones may become impatient with mood swings, lethargy, and irritableness in the sufferer. They see someone who is not the person they knew – but they are the same person, it is just that they are ill and need a lot of support and understanding. Although we have no statistical evidence, we are aware that marriage breakdown is quite common among sufferers.

When talking and writing to sufferers we emphasize that family and friends should read the information we send out and our newsletters. Most people have never heard of thyroid eye disease, so raising awareness of this devastating disease among the public is a priority.

It is a sad fact that there are immense pressures on modem man and woman to conform to an idealized bodily 'norm'. Those who do conform are held to be good and those who do not are shunned. If, through no fault of their own, patients gain or lose weight, have swollen and puffy eyelids and proptotic eyes, they feel angry and alone. If they had a broken leg and hobbled around on crutches they would be the recipient of much sympathy.

There is no easy answer for the problems thyroid eye disease presents, but there is a great deal that can be done. While the disease is in the acute inflammatory stage the patient and family can be given as much information and reassurance as possible. When the disease reaches a stable phase then all the possibilities of surgical rehabilitation should be carefully explained. The prospect of several operations can be very frightening, but we have found that fears can be allayed by giving as much information as possible. Those of our members who set out to become 'experts' in their disease seem to gain much comfort

from amassing as much knowledge as they can. Fear of the unknown can have a debilitating effect, while a positive approach can be very beneficial.

Information and education are the keys to helping patients in dealing with thyroid eye disease. GPs and specialists need to be more familiar with the symptoms and consistent with their information. All too often we receive reports of one doctor opposing the opinion of another; this only leads to confusion. When patients ask why a certain operation or course of treatment is necessary it should be explained to them in a way they can understand. Treatment of a long-term illness is a journey that patients and their doctors make together, and if this is understood barriers will fall and trust will strengthen. Patients and their families need quality information from the medical profession and self-help groups like ours. One of our most important functions is to put patients in touch with each other, which helps to ease their sense of isolation. Whether the last bastion of discrimination, facial disfigurement, will ever be breached is up to us all.

- Thyroid Eye Disease Association (TED,) Solstice, Sea Road, Winchelsea Beach, East Sussex, TN36 4LH. Tel/fax: (+44) (0)1797 222338; E-mail: tedassn@eclipse.co.uk
- British Thyroid Foundation, PO Box 97, Clifford, Wetherby, West Yorkshire, L523 6XD UK
- Thyroid Federation International, 96 Mack Street, Kingston, Ontario, K7L 1 N9 Canada. E-mail: tfi@on.aibn.com

---

Cushing's Syndrome
Karen Campbell, Louise Pace, Mary Brim, Cathy Carbone, and Jane Edwards

CLASSIC FEATURES OF CUSHING'S SYNDROME

The classic features of Cushing's syndrome – truncal obesity, moon-shaped face, and a buffalo hump – are well illustrated in Chapter 15. Because these features develop insidiously in most cases (although in some cases there is a rapid progression), it is not uncommon for patients who have developed Cushing's syndrome to go for years without a diagnosis for their myriad symptoms. Such changes in physical appearance often go unrecognized by physicians (even when they know their patients well), spouses, family, and friends in a society where obesity is endemic and weight gain in middle age is perceived as normal.

In contrast, however, Cushing's patients are painfully aware of all the physical changes, the knowledgable among them often demanding to be tested in spite of the sometimes skeptical protests of their physicians. As one patient related, 'I had only gained 30lbs when I asked to be tested for Cushing's syndrome. My doctor asked me if I knew what someone looked like who had the disease. I pulled out a picture from a textbook, and he said, "It is an extremely rare disorder, and you do not look cushingoid." I replied that I felt I was headed that way.' A careful comparison with earlier photographs can help physicians to distinguish these changes.

Patients with Cushing's syndrome experience a large number of seemingly unrelated symptoms, and these are variable both at the onset and throughout the progression of the disease. While all patients have the same disease, their reasons for seeking a

medical evaluation are often entirely different. One patient recalled neglecting to mention weight gain even though she had gained 90lbs, focusing on other body changes: 'I felt like I was falling apart. I was growing hair where I had never had hair before, I had a buffalo hump between my shoulder blades, and I had bruises all over my arms and legs. The shape of my face had changed, my hair was falling out, and I was very weak.'

Virtually all Cushing's patients suffer from low self-esteem, as physicians, friends, spouses, and partners simply do not believe that their weight gain is not self-induced. Dieting and exercise are futile. Thus, the frustration and emotional impact of the physical deterioration cannot be overestimated. One patient related her frustration: 'I felt so embarrassed about being so ugly and so fat. I tried every diet imaginable. I even tried hypnosis, but I never did lose weight. My husband was convinced that I was a closet eater and wasn't trying very hard.'

Weakness, muscle pain, and low energy are common presentations, as are complaints of poor wound healing, cracking skin, shortness of breath, palpitations, and spontaneous fractures. One patient related 'sitting back in a chair and feeling a jabbing sensation that took my breath away. After weeks of discomfort, I learned that I had spontaneously broken several ribs.' Another recalls 'being so weak that I couldn't get up from a squatting position without difficulty, climb stairs without getting severely out of breath, or hold a glass of water without using both hands.' Complaints of sleeping most of the day are common, as is exhaustion as a result of the insomnia.

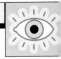

Cushing's syndrome has many deleterious effects on emotional stability and cognitive function. Approximately 61% of patients report feelings of emotional lability, especially depression and suicidal ideation; 49% report cognitive difficulties, most commonly an inability to concentrate and memory loss; and 17% report at least one admission to a mental health facility before diagnosis. In fact, for some patients the emotional upheaval and psychologic disruption caused by cortisol excess are the most difficult aspects of the disease. One patient reported 'being uncontrollably changed, trying desperately to get a grip, but ultimately failing. I was perceived as a hypochondriac by family and friends. I cried for no apparent reason but was just as apt to become enraged for no reason. I had episodes of sheer panic and intense anxiety, which often kept me from my normal activities. I thought about suicide often. My husband was convinced that I was crazy and had me committed to the psychiatric unit of our local hospital. I felt betrayed, angry, and confused.'

Cognitive difficulties often prevent patients from fulfilling their job responsibilities; approximately 56% report work or school difficulties. In some cases, bosses and coworkers are sympathetic and concerned; in other cases, the disease is devastating to professional pursuits. As one patient recalled, 'I lacked my usually proficient verbal skills. I avoided my usual public-speaking responsibilities because I just could not remember the words and had a terrible time concentrating and even completing a thought. I had to write everything down so that I would not forget it. I was once terribly embarrassed because I forgot that I asked colleagues for dinner. I once got lost in a shopping center with which I was very familiar. It was very scary. I thought I was losing my mind.' A lawyer wrote that 'I had to stop practicing law because I was no longer able to concentrate or read what was required. I was physically uncoordinated and thus unable to write.'

Financial hardships resulting from lost work may further strain social and family relationships already damaged by the psychiatric, cognitive, and physical changes wrought by the disease. Marriages dissolve, jobs are lost, professions deteriorate, and schoolwork is neglected, often resulting in repeated failures. Many patients recall being dropped by friends, spouses, and partners not only because of their changed appearance but also because of personality changes. Even outgoing patients may become reclusive and self-conscious. One Cushing mother remembers: 'I felt that I had robbed my children of the stable mother they deserved and my husband of the loving wife he had married. I cannot shake the guilt about being so ill that I destroyed my family. I could not cope with birthday parties, shopping, or just the normal demands put on a mother. My husband asked me, "Where is the wife I married?" I was in the hospital recovering from surgery when my husband took me to court for a divorce and custody of the children.'

Cushing's disease can be particularly devastating for adolescents, whose concern with physical appearance is exaggerated under the best of circumstances. One young woman, who started having symptoms at age 8 but was not diagnosed until she was 24 after surviving many suicide attempts recalls, 'I was picked last for teams. I constantly avoided my friend's entreaties to be social and stayed home alone most weekends, eventually stopping the friendships altogether. I was very self-conscious about my appearance; I felt I looked hideous.'

DIAGNOSIS

There is not only tremendous relief once the diagnosis of Cushing's syndrome is finally made but also often tremendous anger that the correct diagnosis took so long to be made. One patient recalls 'feeling so happy to know that I was not crazy. I felt frightened but also vindicated. All of the devastation in my life was not my fault! However, I soon experienced overwhelming anger and disgust that everyone, even my closest friends, had so readily dismissed my complaints and that no one had taken the time or shown enough interest to help me.'

After elevated cortisol levels are demonstrated, it cannot be emphasized enough how important it is to find the correct cause, which then guides treatment. There are many very distressing cases of numerous surgeries and no cure.

If surgery is deemed the most appropriate treatment, then a surgeon with experience in Cushing's must be chosen. For example, if Cushing's disease, resulting from a pituitary tumor, is diagnosed, the patient should be referred to a neurosurgeon with extensive experience with the transsphenoidal procedure. Not all neurosurgeons are trained appropriately to perform this surgery. A valid question to ask your surgeon is, 'How many pituitary surgeries do you perform a year?' and 'What is your success rate for these surgeries overall?' Patients are often sadly misled by eager but relatively inexperienced surgeons. Recurrences can be prevented and lifelong replacement medications avoided in the hands of a skilled and experienced surgeon who has performed hundreds if not thousands of these operations.

No less care should be taken picking a surgeon for other causes of Cushing's syndrome, where an adrenalectomy is necessary. Surgeons qualified to perform this surgery laparoscopically can often save patients the trauma of a standard open adrenalectomy, where muscles must be severed and ribs must be cut, thereby reducing pain and recovery time.

RECOVERY

After living with high cortisol levels for many years, many patients are unprepared for the effects of steroid withdrawal syndrome, which can accompany successful treatment of Cushing's syndrome. Physicians may have little experience treating Cushing's patients postoperatively, so it is important for patients to know that they need to be tapered back to physiological steroid levels slowly to avoid numerous trips to the emergency room with severe withdrawal symptoms. All patients should be advised to wear a MedicAlert bracelet, be taught how to increase their oral steroid dose during an intercurrent infection or other physical stress, and carry a syringe for injecting a glucocorticoid such as hydrocortisone or dexamethasone in a more severe emergency. This advice should be supplemented by provision of a written leaflet making everything clear. This increase in steroid dosing is necessary for as long as it takes for adrenal function to be restored. While tapering too rapidly is dangerous, tapering too slowly or not tapering at all can lead to lifelong steroid dependence and a decreased quality of life. Patients' reactions to withdrawal are as variable as their presentations of the syndrome.

The reason for the slow recovery of the pituitary–adrenal axis after the high blood levels of hydrocortisone are lowered with successful treatment of Cushing's syndrome, whether due to an adrenocorticotropic hormone (ACTH)-secreting tumor or an adrenal tumor, is because ACTH secretion from the normal pituitary is completely suppressed during the active phase of the disease. Recovery of this secretion is very variable from one person to another and may take years to occur; indeed, occasionally it never recovers. Endocrinologists generally agree that for the hypothalamo–pituitary–adrenal axis to recover, only short-acting steroids, such as prednisone, prednisolone or hydrocortisone, should be used during the tapering process.

Even when an appropriate tapering protocol is followed, patients are often surprised by the duration of the recovery period. It can take years before patients are completely free of replacement therapy and feel more or less 'like themselves'. While some patients experience few problems during this period, others are plagued by debilitating fatigue, muscle and joint pain, depression, and difficulty in concentrating. One patient related: 'It took me 3 years to get back on my feet. I couldn't work, clean my house, or do much of anything but sleep. The "after" period was never discussed by my doctor.' Thus, 'returning to normal' often means reducing work responsibilities and the number of hours spent working. Rest is essential. Physical therapy can help patients to rebuild strength and stamina, and occupational therapy can help patients regain lost skills. A nutritionist can help to provide an adequate diet, perhaps with added protein to help rebuild muscle strength. Psychiatric treatment should be sought for emotional difficulties.

However, most patients are extremely grateful to 'have their life back' once the recovery period is over. One patient's exuberance is unmistakable: 'I've lost 50lbs, my hair has grown back, my blood pressure and blood sugar are normal, I feel strong and energized, and I have gone back to nursing.'

SUPPORT NETWORKS

A patient's personal support network can make an enormous difference in outcome. Family support or religion can be a key to preventing suicide. For example, family members should be encouraged to become involved with physician appointments in order to have a deeper understanding of the disease and its repercussions. Patients who have this support do well. One patient relates: 'My family and friends talked, listened, hugged, and held my hand through all stages of the disease and recovery. My husband held me, let me cry, raced to the emergency room, and stood by, often helpless, but he never gave up on me.'

Patients should be encouraged to seek out support organizations (see below for suggestions). Most Cushing's patients express extreme relief in being able to talk with other Cushing's patients: 'No one can understand Cushing's like another person who has had it.'

SUGGESTED SUPPORT GROUPS

For networking and support services specifically for Cushing's patients

The Cushing's Support and Research Foundation
65 East India Row, #22B
Boston, MA 02110 USA
Tel: +1 (617) 723-3674
Web site: http://www.CSRG.net

ACTH
54 Powney Road
Maidenhead, Berkshire
SL6 6EQ UK
Tel: +44 (0)1628 70389
Provides support and information to Cushing's patients.

Cushing Care
Meadows
Woodplumpton Village
Preston, Lancashire
PR4 OLJ UK
Tel: 01772 690680
Provides information and support to patients and their families.

For support for patients with all types of pituitary tumor

The Pituitary Tumor Network Association
PO Box 1958
Thousand Oaks, CA 91358 USA
Tel: +1 (805) 499-2262

The Pituitary Foundation
PO Box 1944
Bristol
BS99 2UB UK
Telephone: +44 (0)117 927 3355

For support for patients with either Cushing's disease or Addison's disease

The Dutch Addison and Cushing Society
PO Box 52137
2505 CC The Hague Netherlands

FURTHER READING

Brim M. Results of a Cushing's survey by Cushing's Support and Research Foundation (CSRF). Cushing's Newsl. 1999:Spring. (The Cushing's Newsletter is published by CSRF, 65 E India Row, #22B, Boston, MA 02110, USA.)

Gumowski J. Quality of life in Cushing's patients. Paper presented at the Endocrine Nurses Society Symposium, San Diego, CA, 14 June 1999. Cushing's Newsl. 1999;November.

Gotch P. Cushing's syndrome from the patient's perspective. In: Aron DC, Tyrrell JB, eds. Endocrinology and metabolism clinics of North America 23(3). Philadelphia, PA:WB Saunders ; 1994.

Knapen M, Puts P, Hermus A. Cushing patients in the Netherlands. The Hague:Dutch Addison & Cushing Society; 2000:128.

Weiss M. Answers from a pituitary surgeon. Cushing's Newsl. 1997;Spring.

Addison's Disease   Deana Kenward

In May 1983 I had a minor operation. I recovered quickly and carried on with my life. After 5 or 6 weeks I suffered bouts of nausea and often could not face my food. I went to the doctor, who gave me the same medicine I gave my youngest son for his travel sickness, and it did help a little.

During that summer I had lots of things wrong with me, including lethargy, tiredness, muscle weakness, and cramp, none of which were bad enough to bother the doctor with, as they were quite vague to start with.

I went to the doctor when these symptoms worsened but as we have a group practice I never saw the same doctor twice and was told a couple of times that there was nothing wrong and that it was probably the pressure of working and looking after my family. I never did see my own GP during these early stages.

Being of Greek origin my skin had always been fairly dark and I tanned easily in the sunshine but by the end of September I was so dark it was untrue. I'd noticed that my toenails, gums and lips had black marks on them.

By mid-October I was really beginning to feel weak as I had lost about a stone and a half (18 pounds) in weight and had no appetite and I was so cold all of the time, but I looked so well because of the weight loss and my tan, and the doctors still had no explanation for my ailments.

I carried on the best I could, now sleeping downstairs because I could not climb the stairs, and if I rested all morning I had the strength to collect my children from school and cook an evening meal. When I look back I do not know how I ever got through those dark months. I was convinced I was slowly dying but somehow I managed to fool my family I was a lot better than I really was.

November came and I nearly went to meet my maker. I collapsed at my son's playgroup, which was just minutes away from my house. I was brought home and from then on things are a bit blurry.

I remember my own GP coming out and taking blood samples and later I recollect being in an ambulance and the barrage of tests they did in the hospital. I know I cried because I could not keep my legs still and I was so scared of what was happening to me.

Finally, sometime during the night I was told that I had Addison's disease and that it was incurable but treatable with steroids and that I would make a full recovery.

I spent 2 days in intensive care and 10 days on a ward before I was allowed home, just in time for Christmas.

At that time I felt only relief because during the months prior to my diagnosis I had been told that there was nothing wrong. It was later that fear and worry took over as I had never heard of Addison's disease before and I did not want to be dependent on medication for the rest of my life.

I later found out that by the time I got to the hospital I was very close to renal failure and death was just hours away, I thank God for those doctors, especially a wonderful Irish doctor whom I am not allowed to name.

It was at least 3 months before I felt really well and had regained most of the weight I had lost, and then I wanted answers to my questions – what will it be like living with Addison's disease? How will it affect my life? Will my children develop it?

Many more questions and worries filled my mind constantly.

I wrote to magazines and doctors' columns and visited my local library to find out if there was any information about my illness or a charity or group for sufferers of Addison's disease, only to find out that there was nothing at all.

It was suggested to me that I start a self-help group and after much deliberation on my part and encouragement from my family and friends I did just that, founding the Addison's Disease Self Help Group (ADSHG) in July 1984. Now I have 648 group members, 494 females and 154 males, and over the years I have learnt so much about Addison's disease from having the illness myself and from listening to the experiences of my group members.

Those of us who were not diagnosed until we were really ill would like the medical world to be much more aware of Addison's disease and its symptoms. While we think we suffered unnecessarily we do realize how difficult it must be for doctors, who only have a few vague symptoms to go by at the onset of the illness, plus the fact that a great number of doctors have never seen a case of Addison's disease before.

Living with Addison's disease for me is not a problem. I have had two crises but apart from them I am very well. I see my specialist every 6 months and have had a day curve test and a bone density scan quite recently.

I wear a MedicAlert emblem and carry my steroid card at all times. I have an emergency hydrocortisone pack at home and have been told to double up on my steroids in cases of infection or fever. I have been asked if there is really anything wrong with me because I always look so healthy, and I have more energy than some of my friends. I do find, though, along with many others, that mental stress affects me so much more now than prior to diagnosis.

It is always hard for the parents of children with Addison's not to be too overprotective; they must learn along with the child all about the illness and how to cope with it as they grow up.

Not all Addison's patients are as lucky as myself – some have never had a day curve test and rarely see a specialist. However, since joining ADSHG many have told me how they have now had these tests and have had their medication adjusted accordingly; also they say how helpful it is to be able to talk to or even meet someone else with Addison's disease, because it is a rare illness. Some people had never spoken to a fellow sufferer until they joined ADSHG.

We are told that if we are replaced correctly with hydrocortisone there should be no side effects from the illness or drugs but some in my group have osteoporosis and lots have weight-gain problems; some experience mood swings and periods of extreme tiredness.

Diabetes or thyroid problems have developed in some patients since being diagnosed with Addison's disease and it has been difficult for some to achieve the right balance of their different medications.

In an ideal world all Addison's patients would be monitored regularly by their local hospitals and all hospitals would issue an emergency hydrocortisone pack (and teach patients and their families how to use them).

Through my group I help fellow sufferers by listening to their problems and worries, especially if they are newly diagnosed, and give them advice gained through 16 years experience of running the group. I am not medically qualified in any way, so my advice is from a patient's point of view only. I also put group members in touch with each other and many friendships have been made within the group.

I run the only group for Addison's sufferers in Great Britain and Ireland:

Addison's Disease Self Help Group (ADSHG)
E-mail: deana@adshg.freeserve.co.uk
Web site: http://www.surreweb.net/adshgl
Tel/Fax: +44 (0)1483 830673.

There are other organizations in other countries that might be of interest:

- Australian Addison's Disease Association, e-mail: secretary@addisons.orcg.au
- The Canadian Addison Society, e-mail: jsoutham@rogers.com
- New Zealand Addison's Network, e-mail: jeanette@ramhb.co.nz
- NADF (America), e-mail: NADFmail@aol.com
- Addison News – Pleasant Lake, MI, e-mail: hoffmanj@dmci.net
- Addison & Cushing International Federation (ACIF), the Netherlands, e-mail: Holland@addison.nl.

Congenital Adrenal Hyperplasia and Androgen Insensitivity Syndrome

Sherri A Groveman

I embody a cruel and ironic dichotomy. Nature baking a cake with salt instead of sugar. Yes, everything looks right on the outside, but anyone taking a bite to see what I'm really made of would quickly realize there's something terribly wrong with the ingredients.
(Diary entry, 23 June 1983)

I wrote those words 18 years ago, 3 years after diagnosing myself with 'testicular feminization' in a medical school library. At the time, everything on the outside really did look perfect. I was clerking for a powerful judge, having recently graduated near the top of my law school class. I had challenging work, interesting friends, a beautiful home, and a carefully guarded secret I never shared with anyone. Ever.

The secret became a Pandora's box, too dangerous to open for fear its contents would overtake my carefully scripted life. That I had even stumbled across the diagnosis filled me with a sense of shame and dread, as this was a truth my parents and doctors had intended I should never learn. They had told me I had 'twisted ovaries', which had been removed in infancy to prevent them from becoming cancerous. Discovering that in reality I had XY chromosomes, and that my twisted ovaries were really testes, clearly was forbidden information.

As devastating as it was to learn the truth about having androgen insensitivity syndrome – AIS (as I was to later learn that this disorder was now called), my discovery merely reinforced a sense of freakishness that had been instilled by the palpable silences I experienced as my pediatric endocrinologist examined me during annual visits. Such silence was only broken when interns and residents were paraded past my naked body, at which times my genitals were discussed in the third person as I lay supine on an examining table.

Having not been encouraged to seek any kind of counseling, it is perhaps not surprising that my parents' way of helping me cope with the reality of having AIS (or even twisted ovaries, as they intended I believe) was never to discuss it, thinking that by sweeping it under the rug they were protecting me. Indeed, I suspect that their own way of coping with the diagnosis was to consider it merely a fertility problem, rather than appreciating the full truth: that they had an intersex child. We were caught in a tragic dance of deception, my parents and I: they having not told me the truth, and I having not later alerted them that I had discovered it anyway.

I proceeded through my twenties and early thirties convinced that I could never share the truth about myself with either friends or prospective romantic partners for fear they would recoil in horror. On the latter front, I avoided any possibility of sexual intimacy, not only because I feared a partner seeing what I then considered my shameful genitals but also because I had discovered at about age 14 that not even half a tampon could be inserted past the introitus of my vagina. Sadly, neither my parents nor my doctor ever acknowledged this vaginal hypoplasia and thus no guidance was offered about how I might overcome it.

My story could easily have ended there, the remainder of my life merely a continuation of the shame and secrecy that had characterized my first 36 years. But miraculously I found a way out of the corner I had been painted in to. What poetic justice that almost 15 years after making the diagnosis of AIS, I found myself back in a medical library searching the *Index Medicus*. But this time I hit paydirt: tucked among the technical research articles on AIS (to this day indexed in the *Index Medicus* as 'testicular feminization') was a lone human-sounding title, 'Once a Dark Secret'. This entry turned out to be an anonymous letter written to the *British Medical Journal* by a young woman in England recounting her experiences with AIS. This woman, living 6000 miles from my home, described in haunting detail experiences identical to my own. It was the first connection I ever had to another person who understood what my life was about.

I combed later issues of the *British Medical Journal*, hoping that someone else with AIS, or a physician who treated patients with the condition, might respond to this anonymous letter. And to my utter amazement, someone did indeed respond, not only confirming what the author of the original letter recounted but providing the name and contact details of a support group in the UK for women with AIS. I had lived 36 years on a desert island; imagine how overcome I was to be rescued by a 15-digit phone number that held with it the possibility of my being able, for the first time in my life, to look into the eyes of another human being who understood.

Since then, I have gone on to attend dozens of support group meetings, both in the UK and the USA, in the process meeting hundreds of other women with AIS, of all ages, nationalities, and education levels. And despite our demographic differences, there are clear common denominators in our histories. Most of us were not told the truth about AIS, often with tragic consequences such as discovering the diagnosis on their own without any support or learning it by having a family member blurt it out in the heat of an argument. Almost all of us were conditioned to believe there was something shameful about having AIS, reinforced by the palpable silence and discomfort of our parents and doctors.

Part of the difficulty in how our cases were managed was that AIS was considered a 'fertility problem' by both our doctors and our parents. Viewed as such, there was even more reason not to tell us the truth because our doctors assumed that the only real issue attendant on having AIS was our being unable to have biological children. And indeed, infertility is certainly an issue that has caused considerable emotional difficulty for women with AIS. But this doesn't tell the whole story.

What many of our doctors failed to appreciate were the difficulties faced by a young woman who does not have a menstrual cycle (which is a coming-of-age rite on the road to womanhood in most societies) or pubic hair. These seem like such minor losses at one level, and yet they are very real sources of anxiety for those of us who have to face them. I remember all my friends talking about getting their periods and feeling excluded from the discussion, terrified that they would know that I was different.

I still feel a momentary sense of panic and distress when I arrive at my doctor's consulting rooms and continue to be asked by the nurse about when my last period was. Perhaps it seems like a minimal inconvenience to have to respond to this question, and yet I can't help wondering why there isn't better education of nursing staff to prevent the situation from occurring. My sensibilities here are not peculiar. Hundreds of other women I know with AIS report their bodies tensing and their hearts pounding as they are confronted by the same question every time they see doctors who have treated them for years and whose assistants should know better.

I also think that, when the patient is intersexed, it is important that the physician first meet with her while she is still fully clothed, in an office rather than in an examining room. I think physicians often underestimate how just a 5- or 10-minute conversation before an examination can help the patient relax and feel less vulnerable about undressing and submitting to often invasive procedures. Ideally, the examining room will be 'prepped' with child-size specula, given that many women with conditions such as AIS are not able to tolerate adult instruments. But perhaps more than any other preparation, it is essential that the physician conducting the examination be comfortable with intersex, be able to speak in a natural and conversational tone about it rather than hiding behind clinical jargon, and make the patient a 'participant' in such examination.

Perhaps it should go without saying that at such visits no one else besides the physician and an assisting nurse should be present. Too often, intersex individuals (of all ages) report arriving for a physical examination only to discover that they are asked to allow doctors in training to be present in the examining room. It is easy to understand that the justification for this is physician education. What is hard for many doctors to understand is that having your genitals on display in this way, even if your consent is sought and obtained (perhaps a dubious consent when exacted by a well-respected doctor from a patient who has limited options for care), can be emotionally devastating and decimate the patient's sexual self-esteem. It communicates that your genitals have been tested in the crucible of medical science and found wanting. Physician education is important but cannot be justified when the price for such education is paid by a patient who has already has enough difficult issues to work through.

The breach of trust that occurs when a patient feels that she is either being condescended to or treated insensitively will have a direct, and often dire, impact on her medical care. Patients who feel they have no control over their treatment are far more inclined to disobey recommendations for treatment. I routinely discarded my hormone replacement therapy, flushing the pills down the toilet or skipping weeks at a time. It was a foolish choice medically, but psychologically imperative so that I could exercise some element of control. Hindsight is always in focus but I think if I had felt that my endocrinologist and I were on the same team, that I could really trust him, and that there was open and honest dialogue between us, the pills might have made it down my throat.

If the patient does not feel a sense of trust, she will also not reveal her more intimate challenges with being intersexed. For example, many patients with AIS, regardless of whether they have undergone vaginoplasty, experience real problems with penetration, whether because of vaginal hypoplasia, vaginal atresia (the extent of which may not be fully appreciated by physical examination), or a failure to produce adequate lubrication. It should be added that many do not have such problems, and others, for a variety of reasons, may not care about penetrative sex. Yet if there is not an open and honest dialogue between physician and patient, such concerns are often never expressed – and therefore never treated – for decades on end, when something as simple as a prescription for estrogen cream or suppositories can often be of tremendous benefit.

Physicians should also beware of the patient who indicates that she is 'doing fine' in response to inquiries about how she is faring. Some patients are indeed doing well, having adjusted to their diagnosis and not experiencing any physical complications. But many other patients will say they are doing fine either because they think this is what the caregiver needs to hear, or because there is a lack of trust, or because the question is asked at a time when the patient feels awkward (such as when she is naked on an examining table) and is anxious to simply get dressed and beat a hasty retreat. For this reason, I would encourage endocrinologists to employ what I call the 'leading statement'.

For example, to feel the patient out about whether intercourse is painful because of atresia, the physician might say, 'You know, several other women with AIS have reported that it is sometimes painful when they have intercourse because their vagina feels dry and irritated, and I've found that using estrogen cream can sometimes really help them; is that something I can help you with also?' Now the onus is no longer on the patient to raise the subject, the physician has reassured the patient that her experience is not unique, and the patient is given 'permission' to discuss a situation that may be embarrassing or stressful.

The physician should also alert the patient that support groups are available and that other patients have found that the opportunity to discuss their situation with women whose experiences are similar can be quite transforming in the process of coming to terms with being intersexed. International support groups such as the AIS Support Group (AISSG; web site: www.medelp.org/www/ais) provide telephone support, publish a newsletter keeping members abreast of new medical developments as well as providing a forum for them to share their personal histories, and sponsor an annual meeting where both adult members and parents of children with AIS can share mutual support and information. It is especially critical for the adolescent patient to made aware of such resources, because support groups provide an opportunity for young patients to encounter positive role models – adult women with the same medical condition who are building healthy, productive lives. It may be particularly reassuring to these young women to discover that many adult members of the support group have shared their medical histories with romantic partners and that not only has this not been an impediment to sustaining such relationships but it has often been the catalyst to developing a greater sense of intimacy and trust.

Support groups can offer benefits not only to patients but to the endocrinologist as well. With a relatively rare medical condition like AIS, a support group web site can be an excellent source for précis of information on medical journal articles about relevant subject matter. Perhaps even more important, support groups can often provide the anecdotal background to the empirical data contained in such articles. Support groups such as AISSG also vet the medical information they provide to their members. In an age when there is considerable misinformation floating about the Internet, it is even more critical that the patient have an organized way of accessing accurate and up-to-date information.

Resources like a support group can only be accessed, however, if the patient has been told the truth about her medical condition. This suggestion has been met with some resistance from certain physicians, who were trained to deceive their intersex patients. It is difficult to imagine that physicians can ever truly feel a sense of comfort in the presence of a patient they know they have lied to and with whom they therefore must engage in something of a charade concerning treatment. It is even more difficult to imagine that lying makes any practical sense in an era when patients can self-diagnose using resources like the Internet or by watching television programs featuring intersex individuals.

As an attorney, I am tempted to outline all the parameters of informed consent and explain why the approach of lying to intersex patients (or withholding the truth) is legally treacherous. But there is something more important than legalities: patient autonomy.

Intersex isn't a tragedy in much the same way that adoption isn't a tragedy. Both are realities that carry with them personal challenges. Both require the affected individual to parse through a constellation of emotions and make peace with who they are. For both intersex individuals and adoptees there is tremendous meaning and purpose in understanding one's past and working through the difficulties of being different from one's peers. Behavioral scientists have shown that lying to adoptees about their birth parents creates more problems than it solves and that if an adoptee is lied to and later discovers the truth s/he may experience an irreparable breach of trust. There is no reason to believe that the situation is any different for intersex individuals.

How and when to disclose the truth is the question I am asked most frequently by parents of children with AIS. What I generally recommend is that parents begin, even in childhood, to lay the foundation for truthful disclosure. I believe that nothing told to a child should ever be a lie, even if the child isn't yet ready to be told all the facts. If parents promote a spirit of tolerance and appreciation for diversity within the home, it will create a more positive environment for the child to later accept her own differences. Ideally, before parents are at the point at which they will begin the process of disclosure, they should receive counseling to work through their own anxieties, shame, fear, and guilt about having an intersex child. Such counseling should be encouraged as soon as the diagnosis is made, even if such diagnosis occurs in infancy. In the course of counseling, parents can begin to talk openly about intersex, in the process becoming comfortable describing their child's chromosomes and gonads and genitals. They can practice how and what to tell their child about having AIS. This, in turn, will allow them to speak to their child with greater ease. Such parental counseling, perhaps more than any other variable in the medical care of the intersex child, is critical to improving long-term outcomes.

The need for counseling might extend beyond the parents. For example, other family members who might be carriers may require counseling, not only to gain a greater understanding of intersex but also to work through the concerns they might have about potentially bringing an intersex child into the world. Such counseling can have the collateral benefit of transforming such carriers into important emotional resources for both the parents and the individual with AIS.

Care should be taken, however, to ensure that, if such counseling includes a consultation with a geneticist or genetic counselor, such additional healthcare team members also convey a sense of comfort with intersex and do not present it as a family tragedy. The AIS Support Group has heard of unfortunate cases in which genetic counseling for intersex has become little more than abortion counseling. Indeed, a leading geneticist has boasted that he can detect intersex in an 8-week-old fetus. His stated objective was not to use such information to assist families in preparing emotionally for the birth of their intersex child but instead to facilitate early termination of the pregnancy. The specter of eugenics being used to manage intersex is tragic when intersex individuals can and do lead wonderful and productive lives.

This attitude of 'damage control' to manage intersex has, however, unfortunately invaded more than just genetic counseling. It has also formed the basis for how intersex children are frequently treated after their birth. Too often the paradigm of clinical management seeks to make intersex a historical detail of the patient's life. This accomplished by attempting to erase any physical manifestation that the child is intersexed. Thus, it remains an unfortunate practice to engage in early gonadectomy of a child diagnosed with AIS.

While prepubertal gonadectomy might be justified in a child with dysgenetic gonads, in cases such as AIS there are many benefits to retaining the gonads until after puberty. Beyond the physiologic benefit of having a natural source of hormones, there is also the practical benefit of an adolescent not having to comply with taking hormone replacement therapy, particularly when she may be away from home. Moreover, given the relatively small risk of gonadoblastoma or carcinoma-*in-situ* developing in the gonads of an individual with AIS, delaying gonadectomy has the further benefit of allowing the individual to make her own informed medical decisions in later adolescence, thereby respecting her autonomy over her body.

Unfortunately, gonadectomy is often also accompanied by additional surgery, such as vaginoplasty and clitoral rescission. There is no sound reason to perform vaginoplasty on an individual who is not of an age to be sexually active. Moreover, women who have undergone the usual vaginoplasty techniques report an unusually high complication rate, including dyspareunia resulting from the formation of surgically created scar tissue. Most seem to indicate that on 'cost–benefit' analysis the downside outweighs any increase in vaginal length. The use of dilators as an alternative to vaginoplasty seems to offer several potential benefits, and yet this too is not a perfect solution. For example, many women with AIS report having a problem not only with vaginal length but also with an exceptionally narrow introitus. Yet the word 'dilator' is really a misnomer because, while dilators typically graduate in length, commercially available sets that actually dilate are difficult to find, thus failing to address the problem of widening the introitus.

Moreover, endocrinologists appear to underestimate the necessary vaginal length for penetrative sex. Many women with AIS are advised that they can comfortably have intercourse if they have a vagina of 6cm or more. Yet, many women with a vaginal length of 6cm report that intercourse is difficult at best and often impossible, even when they are fairly relaxed with a trusted partner. Other women have tragically not been adequately advised by their endocrinologists about the importance of vaginal length, only to attempt intercourse and wind up in the emergency room hemorrhaging. Given the tremendous

impediment that vaginal hypoplasia can present to the ability to form an intimate relationship, clearly there is a need for more research to improve and expand the available vaginoplasty techniques and alternatives.

While vaginoplasty is not a cosmetic procedure, sadly many intersex individuals born with ambiguous genitalia continue to be subjected to clitoral rescission, purely for cosmetic reasons. While some endocrinologists maintain that such surgery helps to reinforce a female gender assignment for such individuals, much more can be accomplished with therapy rather than a scalpel. Particularly when such surgeries are performed in infancy on a child who cannot give consent, the resulting message is that there is something shameful about the individual's genitals in their original state. A more patient-centered approach would be to instead communicate to young intersex patients that their bodies are healthy and wonderful just as they are. If the patient is experiencing unusual distress about having ambiguous genitalia, and such dysphoria is not aided by counseling, then the patient can always elect to undergo surgery in adulthood. But the message communicated by the endocrinologist prior to that point should be to encourage the patient to view being intersexed as a natural variation that, while presenting personal challenges, is not a shameful tragedy.

I imagine that it is indeed sometimes frustrating for physicians to assist their intersex patients, because physicians cannot offer a 'cure' for intersex. But endocrinologists have a tremendous opportunity to help their intersex patients heal, to assist them in developing a healthy self-esteem, to provide them with the necessary assistance to facilitate their forming positive intimate relationships, and to forge with them a trusted doctor–patient relationship.

Contact the AIS support group via their web site: www.medhelp.org/www/ais. This is a consortium of worldwide AIS support groups and contains AIS support group addresses in many countries.

Klinefelter Syndrome (47,XXY)

Melissa Aylstock

Males with Klinefelter syndrome (47,XXY) often don't appear physically different from their peers. In about 60% of cases, though, they may have cognitive, social/emotional or neurological issues that *may* cause them to seem out of step with others their age.

Our organization has found that many families who learn of the diagnosis early opt to keep it 'hidden'. Some even choose not to tell attending physicians! This may be because of the proliferation of negative press in the 1960s. Yet, as the child ages, the diagnosis becomes a double-edged sword. If parents share the information, there is a very real fear that the child will be treated differently. If parents withhold the information, the possibility that a child will be thought to have a condition brought on by 'poor parenting' is also very real. Children and adolescents may have poor communication skills, which are common in this condition. They may have frustration-based outbursts that make them seem mentally/emotionally unstable. Parents tell us they also suspect that a hormone imbalance may be the underlying cause. Both of these factors point to the need for more research.

Unfortunately, there appears to be a void in research concerning males with Klinefelter syndrome. Dr Harry Klinefelter Jr was working as fellow in Dr Fuller Albright's endocrine clinic at the time the basic set of physical manifestations were first identified. These included breast development, hypogonadism, tall stature, and a female fat pattern. Research during the past 60 years has mainly focused on the endocrine issues that surround hypogonadism. Approximately 10 years after Dr Klinefelter's observations, the patients in the original study were found to have an additional X chromosome. This new development appeared to be only another interesting symptom. With genetics still in its infancy in the early 1950s and the cost of genetic testing prohibitive (especially for screening purposes), not much was done to quantify exactly what effect having an extra X might have on the human condition. This remains true today. This lack of solid scientific research impacts patients who may have other issues brought on by this misunderstood multisystemic condition.

Networking organizations such as ours have the opportunity to communicate with thousands of individuals and families concerning both recent and long-term diagnosis. The common thread seems to be lack of practical information from the medical community on such critical issues as cognition, behavior, neurologic manifestations and socialization within the greater human family.

The two most common themes at networking meetings are: 'If one in 600 males are affected, why wasn't this diagnosed sooner through a screening program?' and 'Why didn't my doctor tell me about the other possible issues we have had to face?' In fact, it may be common for pediatricians and general practitioners to misunderstand what nonphysical symptoms of 47,XXY are related to the condition. Parents have repeatedly been told by their attending physicians that the behavior problems or speech and language delays their children are experiencing are unrelated to having 47,XXY. It is not clear whether this is intentional on the part of the physician, in order to avoid prejudicing the parents' attitude toward such symptoms, or just the result of a lack of solid clinical information on this very common condition.

To date, no formal clinical guidelines for the treatment of Klinefelter syndrome exist. This leaves room for a huge margin of error when treating patients. Those of us who regularly communicate with families and individuals with 47,XXY understand the wide variations in presentation. We readily acknowledge the difficultly of providing guidelines that would apply to all or even most persons with an additional X chromosome. Yet, while we understand that in part this is due to a lack of solid, double-blind studies on the condition, it still leaves families in a constant state of anxiety about how best to help the affected individual.

The anecdotal reality for many families varies. Profiles of the five most common sets of circumstances that a family faces when living with 47,XXY are:

• the prenatal diagnosis;
• the postnatal (early childhood) diagnosis;
• the adolescent diagnosis;
• the adult infertility diagnosis;
• the adult diagnosis not associated with infertility.

THE PRENATAL DIAGNOSIS

The majority of the families in our group with children under 2 years of age were diagnosed via amniocentesis at around 17–19 weeks gestation. The most common profile is a woman over 35 years of age who was screened for other maternal age-related genetic conditions. While an elevated alphafetoprotein level has in some cases lead to amniocentesis in women under 35, it has not been demonstrated that elevated alphafetoprotein levels are common in sex chromosome hyperploidy pregnancies.

Individuals with 47,XXY who are diagnosed via amniocentesis generally have the best outcomes later in life. This is most probably because of the availability of early intervention. Additionally, often the parents are in a generally secure financial situation and are able to aggressively advocate for their sons.

It has been demonstrated that early intervention is effective and can begin as soon as 8 weeks of age in children who display the physical signs of hypotonia and torticollis. By 9 months of age, these children, who generally have greater receptive language skills than the average child, can begin to learn modified forms of

sign language to bridge the gap between expressive and receptive language skills in their preschool years. This compensatory technique is proving to lessen the frustration-based outbursts often reported by parents of children who have trouble with speech and language delay.

While these children are still at risk for speech and language delay and problems with poor muscle tone, many of the cognitive and tonal issues appear to be lessened – or alleviated altogether – through aggressive early intervention. The risk of hormonal difficulties remains constant as a result of the primary hypogonadism.

THE POSTNATAL DIAGNOSIS

When a child is diagnosed during the postnatal period it is almost always in response some type of developmental delay or medical concern. The most frequent issue is lack of developmental milestones, but we have recently come to acknowledge an increase in anecdotally reported seizures in the pediatric population that have subsequently led to a genetic workup revealing the presence of an additional X chromosome.

Early intervention can still successfully be employed in the postnatal diagnosis population. Yet, it appears that children diagnosed because of problems associated with Klinefelter syndrome appear to take longer to compensate than if they had started intervention in the first few months of life. The later the diagnosis, the less certain the outcome of early intervention.

Physicians are usually aware of the benefits of speech and language interventions. They appear to be less aware of the benefits of physical therapy, occupational therapy, or sensory integration for children with 47,XXY.

THE ADOLESCENT DIAGNOSIS

The adolescent diagnosis can come about because of two separate but related issues. In both sets of circumstances; however, most boys report that they were already aware that they were somewhat different from their peers. Thus, a teenager *could* be diagnosed strictly on the size of his testes or the presence of excessive breast tissue – but our observation is that this is seldom the case. Interestingly enough, this type of diagnosis is most frequently reported to the parents not by a physician but by a high-school coach. Adolescents diagnosed strictly because of hypogonadism are usually not as complicated as those diagnosed because of cognitive or behavioral issues. Those diagnosed because of gynecomastia tend to have the expected emotional problems.

However, most of the adolescent diagnoses we are aware of come about in response to either learning disorders such as dyslexia, behavioral issues, or lack of physical/emotional maturation, issues brought to the attention of a primary care physician. At this point, the adolescent diagnosed because of these types of problems has generally missed out on a formal early intervention program. With testosterone levels falling and levels of follicle-stimulating hormone and luteinizing hormone rising, teenage boys can have an emotionally troubled adolescence, often exacerbated by delayed language and social skills.

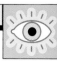

THE ADULT INFERTILITY DIAGNOSIS

When a man is diagnosed with 47,XXY in a fertility workup he is generally quite surprised. Although this diagnosis is almost always accompanied by the diagnosis of primary hypogonadism, the man may have been fully functioning both sexually and cognitively for many years. Although this is a generalization, the wives of these men frequently report that their spouses were always 'perfect gentlemen' prior to marriage. Such men are often in secure marriages and report stable employment. Upon further examination, they may report some of the primary symptoms of hypogonadism, such as fatigue, lack of libido, and poor muscle tone – but not always. Curiously, the men in our group who fit this profile do not always opt for testosterone replacement therapy initially but, as they near 40, many reassess the situation as they become more symptomatic.

Additionally, for men in this group, infertility is what brought them to the attention of the physicians and infertility in the 47,XXY population is being positively addressed. Intracytoplasmic sperm injection, a technique developed to achieve fertilization in cases of poor-quality sperm has proved to be successful in some cases with men who have 47,XXY. Immature sperm can be surgically harvested from the testis of men with 47,XXY. Fertilization can be achieved when only a very small number of sperm are available. Worldwide, there have been over a dozen children born to men who have 47,XXY. All of the liveborn children so far have had normal karyotypes. There is every hope that this procedure will eventually confer fertility on those men with 47,XXY who desire it. Currently, however, it is physically, emotionally, and financially taxing.

THE ADULT DIAGNOSIS NOT ASSOCIATED WITH INFERTILITY

There is a broad span of years when 47,XXY can be diagnosed in an adult. Men who fit this profile often show up at a physician's office with one or more complaints that can be traced to the physical effects of having an extra X chromosome. They may present with some form of breast enlargement – either in one or both breasts. They may complain of extreme fatigue. They may be feeling the effects of low testosterone through falling libido or impotence. They may have leg ulcers. They may have been extraordinarily thin all their lives and then experience rapid weight gain – especially around the stomach. They may be experiencing an increase in hand tremors. Any one of these, or a combination of them, may inspire a man with 47,XXY to seek treatment – but not always. We have men in our organization who were not diagnosed until their 50s or 60s and subsequently report having had all the above symptoms for years without having checked with medical professionals to find out why.

RESEARCH NEEDED

The diagnosis of 47,XXY or Klinefelter's syndrome can occur at a variety of ages and be due to a variety of factors but one thing remain constant – while there are limited treatments and interventions available for all men at all ages who receive the news that they possess an extra X chromosome, more research is needed to target the specific problems endemic to each age and developmental stage of growth. The multisystemic nature of 47,XXY cries out for more specific research in the disciplines of endocrinology, neurology, dermatology, psychology, psychiatry, genetics, cognitive development, and others we may not even be aware of yet.

As the founder of a support organization for males who have 47,XXY, I have been honored to know thousands of men and boys with this genetic condition. One thought based on my observation over the past 10 years that is seldom reported in the literature is that males with 47,XXY have an unusual capacity for empathy and human kindness. As a whole, I have noted that these men are compassionate and observant members of society. They often have an innate sense of benevolence. I believe that, in addition to proper medical treatment, when these empathetic qualities are developed and rewarded society will be the beneficiary.

- **USA**: Klinefelter Syndrome and Associates, PO Box 119, Roseville, CA 95678–0119, USA. Tel: (+1) 916-660-1599; Fax: (+1) 916-660-1899; Website: www.genetic.org; E-mail: ksinfo@genetic.org
- **Australia**: Australian Klinefelter Syndrome Support Group, PO Box 3, Glendenning Mail Centre, NSW 2761, Australia. E-mail: yatesbecks@bigpond.com
- **Germany**: Deutsche Klinefelter-Syndrom Vereinigung, c/o Franz Schorpp, Markusweg 4, 93167 Falkenstein, Germany. Tel: (+3) (0) 94 62 56 73; Fax: (+3) (0) 94 62 91 17 14; Website: www.klinefelter.org/ or www.klinefelter.org
- **UK**:
  United Kingdom Klinefelter Syndrome Association (S. Cook – parent advocate, National Contacts Co-ordinator). Tel: (+44) (0) 1787 237460.
  United Kingdom Klinefelter's Adult Group (Howard Bells – group contact), Woodlands, 31 Ben Bank Road, Silkstone Common, Barnsley, South Yorkshire S75 4PB, UK. Tel/Fax: (+44) (0) 1226 792 442
  United Kingdom Klinefelter Organization, c/o 234 Turton Road, Bradshaw, Bolton BL2 3EE, UK
- **Denmark**: Klinefelter Syndrome Support Group, Psychiatric Hospital Aarhus, Skovagervej 2, DK-8240 Risskov, Denmark. Tel: (+45) 77 89 36 09; Fax: (+45) 77 89 30 90; Website: www.aaa.dk/turner/

Congenital Adrenal Hyperplasia

Julian Pearce

The birth of an infant diagnosed with congenital adrenal hyperplasia (CAH) is often a tumultuous event in the lives of the parents. They often struggle to cope with the implications of having a child with an uncommon genetic disorder and may experience feelings of bewilderment and guilt. After the discharge of their child from hospital parents of a infant with CAH are faced not only with the usual demands of caring for a new baby, but also with caring for one who may have been critically ill prior to diagnosis and who has the potential to become so again. In addition, concerns regarding ambiguous genitalia, reconstructive vaginal surgery, medication regimes and the vigilance required to detect illnesses that warrant prompt medical attention in order to prevent an adrenal crisis can further tax their ability to cope. Thus the dynamics of dealing with CAH on a day-to-day basis is often a source of ongoing emotional strain for parents of an affected child.

As individuals with CAH mature, they have to learn to become self-reliant with medications and to manage the impact of their disorder on their general health, their height and weight, and, for some, their fertility and sexual identity.

DIAGNOSIS AND FOUNDATIONAL KNOWLEDGE

Parents may initially be quite distressed by the diagnosis of CAH and the realization that their child has an incurable genetic disorder. Competent emotional support at the point of diagnosis, accurate information about what to expect, and systematic education regarding the fundamentals of management of CAH are essential. Resources are required to assist parents to explain an uncommon and complex disorder to their extended family and friends, particularly if there has been uncertainty surrounding the infant's gender. Information for parents after the birth of a child with classic CAH typically comes from a variety of sources, which can include a pediatrician, endocrinologist, surgeon, pediatric physician in subspecialty training and nurses. Parents may actually be confused by multiple sources of information and a coordinated approach, with one consistent source of information, is recommended.

MEDICATIONS AND ILLNESS

Discerning the need for doubling or tripling of hydrocortisone doses during periods of physiologic stress caused by illness, commonly referred to as 'stress dosing', presents parents and those affected with CAH with an ongoing challenge. Incremental education concerning management of glucocorticoid and mineralocorticoid medication regimes and the adjustments required during periods of illness will lead to improved health for the child, ease parent's anxiety and empower them to manage the child appropriately.

Even with good care, adrenal crises occur occasionally and, in addition to threatening the child's life, may have significant sequelae in terms of learning disability and overall wellbeing.

Caregivers of children with CAH and adults with CAH need to be vigilant for illnesses with the potential to precipitate an adrenal crisis. With education and experience, most parents understand the need to increase their child's drug doses in response to major physiologic stressors such as bone fracture or diarrhea and vomiting. However, the situation is more difficult in the circumstances of illnesses that commence as somewhat trifling, such as tonsillitis, but then can progress to precipitate an adrenal crisis. Consequently, parents may live in a state of sustained uncertainty regarding illness episodes that can culminate in an adrenal crisis. Families with a baby with CAH who reside some distance from major pediatric centers carry considerable responsibility for decision-making concerning their child's wellbeing, often with minimal support.

An overzealous approach to increasing medication during intercurrent illness has long-term consequences for the individual with CAH such as obesity, advanced bone age and suboptimal final adult height. On balance, however, increased doses of glucocorticoids for the duration of an acute illness are recommended to parents. Fever is commonly used as a marker of physiologic stress sufficient to warrant a temporary increase in glucocorticoids during an illness. Parents of infants with CAH should be instructed in the technique of intramuscular injection of hydrocortisone for emergency situations or circumstances when hydrocortisone cannot be tolerated orally. In such situations a family member should administer an intramuscular hydrocortisone injection prior to evaluation and treatment for adrenal crisis.

GENITAL AMBIGUITY

Virilization of the external genitalia may occur in chromosomal females with CAH, and incorrect sex assignment is possible.[5,6] Uncertainty regarding a neonate's correct gender can be emotionally devastating to parents and has to be resolved quickly. The results of genetic testing and ultrasound investigations to confirm the infant's gender need to be conveyed to parents promptly, accompanied by reassurance that their child will have reproductive capability in adult life. At such times it can be comforting for parents to gain insight into what the future holds for their child by talking to an adult female with CAH or the parents of an older girl with CAH. Such contact can be arranged through a CAH support group. However, even when approached sensitively, gender issues remain an extremely delicate topic for those concerned and women with CAH tend not discuss their concerns regarding genital abnormalities with their doctors.

SUPPORT GROUPS

With infants and children in particular, their caregivers' skills in observation and detection of subtle changes in health and ability to take appropriate action when unwell impact significantly upon the health and wellbeing of the child. The welfare of children with CAH, and their ability to become self-reliant adults,

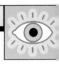

is maximized when parents have a clear understanding of the disorder and receive support in coping with all of the dimensions of life with a child with adrenal insufficiency.

In Australia the mutual support and educational resources provided by the CAH Support Group endeavor to meet the needs of parents of children and affected adults with CAH. The major issues addressed have been the management of medications, strategies for the prevention of adrenal crises, and issues surrounding sexuality.

Mutual support has typically been provided via telephone counseling contacts with parents of older children who are well-experienced in the day-to-day management of the disorder. It was recognized some years ago that much of the medical literature concerning CAH is in a form that is not 'user friendly' to parents. Consequently, CAH support groups have developed materials that better meet layman's needs. These include pamphlets on the management of significant physiologic stressors such as intercurrent illnesses and injuries, and what to do should the child require general anesthesia. A video was produced that frankly discussed the issues surrounding female genital ambiguity and corrective surgery from a parent's perspective. To further meet individuals' educational needs concerning CAH, the Australian CAH support group developed an Internet site, www.vicnet.net.au/-cahsga, in conjunction with pediatric endocrinologists, providing essential information in relatively simple language.

Parental separation from the child with CAH has been perceived as a period of potential vulnerability in terms of whether an injury or the onset of illness would be appropriately managed. Consequently, an advice sheet for caregivers other than parents, such as teachers and family friends, was produced.

Parents have reported that orienting an affected child to CAH has not been problematic. The process has been facilitated by sponsorship of the production of resources such as the excellent publication by Dr Garry Warne, *Your Child with CAH*. Annual Christmas functions have provided a social opportunity for children to meet others with CAH.

Symposia have been organized annually involving those affected by CAH and a variety of specialists, including endocrinologists, pediatricians, gynecologists, geneticists, social workers, and researchers, to provide a forum for education and open discussion with professionals in various health disciplines. The symposia have also emerged as a forum for advocacy for those affected by CAH. For example, they provided the opportunity for members to challenge endocrinologists to defend the practice of routine genital examination of girls during each checkup. Similarly, some mature women within the group have used the symposia as the forum to question the ethics of clitoridectomy, which had been performed during their childhood reconstructive vaginal surgery.

CONCLUSION

In addition to appropriate medical interventions for neonates with CAH, their parents require competent emotional support when the baby is first born, preferably from a single source. They require assistance with strategies to explain an uncommon and complex disorder to their family and friends, particularly when there has been uncertainty surrounding the infant's gender. Systematic and ongoing education regarding the fundamentals of CAH, assistance with management of medication regimes and the home management of typical childhood illnesses is enhanced by membership of a support group. In Australia the Melbourne-based CAH Support Group has made a significant contribution to the ongoing provision of education, emotional support, and advocacy for those affected by CAH.

CONGENITAL ADRENAL HYPERPLASIA SUPPORT GROUPS

Australia

Mr Julian Pearce
PO Box 6036
Highton 3216
Victoria, Australia
Tel: +61 3 5227 8405
Fax: +61 3 5227 8411
E-mail: jcpearce@deakin.edu.au
Web site: www.vicnet.net.au/-cahsga

Netherlands

Dutch Addison and Cushing Society
PO Box 52137, 2505 CC
The Hague,
Netherlands
Web site: www.spin.nl/nvap0300.htm

New Zealand

Ms Helen Mann
22 Oakfield Street
Burnside, Christchurch 5
New Zealand
Tel: 03 3584 505
Fax: 03 3517 265
E-mail: bmann@netaccess.co.nz

UK

Mrs Sue Elford
2 Windrush Close
Flitwick
Beds MK45 1PX
Tel: +44 (0)1525 717536
E-mail via web site on webmaster@cah.org.uk
Web site www.cah.org.uk

Sweden

Riksföreningen för Adrenogentialt Syndrom
c/o Ingela Nilsson
Narvegatan 7
235 35 Vellinge
Sweden
Tel: + / 040 42 18 74
E-mail: fam.i.k.nilsson@telia.com

USA

Marylou Celiberti
National Adrenal Diseases Foundation
505 Northern Boulevard
Great Neck, NY 11021.
+1 516–487–4992
E-mail: nadfmail@aol.com
Web site: www.medhelp.org/nadf

Vietnam

C/o Dr Vo Thi Kim Hue
National Institute of Pediatrics
Giang Vo, Dong Da
Hanoi
Vietnam
E-mail: lilyvo@hotmail.com

FURTHER READING

Pearce J. Congenital adrenal hyperplasia: a potential diagnosis for the neonate in shock. Austr Crit Care. 1995;8(1):16–9.

Donaldson M, Thomas P, Love J, et al. Presentation, acute illness and learning difficulties in salt wasting 21-hydroxylase deficiency. Arch Dis Childh. 1994;7(3):214–8.

Merke D, Cutler G. New approaches to the treatment of congenital adrenal hyperplasia. JAMA. 1997;227(13):1073–7.

New M. Diagnosis and management of congenital adrenal hyperplasia. Annu Rev Med. 1998;49:311–28.

Pang S. Congenital adrenal hyperplasia. Endocrinol Metabol Clin North Am. 1997;26(4):853–89.

White P, Speiser P. Congenital adrenal hyperplasia due to 21-hydroxylase deficiency. Endocrine Rev. 2000;21(3):245–91.

May B, Boyle M, Grant D. A comparative study of sexual experiences. J Health Psychol. 1996;1(4):479–92.

Diabetes

John A Eaddy

There is no other disease that requires of its sufferer such discipline and decision-making each day. Those of us who live with diabetes must, if we are to reach our goals, learn to be our own dietitian, nurse, laboratory technician, exercise coach, physician, and self-motivator. We have learned that to succeed at feeling well and minimizing our risk of both short and long term complications we must become self-managers of our own diabetes. No one can do the daily dance of living with diabetes for us.

This is the bottom-line lesson I've tried to teach to my patients, their families, other diabetics, and physicians during the last 30 years of medical practice. I began learning the lesson for myself when I was diagnosed with type 1 diabetes in 1952. The advent of intensive management tools and techniques, which arrived in 1980, heightened my awareness that patients who could most benefit from these methods were those who demonstrated motivations and skills of self-management behavior. Since then, it has become increasingly clear that the greatest service to be offered by the team of professionals who care for people who live with diabetes is to supply inspired teaching and encouragement for improved self-management of their disease.

Most people who are told of their diagnosis of diabetes experience stages of adjustment to that 'bad' news similar to the stages of dying described by Elizabeth Kubler-Ross. The stages of denial, anger, bargaining, depression, and acceptance will often reappear when patients receive the diagnosis of a major complication of their disease. Patients and families truly appreciate the compassionate caregiver who can recognize the stage of adjustment being expressed and facilitate self-awareness and progress toward acceptance. People often need to be given permission and encouragement to express the anger, resentment, and sadness that accompany living with diabetes. Gratitude and respect are given to physicians and other caregivers who assist patients to turn the liability of diabetes into an asset and ability to manage life's difficulties.

Catherine Feste, a diabetic for 43 years, has addressed the issue of empowering patients with a chronic disease, such as diabetes, to take charge of their health and future wellbeing. Her book *The Physician Within* assists patients to develop a positive attitude, recognize personal resources in their life, and develop skills of self-management. To accomplish the many daily disciplines of good diabetes management requires strong motivation and spiritual strength. Catherine's book *Meditations On Diabetes* can be a strong support for people struggling with the daily tasks of keeping healthy while living with diabetes. Naming the task of living well with diabetes 'a challenge' rather than 'a burden' promotes a positive attitude for the patient and the caregiver.

The physician who demonstrates a positive attitude and is willing to accept/forgive the patient's less than perfect adherence to the treatment plan is likely to observe improved self-management behaviors by the patient. A punitive, reproachful address to the patient intended to produce guilt or fear rarely changes patient behaviors.

It has been my clinical experience that patients want both my advice about improving their health and approval of their efforts to manage their own diabetes. They sometimes don't offer their blood sugar logs for my review but always accept and appreciate feedback about the effort made and possible ways to achieve improved control. I ask each patient to bring their own blood glucose meter at each visit and to perform a test upon being put in the exam room. If the patient forgets to bring the meter the nurse will do a fingerstick glucose for them. Since most patients want to please me, they attempt to reach a normal glucose at the time of their appointment. Frequently, patients arrive with a hypoglycemic value that requires treatment before the visit can proceed. The blood glucose level at the visit deserves discussion as part of the effort to help the patient accept accountability for control. Patients rarely offer histories of hypoglycemic events unless questioned; review of the frequency and severity of events can uncover correctable errors of management and reduce the frequency of future hypoglycemia. Behaviors that embarrass or threaten the patient or their family require discussion, explanation, and planning to prevent future occurrences. Most patients can be taught to minimize severe hypoglycemia by careful planning of insulin dose, meal timing, anticipation of intensity and duration of exercise, and always having sufficient glucose-containing products with them. Encouragement by caregivers to be prepared for hypoglycemia can enhance this part of patient self-management behavior.

Most of us who live with diabetes have specific fears about what the disease may do to us. I have observed that the underlying concern is for loss of independence as a competent, self-sufficient person. The complication of diabetes that leads to dependence may be blindness, amputation, kidney failure, heart attack, or stroke. Each person usually owns a specific fear, which needs to be uncovered and addressed as part of the plan to maximize self-management action. However, attempting to induce behavior changes by using the threat of possible future complications seldom produces positive results. Patients respond to positive feedback about their successes and offers of assistance with the more difficult disciplines of daily management, e.g. making appropriate food choices, blood sugar testing/record-keeping, exercising. People who live with diabetes prefer the carrots of praise and encouragement over the sticks of criticism and blame.

There are millions of people in the world who have diabetes but the individual person who lives with it often feels like a lone sufferer. Attending a summer camp for 2 weeks each year from age 13 to 17 profoundly influenced my acceptance of my disease and my sense of being part of a community of people like me. During the last 19 years as physician for the Tennessee Camp for Diabetic Children, I have observed the growth of attitudes of acceptance and *esprit de corps* of campers as they live, learn, and play with 130 other diabetics for 2 weeks.

Support groups, formal educational courses, attendance at community functions for people who live with diabetes all enhance a sense of community and reduce the loneliness that can accompany diabetes.

The American Diabetes Association (ADA) and national diabetes organizations in many other countries provide an invaluable service to people who have diabetes. The mission of the ADA is to prevent and cure diabetes and to improve the lives of all people affected by diabetes. Patient membership benefits include access to local, regional, and national offices, which provide information, publications, organization of meetings, public and governmental advocacy, and support for diabetes research. Membership includes subscription to the monthly journal *Diabetes Forecast*, which brings to the patient motivational articles by or about other people who are succeeding in managing diabetes, advances in medical treatment/research, discount offers on diabetic supplies, etc. Professional membership provides access to many journals and publications focused on diabetes care and research, options for

membership in working committees, and notices of regional and national meetings. In my life as a diabetic patient and physician the ADA has been a major source of motivation, support, and education. I have strongly recommended membership in the ADA to my patients and peers. Other organizations, such as the Juvenile Diabetes Foundation (JDF), offer support to those who live with diabetes by raising private and public funds for research leading to a cure for diabetes. Patients can find hope and personal satisfaction by participating in JDF functions.

Some people who develop diabetes are blessed with an integration of mind, body, and spirit at the time of diagnosis. Many others struggle to integrate these parts of their self as they learn to live with their diabetes. Physicians and other caregivers who can assess the level of integration and readiness to pursue self-management by the patient are more likely to set realistic goals for disease management. Both the patient and the professional will experience a sense of success when selected goals match the resources of the patient. Physical, psychological, intellectual, social, and spiritual resources are available to those of us who live with diabetes. Diabetics can be helped to recognize and develop these assets to improve their success in self-management.

There are many sources of support for people attempting to achieve goals of disease management and health promotion. Family, friends, co-workers, hobbies, the ADA, spiritual meditation, the health care team are accessible. Frequently the diabetic must teach those from whom support is needed about diabetes, the healthy lifestyle required to maintain wellness, and the kind of help needed for goal attainment. 'You never know until you ask!' is good advice for patients seeking support to enhance self-management of diabetes.

Knowledge is power but ... a little bit of knowledge can be dangerous when it comes to managing the multiple problems of diabetes. Blood glucose, blood pressure, lipid control, abnormal thrombogenesis, weight, and exercise goal attainment all require patient motivation and participation. Those of us who live with diabetes need repeated doses of education about the prescriptions given to enhance our health and protect us from the complications of diabetes. We hope and trust that the professionals we choose to consult accept and honor the obligation to maintain their knowledge and skill. Through continuing education, study of advances in research, and application of new knowledge in their practice, caring for people who live with diabetes can be a mutually exciting and beneficial endeavor. As physician/patient I've come to cherish the 'trickle up' effect when patients teach me the unique nuances they have learned about diabetes management that are not found in medical texts. Each one of us responds to stress, medication, food, exercise, and relaxation with unique physiologic/metabolic patterns and intensity. Listening to patient's stories with a desire to find the true meaning of their experience can lead to a new appreciation for the complexity of living with diabetes.

FURTHER READING

American Diabetes Association. Clinical Practice Recommendations 2002. Diabetes Care. 2002;25(Suppl. 1).

Eaddy J, Lincoln T. Hypoglycemia – living with diabetes. American Diabetes Association; 2001.

Feste C. Meditations on diabetes. Alexandria, VA: American Diabetes Association; 1999.

Feste C. The physician within, 2nd ed. 13911 Ridgeview Drive, Minnetonka, MN:Chronomed Publishing Co.; 1993.

Kubler-Ross E. On death and dying. London:Macmillan; 1969.

Growth Hormone Deficiency in Children and Adults   Tam Fry

THE SAGA

Sarah is one of the two young girls in Figure 43.1. If you've seen this photograph before you will know which one she is and what is wrong with her growth: if you haven't, take 10 seconds to consider the diagnosis. You're right, of course. The little one on the left is growth-hormone-deficient and she is Sarah. You could be forgiven for momentarily thinking that Tamzin, her younger sister by 18 months, might be too tall for her age but on closer scrutiny it is obvious that Sarah has the problem. In the view of the specialist who diagnosed her at the time the picture was taken, her deficiency could have been detected at 100 meters.

Unfortunately for Sarah, for the first 6 years of her life she never got to see a specialist or, indeed, anyone who was remotely interested in her small stature. It wasn't for want of her parents trying. Week after week following her third birthday her mother pleaded with every health-care professional she met to respond to her concern that the baby sibling was outgrowing the older child. Week in, week out, however, she got no more than a pat on the head and reassurance that Sarah had no problem. She was cute, the professionals said, perfectly proportioned and would undoubtedly sprout up when she reached puberty. It was the worst medical advice that any profession could give to a parent who was concerned. I know because I am Sarah's father.

I have been asked that Sarah's story and its sequel in this book should not be too critical of endocrinologists and it won't be. Life is too short to dwell on the unhappy experiences that my family had during those early years, which, of course, have now faded with time. We have nothing but good to say of Professor James Tanner and his colleagues, who subsequently treated Sarah for 8 years with growth hormone. But for them she would not have achieved 155cm instead of the 122cm final height predicted for her. Their care meant that she has been able to lead a life in which she could achieve her full potential as a film and TV costume stylist rather than possibly being a midget dependent on social security. As each year of her life goes by we cannot thank enough the 'system' that allowed Sarah this transformation.

Sarah's growth failure was left undetected because her growth was never monitored. It was neither measured nor assessed in relation to her sister or parents, yet she displayed every clue imaginable to her diminished stature. From her first day at nursery school, although she couldn't reach the clothes pegs or light switches as the other children could, no one questioned why. She played the fairy in the nativity play for 3 years running but only we, her parents, felt that there was something wrong. At junior school she was 'mothered' because of her height but that didn't trigger concern in her teachers. When later she was teased because of it, and the teasing became so brutal that her 'much bigger' little sister had to act as her minder in the playground, no one noticed. Even out of school, friends never asked us if we were happy with her height. Strangers simply gawped at her because they couldn't believe that a girl who looked 3 years old could be reading newspapers. It was only left to a school doctor on the point of retiring who, having read a tabloid article on growth hormone replacement, suggested that we should be referred to Great Ormond Street Hospital for Sick Children. It was the sole

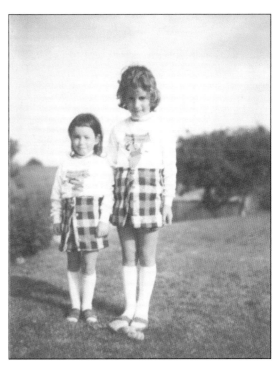

Figure 43.1 Sarah, aged 6 years, is the little girl on the left with her sister Tamzin, aged 4 ¹/₂ years.

positive advice that we ever received and it worked. Professor James Tanner diagnosed growth hormone deficiency in what seems now to be 5 seconds flat although, in reality, it must have been a few weeks before he could confirm his diagnosis with tests.

The tests were, of course, normal for the 1970s but are no longer to be found in 21st century clinical practice. The Bovril tests and exercise tests were year-long before her failure of growth made her eligible for the scarce cadaveric growth hormone. Her treatment couldn't even be authorized by her specialist but had to be sanctioned by a Government Department of Health, Human Growth Hormone Committee, since the hormone was limited in supply and technically still in its research stage. Delivery was not via a nightly subcutaneous injection with a user-friendly, fine-needled pen but by a barbarous, thick, hypodermic needle encased in an undisguised syringe plunged into her frail body three times a week. It was District Nurse Bartelot who had to take charge of the agonizing injection session: neither parent had the stomach to inflict such pain and both needed to remain the caring people to whom Sarah could turn for comfort once the injection was over. Nurse Bartelot was, of course, not only a good nurse but an exceptional one and remained part of the family long after Sarah had finished the beastly growing business.

In the 8 years that she was treated it was spectacular to witness the change that growth hormone made to her and, even with the fact that she may contract Creutzfeldt–Jakob disease still hanging over the family, my wife and I cannot regret the decision that we took on her behalf. She blossomed before our eyes from the 6-year-old who was the height of a 3-year-old to the woman who, although small for her family, is now within the normal range for her gender. The transformation is best described by herself in an interview that she gave as a 17-year-old when, following her treatment, her story was dramatized in a BBC television play, *Being Normal* in 1983.

> Looking back, I think that being mocked and being looked at was the worst part. I hated being picked up because it frightened me. I was afraid I would topple over if they dropped me. I always had this fear of being injured. The worst years were when I was having all those tests in hospital – the smell of hospital food brings back the terror of it all. Dieting is going to be with me for the rest of my life. I have a very slow metabolism and the treatment didn't help my weight. I was a podgy child – it didn't bother me until I was 11 or 12, when you become more conscious of your body. Everybody had boyfriends but I didn't. I hated sport because running was difficult because I had short legs and couldn't keep up. I went to a concert recently and was absolutely ecstatic because I managed to get right up front with all those massive towering people. I had done it – I had overcome my fear of tall people and finally proved that I was normal.

THE SEQUEL

Sarah grew dramatically from 1972 and was on course for her projected adult height when, one day in 1977, a letter arrived from Great Ormond Street. It was to change my life. It invited my wife and I to meet with Professor Tanner and his team to discuss if we could do anything to help finance his NHS clinic, which was subject to increasing financial cutbacks following the oil price increases of the 1970s. Although neither of us had any experience in fundraising it was a request that we couldn't refuse since Sarah's free treatment was therapy that we could never have afforded or taken out insurance to cover. By the creation of the charity envisaged by Tanner we could fundraise to cover not only the Great Ormond Street clinic but other UK clinics too. It would be a way of 'paying back' for all the benefit that Sarah had received. The Child Growth Foundation was born.

I became chairman of the embryonic group more by accident than design. The five other couples handpicked by Tanner families to become co-founders saw to that by clever flattery and playing on my inability to say 'no'. Perceiving that I was an arrogant television producer and suggesting that a little charitable work would be good for my soul, they persuaded me that I could lead a team that would have the fundraising part of the job licked in a couple of years. On top of that, I kidded myself that that my contacts within the media would generate the press coverage necessary to make the fundraising successful. I would show the world how important an issue 'growth' was and the donations would roll in!.

I quickly learned just how arrogant I was. The paltry £2000 ($3300) we managed to raise in the first year as a registered charity showed that, even when told, the public cared little for conditions from which children didn't appear to die. The media showed itself to be universally indifferent and the Foundation was left with only small change from my initial stewardship. My pride couldn't endure the ignominy of delivering neither the cash nor the message and I knew that, if anything was to be accomplished, I was in for a long haul.

The rest, as they say, is history. As this edition goes to press, the Foundation is 25 years old. Hardly a week goes by without a broadcast program, newspaper or magazine covering some aspect of growth and, although it may not always be absolutely correct medically, the underlying message gets through. Hand in hand with the publicity, we now generate more income in a morning's work than our combined 1977–79 revenue and, with a turnover of nearly £500,000 ($0.825m) in our last audited accounts, the Foundation has a secure base on which it can thrive. This is in a country with only 20% of the US population.

These figures would not have been possible if the Foundation had remained merely a self-help group for a relatively small population of families with children in growth outpatient clinics. The income has been achieved only because we have catered for the growth of all British children by marketing the training equipment and charts that are necessary to monitor their growth. In 1984 we made a strategic decision to stretch our charitable objectives to champion the growth of every child and it has paid off.

It is a strategy that has not made us popular. It is not surprising that some people in the medical profession object to outsiders telling them how to do their job but when it became obvious that the growth of the majority of children, like Sarah's, was not being properly monitored, somebody had to. We seized every chance that we could to prove that we were actually on-side but, inevitably, a number of noses were put out of joint by meddlesome parents. Tough.

Although the remaining three paragraphs of this article may sound like a commercial, it is written for the record rather than for advertisement. I apologize if it gives the impression that the Foundation is more an 'industry' than a charity but confirm that we remain dedicated to our initial cause. If we are to ensure that children with growth disorders are quickly identified, promptly referred, and appropriately, we need the cash with which to do it.

For the record, the training began immediately in 1984. Professor Tanner headed an all-star cast for our first 'growth' seminar, a half-day affair at London's Institute of Child Health played out to a packed audience of qualified nurses who had never had any instruction in endocrinology. We were concerned that no one would buy tickets because of the price we had put on them – £2.50 ($4.10)! – and, even then, some of our number thought the price a bit steep. The full-house notices quickly taught us, however, that there was a market ready to be tapped and, although the seminar at the Institute of Child Health in London was the only one we managed in 1984, by 2000 we were staging 80 per year. No longer did we have to worry about finding audiences, or ticketing them, but were invited by primary care managers to put health visitors and school nurses through their paces in their own training centers. The economics favors the managers, even though the per capita cost of training has doubled to £5 ($8.25): since we traveled to the nurses the expense of travel and the traveling time to a seminar elsewhere in the country has been reduced to virtually nothing. The courses will continue into the new century and seek to ensure that every primary practitioner knows everything they need to know to identify abnormal growth.

When considering the marketing of equipment we had no choice but to sell whatever was available. We found, however, that it was expensive and geared to hospital use and, therefore, fairly inappropriate for the community. With the requirement that portability must go hand in hand with accuracy, we set about encouraging manufacturers to produce instruments to our own specifications and, ultimately, took to designing and producing them ourselves. Within a generation of the Growth Foundation being registered, we had reduced the price of height measuring equipment to 5% of its hospital equivalent and brought down the cost of supine measurement by 90%. We won't try to develop scales, since the market is already well served and their cost is rapidly descending dramatically, too.

I hope, however, that it is for our growth charts that the Foundation will be best remembered. Since 1993, every UK child has a set in his or her Personal Child Health Record and, unless something very strange occurs in medical practice, they will continue to be featured there for ever. The Personal Child Health Record charts are produced in the traditional 'distance' formats but other charts are available for specific conditions and community and hospital usage. The UK now has its own Down's syndrome charts, and body mass index charts were introduced in the mid-1990s as an aid to clinicians managing obesity and eating disorders. Thrive Lines, lines that denote a 0.5% weight gain velocity, were introduced in 1999 in an acetate format to assist with the earlier identification of failure to thrive and 'Breast from Birth' acetates followed a year later. The latter were introduced primarily to help mothers recognize that breastfed babies don't keep to the standard centiles and might therefore benefit from having centile charts of their own.

FOOTNOTE

The Foundation is the sequel to a saga that may not yet be quite over. Although Sarah grew up years ago she has not finished with growth hormone itself. She is one of those adults who respond to replacement therapy for its other properties and she would be lost without it. So far she, and every other adult and child who needs treatment, have not been denied the drug by either governmental or administrative directive and the Foundation trusts that this situation will continue. But at the first sign of any attempt to downgrade its indications, the British government and its agencies, and you, will be hearing from me again. Not in a chapter in a book but in person!

GROWTH HORMONE DEFIENCY SUPPORT GROUPS

UK
The Growth Foundation
(formerly The Child Growth Foundation)
2 Mayfield Avenue
Chiswick
London W4 1PW
Tel: +44 (0) 20-8995 0257/8994 7625
Fax: +44 (0) 20-8995 9075

USA
Human Growth Foundation
997 Glen Core Avenue
Glen Head, NY 11545
Tel: +1 800 451 6434
Fax: +1 516 671 4055
Web: www.hgfound.org

Pituitary Diseases

Robert Knutzen

Patients experience pituitary disease from a vastly different perspective from physicians. To ourselves, we are not unusual medical curiosities but too often medical orphans, looking for a home and care in an alien medical world. To us as patients, the emotional, sexual aspects of the disease are just as devastating as (in some cases more than) the other physical manifestations. Since the time of Goliath we have certainly witnessed a number of well-known figures from the Egyptian Pharaoh Akhenaton to contemporary personalities such as Primo Carnera, the Italian boxer, and Andre the Giant, the actor/wrestler, fighting a valiant, but losing battle with acromegaly. Regrettably, there seems to have been no attempt to reconstruct (in a pathologic sense) the lives of any of these individuals in order to know how their personal and family lives were affected by their acromegaly.

Even more regrettable is that there is no history of the 'unsung' pituitary patients with Cushing's syndrome, hyperprolactinemia, Rathke's cleft cyst, nonsecretory adenoma, etc. whose lives in many cases, as we know for certain, were cut short either by suicide (the primary cause of death in Cushing's patients at the turn of the last century), or by intense physical suffering and pain and often a somewhat gruesome death resulting from mismanagement by ignorant but well-meaning surgeons and physicians.

A sense of desperation fills the minds and souls of many patients, who often cry with relief when, after they have made contact with my organization, the Pituitary Network Association, we acknowledge their stories or assure them that, yes indeed, there are experts (however few) who can both properly diagnose and treat hormonal disorders and pituitary disease.

The combination of emotional illness and sexual dysfunction clearly has an enormous influence on a pituitary patient's family life and support system. We focus on these medical arenas simply because the patients who contact us repeatedly complain that these issues trouble them the most and are of greatest concern to their families and loved ones.

It is interesting to note that a large number, perhaps a majority, of pituitary patients say that emotional and psychosocial disorders are the most debilitating aspects of pituitary disease and represent an important component that few physicians ask about. Bipolarity, mood disorders, emotional outbursts, depression, apathy, etc. are present in a great number of pituitary patients, so a large number of them, and family members, come to us for help after release from a suicide watch, mental institution or psychiatric care. Often we hear from them after severe headaches or loss of sight forces the use of magnetic resonance imaging (MRI) to finally seek a solution for their discomfort and pain. Too often, it is only then that their pituitary tumor is discovered. Needless to say, when properly treated, patients can return to their families for care but, at present, they are only intermittently able to resume a working life. Too often we hear of patients who are unable to return to their pre-illness career or job without a major financial 'step-down'. Eventually, they may need disability subsidy or even welfare support. Doctors, lawyers, accountants, nurses, architects, plumbers, actors, and secretaries all too often have their lives and careers permanently interrupted, often before they are diagnosed with a pituitary tumor or hormonal imbalance. (Career, education, and training do not appear to make much difference to the final outcome of pituitary disease.)

Although the discovery of a tumor is a major psychological setback for some patients, it is also an enormous relief for a great number of us. We now know, with an inner sense of intuitive certainty, that we have found the culprit responsible for the insidious symptoms, emotional outbursts, and family break-ups. I would suspect that those physicians and surgeons who attribute 'emotional discomfort' to the actual finding of the tumors or cysts are looking at an 'easy' answer, hard for the patient to dispute at the office visit when informed of the finding of a tumor.

My own conversations with thousands of patients can only, of course, yield anecdotal evidence and insight. However, my own and our staff's conversations with these patients reveal an interesting, and myth-defying, series of concerns.

A startling number of patients turn to us for information to help 'force' a diagnosis from their physicians. They know they are ill but have not yet found anyone to whom they can turn for a definitive diagnosis. We also hear daily from diagnosed but still untreated patients looking for the best medical help, medicines, and treatment options available. They often pour their hearts out to us, needing both to share their feelings and fear and to learn about their disease, the prognosis, what to do and expect next, etc. Sadly, since we are not physicians and healers, we must exchange platitudes and have empathetic, yet nonhelpful conversations, knowing full well that expert care may be denied such people as a result of governmental policies, insurance provider regulations, or because they lack the will and determination to travel to experts in the field and seek help.

Our experiences with these many thousands of patients and their family members have allowed us to categorize the issues facing the patients into four phases:
1. The pre-pituitary-diagnosis period, characterized by a myriad of guesses and the loss of valuable time;
2. The postdiagnostic acute treatment phase;
3. The post-treatment hormone-replacement lifetime medication phase;
4. The gap in care for the remaining psychosocial issues facing both patients and their families and immediate caregivers.

A remarkably high number of patients fill us in on their treatments, recent surgery, triumphs, and disappointments. We learn about medical centers and physicians, side effects of medicines, hormone replacement, etc. It is important to note that our website, www.pituitary.org, alone receives between 15,000 and 40,000 'hits' per day. Patients and family members are as likely to 'visit' from Malta or Qatar as from Australia or Singapore, the USA or Canada. A startling number of them send us e-mails requesting help, referrals, and information and an even larger number develop e-mail 'pals' among themselves. They regularly share intimate and very personal medical information with us, information they may not have even shared with their physicians. A large number of written 'Patient Perspectives' also come into our offices.

We let patients, particularly those with unusual or educational histories, use our resources to publish what we believe is a 'mental catharsis' for them. Some 'physician-bashing' may take place, but we believe some of it is essential to 'tell the whole story' and so we let it alone. Somewhere, hopefully, someone reads it and learns a new perspective on pituitary disorders. Finally, we hear from the 'hopeless'. Sometimes we hear from people who have had surgery three times, two bouts of radiotherapy, and a course of chemotherapy, although obviously these are in the minority. Most often, however, patients are frustrated by a poor response to medication, scarce or unavailable hormone replacement, incomplete or incompetent surgical intervention (e.g. spinal fluid leaks, permanent blindness caused by 'waiting awhile', perforated septum, etc.).

And, regrettably, often little or no attempt is made to help patients recover their mental balance and quality of life. It is often difficult, and sometimes too late, to restore family relationships, long ago destroyed by the effects of hormonal excess or absence. Sadly, psychologists and psychiatrists are often not involved in the treatment plan, nor do physicians refer patients to them as often as they should.

THE PREDIAGNOSIS PERIOD

The bulk of pituitary patients do not see the experts in the field. They must settle for whomever their government, insurance company, or family physician is willing to refer them to. It is clear that tremendous strides in have been made in pituitary knowledge in recent times, yet it is equally clear that this knowledge stays at the top of the medical triangle with the patients caught in the middle, seeking answers from family physicians, urologists, obstetricians, gynecologists, etc., who rarely have the requisite up-to-date knowledge and understanding of pituitary or hormonal disorders (other than diabetes). So they rarely offer much help, let alone help make an accurate and useful diagnosis.

There are two common misconceptions about pituitary disorders. The first is that pituitary disease is 'rare'. We will concede that they are 'rarely' diagnosed but are not willing to agree that they are 'scarce' in the adult human population. Studies looking for intracranial lesions have documented them in up to 20% of 'normals' by MRI and nearly than 25% of autopsied individuals. The other misconception is the classification of pituitary tumors as 'benign', a term that has added a plethora of nonsense to the discussion about pituitary disorders. 'Benign' is a pathological term meant to distinguish metastasizing cancers from non-metastasizing adenomas.

Regrettably, however, some pituitary adenomas are extremely dangerous. Some forms of cancer are easier to treat than some forms of pituitary tumor. And many 'benign' pituitary tumors have devastating emotional and physical effects. The application of the term 'benign' indicates to some medical personnel that a 'wait and see' or 'no intervention needed' approach is sufficient.

This leads to far fewer diagnosed patients and far more unhappiness with medical care. It is still common for patients to be told: 'These things happen with age, you know, it is just stress' (often quite correct as an underlying cause for endocrine problems). Women are most frequently told; 'Oh, it's just in your head!'

We often hear from patients who have been diagnosed and treated for a thyroid condition, fibromyalgia, chronic fatigue syndrome, menstrual problems requiring a hysterectomy to correct 'precancerous ovarian cysts', and, of course, many neurological disorders. Patients often tell of a 20-year search for an accurate diagnosis. We realize that there is an enormous waste of medical expenditure on the multitudes of pituitary patients who not only seek treatment but often undergo extensive and expensive treatment for an un- or underdiagnosed condition.

It is usually women who contact us and discuss their own health, that of their husbands, children, or other relatives, or a friend. Nevertheless, there is still a tendency to consider women as 'too hormonal' and 'too stressed' to discuss these issues rationally. In our experience, this is not usually the case. Women are remarkably open in their discussions and are astute observers of the state of health of their family members and friends.

I would like to emphasize that men, too, are becoming more aware of their own health and are more willing to seek help and assume some responsibility for their own care. In my experience, we hear from very few hypochondriacs or hysterical individuals. Most often they are concerned, frightened, and/or misdiagnosed, mistreated or, worse yet, experiencing severe mental agitation or even psychosis. Sadly, this constantly casts me in a role of a 'scolder' who exhorts these patients to 'fight for their rights' while in fact what I am doing is to look up the world's best hospitals and medical centers and send them to a well-trained professional.

THE POSTDIAGOSTIC, ACUTE TREATMENT PHASE

All too often we hear of what can best be termed 'abdication of responsibility'. By that I mean that treatment during this stage is too often one-dimensional, not meeting anyone's rational expectations of thoughtful intervention. Patients tell us about neurosurgeons who fail to establish a baseline of hormonal levels prior to surgery. Nor are resected tissue samples forwarded to qualified and interested pathologists for a confirming or expanded diagnosis. The result, unfortunately, too often, is a patient who is discharged as 'cured' when in fact s/he may feel worse and be in inferior physical condition than before treatment. Meanwhile, the referring physician sometimes abdicates his/her responsibility to provide the patient with professional and thoughtful care by not staying involved in the case.

We also know that, unfortunately, many surgeons involved in pituitary patient care are not nearly as well versed in pituitary endocrinology as one might hope. So their prescribed hormone replacement therapy may be woefully inadequate for a recently discharged patient who, as far as the world knows, has just come through successful surgery. The opposite also happens rather too often: doctors believe that the patient has a low-level case of hyperprolactinemia because very high prolactin levels have been missed by an inexperienced laboratory or poorly trained technician. Or, as often is the case, a large, invasive, nonsecretory macroadenoma is discovered after many years of treatment for 'mild hyperprolactinemia', which for too long was seen as an inconvenience rather than a destroyer of sexual function, and soon (or already) to be a destroyer of vision.

Within our organization we firmly believe that only a trained team approach to pituitary patient care is an acceptable solution to the myriad symptoms and disorders facing the patient both before and after the acute stage of treatment.

A very personal sense of logic compels me to urge the medical community to look for a baseline of sexual and emotional/psychosocial function also, in order to help the consulting andrologist, fertility expert, or psychiatrist to know where to begin their recuperative treatment in order to achieve near-normal functioning for the patient.

THE POST-TREATMENT, HORMONE-REPLACEMENT STAGE

This is a time of intense trauma for the patient and the family. Will I feel better, am I cured? Again, sadly, a lack of knowledge (or candor?) often leaves the patient and family at odds with each other. Patients, because they are ambulatory, able to walk and urinate on their own, are seen as malingerers and 'crybabies' by their own family. Too often, the attending physician says the same thing when the patient is complaining of being too fatigued, too emotional, and too irrational to return to work and resume other usual societal and family functions and duties. (After all, the surgery was successful, wasn't it?)

The bonds of marriage, love, and family are often strained to breaking-point during the diagnostic and treatment phase. Now they often break permanently because the family thinks the patient should be cured. But the patient often recognizes that s/he is no better off than before. Medical professionals sometimes tend to believe that 'one treatment fits all' and are too often unsympathetic both to the patient and to the immediate family. The seeds are sown for a complete family collapse. The patient again doubts him/herself and the rest of the family believe they are dealing with a less than 'stoutly reliable' person. There are no reserves of love and compassion left and an ongoing deterioration of the family ensues.

Far too often we hear of cases where the doctors fail to test for or give replacement hormones such as testosterone or estrogen. Sometimes patients are left on a continuous (too high) dose of corticosteroids long past the usual time for either reducing or ending use other than in emergencies. Growth hormone replacement is still so controversial, for instance, that we only rarely hear of patients being tested for the deficiency. Sexuality is still such a medical 'taboo' that more men than we ever imagined don't get testosterone. Of course, testosterone replacement for women is still an 'infant' concept!

To us, it is remarkable to discover the thousands of Cushing's patients, for instance, who have never been told to expect that the first 6–12 postoperative months may well be far more frightening and uncomfortable than the last years prior to diagnosis and surgical treatment. Half-hearted attempts to remedy patients' discomfort and often acute symptoms of hormonal deficiency are remarkable to us, not so much because of the degree of discomfort suffered by the patient, but because of the frequency with which they occur. This is often at wide variance with other patient stories we hear of 'caution and awareness' preached by well-informed physicians who take great pains to follow their hormonal 'saga' as it continues to unfold during the weeks, months, and years of their recovery and hormone-replacement therapy (HRT).

This may well be the appropriate place to describe the treatment of the 'average patient' in North America and, indeed, in most countries in the world. How do I know? Through at least 10, often more, e-mails, regular mail, and phone calls per day. Not to mention the postings on our Bulletin Board from almost every country in the world. We have learned this with increasing certainty every year. Most pituitary patients are not treated at centers of excellence. Too often patients are slowly, if ever, diagnosed, and are usually treated half-heartedly by gynecologists or family practitioners with little or no training in endocrinology who believe that 'benign' means 'friendly' or 'harmless'. GPs often make referrals to neurosurgeons on a 'local acquaintance and friendship' basis, without much thought about their training or experience in this particular field of medicine. Follow-up and HRT is too often of a 'cursory' and superficial nature, only enough to sustain life, not enough to enhance or rebuild lost quality of life.

THE PSYCHOSOCIAL REBUILDING STAGE

The famous Dr Harvey Cushing said, as early as 1913: 'It is quite probable that the psychopathology of everyday life hinges largely upon the effects of a ductless gland discharge upon the nervous system.'

At the Pituitary Network Association our experience with thousands of patients tells us that he was remarkably astute. Slow and incomplete diagnosis, half-hearted or misguided treatment, and inadequate or nonexistent HRT are all less important than the medical approach (sometimes almost nonexistent) to psychologic/psychiatric patient and family healing after the years of trauma the patient and the family has lived through.

We have come to the regrettable conclusion that too many patients are 'written off' as hopeless cases not susceptible to modern medical advances and consigned to the human scrapheap as not worthy of, or perhaps beyond, repair and salvation. The societal cost is enormous. Besides paying the disability claims for living expenses, as well as the medical cost of the patient's rest-of-life care, society is also faced with the loss of income and support from a parent, husband, or child. The immediate financial burden of a patient may not be great but the 'ripple effect' through an immediate and extended family may be incalculable. When gifted or trained people are no longer able to contribute to their career or station in life, they are well aware of the enormous loss of social standing, the burden on the family, and the shaken foundation of their identity as human beings. A willingness and ability on the part of society and the medical establishment to recognize the cost of extended care for these people and to take the medical and social steps required to help them and their families to recover completely from the enormous struggle with a 'hormonal challenge' will perhaps, in both the short and long run, be the best medical and societal investment they can make.

Expertise and the required medical and surgical care is available to patients if society and the medical community are only willing to recognize the problem and allocate the requisite resources. The patient deserves it – so does society!

We are very pleased to have acted as a stimulus to the 'birth' of other organizations and are pleased to list some of the organizations we currently know of:

- **UK**: The Pituitary Foundation, PO Box 1944, Bristol B599 2UB, UK
- **Australia**: The Australian Pituitary Foundation, PP Box 4792, North Rocks 2151, NSW, Australia.
- **USA**: PO Box 1958, Thousand Oaks, CA 91358, USA
- **Netherlands**: Bleekvelweg 2, 4695 RJ St Maartensdijk, Netherlands
- **Denmark**: Hypofysennetvaerket, Rebaek Alle 18-B, 2650 Hvidovre, Denmark
- **Sweden**: Stoedforeningen Hypophysis, Hormonella Udda Sjukdomar; Sandhult P1 801, 28040 Skanes Fagerhult, Sweden
- **Germany**: Netzwerk, Medizinische Klinik, Haltenfosstrasse 41, 30167 Hannover, Germany

FURTHER READING

Ezzat S. The Pituitary patient resource guide, 3rd edn. Thousand Oaks, CA: Pituitary Network Association; 1991.

Weitzner MA, Sonino N, Knutzen R, eds. Emotional aspects of pituitary disease. Psychotherapy and psychosomatics. Karger; 1998

Index

Page numbers in *italic* indicate figures and tables